Accession no.

# Essentials of Sports Nutrition and Supplements

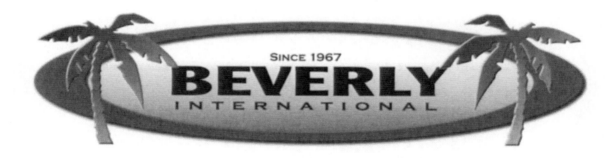

Beverly International is a proud sponsor of the International Society of Sports Nutrition. This textbook was made possible via an educational grant from Beverly International.

# Essentials of Sports Nutrition and Supplements

Edited by

Jose Antonio, PhD
Douglas Kalman, PhD, RD
Jeffrey R. Stout, PhD
Mike Greenwood, PhD
Darryn S. Willoughby, PhD
G. Gregory Haff, PhD

❊ Humana Press

*Editors*

Jose Antonio, PhD
International Society of Sports
  Nutrition
Deerfield Beach, FL, USA

Jeffrey R. Stout, PhD
Department of Health and Exercise
  Science
University of Oklahoma
Norman, OK, USA

Darryn S. Willoughby, PhD
Department of Health, Human
  Performance, and Recreation
Baylor University
Waco, TX, USA

Douglas Kalman, PhD, RD
Division of Nutrition and
  Endocrinology
Miami Research Associates
Miami, FL, USA

Mike Greenwood, PhD
Department of Health, Human
  Performance, and Recreation
Baylor University
Waco, TX, USA

G. Gregory Haff, PhD
Division of Exercise Physiology
West Virginia University
Morgantown, WV, USA

**Additional material to this book can be downloaded from http://extras.springer.com**

ISBN: 978-1-58829-611-5          e-ISBN: 978-1-59745-302-8
DOI: 10.1007/978-1-59745-302-8

Library of Congress Control Number: 2007932994

*Cover illustration*: By Shirley Karina.

Printed on acid-free paper

9 8 7 6 5 4 3 2 1

springer.com

**Dedication**

**In memory of Joseph Allen Chromiak**
**A Father, Husband, Friend, and Scientist**

*This book is dedicated to the memory of Joseph Allen Chromiak, 47, of Starkville, Miss. He passed away after a long battle with cancer. Joseph is survived by his wife, Anna; son, Joseph; parents, Joseph and Bonnie; and his brothers, David and John. Joseph was born in Pennsylvania and earned his B.S. degree from Clarion State College. He continued his education through graduate studies, receiving his M.S. degree from the University of Michigan in 1984, from the Department of Kinesiology, and a Ph.D. degree in physiology from Auburn University in 1990. Joseph was a faculty member of the Department of Sport Health Science at Life University in Georgia and eventually joined the faculty at Mississippi State University in 2000. He rose to the rank of associate professor in the Department of Kinesiology, and served as the department's graduate coordinator and interim head. Joseph touched the lives of many students as a graduate adviser and committee member, mentoring more than 25 students in his discipline. With an always positive attitude, Joseph was a devoted husband, father, and friend to many. He will be missed.*

# Preface

*Essentials of Sports Nutrition and Supplements* brings credible information, research-based education, and validated sports nutrition protocols to the sports nutrition professional and academician. It is the single best resource for anyone interested in the field. This book contains information from the thought leaders in the field, provides the latest scientific (basic and applied in the category) findings, is the culmination of thousands of hours of work, as well as the genesis of an academic society dedicated to sports nutrition. That is, the International Society of Sports Nutrition (ISSN) was founded several years ago to fill the needs of consumers, scientists, and students of sports nutrition. Prior to the genesis of the ISSN, there was no single place that one could go to learn sports nutrition. Certainly, we saw enormous potential in the field of sports nutrition. Advances in the scientific understanding of the link between specific nutritional and supplementation protocols and human performance will make this a tremendously exciting field for decades to come. As scientists, we have dedicated our lives to the sports nutrition field out of passion to see its potential further realized. Many of the current sports nutrition marketing companies work against fulfilling that potential. By featuring physiques that are largely unattainable and unbelievable claims in their advertising, they create an aura of incredibility around their brands. By focusing on hyperbolic advertising instead of clinical research and consumer education, they are failing the professional and serious consumer who simply wants to know the truth. Despite a high level of advertising communications, we think the sports nutrition market (both academic and industrial) is largely underserved. We believe there should be a place that professionals and serious consumers can come for access to the real science and intelligent commentary on sports nutrition. Our goal, via this book as well as the world-class conferences organized by the ISSN, is to bring you scientifically-based information on the sports nutrition and supplement category.

*Essentials of Sports Nutrition and Supplements* should be required reading for all students of exercise physiology and dietetics, and for fitness professionals. As sports nutrition scientists, we are *always* looking for novel breakthroughs in basic and applied sports nutrition. With the introduction of creatine monohydrate in the early 1990s, the sports nutrition industry (both on the research side and the business side) grew rapidly. Not only is the sports supplement industry a $20 billion business, but when you add to the mix the category of functional foods (i.e., foods with supplements added to them), you have an industry that is worth $40 billion or more. With such rapid growth comes consumer confusion (and academic confusion for that matter) regarding what's true and what's marketing hyperbole. Unfortunately, there is no quick way to learn the science of sports nutrition. However, our goal through this textbook is to give you the tools to make an educated and wise decision about the sports nutrition category.

The field of sports nutrition is not "owned" by exercise physiologists or clinical dietitians. It is its own field. It is part exercise, part nutrition, combined with a bit of biochemistry, cell biology, physiology, and anatomy. Thus, with the diverse background of the editors and authors, we truly have accomplished

the gargantuan task of culling the latest science in this new and exciting field
and delivering it to you in a timely fashion.

*Jose Antonio, PhD*
Co-Founder and CEO of the International
Society of Sports Nutrition

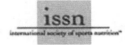

# Contents

# About the Editors and Contributors

**Jose Antonio, PhD**, is the CEO of the International Society of Sports Nutrition (www.theissn.org). He earned his doctorate at the University of Texas Southwestern Medical Center in Dallas, Texas, and completed a postdoctoral fellowship (at UT Southwestern) in Endocrinology and Metabolism. He has coauthored or coedited several books in the sports nutrition field (www.joseantoniophd.com). Contact: DrJoseAntonio@aol.com; Web: www.theissn.org.

**Christopher C. Cheatham, PhD**, is currently an Assistant Professor of Exercise Science in the Department of Health, Physical Education, and Recreation at Western Michigan University. Previously, Dr. Cheatham completed his Bachelor of Science at Miami University, his Master of Science at Ball State University, and his PhD at Kent State University. Before joining the faculty of Western Michigan University, Dr. Cheatham completed a Postdoctoral Fellowship at the John B. Pierce Laboratory, Yale University School of Medicine. His research interests include environmental physiology, the role of exercise and environment on the control of plasma volume, and the impact of nicotine on human performance and thermoregulation. Contact: chris.cheatham@wmich.edu.

**Joseph A. Chromiak, PhD, CSCS, FACSM**, is an Associate Professor in the Department of Kinesiology at Mississippi State University. Dr. Chromiak is a Fellow of the American College of Sports Medicine and is a Certified Strength and Conditioning Specialist. Dr. Chromiak earned a BS degree in biology from Clarion University of Pennsylvania, received an MS degree in kinesiology at the University of Michigan, and earned a PhD in the Interdepartmental Physiology program at Auburn University. Dr. Chromiak was awarded a National Institutes of Health Postdoctoral Fellowship to study with Dr. Herman Vandenburgh at Brown University. His recent research has examined the effects of nutritional supplements and resistance training on body composition and muscular performance. Contact: jchrom@colled.msstate.edu.

**Richard D. Collins, Esq.**, is a lawyer who practices primarily in the area of nutritional supplement law and sports drug defense. He has extensive experience in criminal defense and has successfully tried many serious cases to verdict, including acquittals on a variety of felony charges. He has also conducted civil litigation, including genealogic kinship hearings in Stockholm, Sweden, on behalf of the Public Administrator of Nassau County. He has successfully represented people from all walks of life, from coast to coast, and is known for his thorough and attentive service to all of his clients. A former competitive bodybuilder and certified personal trainer, he often advises legal clients in the strength, health, and fitness community. He is the legal advisor to the International Federation of BodyBuilders and the International Society of Sports Nutrition. Contact: rcollins@cmgesq.com or www.rickcollinsonline.com.

**Suzanne Girard Eberle, MS, RD**, author of *Endurance Sports Nutrition* (Human Kinetics Publishers), is a sports dietitian who practices what she teaches. A former elite runner (4:28 mile/32:40 10 K, 5000-meter national champion, member 3 USA teams), Dr. Eberle lectures, writes and maintains a private practice in Portland, Oregon. She is an avid runner, cyclist, and mountaineer and rock climber. Dr. Eberle holds a master's degree in clinical nutrition from Boston University. She is a member of the American College of Sports Medicine, the American Dietetic Association, and its Sports, Cardiovascular and Wellness Nutritionists Practice Group. Contact: ebcruz@aol.com; www.eat-drinkwin.com.

**Alan H. Feldstein**, JD, brings with him more than a dozen years of advertising and marketing law experience and more than seven years in the dietary supplement industry. His legal career began as a successful civil trial lawyer prosecuting business litigation cases for his clients. He then joined and became a partner in a New York advertising and marketing law firm representing film, television, and music clients, business clients, advertising agencies, direct response television clients, marketing firms, and advertisers. Known for his negotiating skills and business acumen, Dr. Feldstein's clients always have appreciated his business perspective on resolving legal issues affecting their business. Contact: info@cmgesq.com or by phone: 516-294-0300.

**Steven J. Fleck**, PhD, is Chair of the Sport Science Department at Colorado College in Colorado Springs. He earned a PhD in exercise physiology from Ohio State University in 1978. He has headed the physical conditioning program of the U.S. Olympic Committee; served as strength coach for the German Volleyball Association; and coached high school track, basketball, and football. Dr. Fleck is a former vice president of basic and applied research for the National Strength and Conditioning Association (NSCA) and is a Fellow of the American College of Sports Medicine (ACSM). He was honored in 1991 as the NSCA Sport Scientist of the Year. Contact: sfleck@coloradocollege.edu.

**Cassandra Forsythe**, PhD, is a student at the University of Connecticut studying exercise science and nutrition under the supervision of Jeff Volek, PhD, RD. In December 2007, her first diet and weight loss book entitled *The Perfect Body Plan*, written for Women's Health Magazine, was released. Also in December 2007, her second book with Lou Schuler and Alwyn Cosgrove, entitled *The New Rules of Lifting for Women: Lift Like a Man, Look Like a Goddess*, was available on shelves. Contact: cassforsythe@hotmail.com.

**Mike Greenwood**, PhD, is a Professor in the Department of Health, Human Performance, and Recreation at Baylor University. At Baylor he serves as the HHPR Graduate Coordinator as well as the Research Coordinator primarily involved with the Center for Exercise, Nutrition & Preventive Health and the Exercise & Sport Nutrition Laboratory. Dr. Greenwood is a Fellow of ISSN and ACSM and is certified as a strength and conditioning specialist with distinction by the NSCA. He was honored with the NSCA Educator of the Year Award in 2004. He has previously served as a collegiate athletic coach as well as a strength training/conditioning professional. Contact: Mike_Greenwood@baylor.edu.

**G. Gregory Haff**, PhD, is an Assistant Professor of exercise physiology in the medical school at the University of West Virginia. He was awarded the National Strength and Conditioning Association's Young Investigator Award in 2001. He is a member of the National Strength and Conditioning Association's Research Committee and the United States Weightlifting Association's Scientific Committee. Dr. Haff received his PhD from the University of Kansas and his MS from Appalachian State University. Dr. Haff is actively involved in research examining carbohydrate supplements and anaerobic performance. Contact: ghaff@hsc.wvu.edu.

**Disa L. Hatfield**, MA, is currently a Doctoral Fellow in the Department of Kinesiology at the University of Connecticut. She earned her Bachelor of Science degree in Exercise Science from The Pennsylvania State University.

Her first MA was in Health and Human Development Psychology from Antioch University, Santa Barbara, and her second was in Kinesiology from The University of Connecticut. Her research interests are in the areas of resistance training as it relates to exercise endocrinology, children, and nutrition.

**Jennifer Hofheins, MS, RD, LD**, is currently an Exercise and Sports Nutritionist at the Ohio Institute of Health & Human Performance and for the Ohio Research Group (ORG). Research at ORG primarily focuses on the effects of sports and dietary supplements on athletic performance and body composition. She is also active in developing worksite wellness programs as well as disease prevention counseling at local athletic clubs. Jennifer is an active member of the International Society of Sports Nutrition and the American Dietetic Association. She received her Masters in Dietetics from D'Youville College in Buffalo, New York. Contact: jennifer@ohioresearchgroup.com.

**John L. Ivy, PhD, FACSM**, is Chair and Margie Gurley Seay Centennial Professor in the Department of Kinesiology and Health Education, and Professor in the College of Pharmacy, Division of Pharmacology, University of Texas at Austin. He received his PhD in Exercise Physiology from the University of Maryland and his postdoctoral training in physiology and biochemistry from Washington University School of Medicine. He has published more than 140 research and review articles on exercise physiology and the effects of nutrition on physical performance and exercise recovery. He has authored two books on sports nutrition, *Nutrient Timing: The Future of Sports Nutrition* and *The Performance Zone*. Contact: johnivy@mail.utexas.edu.

**Douglas Kalman, PhD, RD**, is the Director at Miami Research Associates in the Nutrition & Endocrinology Division. Mr. Kalman is also a nutrition consultant to NIKE Inc. and the Executive Vice-President of the International Society of Sports Nutrition (www.theissn.org). He is a Fellow of the American College of Nutrition and an original cofounder of the ISSN. He has published extensively in the sports nutrition and supplements field. Contact: dkalman@miamiresearch.com.

**Susan M. Kleiner, PhD, RD, FACN, CNS**, is the owner of HIGH PERFORMANCE NUTRITION™, a consulting firm specializing in media communications, industry consulting, and personal counseling, on Mercer Island, Washington. She is also an Affiliate Assistant Professor in the Department of Medical History and Ethics at The University of Washington School of Medicine. Dr. Kleiner is the author of POWER EATING®, 2nd Edition (Human Kinetics Publishers, 2001). Contact: susan@powereating.com.

**William J. Kraemer, PhD, FACSM, CSCS**, is a Full Professor in the Department of Kinesiology in the Neag School of Education working in the Human Performance Laboratory at the University of Connecticut, Storrs, Connecticut. He also holds an appointment as a full professor in the Department of Physiology and Neurobiology along with an appointment as a Professor of Medicine at the UCONN Health Center/School of Medicine. Contact: william.kraemer@uconn.edu.

**Richard B. Kreider, PhD, FACSM**, is a Professor and Chair of the Department of Health, Human Performance & Recreation at Baylor University and the Director of the Center for Exercise, Nutrition & Preventive Health Research. Dr. Kreider has published more than 100 peer-reviewed articles in the field of sports nutrition and is considered one of the foremost experts in the area of sports nutrition and supplementation. Contact: Richard_Kreider@baylor.edu.

**Jamie Landis, MD, PhD, CSCS**, received a BS in Biology from Ferris State University, an MS in Endocrine Physiology, and a PhD in Neuroscience, both from Bowling Green State University. His MD was earned at the Medical University of Ohio, followed by a residency appointment at the Mayo Clinic. He also holds the CSCS and volunteers his time as a youth weightlifting and football coach. Dr. Landis is currently an Associate Professor of Biology at Lakeland Community College.

**Chris Lockwood, MS, CSCS**, was formerly the Senior Category Director of Diet and Energy for the GNC Corporation (Pittsburgh, PA), and Senior Brand Manager of ABB/Science Foods, formerly a division of Weider Nutrition (Salt Lake City, UT). Mr. Lockwood also worked as the Health and Fitness Writer for *Muscle&Fitness*, and remains an active author and editor of trade publication articles with more than 100 works to his credit, including a scientific review chapter on creatine (*Sports Supplement Encyclopedia*, 2001). Contact: cmlockwood2@yahoo.com.

**Lonnie Lowery, PhD**, holds graduate degrees in both exercise physiology and nutrition and is currently President of Nutrition, Exercise and Wellness Associates, LLC. His company develops academic materials and lay writing regarding exercise and nutrition while providing weight management programs and sports performance services for persons at all levels. Contact: lonman7@hotmail.com.

**Anssi H. Manninen, MHS**, is a well-published research scientist in the sports nutrition field. He holds an MHS in sports medicine from University of Kuopio Medical School. His current position is Senior Science Editor at Advanced Research Press, a publisher of *Muscular Development, FitnessRx for Women,* and *FitnessRx for Men*. He is also an Associate Editor for *Nutrition & Metabolism*, a BioMed Central publication. Contact: sportsnutrition@luukku.com.

**Michael R. McGuigan, PhD**, is currently a Senior Lecturer in Exercise Physiology in the School of Exercise, Biomedical and Health Sciences at Edith Cowan University, Australia. He completed his PhD at Southern Cross University and a postdoctoral research fellowship at Ball State University. His research interests include strength and power development, monitoring training, and the use of resistance training as a health intervention of different populations. Contact: m.mcguigan@ecu.edu.au.

**Ronald W. Mendel, PhD**, holds a doctorate in Exercise Physiology from Kent State University. Dr. Mendel is cofounder of the Ohio Research Group and is the Laboratory Director for the Ohio Institute of Health & Human Performance. He is an active member in the International Society of Sports Nutrition, the American College of Sports Medicine, the National Strength and Conditioning Association, and the American Society of Exercise Physiologists (ASEP) and is the former president of the Ohio Association of Exercise Physiologists. He also maintains adjunct status at several universities. Contact: ron@ohioresearchgroup.com.

**Christopher R. Mohr, PhD, RD, LDN**, is a consultant, author, and freelance writer. He completed his dietetic internship at the University of Delaware, allowing him to sit for the national registration exam to become a Registered Dietitian. From there, Chris attended the University of Massachusetts to pursue a Master of Science in Nutrition Science. While at UMASS, Chris was a Sports Dietitian who worked with most of the 23 Division I teams at the University. He earned a PhD in Exercise Physiology at the University of Pittsburgh. Contact: chris@MohrResults.com.

**Christopher J. Rasmussen, MS, CSCS**, is the Research Coordinator of the Exercise and Sport Nutrition Laboratory within the Center for Exercise, Nutrition and Preventive Health Research at Baylor University. He is also a part-time Lecturer within the Department of Health, Human Performance and Recreation teaching both Human Performance and Health Education courses. Contact: Chris_Rasmussen@baylor.edu.

**Nicholas A. Ratamess, PhD, CSCS**, is currently an Assistant Professor in the Department of Health and Exercise Science at The College of New Jersey. His major research interest is examining how the human body physiologically adapts to resistance training and has authored and coauthored more than 40 scientific and educational publications in the strength and conditioning field. Contact: ratamess@tcnj.edu.

**Timothy P. Scheett, PhD**, is currently an Assistant Professor in the Department of Physical Education and Health at the College of Charleston, South Carolina. Dr. Scheett earned his doctorate at the University of Connecticut. Contact: ScheettT@cofc.edu.

**Christopher B. Scott, PhD**, worked for 5 years at the Cooper Institute for Aerobic Research in Dallas, Texas, and another 5 years in clinical cardiology and pulmonary practice. He is now Assistant Professor in Sports Medicine at the University of Southern Maine. His research focus is on exercise metabolism. Dr. Scott earned his PhD at the University of Wyoming, Laramie. Contact: cscott@usm.maine.edu.

**Rick Seip, PhD, FACSM**, is Senior Scientist in Preventive Cardiology at Hartford Hospital in Hartford, Connecticut. He received the PhD from University of Virginia and completed postdoctoral training in Atherosclerosis, Nutrition, and Lipid Research at Washington University School of Medicine, St. Louis. He has coauthored more than 40 peer-reviewed publications. Contact: rlseip@ aol.com.

**Alan E. Shugarman, MS, RD**, has worked in the nutrition, dietary supplement, and health and fitness industry for more than 15 years. He holds a Bachelor of Science in Chemistry & Biology with a minor in Nutrition, a Master of Science in Food & Nutrition Science, and is a Registered Dietitian. Currently Dr. Shugarman works as a consultant, researcher, product developer, and writer for the nutrition and dietary supplement industry through Discovery Nutrition, Inc. (www.DiscoveryNutrition.com).

**Marie Spano, MS, RD**, is a registered dietitian and holds a BS in Exercise and Sport Science from the University of North Carolina Greensboro and an MS in Foods and Nutrition from the University of Georgia, where she helped run the UGA Sports Nutrition program for the athletic department. Ms. Spano is a Health Scientist working in nutrition and physical activity for the federal government and also works as a freelance writer, consultant, and speaker. Contact: mariespano@comcast.net.

**Jim Stoppani, PhD**, received his doctorate in exercise physiology from the University of Connecticut in 2000 and completed a postdoctoral research fellowship in the prestigious John B. Pierce Laboratory and Department of Cellular and Molecular Physiology at Yale University School of Medicine, where he investigated the effects of exercise and diet on gene regulation in skeletal muscle. He was awarded the Gatorade Beginning Investigator in Exercise Science Award in 2002. Currently, he serves as science editor for *Muscle & Fitness*, *Muscle & Fitness Hers*, and *Flex* magazines at Weider Publications in Woodland Hills, California, and is a science consultant for numerous companies, including Physical magazine, Power Plate, ProSource, StrengthPro, Scivation, and PrimaForce. Contact: jstoppani@amilink.com.

**Jeffrey R. Stout, PhD**, holds a BS degree in Exercise Science from Concordia University, a Masters in Exercise Science, and a PhD in Exercise Physiology from the University of Nebraska in Lincoln. He is a Fellow of the American College of Sports Medicine (FACSM), and Certified Strength and Conditioning Specialist (CSCS). In 2001, Dr. Stout was awarded the leading young scientist of the year by the National Strength and Conditioning Association. Dr. Stout currently teaches and conducts research at the University of Oklahoma. Contact: jeffstoutcscs@aol.com.

**Darin Van Gammeren, MAEd, CSCS**, earned his BS in Exercise Science at the University of Sioux Falls and his master's degree at the University of Nebraska at Kearney (UNK). While at UNK, Mr. Van Gammeren conducted research on various sports supplements and their effects on body composition and athletic performance. Currently, Mr. Van Gammeren is a doctoral candidate in the Exercise Biochemistry Laboratory at the University of Florida studying skeletal muscle plasticity. Specifically, the laboratory is attempting to determine the specific pathways involved in free radical–mediated damage to skeletal muscle. Contact: dgrizz@yahoo.com.

**Jakob L. Vingren, MS,** earned his baccalaureate and master's degrees in the Department of Kinesiology at the University of North Texas. His research interests include resistance exercise as it relates to muscle physiology and endocrinology. Contact: jakob.vingren@uconn.edu.

**Jeff S. Volek, PhD, RD,** received his doctorate from the Pennsylvania State University and is now an assistant professor in the Department of Kinesiology at the University of Connecticut. He has produced more than 100 scientific publications in the area of nutrition and exercise science. His current research focus is on how very-low-carbohydrate diets affect a variety of clinical and performance outcomes including fasting and postprandial lipoproteins, weight loss, body composition, hormonal responses, and adaptations to exercise training. Contact: jvolek@uconnvm.uconn.edu.

**Joe Weir, PhD,** earned his doctorate in exercise physiology from the University of Nebraska and is currently a Professor in the Division of Physical Therapy at Des Moines University–Osteopathic Medical Center. His research interests focus on neuromuscular and autonomic responses to exercise and digital signal processing. Contact: Joseph.Weir@dmu.edu.

**Darryn S. Willoughby, PhD,** holds BS and MEd degrees in Exercise Science from Tarleton State University and a PhD in Neuromuscular Physiology and Biochemistry with a sub-emphasis in Nutritional Biochemistry from Texas A&M University. He is a Fellow of the American College of Sports Medicine and International Society of Sport Nutrition. He is a Certified Strength and Conditioning Specialist through the National Strength and Conditioning Association, and a Certified Nutritional Consultant through the American Fitness Professionals and Associates. Dr. Willoughby is currently an Associate Professor of Exercise and Nutritional Biochemistry and Molecular Physiology at Baylor University in Waco, Texas. Contact: Darryn_Willoughby@baylor.edu.

**Tim N. Ziegenfuss, PhD, CSCS,** is the Chief Executive Officer of The Ohio Research Group of Exercise Science and Sports Nutrition. "Dr. Z" is a well-known author, speaker, and researcher with expertise in exercise training, nutrition, dietary supplements, and sports performance. He is a Fellow of the International Society of Sports Nutrition, a Certified Strength and Conditioning Specialist, and Chair of the exercise physiology and sports nutrition program at Huntington University. Contact: zsciences@yahoo.com.

# Companion CD

This CD-ROM contains a study guide in Adobe PDF format. Adobe Reader® is required to view this document. We have included installers for this free software on this disc for both Mac and PC computers. The application is compatible with most Mac and PC computers.

## PC USERS:

The application "HP_ESN_StudyGuide.exe" should launch automatically on most Windows computers when the disc is inserted into your computer. If the application does not start after a few moments, simply double click the application "HP_ESN_StudyGuide.exe" located on the root of this CD-ROM.

## MAC OSX USERS:

Double click the application "HP_ESN_StudyGuide" after inserting the CD-ROM. The Mac OSX operating system does not support an auto-start feature.

The following hardware and software are the minimum required to use this CD-ROM:

- For Microsoft Windows: An Intel Pentium II with 64 MB of available RAM running Windows 98, or an Intel Pentium III with 128 MB of available RAM running Windows 2000 or Windows XP. A monitor set to 1024 × 768 or higher resolution.
- **For Macintosh OS X**: A Power Macintosh G3 with 128 MB of available RAM running Mac OS X 10.1.5, 10.2.6 or higher. A monitor set to **1024 × 768** or higher resolution.

# PART I

# Basic Exercise Physiology

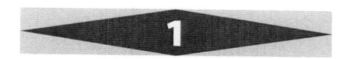

# Thermodynamics, Biochemistry, and Metabolism

## Christopher B. Scott

## OBJECTIVES

On the completion of this chapter you will be able to:

1. Understand the different energy systems used for physical activity.
2. Know how to apply your knowledge of exercise bioenergetics to athletic training programs.
3. Understand how the principle of training specificity relates to exercise bioenergetics.

## ABSTRACT

It is critical for the sports nutritionist to understand the chemical underpinnings of exercise and nutrition. For instance, with the knowledge of the phosphagen energy system, it becomes clear how a dietary supplement such as creatine monohydrate might exert its ergogenic effects. Without such knowledge, you are left to guesswork and speculation. Bioenergetics describes how the continuous exchange of matter and energy through an organism affects energy availability; energy exchange is "costly" in that not all energy is available to perform useful work (e.g., some energy is lost as heat). Energy exchange takes place throughout the anaerobic and aerobic multienzyme metabolic pathways with the breakdown (oxidation) of carbohydrates and fats; the energy held within their molecular bonds is ultimately used to resynthesize adenosine triphosphate (ATP). The chemo-mechanical conversion of ATP (hydrolysis) to allow muscular contraction represents another site of energy exchange. The cycle of ATP hydrolysis and ATP resynthesis is defined as ATP turnover and is described by energy expenditure. Energy expenditure can be interpreted using heat and/or $O_2$ uptake measurements, yet these measures are not always similar; for example, with rapid anaerobic ATP turnover, heat production can exceed $O_2$ uptake. The quantification of total energy expenditure requires estimates or measures of both anaerobic and aerobic ATP turnover during exercise and the recovery from exercise.

*Key Words:* bioenergetics, metabolism, sports-specific, training, biochemistry

Life exploits the natural tendency of energy to be exchanged, undergoing conversion from one form to another and transfer from one place to another. We require this exploitation to interact physically within our environment. What is energy transfer? "Energy" has been traditionally viewed as the capacity to do work or the ability to cause change.[1] The term "transfer" recognizes a removal or shifting from one place to another. The term "conversion" indicates a format change where one type of energy becomes another type of energy. We obtain energy from the environment in the form of food. The environment also withholds what is left over after energy conversion and transfer. Thus,

From: *Essentials of Sports Nutrition and Supplements*
Edited by J. Antonio, D. Kalman, J. R. Stout, M. Greenwood, D. S. Willoughby, and G. G. Haff © Humana Press, a part of Springer Science+Business Media, Totowa, NJ

life changes the environment; these changes can be measured to allow us to interpret the "costs of living" or, in the case of athletes, to determine the costs of training, competing, and recovering from such events. Biologic energy exchange is termed bioenergetics. Bioenergetics invokes the study of thermodynamics, biochemistry, and energy expenditure.

## THERMODYNAMICS

Spontaneity is defined as happening or occurring without external cause. Spontaneous energy exchange requires a gradient. If we place a ball on a ramped surface, for example, the ball will spontaneously roll downhill. Spontaneous energy exchange also takes place in a "downhill" direction, from a source of high energy content to a point of lower energy content (high energy → low energy). Our most basic understanding of this comes in the form of convection as heat flows toward cold (hot → cold). That is one of the 2nd "laws" of thermodynamics. No one has yet witnessed the spontaneous "uphill" flow of energy (heat). It may seem that we are getting ahead of ourselves in terms of the order of learning the thermodynamic laws but in fact the 2nd laws of thermodynamics were founded before the 1st.

One well-known act of energy (heat) exchange is combustion. This occurs when a high-energy fuel that is full of electrons $(e^-)$ and protons $(H^+)$ readily gives them up to oxygen $(O_2)$. The greater the content of $e^-$ and $H^+$ within a fuel, the more energy it is said to contain. Lower-energy products at the completion of combustion can be found in the form of carbon dioxide $(CO_2)$ and water $(H_2O)$. Because combustion involves only a single step during $e^-$ and $H^+$ transfer, it is often a sudden and violent reaction that generates a good deal of heat. Metabolism is the biologic equivalent of combustion. It too entails an act of $e^-$ and $H^+$ transfer along with heat production; albeit, these exchanges are controlled, occurring at a much slower rate than combustion.

Thermodynamics flourished with the study of mechanical motion and heat production or more appropriately, the conversion of heat (energy) to mechanical motion. Heat is an expression of energy; temperature is a measure of intensity or the degree of hotness or coldness of an object. Almost 300 years ago, the first functional steam engines converted heat to mechanical motion with horrendous efficiency, at approximately 6% or worse. Thus, ~94% of the heat (energy) from the fire beneath a steam engine was dissipated into the environment. Currently, engineers design automobiles that operate at approximately 25% efficiency; diesel engines operate at about 35% efficiency. A bicyclist or jogger represents another kind of "machine" that operates with efficiency somewhere in between a gasoline and diesel engine. That is the second half of the 2nd law of thermodynamics; energy conversion and transfer operate with efficiency, the exchange is never perfect. When one form of energy can spontaneously convert to another form, the "value" of that energy is degraded; the transfer of energy from place to place also "costs". This is why perpetual motion machines do not work. As we shall see, both the type of "machine" and the surrounding environment are critical to how engineers and biologists interpret the 2nd law(s) of thermodynamics.

The 1st law of thermodynamics states that energy is conserved. It was Isaac Newton who started conservative thinking with his discovery that momentum was conserved; momentum cannot be spontaneously created from nothing, nor can it be stopped unless acted upon by an outside force. Matter also is conserved; it too cannot be spontaneously created nor destroyed. But make no mistake about it, matter and energy can and do change form. Thermodynamics was the first science to acknowledge, identify, and measure those changes.

## ENERGY EXCHANGE

In an isolated system, within a thermos, for example, no exchange takes place between the system and its environment (a system is any specific quantity of matter or region in space; a thermos, a hot water bottle, and your body are all examples of different types of systems). In a closed system (e.g., a hot water bottle) heat but not matter is exchanged between the system and the environment. Living organisms require a continuous input of nourishment and output of waste, that is, a continuous flux of matter and energy allows us to exist. Cells and athletes all represent open systems as they couple together the forces and flows behind matter and energy exchange.[2] Indeed, life has modified itself from and uses the environment to exploit and create energy gradients (high → low). Living cells do this in a number of ways, for example, by the use of membranes and other structures to create compartments that separate biochemical and electrical gradients, by coupling metabolic pathways that require energy to those that provide energy, and by increasing the flow of substances to and away from active metabolic sites within the cell. Life's modifications are a costly attempt to manipulate the energy exchange potential of a given biochemical reaction.

Because energy can be distributed unequally within or between a system and its immediate environment, the capacity for flow, from high to low, is evident. Scientists are apt to describe ideas with terms and symbols and to substitute these with numbers in an attempt to solve problems. For our discussion, the initial or total energy content within or available to a system will be described as the enthalpy, and has been given the symbol H. By acknowledging the concept of efficiency, it is understood that some of the enthalpy is available to perform work and some is not. The energy that is available to perform work has been given the symbol G in honor of Josiah Gibbs who first described the energy exchanges of chemical reactions. Gibbs also had great appreciation for the energy that was not available to perform work. This nonuseable energy was known as the entropy and was given the symbol S. Expressing these three terms together helps to identify all aspects of energy conversion and transfer:

$$H = G + S$$

The presence of the entropy signifies the grand scheme of energy exchange; useful energy will eventually become useless energy. Other descriptions of the entropy inform us that energy tends to disperse or spread itself out over time (high energy → low energy), randomness is a driving force, and order spontaneously proceeds toward disorder (order → disorder). Taken together, descriptions of the entropy—energy dispersal, inefficiency, useless energy, randomness, disorder—can be difficult to conceptualize. Yet, those who acknowledge and apply entropy production to acts of energy exchange are well rewarded. Indeed, many texts are keen on the following interpretation of useful or available energy because of Gibbs' recognition that enthalpy (H) and entropy (S) are the driving forces behind energy conversion and transfer, respectively:

$$\Delta G = \Delta H - \Delta S$$

Thus, the amount of energy available for use (Gibbs energy, G) is dependent on the total energy within a system and its immediate environment (enthalpy, H) and how much energy is not available (entropy, S). In the above equation, Δ symbolizes to chemists and engineers that there is a beginning and an end to energy exchange so that in a closed system, importance is placed on the difference between the beginning and end points of energy conversion and transfer (Figure 1.1). In a closed system, this difference is not dependent on time so that the rate at which energy exchange takes place is of no concern.

Open systems, however, *must* consider time as matter and energy are exchanged with the environment because an active flux through an open system alters the extent of formation of metabolic products from biochemical reactants.[3,4] In this context, faster rates of energy exchange decrease efficiency. Indeed, all engines operate at a lower efficiency at faster operating speeds and this includes biologic "machines." Moreover, the degree of completion of a biochemical reaction also contributes to the availability of energy. Because of these concerns, open systems are better described not in the context of a beginning and end point, but rather in regard to a particular status in between beginning and end points (Figure 1.1):

$$\partial G \star \partial \xi^{-1}$$

**FIGURE 1.1.** Both figures indicate the Gibbs energy content (G) and concentrations of reactant (r) and product (p) for a hypothetical reaction. On the left is an example of a reaction in a closed system. Closed systems are described by the beginning and end points of the reaction. At the beginning (*) of the reaction there is all reactant (with a high G) and no product. The vertical dotted line and cross (+) signify the end point of the reaction, indicating that less reactant and more product (with a lower G) is present as compared with the start of the reaction; thus, reactant → product. On the right, the reaction takes place within an open system. Gibbs energy availability is represented as the slope of the parabola at any given reactant and product concentration. In an open system, Gibbs energy is degraded and dissipated as the rate of cellular exchange and the product-to-reactant ratio of biochemical reactions both increase. Four different slopes are encircled: (1) at the beginning of the reaction, (2) at about the midpoint of the reaction, (3) at the end point where the reaction is "completed," and (4) under conditions promoting further product formation. Slopes (1) and (2) are negative; this implies a spontaneous reaction. The steeper the negative slope is, the greater the reactant-to-product ratio and the greater is the Gibbs energy availability. Using the energy available from adenosine triphosphate (ATP) as an example, at slope (1) $\partial G = -14\,kcal$, at slope (2) $\partial G = -7\,kcal$, and at a horizontal or zero slope (3) $\partial G = 0\,kcal$ at completion. The parabola indicates that it is advantageous for a cell to keep ATP concentrations relatively higher than adenosine diphosphate so that more energy from ATP is available to the cell. To the right of the "completion" of the reaction (dotted line), the slope is positive (4); it would require the input of energy to make the reaction proceed toward the disappearance of more reactant in the formation of more product. (Adapted from Nicholls and Ferguson.[4])

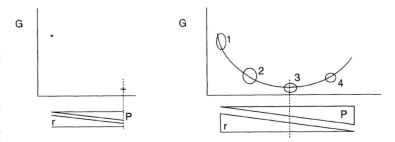

where $\partial$ signifies the rate of exchange, G is Gibbs energy, and $\xi$ is the extent of metabolic product formation from biochemical reactants.[5] The differences between closed and open thermodynamic systems are very real and must be accounted for. Because energy exchange is a nonstop event within an open system, heat and entropy production are the inevitable and continuous result of the irreversible (one-way) flow of matter and energy through a living organism.

In application, life occurs at the expense of the environment.[6] The energy contained within the molecular bonds of the food we eat is described as the enthalpy (H). Life's "costs" are ultimately paid for by the conversion and transfer of energy within food that is made available to us (Gibbs energy, G). The degradation and dissipation of Gibbs energy is measured and calculated as heat and entropy (S) production, respectively.

## BIOCHEMISTRY

Energy is held within the molecular bonds of fats, carbohydrates, and proteins. This energy is exploited as electrons ($e^-$) and protons ($H^+$) from these macronutrients are transferred to a lower-energy end point. Scientists describe $e^-$ and $H^+$ flow as a series of oxidation-reduction (red-ox) reactions where oxidation is the loss of $e^-$ or $H^+$ and reduction is the gain of $e^-$ or $H^+$. The biologic transfer of $e^-$ and $H^+$ within cells is aided by specialized proteins that function as enzymes. Enzymes are catalysts that increase the reaction rate of a spontaneous reaction (enzymes *do not* promote nonspontaneous reactions). Metabolic energy exchanges are typically represented as a series of enzyme-oriented biochemical reactions that are often organized in a flow chart–like manner (Figures 1.2–1.4). Enzyme structure and function and the metabolic intermediates found before, between, and after each enzyme, figure prominently in all contemporary biochemistry textbooks. Biochemists have further recognized that a host of these factors and more can moderate enzyme activity both up (feed-backward) and down (feed-forward) the metabolic pathways. Hormones and other biochemicals can bind to enzymes with the potential to modify enzyme conformation. Slight changes in enzyme shape alter enzyme activity; subsequently, cellular metabolism is affected. The potential influence of a substance on enzyme activity is known as allosteric regulation. Enzyme activity, enzyme concentrations, and enzyme regulators are studied intensely in an attempt to discover how cellular energy exchanges are controlled. As an example, frequent exercise can result in a more efficient energy exchange along the metabolic pathways.

There are a multitude of unique, highly organized metabolic pathways within cells. Some pathways are catabolic in design where food, for example, is broken down and energy is "obtained." Other pathways are anabolic, where energy is utilized, for example, to build cellular materials. Muscular contraction is ultimately fueled by energy conversion and transfer during the biochemical breakdown of fats, carbohydrates, and, to a lesser extent, proteins. There are three types of energy-exchange pathways. Two of these metabolic pathways are anaerobic (without oxygen); the first types utilize a single enzyme, the second requires multiple enzymes. The third metabolic pathway is aerobic (with oxygen) and it too requires multiple enzymes. Importantly, the link

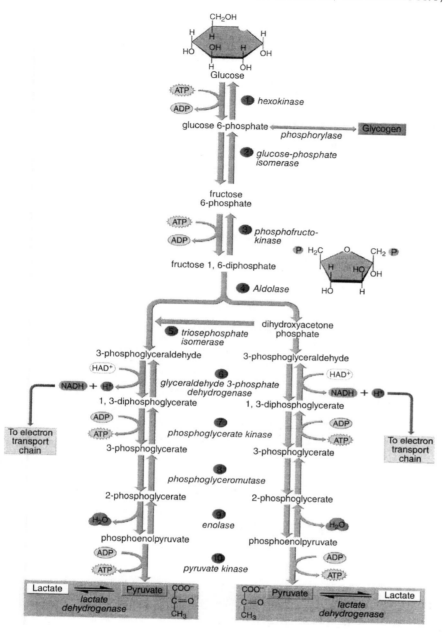

**FIGURE 1.2.** Anaerobic glycolysis occurs in the cellular cytoplasm and includes substrate-level phosphorylation. As its name implies, the metabolic pathway itself does not involve oxygen. Enzymes are numbered and in italic; metabolic intermediates are in bold. In the first half of glycolysis, a 6-carbon glucose molecule is phosphorylated via adenosine triphosphate (ATP) and subsequently cleaved in two. In the last half of glycolysis, the two phosphorylated 3-carbon halves contain enough available energy to resynthesize ATP. If the rate of glycolysis and aerobic respiration are matched, pyruvate enters the Krebs cycle. If the rate of glycolysis exceeds respiration, then the nicotinamide adenine dinucleotide formed in step #6 serves to reduce pyruvate and lactate is subsequently formed. (Reproduced with permission from McArdle, Katch, and Katch, 2001; Figure 6.11.[44])

between the flow of $e^-$ and H$^+$ throughout the multienzyme pathways and muscle contraction is not a direct one. Instead, cells use the metabolic pathways to manufacture a dispensable form of energy in the form of "high-energy" phosphate molecules.

## Adenosine Triphosphate: The "High-Energy" Phosphate

For many cells, immediately available energy comes in the form of the "high-energy" phosphate adenosine triphosphate or ATP. Quotation marks are placed around "high-energy" because the Gibbs energy content of ATP can in fact range from no energy to high energy. A gradient of higher ATP and lower adenosine diphosphate (ADP) concentrations within a cell are kept in an almost 500:1 ratio to maintain a high Gibbs energy availability[7] (Figure 1.1). Yet, even with this high ratio, the concentration of ATP itself within a cell is not large at all. Indeed, the amount of ATP stored within muscle can support contractions for only a few seconds at most. ATP requires a single enzyme, an ATPase,

**FIGURE 1.3.** The first half of the aerobic metabolic pathway is located exclusively within the mitochondria's two membranes and operates to generate electrons ($e^-$) and protons ($H^+$) from the food we eat. All substrate is converted into acetyl-CoA before entry into the cycle. The $e^-$ and $H^+$ carriers NAD and FAD also are depicted. Oxygen is not an immediate part of the Krebs cycle; $O_2$ is present only within the electron transport chain (Figure 1.5). Aerobic metabolic intermediates are in bold; the aerobic enzymes are numbered and in italic. (Reproduced with permission from McArdle, Katch, and Katch, 2001; Figure 6.15.[44])

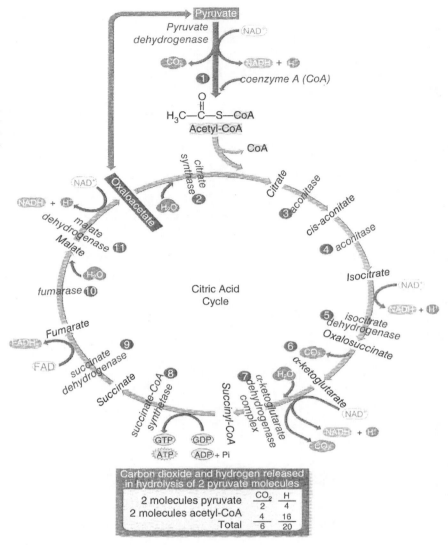

to cleave the last of its three phosphate bonds to form the "lower-energy" products ADP and inorganic phosphate (Pi). ATP cleavage is also known as hydrolysis because it requires water:

$$ATP + H_2O \rightarrow ADP + Pi + H^+ + heat + \Delta S + \partial G$$

ATP hydrolysis also yields a proton ($H^+$; thus, it is a source of metabolic acid), heat, entropy ($\Delta S$), and most importantly useful energy ($\partial G$). Muscle is a chemo-mechanical converter where useful energy is converted from ATP to mechanical motion. The heat and entropy produced during these exchanges represent expenditures, are not recycled and so remain in the environment.

A sedentary human needs about 60–70 kg of ATP to support 1 day of life.[7] It also has been calculated that approximately 60 kg of ATP are required to run the 26 miles of a marathon[8]! How are these rather massive amounts of ATP provided? Accomplishing these feats entails that some of the products of ATP hydrolysis, namely, ADP + Pi, be resynthesized by the metabolic pathways as needed. The energy contained within the molecular bonds of the food we eat is required to resynthesize ATP:

$$ATP + H_2O + heat + \Delta S \leftarrow ADP + Pi + \partial G$$

Heat and entropy production also result from the biochemical-to-biochemical conversion of fats, carbohydrates, and proteins to ATP. As we will see, measurements of energy expenditure attempt to describe biologic ATP turnover that consists of the cycle of 1) ATP hydrolysis fueling cellular work, and 2)

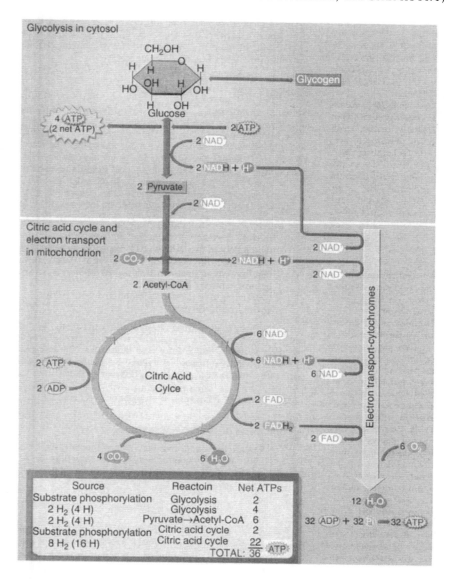

**FIGURE 1.4.** The schematics of the anaerobic and aerobic metabolic pathways are shown where anaerobic energy exchange (i.e., substrate-level phosphorylation) within the cytoplasm (or cytosol) and aerobic energy exchange within mitochondria are joined. Anaerobic glycolysis and the citric acid cycle both oxidize glucose and glycogen and subsequently reduce NAD and FAD which carry $e^-$ and $H^+$ to the electron transport chain. The details of electron transport and the cytochromes are not provided. (Reproduced with permission from McArdle, Katch, and Katch, 2001; Figure 6.16.[44])

ATP resynthesis via the metabolic energy-exchange pathways. It seems that the rate of ATP hydrolysis (i.e., energy demand) best dictates to what degree each of the metabolic pathways contributes to ATP resynthesis (i.e., energy supply).

## More "High-Energy" Phosphates

With extremely rapid rates of ATP hydrolysis, other phosphate molecules act most quickly to resynthesize ATP. Creatine phosphate (CP), for example, contains ample $\partial G$ as it almost instantaneously phosphorylates ADP via the enzyme creatine kinase:

$$CP + ADP + H^+ \rightarrow C + ATP + heat$$

It is of interest that protons ($H^+$) are consumed in the process. Thus, at the very onset of intense muscle contraction, pH can actually increase as the muscle undergoes slight alkalosis. CP is stored in muscle at about 3–4 times the concentration of ATP, but this still is not much. This amount of CP is enough to fuel several seconds of all-out physical work. The rate at which physical work is performed drops off precipitously as CP stores decrease. It was therefore great news when it was discovered that the ingestion of creatine monohydrate could help increase CP stores and enhance muscular strength and endurance.

As intense muscle contraction continues and power output and CP concentrations decrease, the union of two ADP molecules via the enzyme myokinase also contains enough $\partial G$ to resynthesize ATP:

$$2ADP \rightarrow ATP + AMP + heat$$

where AMP is adenosine monophosphate. Recall, however, that the "high-energy" phosphates are a finite energy source; once near depletion, fatigue sets in and normal muscle function ceases. Thankfully, there are other longer-lasting methods that resynthesize ATP to prevent the ATP/ADP ratio from decreasing.

## Glycolysis

During the breakdown of glucose, the transfer of $e^-$ and $H^+$ begins within the cytoplasm of a cell and is known as glycolysis. If glucose is stored for future use instead of immediately being broken apart to obtain useful energy, then another series of biochemical reactions results in glycogen formation; glycogen is the storage form of glucose. Glycogenolysis is the name given to the rapid breakdown of stored glycogen. Glycolysis and glycogenolysis resynthesize ATP as substrate-level phosphorylation.

Glycolysis utilizes several separate enzymes to cleave glucose, a 6-carbon, higher-energy carbohydrate molecule, into two lower-energy, 3-carbon molecules (Figure 1.2). Glycolysis requires two ATP molecules to help accomplish this feat but the investment is well worthwhile. The energy held within the phosphorylated glucose molecules is quickly exchanged to a phosphorylation of four ADP molecules for a net production of two ATPs. The usefulness of substrate-level phosphorylation comes from its rapid rate of ATP resynthesis and the longer time span at which it can perform this function. Glycogenolysis, for example, has the potential to fuel muscle contraction for many seconds longer than the limited stores of "high-energy" phosphates—several minutes or more in a well-motivated athlete. In the example below, glycolysis occurs rapidly where glucose serves as the $e^-$ and $H^+$ donor (oxidation), pyruvate is the $e^-$ and $H^+$ acceptor (reduction), and lactate is subsequently formed.

$$C_6H_{12}O_6 \rightarrow \rightarrow \rightarrow \rightarrow \rightarrow 2e^- + 2H^+ \rightarrow \rightarrow \rightarrow \rightarrow 2C_3H_3O_3^- \rightarrow 2C_3H_5O_3^-$$
Glucose                                          Pyruvate     Lactate

When substrate-level phosphorylation takes place more slowly, then pyruvate remains as the end product of glycolysis and glycogenolysis; that pyruvate may be further broken down to obtain additional energy (see Respiration below). A high concentration of blood and muscle lactate indicates that substrate-level phosphorylation is occurring at an accelerated rate. Lactate has been given a poor reputation from the belief that it is a potent acid that hastens fatigue. This is somewhat misleading because the well-known and excessive formation of metabolic acid (i.e., $H^+$) during heavy/severe exercise actually originates from the rapid hydrolysis of ATP.[9] Unlike CP breakdown and aerobic respiration, however, rapid glycogenolysis does not buffer or reutilize $H^+$. As an ergogenic aid for bouts of heavy/severe exercise, the ingestion of sodium bicarbonate (baking soda) has been used in an attempt to buffer the $H^+$ generated by glycolytically supported ATP turnover and this allows muscle contraction to briefly continue. But be forewarned, the side effects of ingesting baking soda—nausea and diarrhea—can be very real.

# RESPIRATION

Aerobic metabolism does not take place within the cell's cytoplasm and instead requires a compartment or structure of some kind to create an energy-exchange gradient. Cell membranes separate energy gradients. The exchange of $e^-$ and $H^+$ through a cellular membrane is referred to as respiration. The site of aerobic respiration is within the mitochondria. Mitochondria actually possess two membranes. They are often referred to as the "power house" of cells. Mitochondria are where pyruvate and fat undergo aerobic oxidation (proteins too can be oxidized). Mitochondria are known as the powerhouse of cells because of their complete degradation of pyruvate to $CO_2$ and $H_2O$, producing as much as 17 times the ATP of anaerobic glycolysis (that is 34 additional ATPs per molecule of glucose!). Moreover, aerobic metabolism obtains energy from all macronutrients (carbohydrates, fats, and proteins) toward ATP resynthesis; glycolysis and glycogenolysis can only oxidize glucose and glycogen, respectively.

Aerobic metabolism contains two distinct parts: 1) a circular pathway of 11 enzymes that strips $e^-$ and $H^+$ from pyruvate and fat forming carbon dioxide $(CO_2)$ in the process (Figure 1.3), and 1.2) the delivery of $e^-$ and $H^+$ to oxygen $(O_2)$ via the electron transport chain (ETC) that forms ATP and water $(H_2O)$ in the process (Figure 1.4). Below are examples of the aerobic oxidation of lactate and a "typical" fat, palm oil (lactate must be converted back to pyruvate before undergoing aerobic oxidation):

$$2C_3H_5O_3^- + 6O_2 \rightarrow \rightarrow \rightarrow \rightarrow \rightarrow 24e^- + 24H^+ \rightarrow \rightarrow \rightarrow \rightarrow \rightarrow 6CO_2 + 6H_2O$$
Lactate   Oxygen                                      Carbon   Water
                                                      dioxide

$$C_{16}H_{32}O_2 + 23O_2 \rightarrow \rightarrow \rightarrow \rightarrow \rightarrow 92e^- + 92H^+ \rightarrow \rightarrow \rightarrow \rightarrow \rightarrow 16CO_2 + 16H_2O$$
Palm oil  Oxygen                                      Carbon    Water
                                                      dioxide

Aerobic metabolism goes by several names, the Krebs cycle (in honor of its founder Hans Krebs), the citric acid cycle, or the tricarboxylic acid cycle. The word cycle implies a roundabout pathway with the same starting and ending points (Figure 1.3). Before substrate can enter the Krebs cycle it is linked with coenzyme A (Co-A) to become acetyl Co-A. The function of the cycle is to strip $e^-$ and $H^+$ from its 10 metabolic intermediates and attach them to special carrier molecules known as nicotinamide adenine dinucleotide $(NAD^+)$ and flavin adenine dinucleotide $(FAD^+)$. Once reduced, these carriers become NADH and FADH, respectively. The $^+$ sign is missing from NADH and FADH because the positive charges are canceled when carrying two negatively charged electrons. NADH and FADH link the first part of aerobic metabolism to the second.

The ETC is where the $O_2$ part of aerobic metabolism comes into play. Electron flow provides the energy to create a proton $(H^+)$ gradient that ultimately fuels ATP resynthesis (Figures 1.4 and 1.5). Aerobic respiration should be regarded as a marvel of the creation, coupling and exploitation of uphill and downhill energy-exchange gradients. Given the rather immense amounts of $O_2$ we consume during rest, exercise, and the recovery from exercise, a measure of $O_2$ uptake should also serve as an invaluable tool in the estimation of biochemical ATP turnover, and indeed it does.

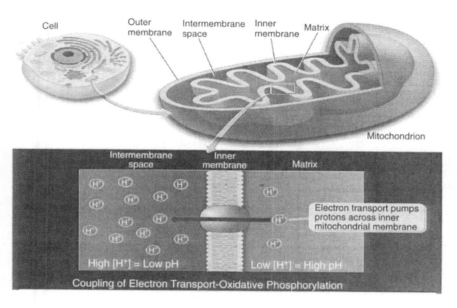

**FIGURE 1.5.** Aerobic respiration provides an excellent example of how cellular compartments separate and subsequently exploit energy exchanges. A gradient exists between the concentration of electrons $(e^-)$ carried by NADH and FADH and oxygen's need for $e^-$; $O_2$ is a strong attractor of $e^-$. The flow of electrons within the electron transport chain from NADH and FADH toward oxygen is exploited to pump protons $(H^+)$ across the inner mitochondrial membrane. This creates a proton gradient where the high concentration of $H^+$ (shown here at bottom, left) is in turn exploited by a mitochondrial enzyme (not shown) to resynthesize ATP from ADP and Pi. (Reproduced with permission from McArdle, Katch, and Katch, 2001; Figure 6.8.[44])

# ENERGY EXPENDITURE

Biologic energy exchanges are described in the context of an open system so that both heat and entropy production (i.e., the degradation and dissipation of Gibbs energy) result from ATP turnover. Thermometers measure temperature, calorimeters measure heat, and the production of the entropy is calculated. $\Delta H$, $\Delta G$, $\Delta S$, work and heat are all measured in units called Joules (1 Joule $\approx$ 0.24 calories; 1 calorie is the "amount" of heat required to increase 1 g of water from 14.5° to 15.5°C). Because heat is a quantifiable expression of energy, direct calorimetry serves as the standard interpretation of energy expenditure. Unfortunately, direct calorimeters are difficult devices to operate. That difficulty resides in the size requirements necessary to house a human subject, the extended length of time required to obtain a meaningful measurement, and the costs involved with building and operating such a device. Thankfully, indirect calorimetry, that is, a measurement of gas exchange—$O_2$ uptake, $CO_2$ production, and ventilation—also can be used to estimate heat production in the estimation of energy expenditure.[10,11]

Technologic advancements have allowed for the measurement of gas exchange to become a universal procedure. Oxygen uptake, $CO_2$ production, and ventilation measurements are now collected by tabletop or handheld devices that can be hooked up to a personal computer to immediately analyze metabolic rate (i.e., energy expenditure). It must be understood, however, that directly measured heat production and the estimate of heat production as provided by $O_2$ uptake are often, but not always, similar (Figure 1.6). Direct and indirect calorimetry are proportional only when an organism resides at a steady state, that is, at maturity, at a stable body weight, and at rest or during low-intensity exercise within a comfortable environment. Gas-exchange measurements at steady state also allow us to determine what substrate is being utilized (oxidized) as a fuel during aerobic respiration.

Determining whether carbohydrate or fat oxidation is taking place requires a division of the number of $CO_2$ molecules exhaled by the number of $O_2$ molecules consumed. When expired air from the mouth and nose is analyzed, this ratio is termed respiratory exchange ratio or RER. At an RER of 1.00, an equal exchange of $CO_2$ and $O_2$ takes place and carbohydrates (e.g., glucose or glycogen) are the exclusive fuel source. The higher the exercise intensity, the greater is the amount of carbohydrate oxidation. Recall that carbohydrate oxidation involves both anaerobic substrate-level phosphorylation and aerobic mitochondrial respiration (Figure 1.4) where heat production has been measured at 21.1 kJ (~5.0 kcals) for every liter of $O_2$ consumed:

$$C_6H_{12}O_6 + 6O_2 \rightarrow 6CO_2 + 6H_2O \qquad 6CO_2 * 6O_2^{-1} = \text{RER of 1.00 Glucose}$$

At an RER of 0.70, an individual is exclusively using fat as a fuel where heat production equals 19.6 kJ (~4.7 kcals) per liter of $O_2$ consumed. Fat is oxidized exclusively within mitochondria; fat oxidation usually fuels resting energy expenditure and energy expenditure at low or easy exercise intensities:

$$C_{16}H_{32}O_2 + 23O_2 \rightarrow 16CO_2 + 16H_2O$$

$$16CO_2 * 23O_2^{-1} = \text{RER of 0.70 Palm oil}$$

**FIGURE 1.6.** These data reveal how measures of direct (heat or $Q_h$; dotted line) and indirect ($O_2$ uptake or M; solid line) calorimetry differentiate throughout a day in an adult sedentary human subject.[39] Between 0500 and 1700 hours, heat production as estimated by $O_2$ uptake exceeds directly measured heat production; the body appears to be storing heat. Between 2300 and 0500 hours, heat production exceeds $O_2$ uptake; the body appears to be "de-storing" heat. Discrepancies in heat production and $O_2$ uptake within this sedentary subject are an indication of the natural fluctuations that occur throughout a day. If rapid glycolysis with lactate production contributes significantly to ATP turnover, a discrepancy also is created between heat production and $O_2$ uptake. A rapid anaerobic metabolism produces heat in excess of aerobic metabolism so that the interpretation of total energy expenditure requires an estimate and/or measure of both anaerobic and aerobic metabolic contributions to ATP turnover.

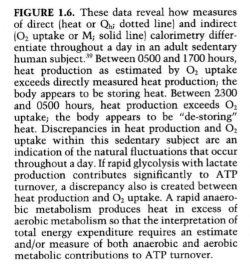

The slight difference in heat production per oxygen equivalent has been traditionally explained by the hydrogen/carbon ratio of the substances being oxidized.[12] Yet this ratio (2 hydrogens/1 carbon) is identical for both palm oil and glucose. Thus, the 1.5-kJ difference between fat and carbohydrate oxidation, although small, is perhaps better attributed to anaerobic energy exchange (entropy and heat production). Substrate-level phosphorylation contributes ~2 of ~36 mol of ATP resynthesis during the oxidation of 1 mol of glucose and this too suggests a small portion of energy exchange from anaerobic sources. In fact, $O_2$ uptake as part of mitochondrial heat production[10] (at 19.6 kJ per liter of $O_2$ consumed) is similar to $O_2$ uptake during combustion;[13] in both instances, there is no anaerobic component. During combustion, the ratio of heat flux to $O_2$ flux has been measured at –450 kJ per mole of $O_2$ uptake (~19.6 kJ per liter of $O_2$ uptake).[10,12] However, in cultivated mammalian cells, heat production can exceed –800 kJ·mol $O_2^{-1}$ and the rather extensive additional heat production is best related to the amount of lactate produced.[14,15]

Heavy/severe exercise requires a rapid need for ATP. Significant amounts of ATP are resynthesized anaerobically because substrate-level phosphorylation with lactate production can proceed at a rate that is *several hundred-fold faster* than that of mitochondrial ATP resynthesis.[16] It is important to note, therefore, that the heat produced by rapid anaerobic ATP turnover can go unaccounted for if $O_2$ uptake measurements alone are used as the sole interpretation of all energy exchanges; a measurement of anaerobic energy expenditure also is required to properly estimate exercise energy expenditure. Unfortunately, anaerobic measurements are fraught with validity problems. For example, although blood lactate concentrations are an excellent indication that rapid glycolysis or glycogenolysis has taken place, they also can poorly reflect the extent of glycolytic ATP turnover.

In fact, *all* current measures of anaerobic metabolism have validity problems so that no "gold standard" exists for proper comparison. Measurement problems arise because of the difficulties inherent to the collection of metabolic markers from within an active muscle mass. In addition, repeated bouts of intermittent exercise have an increasingly larger aerobic and a continuously diminishing anaerobic component.[16] Moreover, anaerobic and aerobic metabolic efficiencies are different and can change over time.[17,18] Even so, the largest error in estimating energy expenditure may not reside among any one measure of anaerobic energy expenditure, but rather from the absence of an anaerobic energy expenditure measure itself[19] (recall that $O_2$ uptake also serves to *estimate* heat production only under specific conditions). The estimation of energy expenditure requires a *reasonable estimate* of the anaerobic component.

A reasonable estimate of rapid substrate-level ATP turnover has been interpreted in the context of an $O_2$ equivalent measurement where every millimole of blood lactate above resting levels equals an energy expenditure of 3 mL of $O_2$ uptake per kilogram of body weight (3 mL $O_2$ kg per mmol of Δblood lactate[20]). The oxygen deficit at the start of exercise also can be used to reasonably estimate anaerobic energy expenditure.[21,22] The oxygen deficit is described as the difference between a measure or estimate of steady-state $O_2$ uptake and actual $O_2$ uptake (Figure 1.7).

**FIGURE 1.7.** In the top example, the task being performed is an abruptly started 5-minute walk on a horizontal treadmill. The small black area at the start of exercise is the oxygen deficit. The oxygen deficit exists because it takes time (~2 minutes or so) for exercise $O_2$ uptake to reach the steady-state energy requirement of the walk. After the walk is finished, the excess post-exercise oxygen consumption (EPOC) gradually returns to resting level. Anaerobic energy expenditure during the oxygen deficit is provided by anaerobic glycolysis and the use of the ATP and CP stores. For this easy walk, anaerobic glycolysis contributes little to total energy expenditure (TEE). The bottom figures represent a 1-minute sprint up a steep hill. In this example, anaerobic glycolysis and EPOC are both large and contribute significantly to TEE. On the bottom left, without an estimate of anaerobic glycolysis, $O_2$ uptake measures alone (exercise $O_2$ uptake and EPOC) do not accurately reflect exercise energy expenditure or TEE. On the bottom right, an estimate of anaerobic glycolysis and a measurement of exercise $O_2$ uptake provide a reasonable estimation of exercise energy expenditure, but without an EPOC measurement, TEE is misrepresented. If a 75-kg person performed each exercise then TEE may be estimated as follows:

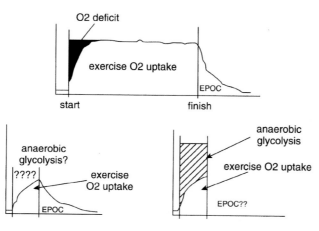

| *5-minute walk and recovery* | *1-minute all-out sprint and recovery* |
|---|---|
| 1 mmol of Δlactate ≈ 4.7 kJ | 12 mmol Δlactate ≈ 57 kJ |
| 2 L of exercise $O_2$ uptake ≈ 42.2 kJ | 1.5 L of exercise $O_2$ uptake ≈ 31.7 kJ |
| 1 L of EPOC ≈ 19.6 kJ | 5 L of EPOC ≈ 98.0 kJ |
| TEE ≈ 66.5 kJ | TEE ≈ 186.7 kJ |

The interpretation of total energy expenditure (TEE) requires an additional measure of ATP turnover during the recovery from exercise (especially after heavy/severe exercise). Energy expenditure during recovery is mostly aerobic and has been termed excess postexercise oxygen consumption or EPOC.[23] The physiologic causes behind EPOC have not all been identified, yet it is important to keep in mind that the ATP and CP stores that were used during exercise are replenished as a part of EPOC.[24] Lactate and fat are the principle nutrients that are oxidized during EPOC[25] (at 19.6 kJ per liter of $O_2$ uptake).

In practice then, the estimation of TEE for a period of exercise and recovery should include three separate measures: 1) a reasonable estimate of rapid glycogenolysis, 2) an exercise $O_2$ uptake measurement, and 3) an EPOC measurement.

## SUMMARY

Biologic energy exchange or bioenergetics invokes the study of thermodynamics (H = G + $S$), biochemistry (ATP turnover), and energy expenditure (entropy and heat production). Bioenergetics describes how the continuous exchange of matter and energy through an organism affects energy availability; energy exchanges are "costly" in that not all energy is available to perform useful work. Energy undergoes conversion and transfer throughout the anaerobic and aerobic multienzyme metabolic pathways with the breakdown (oxidation) of carbohydrates and fats; the energy held within their molecular bonds is ultimately used to resynthesize ATP. The chemo-mechanical conversion of ATP (hydrolysis) to allow muscular contraction represents another site of energy exchange. The cycle of ATP hydrolysis (energy demand) and ATP resynthesis (energy supply) is defined as ATP turnover and is described by energy expenditure. Energy expenditure can be interpreted utilizing heat and/or $O_2$ uptake measurements, yet these measures are not always similar; for example, with rapid anaerobic ATP turnover, heat production can exceed $O_2$ uptake. The quantification of TEE requires estimates or measures of both anaerobic and aerobic ATP turnover during exercise and ATP turnover in the recovery from exercise.

## Sidebar 1.1. New and Improved Metabolic Descriptions

Cells have traditionally been described as watery bags of enzymes where reactants and products diffuse from enzyme to enzyme.[26] Likewise, the diffusion of metabolites around and about the enzymes was thought to represent the end-all-and-be-all of metabolic regulation. This view may have arisen in part from the explosive developments in biochemistry to locate, isolate, and subsequently uncover what does and does not influence enzyme activity. As biochemistry blossomed, cell biology grew more slowly. Cell biology is now undergoing an explosive growth of its own and with it has come new hypotheses that suggest cellular infrastructure as another possible mechanism of metabolic control and regulation.

Cells are much more structured and organized than was previously thought. We know now for, example, that an intricate and highly modifiable internal arrangement of protein fibers known as the cytomatrix exists within each cell. These fibers certainly serve in the capacity of an internal skeleton but also seem to have a role in biochemical energy exchange. For example, the activity of lactate dehydrogenase (the enzyme that reduces pyruvate to lactate) is almost doubled when in contact with actin, a chief protein of the cytomatrix.[27] Indeed, many if not all of the 11 glycolytic enzymes have been found to not only associate with the cytomatrix but also to be organized in multienzyme associations whose aggregation also may influence metabolic rate.[28,29]

Other contemporary hypotheses promote the idea that extra- and intracellular metabolites and intermediates undergo convection toward and away from enzymes along predetermined routes or tunnels created by the cytomatrix.[30–32] The concept that reactant and product undergo transfer by means of enzyme–enzyme interaction and convective routing is a far cry from the traditional concept of random diffusion and helps explain how some reactions within a cell are promoted. These ideas will certainly influence our current interpretations of enzyme control and regulation and, perhaps, disease pathology and athletic performance as well. Faster versus slower metabolic rates, for example, may be based as much on cellular infrastructure as on enzyme kinetics.

## Sidebar 1.2. Useful Conversions

1 mole or mol = $6 \times 10^{23}$ molecules, that is, the number of molecules per gram weight of a substance.

A mol is numerically equal to the molecular weight of 1 g of a substance.

1 mol of an ideal gas (e.g., $O_2$) has a volume $\approx 22.4–24.5$ L, dependent on environmental conditions

1 L of $O_2 \approx 0.04$ mol

1 L of $O_2$ for respiration $\approx 19.6$ (fats) – 21.1 (glucose) kJ (or 4.7 – 5.0 kcal)

1 L of $O_2$ for combustion $\approx 19.6$ kJ (or 4.7 kcal)

1 L of EPOC $\approx 19.6$ kJ

1 mol ATP $\approx 3.45$ L of $O_2$

1 mol ATP $\approx 29–59$ kJ (7–14 kcal)

1 L of $O_2 \approx 0.136$ kg of ATP

1 mol of glucose $\approx 2870$ kJ (686 kcal)

1 mol of glucose $\approx 30–36$ mol ATP

1 mol of glucose ($\sim180$ g) reacts with $\sim6$ mol of $O_2$ ($\sim134–147$ L) to yield $\approx 2870$ kJ

1 mmol lactate (blood lactate is measured in millimoles) $\approx 1.5–2.0$ mmol ATP

1 mmol blood lactate $\approx 3$ mL of $O_2$ (equivalents) per kilogram of body weight

## Sidebar 1.3. Anaerobic Exercise?

The word "anaerobic" literally means without oxygen. This is true of "anaerobic" glycolysis where oxygen is not a part of substrate-level phosphorylation. So does the term "anaerobic exercise" indicate that no oxygen is utilized during such activity? Perhaps the most common examples of anaerobic exercise are found with weightlifting, sprinting, and other heavy, severe, or intense activity that is performed at work levels that can exceed maximal oxygen uptake (i.e., $VO_2$ max).

It is apparent that the term "anaerobic exercise" and its literal "anaerobic" meaning were coined well before adequate measurements could be taken to indicate the absolute presence or absence of oxygen at the mitochondrial level. It is unfortunate that current technology has not yet been able to directly and conclusively prove or disprove a continuous flow of oxygen to and from the ETC during heavy/severe/intense exercise. Be that as it may, there is plenty of indirect evidence to support both aerobic (oxygen is available) and anaerobic (oxygen is not available) viewpoints.[33,34] Indeed, if one were to hold an all-out isometric contraction for an extended period of time, then the force of that contraction could compress arterial and capillary blood flow and prevent adequate oxygenation of the muscle. However, the rate at which anaerobic glycolysis can proceed easily exceeds that of mitochondrial respiration, even at rest, so that lactate production is often found even when plenty of oxygen is available. Excluding those activities at the extreme range of exercise (i.e., the absolute easiest versus the most intense exercise), increases in energy expenditure usually invoke the utilization of all metabolic systems; that is, the stored high-energy phosphates, "anaerobic" glycolysis and oxygen uptake all contribute, albeit to different extents, during most forms of exercise.

## Sidebar 1.4. Which Energy System(s) Does Your Sports Use?

Although it is regularly implied that the stored "high-energy" phosphates (ATP and CP) contribute mostly to exercise lasting a few seconds, that rapid glycolysis with lactate production contributes more to exercise lasting several seconds to a few minutes, and that oxygen uptake fuels exercise lasting several minutes or longer, the specific contribution by each metabolic pathway can be difficult to determine within an individual athlete for any given sport.

For example, it has been shown that elite 100-meter sprinters deplete about 88% of CP stores within 5.5 seconds of an 11-second sprint.[35] The better the sprinter, the more CP is utilized at the beginning of the sprint. For all sprinters, lactate accumulation was similar at distances of 40, 60, 80, and 100 meters. Yet, because CP stores contribute less and less to sprinting as more distance is covered, glycolysis seems to contribute more to energy supply at the end of the sprint. An all-out sprint lasting 75 seconds has an equal (50–50) contribution of both anaerobic and aerobic energy systems.[36] Thus, as continuous all-out exercise exceeds 75 seconds, aerobic metabolism seems to dominate energy expenditure.

Contributions of the metabolic systems to intermittent activities such as racket sports (e.g., tennis, badminton, racquetball) and team sports (e.g., baseball, American football, soccer) are still somewhat of a mystery although we can make educated guesses based on how much time is spent sprinting about versus walking or jogging around. Track and field offers the best insight into the contributions by each metabolic system.

*"High-energy" phosphates*

| Short sprints and field events: | Sprints (100-meter dash and hurdles)<br>Jumps (high, long, and triple jumps)<br>Throws (shot, discus, hammer, javelin) |
|---|---|

*Glycolysis with lactate production*

| Sprints to middle distances | 100, 200, 400 (sprints and hurdles)<br>800- and 1500-meter runs |
|---|---|

*Oxygen uptake*

| Longer distances | 1500 meters to the marathon |
|---|---|

## PRACTICAL APPLICATIONS

### Sufficient Caloric Intake

When quantifying the caloric needs of individuals involved with heavy/severe training regimens, supplemental food intake should be based on TEE. In this regard, athletes need to compensate for any energy expenditure over-and-above resting $O_2$ uptake that is associated with anaerobic glycolysis, exercise $O_2$ uptake, and EPOC. If energy intake is based on resting or exercise steady-state $O_2$ uptake alone, hard-working individuals may become calorie deficient.

### Promoting Weight Loss

Weight-loss strategies that focus on energy expenditure (i.e., exercise) should use repeated bouts of heavy/severe work to increase TEE; heavy/severe exercise periods should be coupled to an active rather than a passive recovery. The type of activities that would be most "costly" would involve high-power outputs using large muscle masses to exploit anaerobic glycogenolysis, exercise $O_2$ uptake, and EPOC.

In terms of both energy intake and energy expenditure, there is evidence that the type of macronutrients ingested may promote acute weight loss. In this regard, high protein/low carbohydrate diets are thought to promote protein turnover (a costly undertaking) and fat breakdown.[37]

### Measuring Metabolic Efficiency

Recent measurements at the onset of muscle contraction have indicated that heat production is lower during anaerobic metabolism than for aerobic metabolism.[18] This finding is partly attributable to the hydrolysis and heat production of the stored high-energy phosphates (ATP and CP) at the onset of muscle contraction as representing only half of the ATP turnover.[18] The other half of this turnover—resynthesis of the ATP and CP stores—also results in heat production, yet this takes place during the recovery from muscle contraction (i.e., EPOC) and so is not accounted for at exercise onset. Measures or estimates of $\partial G$ degradation and dissipation (i.e., heat and entropy production) for both anaerobic and aerobic metabolism are required to better interpret efficiency and energy expenditure throughout both exercise and recovery.

### Interpreting Exercise Economy

Exercise economy is typically identified by the sole measure of $O_2$ uptake. During hard-to-severe continuous steady-state exercise, $O_2$ uptake tends to slowly but steadily increase rather than remain at a steady rate value.[38] This increased or "extra" energy expenditure has been described solely in the context of a slow $O_2$ component. Because the slow $O_2$ component occurs at exercise rates that are above the lactate threshold—where lactate production exceeds lactate removal—there also is likely to be an "anaerobic" component to continuous heavy/severe exercise.[39] Better measures of anaerobic metabolism are required and need to be included with exercise $O_2$ uptake in the interpretation of exercise economy.

## Improving Patient Diagnosis and Prognosis

Exercise stress tests typically focus on the electrocardiogram to diagnose cardiopulmonary disease. Some facilities also make use of gas-exchange measurements to aid in the interpretation of the underlying cause of why a patient stops their exercise test, that is, to help describe whether the patient has a cardiac, pulmonary, or skeletal muscle limitation to exercise. Gas-exchange measurements taken during an exercise stress test often focus on exercise $O_2$ uptake (e.g., VO$_2$ max). It is of interest to determine whether estimates of anaerobic energy expenditure and measurements of EPOC could improve exercise test sensitivity and specificity in terms of the diagnosis and prognosis of heart, pulmonary, and skeletal muscle disorders.

# QUESTIONS

## Thermodynamics

1. What is the 1st law of thermodynamics?
   a. Matter is conserved
   b. Energy is conserved
   c. $E = MC^2$
   d. Heat and temperature are not equivalent

2. What are the 2nd laws of thermodynamics?
   a. Heat flows in one direction only, toward cold
   b. Energy transfer takes place at less than 100% efficiency
   c. Heat and temperature are equivalent
   d. Energy expenditure is linear

3. What form of energy best describes why perpetual motion machines do not exist?
   a. Enthalpy
   b. Gibbs energy
   c. Entropy
   d. High energy

4. The total energy content of a system and its immediate environment is termed:
   a. Enthalpy (H)
   b. Gibbs energy (G)
   c. Entropy (S)
   d. Heat (Q)

5. What is a major difference between chemical reactions in an open as compared with a closed system?
   a. High-energy → low-energy flow
   b. Heat is exchanged
   c. Entropy production
   d. Reaction rate must be accounted for

6. Which condition best describes energy conversion and transfer in an open system?
   a. The continuous exchange of matter and energy with the environment
   b. Biochemical reactions that are reversible
   c. The disappearance of the entropy (S)
   d. ΔG

7. In what form does the degradation and dissipation of Gibbs energy take?
   a. Heat
   b. entropy
   c. Both heat and entropy
   d. Neither heat nor entropy

8. Heat is an expression of energy.
   a. True
   b. False

9. Life occurs at the expense of the environment.
   a. True
   b. False

10. The molecular bonds within the food you eat are interpreted as Gibbs energy (G).
    a. True      b. False

## Biochemistry

1. Enzymes are best known as:
   a. Energy-exchange agonists      b. Biologic catalysts
   c. Equilibrium constant inhibitors      d. Equilibrium promoters

2. Substrate-level phosphorylation is a part of:
   a. Glycolysis      b. Glycogenolysis
   c. Anaerobic energy expenditure      d. All answers

3. Energy exchange via the use of a cellular membrane is referred to as:
   a. Respiration      b. Oxidation
   c. Phosphorylation      d. Hydrolysis

4. Select an answer that reveals how cells keep the energy availability within ATP at a "high" level.
   a. Attaching additional phosphates to ATP
   b. Operating glycolysis and respiration at faster rates
   c. Maintaining a greater ATP concentration as compared with ADP concentration
   d. Increasing enzyme concentrations

5. What two answers best describe oxidation reduction.
   a. Oxidation is the loss of electrons or protons
   b. Reduction is the loss of electrons or protons
   c. Oxidation is the gain of electrons or protons
   d. Reduction is the gain of electrons or protons

6. What enzymes are directly associated with the "high-energy" phosphates?
   a. ATPase
   b. Creatine kinase
   c. Myokinase
   d. All answers

7. Oxygen uptake is associated with what specific part of aerobic metabolism?
   a. Substrate-level phosphorylation
   b. Krebs cycle
   c. Electron transport chain
   d. Mitochondrial ATPase

8. ATP turnover consists of both ATP hydrolysis and ATP resynthesis.
   a. True      b. False

9. A molecule of glucose has many more electrons and hydrogen ions than does a molecule of fat.
   a. True      b. False

10. Respiration operates at a much faster rate than substrate-level phosphorylation.
    a. True      b. False

## Energy Expenditure

1. The "gold standard" interpretation of energy expenditure is measured by:
   a. Direct calorimetry      b. Indirect calorimetry
   c. $O_2$ uptake      d. Lactate concentration

2. Substrate (fuel) utilization is determined by measuring gas exchange at steady state as:
   a. $CO_2$ output ÷ $O_2$ uptake      b. $O_2$ uptake ÷ $CO_2$ output
   c. $CO_2$ uptake ÷ $O_2$ output      d. $O_2$ output ÷ $CO_2$ uptake

3. During heavy/severe exercise, the ratio of heat production to $O_2$ uptake increases. What is most responsible for this increase?
   a. Decreased metabolic efficiency    b. Decreased economy
   c. Increased lactate production       d. Increased entropy production

4. Anaerobic energy expenditure can be reasonably estimated using:
   a. Blood lactate concentration    b. Oxygen deficit
   c. Heat measurements               d. All answers

5. A proper estimation of total energy expenditure consists of what component(s)?
   a. Exercise $O_2$ uptake                b. Anaerobic glycogenolysis
   c. Excess postexercise $O_2$ consumption    d. All answers

6. What two nutrients are primarily used to fuel the recovery from heavy/severe exercise?
   a. Fatty acids    b. Glucose
   c. Protein         d. Lactate

7. Bioenergetics invokes the study of:
   a. Thermodynamics    b. Biochemistry
   c. Energy expenditure    d. All answers

8. The heat produced from the oxidation of 1 g of fat is equivalent between mitochondrial respiration and combustion.
   a. True    b. False

9. Direct and indirect calorimetry are always equivalent.
   a. True    b. False

10. Energy expended to the environment is best described in the context of an open thermodynamic system as heat and entropy production.
    a. True    b. False

## REFERENCES

1. Cengel YA, Boles MA. Thermodynamics: An Engineering Approach. New York: McGraw-Hill; 1989:2.
2. Schneider ED, Kay JJ. Life as a manifestation of the second law of thermodynamics. Math Comp Model 1994;19:25–48.
3. Gnaiger E. Efficiency and power strategies under hypoxia. Is low efficiency at high glycolytic ATP production a paradox? In: Hochachka PW, Lutz PL, Sick T, Rosenthal M, van den Thillart G, eds. Surviving Hypoxia: Mechanisms of Control and Adaptation. Boca Raton, FL: CRC Press; 1993:78–109.
4. Nicholls DG, Ferguson SJ. Bioenergetics 3. Amsterdam: Academic Press; 2002.
5. Welch GR. Some problems in the usage of Gibbs free energy in biochemistry. J Theor Biol 1985;114:433–446.
6. Toussaint O, Schneider ED. The thermodynamics and evolution of complexity in biological systems. Comp Biochem Physiol A 1994;120:3–9.
7. Bender DA. Introduction to Nutrition and Metabolism. 3rd ed. London: Taylor & Francis; 2002.
8. Buono MJ, Kolkhorst FW. Estimating ATP resynthesis during a marathon run: a method to introduce metabolism. Adv Physiol Edu 2001;25:142–143.
9. Dennis SC, Gevers W, Opie LH. Protons in ischemia: where do they come from; where do they go to? J Mol Cell Cardiol 1991;23:1077–1086.
10. Kleiber M. The Fire of Life: An Introduction to Animal Energetics. Malabar, FL: Krieger Publishing; 1975.
11. McLean JA, Tobin G. Animal and Human Calorimetry. Cambridge: Cambridge University Press; 1987.
12. Huggett C. Estimation of rate of heat release by means of oxygen consumption measurements. Fire Mater 1980;4:61–65.
13. Thornton WM. The relation of oxygen to the heat of combustion of organic compounds. Philos Mag Ser 1917;33:196–203.
14. Gnaiger E, Kemp RB. Anaerobic metabolism in aerobic mammalian cells: information from the ratio of calorimetric heat flux and respirometric oxygen flux. Biochim Biophys Acta 1990;1016:328–332.
15. Scott CB, Kemp RB. Direct and indirect calorimetry of lactate oxidation: implications for whole-body energy expenditure. J Sports Sci 2005;23:15–19.

16. Spreit LL. Anaerobic metabolism during high-intensity exercise. In: Hargreaves H, ed. Exercise Metabolism. Champaign, IL: Human Kinetics Publishers; 1995:1–40.

17. Krustup P, Ferguson RA, Kjaer M, Bangsbo J. ATP and heat production in skeletal muscle during dynamic exercise: higher efficiency of anaerobic than aerobic ATP resynthesis. J Physiol 2003;549:255–269.

18. Pahud P, Ravussin E, Jequier E. Energy expended during oxygen deficit period of submaximal exercise in man. J Appl Physiol 1980;48:770–775.

19. Scott CB. Interpreting anaerobic and total energy expenditure for brief non-exhaustive exercise and recovery. Med Sci Sports Exerc 2004;36:S278.

20. Di Prampero PE, Ferretti G. The energetics of anaerobic muscle metabolism: a reappraisal of older and recent concepts. Respir Physiol 1999;118:103–115.

21. Scott CB. Energy expenditure of heavy to severe exercise and recovery. J Theor Biol 2000;207:293–297.

22. Medbo JI, Mohn A-C, Tabata I, Bahr R, Vaage O, Sejersted OM. Anaerobic capacity determined by maximal accumulated O2 deficit. J Appl Physiol 1988;64:50–60.

23. Gaesser G A, Brooks GA. Metabolic bases of excess post-exercise oxygen consumption: a review. Med Sci Sports Exerc 1984;16:29–43.

24. Bangsbo J, Gollnick PD, Graham TE, et al. Anaerobic energy production and O2 deficit-debt relationships during exhaustive exercise in humans. J Physiol 1990;422:539–559.

25. Bahr R. Excess post-exercise oxygen consumption—magnitude, mechanisms and practical implications. Acta Physiol Scand 1992;144(Suppl 605):1–70.

26. Weiss JN, Korge P. The cytoplasm: no longer a well-mixed bag. Circ Res 2001;89:108–110.

27. Bereiter-Hahn J, Airas J, Blum S. Supramolecular associations with the cytomatrix and their relevance in metabolic control: protein synthesis and glycolysis. Zoology 1997;100:1–24.

28. Srivastava DK, Bernhard SA. Metabolite transfer via enzyme-enzyme complexes. Science 1986;234:1081–1086.

29. Spivey HO. Evidence of NADH channeling between dehydrogenases. J Theor Biol 1991;152:103–107.

30. Coulson RA. Metabolic rate and the flow theory: a study in chemical engineering. Comp Biochem Physiol 1986;84A:217–229.

31. Wheatley DN. Diffusion theory, the cell and the synapse. Biosystems 1998;45:151–163.

32. Hochachka PW. Intracellular convection and metabolic regulation. J Exp Biol 2003;206:2001–2009.

33. Connett RJ, Honig CR, Gayeski TEJ, Brooks GA. Defining hypoxia: a systems view of VO2, glycolysis, energetics and intracellular PO2. J Appl Physiol 1990;68:833–842.

34. Tschakovsky ME, Hughson RL. Interaction of factors determining oxygen uptake at the onset of exercise. J Appl Physiol 1999;86:1101–1113.

35. Hirvonen J, Rehunen S, Rusko H, Harkonen M. Breakdown of high-energy phosphate compounds and lactate accumulation during short supramaximal exercise. Eur J Appl Physiol 1987;56:253–259.

36. Gastin PB. Energy system interaction and relative contribution during maximal exercise. Sports Med 2001;31:725–741.

37. Fine EJ, Feinman RD. Thermodynamics of weight loss diets. Nutrition & Metabolism 2004, 1:15 (8 December 2004).

38. Gaesser GA, Poole DC. The slow component of oxygen uptake kinetics in humans. Exerc Sport Sci Rev 1996;24:35–70.

39. Scott CB. Oxygen deficit and slow oxygen component relationships between intermittent and continuous exercise. J Sports Sci 1999;17:951–956.

40. Webb P. The physiology of heat regulation. Am J Physiol 1995;268:R838–R850.

41. McArdle WD, Katch FI, Katch VL. Exercise Physiology. Energy, Nutrition and Performance-Baltimore: Williams & Wilkins, 2001.

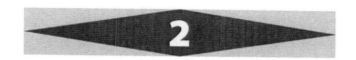

# Skeletal Muscle Plasticity

## Joseph A. Chromiak and Jose Antonio

## OBJECTIVES

On the completion of this chapter you will be able to:
1. Define the basic definitions associated with bioenergetics.
2. Understand the basic principles behind thermodynamics.
3. Develop an understanding of the concept of energy transfer.
4. Describe the biochemical reactions associated with various energy-transfer pathways in the body.
5. Explain the basics of energy expenditure, the methods for measuring energy expenditure, and the relationship of energy expenditure to exercise.

## ABSTRACT

Skeletal muscle is a highly organized tissue designed to produce force for postural control, movement, and even breathing. Various architectural designs, varying amounts of muscle proteins (e.g., enzymes or myosin), and different isoforms of many muscle proteins provide for a wide range of force-producing, biochemical, and metabolic characteristics. Additionally, the ability of skeletal muscle to adapt to the demands placed upon it, such as increased mitochondrial volume associated with endurance training or increased muscle fiber cross-sectional area as a result of strength training, demonstrates a tremendous plasticity. For the sports nutritionist, a fundamental understanding of the structure and function of skeletal muscle is important inasmuch as the adaptive response to various contractile and nutritional perturbations are manifest in this tissue. It should be noted that there is a large variation among individuals with regard to the magnitude of muscle adaptability to various types of training. Differing muscle characteristics, such as muscle pennation and fiber type, and variation in degree of adaptability among individuals partially explain the wide range of differences in aspects of exercise performance, such as muscular endurance or strength.

*Key Words*: **skeletal muscle, muscle, fiber types, fiber composition, slow twitch, fast twitch, myosin, isoforms, myosin heavy chain, muscle plasticity**

Skeletal muscle has a large capacity to adapt to the demands imposed on it, which is termed plasticity. As a result of repeated bouts of endurance or aerobic exercise training, there are increases in the number and size of the mitochondria, as well as increases in the content of various enzymes involved with oxidative energy metabolism. In contrast, skeletal muscle adapts to repeated bouts of resistance exercise by increasing in size. This increase in size, termed

From: *Essentials of Sports Nutrition and Supplements*
Edited by J. Antonio, D. Kalman, J. R. Stout, M. Greenwood, D. S. Willoughby, and G. G. Haff © Humana Press, a part of Springer Science+Business Media, Totowa, NJ

hypertrophy, is the result of an increase in the amount of contractile proteins in each muscle fiber. Consider that any given muscle may be contracting during strength training workouts for a small fraction (<1%) of the total time in a week and that the other 99% of the time the muscle is not contracting forcefully. Despite the rather small proportion of the time that most muscles are developing very high amounts of tension, muscle hypertrophy occurs.[1] In this chapter, the structure and function of skeletal muscle are described followed by a discussion about the regulation of muscle action. Depending on the type of exercise training performed, additional adaptations occur that are discussed in this chapter. It is hoped that the reader will gain an appreciation for the amazing plasticity of skeletal muscle.

## SKELETAL MUSCLE STRUCTURE

### Skeletal Muscle Has Several Layers of Connective Tissue

Each muscle is surrounded by a layer of connective tissue called the epimysium (Figures 2.1 and 2.2). Muscles are typically divided in bundles of fibers that are referred to as fasciculi. Each fasciculus is surrounded by a tough connective tissue layer known as the perimysium. It is through this layer that the nerves and blood vessels running through the muscle are found. Each muscle fiber is surrounded by a basal lamina and a mesh-like sheath of connective tissue called the endomysium. The basal lamina serves as a scaffold for muscle fiber formation and recovery from injury. A major component of each connective tissue layer is the protein collagen although the organization of the collagen fibrils is different at each level. These connective tissue layers merge at the junction of the muscle and tendon, referred to as the myotendinous junction. The various

**FIGURE 2.1.** Cross-section of skeletal muscle structures and arrangement of the various connective tissue layers. The epimysium surrounds the entire muscle, the perimysium envelopes bundles of muscle fibers called fasciculi, and the endomysium surrounds each muscle fiber. (From McArdle, WD, Katch FI, Katch VL. Exercise Physiology: Energy, Nutrition, and Human Performance. 5th ed. Baltimore: Lippincott Williams & Wilkins: 2001. Reprinted with permission of Lippincott Williams & Wilkins.)

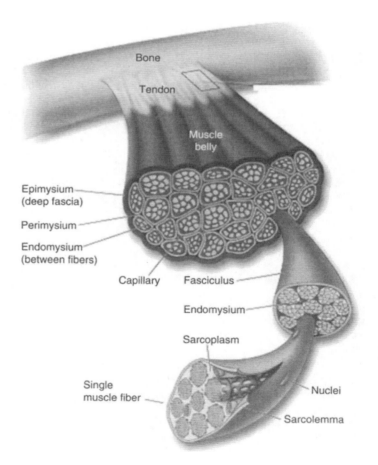

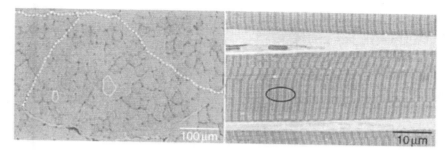

**FIGURE 2.2.** Muscle fibers in longitudinal view showing striated appearance and in cross-section showing polygonal shape of muscle fibers. Cross-section (left) and longitudinal section (right) of a tibialis anterior biopsy specimen. The alternating light and dark regions correspond to the A and I bands of the sarcomere. The cross-sectional view shows the polygonal shape of the densely packed muscle fibers. Each muscle fiber is surrounded by a connective tissue layer called the endomysium, which is outlined for two fibers as solid white lines. Muscle fibers are organized into fascicles that are surrounded by another layer of connective tissue referred to as the perimysium and is identified by the dashed lines. (From Lieber.[27] Modified and reprinted with permission of Lippincott Williams & Wilkins.)

connective tissue layers have an important function in transmission of force from the muscle fibers to the tendons.

## Muscle Fibers and Muscle Architecture

Each muscle fiber is a single cell that is composed of tens to hundreds of nuclei. The terms muscle fiber and muscle cell are used interchangeably, and the term myofiber can be used also. An important characteristic of skeletal muscle fibers is that they have a polygonal shape rather than the circular or cylindrical shapes used in many textbook illustrations (Figure 2.2). This allows many more myofibers to be packed into a given volume of muscle. Another unique feature of skeletal muscle fibers is their striated appearance. The alternating dark and light bands across the surface of the myofiber are attributed to the highly organized arrangement of muscle proteins within the cell.

It is a common conception that muscle fibers run the entire length of the muscle, but this is seldom the case. In some muscles, the muscle fibers are arranged in parallel to the long axis or force-generating axis of the muscle. These muscles are referred to as fusiform muscles (Figure 2.3). Even in fusiform muscles, the myofibers frequently do not extend the length of the muscle. In some long, strap-like muscles, the myofibers often are divided into compartments by transverse bands of connective tissue called inscriptions. These inscriptions add elasticity to very long muscles and also allow for more efficient depolarization and contraction. In other muscles, muscle fibers begin at the proximal tendon and end somewhere within the belly of the muscle, whereas other myofibers begin and terminate within the belly of the muscle, and still others begin within the muscle belly and run to the distal tendon. This type of muscle architecture is referred to as serially arranged fibers. Serially arranged fibers may add elasticity to the muscle and enhance force transmission from the individual muscle fibers to the tendon.

In many muscles, the muscle fibers are oriented transversely to the long or force-generating axis of the muscle. This is referred to as a pennate fiber

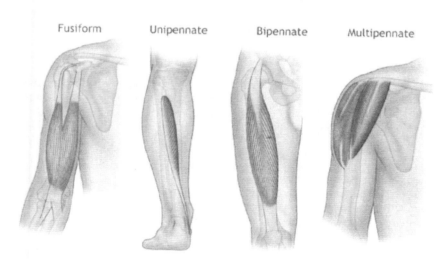

Fusiform     Unipennate     Bipennate     Multipennate

**FIGURE 2.3.** Various architectural arrangements of muscle fibers within human skeletal muscles. In fusiform muscles, the myofibers run parallel to the long axis or force-generating axis of the muscle. In a unipennate muscle, the fibers run transversely to the long axis of the muscle, in bipennate muscles two sets of myofibers are oriented transversely to the long axis of the muscle, and in multipennate muscles three of more sets of myofibers are oriented transversely to the muscle's force-generating axis. (From McArdle, WD, Katch FI, Katch VL. Exercise Physiology: Energy, Nutrition, and Human Performance. 5th ed. Baltimore: Lippincott Williams & Wilkins: 2001. Reprinted with permission of Lippincott Williams & Wilkins.)

arrangement. Pennation allows for more myofibers to be packed into a given volume of muscle. This increases the functional cross-sectional area of the muscle and the muscle's capacity for force generation. In some muscles, there may be two (bipennate) or more (multipennate) groups of muscle fibers each oriented transversely to the long axis of the muscle. This further increases the force-generating capacity of the muscle.

## THE SKELETAL MUSCLE FIBER

### The Sarcolemma

The plasma membrane of the muscle fiber is referred to as the sarcolemma. The sarcolemma is largely composed of phospholipids and some cholesterol. Many different proteins, such as channels, pumps and receptors, are embedded within the sarcolemma or span across the sarcolemma. Channels and pumps control the movement of various substances into and out of the cell. Receptor proteins allow substances outside the cell, such as epinephrine or insulin, to communicate with the interior of the cell. The $Na^+$- $K^+$-adenosine triphosphatase (ATPase) pumps and channels, primarily $Na^+$ and $K^+$ channels, are responsible for the development of a difference in electrical potential across the cell membrane and enable the sarcolemma to conduct a change in electric potential. The ability of the sarcolemma to propagate an action potential is very important for excitation of the cell during muscle actions.

### The Neuromuscular Junction

Each muscle fiber in adult human skeletal muscle is innervated by a single motor neuron. As a motor neuron nears its target muscle fibers, the neuron branches and gives rise to the axon terminal. The ends of the neuron at the axon terminal are expanded to form the synaptic knobs of boutons. The synaptic knobs are filled with vesicles, known as the synaptic vesicles that contain the neurotransmitter acetylcholine (ACh). The motor neuron and muscle fiber are separated by a very small space referred to as the synaptic cleft. The region of the muscle fiber across from the axon terminal is highly invaginated and contains many receptors for responding to the ACh that is released from the motor neuron. This region of the myofiber is termed the motor end plate. The region of the axon terminal, synaptic cleft, and motor end plate is termed the neuromuscular junction.

### The Transverse Tubules and the Sarcoplasmic Reticulum

Skeletal muscle fibers have an elaborate system of channels that are essential for activating the entire myofiber. The two components of this system of channels are the transverse or T tubules and the sarcoplasmic reticulum (Figure 2.4). At regular intervals along the muscle fiber, specifically at each A–I band junction, the sarcolemma gives rise to the transverse tubules. The T tubules, which are invaginations of the sarcolemma, enable the action potential to be propagated deep into the core of the muscle fibers. In the region where the sarcoplasmic reticulum nears the T tubules, the sarcoplasmic reticulum becomes enlarged to form the terminal cisternae. The T tubule and sarcoplasmic reticulum on either side are referred to as a triad, but the membranes of the T tubules and sarcoplasmic reticulum do not touch. Voltage-sensing proteins in the T tubule membrane known as dihydropyridine receptors trigger the release of calcium through channels on the membrane of the sarcoplasmic reticulum termed the ryanodine receptors.[2]

The sarcoplasmic reticulum is an extensive series of channels that run primarily with the longitudinal axis of the fibers and surround each myofibril. The sarcoplasmic reticulum also has extensive cross-connections, especially in fast-twitch fibers. The sarcoplasmic reticulum is a large reservoir for calcium

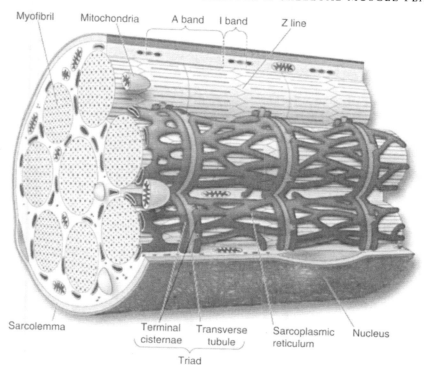

Myofibril | Mitochondria | A band | I band | Z line

Sarcolemma | Terminal cisternae | Transverse tubule | Sarcoplasmic reticulum | Nucleus

Triad

**FIGURE 2.4.** Cross-sectional and longitudinal illustration showing the transverse tubules and sarcoplasmic reticulum that surround each myofibril within the myofiber. The transverse tubules are invaginations of the sarcolemma that run into the core of the myofiber and are located at the A–I band junctions of the sarcomeres. The sarcoplasmic reticulum serves as a reservoir for calcium. (From McArdle, WD, Katch FI, Katch VL. Exercise Physiology: Energy, Nutrition, and Human Performance. 5th ed. Baltimore: Lippincott Williams & Wilkins: 2001. Reprinted with permission of Lippincott Williams & Wilkins.)

ions. The ryanodine receptors allow calcium to diffuse rapidly into the sarcoplasm during muscle activation. During muscle relaxation, SERCA (sarcoplasmic-endoplasmic reticulum, calcium-ATPase) pumps in the membrane of the sarcoplasmic reticulum remove the calcium from the sarcoplasm by pumping it back into the sarcoplasmic reticulum.

## Sarcoplasm and Cellular Organelles

Various organelles, such as ribosomes and mitochondria, are located in the sarcoplasm of the muscle cell. The sarcoplasm is the gel-like fluid within the myofiber containing various ions, glycogen granules, and organelles. Mitochondria, which are often referred to as the "powerhouses of the cell," are the site for oxidative metabolism within the myofiber.

## Myofibrils and Sarcomeres: The Working Contractile Units of the Muscle Fiber

Long, cylindrical filaments known as myofibrils, which literally means "muscle thread," extend the length of the muscle fibers (Figure 2.5). Myofibrils are the largest functional unit of a myofiber and hundreds of myofibrils may constitute a muscle fiber. A myofibril is formed by sarcomeres lined up end to end or "in series." Sarcomeres, literally "muscle unit," are the smallest functional unit of skeletal muscle fibers (Figure 2.5C and E). Sarcomeres are composed of the thick and thin contractile filaments (discussed below), as well as many cytoskeletal proteins. Structures termed Z lines serve as a skeleton or scaffold for the sarcomere and are located at each end of the sarcomere. The major protein of the Z lines is α-actinin. Sarcomeres are lined up end to end as the Z line of one sarcomere also serves as a Z line for the next sarcomere in series. Sarcomeres of adjacent myofibrils are said to be arranged in parallel. The number of sarcomeres in parallel within a muscle fiber is directly related to the capacity of the myofiber to produce force.

**FIGURE 2.5.** The gross and subcellular organization of skeletal muscle. **A:** Skeletal muscle is composed of individual muscle fibers. **B:** Muscle fibers consist of many myofibrils that are composed of numerous proteins including actin and myosin. **C:** Myofibrils are composed of sarcomeres arranged in series. **D:** Sarcomeres are composed of thick and thin filaments. **E:** Microscopic view of a sarcomere. **F:** Cross-sectional view of the thick and thin filaments showing their arrangement at different regions along the sarcomere. (From McArdle, WD, Katch FI, Katch VL. Exercise Physiology: Energy, Nutrition, and Human Performance. 5th ed. Baltimore: Lippincott Williams & Wilkins: 2001. Reprinted with permission of Lippincott Williams & Wilkins.)

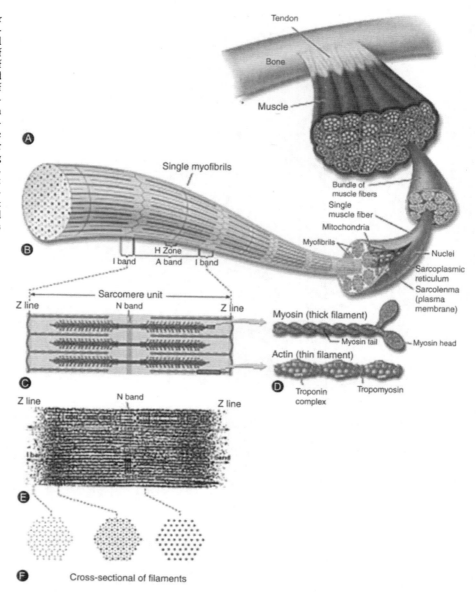

## MUSCLE CONTRACTILE AND REGULATORY PROTEINS

### The Thick or Myosin Filament

The thick filament is often referred to as the myosin filament because myosin is the only protein present (Figure 2.5D). An intact myosin molecule actually consists of two molecules of myosin heavy chain (MHC) and four myosin light chain molecules. The tail regions of the two MHC molecules coil around each other. The tail regions of about 200–250 pairs of MHC molecules are intertwined to form the thick filament, with approximately half of the myosin cross-bridges extending toward one Z line with the other half extending toward the other Z line. Each MHC molecule has a hinge region that gives rise to a globular head. The globular head is also known as the myosin cross-bridge, because it is this portion of the molecule that projects outward toward the thin filament and will bind to the actin molecules of the thin filament. An intrinsic part of the globular head of MHC is myosin ATPase activity. This enzymatic activity hydrolyzes ATP to provide energy for movement of the myosin cross-bridge, which is called the power stroke. The thick filament is highly organized, such that every 14.3 nm along the thick filament, three pairs of myosin heads rotated 120 degrees from each other project toward the thin filament. A complete myosin molecule also consists of two regulatory and two essential myosin light chain molecules. The light chains are located near the hinge region of the MHC molecules with the two essential myosin light chain molecules located just below the globular head of the MHCs. Although the role of the myosin light chains is not completely understood, they apparently affect the power stroke by modulating the interaction between myosin and actin.[3] The essential myosin light chains are believed to influence the maximal shortening velocity of the myofibers. The regulatory light chains, which can be phosphorylated, may affect force production during submaximal contractions. Phosphorylation of these light chains may increase the sensitivity of the contractile proteins to calcium, thus enhancing force generation at low, but not maximal, stimulation frequencies.[4]

## The Thin Filament: Actin, Troponin, and Tropomyosin

Thin filaments begin at the Z lines and run out toward the center of the sarcomere where they interdigitate with the thick filaments to form a hexagonal lattice (Figure 2.5E). The thin filaments are often called the actin filaments because actin is the major contractile protein of this filament. The thin filament also consists of two proteins, troponin and tropomyosin, that have regulatory functions (Figure 2.5D). The actin filaments consist of long chains of individual actin molecules that have a globular shape, and are sometimes referred to as G-actin, with the "G" denoting "globular." The long chains of G-actin molecules form a strand-like protein called filamentous or F-actin. Two F-actin strands coil around each other in an α-helix to form a thin filament. Tropomyosin runs alongside the F-actin and in the resting state fits into a groove formed by the α-helical arrangement of the two F-actin strands. The groove of the thin filament contains the active sites that myosin cross-bridges will bind during muscle contraction. Each tropomyosin molecule runs the length of seven G-actins and is closely associated with troponin. An intact troponin (Tn) molecule consists of three subunits. The troponin-tropomyosin (Tn-T) subunit links to tropomyosin. The other subunits are Tn-inhibitory (Tn-I) and Tn-calcium (Tn-C). When calcium levels in the sarcoplasm increase during muscle activation, up to four calcium molecules bind each Tn-C, inducing a change in the conformation of Tn-I. As Tn-I changes shape, it pulls on Tn-T, which in turn tugs on tropomyosin, thus rotating it away from the active sites on actin. This movement of tropomyosin out of the actin groove is called the "tropomyosin shift." Now myosin cross-bridges can bind with actin in a "strong binding state."

The highly organized arrangement of thick and thin filaments gives myofibers their striated appearance of light and dark bands. These regions are named based on their appearance. The A band is the region of the sarcomere where there is thick filament, which includes a region where the thick and thin filaments overlap and a region where there is only thick filament (Figure 2.5E). This latter portion is referred to as the H-zone. The I band is the region where there is only thin filament and it extends out from both sides of the Z line. Because of the nature of muscle fiber action, which is discussed below, the regions of the H-zone and I band change length during muscle contraction, but the length of the A band does not change.

# THE CYTOSKELETON: THE SCAFFOLD OF THE CELL

## The Endosarcomeric Cytoskeleton

To maintain the highly organized arrangement of thick and thin filaments, each sarcomere has many proteins that serve as a supporting framework (Figure 2.6). The Z line, which is composed primarily of α-actinin, can be

**FIGURE 2.6.** Cytoskeletal proteins associated with skeletal muscle fibers. Some of the major endosarcomeric and exosarcomeric cytoskeletal proteins are shown in relationship to the sarcomeres. (From McArdle, WD, Katch FI, Katch VL. Exercise Physiology: Energy, Nutrition, and Human Performance. 5th ed. Baltimore: Lippincott Williams & Wilkins: 2001. Adapted and reprinted with permission of Lippincott Williams & Wilkins.)

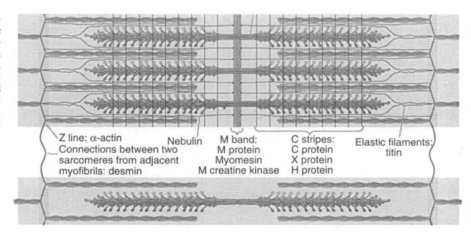

considered part of this endosarcomeric cytoskeleton. Titin, as the name implies, is an extremely large protein that begins at the Z line, runs parallel to the thick filaments, and may link to myosin at the M line of the sarcomere. In the region of the sarcomere where only F-actin is present (I-band region), the titin molecule is highly extensible, but as titin runs alongside the thick filament it becomes more rigid. Titin is largely responsible for the passive tension within muscle fibers and is thought to hold the myosin filament in the center of the sarcomere during muscle contraction. Additionally, titin may regulate the number of myosin molecules in the thick filament.

Nebulin extends out from the Z line, running alongside the thin filament. Nebulin may provide structural support for the thin filament, as well as regulate the number of G-actin monomers in F-actin. In the center of the sarcomere, additional proteins run perpendicular to the direction of the thick and thin filaments. These proteins constitute the M-line proteins and center the thick filaments within the sarcomere during contraction. Additional proteins referred to as the C stripes run perpendicular across the sarcomere and also may have a role in keeping the thick filaments centered within the sarcomere during muscle action.

## The Exosarcomeric Cytoskeleton

Skeletal myofibers also have many cytoskeletal proteins that link adjacent sarcomeres together and connect the myofibrils at the periphery of the cell to the sarcolemma. A complete discussion of all the cytoskeletal proteins is beyond the scope of this chapter, but a few prominent proteins will be mentioned here. Desmin is part of a group of proteins termed intermediate filaments. Desmin links adjacent sarcomeres at their Z lines. Actin, which is an important contractile protein, also serves as an important cytoskeletal protein linking peripheral myofibrils to the sarcolemma.

Dystrophin is located near the sarcolemma and has a role in stabilizing the membrane during contraction.[5] The extremely large dystrophin protein is part of a network of proteins that are essential for maintaining the integrity of the cell. A mutation of the gene that codes for dystrophin results in the well-known disease Duchenne muscular dystrophy.[6] Muscle fibers lacking dystrophin are readily damaged during muscle use and undergo repeated cycles of degeneration and regeneration. These repetitive cycles of degeneration and repair are associated with a progressive decline in the functional capacity of the muscle because of a loss of myofibers and an accumulation of connective tissue and fat cells within the muscle.

## SKELETAL MUSCLE ACTION: TYPES OF MUSCLE CONTRACTIONS

Muscles are capable of several different types of actions that can be categorized as static or dynamic. It should be noted that some sports scientists prefer the term "muscle action" rather than "contraction" (which implies shortening), because muscles may lengthen or change little in length in addition to shortening when the myofibers develop tension. Others argue that it is widely understood that "contraction" does not refer only to shortening with respect to muscle actions. "The term 'contraction' refers to the state of muscle activation in which cross-bridges are cycling in response to an action potential"[7]; therefore, both terms will be used interchangeably. During static, or isometric, contractions the muscle fibers develop tension with little change in length, and the angle about the involved joints remains constant as the myofibers develop force that is equal to the external resistance, or the external resistance is stationary. Static muscle actions are common for the postural muscles of the body that act to maintain a constant position during standing.

Most muscle actions in athletics require movement and are dynamic in nature. Dynamic muscle actions include concentric, eccentric, and plyometric contractions. During concentric muscle actions, the force developed by the muscle fibers is greater than the external resistance so myofiber shortening and movement occur. During eccentric muscle actions, the myofibers lengthen while developing force. The force developed by the muscle fibers is less than the external resistance. Eccentric contractions, which are sometimes referred to as "negatives," are popular with many athletes including bodybuilders because more weight or external resistance can be use compared with static and concentric muscle actions. Finally, during many of the rapid and powerful movements performed in sports, eccentric muscle actions are followed rapidly by concentric muscle actions. These types of actions are referred to as plyometric muscle actions. It is well known that a concentric muscle contraction is more powerful when preceded by an eccentric muscle action. Many coaches and athletes incorporate specific plyometric exercises into training programs to mimic many of the actions used in sports.

## SKELETAL MUSCLE ACTION: INITIATION OF MUSCLE FIBER ACTIVATION AND EXCITATION-CONTRACTION COUPLING

Muscle actions are initiated when motor neurons within the central nervous system are excited sufficiently to develop action potentials. When depolarization of the motor neuron reaches the axon terminals, the synaptic vesicles within the synaptic knobs release their ACh into the synaptic cleft (Figure 2.7). ACh diffuses across the synaptic cleft and binds to specific ACh receptors on the motor end plate. This initiates the myofiber action potential that rapidly propagates along the sarcolemma in all directions.

Excitation-contraction coupling refers to the process of an electrical event, depolarization of the sarcolemma, inducing a mechanical event, muscle contraction. The electrical and mechanical events are coupled by the release of calcium from the sarcoplasmic reticulum. The propagation of the action potential down the T tubules triggers the release of calcium through the ryanodine receptor channels in the adjacent terminal cisternae of the sarcoplasmic reticulum. Calcium binds to troponin, inducing the tropomyosin shift allowing myosin to enter a strong binding state with actin. From the time that calcium is released into the sarcoplasm until the calcium has been resequestered in the sarcoplasmic reticulum, the muscle fiber is in the active state and tension development can occur.

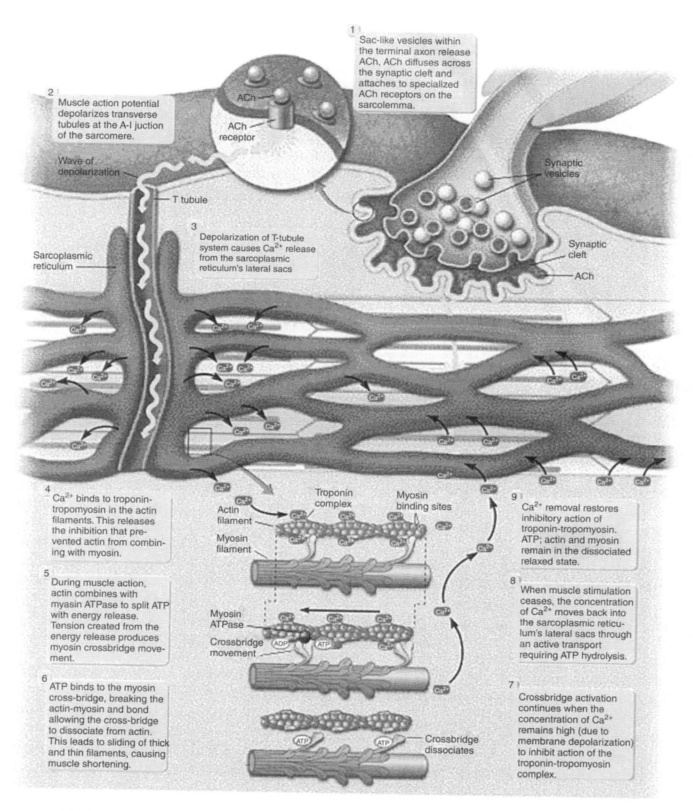

**FIGURE 2.7.** Illustration of the major events in muscle contraction and relaxation. The neurotransmitter acetylcholine (ACh) is released from the synaptic vesicles of the axon terminal (1). ACh diffuses across the synaptic cleft and initiates the action potential on the sarcolemma (2). Depolarization of the sarcolemma and T tubules induces calcium release from the sarcoplasmic reticulum (3). $Ca^{2+}$ binding to troponin leads to the tropomyosin shift (4) allowing for stronger myosin-actin binding and muscle contraction.[5-7] Muscle relaxation occurs when $Ca^{2+}$ is resequestered in the sarcoplasmic reticulum.[8,9] (From McArdle, WD, Katch FI, Katch VL. Exercise Physiology: Energy, Nutrition, and Human Performance. 5th ed. Baltimore: Lippincott Williams & Wilkins; 2001. Reprinted with permission of Lippincott Williams & Wilkins.)

# SKELETAL MUSCLE ACTION:
# THE SLIDING FILAMENT THEORY AND THE
# CROSS-BRIDGE CYCLE

The sliding filament theory best explains the mechanism by which sarcomeres, and therefore muscle fibers, change length during muscle contraction. The thick and thin filaments do not change length, rather sarcomeres shorten or lengthen as the thin (actin) filaments slide over the thick (myosin) filaments (Figure 2.8).[8]

Recent evidence suggests that myosin cross-bridges are always attached to actin. When the muscle fibers are not contracting, the myosin cross-bridges are weakly bound to actin, the "weak binding state." When the muscle fiber is developing tension, myosin is bound in a "strong binding state" with actin. During this strong binding state, the orientation of the myosin cross-bridges is such that when attached to actin they attempt to pull the thin filament over the thick filament.

The series of events whereby the myosin cross-bridge enters the strong binding state with actin, undergoes the power stroke, and reenters the weak binding state while the myosin cross-bridge returns to its initial orientation is termed the cross-bridge cycle. The energy for the power stroke during this cycle comes from the hydrolysis of adenosine triphosphate (ATP) by myosin ATPase. Myosin exists in an "energized" state, which means that the ATP has already been hydrolyzed to adenosine diphosphate and Pi to release energy. However, the "energized" myosin cross-bridge does not use this energy for the power stroke until it enters the strong binding state with actin. After completion of the power stroke, attachment of another ATP to the myosin cross-bridge causes it to enter the weak binding state and return to its original position. Because the total distance that a myosin cross-bridge moves the thin filament with a single power stroke is very minute, each myosin head likely undergoes multiple cross-bridge cycles during a single muscle contraction.[9]

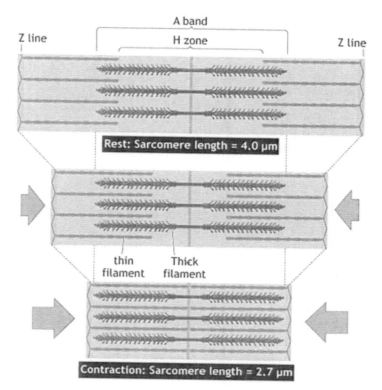

FIGURE 2.8. The sliding filament theory and sarcomere shortening. Schematic view of a sarcomere showing that shortening of the sarcomere occurs as the thin filaments are pulled closer to the center of the sarcomere by the thick filaments. (From McArdle, WD, Katch FI, Katch VL. Exercise Physiology: Energy, Nutrition, and Human Performance. 5th ed. Baltimore: Lippincott Williams & Wilkins: 2001. Reprinted with permission of Lippincott Williams & Wilkins.)

## MUSCLE RELAXATION

Skeletal muscle fibers continue contracting until impulses from the motor neuron at the neuromuscular junction stop so that no more ACh is bound to ACh receptors at the motor end plate. Muscle relaxation occurs when the SERCA pumps have transported sufficient calcium into the sarcoplasmic reticulum to end the active state, so that tropomyosin returns to its original position over the myosin cross-bridge binding sites on actin.

## THE CLASSIFICATION OF MUSCLE FIBER AND MOTOR UNIT TYPES

Several systems of categorizing muscle fibers and motor units have been developed. Three of the most frequently used schemes are presented in this chapter. Before introducing the first classification scheme, it is important to note that, although muscle fibers and motor units are placed into categories, myofibers and motor units possess a broad and nearly continuous range of contractile and metabolic properties.

Drs. James Peter, James Barnard, Reggie Edgerton and their colleagues[10] collaborated to develop a classification system based on the contractile and metabolic properties of the myofibers. Fiber types designated as slow or fast contracting were identified. The slow-contracting fibers also had a very high oxidative capacity and were designated SO fibers (Table 2.1). The fast-twitch fibers were further subdivided into those with moderate to high oxidative and glycolytic capacities (FOG fibers) and fibers that had a substantial capacity for glycolytic metabolism but a low capacity for oxidative metabolism (FG fibers).

Another common classification system is based on the differential sensitivities of myosin ATPase to solutions of varying pH[11,12] (Figure 2.9). The underlying basis for this scheme is the primary type of MHC present within the myofiber. There are three isoforms of MHC in adult, human skeletal muscle that are designated MHC I, MHC IIa, and MHC IIx.[13] Preincubation in an acidic solution (pH 4.3) denatures the portion of the MHC IIa and IIx proteins that has the ATPase activity, so when the myofibers are stained for myosin ATPase, only those containing the MHC I isoform will stain darkly. By using solutions of various pH, three primary types of fibers labeled I, IIa, and IIx are identified. Preincubation in an alkaline solution results in the type IIa and IIx myofibers staining darkly, whereas the type I fibers stain lightly. The type of

TABLE 2.1. Biochemical, contractile, and structural properties of the three major classes of muscle fibers.

|  | Slow oxidative | Fast oxidative-glycolytic | Fast glycolytic |
|---|---|---|---|
| Biochemical properties |  |  |  |
| Myosin ATPase activity | Low | Moderately high | Highest |
| Oxidative capacity | High | Moderate to high | Low |
| Glycolytic capacity | Low | Moderate to high | High |
| Resistance to fatigue | High | Moderate to high | Low |
| Contractile properties |  |  |  |
| Shortening velocity | Slow | Fast | Fastest |
| Relaxation | Slow | Fast | Fast |
| Specific tension | Moderate | High | High |
| Power | Low | High | Very high |
| Structural properties |  |  |  |
| Mitochondrial density | High | Moderately high | Low |
| Z-line thickness | Wide | Intermediate | Narrow |
| M-line thickness | 5 M-bridges | 3 prominent and 2 less-prominent M-bridges | 3 M-bridges |
| Sarcoplasmic reticulum | Not extensive | Extensive | Extensive |

ATPase = adenosine triphosphatase.

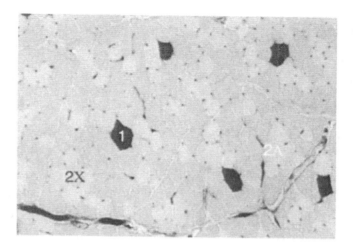

**FIGURE 2.9.** Myofibrillar ATPase stain using acid preincubation. Cross-section of a rabbit tibialis anterior biopsy sample showing the differential staining of type I and II fibers. Slow type I fibers stain darkly whereas the fast type IIa and IIx fibers stain lightly. (From Lieber.[27] Reprinted with permission of Lippincott Williams & Wilkins.)

MHC is a very important component in determining the contractile properties of the muscle fiber. The maximal velocity of muscle fiber shortening, termed $V_{max}$, is determined by the rate at which the myosin ATPase hydrolyzes ATP to provide energy for the power stroke. Slow-twitch fibers expressing type I MHC have a low $V_{max}$, whereas fast-twitch fibers expressing type IIa or IIx have high $V_{max}$ values.

Another important classification method categorizes motor units.[14] A motor unit consists of an α-motor neuron and all the muscle fibers that it innervates. In adult, human skeletal muscle, each muscle fiber is innervated by only one motor neuron. This scheme is based on the contractile properties of the motor unit and their resistance to fatigue. Using this scheme, slow contracting motor units that are highly resistant to fatigue are designated with an S. Fast contracting motor units that have a moderately high resistance to fatigue are denoted as FR, and fast contracting but highly fatigable motor units are labeled FF. The fatigue characteristics are related to the biochemical properties of the motor unit (Figure 2.10).

In general, there is a significant amount of overlap between these three classification systems. For example, the S motor units that have a high resistance to fatigue also have a very high oxidative capacity, which provides them with this fatigue resistance. Most likely, fibers classified as SO or type I would be part of S motor units. Fibers expressing either IIa or IIx MHC are likely to be FOG or FG fibers and belong to FR or FF motor units, respectively. However, caution should be used in going between the classification systems especially when categorizing the fast-contracting fibers. Remember, most properties of

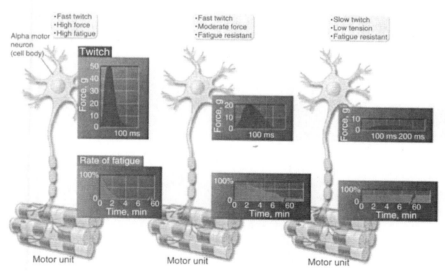

**FIGURE 2.10.** The contraction velocity, force, and fatigue characteristics of the fast fatigable (left), fast fatigue resistant (center), and slow (right) motor units. The upper graphs depict the twitch response to a single stimulus and the lower graphs show the fatigability of the motor units. (From McArdle, WD, Katch FI, Katch VL. Exercise Physiology: Energy, Nutrition, and Human Performance. 5th ed. Baltimore: Lippincott Williams & Wilkins: 2001. Reprinted with permission of Lippincott Williams & Wilkins.)

## Sidebar 2.1. Muscle Fiber Types, Fiber-Type Transitions, and Athletic Performance

Although muscle fiber type may be an important contributor to success in many sports, it should be recognized that many other factors including biomechanics, cardiorespiratory capacity, biochemical and psychologic characteristics determine successful athletic performance. Clearly, skeletal muscle demonstrates an enormous capacity for adaptation.[15-19] The fast-twitch or type II muscle fibers are capable of producing greater force, especially for higher-velocity movements, compared with slow-twitch or type I fibers, and sprint performance has been correlated with the proportion of type II fibers.[20] Successful weightlifting performances and vertical jump power were correlated with type II fiber characteristics.[21] In general, most muscles of elite sprinters are composed of approximately 75% fast-twitch fibers (Table 2.2). The slow-twitch or type I muscle fibers have a very high resistance to fatigue, and most successful endurance athletes have high percentages of slow-twitch fibers. However, it is possible that on occasion an athlete might be successful in endurance events with a lower proportion of slow-twitch fibers. Don Kardong was a member of the United States men's Olympic marathon team in 1976, and he was typed as having 50% slow-twitch fibers.[22,23]

The primary factor that regulates the characteristics of muscle fibers is the motor neuron that innervates them. Experiments performed nearly 50 years ago demonstrated that when the motor nerve to a muscle that is primarily composed of slow-twitch fibers is redirected toward a muscle consisting of a majority of fast-twitch fibers that the myofibers take on the characteristics of slow-twitch fibers.[15] Experiments since then have clearly demonstrated that over time, all of the biochemical, contractile, and structural characteristics of muscle fibers change when innervated by a different type of motor neuron or electrically stimulated in a manner similar to the other motor neuron type.[17] Although these experiments do not truly mimic the exercise training of athletes, they do show the tremendous plasticity of muscle fibers.

Both endurance- and strength-training studies have shown that the IIx fibers readily transition to IIa fibers. In fact, a significant decrease in the proportion of IIb myofibers in the vastus lateralis muscle of women occurred after only 2 weeks (4 workouts) of strength training.[19] (Recent research shows that the IIb myosin isoform is not expressed in human skeletal myofibers. So fibers that were typed previously as IIb myofibers are truly IIx myofibers.)

The extent of transitions between the type I and IIa myofibers in response to exercise training is more controversial. An increase in the proportion of type I fibers and decline in the percentage of type II fibers during endurance training consistent with a transition from IIa to I fibers has been reported.[16] It might be significant to note that these studies are relatively short in duration compared with the years of training for many elite athletes. A progressive increase in the percentage of type I fibers with years of training has been reported in professional road cyclists.[24] It is likely that the very high percentage of type I myofibers in the muscles of some elite endurance athletes is attributable primarily to genetics with some contribution from training-induced fiber-type transitions (Table 2.2). The extent of this transition to type I fibers is unclear, but may depend on the total amount of endurance training performed as well as the underlying genetic potential or resistance of the fibers to transition. Whether significant transition of slow-twitch to fast-twitch fibers occurs in sprinters is even less clear, because there are few reports of type I to type II transitions in humans.[25] Finally, the fiber-type composition of athletes in many sports, such as soccer, hockey, and football, has not been studied to a large extent. The effect of any fiber-type transitions on performance is unclear, but at the elite levels of sport, small differences may have a large impact on athletic success.

TABLE 2.2. Fiber type percentages for elite endurance athletes, sprinters, and untrained individuals.

| Study | Sport and group | Muscle | % Type I | % Type IIa | % Type IIx |
|---|---|---|---|---|---|
| Costill et al.,[17] 1976 | Best American distance runners | Gastrocnemius | 79.0 | 21.0 (all type II fibers) | |
| | Untrained men | | 57.7 | 42.3 (all type II fibers) | |
| Costill et al.,[17] 1976 | Sprinters, male | Gastrocnemius | 24.0 | 76.0 (all type II fibers) | |
| | Sprinters, female | | 27.4 | 72.6 (all type II fibers) | |
| Howald et al.,[16] 1982 | Distance runners | Vastus lateralis | 78.0 | 19.0 | 2.5 |
| | Controls | | 51.0 | 41.0 | 7.1 |
| Baumann et al., 1987[26] | Professional cyclists | Vastus lateralis | 80.0 | 17.0 | 0.6 |
| | Sedentary controls | | 53.0 | 33.0 | 13.0 |

myofibers and motor units are a continuum rather than discrete points, so myofibers and motor units might not always fit neatly into a given category.

## FACTORS DETERMINING MUSCULAR STRENGTH: BIOMECHANICS

Various biomechanical and biochemical factors affect a muscle's ability to produce force and move or lift objects. Skeletal muscles along with the bones to which they attach operate as levers. The length of a limb and the point of tendon attachment on a bone are important determinants of an individual's ability to exert force and move objects. Elbow flexion involving the biceps brachii muscle and the radius provides a good example of how limb length and tendon insertion points affect the ability to lift a weight. During an arm curl, the biceps brachii must develop tension and shorten in order to cause rotation at the elbow joint resulting in flexion. For this movement, the axis of rotation is at the elbow and the resistance, such as a dumbbell, is held in the hand. The longer the limb, the greater the force that muscles would need to produce in order to lift an object at the end of the limb. Also, the further out on the limb that the biceps tendon attaches to the radius, the heavier the resistance that can be moved for a given amount of force the muscle produces.

## FACTORS DETERMINING MUSCULAR FORCE PRODUCTION: SARCOMERE LENGTH–TENSION RELATIONSHIP

The ability of a muscle to produce force throughout a range of motion is dependent on muscle length. For each muscle, there is a range of muscle lengths that are optimal for force production based on sarcomere length. Sarcomeres produce the greatest amount of force when there is the greatest possible number of myosin cross-bridge interactions with action. This is termed optimal length and designated as $L_0$ (Figure 2.11). When the muscle is

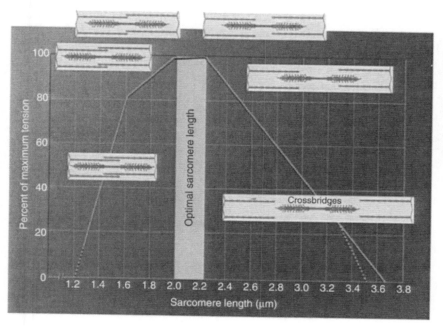

**FIGURE 2.11.** The relationship between sarcomere length and tension development under static conditions. Optimal sarcomere length (2.0–2.25 μm) results in the maximal tension production because the greatest number of myosin cross-bridges can bind to actin. Tension output decreases as sarcomere length decreases or increases beyond optimal length. (From McArdle, WD, Katch FI, Katch VL. Exercise Physiology: Energy, Nutrition, and Human Performance. 5th ed. Baltimore: Lippincott Williams & Wilkins: 2001. Reprinted with permission of Lippincott Williams & Wilkins.)

lengthened beyond $L_0$, force production decreases as the thin filaments are pulled away from the thick filaments and the potential number of myosin–actin interactions declines. When the muscle is shortened to less than $L_0$, force also declines as the thin filaments from the opposing Z lines of the sarcomere overlap. This overlap may interfere with the binding of myosin to actin.

## FACTORS DETERMINING MUSCULAR FORCE PRODUCTION: FORCE–VELOCITY RELATIONSHIP

The force that a muscle can produce is a function of the type of contraction and the velocity of movement. The velocity at which a muscle can contract is determined by the force acting against it. The force–velocity relationship is often described with reference to a static muscle action. For concentric muscle actions, there is a decline in muscle force production as the velocity of shortening increases. Initially, rather small increases in shortening velocity result in a dramatic decrease in force production (Table 2.3). For example, the force produced by a muscle declines by 25% or more when going from a static muscle contraction to a velocity of shortening that is only 6% of the maximum shortening velocity. When resistances greater than the maximal force-producing capacity of the muscle are used, an eccentric muscle action results. Initially, as the velocity of lengthening increases a small amount, there is a fairly large increase in muscle force production. Finally, as lengthening velocity continues to increase, muscle force production levels off.

The force–velocity curve differs among the three major myofiber types. Specific tension is the amount of force produced per unit cross-sectional area of muscle, and allows for comparison of the force-production capabilities of muscle fibers of different sizes. Recent research using rat muscle shows that for static muscle actions, fast-twitch fibers are capable of producing greater specific tension than slow-twitch fibers.[28] Secondly, the slope of the initial decline in force as shortening velocity increases is greatest for type I fibers, intermediate for type IIa fibers, and least for IIx fibers. Therefore, for any given velocity of shortening, type IIx fibers produce the greatest amount of force and type I fibers produce the lowest force.

Power is the product of force and velocity and is a very important factor determining successful performance in many sports. The peak power generated by a muscle or muscle fibers is related to the velocity as well as the force of muscle contraction. Maximal power production occurs at approximately one third of maximal force production as well as one third of maximal shortening velocity. Because fast-twitch fibers are capable of greater force production at any given contraction velocity compared with slow-twitch fibers, the fast-

TABLE 2.3. Relative muscle force at various relative contraction velocities.

| Muscle force (% of maximal static contraction) | Velocity of shortening (% of maximal shortening velocity) |
|---|---|
| 100 | 0 |
| 95 | 1 |
| 90 | 2.2 |
| 75 | 6.3 |
| 50 | 16.6 |
| 25 | 37.5 |
| 10 | 64.3 |
| 5 | 79.1 |
| 0 | 100 |

*Source:* Adapted from Lieber.[27]

twitch fibers are capable of greater power production than slow-twitch fibers.

# REGULATION OF MUSCLE FORCE PRODUCTION

Muscle fibers are recruited as groups known as motor units, which are the functional units of the neuromuscular system. When an α motor neuron is excited sufficiently to develop an action potential, all myofibers that are innervated by the motor neuron are activated. This is referred to as the all-or-none principle. In general, the slow (S) motor units are the smallest having the lowest innervation ratios, which is the number of fibers innervated per motor neuron. The neurons of S motor units typically have the least synaptic input and the smallest soma and axon diameters. Fast, fatigue-resistant (FR) motor units have intermediate innervation ratios, and the soma and axon are intermediate in size. Typically, fast fatigable (FF) motor units have the greatest innervation ratios, their neurons have the greatest synaptic input, and the soma and axon diameters are the largest.

For static and concentric muscle actions, motor units are recruited on the basis of size beginning with the smallest motor units and as more force is needed larger motor units are recruited. This is known as Henneman's size principle of motor unit recruitment. It should be noted that this orderly recruitment of motor units is both sequential and additive. More recent evidence suggests that motor unit recruitment occurs in reverse order beginning with larger motor units for eccentric muscle actions.[29] Also noteworthy is that motor unit recruitment has been studied primarily for contractions and movements much less powerful and complex than many of the ballistic, multi-joint movements observed in sports. Many contractions in sports are plyometric in nature. The manner of motor unit recruitment for these types of actions is not entirely clear.

Force production by a muscle can vary over a very wide range, which is essential for smooth, coordinated movements. The neuromuscular system uses two major strategies to regulate force production during muscular contractions. The first strategy involves the recruitment of motor units in an orderly manner as described above and is called multiple motor unit summation. Simply stated, as more force is needed, additional motor units are recruited. A second strategy involves rate coding or recruiting motor units at various frequencies in order to vary the force output by the muscle fibers of that motor unit. This strategy is termed wave summation.

To better understand wave summation, an understanding of the response of muscle fibers to neural stimulation is essential. When the myofibers of a motor unit are stimulated, they develop tension then relax. This is referred to as a twitch (see Figure 2.13). If a second stimulus occurs before complete myofiber relaxation, then the second twitch results in greater force than the first twitch. As the frequency of motor unit stimulation increases, the force of the individual twitches begins to add up or summate. If the frequency of motor unit firing is sufficient, the individual twitches merge and force output increases to a maximal value. The increased force in response to a series of stimuli is referred to as tetanus. The underlying physiologic explanation of wave summation is related to the amount of time needed for the SERCA pumps to resequester calcium into the sarcoplasmic reticulum. With increasing frequencies of neuromuscular stimulation, there is inadequate time to pump the calcium that had been released back into the sarcoplasmic reticulum. With each additional stimulus, additional calcium is released into the sarcoplasm. As calcium concentrations in the sarcoplasm increase, the amount of calcium bound to troponin increases, which exposes more binding sites on actin so more force can be produced. It is important to note that even though muscle twitches are discussed, muscle contractions during human movements involve repeated and sustained contractions rather than twitches.

An increased synchronization of motor unit firing has been observed in strength-trained individuals[30,31]; therefore, it has been speculated that motor unit synchronization is a third strategy used by the neuromuscular system to increase force production. Synchronization refers to an increased temporal coincidence of action potentials by the motor neurons. Research suggests that this strategy does not change maximal muscle tension during static contractions.[32] Synchronization may increase the rate of muscle force production thus allowing the muscle to achieve maximal force output more rapidly or it may serve as a mechanism to coordinate the activity of multiple muscles synergistically.[33]

Based on the current understanding of motor unit recruitment, some important applications to the training of athletes can be made. Athletes need to incorporate contraction types and movement patterns into their training that are as similar as possible to those in their sport in order to optimize neuromuscular recruitment. Concentric, eccentric, and plyometric muscle actions must be included in the training of athletes to induce neuromuscular adaptations that result in optimal motor unit recruitment for these various contraction types. Maximal muscle contractions need to be incorporated into strength-training workouts in order to recruit and thus induce adaptations of all motor units and muscle fibers.

## MUSCULAR FATIGUE

Fatigue is defined as an inability to maintain the desired intensity of exercise. Fatigue can result from many factors that can be categorized as central or peripheral. Also, the factors contributing to fatigue vary depending on the intensity and duration of exercise. With regard to central fatigue, many factors such as decreased blood glucose concentrations or sensation of pain may increase the difficulty of voluntarily exciting the motor nerves in the motor cortex of the brain sufficiently. At the muscular level, several factors may contribute to an inability to maintain a given effort during very-high-intensity exercise. The depletion of ATP and phosphocreatine (PCr) during supramaximal exercise causes a decline in exercise intensity. Lactic acid, or more accurately the $H^+$ ions associated with it, has long been considered the major cause of fatigue during high-intensity, anaerobic exercise. This view has been challenged by evidence demonstrating that inorganic phosphate (Pi) is the major contributor to fatigue at the level of the myosin cross-bridge.[34,35] A role for $H^+$ as a contributor to fatigue cannot be completely discounted because buffering $H^+$ ions by bicarbonate loading has been shown to improve run times for races ranging from 400 to 1500 meters.[36–38]

During longer-duration aerobic exercise, the almost complete depletion of intramuscular glycogen is a dramatic cause of fatigue. In highly trained athletes, whose nutritional practices are sound, complete depletion of intramuscular glycogen rarely occurs. However, depletion of glycogen within individual fibers may occur. When this happens, myofibers associated with larger motor units must be recruited to maintain intensity. These larger motor units are more difficult to excite voluntarily, thus increasing the difficulty of maintaining the desired intensity of exercise. Because carbohydrates are the primary substrate for high-intensity exercise, carbohydrate consumption during exercise prolongs time to exhaustion.[39,40]

The inability of elite athletes to maintain a given level of effort during long-distance races is likely attributable to multiple peripheral and central factors. One interesting factor that may be involved is excitation-contraction coupling failure induced by an accumulation of $K^+$ ions with the lumen of the T tubules. A buildup of $K^+$ may result in failure of action potentials to propagate down the T tubules resulting in a reduction in the amount of calcium released from the sarcoplasmic reticulum. Decreased calcium release results in fewer myosin cross-bridges interacting with actin in the strong binding state, thus reducing force production.

## Sidebar 2.2. Sensory Receptors in Skeletal Muscle

There are several types of sensory receptors associated with skeletal muscle that are responsive to various types of stimuli including chemicals (chemoreceptors), mechanical forces (mechanoreceptors), pain-producing substances (nociceptors), and temperature (thermoreceptors).

**Free nerve endings:** Free nerve endings are the simplest type of sensory receptor and are found in most tissues of the body. Different types of free nerve endings are sensitive to each of the categories of stimuli listed above. Free nerve endings that are responsive to chemicals include those that are sensitive to changes in the level of extracellular $H^+$, $K^+$, $O_2$, and $CO_2$. Chemoreceptors send information about the local chemical environment via afferent or sensory neurons to the central nervous system. Chemoreceptors may be involved in the sensation of muscular discomfort and in cardiorespiratory responses during exercise.

**Proprioception:** Muscles and their associated joints contain several types of receptors that relay information about muscular dynamics and limb movements to the central nervous system. Proprioception enables the central nervous system to track a sequence of movements and provides a means for modifying subsequent motor behavior if needed. In skeletal muscle, Golgi tendon organs (GTOs) and muscle spindles are important proprioceptors.

**Golgi tendon organs:** GTOs are a type of mechanoreceptor that are located at the musculotendinous junction and are very sensitive to force development by the muscle fibers (Figure 2.12). GTOs act to protect the myofibers from damage that might occur from excessive muscular force output. When excited by high force production, GTOs transmit an inhibitory signal via a type Ib sensory or afferent neuron to the spinal column. Within the spinal column, this inhibitory input depresses motor neuron excitability, thus increasing the amount of excitatory input necessary to stimulate the motor neuron sufficiently to develop an action potential. This is likely to cause a decrease in muscle force production. One of the early neural adaptations to strength training is the ability to more readily overcome the inhibitory effects of the GTOs.

**Muscle spindles:** Muscle spindles are referred to as stretch receptors and are the most complex sensory receptors in skeletal muscle (Figure 2.13). In response to rapid lengthening of the muscle, they can trigger a reflex muscle contraction, which is called a stretch or myotatic reflex. Muscle spindles are mechanoreceptors that contain specialized muscle fibers called intrafusal fibers encapsulated within a connective tissue sheath. Muscle spindles are located throughout the muscle and run in parallel with the other myofibers, which are referred to as extrafusal fibers. Muscle spindles contain two types of sensory nerve endings. Primary nerve endings are sensitive to dynamic changes in muscle length, whereas secondary nerve endings provide information about muscle length. Muscle spindles are even more complex because they are innervated by γ-motor neurons. When α motor neurons stimulate the extrafusal fibers to contract, γ-motor neurons stimulate the intrafusal fibers to contract in order to keep them at a length consistent with that of the muscle and thus sensitive to further length changes. When the primary nerve endings are excited by muscle lengthening, they transmit an excitatory impulse to the spinal cord. At the spinal level, the sensory neuron excites the motor neurons innervating the same muscle, which can initiate a reflex contraction of the muscle. Muscle spindles have important roles in postural control and regulation of movement.

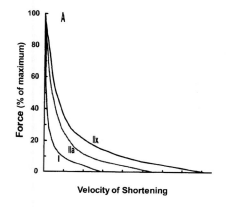

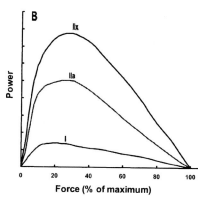

**FIGURE 2.12.** The relationship of (**A**) force and velocity and (**B**) power and force for the three adult human fiber types. **A:** Muscle fiber force production decreases rapidly from a static muscle action (0 velocity) to slow shortening velocities. For any given velocity of shortening, type IIx fibers are capable of the greatest force output and type I fibers produce the lowest force. **B:** Type IIx fibers are capable of greater power production than type IIa or I fibers, and type I fibers produce the lowest power outputs.

**FIGURE 2.13.** A twitch response and wave summation. A single stimulation of a muscle (shown as ↑) results in a twitch response. Repetitive stimuli result in summation until maximal force output by the muscle is achieved at tetanus.

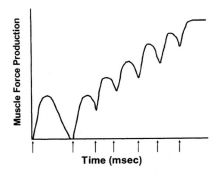

# RESPONSES AND ADAPTATION OF SKELETAL MUSCLE TO EXERCISE TRAINING

## Delayed-Onset Muscle Soreness

A common experience for fitness enthusiasts and athletes alike is the sensation of muscular pain or discomfort beginning approximately 16–24 hours after a workout. This delayed-onset muscle soreness (DOMS) usually peaks about 24–48 hours postexercise before beginning to subside. Depending on the training status of the individual and the rigor of the workout, the pain may have dissipated within 72 hours, but in cases of more severe damage can last several days. DOMS is accompanied by decreases in the maximum force capabilities of the muscle.[41]

The primary cause of DOMS is muscle fiber damage that may include tension-induced disruption of the sarcomeres and sarcolemma, as well as increased intracellular calcium, which activates enzymes that degrade muscle proteins.[42–46] Eccentric contractions are much more likely to cause myofiber damage and DOMS than static or concentric muscle actions. Although DOMS is most often associated with strength-training exercises, endurance-type exercise with a significant eccentric component, such as running downhill, can cause DOMS also. The most common finding after eccentric exercise-induced muscle damage is disruption of the myofibrillar material, especially at the Z disk[41,43] (Figure 2.14). Studies also show that there is disruption of the proteins

**FIGURE 2.14.** The Golgi tendon organ and its neural connections. Golgi tendon organs are responsive to muscle tension development. Golgi tendon organs function as a protective sensory mechanism to detect and subsequently reduce excess strain at the musculotendinous junction. Excessive tension within the muscle activates the Golgi tendon organs inducing a reflex inhibition of the muscle. (From McArdle, WD, Katch FI, Katch VL. Exercise Physiology: Energy, Nutrition, and Human Performance. 5th ed. Baltimore: Lippincott Williams & Wilkins: 2001. Reprinted with permission of Lippincott Williams & Wilkins.)

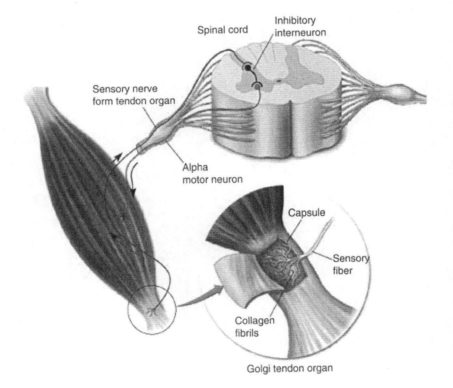

Sidebar 2.3. Reducing Delayed-Onset Muscle Soreness: Regular Exercise Is Recommended But Long-Term Use of Nonsteroidal Antiinflammatory Drugs Should Be Avoided

Anytime an individual performs exercise to which they are not accustomed, DOMS is likely to occur. Mild DOMS is not uncommon for athletes and fitness enthusiasts who perform strenuous workouts, but the soreness is not usually as great as the first time that DOMS is experienced. The most effective means of reducing DOMS is to exercise on a regular basis. Even a single bout of exercise has a significant protective effect against muscle soreness during subsequent bouts of similar exercise.[48,49] This phenomenon is called the repeated bout effect.

Aspirin and other nonsteroidal antiinflammatory drugs (NSAIDs) reduce the sensation of muscular pain; however, longer-term use may slow recovery. Drs. Jan Friden, Richard Lieber, and colleagues induced muscle damage in rabbits by repetitive stretching of the contracting muscles of the anterior compartment of the leg.[50] Initially, there was a more rapid recovery of contractile strength by the leg muscles of rabbits treated with the NSAID flurbiprofen, but there was a longer-term deficit in muscle force production compared with untreated rabbits. Based on histologic observation, muscles from the treated animals showed a less effective regenerative response. Although the use of NSAIDs may reduce DOMS, their routine use for reducing soreness should be avoided.

that make up the cytoskeleton.[44,47] Muscle damage leads to an inflammatory process and the accumulation of fluid and pain-producing substances within the muscle. It is important to realize that the actual amount of damage to the muscle fibers that causes significant muscular discomfort is quite small. Often, the damage within a myofiber extends for only a few sarcomeres. These localized areas of damage are readily repaired if adequate time is allowed for recovery.

## Muscle Satellite Cells: Role in Muscle Repair, Regeneration, and Adaptation

Satellite cells of skeletal muscle are quiescent, myogenic stem cells located outside the myofiber sarcolemma but within its basement membrane. Approximately 1%–5% of the nuclei associated with a myofiber are satellite cell nuclei,[51] and it seems that more oxidative muscle fibers have a greater density of satellite cell nuclei compared with more glycolytic myofibers.[52] The greater percentage of satellite cell nuclei associated with oxidative or slow-twitch fibers may be attributable to their greater use (e.g., maintenance of posture, light activity), and thus greater wear and tear. Satellite cells are important for the repair of myofiber damage and regeneration of necrotic myofibers.[51,53] Skeletal muscle fiber damage induces satellite cell activation by various mitogens that have not been clearly defined. Activated satellite cells undergo one or more cycles of mitosis to give rise to daughter cells. The fate of these additional cells depends on the chemical signals acting on the cell. Daughter cells may undergo additional cycles of mitosis, fuse with damaged fibers or with other satellite cells to form a myotube, or return to a state of quiescence. Whether myofiber damage must occur for satellite cell activation is unclear, but recent experimental work shows that satellite cells are likely to contribute additional nuclei during myofiber hypertrophy in response to strength training.[52–54] Also, recent evidence shows that satellite cells are activated during fiber-type transformation.[53]

## Adaptations of Skeletal Muscle to Endurance Training

Repeated bouts of endurance exercise increase an individual's maximal oxygen uptake, which indicates a greater ability for the cardiorespiratory system to deliver oxygenated blood to the working skeletal muscles and for muscle fibers to extract and use the oxygen for energy production. Within skeletal muscle, several important adaptations occur that increase the oxidative capacity of muscle, including an increased number and size of mitochondria and increases in the enzymes of metabolic pathways involved in oxidative metabolism.[55–57] These enzymes include succinate dehydrogenase and malate dehydrogenase, which are enzymes in Krebs tricarboxylic acid cycle. Endurance exercise also induces a shift toward a greater reliance on lipid metabolism. As discussed earlier, a transition of type IIx fibers to type IIa fibers occurs quite readily in response to endurance training. Transitions from type II fibers to type I fibers have been reported in some studies, but the extent of these transitions is unclear.

## Skeletal Muscle Adaptations to Strength Training

Increases in muscular strength and size occur as a result of resistance or strength training.[58–61] Strength gains during the first few weeks of strength training are largely the result of adaptations within the nervous system. Some of the adaptations include reduced activation of antagonistic muscles and enhanced ability to overcome the inhibitory effects of the GTOs. These neural adaptations allow the individual to use heavier resistances during a training session, thus loading the muscle to a greater degree.

Longer-term increases in muscle strength result primarily from muscle hypertrophy, although nervous system adaptations are always important. Increased muscle size is important because the force that a muscle can produce is directly related to its cross-sectional area. The primary way that muscle hypertrophy occurs is by growth of individual muscle fibers. This is a result of altering protein turnover in favor of net protein synthesis (Figures 2.15 and 2.16). Strength training causes a short-term increase in protein degradation, but a longer-term increase in protein synthesis (Figure 2.17). Adequate protein and carbohydrate consumption before or after a strength-training workout can shift protein turnover further toward a positive protein balance by reducing degradation and increasing protein synthesis.[62,63] Several studies show a greater rate of myofiber hypertrophy for the type II fibers compared with the type I fibers.[64,65] Individuals who have a higher proportion of type II myofibers may increase muscle mass at a greater rate compared with individuals with a higher proportion of type I myofibers. This may explain the observation of many fitness enthusiasts who seem to have a difficult time increasing muscle size whereas other individuals seem to gain muscle mass more readily.

Although the primary means by which muscle size increases as a result of resistance training is myofiber hypertrophy,[64] increasing evidence suggests that some increase in the number of muscle fibers, termed myofiber hyperplasia, is possible.[66–69] Initially, evidence showing that hyperplasia could occur was from experimental animal models, such as the compensatory hypertrophy of muscles

FIGURE 2.15. Structure of the muscle spindle including a detailed view of the intrafusal fibers and neural connections. The muscle spindles are stretch receptors within skeletal muscle. The two different types of intrafusal fibers within the muscle spindle are responsive to length changes or changes in the rate of change of length. (From McArdle, WD, Katch FI, Katch VL. Exercise Physiology: Energy, Nutrition, and Human Performance. 5th ed. Baltimore: Lippincott Williams & Wilkins: 2001. Modified and reprinted with permission of Lippincott Williams & Wilkins.)

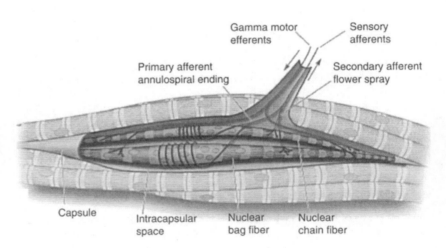

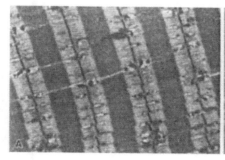
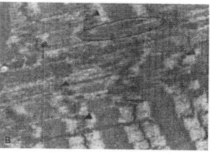

**FIGURE 2.16.** Ultrastructural changes in human vastus lateralis muscle after eccentric contractions. **A:** Normal muscle. **B:** Muscle obtained 3 days after eccentric contraction-induced injury. It is important to note that the disruptions are localized and primarily in the region of the Z disk. (From Lieber.[27] Reprinted with permission of Lippincott Williams & Wilkins.)

that occurred after ablation (removal) of the synergists and the wing-stretch model in chickens and quail. Although these models were criticized for not being similar to strength training in humans, they did demonstrate that muscle fiber formation was possible in adult animals. The research of Dr. William Gonyea and colleagues[69] in which cats were trained to perform resistance-training exercise in order to obtain a food reward added additional support for myofiber hyperplasia. Cats that performed resistance-training exercise for an average of 101 weeks had a 9% greater myofiber number in the flexor carpi radialis muscle of their trained limb compared with their untrained limb. Obviously, these types of experiments cannot be done for ethical reasons in humans; however, a substantial body of indirect evidence supports the likelihood of muscle fiber hyperplasia in humans as a result of strength training,[70,71] although the extent of the hyperplasia is unclear.

With regard to fiber-type transitions, a shift of type IIx fibers to IIa fibers occurs quite rapidly in response to heavy strength training. In women performing strength-training exercises, a shift from type IIx to IIa fibers was observed after only four workout sessions.[19] A shift of type II to type I fibers or vice versa has not been reported with resistance training.

## Skeletal Muscle Adaptations to Sprint Training

A variety of sprint-training workouts can be achieved by altering the duration or distance of the sprint, workout intensity, the duration of the recovery interval, and training frequency. Energy for sprinting exercise is derived largely from the ATP/PCr and glycolytic/glycogenolytic energy systems.[72–74] However, when repetitive sprints are performed with short recovery intervals or when sprint duration is increased, the contribution of aerobic energy metabolism increases.[73,75]

Although there is substantial variation among studies, adaptations to sprint exercise training include increases in enzymes associated with all three energy systems and improved muscle buffering capacity.[76] Differences among studies may be attributable in part to differences in sprint duration, duration of the

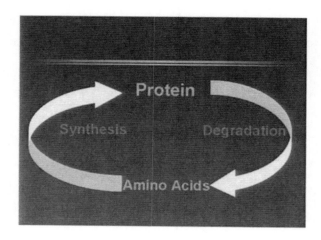

**FIGURE 2.17.** Schematic representation of the relationship of protein synthesis and degradation with muscle protein and amino acids. Muscle hypertrophy associated with strength training results largely from an increase in protein synthesis. Postexercise nutrition may promote greater increases in protein synthesis and reduce degradation.[62,63]

recovery interval, and training volume. Increases in the activities of enzymes of the phosphagen energy system, myokinase and creatine phosphokinase, have been reported after sprint training.[76] Interestingly, the majority of studies have shown no increase in the amount of intramuscular ATP and PCr after sprint training; however, the ability to resynthesize ATP may be more important than the absolute muscle content.[76] Increases in the enzymes of the glycolytic/glycogenolytic pathway are often observed after sprint training. For example, significant increases in the activity of hexokinase (+56%) and phosphofructokinase (+49%) were observed in vastus lateralis muscle after training with repeated bouts of 30-second sprints on a cycle ergometer for 7 weeks.[77] Other studies have reported increases in the rate-limiting enzyme of glycolysis, phosphofructokinase, as well as glycogen phosphorylase and lactate dehydrogenase.[76]

It is important to point out that increases in maximal oxygen consumption[78] as well as increases in enzymes involved in oxidative metabolism have been reported after sprint or interval-type training.[76] This is significant for the conditioning of athletes in sports that require high degrees of strength and power, because aerobic-type training can attenuate training-induced gains in strength and power.[79-81] The necessary degree of aerobic conditioning for athletes in many sports characterized by strength–power or a high anaerobic component might be achieved by repeated bouts of short duration and very-high-intensity exercise.

In addition to the metabolic changes that have been discussed, adaptations in fiber size, fiber type, and morphology have been observed in response to sprint training. Increases in myofiber cross-sectional area of 5%–16% have been reported for type I and II fibers after 8 weeks to 8 months of sprint training.[76] The volume of the sarcoplasmic reticulum may increase in response to sprint training.[76,82] Finally, transition of type IIx fibers to IIa frequently occurs after sprint training. A decrease in the proportion of type I fibers and increase in the percentage of type IIa fibers suggests that sprint training can induce a type I to IIa fiber-type transition.[25,76] However, changes suggestive of a IIa to I shift have been reported also.[83,84] Differences among studies may be related to longer sprint durations or a greater training frequency.[76]

## Concurrent Strength and Endurance Training: Beneficial for Endurance Athletes But Not Strength–Power Athletes

A frequently asked question in sports is whether athletes competing in sports requiring a large amount of strength and power should establish a conditioning base with aerobic-type exercise. The classic work of Dr. Robert Hickson[80] clearly demonstrated that endurance exercise can hinder the development of muscular strength. It is possible that adaptations and responses necessary for improving strength and power, including neuromuscular recruitment,[85] myofiber hypertrophy,[86] and hormonal levels,[86] are compromised when concurrent strength and endurance exercise is performed.[79] Athletes participating in strength–power sports can improve aerobic capacity through the use of high-intensity, short-duration work intervals with short rest periods.[76]

Interestingly, endurance athletes may benefit from strength training. After 10 weeks of training, individuals performing concurrent endurance and strength training had increased running or cycling times to exhaustion despite no increase in aerobic capacity.[81,87] The addition of strength training improves running and cycling performance by enhancing movement economy.[88,89] Also, the addition of explosive-strength training that included sprints and plyometric exercises to an endurance training program improved 5-kilometer time in well-trained endurance athletes without changes in their maximal oxygen uptake. This improvement was attributed to improved neuromuscular characteristics and enhanced running economy.[90] Interestingly, strength training does not seem to substantially improve swim performance.[91] It is important to note that endurance athletes should avoid a substantial increase in lean body mass, because the additional body weight is likely to have a detrimental impact on performance.

Because most research has been done on sedentary or moderately trained individuals who are not elite, there is some debate as to whether highly trained or elite athletes can benefit from strength training. It has been suggested that the neuromuscular recruitment patterns of elite athletes are so efficient that strength training will not improve movement economy.[92] At this time, it can be concluded that the addition of an appropriately designed strength-training program can improve the performance of many fitness enthusiasts and athletes. However, additional research is necessary to determine whether the appropriate application of strength training can enhance the performance of elite athletes.

## SUMMARY

Skeletal muscle is a highly organized tissue designed to produce force for postural control, movement, and even breathing. Various architectural designs, varying amounts of muscle proteins (e.g., enzymes or myosin), and different isoforms of many muscle proteins provide for a wide range of force-producing, biochemical, and metabolic characteristics. Additionally, the ability of skeletal muscle to adapt to the demands placed on it, such as increased contractile activity associated with endurance training or increased loading attributable to strength training, demonstrates a tremendous plasticity. It should be noted that there is a large variation among individuals with regard to the magnitude of muscle adaptability to various types of training. Differing muscle characteristics, such as muscle pennation and fiber type, and variation in degree of adaptability among individuals partially explains the wide range of differences in aspects of exercise performance, such as muscular endurance or strength.

## PRACTICAL APPLICATIONS

Effective exercise training programs must be designed to induce adaptations necessary for success in a given sport or achieving individual goals. The specificity of training principle states that training should be as specific as possible to the event in which an athlete competes. For example, for increasing strength and power, athletes must include maximal muscle contractions using movement patterns that are as similar as possible to those in their sport in order to recruit all motor units and to optimize neuromuscular recruitment. Also, endurance, strength, and sprint training tend to induce different adaptations in skeletal muscle although there is some degree of overlap depending on the design of the training program. For example, repeated bouts of very-high-intensity exercise (sprinting) with short rest periods will increase the oxidative capacity of skeletal muscle.[93, 94] Familiarity with the characteristics of skeletal muscle that contribute to success in various types of athletic events, as well as knowledge of the adaptations of skeletal muscle to different types of exercise training programs enables athletes, coaches, and sports nutritionists to design more effective training programs.

## QUESTIONS

1. What is the innermost layer of connective tissue that surrounds each individual muscle fiber?
   a. Endomysium
   b. Perimysium
   c. Epimysium
   d. Myomysium

2. Which of the following is the type of muscle action during which the muscle develops tension and lengthens?
   a. Concentric
   b. Static
   c. Eccentric
   d. Isometric

3. Skeletal muscles are divided in bundles of muscle fibers. Which term refers to these bundles of muscle fibers?
   a. Sarcomeres
   b. Myofibrils
   c. Synergists
   d. Fasciculi

4. What is the name of a very large protein in muscle fibers that keeps myosin centered within the sarcomere?
   a. Z disk
   b. Titin
   c. Troponin
   d. Sarcoplasmic reticulum

5. If a football player begins a strength-training program, which of the following is most accurate regarding muscle hypertrophy?
   a. The type I muscle fibers will hypertrophy at the greatest rate.
   b. The type II muscle fibers will hypertrophy at the greatest rate.
   c. Usually the type I and II muscle fibers hypertrophy at the same rate.
   d. The primary means by which muscle hypertrophy occurs is muscle fiber hyperplasia.

6. The thick filaments of the sarcomere are composed of which of the following?
   a. Myelin
   b. Actin
   c. Myosin
   d. Tropomyosin

7. Justin Gatlin won the gold medal in the 100-meter sprint at the recent Olympic games. If you could study his leg muscles, you would likely find which of the following?
   a. His muscles have a very high percentage of slow-twitch muscle fibers.
   b. His muscles have a very high percentage of fast-twitch muscle fibers.
   c. His muscles have about 50% fast-twitch muscle fibers.
   d. There is no relationship between muscle fiber type and sprinting performance.

8. Which term refers to the most basic contractile element of skeletal muscle?
   a. Myofibrils
   b. Sarcomeres
   c. Filaments
   d. Mitochondria

9. Which of the following is the best description of how muscle fibers shorten during a concentric muscle action?
   a. Muscle shortening occurs as the thick (myosin) filaments shorten and pull the thin filaments toward the center of the sarcomere.
   b. Muscle shortening occurs as the thin filaments shorten.
   c. Muscle shortening occurs as the myosin cross-bridges slide the thin filaments over the thick filaments.
   d. Muscle shortening occurs as the thin filaments are pulled away from the thick filaments.

10. When calcium is released, what is the protein on the thin filament with which it interacts?
    a. Actin
    b. Titin
    c. Troponin
    d. Tropomyosin

11. Which of the following group of athletes would be expected to have the highest percentage of slow-twitch fibers in the muscles of their legs?
    a. Sprinters
    b. Shot putters

    c. Football players
    d. Soccer players
    e. Long-distance runners

12. Which of the following is not a factor in determining the amount of force that a muscle can produce?
    a. The size of the muscle
    b. The number of motor units activated
    c. The amount of mitochondria within the muscle
    d. The speed of the muscle contraction

13. Which of the following statements most accurately describes strength gains during the initial 6–8 weeks of resistance training?
    a. Strength gains are attributable largely to neural adaptations
    b. Strength gains are attributable largely to muscle fiber hypertrophy
    c. Strength gains are attributable almost equally to neural adaptations and muscle fiber hypertrophy
    d. Strength gains are minimal during the initial 6–8 weeks of strength training

14. Which of the following is the type of muscle contraction that is most likely to cause delayed-onset muscle soreness?
    a. Concentric
    b. Static
    c. Eccentric
    d. Isometric

15. Which of the following is the most likely cause of delayed-onset muscle soreness?
    a. Structural damage to the muscle
    b. High levels of lactic acid in the muscle
    c. Depletion of muscle glycogen
    d. Increased muscle spindle activity

16. In human adult skeletal muscle, each muscle fiber is typically innervated by which number of motor neurons?
    a. One
    b. Two or three
    c. About five
    d. More than ten

17. Which of the following terms is used to refer to the order in which motor units are recruited during a concentric muscle action?
    a. Size principle
    b. Saltatory conduction
    c. Principle of contraction-type specificity
    d. Static recruitment

18. Which of the following muscle fiber types has the greatest oxidative (aerobic) capacity?
    a. Type I
    b. Type Ib
    c. Type IIa
    d. Type IIx

19. What is the extensive series of channels that run throughout the skeletal muscle fiber and is a site for calcium storage?
    a. Transverse tubules
    b. Myofibrils
    c. Sarcolemma
    d. Sarcoplasmic reticulum

20. What is the type of muscle contraction during which the muscle develops force but there is no rotation about a joint?
    a. Eccentric
    b. Static

c. Plyometric
d. Concentric

21. What is the structure within a muscle cell that is formed by lining up sarcomeres end to end?
a. Myofibrils
b. Fasciculi
c. Z lines
d. Sarcoplasmic reticulum

22. Which of the following types of muscle sensory receptor is responsive to force (tension) development by the muscle?
a. Muscle spindles
b. Golgi tendon organs
c. Free nerve endings
d. Nociceptors

23. Which of the following is an example of a skeletal muscle adaptation that occurs in response to endurance training?
a. Increased muscle fiber size
b. Decreased percentage of type I fibers
c. Increased number of myofibrils
d. Increased size and number of mitochondria

24. Which of the following types of receptors is sensitive to painful stimuli or chemicals?
a. Nociceptors
b. Mechanoreceptors
c. Thermoreceptors
d. Golgi tendon organs

25. Which term refers to an increase in the number of muscle fibers within a muscle?
a. Hypoplasia
b. Hypertrophy
c. Hyperplasia
d. Atrophy

26. Which of the following proteins link the Z lines of adjacent sarcomeres together?
a. α-Actinin
b. Dystrophin
c. Nebulin
d. Desmin

27. What is the chemical that is found in the numerous synaptic vesicles located in the axon terminals of motor neurons?
a. Epinephrine
b. Calcium
c. Acetylcholine
d. Norepinephrine

28. Which of the following factors is a major determinant of the velocity of muscle fiber shortening?
a. The number of mitochondria within the muscle fiber
b. The type of myosin ATPase activity
c. The amount of calcium released from the sarcoplasmic reticulum
d. The size of the muscle fiber

29. Based on recent research, which of the following is the most likely cause of muscle fatigue during very-high-intensity exercise?
a. $H^+$ ions from lactic acid
b. Depletion of muscle glycogen
c. Low blood glucose levels
d. Accumulation of inorganic phosphate within the muscle fiber

30. Which of the following statements most accurately represents muscle fiber type alterations with exercise training?
    a. Transitions from type IIx to type IIa occur with either aerobic training or strength training
    b. Transitions from type IIx to type IIa occur with aerobic training, but not with strength training
    c. Transitions from type IIa to type IIx occur with either aerobic training or strength training
    d. Transitions from type IIa to type IIx occur with strength training, but not with aerobic training

## REFERENCES

1. Wong TS, Booth FW. Protein metabolism in rat tibialis anterior muscle after stimulated chronic eccentric exercise. J Appl Physiol 1990;69:1718–1724.
2. Franzini-Armstrong C. The sarcoplasmic reticulum and the control of muscle contraction. Faseb J 1999;13(Suppl 2):S266–270.
3. Lowey S, Waller GS, Trybus KM. Skeletal muscle myosin light chains are essential for physiological speeds of shortening. Nature 1993;365:454–456.
4. Sweeney HL, Bowman BF, Stull JT. Myosin light chain phosphorylation in vertebrate striated muscle: regulation and function. Am J Physiol 1993;264:C1085–1095.
5. Petrof BJ, Shrager JB, Stedman HH, Kelly AM, Sweeney HL. Dystrophin protects the sarcolemma from stresses developed during muscle contraction. Proc Natl Acad Sci USA 1993;90:3710–3714.
6. Hoffman EP, Brown RH Jr, Kunkel LM. Dystrophin: the protein product of the Duchenne muscular dystrophy locus. Cell 1987;51:919–928.
7. Enoka RM. Activation order of motor axons in electrically evoked contractions. Muscle Nerve 2002;25:763–764.
8. Huxley AF, Niedergerke R. Structural changes in muscle during contraction: interference microscopy of living muscle fibres. Nature 1954;173:971–973.
9. Kitamura K, Tokunaga M, Iwane AH, Yanagida T. A single myosin head moves along an actin filament with regular steps of 5.3 nanometres. Nature 1999;397:129–134.
10. Peter JB, Barnard RJ, Edgerton VR, Gillespie CA, Stempel KE. Metabolic profiles of three fiber types of skeletal muscle in guinea pigs and rabbits. Biochemistry 1972;11:2627–2633.
11. Brooke MH, Kaiser KK. Three "myosin adenosine triphosphatase" systems: the nature of their pH lability and sulfhydryl dependence. J Histochem Cytochem 1970;18:670–672.
12. Brooke MH, Kaiser KK. Muscle fiber types: how many and what kind? Arch Neurol 1970;23:369–379.
13. Smerdu V, Karsch-Mizrachi I, Campione M, Leinwand L, Schiaffino S. Type IIx myosin heavy chain transcripts are expressed in type IIb fibers of human skeletal muscle. Am J Physiol 1994;267:C1723–1728.
14. Burke RE, Levine DN, Zajac FE 3rd. Mammalian motor units: physiological-histochemical correlation in three types in cat gastrocnemius. Science 1971;174:709–712.
15. Buller AJ, Eccles JC, Eccles RM. Interactions between motoneurones and muscles in respect of the characteristic speeds of their responses. J Physiol 1960;150:417–439.
16. Howald H, Hoppeler H, Claassen H, Mathieu O, Straub R. Influences of endurance training on the ultrastructural composition of the different muscle fiber types in humans. Pflugers Arch 1985;403:369–376.
17. Pette D. Historical perspectives: plasticity of mammalian skeletal muscle. J Appl Physiol 2001;90:1119–1124.
18. Pette D, Staron RS. Transitions of muscle fiber phenotypic profiles. Histochem Cell Biol 2001;115:359–372.
19. Staron RS, Karapondo DL, Kraemer WJ, et al. Skeletal muscle adaptations during early phase of heavy-resistance training in men and women. J Appl Physiol 1994;76:1247–1255.
20. Esbjornsson M, Sylven C, Holm I, Jansson E. Fast twitch fibres may predict anaerobic performance in both females and males. Int J Sports Med 1993;14:257–263.
21. Fry AC, Schilling BK, Staron RS, Hagerman FC, Hikida RS, Thrush JT. Muscle fiber characteristics and performance correlates of male Olympic-style weightlifters. J Strength Cond Res 2003;17:746–754.

22. Costill DL, Daniels J, Evans W, Fink W, Krahenbuhl G, Saltin B. Skeletal muscle enzymes and fiber composition in male and female track athletes. J Appl Physiol 1976;40:149–154.

23. Costill DL, Fink WJ, Pollock ML. Muscle fiber composition and enzyme activities of elite distance runners. Med Sci Sports 1976;8:96–100.

24. Rodriguez LP, Lopez-Rego J, Calbet JA, Valero E, Varela E, Ponce J. Effects of training status on fibers of the musculus vastus lateralis in professional road cyclists. Am J Phys Med Rehabil 2002;81:651–660.

25. Jansson E, Esbjornsson M, Holm I, Jacobs I. Increase in the proportion of fast-twitch muscle fibres by sprint training in males. Acta Physiol Scand 1990;140:359–363.

26. Baumann H, Jaggi M, Soland F, Howald H, Schaub MC. Exercise training induces transitions of myosin isoform subunits within histochemically typed human muscle fibres. Pflugers Arch 1987;409:349–360.

27. Lieber RL. Skeletal Muscle Structure, Function, and Plasticity: The Physiological Basis of Rehabilitation. 2nd ed. Baltimore: Lippincott Williams & Wilkins; 2002.

28. Bottinelli R, Canepari M, Reggiani C, Stienen GJ. Myofibrillar ATPase activity during isometric contraction and isomyosin composition in rat single skinned muscle fibres. J Physiol 1994;481(Pt 3):663–675.

29. Nardone A, Romano C, Schieppati M. Selective recruitment of high-threshold human motor units during voluntary isotonic lengthening of active muscles. J Physiol 1989;409:451–471.

30. Milner-Brown HS, Stein RB, Yemm R. The contractile properties of human motor units during voluntary isometric contractions. J Physiol 1973;228:285–306.

31. Semmler JG, Nordstrom MA. Motor unit discharge and force tremor in skill- and strength-trained individuals. Exp Brain Res 1998;119:27–38.

32. Yao W, Fuglevand RJ, Enoka RM. Motor-unit synchronization increases EMG amplitude and decreases force steadiness of simulated contractions. J Neurophysiol 2000;83:441–452.

33. Semmler JG. Motor unit synchronization and neuromuscular performance. Exerc Sport Sci Rev 2002;30:8–14.

34. Stackhouse SK, Reisman DS, Binder-Macleod SA. Challenging the role of pH in skeletal muscle fatigue. Phys Ther 2001;81:1897–1903.

35. Westerblad H, Allen DG, Lannergren J. Muscle fatigue: lactic acid or inorganic phosphate the major cause? News Physiol Sci 2002;17:17–21.

36. Bird SR, Wiles J, Robbins J. The effect of sodium bicarbonate ingestion on 1500-m racing time. J Sports Sci 1995;13:399–403.

37. Goldfinch J, McNaughton L, Davies P. Induced metabolic alkalosis and its effects on 400-m racing time. Eur J Appl Physiol Occup Physiol 1988;57:45–48.

38. Wilkes D, Gledhill N, Smyth R. Effect of acute induced metabolic alkalosis on 800-m racing time. Med Sci Sports Exerc 1983;15:277–280.

39. Ivy JL. Role of carbohydrate in physical activity. Clin Sports Med 1999;18:469–484.

40. Jacobs KA, Sherman WM. The efficacy of carbohydrate supplementation and chronic high-carbohydrate diets for improving endurance performance. Int J Sport Nutr 1999;9:92–115.

41. Friden J, Sjostrom M, Ekblom B. Myofibrillar damage following intense eccentric exercise in man. Int J Sports Med 1983;4:170–176.

42. Morgan DL. New insights into the behavior of muscle during active lengthening. Biophys J 1990;57:209–221.

43. Friden J. Delayed onset muscle soreness. Scand J Med Sci Sports 2002;12:327–328.

44. Lieber RL, Friden J. Morphologic and mechanical basis of delayed-onset muscle soreness. J Am Acad Orthop Surg 2002;10:67–73.

45. Crenshaw AG, Karlsson S, Styf J, Backlund T, Friden J. Knee extension torque and intramuscular pressure of the vastus lateralis muscle during eccentric and concentric activities. Eur J Appl Physiol Occup Physiol 1995;70:13–19.

46. Crenshaw AG, Thornell LE, Friden J. Intramuscular pressure, torque and swelling for the exercise-induced sore vastus lateralis muscle. Acta Physiol Scand 1994;152:265–277.

47. Lieber RL, Thornell LE, Friden J. Muscle cytoskeletal disruption occurs within the first 15 min of cyclic eccentric contraction. J Appl Physiol 1996;80:278–284.

48. Evans WJ, Meredith CN, Cannon JG, et al. Metabolic changes following eccentric exercise in trained and untrained men. J Appl Physiol 1986;61:1864–1868.

49. Newham DJ, Jones DA, Clarkson PM. Repeated high-force eccentric exercise: effects on muscle pain and damage. J Appl Physiol 1987;63:1381–1386.

50. Mishra DK, Friden J, Schmitz MC, Lieber RL. Anti-inflammatory medication after muscle injury. A treatment resulting in short-term improvement but subsequent loss of muscle function. J Bone Joint Surg Am 1995;77:1510–1519.

51. Allbrook D. Skeletal muscle regeneration. Muscle Nerve 1981;4:234–245.

52. Schultz E. Satellite cell behavior during skeletal muscle growth and regeneration. Med Sci Sports Exerc 1989;21:S181–186.

53. Russell B, Dix DJ, Haller DL, Jacobs-El J. Repair of injured skeletal muscle: a molecular approach. Med Sci Sports Exerc 1992;24:189–196.

54. Vierck J, O'Reilly B, Hossner K, et al. Satellite cell regulation following myotrauma caused by resistance exercise. Cell Biol Int 2000;24:263–272.

55. Holloszy JO, Booth FW. Biochemical adaptations to endurance exercise in muscle. Annu Rev Physiol 1976;38:273–291.

56. Hawley JA. Adaptations of skeletal muscle to prolonged, intense endurance training. Clin Exp Pharmacol Physiol 2002;29:218–222.

57. Hoppeler H, Fluck M. Plasticity of skeletal muscle mitochondria: structure and function. Med Sci Sports Exerc 2003;35:95–104.

58. Tesch PA, Larsson L. Muscle hypertrophy in bodybuilders. Eur J Appl Physiol Occup Physiol 1982;49:301–306.

59. Dudley GA, Tesch PA, Miller BJ, Buchanan P. Importance of eccentric actions in performance adaptations to resistance training. Aviat Space Environ Med 1991;62:543–550.

60. Tesch PA, Thorsson A, Essen-Gustavsson B. Enzyme activities of FT and ST muscle fibers in heavy-resistance trained athletes. J Appl Physiol 1989;67:83–87.

61. Tesch PA. Skeletal muscle adaptations consequent to long-term heavy resistance exercise. Med Sci Sports Exerc 1988;20:S132–134.

62. Lemon PW, Berardi JM, Noreen EE. The role of protein and amino acid supplements in the athlete's diet: does type or timing of ingestion matter? Curr Sports Med Rep 2002;1:214–221.

63. Wolfe RR. Protein supplements and exercise. Am J Clin Nutr 2000;72:551S–557S.

64. McCall GE, Byrnes WC, Dickinson A, Pattany PM, Fleck SJ. Muscle fiber hypertrophy, hyperplasia, and capillary density in college men after resistance training. J Appl Physiol 1996;81:2004–2012.

65. Antonio J, Gonyea WJ. Skeletal muscle fiber hyperplasia. Med Sci Sports Exerc 1993;25:1333–1345.

66. Antonio J, Gonyea WJ. Progressive stretch overload of skeletal muscle results in hypertrophy before hyperplasia. J Appl Physiol 1993;75:1263–1271.

67. Antonio J, Gonyea WJ. Muscle fiber splitting in stretch-enlarged avian muscle. Med Sci Sports Exerc 1994;26:973–977.

68. Alway SE, Winchester PK, Davis ME, Gonyea WJ. Regionalized adaptations and muscle fiber proliferation in stretch-induced enlargement. J Appl Physiol 1989;66:771–781.

69. Gonyea WJ, Sale DG, Gonyea FB, Mikesky A. Exercise induced increases in muscle fiber number. Eur J Appl Physiol Occup Physiol 1986;55:137–141.

70. Larsson L, Tesch PA. Motor unit fibre density in extremely hypertrophied skeletal muscles in man. Electrophysiological signs of muscle fibre hyperplasia. Eur J Appl Physiol Occup Physiol 1986;55:130–136.

71. MacDougall JD, Sale DG, Elder GC, Sutton JR. Muscle ultrastructural characteristics of elite powerlifters and bodybuilders. Eur J Appl Physiol Occup Physiol 1982;48:117–126.

72. Gaitanos GC, Williams C, Boobis LH, Brooks S. Human muscle metabolism during intermittent maximal exercise. J Appl Physiol 1993;75:712–719.

73. Bogdanis GC, Nevill ME, Boobis LH, Lakomy HK. Contribution of phosphocreatine and aerobic metabolism to energy supply during repeated sprint exercise. J Appl Physiol 1996;80:876–884.

74. Bogdanis GC, Nevill ME, Lakomy HK, Boobis LH. Power output and muscle metabolism during and following recovery from 10 and 20 s of maximal sprint exercise in humans. Acta Physiol Scand 1998;163:261–272.

75. McCartney N, Spriet LL, Heigenhauser GJ, Kowalchuk JM, Sutton JR, Jones NL. Muscle power and metabolism in maximal intermittent exercise. J Appl Physiol 1986;60:1164–1169.

76. Ross A, Leveritt M. Long-term metabolic and skeletal muscle adaptations to short-sprint training: implications for sprint training and tapering. Sports Med 2001;31:1063–1082.

77. MacDougall JD, Hicks AL, MacDonald JR, McKelvie RS, Green HJ, Smith KM. Muscle performance and enzymatic adaptations to sprint interval training. J Appl Physiol 1998;84:2138–2142.

78. Dawson B, Fitzsimons M, Green S, Goodman C, Carey M, Cole K. Changes in performance, muscle metabolites, enzymes and fibre types after short sprint training. Eur J Appl Physiol Occup Physiol 1998;78:163–169.

79. Chromiak JA, Mulvaney DR. The effects of combined strength and endurance training on strength development. J Appl Sport Sci Res 1990;4:55–60.

80. Hickson RC. Interference of strength development by simultaneously training for strength and endurance. Eur J Appl Physiol Occup Physiol 1980;45:255–263.

81. Hickson RC, Rosenkoetter MA, Brown MM. Strength training effects on aerobic power and short-term endurance. Med Sci Sports Exerc 1980;12:336–339.

82. Ortenblad N, Lunde PK, Levin K, Andersen JL, Pedersen PK. Enhanced sarcoplasmic reticulum Ca(2+) release following intermittent sprint training. Am J Physiol Regul Integr Comp Physiol 2000;279:R152–160.

83. Cadefau J, Casademont J, Grau JM, et al. Biochemical and histochemical adaptation to sprint training in young athletes. Acta Physiol Scand 1990;140:341–351.

84. Simoneau JA, Lortie G, Boulay MR, Marcotte M, Thibault MC, Bouchard C. Human skeletal muscle fiber type alteration with high-intensity intermittent training. Eur J Appl Physiol Occup Physiol 1985;54:250–253.

85. Dudley GA, Djamil R. Incompatibility of endurance- and strength-training modes of exercise. J Appl Physiol 1985;59:1446–1451.

86. Kraemer WJ, Patton JF, Gordon SE, et al. Compatibility of high-intensity strength and endurance training on hormonal and skeletal muscle adaptations. J Appl Physiol 1995;78:976–989.

87. Hickson RC, Dvorak BA, Gorostiaga EM, Kurowski TT, Foster C. Potential for strength and endurance training to amplify endurance performance. J Appl Physiol 1988;25:191–200.

88. Millet GP, Jaouen B, Borrani F, Candau R. Effects of concurrent endurance and strength training on running economy and VO(2) kinetics. Med Sci Sports Exerc 2002;34:1351–1359.

89. Johnston RE, Quinn TJ, Kertzer R, Voman NB. Strength training in female distance runners: impact on running economy. J Strength Cond Res 1997;11:224–229.

90. Paavolainen L, Hakkinen K, Hamalainen I, Nummela A, Rusko H. Explosive-strength training improves 5-km running time by improving running economy and muscle power. J Appl Physiol 1999;86:1527–1533.

91. Tanaka H, Swensen T. Impact of resistance training on endurance performance. A new form of cross-training? Sports Med 1998;25:191–200.

92. Hawley J, Burke L. Peak Performance. Training and Nutritional Strategies for Sport. St. Leonards, Australia: Allen & Unwin; 1998.

93. Burgomaster KA, Hughes SC, Heigenhauser GJ, Bradwell SN, Gibala MJ. Six sessions of sprint interval training increases muscle oxidative potential and cycle endurance capacity in humans. J Appl Physiol 2005;98:1985–1990.

94. Gibala MJ, Little JP, van Essen M, Wilkin GP, Burgomaster KA, Safdar A, Raha S, Tarnopolsky MA. Short-term sprint interval versus traditional endurance training: similar initial adaptations in human skeletal muscle and exercise performance. J Physiol 2006;575:901–911.

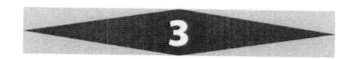

# The Endocrinology of Resistance Exercise and Training

William J. Kraemer, Nicholas A. Ratamess, Disa L. Hatfield, and Jakob L. Vingren

## OBJECTIVES

On completion of this chapter you will be able to:

1. Describe the basic relationship between exercise training and the endocrine system.
2. Understand the role of testosterone and how acute and chronic resistance training affects testosterone concentrations.
3. Describe the factors that affect the androgen receptor ability to induce muscular changes.
4. Explain the effect of carbohydrate/protein supplementation on the hormonal responses to a resistance training bout.
5. Understand the effects of resistance training on luteinizing hormone, sex hormone binding globulin.
6. Discuss the effects of supplementation with testosterone precursors.
7. Describe the acute and chronic growth hormone adaptations associated with resistance training.
8. Describe the resistance training factors that are associated with alterations in growth hormone concentrations.
9. Discuss the acute and chronic effects of resistance training on glucocorticoid release.
10. Discuss the importance of the testosterone/cortisol ratio.
11. Understand the effects of acute and chronic resistance training on insulin-like growth factors.
12. Explain the effects of resistance training and carbohydrate and protein supplements on insulin release.
13. Discuss the acute and chronic effects of resistance training on catecholamines, β-endorphins, thyroid hormones, leptin, peptide F, and fluid regulatory hormones.
14. Differentiate between overtraining and overreaching.
15. Describe the hormonal effects of short- and long-term detraining.

## ABSTRACT

Resistance exercise elicits an array of hormonal responses critical to acute muscular force and power production as well as subsequent tissue growth and remodeling. In general, the acute response is dependent upon the stimulus and may be the most critical element to tissue remodeling. Thus, modifications of training intensity, volume (or total work), muscle mass involvement, rest intervals, and frequency can impact the acute hormonal response. Long-term adaptations in neuroendocrine function seem minimal but may be related to

From: *Essentials of Sports Nutrition and Supplements*
Edited by J. Antonio, D. Kalman, J. R. Stout, M. Greenwood, D. S. Willoughby, and G. G. Haff © Humana Press, a part of Springer Science+Business Media, Totowa, NJ

the current intensity/volume of the training stimulus. The significance of these hormonal responses is not entirely known. For the sports nutritionist, the effect of various nutritional/supplemental strategies can indeed have an effect on the hormonal milieu. For instance, the timing of supplementation/feeding pre- and postexercise may affect the endocrine response to resistance exercise. Also, the consumption of various macronutrients can impact the basal concentration of various hormones.

*Key Words:* **hormone, endocrine response, testosterone, insulin, resistance exercise, endocrinology**

The neuroendocrine system has a vital role in the homeostatic regulation of metabolism. Resistance exercise and/or training elicits a milieu of acute physiologic responses and chronic adaptations that are critical for increasing muscular strength, power, hypertrophy, and local muscular endurance.[1] The neuroendocrine system is of primary importance to acute exercise performance and subsequent tissue remodeling.[2] Neuroendocrine responses to resistance exercise take place in a unique physiologic environment and are a result of either increased secretion, reduced hepatic clearance, plasma volume reductions, and/or reduced degradation rates. Acute elevations in circulating blood hormone concentrations observed during and immediately after a resistance exercise protocol increase the molar exposure of a hormone to its receptor on either the target tissue cell membrane (e.g., peptides) or with nuclear/cytoplasmic receptors located within the target tissue (e.g., steroid receptors) and increase receptor availability for binding and subsequent cellular changes. Receptor response from this interaction initiates events ultimately leading to a specific response, such as an increase in muscle protein synthesis or the use of a particular metabolic substrate.

Proper resistance exercise prescription and manipulation of the acute program variables (i.e., choice of exercise, order of exercise, rest period lengths, resistance used, and number of sets) are perhaps the most influential mediating factors in the acute responses and subsequent adaptations of the hormonal response pattern.[2,3] Program design will incorporate three fundamental concepts of progression: 1) progressive overload, 2) variation, and 3) specificity, which attempt to optimize adaptations of the neuromuscular system (i.e., increases in motor unit recruitment).[1,4] Furthermore, tissue activation is a precursor to anabolism. Based on size principle, recruitment of a greater number of motor units enables greater hormone–tissue interaction in a larger percentage of total muscle mass. Genetic predisposition, gender, fitness level, and the potential for adaptation also have significant roles in the hormonal responses to resistance exercise.

The focus of this chapter relates to the classic responses of anabolic and catabolic hormones most relevant to tissue remodeling and repair in response to resistance exercise training. Thus, adaptations to resistance training entail four general classifications:

1. Acute changes during and after resistance exercise.
2. Chronic changes in resting concentrations.
3. Chronic changes in the acute response to a resistance exercise stimulus.
4. Changes in receptor content and binding proteins.

Other factors such as nutritional intake, training experience, gender, age and/or maturity, interaction with other modalities of exercise, and diurnal variations affecting the endocrine response are also discussed.

## TESTOSTERONE

### Acute Responses to Resistance Exercise

Testosterone has an important role in the signaling phenomenon for protein synthesis and obviates the impact of catabolic hormones. Resistance exercise has been shown to acutely increase total testosterone concentrations in men,[5–12] whereas in young women no change[8] or an elevation[13,14] may occur. In a classic view of the endocrine system, elevations in testosterone have been attributed to plasma volume reductions, adrenergic stimulation,[15] lactate-stimulated secretion,[16,17] and potential adaptations in testosterone synthesis and/or secretory capacity of the Leydig cells.[18] Testosterone's role in augmentation of other hormonal mechanisms [e.g., growth hormone(s) (GH), insulin-like growth factor (IGF)-1] in anabolic processes,[19] and on the nervous system (i.e., interaction with receptors on neurons can increase the amount of neurotransmitters released, regenerate nerves, increase cell body size and dendrite length/diameter)[20,21] may be of primary interest in enhancing force production.

The concept of the "free hormone" hypothesis remains controversial because the total concentration impacts the absolute amount of unbound hormone in the blood. The unbound fraction of testosterone is what has been classically thought to be biologically active and able to interact with androgen receptors (ARs). However, it is the total amount of hormone available that may well dictate the free hormone available, leading many to think that total production is still what mediates the absolute magnitude of free hormone response. Thus, the response of free testosterone has been shown to parallel total testosterone in some studies,[11,12,22] whereas a lack of response or reductions have been demonstrated in others.[23,24] Tremblay et al.[11] reported the acute elevation of free testosterone concentrations after resistance exercise was greater in resistance-trained men than endurance-trained men, thereby indicating a beneficial chronic adaptation from resistance training. These data partially support Kraemer et al.[25] who reported significant elevations in serum free testosterone in both young and elderly men. The magnitude of elevation was greater after 10 weeks of periodized strength training compared with the pretraining response, suggesting that a resistance training base may enhance the acute response to a workout. Free testosterone has been shown to be elevated by 25% in young women after acute resistance exercise [e.g., 6 sets of 10-repetition maximum (RM) squats with 2-minute rest intervals[14]]; however, no changes have been observed after resistance exercise in middle-aged and elderly women.[26] It may be that the changes in the free testosterone available in greater concentrations in younger people may mediate the greater magnitude of muscle mass development.

From what we know, the choice of exercise would be best served by using large muscle mass exercises with enough volume to elicit a testosterone response in men or in women. Thus, several factors seem to influence the acute serum total testosterone responses to resistance exercise. The magnitude of elevation during resistance exercise is affected by the muscle mass involved (i.e., exercise selection),[27,28] intensity and volume,[29–36] nutritional intake,[9] and training experience,[11,37] and is independent of the individual's absolute level of muscular strength.[37] A strong metabolic component may be a stimulus for testosterone release.[16] Large muscle mass exercises, such as the Olympic lifts,[38] deadlift,[39] and jump squats,[27] have been shown to be potent metabolic stressors and produce large elevations in testosterone compared with small-mass exercises.[35,40]

Little is known concerning the testosterone response to varying the sequence of exercises during resistance training. It has been suggested that large muscle mass exercises be performed before small muscle mass exercises.[1] The hypothesis is that performing large muscle mass exercises (i.e., squat, deadlift, power clean) first may produce significant elevations in testosterone, thus exposing smaller muscles to a greater response than that resulting from performance of small muscle mass exercises only. To examine this hypothesis, Hansen et al.[28] measured muscle strength changes in the elbow flexor muscles after 9 weeks of resistance training. One group performed a workout consisting of elbow flexion exercises only and a second group performed lower-body exercises before the elbow flexion exercises. Performing elbow flexion exercises only failed to acutely elevate testosterone significantly (see Figure 3.1).

However, testosterone was significantly elevated when lower-body exercises were performed first, and muscle strength increased to a greater extent when both lower- and upper-body exercises were performed. These data provide support for performing large muscle mass, multiple-joint exercises early in a workout when training to enhance muscle strength.

The acute testosterone response is affected by the intensity and volume of the resistance training program. A threshold of sufficient intensity and volume

**FIGURE 3.1.** The effect of muscle mass involvement on the testosterone response to a bout of resistance exercise. (Data from Hansen et al.[28])

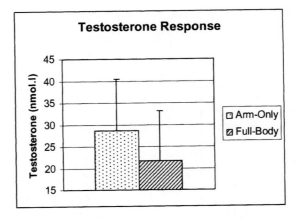

exists for substantial elevations in total testosterone to be observed (see Table 3.1). Schwab et al.[32] reported significant elevations in testosterone during two squat protocols. However, testosterone did not significantly increase until after the fourth set was completed. When resistance is held constant, the larger acute testosterone response is observed in the protocol consisting of a higher number of sets.[34–36] Similarly, if repetitions are held constant, then the protocol with higher loading tends to produce the greatest acute testosterone response in most studies[31] but not all.[12]

The interaction between these training-related variables has yielded interesting results favoring those programs with a higher glycolytic component (e.g., moderate intensity, high volume, relative short rest intervals) versus higher-load, low-volume training with long rest periods (3 minutes).[29,30] Guezennec et al.[41] reported minor elevations in testosterone during conventional strength training (i.e., 3–4 sets of 3–10 repetitions at 70%–95% of 1 RM, 2.5-minute rest periods). However, when load was increased and repetitions decreased to 3, a limited testosterone response was observed. Also, Kraemer et al.[42] reported significant elevations in testosterone after 5 sets of 15–20 repetitions of the squat despite using loads of 50% of 1 RM.

The effect of training frequency on the acute testosterone response is less clear. Häkkinen et al.[24] reported a greater testosterone response during afternoon sessions compared with morning sessions in elite weightlifters performing multiple training sessions per day. However, diurnal variation influences make it difficult to interpret hormonal data at different times of day. In addition, total training volume is influential because serum testosterone concentrations returned to normal when training frequency was reduced to one workout per day.[43]

Age, training experience, gender, and baseline values have been shown to affect the acute response of testosterone. College-aged men typically display a

**TABLE 3.1. The effects of intensity and volume on the acute testosterone response.**

| Reference | Protocol | Results |
|---|---|---|
| Weiss et al.[7] | 3 sets of 4 exercises to failure, 80% of 1 RM with 2-min rest interval | Sig. ↑ in T |
| Ratamess et al.[35] | 1 × 10 squats, 80%–85% 1 RM<br>6 × 10 squats, 80%–85% 1 RM, 2-min rest interval | No change<br>Sig. ↑ in T |
| Raastad et al.[31] | 70% of 3–6 RM vs. 100% of 3–6 RM | Sig. ↑ in T; 100% > 70% |
| Schwab et al.[32] | 4 × 6 squats (90%–95% of 6 RM)<br>4 × 9–10 (60%–65% of load used for high-intensity) | 31% ↑ in T<br>27% ↑ in T |
| Bosco et al.[34] | 20 sets of 2–4 repetitions vs.<br>10 sets of 2–3 repetitions of half squats | Sig. ↑ in T<br>No change |
| Häkkinen and Pakarinen[33] | 20 sets of 1 RM squats<br>10 sets of 10 reps with 70% of 1 RM | No change<br>Sig. ↑ in T |
| Gotshalk et al.[36] | 1 vs. 3 sets of 10 RM for 8 exercises | Sig. ↑ in T; 3 > 1 |
| Kraemer et al.[29,30] | 8 exercises, 3–5 × 5 RM vs. 10 RM with 1- and 3-min rest intervals | Sig. ↑ in T; T ↓ as load ↓ and rest intervals ↑ |

RM = repetition maximum, T = testosterone.

significant acute response, whereas the response in high school–aged men is limited.[39] Junior weightlifters (14–18 years of age) with more than 2 years of lifting experience have been shown to produce a greater acute testosterone response than those with fewer than 2 years of experience.[38] However, these results have not been seen in adults.[44] Ahtiainen et al.[45] reported no differences in the acute response between strength-trained and non–strength-trained men before and after 21 weeks of training. Older individuals have been shown to produce significant elevations of testosterone; however, the absolute concentrations are significantly lower than that of younger individuals.[25] The acute testosterone response in women seems limited[8,34,46,47] because only few studies have shown significant elevations.[13,14] In direct comparison, men, but not women, have shown acute elevations in testosterone immediately after the same protocol.[7,8] It seems other anabolic hormones, e.g., GH, may be more influential for promoting muscle hypertrophy in women.

The acute testosterone response to resistance exercise seems to be influenced by nutritional supplementation. Carbohydrate/protein supplementation has been shown to limit the testosterone response to resistance exercise.[9] The rationale is unclear but a previous study reported reduced circulating concentrations of testosterone in response to low dietary fat intake and a diet with a high protein/carbohydrate ratio.[27] Elevations in insulin concentrations have coincided with decreased testosterone in another study examining protein/carbohydrate supplementation.[6] Thus, a possible interaction between insulin and testosterone warrants further study.

## Chronic Changes in Resting Concentrations of Testosterone

Reported changes in resting testosterone concentrations during resistance training have been inconsistent in men and women[48–51] with elevations,[25,45,52–54] no differences,[5,23,26,49,55–57] and reductions[45,58] in resting testosterone concentrations reported. However, significant elevations have been reported in both prepubertal and pubertal boys.[59] It seems that resting concentrations may reflect the response of muscle tissue in its current state to changes in the volume and intensity of training.[45,52] Examination of elite Olympic weightlifters has shown no significant differences occurring over a 1-year period,[23] with elevations reported after a second year of training.[52] Ahtiainen et al.[45] reported significantly higher free and total testosterone concentrations during a 7-week high-volume training phase compared with pretraining values. However, reductions were observed when volume was reduced and intensity was increased over a subsequent 7-week training period. These findings have been replicated during 2 weeks of high-volume overreaching and a subsequent 2-week high-intensity, lower-volume phase.[58] In addition, Raastad et al.[60] reported 12% reductions in resting testosterone concentrations during a heavy training phase. Thus, substantial changes in volume and intensity may elicit transient changes in resting testosterone concentrations and values may return to baseline when the individual returns to "normal" training.

## Modification of Androgen Receptor Content

The presence of ARs in tissues has been shown to correlate highly with the known functions of androgens and depends on several factors including muscle fiber type, contractile activity, testosterone concentrations, and resistance training status.[61–64] In rats, resistance training elicits a significant increase in androgen binding capacity in the extensor digitorum longus muscle but reduces androgen binding capacity in the soleus, demonstrating a fiber-type specific effect of training.[65] Electrical stimulation of the rat gastrocnemius increased AR content by 25% within 3 days (with a concomitant increase in muscle mass) but plateaued at 5 days when the stimulation remained the same.[66] However, administration of an AR antagonist in rats (i.e., oxendolone) during 2 weeks of electrical stimulation attenuated 70% of the stimulation-induced hypertrophy observed in comparison to a vehicle control group.[67] Collectively, these data demonstrate the importance of the androgen–AR interaction during training to maximize hypertrophy.

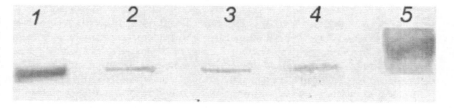

**FIGURE 3.2.** Representative Western blot. Western blot analysis for determination of androgen protein content in muscle. Lane 1: rat prostrate positive control; lane 2: individual baseline sample; lane 3: individual single-set sample; lane 4: individual multiple-set sample; lane 5: prestained molecular-weight standard (β-galactosidase, 128 kDa) used in androgen receptor identification. (Courtesy of Dr. Kraemer's Laboratory.)

Resistance training has been shown to up-regulate AR content after resistance exercise. Bamman et al.[68] reported that AR mRNA in the vastus lateralis increased 63% and 102%, respectively, 48 hours after 8 sets of 8 repetitions of eccentric (~110% of 1 RM) and concentric (~85% of 1 RM) squats. Kadi et al.[69] cross-sectionally examined 17 power lifters, 9 of whom were cycling anabolic steroids, and reported that power lifters had a higher percent of AR-positive myonuclei in the trapezium muscles compared with untrained controls. Power lifters using anabolic steroids had a greater percent of AR-positive myonuclei than drug-free power lifters. Interestingly, no differences were observed between power lifters and controls for percent of AR-positive myonuclei in the vastus lateralis muscle during baseline measurements. However, significant correlations have been reported between baseline AR content in the vastus lateralis and 1 RM squat thereby suggesting that AR content assists in mediating strength changes during resistance training.[35]

The resistance exercise stimulus seems to mediate the magnitude of acute AR content modifications. Ratamess et al.[35] compared two squat exercise protocols (1 versus 6 sets of 10 repetitions) to examine acute modifications in AR content 1 hour after exercise. No differences were observed in AR content after the single-set protocol. However, the higher-volume protocol elicited significant down-regulation of AR content. Considering that ARs are protein molecules and protein catabolism increases during resistance exercise,[70] these data suggest that when sufficient volume is reached, AR protein content may initially down-regulate (despite large elevations in circulating testosterone) before the up-regulation that has been observed in other studies.[68] However, this relationship warrants further investigation.

Nutritional intervention may also have a role in AR modification after resistance exercise. It has been observed that the ingestion of a protein/carbohydrate supplement before and after the workout attenuates the AR down-regulation with higher-volume resistance exercise observed 1-hour after `exercise (unpublished observation). Androgen protein content has an important role in determining changes at the target level. An example of androgen protein content is shown in Figure 3.2.

## Response of Luteinizing Hormone

Luteinizing hormone (LH) is a protein hormone secreted from the basophilic cells of the anterior pituitary which is the primary regulator of testosterone secretion from the Leydig cells of the testes.[18] Blood concentrations of LH are positively related to the intensity and volume of resistance training.[23,71] Resting concentrations of LH did not change significantly in men and women during 16–24 weeks of strength and power training[50,55] but slight elevations have been shown in strength athletes during intense training periods[72] and in resistance-trained men compared with endurance-trained men.[11] Busso et al.[71] compared a 4-week intensive training program in elite weightlifters with a 2-week reduced training period and reported a reduction in testosterone concentrations with a concurrent elevation in LH during the intense training phase. It was hypothesized that the decrease in testosterone contributed to the elevation in LH. An acute bout of resistance exercise does not induce LH secretion[43]; however, a delayed response has been demonstrated later into the recovery period[11] suggesting that acute elevations in serum testosterone concentrations during resistance exercise are attributable to other regulatory mechanisms. The importance of LH has become even more important as a possible pulse generator for many hormones including leptin so closely involved in fat cell metabolism and signals.

## Testosterone Precursors

The biosynthetic pathway of testosterone contains many steps. Theoretically, supplementation with testosterone precursors may enhance testosterone concentrations (by reducing the number of conversion steps) and subsequent acute resistance exercise performance. Precursor molecules that have been investigated include dehydroepiandrosterone (DHEA), 4-androstendione, 4-androstenediol, 5-androstenediol, 19-norandrostenediol, 19-norandrostenedione, and 1-androstene-3β-17β-diol.[73,74] Studies have shown that low doses (50–100 mg/day) of these prohormones do not increase circulating testosterone concentrations in young, healthy men,[75–79] although dosages used may have been too low.[73] However, elevations of DHEA, androstenedione, and LH have been observed in addition to less desirable responses such as elevations in estrone and estradiol and reductions in high density lipoproteins, the magnitude of which seems to be dose dependent.[79] Interestingly, low-dose supplementation of androstenedione has been shown to elevate testosterone in postmenopausal women[80] and higher doses (~300 mg) have been shown to elevate free testosterone by 37% in middle-aged men.[81] However, in young men, supplementation with 200–300 mg/day of 4-androstenediol, 4-androstenedione, and/or supplements consisting of multiple prohormones (i.e., 300 mg of androstenedione + 150 mg of DHEA) has shown acute elevations[79,82] and no acute elevation in testosterone.[83] Leder et al.[84] have shown that during small (i.e., 100 mg) and large (i.e., 300 mg) administered doses of oral androstenedione, the majority of androstenedione undergoes hepatic metabolism to testosterone and then to testosterone metabolites before release into systemic circulation. The net effect is a large production of testosterone metabolites despite only no or small elevations in testosterone. Further support for these data were provided by Brown et al.[85] who examined a low dose of sublingual androstenediol administration (60 mg) and reported significant elevations of both total and free testosterone (that were not observed during oral administration) for 180 minutes (with a peak occurring at 60 minutes) after administration. These data indicate that small to moderate oral doses of prohormones produce minimal, if any, elevations in testosterone in young men. However, the subsequent elevations in testosterone metabolites, estradiol, estrone, and reductions in high density lipoproteins potentially pose health risks that need to be considered before prohormone use.

Long-term studies have shown no further improvement in muscle strength or hypertrophy with DHEA/androstenedione/androstenediol supplementation (150–300 mg/day) over 8–12 weeks of resistance training.[75,78,83,86–88] Baseline testosterone values measured during this time did not change significantly; although significant elevations in androstenedione/androstenediol, DHEA sulfate, estrone, and estradiol were reported.[86] In addition, 5 days of oral androstenedione supplementation (100 mg/day) did not elevate protein synthesis.[89] Therefore, the potential ergogenic effects of precursor hormones remain to be seen and require further examination.

## Sidebar 3.1. Food and Drug Administration Warns Manufacturers to Stop Distributing Andro-Containing Products

On March 11, 2004, the Food and Drug Administration (FDA) announced a crackdown on companies that manufacture, market, and distribute products containing androstenedione. Despite conflicting evidence, the FDA stated that these products act similar to a steroid once they are metabolized by the body and therefore can pose similar kinds of health risks as steroids. The FDA concluded that because there is inadequate information to establish that a dietary supplement containing androstenedione will reasonably be expected to be safe, the ban of products containing andro is necessary. The majority of concern was focused on increasing use of these products in teenagers. The FDA press release cited a 2002 survey by the National Institute on Drug Abuse that reported 1 of 40 high school seniors and 1 of 50 10th graders used andro in the past year.

Few studies have examined the acute response of precursors without corresponding supplementation to resistance exercise. Weiss et al.[7] reported 8%–11% elevations in circulating androstenedione in both men and women after a program consisting of 4 exercises for 3 sets to failure with 80% of 1 RM and 2-minute rest intervals. Tremblay et al.[11] reported elevations in DHEA sulfate during resistance exercise and this response was greater in resistance-trained men than endurance-trained men. No changes[26] and reductions[48] in baseline concentrations of androstenedione, DHEA, and DHEA sulfate have been reported during 24 weeks of resistance training. However, baseline concentrations of DHEA sulfate were elevated after 8 weeks of resistance training in young women and this elevation correlated significantly to increases in lean body mass.[90]

Adrenal androgens may have a greater role in women, considering the low levels of testosterone present. Women tend to have a slightly larger conversion percentage of circulating DHEA and its precursor DHEA sulfate to androstenedione and testosterone at the tissue level,[91] and typically have higher baseline concentrations of androstenedione than men.[7] However, androstenedione is significantly less potent than testosterone. The impact of acute and chronic changes in the concentrations of testosterone precursors warrants further investigation.

## Sex Hormone-Binding Globulin

Circulating androgens are predominately bound to the transport protein sex hormone-binding globulin (SHBG). A change in SHBG concentrations may influence the binding capacity of testosterone and the magnitude of free testosterone available for diffusion across the cell membrane to interact with membrane-bound ARs. Recent studies have identified SHBG receptors on cell membranes and a possible receptor-mediated role for SHBG in mediating androgen actions through a cyclic adenosine monophosphate mechanism.[92] Differential responses have been observed during resistance training. Acute elevations have been reported[35,37] in some but not all studies,[24] whereas reductions[23] and no changes in resting SHBG concentrations have been reported after 3–24 weeks of resistance training,[26,50,51,55,57] after 1 week of intensive Olympic weightlifting,[43] and over a 2-year period in elite Olympic weightlifters.[52]

## GROWTH HORMONE SUPER FAMILY

The acidophilic cells of the anterior pituitary secrete molecules that make up the family of GH polypeptides. The most frequently studied GH isoform, the 22-kD molecule, consists of 191 amino acids.[18] Other biologically active spliced fragments are also released such as a 20-kD isoform missing residues 32–46; a 5-kD isoform consisting of residues 1–43; and a 17-kD isoform consisting of residues 44–191.[93] In addition, other monomeric, dimeric, protein-bound GHs, and aggregates of GH have been identified which are included this GH superfamily.[93] The physiologic roles of these variants are now under investigation but seem to function similarly to the 22-kD molecule in promoting tissue anabolism.

## Acute Response to Resistance Exercise

The 22-kD GH molecule has been the focus of most resistance exercise studies. Exercise,[94–96] especially resistance exercise,[97] has been shown to acutely elevate many of the GH variants. However, Hymer et al.[98] reported significant elevations in GH variants <30 kD and 30–60 kD in size in women after 6 sets of 10 repetitions of the squat with 75% of 1 RM with 2-minute rest intervals. Using the same protocol, Kraemer et al.[99] reported differential acute responses in GH variants based on muscular strength in women. A subgroup of the 10 strongest women showed the highest resting concentrations of all GH fractions, whereas the 10 weakest women displayed the highest concentrations of the <30-kD fractions. Similar acute responses were observed in strong and weak women in >30-kD fractions although the weaker women showed a greater <30-kD response. These results indicate that molecular-weight variants of GH seem responsive to resistance exercise; however, further research is warranted to elucidate the impact of these elevations. The remainder of this section focuses on the often-studied 22-kD GH molecule.

Resistance exercise elevates the concentrations of human GH through 30 minutes after exercise similarly in men and women; however, the resting concentrations of GH are significantly higher in women.[46] The magnitude seems dependent on exercise selection and subsequent amount of muscle mass recruited,[28,38] muscle actions used (i.e., greater response during concentric than eccentric muscle actions),[22] intensity,[12,100,101] volume,[36,102] rest intervals between sets,[29,30] total work (i.e., greater responses seen with multiple-set protocols),[36,103,104] and training status (e.g., greater acute elevations based on individual strength and the magnitude of total work performed).[45,105,106] Also, protocols eliciting high blood lactate values (e.g., those programs moderate to high in intensity, high in volume, that stress large muscle mass, and use relative short rest intervals) tend to produce the most substantial GH responses.[29,30,36,42,102] High correlations between blood lactate and serum GH concentrations have been reported,[33] and it has been proposed that $H^+$ accumulation produced by lactic acidosis may be the primary factor influencing GH release.[46] This finding was supported by an attenuated GH response after induced alkalosis during high-intensity cycling.[107] Hypoxia, breath holding, acid-base shifts, and protein catabolism have been reported to influence GH release.[46] Thus, resistance exercise is a potent stimulus for elevating GH so long as the threshold of volume and intensity are met.[100] Several investigations have given support to the association between acidosis resulting from resistance exercise, total work (i.e., moderate- to high-intensity, high-volume programs), and the acute GH response[29,30]; however, the attenuated GH response to a low-volume strength protocol may be enhanced by the addition of one high-volume set at the end of the workout.[108] Table 3.2 offers a synopsis of recent investigations comparing high- and low-volume acute exercise protocols.

It has been shown that the acute GH response is somewhat limited in older individuals.[25,44,101] However, it has been suggested that a major factor contributing to this limited GH response may be the magnitude of exertion displayed. Pyka et al.[101] reported lower blood lactates in the elderly during resistance exercise, thereby supporting the hypothesis that maximal effort is necessary for optimizing the exercise-induced secretion of GH. Interestingly, resistance training over 12 weeks in the elderly has been shown to promote greater acute GH response to a resistance exercise protocol,[44] possibly indicating that the greater response was attributable to an increased ability to exert oneself.

The specificity of muscle action selection during resistance training may affect the acute GH response to resistance exercise. Kraemer et al.[109] reported that the GH response was highest for an eccentric protocol after 19 weeks of training with eccentric and concentric repetitions; however, significant elevations in GH were seen with a concentric protocol in a group that trained with concentric repetitions only.

The anterior pituitary may be directly innervated by nerve fibers mostly with synapses on corticotroph and somatotroph cells.[110] In the "neural-humoral" regulation of GH secretion, a rapid neural response is observed during the initial stress with the humoral phase subsequently occurring.[110] Thus, higher brain centers, e.g., motor cortex, may have an active role in regulating GH secretion during resistance exercise and this regulatory mechanism may be sensitive to specific muscle actions used during resistance training.

## Chronic Changes in Resting Growth Hormone Concentrations

Traditional resistance training does not seem to affect resting concentrations of GH. This may be attributable to the lack of real regulatory roles for the 22-kD monomer of GH, and unpublished observations from our laboratory now

TABLE 3.2. Growth hormone response to acute low-volume versus high-volume exercise.

| Reference | Exercise(s) | Sets | Reps | Intensity (% of 1RM) | Rest (min) | Result (after exercise) |
|-----------|-------------|------|------|----------------------|------------|-------------------------|
| Häkkinen & Pakarinen[33] | Squat | 10 vs. 20 | 10 vs. 1 | 70% vs. 100% | 3 | Significant ↑ vs. slight ↑ |
| Hoffman et al.[102] | Squat | 5 | 15 vs. 4 | 60% vs. 90% | 3 | Significant ↑ for both, but higher volume was significantly ↑ than lower volume |
| Zafeiridis et al.[116] | Squat, Bench Press, Lat Pulldown, Overhead Press | 4 | 15 vs. 10 vs. 5 | 60% vs. 75% vs. 88% | 1 vs. 2. vs.3 | Significant ↑ for all groups, but the moderate and high volume groups were significantly ↑ compared to low volume, with highest values seen in the high volume group |
| Smilios et al.[117] | Squat, Bench Press, Lat Pulldown, Overhead Press | 2 & 4 vs. 2, 4, & 6 vs. 2, 4, & 6 | 15 vs. 10 vs. 5 | 60% vs. 68–75% vs. 80–88% | 1 vs. 2 vs. 3 | Significant ↑ for in moderate and high volume protocols for 4 sets vs. 2 sets and vs. low volume protocol, with highest values seen after the high volume protocol, No difference in 6 vs. 4 sets, No difference for 2 sets in low and moderate protocols |
| Ahtiainen et al.[12] | Leg press, Squat, Leg Extension | 4, 2, 2, respectively | 12 vs. 12 | 12 RM vs. 12 RM weight + 15%, forced reps | 2 (4 min between exercises) | Significant ↑ for both, but 12 RM + 15% loading with forced reps protocol showed significant ↑ after the first exercise and throughout the remainder of the protocol vs. 12 RM |
| Williams et al.[118] | 8 exercises (full body) vs. Leg Extension vs. Leg Extension | 3 vs. 15 vs. 3 | 10 | 10 RM | 1 | Significant ↑ only seen in the full body exercise group |
| Goto et al.[108] | Knee Extension | 5 vs. 5+1 | 1 vs. 1+ | 90% vs 90% + 50% vs. 90% + 70% vs. 90% + 90% | 3 | Low response with high intensity and low volume; however, significant ↑ seen with one addition set for as many reps as possible at 50% of 1 RM |

show that the larger molecular variants and binding proteins may be the more responsive elements related to training adaptations (unpublished observations). No changes in resting GH concentrations have been observed in men and women of various ages.[25,26,54,57] This contention is also supported by data demonstrating similar resting concentrations of GH in elite Olympic weightlifters[52] and strength athletes (i.e., body builders, power lifters, weightlifters)[45] compared with lesser-trained individuals. These findings are consistent with dynamic feedback mechanisms of GH and its roles in the homeostatic control of other variables, e.g., glucose. In addition, the exercise-induced increase has been highly correlated with the magnitude of type I and type II muscle fiber hypertrophy (r = 0.62–0.74).[57] These relationships could be indicative of a role for repeated acute resistance exercise-induced GH elevations on cellular adaptations in trained muscle. Changes in receptor sensitivity, differences in feedback mechanisms, IGF-1 potentiation, and diurnal variations may also have significant roles.

## Growth Hormone Binding Protein

Circulating GH is complexed to mostly high-affinity GH-specific binding proteins (GHBPs) that greatly extend its half-life and enhance the overall biologic effects of GH. The human high-affinity GHBP arises from proteolytic cleavage of the extracellular domain of the GH receptor.[111] This process is thought to occur principally at the liver, which is the most GH receptor–rich tissue, but could occur wherever the GH receptor exists. Little is known concerning GHBP and resistance exercise. Rubin et al.[106] recently reported that acute resistance exercise (6 sets of squats with 80%–85% of 1 RM for 10 repetitions with 2-minute rest intervals) resulted in significant elevations of GHBP; however, no differences were observed between resistance-trained and untrained individuals suggesting that chronic resistance training does not alter circulating GHBP or change GH receptor expression.

# CORTISOL

The adrenal cortex releases glucocorticoids in response to the stress of exercise. Of these, cortisol accounts for approximately 95% of all glucocorticoid activity. The primary functions of cortisol are catabolic; in peripheral tissues, cortisol stimulates lipolysis in adipose cells and increases protein degradation and decreases protein synthesis in muscle cells. Thus, the action of cortisol results in greater release of lipids and amino acids into circulation. The effects of cortisol are greater in fast-twitch as compared with slow-twitch muscle fibers.[2] The majority of circulating cortisol is bound to binding proteins (~75% to corticosteroid-binding globulin and ~15% to albumin), whereas only ~10% is unbound. The unbound cortisol is the most bioactive fraction of cortisol. The major role of cortisol in tissue remodeling has made it a prime target of investigation with regard to both acute and chronic changes in response to resistance training. It is interesting to note that cortisol's role also is to protect glycogen stores which are limited in the body. Elevations in cortisol shunts metabolism to other energy sources (e.g., shift to protein degradation for gluconeogenesis and inhibition of immune cells that only use glucose for metabolism) in order to delay glycogen depletion. It is also interesting that the uninhibition of the cortisol effect can also occur with training in that the receptor no longer interacts with the same intensity of binding as in the untrained state (unpublished observations).

## Acute Response to Resistance Exercise

Acutely, a bout of resistance exercise elevates both cortisol and the cortisol-releasing hormone adrenocorticotropic hormone (ACTH).[10,24,25,38,41,46] The response seems to be similar in men and women,[46] although one study found that the same protocol elicited cortisol increases in men but not in women.[8] The acute cortisol response seems to be independent of training status at least in adolescent weightlifters[38]; however, a recent study showed that endurance athletes had a smaller cortisol response compared with resistance-trained men performing the same resistance exercise protocol.[11] In addition, it has been reported that the acute increase in cortisol secretion during resistance exercise may be attenuated by anabolic steroid use.[112]

Acute resistance exercise–induced elevations in serum cortisol have been reported to have a significant positive correlation with both blood lactate[35,113] and 24-hour postexercise serum creatine kinase concentrations.[114] The greatest acute lactate and cortisol response is elicited by metabolically demanding protocols high in total work, i.e., high-volume and moderate-to-high intensity with short rest periods, whereas conventional strength/power training induces little change.[33,46,115] In fact, in the same group of participants, hypertrophy and endurance (i.e., high work) protocols elicited substantial acute elevations in serum cortisol concentrations through 30 minutes postexercise whereas strength protocols elicited no significant cortisol response.[116,117] In most studies, the acute cortisol response is influenced by 1) the number of sets per exercise, 2) total training volume, and/or 3) length of rest intervals.[46,115,118] We recently found that 6 sets of 10 RM squats with 2-minute rest intervals increased serum cortisol concentrations substantially whereas only 1 set did not elicit any response.[35] Similarly, 4–6 sets of resistance exercise induced a significantly larger cortisol response compared with 2 sets.[117] With respect to volume, higher-intensity sets using forced repetitions have been found to elicit a larger cortisol response than the same protocol performed with less loading and no forced repetitions.[12] The acute cortisol response to 8 sets of 10 RM leg press with 1-minute rest intervals was found to be significantly greater than to the same protocol using 3-minute rest periods.[119] Although chronic high levels of cortisol have adverse effects, acute elevations may be important in the muscle tissue remodeling process from resistance exercise.

The acute cortisol response to resistance exercise can be influenced by nutritional intake. Some evidence suggests that carbohydrate supplementation can limit the acute cortisol response to resistance exercise. Consumption of a 6% carbohydrate solution during resistance exercise limited the acute cortisol response and led to greater gains in hypertrophy over 12 weeks of resistance training.[120] Kraemer et al.[9] reported that during 3 days of carbohydrate supplementation and resistance training, the cortisol response was blunted. However, carbohydrate supplementation has also been reported to have no effect on the acute cortisol response to resistance exercise.[118] Carbohydrate supplementation during resistance exercise has been suggested to reduce the demand for gluconeogenesis, thereby reducing the need for cortisol.[121] In contrast to the potential down-regulation by carbohydrate supplementation, alcohol consumption directly after resistance exercise has been found to prolong the exercise-induced elevation of cortisol, thus potentially prolonging the catabolic phase of recovery.[122]

## Chronic Adaptations in Resting Cortisol Concentrations

Resting cortisol concentrations generally reflect long-term training stress. The resting cortisol response to long-term resistance training does not seem to produce consistent patterns because elevations,[72] reductions,[37,48,54,55,57] and no change,[23,26,45,49–52,58,124] have been found with normal strength and power training in men and women and during short-term overreaching. In animals, cortisol concentrations have explained a substantial amount of the variance observed

## Sidebar 3.2. Alcohol and Resistance Exercise

Alcohol abuse has been found to influence the resting concentrations of many different hormones. Several of these hormones are also influenced by resistance exercise. From the high school level and up, athletes have been found to consume alcohol in amounts equal to or even exceeding their nonathletic peers. Investigations on the effect of alcohol ingestion after resistance exercise have revealed several findings that may be important to individuals that consume alcohol and are concomitantly involved in resistance training.

When resistance exercise was followed by alcohol ingestion leading to a peak blood alcohol concentration of ~22 mmol·L$^{-1}$ (0.10 g·dL$^{-1}$), changes were found in the postexercise response of cortisol,[122] total testosterone,[122] and free testosterone,[123] whereas no changes were found for catecholamines,[122] LH,[122] or adrenal corticotropin-releasing hormone.[122] Interestingly, alcohol intoxication both prolonged the exercise-induced elevation in cortisol and prevented a depression in free and total testosterone response after the initial exercise-induced elevation. Thus, alcohol contributed to higher levels of both cortisol and testosterone 60–120 minutes postexercise. The latter was a surprising finding because acute alcohol intoxication usually decreases circulating testosterone concentrations. It was suggested that the higher postexercise concentrations of free testosterone seen with alcohol intoxication could be attributable to either reduced levels of ARs or inhibition of these receptors.[123] It seems that alcohol consumption may interfere with some of the desired effects of resistance exercise.

in muscle mass changes.[125] Thus, the acute cortisol response may reflect metabolic stress, whereas chronic changes (or lack of change) may be important to tissue homeostasis involving protein metabolism. Again, how it relates to overtraining or overuse syndromes in tissues is relevant to the interactions with anabolic hormones and as to which receptor predominates in the interaction of the two opposing signals.

## Testosterone/Cortisol Ratio

Although oversimplistic in nature, the anabolic/catabolic status of skeletal muscle resistance training has been suggested to be reflected by the testosterone/cortisol (T/C) ratio and/or free T/C ratio.[126] Either an increase in testosterone or a decrease in cortisol, or both, would indicate an increased anabolic state. This ratio, however, seems to be an oversimplification and is at best only an indirect measure of the anabolic/catabolic properties of skeletal muscle.[18] Changes in the T/C ratio during strength and power training have been reported in some studies, and this ratio has been positively related to performance improvements,[48,55] whereas other studies have shown no change.[45] It seems that the T/C ratio is affected by the training protocol. Periodized, higher-volume programs have been shown to elucidate a significantly greater increase in the T/C ratio than a low-volume, single-set program,[54] and the T/C ratio decreased in elite weightlifters involved in stressful training (overreaching).[23] The use of the T/C ratio, however, remains questionable. In an animal study where the T/C ratio was manipulated to examine muscle hypertrophy, the T/C ratio was not a useful indicator of tissue anabolism.[125]

## The Glucocorticoid Receptor and Resistance Training

Cortisol's catabolic effects are mediated by its interaction with glucocorticoid receptors. The regulation of glucocorticoid receptors seem to be determined by the cortisol and possibly androgen concentrations. It has been suggested that anabolic steroids may have anticatabolic properties as a result of competition with cortisol in binding to the glucocorticoid receptor.[127] Although there is evidence to support this contention,[128] additional research is needed to elucidate the suggested anticatabolic nature of androgens by binding to glucocorticoid receptors. Long-term resistance training may down-regulate the glucocorticoid receptor content thus reducing the catabolic influence of cortisol on skeletal muscle tissue. In contrast, eccentric resistance exercise has been shown to up-regulate glucocorticoid receptor content and myofibrillar proteolysis.[129] Recently, Willoughby et al.[129] reported significant up-regulation of glucocorticoid receptor content and mRNA 6 and 24 hours after 2 identical eccentric resistance exercise protocols (7 sets of 10 repetitions of knee extensions with 150% of 1 RM) separated by 3 weeks. The up-regulation, however, was significantly lower after the second bout indicating a protective training effect from previous exposure to eccentric exercise. These changes were paralleled by serum cortisol that showed greater elevations 0–48 hours after bout 1 than after bout 2. The reduced up-regulation in glucocorticoid receptor content and mRNA after bout 2 also coincided with reduced up-regulation of factors of the adenosine triphosphate–dependent ubiquitin proteolytic pathway. Combined, these data suggest that a repeated bout of eccentric resistance training provides a protective effect by reducing tissue catabolism and thereby muscle damage via a modification in glucocorticoid receptor content.

## INSULIN-LIKE GROWTH FACTORS

IGFs are small polypeptide hormones (70 and 67 amino acid residues for IGF-1 and IGF-2, respectively) that are secreted by the liver in response to GH-stimulated DNA synthesis.[92] Structurally, IGFs are related to insulin and serve to mediate many of the actions of GH. IGFs increase protein synthesis during resistance training and thus enhance muscle hypertrophy.[92] The importance of these hormones, in particular IGF-1, has recently been demonstrated because immunization to IGF-1 in diabetic rats prevented protein synthesis after resistance exercise.[130] Of the IGFs, IGF-1 has been most extensively studied and is discussed below.

### Acute Insulin-Like Growth Factor 1 Response to Resistance Exercise

The acute resistance exercise response of IGF-1 is still unclear. Most studies have found no change in IGF-1 during or immediately after a bout of resistance exercise,[6,9,131] whereas other studies have found acute elevations during and after resistance exercise.[29,30,106] The secretion of IGF-1 is delayed, i.e., 3–9 hours, after GH-stimulated messenger RNA synthesis and this delay has been suggested to account for the lack of acute changes,[46] because peak values may not be achieved until 16–28 hours after stimulated GH release.[6] Thus, IGF-1 elevation after an acute bout of resistance exercise may be delayed until GH-stimulated synthesis and secretion from the liver can take place.

### Chronic Circulating Insulin-Like Growth Factor 1 Adaptations to Resistance Training

Short-term resistance training[25,57] or overreaching,[58] does not seem to change resting levels of IGF-1 unless they are concurrent with carbohydrate/protein supplementation.[9] However, with long-term resistance training, resting IGF-1 concentrations have been found to be higher in trained than untrained men[106] and similar results have been found in women, particularly during high-volume training.[54,132] Six months of training in previously untrained women was found to significantly increase resting IGF-1 concentrations, and the magnitude was greater when a high-volume, multiple-set program was used.[57] Borst et al.[133] reported significant elevations in resting serum IGF-1 after 13 weeks of resistance training; however, these elevations were similar between single-set and multiple-set training groups despite a significantly larger increase in strength for the multiple-set group. Reductions in IGF-1 (~11%) have also been reported during high-volume and intensity overreaching; however, IGF-1 concentrations returned to baseline once the overreaching phase subsided.[60,134] It seems that the intensity and volume of training significantly impact the chronic IGF-1 adaptations.

### Muscle Isoforms of Insulin-Like Growth Factor 1 and Adaptations to Resistance Training

Within muscle cells, IGF-1 has autocrine/paracrine functions.[135,136] Two independently functioning nonhepatic isoforms have been identified in skeletal muscle.[137] One muscle-specific isoform is similar to the circulating hepatic IGF-1 (IGF-1Ea) whereas the other muscle-specific isoform of IGF-1 called mechano growth factor (MGF), only differs from the liver isoform by the presence of the first 49 bp from exon 5.[136,137] Both muscle isoforms seem to increase protein synthesis and promote satellite cell activation.[137] Bamman et al.[68] reported significant elevations in muscle IGF-1 mRNA after resistance exercise, particularly during eccentric resistance exercise. Thus, it seems that overloaded muscle and subsequent mechanical damage, as can occur with resistance training, is a prominent stimuli for muscle IGF-1 isoform production/release.[68,136] However, 2.5 hours after a lower-body workout (10 sets of 6 repetitions using 80% of 1 RM with 2-minute rest intervals), IGF-1Ea mRNA did not change significantly in either young or older men and MGF mRNA only increased substantially in young men.[137] In addition, Brahm et al.[138] found that during intensive exercise, arterial concentrations of IGF-1 remained constant. However, venous concentrations of IGF-1 did increase, suggesting that a circulating elevation may be accounted for by greater release from the muscles (i.e., via cell disruption and greater blood flow). Thus, it seems that the IGF-1 muscle isoforms have an important role during tissue remodeling.

## Insulin-Like Growth Factor Binding Proteins

Nearly all circulating IGFs are bound to IGF binding proteins (IGFBPs) which regulate IGF availability and thus prolong IGF in the circulation.[92] Acute resistance exercise has been shown to elevate IGFBP-3 (the most common IGFBP)[42,139] and this response was further elevated when resistance exercise was combined with L-carnitine L-tartrate supplementation.[42] Nindl et al.[139] found that one effect of an acute bout of resistance exercise was a change in the way IGF-1 was partitioned among the different IGFBPs and not a change in the IGF-1 directly. After resistance exercise, IGFBP-3 was elevated for the first hour but did not differ overnight, whereas IGFBP-2 was elevated overnight.[139] The effect of chronic resistance training on circulating concentrations of IGFBPs remains unclear; however, Borst et al.[133] have reported that IGFBP-3 declined significantly from weeks 13 to 25 of a resistance-training program.

## INSULIN

Insulin has a potent up-regulating effect on muscle protein synthesis when adequate amino acids are available.[140,141] Serum insulin concentrations parallel changes in blood glucose, and its response is enhanced by protein/carbohydrates ingestion before, during, or immediately after the workout.[6,9,140-143] Without such ingestion before exercise, serum insulin concentrations have been shown to decrease during an acute bout of resistance exercise.[31] We have also reported that during 4 weeks of resistance training, overreaching fasted insulin values were depressed.[58,144] Although a potent anabolic hormone when in its normal physiologic range of concentrations, insulin seems to be significantly more affected by blood glucose concentrations and/or dietary intake than by exercise. Thus, ingestion of carbohydrates, amino acids, or combinations of both before, during, and/or immediately after the resistance exercise protocol is recommended for maximizing insulin's anabolic effect on muscle tissue. Ingestion of these nutrients before or during resistance exercise is especially important to maximize protein synthesis because the large increase in muscular blood flow will lead to increased amino acid delivery.

## CATECHOLAMINES

Catecholamines reflect the acute stress of the resistance exercise protocol and are important for increasing energy availability, force production, muscle contraction rate, and for several other functions including the augmentation of hormones such as testosterone.[2] Plasma concentrations of epinephrine,[10,41,115,145] norepinephrine,[10,41,115] and dopamine[10,115] have been shown to be increased by an acute bout of resistance exercise and the magnitude may be dependent upon the force of muscle contraction, amount of muscle stimulated, volume of exercise, and rest intervals.[115,145] Significant elevations in plasma epinephrine and norepinephrine have also been observed immediately before intense exercise.[10,30] This "anticipatory rise" may be part of the body's psychophysiologic adjustment in preparation to exert maximal effort during resistance exercise. Chronic adaptations remain unclear although it has been suggested that training reduces the catecholamine response to resistance exercise.[41] However, alterations in the acute response may reflect the demands of the program such that systematic variation and progressive overload may obviate a chronic decrease.

## Sidebar 3.3. Dietary Nutrients and Resistance Exercise in Relationship to Testosterone and Cortisol

Testosterone has both anabolic and anticatabolic effects on muscle tissue, whereas cortisol has catabolic effects. Therefore, the resting and exercise-induced levels of these hormones are of importance to individuals engaged in resistance training. Dietary intake has been found to influence the resting levels of the testosterone and cortisol, but the knowledge of dietary influence on postexercise levels is limited.

To increase the knowledge of this area, Volek and colleagues[27] investigated the relationship between resting and exercise-induced concentrations of testosterone and cortisol and selected dietary nutrients. Twelve healthy, resistance-trained men (23.8 ± 1.1 years, 172.3 ± 2.2 cm, 75.6 ± 2.4 kg) completed a detailed 17-day dietary record before performing 2 different exercises on consecutive days: 1) bench press (5 sets to failure using 10-repetition max load), and 2) jump squat (5 sets of 10 repetitions with 30% of 1-repetition max load). Sets were separated by a 2-minute rest period. Blood samples were collected pre- and 5 minutes postexercise for testosterone and cortisol analysis.

Both exercises significantly increased testosterone 5 minutes postexercise, whereas no changes were found for cortisol. It was also found that resting (pre) testosterone concentrations were significantly positively correlated with fatty acids, monounsaturated fatty acids, and percent energy from fat in the diet for the 17 days preceding the exercise. Resting testosterone was also found to be significantly negatively correlated with percent energy from protein, the protein/carbohydrate ratio, and the polyunsaturated/saturated fatty acid ratio. No significant correlations were found between any of the nutrient variables measured and resting cortisol, or absolute postexercise increases in cortisol and testosterone.

From the findings of this study, it seems that the dietary amount and composition of macronutrients influence resting concentrations of testosterone but not of cortisol in young healthy resistance-trained men. In addition, testosterone and cortisol concentrations 5 minutes postexercise do not seem to be influenced by nutrient intake 17 days before exercise. The authors suggest that this may be important for athletes experiencing overtraining which is frequently accompanied by down-regulations in resting testosterone. For such athletes, a low-calorie, low-fat diet may exacerbate this down-regulation in resting testosterone concentrations.[27]

## OTHER HORMONES

### β-Endorphins

The role of β-endorphins during resistance training remains elusive. Acutely, resistance exercise has been reported to lead to elevations in men and women,[38,146,147] no changes,[148,149] or postexercise reductions.[150] This apparent discrepancy may be explained by a minimum threshold of intensity and volume that must be reached for acute elevations to occur. Such a scenario, as has been reported for aerobic exercise,[151] may be observed during resistance exercise because protocols that have shown no acute elevation in β-endorphins have also failed to result in acute elevations of cortisol.[148] The acute elevation in β-endorphins has been attributed to the magnitude of muscle mass used, rest interval length, intensity, and volume of the resistance exercise program,[38,114] and was highly correlated with blood lactate concentrations in those studies that reported elevations.[113,114] Furthermore, the response does not seem related to training experience or muscle strength[38] and is greater and longer in duration when resistance exercise is performed by individuals in negative energy balance.[147] Bodybuilding-type workouts (high volume, moderate load, short rest periods) elicit the most substantial elevations in plasma β-endorphin concentrations compared with traditional strength training (high load, low repetitions, long rest periods).[114] Thus, acute elevations may occur during resistance exercise; however, further research is needed to elucidate the role(s) of β-endorphins during resistance training.

### Thyroid Hormones

The role of thyroid hormones during resistance training remains unclear but may be permissive in its interaction with other hormones. In animals, the interaction of triiodothyronine (T3) with its receptor has been shown to up-regulate AR mRNA with this effect potentiated by higher androgen concentrations.[152] Pakarinen et al.[153] reported significant reductions in thyroid-stimulating hormone (TSH), T3, and thyroxine (T4) during 1 week of intensive resistance training (2 workouts per day) in elite weightlifters. However, over the course of 1 year of training in elite weightlifters no changes were observed for any thyroid hormone until the precompetition period, i.e., lower volume of training, where significant increases in free T4 and T3 were reported.[154] These hormonal changes returned to baseline when the intensity increased during the next training phase. In moderately trained men and highly trained rowers, significant resting reductions in T4,[155] free T4,[155] free T3,[156] and TSH[156] were reported whereas no changes in T3[155] or T4[156] were also reported. It seems that resistance training may alter thyroid function; however, the impact of these alterations remains speculative. Because of the tight homeostatic control of thyroid hormones, elevations during resistance training are not expected.

## Fluid Regulatory Hormones

Although fluid homeostasis is critical to acute exercise performance in general, the majority of the literature has examined aerobic modalities of exercises. Fluid regulatory hormones such as arginine vasopressin, atrial peptide, renin, aldosterone, and angiotensin II have been shown to increase in response to exercise with the magnitude dependent on exercise intensity, duration, and hydration status.[157,158] Resistance exercise has been shown to reduce plasma volume[35,159] comparable to changes elicited by running and/or cycling at 80%–95% of maximal oxygen uptake ($VO_2$ max).[160] In competitive power lifters who performed 1 set of leg press at 80% of their 1 RM to exhaustion, plasma osmolality, atrial peptide, renin activity, and angiotensin II were elevated from immediately after exercise to 5 minutes after exercise.[10] These data were the first to demonstrate that fluid balance and the subsequent hormonal response may already be affected after the first set of a resistance exercise workout.

## Leptin

Leptin, a product of the ob gene arising from adipose tissue, is a protein hormone thought to relay satiety signals to the hypothalamus to regulate energy balance and appetite.[161] Leptin concentrations are highly correlated to body fat mass such that obese humans have on average 4 times more serum leptin than lean individuals.[162] Serum leptin concentrations may be influenced by gender, metabolic hormones, e.g., stimulated by insulin and cortisol and inhibited by β-adrenergic agonists, and current energy requirements.[163]

Many studies have shown no direct impact of exercise on leptin concentrations independent of its effect on adipose tissue or body composition.[116,163,164] Rather than resistance exercise, fasting and/or diurnal variation seem to be critical factors; this was supported by our recent findings in fasted subjects after resistance exercise.[106] Although resistance exercise seems to have no acute effect on leptin, high levels of energy expenditure may lead to a delayed reduction. Simsch et al.[156] found reductions in resting leptin concentrations after high-intensity resistance training in highly trained rowers. Nindl et al.[165] reported a high-volume protocol (i.e., 50 total sets) led to no acute changes in leptin concentrations; however, a delayed reduction (9–13 hours) was observed and this was accompanied by a 12% increase in resting energy expenditure. This suggests that a large disruption in metabolic homeostasis (e.g., >800 kcals of exercise) could elicit reductions in leptin independent of changes in fat mass. These data indicate that the resistance exercise stimulus (i.e., interaction of volume, intensity, rest intervals, total work, etc.) does not influence the acute leptin response; however, if a protocol high enough in volume is performed, then a delayed response may be observed.

Leptin has a critical role in several of the endocrine pathways pertinent to resistance training. One such pathway regulated by leptin is testicular steroidogenesis. Leptin has been shown to directly reduce steroidogenesis by reducing enzymatic conversion to 17-OH progesterone, and through inhibition of steroidogenic acute regulatory protein, cytochrome P450 cholesterol side-chain cleavage enzyme, and steroidogenic factor 1,[166] whereas only having small negative effects on LH and follicle-stimulating hormone pulse amplitude.[167] Men who are obese (i.e., with high serum concentrations of leptin) have been shown to have low concentrations of total and free testosterone (i.e., 22%–45%), SHBG, and SHBG binding capacity with the magnitude directly related to the level of body fat.[167,168] Thus, high levels of leptin may be associated with reduced androgen production. The impact of reduced steroidogenesis on subsequent adaptations to resistance training requires further study but does seem to be a potential limiting factor.

## Peptide F

Peptide F is one of many proenkephalin fragments secreted from chromaffin cells of the adrenal medulla along with epinephrine.[18] Although the physiologic function of peptide is not entirely elucidated, it is known that it improves the B cell helper function of T lymphocytes.[169] Kraemer et al.[170] first isolated this preproenkephalin fragment in blood in 1985 and, although exercise has been shown to increase concentrations of peptide F, little is known concerning the effect of resistance training. High-intensity resistance exercise-induced overtraining does not change circulating peptide F concentrations at rest or after exercise[171]; however, acute heavy resistance exercise has been shown to depress peptide F 4 hours into the recovery period.[145] Interestingly, changes in the ratio of peptide F to epinephrine were observed suggesting that overtraining may alter the secretory patterns of chromaffin cells.[171]

## OVERTRAINING

Overtraining is defined as any increase in training volume and/or intensity resulting in long-term performance decrements.[18] In contrast, overreaching is a short-term increase in volume and/or intensity that is often planned in resistance training programs and thought to increase performance via a "rebound effect."[124,144] Repeated overreaching may lead to overtraining and subsequent performance decrements in addition to neuroendocrine changes. Resting concentrations of testosterone and IGF-1 have been shown to be reduced after 1 and 2 weeks of overreaching,[43,60] and the decreases were significantly correlated to strength decrements.[60] We have reported that 4 weeks of overreaching with and without amino acid supplementation did not alter resting concentrations of IGF-1 and cortisol[58]; however, the free androgen index (total testosterone/SHBG) was reduced and this effect was more notable in the placebo group.[58] Although a significant elevation in cortisol was observed in a group supplementing with creatine after 1 week of high-volume overreaching,[144] it seems that short-term overreaching may not result in elevated resting cortisol and may augment the acute testosterone response to resistance exercise when the individual has at least 1 year of weightlifting training and previous exposure to the overreaching stimulus.[124] Thus, depending on the volume/intensity of the training stimulus as well as nutritional supplementation, overreaching may either reduce or not change the resting concentrations of some anabolic hormones, and increase or not change cortisol concentrations.

Overtraining, resulting from a chronic large increase in volume, has been shown to result in elevated cortisol and reductions in resting LH, total and free testosterone concentrations with free testosterone being the most sensitive to overtraining stimuli.[18,72] In addition, the exercise-induced elevation in total testosterone is attenuated during volume-related overtraining.[23] Intensity-related overtraining does not seem to alter resting concentrations of hormones thus demonstrating a differential response in comparison to large increases in training volume.[18] Fry et al.[171] reported no changes in circulating total or free testosterone, cortisol, GH, or peptide F concentrations during high-intensity overtraining, e.g., ten 1 RM lifts of the squat every day for 2 weeks. In a similar study, Fry et al.[172] reported no change in resting concentrations of epinephrine or norepinephrine; however, the acute catecholamine response to resistance exercise was larger in overtrained men. It seems that intensity-related overtraining does not alter resting hormonal concentrations significantly corresponding to a decrease in performance, whereas volume-related overtraining seems to significantly alter circulating hormone concentrations.

## DETRAINING

Detraining is the cessation of resistance training or significant reduction of training volume, intensity, or frequency resulting in reduced performance, e.g., reduced muscle strength, power, hypertrophy, and/or local muscle endurance.[2] In addition to alterations in neural and muscle function, changes in hormonal activity may also occur. The duration of the detraining period seems to be important for the magnitude of change as well as the training status of the individual. After 2 weeks of detraining in highly trained power lifters and football players, resting concentrations of GH, testosterone, and the T/C ratio were significantly increased, whereas cortisol was significant reduced.[173] It was hypothesized that these changes were related to the body's ability to combat the catabolic processes associated with detraining and suggested that short-term detraining may represent an augmented stimulus for tissue remodeling and repair. These increases, however, have only been found during short-term detraining. Recently, we reported no significant changes in testosterone, GH, LH, SHBG, cortisol, or ACTH after 6 weeks of detraining in recreationally trained men.[174] Similarly, 8 weeks of detraining in women did not change concentrations of cortisol, SHBG, or LH.[50] Detraining periods longer than 8 weeks have shown significant reductions in the T/C ratio which correlated highly to strength decrements[48,55] and elevations in T4.[155] These hormonal changes coincide with periods of muscle atrophy[173] indicating a hormonal role in muscle size and strength reductions observed during periods of detraining.

## CIRCADIAN PATTERNS

Several hormones are secreted in various pulses throughout the day in a circadian pattern. Salivary testosterone secretion has been shown to be secreted in a circadian manner with the greatest elevations observed early in the morning and less throughout the rest of the waking day.[175] Because of circadian patterns, it is essential that researchers examining resistance exercise measure hormonal concentrations at the same time of day or use control, nonexercised subjects for multiple sampling periods throughout the day for circadian control. Considering that resistance exercise stimulates acute alterations in hormone concentrations, it is of interest whether or not resistance exercise changes circadian patterns. Kraemer et al.[175] reported that resistance exercise did not affect circadian patterns of testosterone secretion over a 16-hour waking period in resistance-trained men. However, resistance exercise performed in the afternoon has been found to sometimes induce greater elevations in testosterone than when performed in the morning.[72] Despite acute hormone concentration changes after a resistance exercise workout, it seems that regulatory mechanisms are quickly reengaged such that homeostasis is maintained within 1 hour after exercise.

The nocturnal hormonal response after resistance exercise may differ. McMurray et al.[176] trained individuals using 3 sets of 6 exercises to exhaustion at 1900–2000 hours and sampled blood before, and at 20-minute intervals after exercise from 2100 to 0700 hours. Resistance exercise did not alter nocturnal patterns of GH or cortisol secretion, whereas testosterone secretion was greater between 0500 and 0700 hours and nocturnal secretion of T4 lower in the resistance exercise group. Nindl et al.,[177] however, examined GH pulsatility at 10-minute intervals (e.g., shorter intervals than McMurray et al.[176]) after high-volume resistance exercise and reported that a differential pattern during sleep in which GH was lower during the first half of sleep and higher during the last half of sleep. Total and free IGF-1 did not differ overnight, but IGFBP-2 was elevated suggesting that heavy-resistance exercise may alter the partitioning of IGF-1 to its binding proteins overnight.[139] The circulating IGF-1 response beyond the overnight period remains to be elucidated but would be of interest to study because of the late pulsatile bursts of GH observed the day of heavy-resistance exercise. Thus, nocturnal changes in these hormones may have implications for tissue anabolism.

## CONCURRENT STRENGTH AND ENDURANCE TRAINING

Several studies have indicated that simultaneous high-intensity strength and endurance training seems to limit maximal strength and power,[178,179] whereas the neuroendocrine system may or may not be altered. Kraemer et al.[178] reported that 4 days per week of endurance training along with a total-body, high-volume resistance training program 4 days per week for 12 weeks substantially increased exercise-induced cortisol concentrations. Although greater urinary cortisol was observed in women, 12 weeks of combined strength and endurance training did no change resting concentrations of testosterone, SHBG, or GH.[179] These data indicate that the incompatibility may also be the result of overtraining which in itself may produce a catabolic hormonal environment.

## SUMMARY

Resistance exercise elicits an array of hormonal responses critical to acute muscular force and power production as well as subsequent tissue growth and remodeling. In general, the acute response is dependent upon the stimulus and may be the most critical element to tissue remodeling. Thus, modifications of training intensity, volume (or total work), muscle mass involvement, rest intervals, and frequency can impact the acute hormonal response. Long-term adaptations in neuroendocrine function seem minimal but may be related to the current intensity/volume of the training stimulus.

## PRACTICAL APPLICATIONS

- Timing of supplementation/feeding pre- and postexercise affects the endocrine response to resistance exercise.
- Carbohydrate/protein should be ingested immediately before, during, or immediately after resistance exercise in order to increase the testosterone response and decrease the cortisol response.
- Alcohol intoxication should be avoided in individuals involved in resistance exercise.
- Acutely, alcohol intoxication may impair desired resistance exercise-induced endocrine responses.
- Gender and age-related differences to resistance exercise.
- Strength gain in females and older individuals of both genders results from neuromuscular adaptation and less from androgens.
- Hormonal responses are interrelated, thus changes in one hormone may affect other hormones.
- Increases in circulating concentrations of LH, for example, may lead to greater testosterone release in men.
- Acute variables of resistance exercise, such as volume, load, sets, and intensity will affect the hormonal response to exercise.
- For β-endorphins, a minimum intensity and load is required for a resistance exercise-induced increase.
- Multiple sets elicit larger increases in several hormones, such as testosterone, cortisol, and GH, than one set alone.

# QUESTIONS

1. What is the acute circulating testosterone response in men to a bout of resistance exercise?
   a. Elevation
   b. Suppression
   c. Seems to be limited
   d. A suppression followed by an elevation
   e. Results are equivocal with elevation, no change, and suppression reported

2. The acute circulating testosterone response in men to resistance exercise is affected by:
   a. The muscle mass involved (i.e., exercise selection)
   b. Nutritional intake
   c. Intensity and volume
   d. All of the above
   e. There is no acute testosterone response to resistance exercise

3. What is the acute circulating testosterone response in women to a bout of resistance exercise?
   a. Elevation
   b. Suppression
   c. Seems to be limited
   d. A suppression followed by an elevation
   e. None of the above

4. What is the effect of resistance training on resting circulating testosterone concentrations in men and women?
   a. Elevation
   b. Suppression
   c. No change
   d. Only a change in women
   e. Results are equivocal, with elevation, no change, and suppression reported

5. What is the effect of a bout of resistance exercise on skeletal muscle androgen receptor content?
   a. Elevation
   b. Suppression
   c. Seems to be limited
   d. Elevations only with 1 set
   e. None of the above

6. The skeletal muscle androgen receptor content response to resistance exercise may depend on:
   a. Carbohydrate ingestion
   b. Protein ingestion
   c. Sets performed during the exercise session
   d. All of the above
   e. b and c only

7. What is the acute circulating growth hormone response to a bout of resistance exercise?
   a. Elevation
   b. Suppression
   c. Seems to be limited
   d. A suppression followed by an elevation
   e. None of the above

8. What seems to be the main fate(s) of exogenous prohormones, such as androstenedione?
   a. Conversion to testosterone, leading to significantly increased circulating concentration of testosterone

   b. Conversion to estradiol, leading to significantly increased circulating concentration of estradiol
   c. Metabolized in the liver to testosterone metabolites
   d. b and c only
   e. All of the above

9. Prohormone supplementation (DHEA, androstenedione, androstenediol, etc.) seems to lead to:
   a. Increased hypertrophy
   b. Increased strength
   c. Increased circulating testosterone concentration
   d. All of the above
   e. None of the above

10. Most resistance exercise studies have focused on the _____ growth hormone molecule fraction(s).
   a. 17 kD
   b. 22 kD
   c. 30–60 kD
   d. All of the above
   e. None of the above

11. What is/are the main benefit(s) of carbohydrate ingestion immediately before, during, or immediately after a resistance exercise session?
   a. Increases catabolism
   b. Increases protein synthesis
   c. Replenishes depleted free fatty acid stores
   d. There is no benefit
   e. a and c only

12. What is/are the main benefit(s) of amino acid ingestion immediately before, during, or immediately after a resistance exercise session?
   a. Increases catabolism
   b. Increases protein synthesis
   c. Directly prevents muscle damage
   d. There is no benefit
   e. b and c only

13. Insulin-like growth factor 1 (IGF-1) is produced in which tissue?
   a. Liver
   b. Adipose tissue
   c. Bone
   d. Muscle
   e. a and d only

14. Which of the following is NOT a hormone with major anabolic properties?
   a. Growth hormone (GH)
   b. Insulin-like growth factor 1 (IGF-1)
   c. Testosterone
   d. Insulin
   e. None of the above; they all have major anabolic properties

15. What is the acute circulating response in cortisol to a bout of resistance exercise?
   a. Elevation
   b. Suppression
   c. No change
   d. A suppression followed by an elevation
   e. Elevation in men, suppression in women

16. What is the effect of long-term resistance training on resting insulin-like growth factor 1 (IGF-1) concentrations in the circulation?
   a. Elevation
   b. Suppression
   c. No change

    d. Elevation in men, suppression in women

    e. The effect is not known at present time

17. What is the acute circulating response of the catecholamines to a bout of resistance exercise?

    a. Elevation

    b. Suppression

    c. No change, catecholamines follow fasting and/or diurnal variation

    d. A suppression followed by an elevation

    e. Elevation in men, suppression in women

18. What is the acute response of the leptin to a bout of medium-volume resistance exercise?

    a. Elevation

    b. Suppression

    c. No change, leptin follows fasting and/or diurnal variation

    d. Elevation, but only with upper-body exercise

    e. Elevation, but only when including isometric exercises

19. Alcohol ingested immediately after a bout of resistance exercise:

    a. Reduces cortisol concentration to baseline almost immediately

    b. Elevates cortisol concentration to baseline almost immediately

    c. Prolongs the elevation of cortisol concentration

    d. Prolongs the suppression of cortisol concentration

    e. Has no effect on cortisol

20. What has been suggested regarding the circulating β-endorphin response to acute resistance exercise?

    a. It is elevated

    b. It is decreased

    c. There is no response

    d. The response occurs only in women

    e. A minimum threshold of training intensity and volume must be reached to elicit a β-endorphins response

21. Circulating insulin-like growth factor 1 (IGF-1) elevation after an acute bout of resistance exercise may be delayed until GH-stimulated synthesis and secretion from the liver of IGF-1 can take place.

    a. True

    b. False

22. Chronic adaptations to resistance training may include a down-regulation of resting glucocorticoid receptor content.

    a. True

    b. False

23. Resistance exercise performed in the morning induces greater elevations in circulating testosterone concentrations than when performed in the afternoon.

    a. True

    b. False

24. An acute bout of resistance exercise increases circulating concentrations of insulin regardless of diet.

    a. True

    b. False

25. The majority of circulating insulin-like growth factor 1 (IGF-1) is bound to binding proteins.

    a. True

    b. False

26. The role of thyroid hormones during resistance training remains unclear.

    a. True

    b. False

27. Testosterone is a major catabolic hormone.
    a. True
    b. False

28. Resistance exercise induces the same acute circulating testosterone response in men and women.
    a. True
    b. False

29. Hormone binding proteins increase hormone biologic activity.
    a. True
    b. False

30. Programs designed to stimulate testosterone secretion should be structured around large muscle mass exercises.
    a. True
    b. False

# REFERENCES

1. Kraemer WJ, Ratamess NA. Physiology of resistance training: current issues. Orthop Phys Ther Clin North Am Exerc Technol 2000;9:467–513.
2. Kraemer WJ, Ratamess NA. Endocrine responses and adaptations to strength and power training. In: Komi PV, ed. Strength and Power in Sport. 2nd ed. Malden, MA: Blackwell Scientific Publications; 2003:361–386.
3. Kraemer WJ, Ratamess NA, Rubin MR. Basic principles of resistance exercise. In: Jackson CR, ed. Nutrition and the Strength Athlete. Boca Raton, FL: CRC Press; 2000:1–29.
4. Sale DG. Neural adaptations to resistance training. Med Sci Sports Exerc 1988; 20(Suppl):S135–145.
5. Hickson RC, Hidaka K, Foster C, et al. Successive time courses of strength development and steroid hormone responses to heavy-resistance training. J Appl Physiol 1994;76:663–670.
6. Chandler RM, Byrne HK, Patterson JG, Ivy JL. Dietary supplements affect the anabolic hormones after weight-training exercise. J Appl Physiol 1994;76:839–845.
7. Weiss LW, Cureton KJ, Thompson FN. Comparison of serum testosterone and androstenedione responses to weight lifting in men and women. Eur J Appl Physiol 1983;50:413–419.
8. Häkkinen K, Pakarinen A. Acute hormonal responses to heavy resistance exercise in men and women at different ages. Int J Sports Med 1995;16:507–513.
9. Kraemer WJ, Volek JS, Bush JA, et al. Hormonal responses to consecutive days of heavy-resistance exercise with or without nutritional supplementation. J Appl Physiol 1998;85:1544–1555.
10. Kraemer WJ, Fleck SJ, Maresh CM, et al. Acute hormonal responses to a single bout of heavy resistance exercise in trained power lifters and untrained men. Can J Appl Physiol 1999;24:524–537.
11. Tremblay MS, Copeland JL, Van Helder W. Effect of training status and exercise mode on endogenous steroid hormones in men. J Appl Physiol 2003;96:531–539.
12. Ahtiainen JP, Pakarinen A, Kraemer WJ, Häkkinen K. Acute hormonal and neuromuscular responses and recovery to forced vs maximum repetitions multiple resistance exercises. Int J Sports Med 2003;24:410–418.
13. Cumming DC, Wall SR, Galbraith MA, Belcastro AN. Reproductive hormone responses to resistance exercise. Med Sci Sports Exerc 1987;19:234–238.
14. Nindl BC, Kraemer WJ, Gotshalk LA, et al. Testosterone responses after resistance exercise in women: influence of regional fat distribution. Int J Sport Nutr Exerc Metab 2001;11:451–465.
15. Jezova D, Vigas M. Testosterone response to exercise during blockade and stimulation of adrenergic receptors in man. Horm Res 1981;15:141–147.
16. Lu SS, Lau CP, Tung YF, et al. Lactate and the effect of exercise on testosterone secretion: evidence for the involvement of a cAMP-mediated mechanism. Med Sci Sports Exerc 1997;29:1048–1054.
17. Lin H, Wang SW, Wang RY, Wang PS. Stimulatory effect of lactate on testosterone production by rat Leydig cells. J Cell Biochem 2001;83:147–154.
18. Fry AC, Kraemer WJ. Resistance exercise overtraining and overreaching. Neuroendocrine responses. Sports Med 1997;23:106–129.
19. Giustina A, Veldhuis JD. Pathophysiology of the neuroregulation of growth hormone secretion in experimental animals and the human. Endocr Rev 1998;19:717–797.

20. Nagaya N, Herrera AA. Effects of testosterone on synaptic efficacy at neuromuscular junctions in asexually dimorphic muscle of male frogs. J Physiol 1995;483:141–153.

21. Brooks BP, Merry DE, Paulson HL, et al. A cell culture model for androgen effects in motor neurons. J Neurochem 1998;70:1054–1060.

22. Durand RJ, Castracane VD, Hollander DB, et al. Hormonal responses from concentric and eccentric muscle contractions. Med Sci Sports Exerc 2003;35:937–943.

23. Häkkinen K, Pakarinen A, Alen M, et al. Relationships between training volume, physical performance capacity, and serum hormone concentrations during prolonged training in elite weight lifters. Int J Sports Med 1987;8(Suppl):61–65.

24. Häkkinen K, Pakarinen A, Alen M, et al. Neuromuscular and hormonal responses in elite athletes to two successive strength training sessions in one day. Eur J Appl Physiol 1988;57:133–139.

25. Kraemer WJ, Häkkinen K, Newton RU, et al. Effects of heavy-resistance training on hormonal response patterns in younger vs. older men. J Appl Physiol 1999;87:982–992.

26. Häkkinen K, Pakarinen A, Kraemer WJ, et al. Basal concentrations and acute responses of serum hormones and strength development during heavy resistance training in middle-aged and elderly men and women. J Gerontol A Biol Sci Med Sci 2000;55:B95–105.

27. Volek JS, Kraemer WJ, Bush JA, et al. Testosterone and cortisol in relationship to dietary nutrients and resistance exercise. J Appl Physiol 1997;8:49–54.

28. Hansen S, Kvorning T, Kjaer M, Szogaard G. The effect of short-term strength training on human skeletal muscle: the importance of physiologically elevated hormone levels. Scand J Med Sci Sport 2001;11:347–354.

29. Kraemer WJ, Marchitelli L, Gordon SE, et al. Hormonal and growth factor responses to heavy resistance exercise protocols. J Appl Physiol 1990;69:1442–1450.

30. Kraemer WJ, Gordon SE, Fleck SJ, et al. Endogenous anabolic hormonal and growth factor responses to heavy resistance exercise in males and females. Int J Sports Med 1991;12:228–235.

31. Raastad T, Bjoro T, Hallen J. Hormonal responses to high- and moderate-intensity strength exercise. Eur J Appl Physiol 2000;82:121–128.

32. Schwab R, Johnson GO, Housh TJ, et al. Acute effects of different intensities of weight lifting on serum testosterone. Med Sci Sports Exerc 1993;25:1381–1385.

33. Häkkinen K, Pakarinen A. Acute hormonal responses to two different fatiguing heavy-resistance protocols in male athletes. J Appl Physiol 1993;74:882–887.

34. Bosco C, Colli R, Bonomi R, et al. Monitoring strength training: neuromuscular and hormonal profile. Med Sci Sports Exerc 2000;32:202–208.

35. Ratamess NA, Kraemer WJ, Volek JS, et al. Androgen receptor content following heavy resistance exercise in men. J Steroid Biochem Mol Biol 2005;93(1):35–42.

36. Gotshalk LA, Loebel CC, Nindl BC, et al. Hormonal responses to multiset versus single-set heavy-resistance exercise protocols. Can J Appl Physiol 1997;22:244–255.

37. Kraemer WJ, Staron RS, Hagerman FC, et al. The effects of short-term resistance training on endocrine function in men and women. Eur J Appl Physiol 1998;78:69–76.

38. Kraemer WJ, Fry AC, Warren BJ, et al. Acute hormonal responses in elite junior weightlifters. Int J Sports Med 1992;13:103–109.

39. Fahey TD, Rolph R, Moungmee P, et al. Serum testosterone, body composition, and strength of young adults. Med Sci Sports Exerc 1976;8:31–34.

40. Ballor DL, Becque MD, Katch VL. Metabolic responses during hydraulic resistance exercise. Med Sci Sports Exerc 1987;19:363–367.

41. Guezennec Y, Leger L, Lhoste F, et al. Hormone and metabolite response to weight-lifting training sessions. Int J Sports Med 1986;7:100–105.

42. Kraemer WJ, Volek JS, French DN, et al. The effects of L-carnitine L-tartrate supplementation on hormonal responses to resistance exercise and recovery. J Strength Cond Res 2003;17:455–462.

43. Häkkinen K, Pakarinen A, Alen M, et al. Daily hormonal and neuromuscular responses to intensive strength training in 1 week. Int J Sports Med 1988;9:422–428.

44. Craig BW, Brown R, Everhart J. Effects of progressive resistance training on growth hormone and testosterone levels in young and elderly subjects. Mech Ageing Dev 1989;49:159–169.

45. Ahtiainen JP, Pakarinen A, Alen M, et al. Muscle hypertrophy, hormonal adaptations and strength development during strength training in strength-trained and untrained men. Eur J Appl Physiol 2003;89:555–563.

46. Kraemer WJ, Fleck SJ, Dziados JE, et al. Changes in hormonal concentrations after different heavy-resistance exercise protocols in women. J Appl Physiol 1993;75: 594–604.

47. Stoessel L, Stone MH, Keith R, et al. Selected physiological, psychological and performance characteristics of national-caliber United States women weightlifters. J Appl Sport Sci Res 1991;5:87–95.

48. Alen M, Pakarinen A, Häkkinen K, Komi PV. Responses of serum androgenic-anabolic and catabolic hormones to prolonged strength training. Int J Sports Med 1988;9:229–233.

49. Potteiger JA, Judge LW, Cerny JA, Potteiger VM. Effects of altering training volume and intensity on body mass, performance, and hormonal concentrations in weight-event athletes. J Strength Cond Res 1995;9:55–58.

50. Häkkinen K, Pakarinen A, Kyrolainen H, et al. Neuromuscular adaptations and serum hormones in females during prolonged power training. Int J Sports Med 1990;11:91–98.

51. Häkkinen K, Pakarinen A, Kallinen M. Neuromuscular adaptations and serum hormones in women during short-term intensive strength training. Eur J Appl Physiol 1992;64:106–111.

52. Häkkinen K, Pakarinen A, Alen M, et al. Neuromuscular and hormonal adaptations in athletes to strength training in two years. J Appl Physiol 1988;65:2406–2412.

53. Staron RS, Karapondo DL, Kraemer WJ, et al. Skeletal muscle adaptations during early phase of heavy-resistance training in men and women. J Appl Physiol 1994; 76:1247–1255.

54. Marx JO, Ratamess NA, Nindl BC, et al. Low-volume circuit versus high-volume periodized resistance training in women. Med Sci Sports Exerc 2001;33:635–643.

55. Häkkinen K, Pakarinen A, Alen M, Komi PV. Serum hormones during prolonged training of neuromuscular performance. Eur J Appl Physiol 1985;53:287–293.

56. Reaburn P, Logan P, Mackinnon L. Serum testosterone response to high-intensity resistance training in male veteran sprint runners. J Strength Cond Res 1997;11: 256–260.

57. McCall GE, Byrnes WC, Fleck SJ, et al. Acute and chronic hormonal responses to resistance training designed to promote muscle hypertrophy. Can J Appl Physiol 1999;24:96–107.

58. Kraemer WJ, Ratamess NA, Volek JS, Häkkinen K, Rubin MR, French DN, Gómez AL, McGuigan MR, Scheett TP, Newton RU, Spiering BA, Izquierdo M, Dioguardi FS. The effects of amino acid supplementation on hormonal responses to resistance training overreaching. Metabolism 2006;55(3):282–291.

59. Tsolakis C, Messinis D, Stergioulas A, Dessypris A. Hormonal responses after strength training and detraining in prepubertal and pubertal boys. J Strength Cond Res 2000;14:399–404.

60. Raastad T, Glomsheller T, Bjoro T, Hallen J. Changes in human skeletal muscle contractility and hormone status during 2 weeks of heavy strength training. Eur J Appl Physiol 2001;84:54–63.

61. Dorlochter M, Astrow SH, Herrera AA. Effects of testosterone on a sexually dimorphic frog muscle: repeated in vivo observations and androgen receptor distribution. J Neurobiol 1994;25:897–916.

62. Bricout VA, Serrurier BD, Bigard AX, Guezennec CY. Effects of hindlimb suspension and androgen treatment on testosterone receptors in rat skeletal muscles. Eur J Appl Physiol 1999;79:443–448.

63. Bricout VA, Germain PS, Serrurier BD, Guezennec CY. Changes in testosterone muscle receptors: effects of an androgen treatment on physically trained rats. Cell Mol Biol 1994;40:291–294.

64. Lu Y, Tong Q, He L. The effects of exercise on the androgen receptor binding capacity and the level of testosterone in the skeletal muscle. Zhongguo Ying Yong Sheng Li Xue Za Zhi 1997;13:198–201.

65. Deschenes MR, Maresh CM, Armstrong LE, et al. Endurance and resistance exercise induce muscle fiber type specific responses in androgen binding capacity. J Steroid Biochem Mol Biol 1994;50:175–179.

66. Inoue K, Yamasaki S, Fushiki T, et al. Rapid increase in the number of androgen receptors following electrical stimulation of the rat muscle. Eur J Appl Physiol 1993;66:134–140.

67. Inoue K, Yamasaki S, Fushiki T, et al. Androgen receptor antagonist suppresses exercise-induced hypertrophy of skeletal muscle. Eur J Appl Physiol 1994;69: 88–91.

68. Bamman MM, Shipp JR, Jiang J, et al. Mechanical load increases muscle IGF-1 and androgen receptor mRNA concentrations in humans. Am J Physiol 2001;280: E383–390.

69. Kadi F, Bonnerud P, Eriksson A, Thornell LE. The expression of androgen receptors in human neck and limb muscles: effects of training and self-administration of androgenic-anabolic steroids. Histochem Cell Biol 2000;113:25–29.
70. Biolo G, Maggi SP, Williams BD, et al. Increased rates of muscle protein turnover and amino acid transport after resistance exercise in humans. Am J Physiol 1995;268: E514–520.
71. Busso T, Häkkinen K, Pakarinen A, et al. Hormonal adaptations and modeled responses in elite weightlifters during 6 weeks of training. Eur J Appl Physiol 1992;64:381–386.
72. Häkkinen K, Pakarinen A. Serum hormones in male strength athletes during intensive short term strength training. Eur J Appl Physiol 1991;63:191–199.
73. Broeder CE. Oral andro-related prohormone supplementation: do the potential risks outweigh the benefits? Can J Appl Physiol 2003;28:102–116.
74. Delbeke FT, Van Eenoo P, Van Thuyne W, Desmet N. Prohormones and sport. J Steroid Biochem 2003;83:245–251.
75. King DS, Sharp RL, Vukovich MD, et al. Effect of oral androstenedione on serum testosterone and adaptations to resistance training in young men: a randomized controlled trial. JAMA 1999;281:2020–2028.
76. Ballantyne CS, Phillips SM, MacDonald JR, et al. The acute effects of androstenedione supplementation in healthy young males. Can J Appl Physiol 2000;25: 68–78.
77. Wallace MB, Lim J, Cutler A, Bucci L. Effects of dehydroepiandrosterone vs androstenedione supplementation in men. Med Sci Sports Exerc 1999;31:1788–1792.
78. Brown GA, Vukovich MD, Sharp RL, et al. Effect of oral DHEA on serum testosterone and adaptations to resistance training. J Appl Physiol 1999;87:2274–2283.
79. Leder BZ, Longscope C, Catlin DH, et al. Oral androstenedione administration and serum testosterone concentrations in young men. JAMA 2000;283:779–782.
80. Leder BZ, Leblanc KM, Longscope C, et al. Effects of oral androstenedione administration on serum testosterone and estradiol levels in postmenopausal women. J Clin Endocrinol Metab 2002;87:5449–5454.
81. Brown GA, Vukovich MD, Martini ER, et al. Endocrine and lipid responses to chronic androstenediol-herbal supplementation in 30 to 58 year old men. J Am Coll Nutr 2001;20:520–528.
82. Earnest CP, Olson MA, Broeder CE, et al. In vivo 4-androstene-3,17-dione and 4-androstene-3β,17β-diol supplementation in young men. Eur J Appl Physiol 2000; 81:229–232.
83. Brown GA, Vukovich MD, Reifenrath TA, et al. Effects of anabolic precursors on serum testosterone concentrations and adaptations to resistance training in young men. Int J Sport Nutr Exerc Metab 2000;10:340–359.
84. Leder BZ, Catlin DH, Longscope C, et al. Metabolism of orally administered androstenedione in young men. J Clin Endocrinol Metab 2001;86:3654–3658.
85. Brown GA, Martini ER, Roberts BS, et al. Acute hormonal response to sublingual androstenediol intake in young men. J Appl Physiol 2002;92:142–146.
86. Broeder CE, Quindry J, Brittingham K, et al. The Andro project: physiological and hormonal influences of androstenedione supplementation in men 35 to 65 years old participating in a high-intensity resistance training program. Arch Intern Med 2000;160:3093–3104.
87. Van Gammeren D, Falk D, Antonio J. The effects of supplementation with 19-nor-4-androstene-3,17-dione and 19-nor-4-androstene-3,17-diol on body composition and athletic performance in previously weight-trained male athletes. Eur J Appl Physiol 2001;84:426–431.
88. Van Gammeren D, Falk D, Antonio J. Effects of norandrostenedione and norandrostenediol in resistance-trained men. Nutrition 2002;18:734–737.
89. Rasmussen BB, Volpi E, Gore DC, Wolfe RR. Androstenedione does not stimulate muscle protein anabolism in young healthy men. J Clin Endocrinol Metab 2000;85:55–59.
90. Aizawa K, Akimoto T, Inoue H, et al. Resting serum dehydroepiandrosterone sulfate level increases after 8-week resistance training among young females. Eur J Appl Physiol 2003;90:575–580.
91. Longscope C. Dehydroepiandrosterone metabolism. J Endocrinol 1996;150:S125–127.
92. Kahn SM, Hryb DJ, Nakhla AM, et al. Sex hormone-binding globulin is synthesized in target cells. J Endocrinol 2002;175:113–120.
93. Kraemer WJ, Mazzetti SA. Hormonal mechanisms related to the expression of muscular strength and power. In: Komi PV, ed. Strength and Power in Sport. 2nd ed. Malden, MA: Blackwell Scientific Publications; 2003:73–95.

94. Wallace JD, Cuneo RC, Bidlingmaier M, et al. The response of molecular isoforms of growth hormone to acute exercise in trained adult males. J Clin Endocrinol Metab 2001;86:200–206.

95. McCall GE, Goulet EC, Grindeland RE, et al. Bed rest suppresses bioassayable growth hormone release in response to muscle activity. J Appl Physiol 1997;83: 2086–2090.

96. McCall GE, Grindeland RE, Roy RR, Edgerton VR. Muscle afferent activity modulates bioassayable growth hormone in human plasma. J Appl Physiol 2000;89: 1137–1141.

97. Nindl BC, Kraemer WJ, Hymer WC. Immunofunctional vs immunoreactive growth hormone responses after resistance exercise in men and women. Growth Horm IGF Res 2000;10:99–103.

98. Hymer WC, Kraemer WJ, Nindl BC, et al. Characteristics of circulating growth hormone in women after acute heavy resistance exercise. Am J Physiol Endocrinol Metab 2001;281:E878–887.

99. Kraemer WJ, Rubin MR, Häkkinen K, et al. Influence of muscle strength and total work on exercise-induced plasma growth hormone isoforms in women. J Sci Med Sport 2003;6:295–306.

100. Vanhelder WP, Radomski MW, Goode RC. Growth hormone responses during intermittent weight lifting exercise in men. Eur J Appl Physiol 1984;53:31–34.

101. Pyka G, Wiswell RA, Marcus R. Age-dependent effect of resistance exercise on growth hormone secretion in people. J Clin Endocrinol Metab 1992;75:404–407.

102. Hoffman JR, Im J, Rundell KW, et al. Effect of muscle oxygenation during resistance exercise on anabolic hormone response. Med Sci Sports Exerc 2003;35:1929–1934.

103. Craig BW, Kang H. Growth hormone release following single versus multiple sets of back squats: total work versus power. J Strength Cond Res 1994;8:270–275.

104. Mulligan SE, Fleck SJ, Gordon SE, et al. Influence of resistance exercise volume on serum growth hormone and cortisol concentrations in women. J Strength Cond Res 1996;10:256–262.

105. Taylor JM, Thompson HS, Clarkson PM, et al. Growth hormone response to an acute bout of resistance exercise in weight-trained and non-weight-trained women. J Strength Cond Res 2000;14:220–227.

106. Rubin MR, Kraemer WJ, Maresh CM, et al. High-Affinity growth hormone binding protein and acute heavy resistance exercise. Med Sci Sports Exerc 2005;37(3): 395–403.

107. Gordon SE, Kraemer WJ, Vos NH, et al. Effect of acid-base balance on the growth hormone response to acute high-intensity cycle exercise. J Appl Physiol 1994;76: 821–829.

108. Goto K, Sato K, Takamatsu K. A single set of low intensity resistance exercise immediately following high intensity resistance exercise stimulates growth hormone secretion in men. J Sports Med Phys Fitness 2003;43:243–249.

109. Kraemer WJ, Dudley GA, Tesch PA, et al. The influence of muscle action on the acute growth hormone response to resistance exercise and short-term detraining. Growth Horm IGF Res 2001;11:75–83.

110. Ju G. Evidence for direct neural regulation of the mammalian anterior pituitary. Clin Exp Pharmacol Physiol 1999;26:757–759.

111. Zhang Y, Jiang J, Black RA, et al. Tumor necrosis factor-α converting enzyme (TACE) is a growth hormone-binding protein (GHBP) sheddase: the metalloprotease TACE/ADAM-17 is critical for (PMA-induced) GH receptor proteolysis and GHBP generation. Endocrinology 2000;141:4342–4348.

112. Boone JB, Lambert CP, Flynn MG, et al. Resistance exercise effects on plasma cortisol, testosterone and creatine kinase activity in anabolic-androgenic steroid users. Int J Sports Med 1990;11:293–297.

113. Kraemer WJ, Fleck SJ, Callister R, et al. Training responses of plasma beta-endorphin, adrenocorticotropin, and cortisol. Med Sci Sports Exerc 1989;21:146–153.

114. Kraemer WJ, Dziados JE, Marchitelli LJ, et al. Effects of different heavy-resistance exercise protocols on plasma β-endorphin concentrations. J Appl Physiol 1993;74: 450–459.

115. Kraemer WJ, Noble BJ, Clark MJ, Culver BW. Physiologic responses to heavy-resistance exercise with very short rest periods. Int J Sports Med 1987;8:247–252.

116. Zafeiridis A, Smilios I, Considine RV, Tokmakidis SP. Serum leptin responses after acute resistance exercise protocols. J Appl Physiol 2003;94:591–597.

117. Smilios I, Pilianidis T, Karamouzis M, Tokmakidis SP. Hormonal responses after various resistance exercise protocols. Med Sci Sports Exerc 2003;35:644–654.

118. Williams AG, Ismail AN, Sharma A, Jones DA. Effects of resistance exercise volume and nutritional supplementation on anabolic and catabolic hormones. Eur J Appl Physiol 2002;86:315–321.

119. Kraemer WJ, Clemson A, Triplett NT, et al. The effects of plasma cortisol elevation on total and differential leukocyte counts in response to heavy-resistance exercise. Eur J Appl Physiol 1996;73:93–97.

120. Tarpenning KM, Wiswell RA, Hawkins SA, Marcell TJ. Influence of weight training exercise and modification of hormonal response on skeletal muscle growth. J Sci Med Sport 2001;4:431–446.

121. Haff GG, Lehmkuhl MJ, McCoy LB, Stone MH. Carbohydrate supplementation and resistance training. J Strength Cond Res 2003;17:187–196.

122. Koziris LP, Kraemer WJ, Gordon SE, Incledon T, Knuttgen HG. Effect of acute postexercise ethanol intoxication on the neuroendocrine response to resistance exercise. J Appl Physiol 2000;88:165–172.

123. Vingren JL, Koziris LP, Ben-Ezra V, Kraemer WJ. Post-exercise ethanol intoxication and serum free testosterone concentration following resistance exercise. Med Sci Sports Exerc 2003;35(Suppl):S330.

124. Fry AC, Kraemer WJ, Stone MH, et al. Endocrine responses to overreaching before and after 1 year of weightlifting. Can J Appl Physiol 1994;19:400–410.

125. Crowley MA, Matt KS. Hormonal regulation of skeletal muscle hypertrophy in rats: the testosterone to cortisol ratio. Eur J Appl Physiol 1996;73:66–72.

126. Häkkinen K. Neuromuscular and hormonal adaptations during strength and power training. A review. J Sports Med Phys Fitness 1989;29:9–26.

127. Hickson RC, Czerwinski SM, Falduto MT, Young AP. Glucocorticoid antagonism by exercise and androgenic-anabolic steroids. Med Sci Sports Exerc 1990;22:331–340.

128. Mayer M, Rosen F. Interaction of anabolic steroids with glucocorticoid receptor site in rat muscle cytosol. Am J Physiol 1975;229:1381–1386.

129. Willoughby DS, Taylor M, Taylor L. Glucocorticoid receptor and ubiquitin expression after repeated eccentric exercise. Med Sci Sports Exerc 2003;35:2023–3201.

130. Fedele MJ, Lang CH, Farrell PA. Immunization against IGF-1 prevents increases in protein synthesis in diabetic rats after resistance exercise. Am J Physiol Endocrinol Metab 2001;280:E877–885.

131. Kraemer WJ, Aguilera BA, Terada M, et al. Responses of IGF-1 to endogenous increases in growth hormone after heavy-resistance exercise. J Appl Physiol 1995;79:1310–1315.

132. Koziris LP, Hickson RC, Chatterton RT, et al. Serum levels of total and free IGF-1 and IGFBP-3 are increased and maintained in long-term training. J Appl Physiol 1999;86:1436–1442.

133. Borst SE, De Hoyos DV, Garzarella L, et al. Effects of resistance training on insulin-like growth factor-I and IGF binding proteins. Med Sci Sports Exerc 2001;33:648–653.

134. Raastad T, Glomsheller T, Bjoro T, Hallen J. Recovery of skeletal muscle contractility and hormonal responses to strength exercise after two weeks of high-volume strength training. Scand J Med Sci Sports 2003;13:159–168.

135. Adams GR. Role of insulin-like growth factor-I in the regulation of skeletal muscle adaptation to increased loading. Exerc Sports Sci Rev 1998;26:31–60.

136. Goldspink G. Changes in muscle mass and phenotype and the expression of autocrine and systemic growth factors by muscle in response to stretch and overload. J Anat 1999;194:323–334.

137. Hameed M, Orrel RW, Cobbold G, et al. Expression of IGF-1 splice variants in young and old human skeletal muscle after high resistance exercise. J Physiol 2003;547:247–254.

138. Brahm H, Piehl-Aulin K, Saltin B, Ljunghall S. Net fluxes over working thigh of hormones, growth factors and biomarkers of bone metabolism during short lasting dynamic exercise. Calcif Tissue Int 1997;60:175–180.

139. Nindl BC, Kraemer WJ, Marx JO, et al. Overnight responses of the circulating IGF-1 system after acute heavy-resistance exercise. J Appl Physiol 2001;90:1319–1326.

140. Biolo G, Tipton KD, Klein S, Wolfe RR. An abundant supply of amino acids enhances the metabolic effect of exercise on muscle protein. Am J Physiol Endocrinol Metab 1997;273:E122–129.

141. Wolfe RR. Effects of insulin on muscle tissue. Curr Opin Clin Nutr Metab Care 2000;3:67–71.

142. Borsheim E, Cree MG, Tipton KD, et al. Effect of carbohydrate intake on net muscle protein synthesis during recovery from resistance exercise. J Appl Physiol 2004;96:674–678.

143. Thyfault JP, Carper MJ, Richmond SR, et al. Effects of liquid carbohydrate ingestion on markers of anabolism following high-intensity resistance exercise. J Strength Cond Res 2004;18:174–179.

144. Volek JS, Ratamess NA, Rubin MR, et al. The effects of creatine supplementation on muscular performance and body composition responses to short-term resistance training overreaching. Eur J Appl Physiol 2004;91(5–6):628–637.

145. Bush JA, Kraemer WJ, Mastro AM, et al. Exercise and recovery responses of adrenal medullary neurohormones to heavy resistance exercise. Med Sci Sports Exerc 1999;31:554–559.

146. Elliot DL, Goldberg L, Watts WJ, Orwoll E. Resistance exercise and plasma beta-endorphin/beta-lipotrophin immunoreactivity. Life Sci 1984;34:515–518.

147. Walberg-Rankin J, Franke WD, Gwazdauskas FC. Response of beta-endorphin and estradiol to resistance exercise females during energy balance and energy restriction. Int J Sports Med 1992;13:542–547.

148. Kraemer RR, Acevedo EO, Dzewaltowski D, et al. Effects of low-volume resistive exercise on beta-endorphin and cortisol concentrations. Int J Sports Med 1996;17: 12–16.

149. Pierce EF, Eastman NW, Tripathi HT, et al. Plasma beta-endorphin immunoreactivity: response to resistance exercise. J Sports Sci 1993;11:499–502.

150. Pierce EF, Eastman NW, McGowan RW, et al. Resistance exercise decreases beta-endorphin immunoreactivity. Br J Sports Med 1994;28:164–166.

151. Goldfarb AH, Hatfield BD, Armstrong D, Potts J. Plasma beta-endorphin concentration: response to intensity and duration of exercise. Med Sci Sports Exerc 1990;22: 241–244.

152. Cardone A, Angelini F, Esposito T, et al. The expression of androgen receptor messenger RNA is regulated by tri-iodothyronine in lizard testis. J Steroid Biochem Mol Biol 2000;72:133–141.

153. Pakarinen A, Häkkinen K, Alen M. Serum thyroid hormones, thyrotropin, and thyroxine binding globulin in elite athletes during very intense strength training of one week. J Sports Med Phys Fitness 1991;31:142–146.

154. Alen M, Pakarinen A, Häkkinen K. Effects of prolonged training on serum thyrotropin and thyroid hormones in elite strength athletes. J Sports Sci 1993;11:493–497.

155. Pakarinen A, Alen M, Häkkinen K, Komi P. Serum thyroid hormones, thyrotropin and thyroxine binding globulin during prolonged strength training. Eur J Appl Physiol 1988;57:394–398.

156. Simsch C, Lormes W, Petersen KG, et al. Training intensity influences leptin and thyroid hormones in highly trained rowers. Int J Sports Med 2002;23:422–427.

157. Mannix ET, Palange P, Aronoff GR, et al. Atrial natriuretic peptide and the renin-aldosterone axis during exercise in man. Med Sci Sports Exerc 1990;22:785–789.

158. Convertino VA, Keil LC, Bernauer EM, Greenleaf JE. Plasma volume, osmolality, vasopressin, and renin activity during graded exercise in man. J Appl Physiol 1981;50:123–128.

159. Gordon NF, Russell HMS, Krüger PE, Cilliers JF. Thermoregulatory responses to weight training. Int J Sports Med 1985;6:145–150.

160. Collins MA, Hill DW, Cureton KJ, DeMello JJ. Plasma volume change during heavy-resistance weight lifting. Eur J Appl Physiol 1986;55:44–48.

161. Kalra SP, Dube MG, Pu S, et al. Interacting appetite-regulating pathways in the hypothalamic regulation of body weight. Endocr Rev 1999;20:68–100.

162. Considine RV, Sinha MK, Heiman ML, et al. Serum immunoreactive-leptin concentrations in normal-weight and obese humans. N Engl J Med 1996;334:292–295.

163. Considine RV. Weight regulation, leptin and growth hormone. Horm Res 1997; 48(Suppl 5):116–121.

164. Gippini A, Mato A, Peino R, et al. Effect of resistance exercise (body building) training on serum leptin levels in young men. Implications for relationship between body mass index and serum leptin. J Endocrinol Invest 1999;22:824–828.

165. Nindl BC, Kraemer WJ, Arciero PJ, et al. Leptin concentrations experience a delayed reduction after resistance exercise in men. Med Sci Sports Exerc 2002;34:608–613.

166. Tena-Sempere M, Manna PR, Zhang FP, et al. Molecular mechanisms of leptin action in adult rat testis: potential targets for leptin-induced inhibition of steroidogenesis and pattern of leptin receptor messenger ribonucleic acid expression. J Endocrinol 2001;170:413–423.

167. Isidori AM, Caprio M, Strollo F, et al. Leptin and androgens in male obesity: evidence for leptin contribution to reduced androgen levels. J Clin Endocrinol Metab 1999;84:3673–3680.

168. Lima N, Cavaliere H, Knobel M, et al. Decreased androgen levels in massively obese men may be associated with impaired function of the gonadostat. Int J Obes Relat Metab Disord 2000;24:1433–1437.

169. Triplett-McBride NT, Mastro AM, McBride JM, et al. Plasma proenkephalin peptide F and human B cell responses to exercise stress in fit and unfit women. Peptides 1998;19:731–738.

170. Kraemer WJ, Noble B, Culver B, Lewis RV. Changes in plasma proenkephalin peptide F and catecholamine levels during graded exercise in men. Proc Natl Acad Sci USA 1985;82:6349–6351.
171. Fry AC, Kraemer WJ, Ramsey LT. Pituitary-adrenal-gonadal responses to high-intensity resistance exercise overtraining. J Appl Physiol 1998;85:2352–2359.
172. Fry AC, Kraemer WJ, Van Borselen F, et al. Catecholamine responses to short-term high-intensity resistance exercise overtraining. J Appl Physiol 1994;77:941–946.
173. Hortobagyi T, Houmard JA, Stevenson JR, et al. The effects of detraining on power athletes. Med Sci Sports Exerc 1993;25:929–935.
174. Kraemer WJ, Koziris LP, Ratamess NA, et al. Detraining produces minimal changes in physical performance and hormonal variables in recreationally strength-trained men. J Strength Cond Res 2002;16:373–382.
175. Kraemer WJ, Loebel CC, Volek JS, et al. The effect of heavy resistance exercise on the circadian rhythm of salivary testosterone in men. Eur J Appl Physiol 2001;84:13–18.
176. McMurray RG, Eubank TK, Hackney AC. Nocturnal hormonal responses to resistance exercise. Eur J Appl Physiol 1995;72:121–126.
177. Nindl BC, Hymer WC, Deaver DR, Kraemer WJ. Growth hormone pulsatility profile characteristics following acute heavy resistance exercise. J Appl Physiol 2001;91:163–172.
178. Kraemer WJ, Patton JF, Gordon SE, et al. Compatibility of high-intensity strength and endurance training on hormonal and skeletal muscle adaptations. J Appl Physiol 1995;78:976–989.
179. Bell GJ, Syrotuik D, Martin TP, et al. Effect of concurrent strength and endurance training on skeletal muscle properties and hormone concentrations in humans. Eur J Appl Physiol 2000;81:418–427.

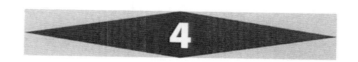

# Cardiovascular and Pulmonary Responses to Exercise

## Rick Seip

## OBJECTIVES

On the completion of this chapter you will be able to:

1. Explain the steps associated with ventilation and pulmonary circulation.
2. Describe the difference between ventilation during resting and exercise conditions.
3. Understand the consequences of the Valsalva maneuver.
4. Describe the membranes that must be crossed in order to get oxygen from the lungs into the blood.
5. Explain the blood-carrying capacity and how erythropoietin affects this capacity.
6. Understand the steps associated with moving blood through the systemic circulation.
7. Describe the acute and chronic effects of endurance and resistance training on the cardiovascular system.
8. Explain the differences in $\dot{V}O_2$ max between men and women and athletes in a variety of sports.
9. Understand the effects of different genetic characteristics on endurance and resistance training performance.

## ABSTRACT

Voluntary contraction of skeletal muscle increases the demand for oxygen and fuels such as glycogen and fatty acids. Whereas fuels are conveniently stored within muscle cells close to the mitochondria and contractile machinery, there is practically no oxygen reserve in muscle cells and the small amount found in the blood can sustain resting aerobic metabolism only for a few minutes. When muscles contract, they need more oxygen, and whole body oxygen consumption can increase by 10- to 20-fold. The circulatory and the pulmonary systems work together to increase oxygen transport in a highly responsive and coordinated manner. By performing specific exercises consistently for weeks, months, or years, an athlete can stimulate the cardiovascular system to adapt specifically to them. Presented in this chapter is a discussion of the cardiopulmonary responses to a single exercise bout, called the acute response to exercise, as well as chronic adaptations of the cardiovascular system to the many different demands of sport.

*Key Words:* heart, cardiac, cardiovascular, maximal oxygen uptake, oxygen, $\dot{V}O_2$ max, cardiac output, stroke volume, heart rate

From: *Essentials of Sports Nutrition and Supplements*
Edited by J. Antonio, D. Kalman, J. R. Stout, M. Greenwood, D. S. Willoughby, and G. G. Haff © Humana Press, a part of Springer Science+Business Media, Totowa, NJ

**FIGURE 4.1.** Links of the oxygen transport chain including pulmonary ventilation, blood hemoglobin, the heart, systemic circulation, and muscles themselves, where mitochondria utilize oxygen in energy transfer.

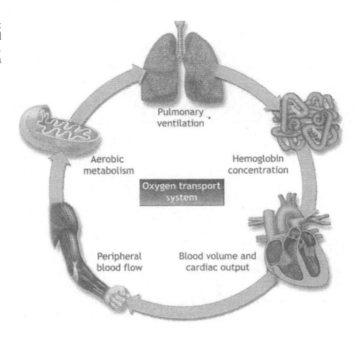

## THE OXYGEN TRANSPORT SYSTEM

Oxygen is transported from room air to the working muscles, 24 hours a day, 7 days per week, for life! This tireless transport system can be thought of as a chain with five links, including 1) ventilation, 2) perfusion of the pulmonary circulation, 3) pumping of the blood by the heart, 4) transport via the systemic circulation to organs and tissues including muscles, and 5) the muscles themselves. To obtain a good working knowledge of pulmonary and circulatory anatomy, consult basic anatomy and physiology texts. To gain a broader, deeper appreciation of the oxygen transport system, consult a current exercise physiology text.[1-4] Assuming this background, herein is described the path taken by oxygen from outside the body, through the circulation, and to the mitochondria of the muscle (Figure 4.1).

### Ventilation and the Pulmonary Circulation

Ventilation is the movement of air in and out of the lungs. It is accomplished by forcibly and reversibly changing the size of the pulmonary cavity through contraction of specialized muscles. Inhalation increases the cavity size, causing environmental air to flow into the lungs, whereas exhalation compresses the pulmonary cavity, forcing air up and out through the airways. From rest to exercise, the mechanics of ventilation change. At rest, inhalation includes contraction of both the diaphragm muscle and the external intercostal muscles of the rib cage. Contraction of the diaphragm moves it downward, lowering the floor of the pulmonary cavity. Contraction of the external intercostal muscles pulls the rib cage upward and outward, enlarging the pulmonary cavity. Exhalation is passive. The weight of the rib cage bears down on the cavity, compressing it, and the diaphragm muscle relaxes and moves upward to its resting position, raising the floor of the cavity. During exercise, ventilation increases via increased respiratory rate (number of breaths/minute) and tidal volume (volume of air exhaled in each breath). Exercise exhalation calls into play the internal intercostal muscles. Their contraction pulls the ribs closer together and squeezes the pulmonary cavity, increasing pressure and forcing air upward through the airways. In maximal aerobic exercise, the abdominal muscles may contract to compress the abdominal cavity and assist exhalation.

Ventilation brings to the alveolar space air that is higher in $O_2$ concentration and lower in $CO_2$ concentration compared with that of the blood entering

## Sidebar 4.1. Should Athletes Control Breathing to Improve Performance?

Momentarily suspending ventilation by "holding one's breath"—called the Valsalva maneuver—during maximal isometric contractions stabilizes the torso, providing an anchor for maximal strength performance. This conscious maneuver can pose an immediate health risk in persons with cardiovascular disease. In rhythmic aerobic exercise such as running, rowing, swimming, and cross-country skiing, a sustained high rate of ventilation is very important. Should the athlete try to control breathing? Ventilation accounts for 3%–15% of the energy used during such work.[5] Fortunately, the natural rate and depth of breathing are usually very efficient, as shown by laboratory studies of runners. Perhaps the best advice to endurance athletes is to ignore any conscious effort to breathe a certain way. Instead, good advice would be to consciously relax the abdominal muscles to allow free, easy, and natural movement of the diaphragm.

the lungs from the heart via the pulmonary artery. By simple chemical diffusion, $O_2$ traverses, in order, the following barriers: the alveolar membrane, the extravascular fluid space, pulmonary capillary membrane, intravascular fluid space, and finally the red blood cell membrane where the hemoglobin protein binds and stores the $O_2$ during transport. Obstructed airways, or constricted bronchioles as in asthma, impair ventilation and prevent adequate oxygenation of the blood. At rest, the transit time of blood passing through the lungs is 0.8–1.0 second, long enough for complete oxygenation of the blood. In elite endurance athletes with high maximal cardiac output, the pulmonary transit time may be reduced to 0.4 second, possibly preventing oxygen saturation of the blood.

### Blood Oxygen-Carrying Capacity

Fully oxygenated blood carries about $20\,mL\,O_2 \cdot 100\,mL^{-1}$, most of which is bound to hemoglobin. Because hemoglobin requires iron to carry oxygen, dietary iron is important for oxygen transport capacity and good exercise performance depends on sufficient hemoglobin concentration.[6] The lower hemoglobin concentration in women is one reason for the maximal oxygen uptake ($\dot{V}O_2$ max) differences between male and female athletes. A surrogate measure for hemoglobin is the hematocrit, which is the percent of total blood volume that is red blood cell mass. Hemoglobin concentrations range from 12 to 15 g/dL in women and 13.6 to 17.2 g/dL in men. Equivalent hematocrit levels are 35%–47% and 42%–52% for women and men, respectively.[7]

### The Heart and Systemic Circulation

Oxygenated blood returns from the lungs to the heart via the pulmonary vein to the left atrium of the heart. The atrium then contracts. Rising atrial pressure closes the pulmonary valve, and opens the arteriovenous (AV) valve and pushes blood into the left ventricle (LV), causing it to expand slightly. The LV quickly contracts, increasing LV pressure, opening the aortic valve and closing the AV valve. A volume of blood [the stroke volume (SV)] exits the heart and enters the aorta before the aortic valve closes again. The systemic arterial circulation carries blood to the muscles (and of course to all other organs) via large arteries that become smaller as they branch into progressively smaller arteries. In going from larger to smaller arteries, the sensitivity of the control of the arterial cross-sectional area by smooth muscle constriction and relaxation increases. Contraction of the smooth muscle encircling arterioles closes them and restricts local blood flow. Through neural and chemical influences on the tiniest arterioles and precapillary sphincters, the body directs blood flow to muscle tissue that requires it, and restricts flow from the muscle and tissues not requiring it.

## Sidebar 4.2. Erythropoietin and Blood Doping Increase the Oxygen Transport Capacity of the Blood

Erythropoietin (EPO), a naturally occurring hormone produced by the kidneys, stimulates the body to produce more red blood cells. Increasing the red cell content of the blood can increase aerobic performance. EPO has been used as a performance-enhancing drug in endurance athletes including some cyclists (in the Tour de France), long-distance runners, speed skaters, and Nordic (cross-country) skiers. When misused in such situations, EPO is thought to be especially dangerous (perhaps because dehydration can further increase the viscosity of the blood, increasing the risk for heart attacks and strokes).[8] EPO has been banned by the Tour de France, the Olympics, and other sports organizations. However, it is difficult or impossible to detect EPO with urine or blood testing because athletes stop taking EPO long before competition, knowing that the red cell mass increase will linger for weeks after stopping EPO intake. During the 2004 Summer Olympics, more than 3000 drug tests were conducted in Athens, a 25% increase from the 2000 Sydney Games.[9]

## Muscle

The final link in the oxygen transport chain is muscle. One might think of exercising muscle as a "sink" with a capacity to drain the blood of oxygen. Muscle capacity to utilize oxygen is directly related to mitochondrial volume and the levels of enzymes of glycolysis and β-oxidation.[10] Glycolysis and β-oxidation are cellular processes that utilize oxygen to synthesize adenosine triphosphate, which is a high-energy molecule containing the energy for muscle contraction. Glycolysis refers to the breakdown of glucose, and β-oxidation to the breakdown of fats. The enzymes catalyze reactions in which oxygen is combined with carbon to form $CO_2$ and with hydrogen to form $H_2O$. Aerobic enzyme activities are higher in slow (Type I) compared with fast twitch (Type II) fibers.[11] Capillaries are found throughout muscle, often running parallel to individual fibers. The number of capillaries can increase with months of aerobic training at high intensity. In endurance athletes, the higher ratio of capillaries to muscle fibers facilitates $O_2$ delivery to muscle fibers. Myoglobin found within the cells shuttles $O_2$ from the sarcolemma (cell membrane) to the mitochondria. Muscles comprise on the average 40% of the body mass and, through voluntary exercise, can increase oxygen consumption by 100-fold![12] This ability far exceeds that of any other organ. The muscles, therefore, have great capacity to dictate the cardiopulmonary response.

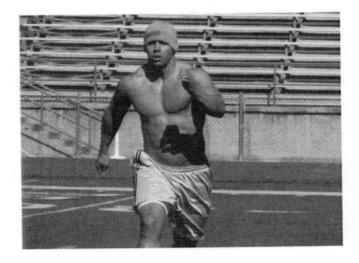

# CARDIOVASCULAR RESPONSES TO ACUTE EXERCISE AND CHRONIC EXERCISE

It is useful to think of the body's adaptations to exercise in two ways. The immediate changes within the cardiovascular and pulmonary systems from rest to exercise such as the increase in ventilation, heart rate, cardiac output, and systolic blood pressure, are termed acute responses. Adaptations to repeated exercise training bouts—such as the increases in maximal oxygen uptake, capillaries, heart size, and blood volume; the thickening of heart walls (myocardium); and the decrease in resting heart rate—are called responses to chronic exercise. This section briefly outlines cardiovascular responses to acute voluntary exercise, and describes adaptations to chronic resistance training and aerobic training.

## ACUTE EXERCISE

Ventilation at rest is $6 L \cdot min^{-1}$ and may increase to $150 L \cdot min^{-1}$ at maximal aerobic exercise. Although ventilation at maximal exercise may approach 200 L/min in a well-trained endurance athlete,[13] the ventilation recorded during maximal treadmill exercise is less than the maximal forced voluntary ventilation that is possible at rest.[5] Ventilation normally does not limit maximal aerobic exercise performance. However, in a few elite athletes with a high maximal cardiac output, the transit time of blood passing through the lungs may be insufficient for complete $O_2$ saturation of blood. In this case, less $O_2$ is delivered to muscle and this may limit maximal aerobic performance (discussed in ref. 2, p. 206).

The level of ventilation associated with sports performance varies with the demands of the activity. Breathing increases slowly and in proportion to increasing oxygen uptake until 50%–75% of maximal intensity, at which point the increase becomes greater or curvilinear. This inflection point, called the ventilatory threshold, is illustrated in Figure 4.2A. Below the ventilatory threshold, the energy cost of ventilation is modest (3%–8% of whole body $\dot{V}O_2$) but it increases to 10%–15% at maximal exercise.[5] Other parameters typically measured during exercise are shown in Figure 4.2.

Heart rate increases from an average of 60 beats·min$^{-1}$ at rest to $200 \pm 10$ beats·min$^{-1}$ at maximal exercise in a 20-year-old man or woman, as shown in Figure 4.2B. Maximal exercise heart rate can be predicted by calculating 220 – age.

## Sidebar 4.3. Stroke Volume in Elite Endurance Athletes

Many studies support the conclusion that SV increases up to 40% of maximal exercise intensity, where it remains through 100% intensity. This plateau occurs at about 110–120 mL for sedentary and about 130–140 mL for endurance athletes. But the truly elite endurance athlete may have an SV advantage. Five runners capable of running 2:15 in the marathon or 28:00 in the 10-km races were found to have a maximal SV = $187 \pm 15$ mL.[14] For these athletes, SV did not plateau at submaximal exercise, instead continuing to increase throughout, supporting an earlier study that also concluded no plateau in SV for elite endurance athletes.[15] A longer time for diastolic filling,[15] reduced pericardial resistance to filling of the LV between beats,[16] and larger heart size have been postulated as mechanisms. Could there be subtle, genetically determined factors that separate elite from nonelite runners?

Cardiac output, which is the product of heart rate (beats/min) × SV (mL of blood pumped per heartbeat), increases from about $5 L \cdot min^{-1}$ at rest to $20 L \cdot min^{-1}$ in an untrained person. A highly trained endurance athlete may attain $35–40 L \cdot min^{-1}$.[17] Cardiac output (in L/min) increases in proportion to the oxygen uptake (in L/min) in the ratio of 6:1 for sedentary as well as trained athletes.

**FIGURE 4.2.** Physiologic responses to acute exercise in a healthy young adult. **A:** Ve vs. work; **B:** HR vs. work; **C:** SV vs. work; **D:** V̇O₂ vs. work; **E:** CO vs. work; and **F:** BP vs. work.

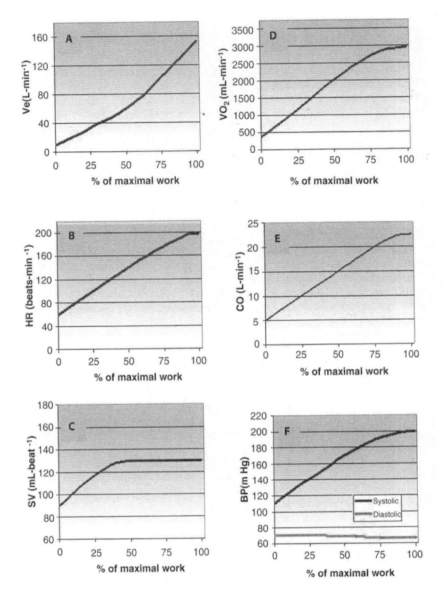

## The Distribution of Cardiac Output

At rest, the cardiac output is distributed evenly among many tissues (see Figure 4.3A), but during exercise, blood flow to muscle and the heart is dramatically increased (Figure 4.3B) compared with other organs. Note that some tissues (e.g., kidney and liver) actually receive less blood flow than at rest, because the vascular system can redirect arterial blood flow away from nonworking tissues.

Hot weather imposes an additional demand to increase blood flow to the skin to dissipate the heat generated by exercise. Aerobic sport performance suffers because a portion of the cardiac output ordinarily destined for muscle is diverted to the skin for cooling. Dehydration caused by sweat loss further impairs aerobic performance because it decreases blood volume, lowers SV, lowers cardiac output, and decreases oxygen delivery to muscle.

## MAXIMAL OXYGEN UPTAKE TESTING

V̇O₂ max refers to the maximal oxygen uptake and is a measure of the maximal aerobic exercise capacity. Most exercise physiologists believe that V̇O₂ max is

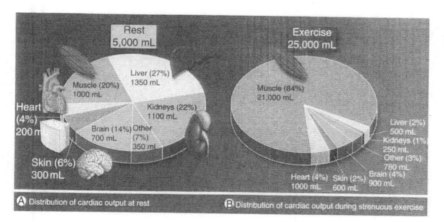

**FIGURE 4.3.** The distribution of cardiac output to tissues (**A**) at rest and (**B**) during exercise. During exercise, skeletal muscles receive >80% of the cardiac output.

the single best indicator of physical fitness because achievement of a high $\dot{V}O_2$ max is only possible when both the cardiac output and muscle aerobic capacity are high. It is expressed in absolute terms as liters of oxygen consumed per minute ($LO_2 \cdot min^{-1}$) or in terms relative to body size ($mLO_2 \cdot kgBW^{-1} \cdot min^{-1}$). The latter permits comparisons between athletes of different sizes. The laboratory $\dot{V}O_2$ max test employs exercise in a mode that uses a large fraction of the muscle mass such as treadmill running, cycling, Nordic skiing, or, where swimming flume facilities exist, swimming (Figure 4.4). Exercise progresses in timed stages from light to moderate to heavy, until the athlete's cardiorespiratory limit is reached. The measurement of oxygen uptake is made possible throughout the test by measuring exhaled gases for volume (i.e., ventilation), and the content of oxygen and carbon dioxide. The maximal oxygen uptake is the highest level of oxygen uptake attained during exhaustive exercise. Many protocols exist and are found in a handbook published by the American College of Sports Medicine.[18] Figure 4.5 shows that $\dot{V}O_2$ max is higher after aerobic training in part because of the increased cardiac output. Training also induces structural and biochemical changes in the muscle that increase muscle's ability to utilize oxygen, as discussed later.

$\dot{V}O_2$ max values in athletes vary depending on the sport (see Figure 4.6). Endurance athletes demonstrate the highest values. $\dot{V}O_2$ max values expressed in terms relative to body weight are 5%–10% lower in women than men, because of lesser hemoglobin concentration, a slightly smaller heart size relative to the size of the chest cavity, less plasma volume, and greater body fat.

**FIGURE 4.4.** Examples of laboratory methods to measure oxygen uptake during (**A**) cycling and (**B**) box loading and unloading.

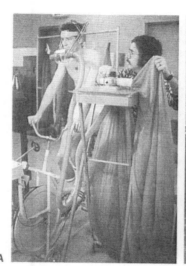

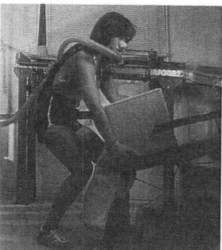

A                                                                              B

**FIGURE 4.5.** Relationship between maximal cardiac output and maximal oxygen uptake in untrained and trained individuals.

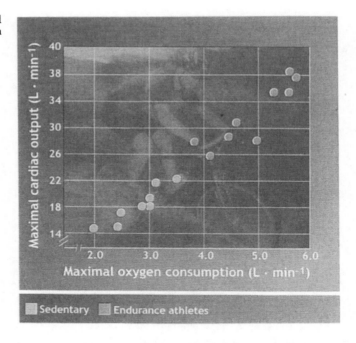

## ADAPTATIONS TO CHRONIC EXERCISE

How different are the cardiopulmonary demands of endurance exercise compared with resistance exercise? One can picture a continuum, with a lean, long-distance cyclist (Figure 4.7), photo of runner and lifter runner, skier, or swimmer standing at one end, and at the other end, a muscular Olympic weightlifter. The range of adaptations can be shown by physiologic measurements taken in men who have trained at the extreme ends of the training continuum. A resistance training regimen consisting of, say, 8–10 exercises, each done for 3–5 sets of 10–12 reps, completed in 60–75 minutes is relatively aerobic and would fall in the middle of the continuum.

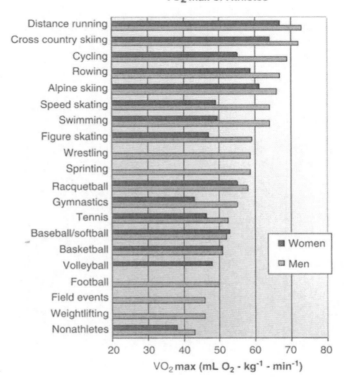

**FIGURE 4.6.** $\dot{V}O_2$ max of athletes.

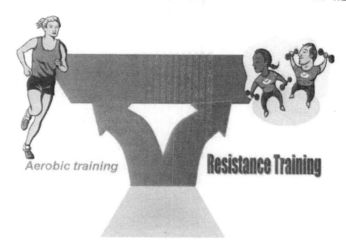

**FIGURE 4.7.** Training for cardiorespiratory endurance and training for muscle power and hypertrophy lead to different kinds of adaptations in skeletal muscle and the cardiovascular system.

## RESTING CARDIOPULMONARY FUNCTION: EFFECTS OF TRAINING

Some common measures of cardiovascular function are shown for 18- to 45-year-old men in Table 4.1. Typical values for a sedentary but not overweight man are compared with those for a highly trained endurance athlete and a highly trained resistance athlete.

### Endurance Training Effects

Endurance exercise involves many repeated muscle contractions at a low percentage of maximal voluntary contraction (MVC). The low resistance to flow through the exercising muscles creates a "volume flow" type demand to which the cardiovascular system adapts. The pump becomes larger and stronger, and muscles portray greater capillary density and aerobic enzyme activity. Endurance training decreases the resting heart rate and increases SV, but has little effect on resting cardiac output. This is not surprising because tissues of the well-rested endurance athlete have no need for extra blood supply. Blood volume is greater in the endurance athlete, because of increased plasma volume. The red blood cell mass is maintained resulting in hematocrit that is lower. Arterial blood pressure is generally lower. At the microcirculatory level, the capillary-to-muscle fiber ratio is increased. The heart dimensions are changed to reflect larger chambers and proportionately thickened LV wall muscle.

At maximal exercise, cardiac output is increased as a result of greater SV, whereas heart rate remains unchanged or slightly lower in the endurance athlete. The AV difference in oxygen content may be larger compared with the sedentary man, which means that the athlete extracts slightly more oxygen from the arterial blood.

**TABLE 4.1.** Heart dimensions in sedentary men and endurance-trained or resistance-trained athletes

| Variable | Nonathletes N = 16 | College runners N = 15 | World class runners N = 10 | College wrestlers N = 12 | World class shot putters N = 4 |
|---|---|---|---|---|---|
| LVIDd, mm | 46 | 54 | 48–59 | 48 | 43–52 |
| LVV, mL | 101 | 160 | 154 | 110 | 122 |
| SV, mL | — | 116 | 113 | 75 | 68 |
| LVWT, mm | 10.3 | 11.3 | 10.8 | 13.7 | 13.8 |
| Septal thickness, mm | 10.3 | 10.9 | 10.9 | 13.0 | 13.5 |
| LV mass, g | 211 | 302 | 283 | 335 | 348 |

*Source:* Data from McArdle et al.[4]

LVIDd = left ventricular internal diameter at diastole, LVV = left ventricular volume, SV = stroke volume, LVWT = left ventricular wall thickness, LV = left ventricle.

## Sidebar 4.4. Oxygen Extraction from the Arterial Blood

Any chain is only as strong as its weakest link and the oxygen transport system is no exception. In many Western nations, cardiovascular disease is the number one cause of death. The heart, or pump, is the link most likely to be broken. Whereas maximal cardiac output in elite endurance athletes exceeds $30\,L\cdot min^{-1}$ and $\dot{V}O_2$ max exceeds $75$–$80\,mLO_2\cdot kg^{-1}\cdot min^{-1}$, in a cardiac rehabilitation patient at max exercise, the pump may only be capable of a maximal CO = $10\,L/min$. Interestingly, patients in cardiac rehabilitation programs can still increase their $\dot{V}O_2$ max! How? They can extract more oxygen from the arterial blood. The AV $O_2$ difference at maximal exercise is normally $15\,mLO_2\cdot min^{-1}$ at max exercise but may be $17$–$18\,mLO_2\cdot min^{-1}$ in cardiac patients. The highly adaptable cardiovascular system learns to temporarily shunt blood to the working muscles and away from those tissues less in need.

### Resistance Training Effects

The demands of resistance training vary depending on the nature of the training program. Variation in the number of sets, reps, and overall caloric costs can lead to differing cardiovascular effects. Low-repetition, heavy weightlifting done for years leads to great skeletal muscularity. High-repetition exercise with many sets and with little rest between sets leads to aerobic endurance-like cardiovascular adaptations. Resistance exercises are typically performed at a high percentage of 1 repetition maximum (RM), and arterial blood pressures are elevated creating a "pressure" demand on the cardiovascular system. The resistance-trained athlete adapts with thickened heart walls and a cardiac mass that has increased in proportion to the lean mass that has been added by training. Neither muscle aerobic activity nor muscle capillarity is increased (Table 4.2).

TABLE 4.2. Resting and maximal cardiorespiratory physiologic responses in sedentary, endurance-trained, and resistance-trained athletes.

|  | Sedentary* | Resistance trained† | Endurance trained‡ |
|---|---|---|---|
| **AT REST:** | | | |
| Heart rate | 60–90 beats/min | No change or decrease | Decrease |
| Stroke volume | $100\,mL\cdot beat^{-1}$ | No change or increase | Increase |
| Cardiac output | $5\,LO_2\cdot min^{-1}$ | No change | No change |
| $\dot{V}O_2$ | $3.5\,mLO_2\cdot kg^{-1}\cdot min^{-1}$ | No change or increase§ | No change |
| Systolic blood pressure | $120 \pm 10\,mmHg$ | No change or small decrease | No change or small decrease |
| Diastolic blood pressure | $80 \pm 10\,mmHg$ | No change or small decrease | No change or small decrease |
| **MAXIMAL EXERCISE:** | | | |
| Heart rate | $200\,beats\cdot min^{-1}$ | No change | No change or decrease |
| Stroke volume | $120\,mL$ | No change | Increase |
| Cardiac output | $15$–$20\,L/min$ | No change | Increase |
| $VO_2$ | $35\,mLO_2\cdot kg^{-1}min^{-1}$ | No change or slight increase | Increase |
| Systolic blood pressure | $200 \pm 15\,mmHg$ | No change | No change |
| Diastolic blood pressure | $75 \pm 15\,mmHg$ | No change | No change |

*A man between ages 18–45 years, height = 175 cm, weight = 70 kg, % body fat = 20%.
†Data modified from Fleck and Kraemer,[21] pp. 117–127.
‡Data modified from McArdle et al.[4]
§Significantly higher in resistance trained on high protein, low carbohydrate, low fat diet.

## Sidebar 4.5. Blood Flow Through the Working Muscle

In a classic experiment, Barcroft and Millen (1939)[19] showed that blood flow through the calf muscles is obstructed by muscular contraction. When muscles contract, sarcomeres shorten, myofibrils increase in diameter and exert pressure on adjacent capillaries and arterioles. If the pressure exceeds the intravascular pressure, the vessels are squeezed shut, and flow stops. This occurs at 30% of maximal force. Thus, isometric exercise is virtually entirely anaerobic, and dynamic exercise using free weights is anaerobic during the time that force exceeds 30% MVC.

## Sidebar 4.6. Blood Pressure During Resistance Exercise

Very high blood pressures can occur during resistance exercise. Direct arterial measurement in five experienced male bodybuilders revealed mean systolic blood pressure of 320 mm Hg and diastolic blood pressure of 250 during performance of double leg press at 90% 1 RM to failure.[20] Mean pressures were lower during one-arm curls (235/170), showing that the increase in blood pressure is proportional to the amount of muscle mass exerting force. In another study, continuous blood pressure monitoring during 3 sets of a 10-RM double leg press exercise showed increased blood pressure with each set. The highest pressures during the leg press were achieved as the lift was initiated from the flexed position. Average peak systolic blood pressures were: set 1, $238 \pm 18$; set 2, $268 \pm 18$; set 3, $293 \pm 21$ mm Hg. These pressures demonstrate the severity of the stress to which the cardiovascular system can adapt.

### Heart Size

Echocardiography reveals LV dimensions that differ according to athletic history (Table 4.3). Aerobic athletes show an enlarged LV internal diameter at diastole (LVIDd) and greater LV volume (LVV) versus nonathletes. The increase in LV cavity size goes hand in hand with increased blood volume of 5%–10%. Both are necessary for the greater SV at rest and during exercise in endurance athletes. The LV posterior (LVW) and septal walls are thickened in proportion to the cavity enlargement and this is called eccentric hypertrophy. Contractile power of the LV walls is also enhanced. Resistance-trained power athletes show little change in LVIDd or LVV. However, LV wall thicknesses can increase by 20%–30% and LV mass by 30% compared with nonathletes. In power athletes, the greater thickening of walls relative to the LV cavity dimensions is an adap-

TABLE 4.3. Muscle adaptations that reflect oxidative capacity in endurance- and resistance-trained athletes.

| | Resistance trained* | Endurance trained |
|---|---|---|
| Energy system enzyme capacity: | | |
| Phosphagen | Increase | Increase |
| Short-term glycolytic | Increase | Increase |
| Aerobic | No change | Increase |
| Mitochondrial volume | Decreased, when expressed per unit muscle fiber[24] | Increased by 40% or more[10] |
| Capillary-to-muscle fiber ratio | Slight or no increase† | Increased by 10%–20%[25] |

*Data modified from Fleck and Kraemer.[21]

†Dependent on total training volume (see ref. 21, p. 82).

tive response to the increased stress on the LV walls as they contract against the systemic pressure created during resistance exercise. This type of growth, called concentric hypertrophy, is proportional to the overall increase in skeletal muscle mass (see ref. 21, p.117). When a trained endurance athlete stops training for an extended time, the myocardium returns to normal size.[22] It is not known if hypertrophy reverses with cessation of resistance training. In summary, exercise training–associated changes in the LV are thought to be adaptive rather than harmful (Table 4.1).[23]

## Muscle Changes

Muscles adapt to endurance training by increasing oxidative energy-producing capacity. Aerobic system enzyme activities increase within the cells, and capillary density, defined as the number of capillaries relative to the number of muscle fibers, increases. Little change in fiber size occurs. In resistance training, the muscle fibers increase in cross-sectional area primarily with little change in oxidative capacity.

## Genetic Influence on Training

Anyone who persists with exercise training will adapt to it. Yet scientific evidence shows that training responses vary from athlete to athlete and it has been hypothesized that heredity explains a significant part of adaptive variation. However, such genetic research is in its infancy. So far, only tiny pieces of what promises to be an enormous polygenic puzzle are known.

## Sidebar 4.7. Genetics of Aerobic Endurance

Angiotensin-converting enzyme (ACE) catalyzes the conversion of angiotensinogen to angiotensin, which is a potent vasoconstrictor. A common variant in the ACE gene is the presence (I, insertion) or absence (D, deletion) of a 287 base pair segment in a noncoding part of the gene. Approximately 50% of the population carries the I/D genotype, others have either I/I or D/D. The amino acid sequence of the ACE protein is not affected by the presence/absence of the I allele, but blood concentrations are highest in the D/D genotype and lowest in I/I. An early study showed that the persons with two I alleles (I/I genotype) seem to have better endurance performance capacity than those with the D/D genotype,[26] but this is not always the case.[27] More studies are needed to confirm the physiologic consequences of such genetic variants and exactly how they exert their effects.

## SUMMARY

The need for increased oxygen transport to working muscles is the basis for the changes in the cardiovascular system that accompany endurance training. The following central (heart size and blood volume) and peripheral (muscle-based) factors contribute to the increase in $\dot{V}O_2$ max: 1) muscle cells increase their aerobic energy-producing capacity, 2) the maximal cardiac output increases to provide increased oxygen-delivery capacity, and 3) vascular system adjustments occur that direct flow to the specific muscles in need of increased oxygen. In resistance training, the muscles contract at a high percentage of maximal force, reducing or stopping blood flow. The cardiovascular system experiences high pressures for the short duration of resistance exercise, and, if training at high volume continues for months, cardiac adaptations occur. Probably systemic vascular changes occur in resistance training but these need to be studied more. The aerobic capacity of resistance-trained muscles is not changed.

## PRACTICAL APPLICATIONS

The sports nutritionist should be knowledgeable about acute exercise responses and adaptations to long-term training.

1. Acute exercise response—the demands of exercise on the circulation are great.
   1.1 Athletes should have a physical examination before beginning demanding sport training. An important component of the physical examination is the detection of heart abnormalities.
   1.2 Because circulatory adjustments may compromise blood flow to the gastrointestinal system, it is prudent to restrict meal intake to >3 hours before competition or a heavy training bout.
   1.3 Stroke volume is dependent on venous return, which is dependent, in part, on blood volume. Three volume-related factors impair intravascular pressure:
      1.3.1 Blood pressure drives fluid out of the vascular space
      1.3.2 Diversion of blood to the skin during exercise
      1.3.3 Loss of fluid as a result of sweating

Therefore, hydration before, during, and after acute exercise, especially of long duration, is critical.

2. Adaptations to training:
   2.1 Structural adaptations (growth of capillaries, increased muscle mass, increased heart size) require weeks to months to occur. Diet should provide nutrition to support the structural changes.
   2.2 Enzymatic adaptations (for example, muscle enzymes of beta oxidation, glycolysis) occur quickly and require little in the way of dietary measures.
   2.3 Rest is important to allow the body time to synthesize proteins that comprise the structural changes.
   2.4 Refueling is important to maintain training quality so that training adaptations may occur as expected.
   2.5 Hydration should be monitored during endurance training because chronic dehydration is possible with repeated endurance bouts.
   2.6 Anemia and endurance—iron is a component of hemoglobin and the importance of dietary iron cannot be overstated. Female athletes are at risk for anemia, and anemia will decrease aerobic endurance performance.

## QUESTIONS

1. Probably the best single indicator of physical fitness is:
   a. $\dot{V}O_2$ max
   b. The ventilatory threshold
   c. Resting heart rate
   d. Blood pressure at maximal exercise

2. Resting ventilation is:
   a. Usually <10 L/min
   b. Usually >10 L/min
   c. Greater than $\dot{V}O_2$ max
   d. None of these

3. Which of the following increases during progressive exercise to maximal capacity?
   a. Systolic blood pressure
   b. Diastolic blood pressure
   c. Ventilation
   d. Oxygen uptake
   e. All but b

4. A typical value for $\dot{V}O_2$ max in a young adult who is untrained is:
  a. $15\,mL\cdot kg^{-1}\cdot min^{-1}$
  b. $35\,mL\cdot kg^{-1}\cdot min^{-1}$
  c. $55\,mL\cdot kg^{-1}\cdot min^{-1}$
  d. $75\,mL\cdot kg^{-1}\cdot min^{-1}$

5. The main components of the oxygen transport system are:
  a. The neural system and the muscles
  b. The pulmonary system, its capillaries, and the pulmonary vein
  c. The pulmonary system, the pulmonary vein, the heart, the systemic arterial system, blood oxygen transport capacity, and the muscle
  d. The heart, the aorta, and the major vessels that branch from it to the limbs

6. Men and women differ in $\dot{V}O_2$ max because of:
  a. Traditional differences in the approach to training
  b. Differences in blood hemoglobin concentration
  c. Lower center of gravity in women
  d. Decreased blood pressure in women

7. Cardiac output refers to:
  a. The total amount of blood pumped per minute
  b. The amount of blood pumped during a single ventricular contraction
  c. The amount of oxygen consumed per minute
  d. The blood volume × hemoglobin concentration

8. Endurance athletes have ____ compared with resistance-trained athletes.
  a. Higher resting blood pressure
  b. Higher resting cardiac output
  c. Higher $\dot{V}O_2$ max
  d. Lower ventilation rate

9. Capillary density refers to:
  a. The amount of protein in the walls of the capillaries
  b. The number of capillaries per unit of muscle
  c. The mean distance from an arteriole to the muscle mitochondria

10. The highest $\dot{V}O_2$ max values have been recorded in which groups of athletes?
  a. Golfers and skateboarders
  b. Power lifters and bodybuilders
  c. Dancers and basketball players
  d. Football players
  e. Distance runners and triathletes

11. During ventilation, which actions expand the pulmonary cavity?
  a. Contraction of the diaphragm
  b. Contraction of the external intercostals muscles
  c. Contraction of the internal intercostals muscles
  d. Both a and b

12. What is the Valsalva maneuver?
  a. Rapid shallow breathing
  b. Maximal exhalation which collapses the lungs
  c. Slow deep breathing
  d. A conscious breathing maneuver often used during maximal weight-lifting

13. Which is the correct pathway traveled by oxygen from outside the body to the muscle?
  a. Systemic arteries, heart, lungs
  b. Lungs, pulmonary artery, heart, systemic arteries, muscles
  c. Lungs, pulmonary artery, heart, veins, muscles
  d. Lungs, pulmonary vein, heart, systemic arteries, muscles
  e. None of the above

14. Blood levels of hemoglobin and hematocrit are:
    a. Vital to oxygen transport
    b. Often higher in women than men
    c. Unimportant for attainment of a high $\dot{V}O_2$ max
    d. Determined by the number of muscle fibers present in the body

15. What is erythropoietin?
    a. A strength-increasing substance that is a member of the family of steroid hormones
    b. An oxygen-carrying hormone
    c. A hormone produced by the kidneys that stimulates red blood cell production
    d. A hormone produced by the liver that increases slow twitch muscle fibers

16. What qualities of muscle are needed for a high $\dot{V}O_2$ max?
    a. High mitochondrial volume and high aerobic enzyme activities
    b. Low levels of myoglobin and small mitochondrial volume
    c. Increased capillary number
    d. More than one of the above

17. Ventilation at maximal exercise may be ____ times higher than rest.
    a. 10
    b. 20–30
    c. 100
    d. 200

18. Which is NOT a rapidly occurring cardiovascular response to acute exercise?
    a. Increase in stroke volume
    b. Increase in the mitochondrial volume
    c. Increase in blood pressure
    d. Increase in ventilation

19. What is the ventilatory threshold?
    a. The ventilation at maximal exercise
    b. During gradually increasing exercise, the point at which the increase in ventilation becomes curvilinear
    c. During gradually increasing exercise, the point at which ventilation stabilizes
    d. During gradually increasing exercise, the point at which ventilation decreases

20. Which is the only systemic cardiovascular response that is not expected to increase with exercise?
    a. Diastolic blood pressure
    b. Oxygen uptake
    c. Ventilation
    d. Systolic blood pressure
    e. More than one of the above

21. Which is higher in the trained runner compared with the sedentary person?
    a. $\dot{V}O_2$ max
    b. Resting ventilation
    c. Maximal ventilation
    d. Heart size
    e. All but one of the above

22. Why might aerobic athletic performance be decreased in hot weather?
    a. Muscles become too warm to function
    b. Dehydration may decrease blood volume and cardiac output
    c. Cardiac output is diverted away from muscle and to the skin for cooling
    d. Because most athletes feel sluggish in warm weather
    e. Both c and d are true

23. What physiologic differences exist in the trained endurance athlete compared with the sedentary person?
    a. Higher resting cardiac output
    b. Lower stroke volume
    c. Larger left ventricle
    d. Fewer capillaries in the muscle

24. Blood flow through a muscle is momentarily suspended when the muscle contracts at ____ or more of its maximal force-generating capacity.
    a. 10%
    b. 20%
    c. 30%
    d. None of the above

25. During performance of resistance exercise:
    a. Blood pressure typically decreases
    b. Systolic pressure increases whereas diastolic decreases
    c. Systolic pressure and diastolic pressure increase
    d. Systolic pressure decreases and diastolic increases

26. Maximal heart rate:
    a. Is higher in trained athletes
    b. Is generally unchanged in athletes or slightly decreased
    c. Is higher in truly elite runners
    d. Is higher in truly elite bodybuilders

27. The left ventricular internal diameter at diastole is greatest in:
    a. Sedentary persons
    b. Runners
    c. Wrestlers
    d. Power athletes such as shot putters

28. The left ventricular wall thicknesses are greatest in:
    a. Sedentary persons
    b. Runners
    c. Power athletes such as shot putters

29. Which is true about the quality of muscle in resistance-trained versus endurance-trained athletes?
    a. Mitochondrial volume is decreased
    b. Contractile proteins are increased
    c. Capillaries are increased
    d. The aerobic energy system has less capacity
    e. All are true except c

30. Genetic research on exercise performance:
    a. Suggests that genes determine, to some extent, who becomes a great athlete
    b. Suggests that many, many genes have a role in determining how well an athlete responds to training
    c. Has shown that angiotensin-converting enzyme gene variants may affect endurance performance
    d. Is in its infancy
    e. All of the above are true

# REFERENCES

1. Wilmore JH, Costill DL. Physiology of Sport and Exercise. Champaign, IL: Human Kinetics; 1999.
2. Powers SK, Howley ET. Exercise Physiology. Theory and Application to Fitness and Performance. New York: McGraw-Hill; 2001.
3. Plowman SA, Smith DL. Exercise Physiology for Health, Fitness, and Performance. San Francisco: Benjamin Cummings; 2003.
4. McArdle WD, Katch FI, Katch VL. Exercise Physiology. Energy, Nutrition, Performance. Baltimore: Lippincott, Williams & Wilkins; 2001.

5. Aaron EA, Seow KC, Johnson BD, Dempsey JA. Oxygen cost of exercise hyperpnea: implications for performance. J Appl Physiol 1992;72:1818–1825.

6. Gardner GW, Edgerton VR, Barnard RJ, Bernauer EM. Cardiorespiratory, hematological and physical performance responses of anemic subjects to iron treatment. Am J Clin Nutr 1975;28:982–988.

7. Chernecky CC, Berger BJ. Laboratory Tests and Diagnostic Procedures. Philadelphia: W.B. Saunders; 2004.

8. Tokish JM, Kocher MS, Hawkins RJ. Ergogenic aids: a review of basic science, performance, side effects, and status in sports. Am J Sports Med 2004;32:1543–1553.

9. Anonymous. Olympics: tests throw up six more drug cases. New Zealand Herald; 2004.

10. Holloszy JO. Biochemical adaptations in muscle. Effects of exercise on mitochondrial oxygen uptake and respiratory enzyme activity in skeletal muscle. J Biol Chem 1967;242:2278–2282.

11. Essen B, Jansson E, Henriksson J, Taylor AW, Saltin B. Metabolic characteristics of fibre types in human skeletal muscle. Acta Physiol Scand 1975;95:153–165.

12. Andersen P, Saltin B. Maximal perfusion of skeletal muscle in man. J Physiol 1985;366:233–249.

13. Dempsey JA, Harms CA, Ainsworth DM. Respiratory muscle perfusion and energetics during exercise. Med Sci Sports Exerc 1996;28:1123–1128.

14. Zhou B, Conlee RK, Jensen R, Fellingham GW, George JD, Fisher AG. Stroke volume does not plateau during graded exercise in elite male distance runners. Med Sci Sports Exerc 2001;33:1849–1854.

15. Gledhill N, Cox D, Jamnik R. Endurance athletes' stroke volume does not plateau: major advantage is diastolic function. Med Sci Sports Exerc 1994;26:1116–1121.

16. Rowell LB, O'Leary DS, Kellogg DL Jr. Integration of Cardiovascular Control Systems in Dynamic Exercise. New York: Oxford University Press; 1996.

17. Blomqvist CG, Saltin B. Cardiovascular adaptations to physical training. Annu Rev Physiol 1983;45:169–189.

18. American College of Sports Medicine. Guidelines for Exercise Testing and Prescription. Baltimore: Williams & Wilkins; 2000.

19. Barcroft H, Millen JLE. Blood flow through the muscle during sustained contractions. J Physiol 1939;97:17–27.

20. MacDougall JD, Tuxen D, Sale DG, Moroz JR, Sutton J. Arterial blood pressure response to heavy resistance exercise. J Appl Physiol 2000;58(3):785–790.

21. Fleck SJ, Kraemer WJ. Designing Resistance Training Programs. Champaign, IL: Human Kinetics Publishers; 2004.

22. Hickson RC, Foster C, Pollock ML, Galassi TM, Rich S. Reduced training intensities and loss of aerobic power, endurance, and cardiac growth. J Appl Physiol 1985;58(2):492–499.

23. Puffer JC. Overview of the athletic heart syndrome. In: Thompson PD, ed. Exercise and Sports Cardiology. New York: McGraw-Hill; 2001:30–42.

24. Chilibeck PD, Syrotuik DG, Bell GJ. The effect of strength training on estimates of mitochondrial density and distribution throughout muscle fibres. Eur J Appl Physiol Occup Physiol 1999;80:604–609.

25. McCall GE, Byrnes WC, Dickinson A, Pattany PM, Fleck SJ. Muscle fiber hypertrophy, hyperplasia, and capillary density in college men after resistance training. J Appl Physiol 1996;81:2004–2012.

26. Montgomery HE, Marshall R, Hemingway H, et al. Human gene for physical performance. Nature 1998;393:221–222.

27. Frederiksen H, Bathum L, Worm C, Christensen K, Puggaard L. ACE genotype and physical training effects: a randomized study among elderly Danes. Aging Clin Exp Res 2003;15:284–291.

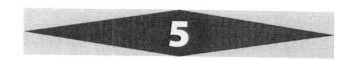

# Molecular Biology of Exercise and Nutrition

## Darryn S. Willoughby

## OBJECTIVES

On the completion of this chapter you will be able to:

1. Understand the basic steps associated with the flow of genetic information.
2. Explain how genes regulate the adaptive processes associated with exercise.
3. Describe different regulatory proteins and how they activate or inhibit specific signaling pathways.
4. Understand the interaction between a ligand and a receptor complex.
5. Describe how signals are passed through cell membrane to initiate specific signaling pathways.
6. Explain how a polypeptide is initiated.
7. Describe how a polypeptide is translated into a functional protein.
8. Understand how newly synthesized proteins are manipulated.
9. Explain the specific mechanisms associated with the degradation of proteins.
10. Describe specific proteolytic pathways.
11. Understand the balance between anabolism and catabolism.
12. Explain the relationship between anabolic and catabolic hormones and how they relate to protein turnover.

## ABSTRACT

The basis for improvements in exercise performance typically revolves around the systemic processes, that is, what happens at the molecular level, that govern our body's ability to adapt to various methods of training and nutritional intervention. It is a well-known and accepted fact that many of these processes of adaptation are governed by regulatory signals centered at the molecular level; however, at present, many of these signals are not well elucidated. For instance, these signals are many times responsible for regulating the activity of protein synthesis. Furthermore, protein synthesis is, in many ways, completely dependent on the expression patterns of various genes which, when up-regulated, are responsible for initiating the cascade of events leading to the synthesis of a respective protein. This being the case, exercise and nutrition provide potent stimuli through which many exercise-responsive genes are expressed. Additionally, a person's nutritional status and dietary habits can oftentimes have significant roles in regulating the molecular regulatory mechanisms that seem to govern many of the processes of physiologic adaptation to exercise. Because of the overwhelming complexity of this topic, it should be understood by the

From: *Essentials of Sports Nutrition and Supplements*
Edited by J. Antonio, D. Kalman, J. R. Stout, M. Greenwood, D. S. Willoughby, and G. G. Haff © Humana Press, a part of Springer Science+Business Media, Totowa, NJ

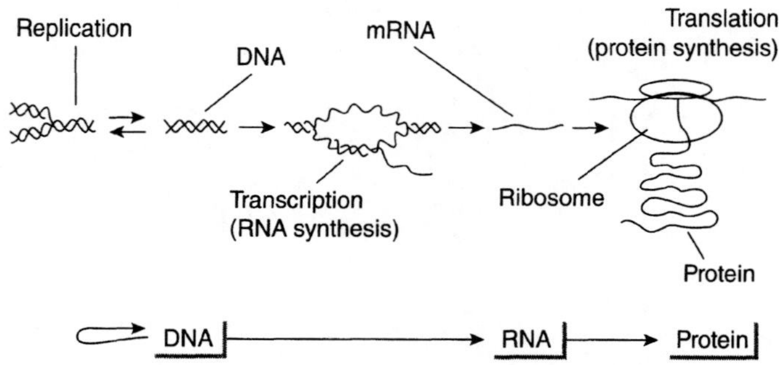

**FIGURE 5.1.** An illustration of the central dogma of molecular biology.

reader that information contained in this chapter will only provide a general overview of the molecular aspects of exercise and nutrition. Also, many of the molecular principles discussed herein occur in many different cell and tissue types. However, because of the nature of this textbook, bias will primarily be given to skeletal muscle because it is a tissue highly susceptible to exercise adaptation. Also, because the central dogma of molecular biology is based on the premise that molecular responses are primarily involved in protein synthesis, this chapter focuses more on the role of protein rather than the other macronutrients, carbohydrates and fats.

*Key Words:* **gene expression, protein synthesis, transcription, translation, muscle adaptation, myogenic regulatory factors**

## THE CENTRAL DOGMA OF MOLECULAR BIOLOGY

The central dogma of molecular biology is based on the principle that the flow of genetic information travels from DNA to RNA and finally to the translation of proteins. Figure 5.1 presents an oversimplified illustration of this process. DNA can self-replicate in the nucleus of a cell by using one strand of the double helix as a template and the enzyme DNA polymerase. The DNA also codes for mRNA (messenger RNA) in a process called transcription. The mRNA is then transported out of the nucleus and into the cytoplasm where proteins are formed through a process called translation.

Translation utilizes the 20 different amino acids (9 essential and 11 nonessential) to synthesize proteins. All of the genes contained within our DNA are called the genome. The central dogma relies on the premise that one gene encodes for one protein and therefore the human genome defines the complement of all the expressed proteins of an individual, or the proteome. Not surprisingly, the synthesis of a protein from a gene sequence is subject to complex processes. Subsequently, further posttranslational modifications (changes in the protein's structure that occur after a protein has been produced from its mRNA) are oftentimes essential for the appropriate function of many proteins. Furthermore, proteins interact with each other (and other macromolecules) in complex ways, which typically have various regulatory consequences on intracellular metabolism.

## GENE EXPRESSION: THE FOUNDATION OF PHYSIOLOGIC ADAPTATION TO EXERCISE

Some genes are expressed, or turned on to produce their specific proteins, in some parts of our bodies and not in others. Another set of genes code for proteins that regulate the expression of genes. These regulatory genes and their protein products form complex interacting systems that ultimately control the mechanisms involved in instigating, controlling, and maintaining various physiologic adaptations to exercise. There are data showing that heavy resistance training increases the gene expression of various muscle-specific genes, most notably myosin heavy chain isoforms.[1] Gene expression, however, is

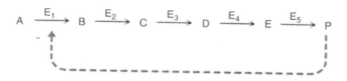

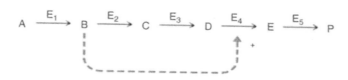

**FIGURE 5.2.** Diagrammatic representation of the processes of feedback (top) and feedforward (bottom) regulation involved in regulating gene expression.

highly controlled and regulated as a result of various feedback and feedforward mechanisms (Figure 5.2) involved in signal transduction and, in many cases, are still not well understood.

An example of regulatory proteins that control the expression of various skeletal-muscle specific genes, such as myosin heavy chain, troponin, actin, and creatine kinase, is the family of so-called DNA binding proteins known as the myogenic regulatory factors. These proteins, named individually as Myo-D, myogenin, MRF-4, and myf-5 are transcription factors known to bind to DNA sequences at specific points along the gene's promoter (a gene's ignition switch) and up-regulate gene expression. Therefore, the binding of a regulatory protein to the DNA of a gene can either activate the gene (promoting its expression) or block it (thereby preventing or blunting expression), as in the case of the DNA binding protein Id-1. That is to say, there are "ON" switches and there are "OFF" switches within muscle-specific genes that are referred to as enhancers and silencers, respectively (Figure 5.3). It has been shown that exercise and certain types of nutritional intervention can change the activity of these myogenic regulatory factors. For instance, even single bouts of resistance exercise can increase the expression and subsequent binding of Myo-D, myogenin, and MRF-4, while subsequently decreasing the activity of Id-1. These changes are correlated to the increased expression of the genes encoding both the slow and fast types of the myosin heavy chain.[2] In addition, it was shown that creatine supplementation in conjunction with a heavy-resistance training protocol preferentially up-regulated the expression of the gene encoding the slow and fast types of myosin heavy chain[3] and the enzyme creatine kinase.[4]

# SIGNALING CONTROL OF TRANSCRIPTION

Transcription is typically activated when a transcription factor protein binds to the specific sequence called the promoter within a gene and activates the enzyme RNA polymerase. What happens next is that the bound protein

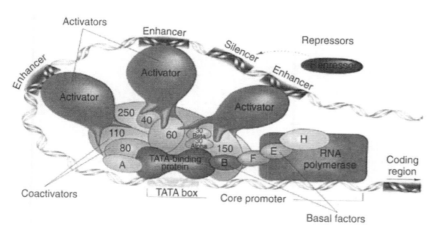

**FIGURE 5.3.** Illustration of a transcription complex highlighting the basal transcription factors along with the regulatory control elements factors such as enhancers and silencers involved in regulating gene expression.

**FIGURE 5.4.** Illustration of testosterone (ligand) and androgen receptor interaction and its downstream effects on gene transcription. T = testosterone, AR = androgen receptor, HSP = heat shock protein, DHT = dihydrotestosterone, ARE = androgen response element, TF = transcription factor.

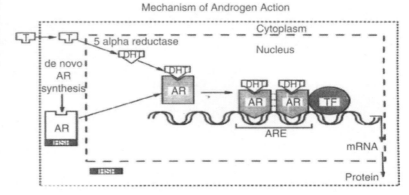

undergoes a change that eventually results in the activation of transcription. In many cases, intracellular receptor proteins also serve as a transcription factor when they become bound with their respective signaling protein. The molecule that binds a receptor protein is called a ligand, and once bound forms a ligand–receptor complex. Ligands can be small molecules such as protein or a steroid hormone such as testosterone that pass through the cell membrane, bind with the androgen receptor, and activate transcription directly, as illustrated in Figure 5.4. However, there are also protein molecules that cannot move through the cell membrane, either because of their size, electrical charge, or solubility, and must find a receptor protein that resides in the cell membrane. Once the membrane receptor becomes bound with its ligand, then signaling transduction pathways are activated in which transcription is initiated somewhat indirectly (not as direct result of ligand–receptor complex binding with DNA), as illustrated in Figure 5.5. An example of this process is insulin binding with the insulin receptor and facilitating the uptake of glucose into the muscle cell. It is well established that various forms of exercise, nutritional intervention, and supplementation can have profound effects on the extent to which transcriptional control mechanisms are regulated.

## ACTIVATION OF TRANSCRIPTION VIA SIGNAL TRANSDUCTION PATHWAYS

If the receptor is found in the membrane of the cell, a series of signals must be passed through the membrane to intercellular molecules, which in turn activate transcription. This series of signals is called a signal transduction pathway. Receptor kinases are a class of membrane-bound receptor proteins and have the ability to phosphorylate (add phospate groups) other proteins. This receptor protein binding and activation can be the beginning of the signaling pathway that eventually results in the activation of transcription. There are also intra-

**FIGURE 5.5.** Illustration of the insulin-signaling pathway regulating cellular glucose uptake.

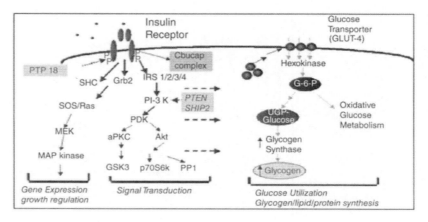

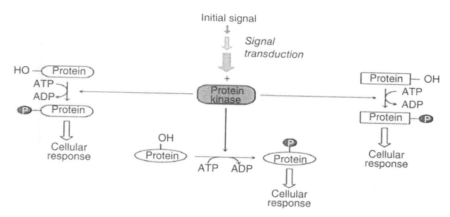

**FIGURE 5.6.** Diagrammatic representation of the role of a protein kinase enzyme involved in a signal transduction pathway. ATP = adenosine triphosphate, ADP = adenosine diphosphate.

cellular kinase enzymes that will cause phosphorylation within the pathway, whereas phosphatase enzymes result in dephosphorylation (removal of a phosphate group). This intermittent signal process of phosphorylation and dephosphorylation is known as covalent modification and serves as a type of activation and deactivation of the signaling proteins. Figures 5.5 and 5.6 illustrate that this signal is passed through several intracellular proteins where eventually a transcription factor is modified such that it activates transcription. An example of this is the insulin-signaling pathway mediated by increases in the levels of carbohydrate (glucose) in the blood. The increased pancreatic secretion of the peptide hormone insulin binds with glucose and then inevitably insulin receptors. This binding generates a response that facilitates a process of signal transduction that elicits a cascade of physiologic effects, many resulting in gene expression, in skeletal muscle and adipose tissue.

## PROTEIN TRANSLATION: THE BIRTH OF A POLYPEPTIDE

Translation is the process by which the information contained in the nucleotide sequence of mRNA instructs the synthesis of a particular polypeptide (a molecule consisting of amino acids connected by peptide bonds). This process, outlined in Figure 5.7, has been divided into three phases: initiation, elongation, and termination, and it is regulated by soluble proteins called initiation factors, elongation factors, and termination factors.

Initiation consists of the reactions wherein the first aminoacyl-transfer RNA and the mRNA are bound to the ribosome and carries the amino acid methionine. The first reactions involve the formation of an initiation complex consisting of methionyl-initiator tRNA bound to the 40S ribosomal subunit. This reaction is catalyzed by initiation factor 2 (eIF2), which binds the initiator methione-tRNA to the 40S ribosomal subunit. Initiation factor 4 (eIF4) IF4E then unwinds the helical shape of mRNA. The 40S ribosomal subunit then travels down the message until it reaches a termination signal. Only after the

**FIGURE 5.7.** An illustration of the three steps involved in protein translation.

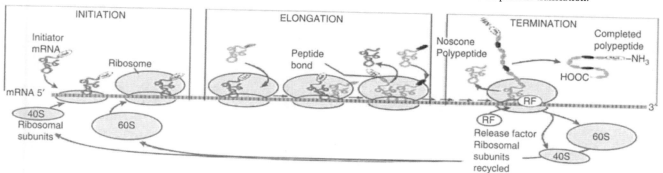

mRNA has been properly positioned on the small ribosomal subunit can the 60S ribosomal subunit bind. This completes the initiation reaction.

During elongation, as amino acids are joined together, the ribosome travels down the mRNA. This allows another ribosome to bind to the mRNA and also begin initiation. Thus, any mRNA usually will have several ribosomes attached to it. This structure is then called a polyribosome or, more commonly, a polysome. The termination of protein synthesis takes place when a termination signal on the mRNA is exposed on the ribosome. The ribosome then separates into its two subunits, and the cycle of translation repeats itself if the appropriate signals are present.

## OUTCOME OF PROTEIN TRANSLATION: THE SYNTHESIS OF A FUNCTIONAL PROTEIN

During translation, once signaling sequences are recognized, they terminate the translation of polypeptides. Once polypeptides are synthesized, many will need to undergo additional processing, known as posttranslational modification, in which the polypeptide's primary structure (sequence of attached amino acids) will need to undergo changes in its structure to assume a shape that will allow the polypeptide to become a fully active protein. Proteins have four primary structures and are primary, secondary, tertiary, and quaternary (Figure 5.8). The primary structure of peptides and proteins refers to the linear number and order of the amino acids present. The convention for the designation of the order of amino acids is that the structure contains an N-terminal end (end bearing the residue with the free amino group) and a C-terminal end (end with the residue containing a free carboxyl group). The outcome of this process is to create a fully functional protein.

The ordered array of amino acids in a protein confers regular conformational forms upon that protein. These conformations constitute the secondary structures of a protein. In general, there are two categories of secondary structure for proteins termed globular or fibrous proteins. Globular proteins typically contain an α-helix and are compactly folded and coiled, whereas fibrous proteins are more filamentous or elongated. Whereas an α-helix is composed of a single linear array of helically disposed amino acids, β-sheets are composed of two or more different regions of "sheet-like" stretches of at least 5–10 amino acids. Within a single protein, different regions of the polypeptide chain may assume different conformations determined by the primary sequence of the amino acids.

Tertiary structure refers to the complete three-dimensional structure of the polypeptide units of a given protein. Included in this description is the spatial relationship of different secondary structures to one another within a polypeptide chain and how these secondary structures themselves fold into the three-dimensional form of the protein. Many proteins contain two or more different

**FIGURE 5.8.** An illustration of the four different types of protein structures.

(a) Primary structure

– Ala – Glu – Val – Thr – Asp – Pro – Gly –

(b) Secondary structure

α helix

β sheet

(c) Tertiary structure

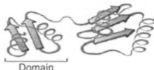

Domain

(d) Quaternary structure

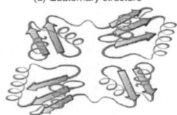

polypeptide chains that are held in association by the same noncovalent forces that stabilize the tertiary structures of proteins. Proteins with multiple polypeptide chains are termed oligomeric proteins. The structure formed by monomer–monomer interaction in an oligomeric protein is known as quaternary structure. Oligomeric proteins can be composed of multiple identical polypeptide chains or multiple distinct polypeptide chains. The inevitable outcome of translation is the synthesis of proteins with a variety of specific functions.

## MOLECULAR CHAPERONES

The folding of many newly synthesized proteins in the cell depends on a set of conserved proteins known as molecular chaperones. These prevent the formation of misfolded protein structures, both under normal conditions and when cells are exposed to stresses such as high temperature. Most, but not all, heat shock proteins are molecular chaperones. Molecular chaperones bind and stabilize proteins at intermediate stages of folding, assembly, translocation across membranes, and degradation. Heat shock proteins have been classified by molecular weight, for example, HSP-70 for the 70-kDa heat shock protein. HSP-70 is expressed at a much reduced level in unstressed conditions, but it has an important role in the export of proteins to the cytoplasm and in protein degradation during periods of physiologic stress. The inducible or activated version of cytosolic HSP-70, known as HSP-72, is now better described as a stress protein because it is known to be expressed at temperatures that deviate from the norm and also during periods of cell stress that are known to result in proteolysis (such as with intense exercise or significant caloric restriction). It has been shown that HSP-72 is significantly expressed during periods of high-intensity eccentric exercise and muscle injury[5] and denervation resulting from spinal cord injury.[6] Along with HSP-72 exists a constitutively expressed heat shock protein cognate (HSC-70 or HSP-73) which participates in protein translocation across membranes and other functions.

Molecular chaperones such as HSP-72 interact with unfolded or partially folded protein subunits (e.g., nascent chains emerging from the ribosome, or extended chains being translocated across subcellular membranes) to stabilize nonnative conformation and facilitate correct folding of protein subunits. They do not interact with native proteins, nor do they form part of the final folded structures. Some chaperones are nonspecific, and interact with a wide variety of polypeptide chains, but others are restricted to specific targets. They often couple adenosine triphosphate (ATP) binding/hydrolysis to the folding process (Figure 5.9). Essential for viability, the expression of molecular chaperones is often increased by cellular stress where their primary role seems to be to stabilize unfolded proteins, unfold them for translocation across membranes or for degradation, and/or to assist in their correct folding and assembly (Figure 5.10). In general, molecular chaperones prevent inappropriate association or aggregation of exposed hydrophobic surfaces and direct their substrates into productive folding, transport, or degradation pathways.

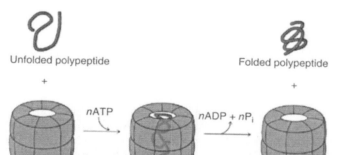

**FIGURE 5.9.** A generalized view of the role of a molecular chaperone in protein folding. ATP = adenosine triphosphate, ADP = adenosine diphosphate.

Unfolded polypeptide

Folded polypeptide

$nATP$

$nADP + nP_i$

Chaperone

**FIGURE 5.10.** Diagrammatic representation of a specific molecular chaperone (heat shock protein 72) and its role in posttranslational modification of protein structure. ATP = adenosine triphosphate.

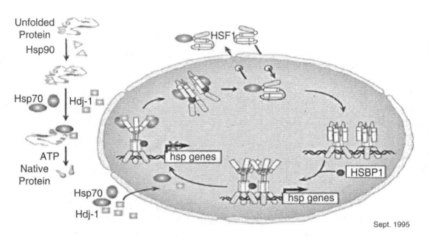

# MECHANISMS OF INTRACELLULAR PROTEIN DEGRADATION

Protein molecules are continuously synthesized and degraded in all living organisms. The concentration of individual cellular proteins is determined by a balance between the rates of synthesis and degradation, which in turn are controlled by a series of regulated biochemical mechanisms. Differences in the rates of protein synthesis and breakdown result in an imbalance in the anabolism/catabolism ratio. The degradation rates of cellular proteins are highly regulated but critically important in helping to establish and maintain an appropriate cellular concentration for the given cellular environment at that particular time. For instance, cellular concentrations vary greatly in the same individual whether they are sedentary, involved in an exercise-training program, or detraining. If an individual consistently consumes a hypocaloric diet, particularly coupled with exercise, then the likelihood of them inducing varying levels of intracellular protein degradation is significant. An individual also assumes the same risk if they consistently consume too little protein in their diet while also participating in an exercise program.

Protein degradation is energy dependent, requiring ATP, and is limited by the concentration of the reactants, whereas protein synthesis cannot be completed in the absence of any one of the necessary reactants. Protein can degrade at rates ranging from 100% per hour during periods of extreme physiologic and/or pathologic stress to less than 10% per hour, and their half-lives (time taken for loss of half the protein molecules) may vary anywhere between the order of 24 to 72 hours. Regulatory enzymes and proteins have much shorter half-lives of the order of 5 to 120 minutes and protein breakdown can take place in the mitochondria and endoplasmic reticulum, but occurs mainly in one of two major sites of intracellular proteolysis, lysosomes and the cytosol. Short-lived regulatory proteins are degraded in the cytosol by local proteolytic mechanisms. All short-lived proteins are thought to contain recognition signals that mark them for early degradation. The individual degradation rates of proteins vary within a single organelle or cell compartment and also from compartment to compartment, because of either differing sensitivity to local proteases or differing rates of transfer to the cytosol or lysosomes.

Because proteins exist as a linear chain of amino acids (polypeptide), they can degrade over time in response to various physiologic elements such as heat, acid, and enzymes. When proteins degrade over time, this is called protein turnover. It is the balance between a protein's degradation and its synthesis that determines the concentration of that protein inside the cell. Protein turnover rates have shown that some proteins are short-lived whereas others are long-lived. Long-lived proteins constitute the majority of proteins in the cell. Short-lived proteins are typically key regulatory proteins.

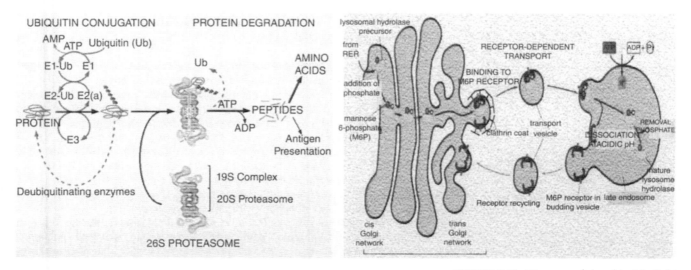

**FIGURE 5.11.** Diagrams of the ubiquitin (left) and lyosomal (right) proteolytic pathways. ATP = adenosine triphosphate, ADP = adenosine diphosphate.

There are three well-characterized intracellular proteolytic systems in skeletal muscle. One system is the lysosomal pathway (Figure 5.11). Lysosomes are responsible for the nonselective degradation of many macromolecules, including proteins, and mostly degrade soluble and extracellular proteins. Lysosomes are organelles that contain a powerful mixture of proteases, peptidases, and other hydrolases capable of degrading most intracellular and extracellular macromolecules. The proteases responsible for the degradation of proteins inside lysosomes are called cathepsins. In general, lysosomes have been considered to be responsible for the continuous basal turnover of most intracellular proteins (mainly long-lived proteins) in liver, kidney, and certain other tissues. The lyosomal pathway is not thought to be significantly involved in the degradation of myofibrillar protein and has only a minor role in the overall proteolytic activity in skeletal muscles. The rates of lysosomal degradation can vary greatly with cell type and conditions.

Another system is the calcium-dependent proteases (calpains), which primarily degrade cytoskeletal but not myofibrillar proteins and are mostly involved in limited proteolysis of some specific target proteins. Calpains constitute a major cytosolic proteolytic system. The activity of these neutral, thiol proteases is tightly regulated by intracellular calcium levels. Calpains are translocated to the cell membrane where they are able to partially degrade membrane and cytoskeletal proteins and several membrane-associated enzymes.

The third system is the ATP-dependent ubiquitin pathway in which proteins are degraded by multiple enzymes requiring ATP (Figure 5.11). This system involves the selective breakdown of abnormal and short-lived regulatory proteins but seems to be the primary system for degradation of the majority of myofibrillar proteins. Whereas the ubiquitin system seems mainly responsible for myofibrillar protein degradation, the calpain system has an important role in initiating muscle protein degradation. This is attributed to the fact that the ubiquitin system does not degrade intact myofibrils. Therefore, the calpain system is able to release myofibrillar proteins for degradation by the ubiquitin system. In the absence of changes in the proteasome activity, a reduction in protein ubiquitination could also result in reduced intracellular protein breakdown. The fact that changes in protein ubiquitination do not always indicate changes in protein degradation rates may reflect the participation of ubiquitin in intracellular processes other than protein degradation. The ubiquitin pathway is often up-regulated in response to physiologic stressors. It has been shown that various crucial components of the ubiquitin pathway such as free ubiquitin, the E2 ubiquitin conjugating enzyme, the E3 ubiquitin protein ligase, and the 20S proteasome are up-regulated in response to muscle injury caused by eccentric contractions,[5] during periods of muscle immobilization,[7] and muscle paralysis caused by spinal cord injury.[6,8]

## ANABOLISM VERSUS CATABOLISM ...
## AN ONGOING RATIO

The numerous and complex biochemical processes that comprise the body's metabolism can be generally classified as either anabolism or catabolism. In very simplistic rationale, this can be thought of as the anabolism/catabolism ratio. Anabolism is the building up of complex molecules, whereas catabolism is their breakdown. Figure 5.12 illustrates that to synthesize biomolecules and sustain life, the body requires energy in the form of ATP. This energy is liberated from the breakdown of nutrients such as glucose and fatty acids. So, for molecular construction to occur, molecular destruction must go on at the same time to release the energy required to drive the biochemical reactions. When anabolism exceeds catabolism, net growth occurs. Therefore, there is an increased anabolism/catabolism ratio. For example, with resistance training when muscle protein synthesis exceeds protein degradation, muscle hypertrophy (increases in muscle mass) occurs.[9] However, with a decreased anabolism/catabolism ratio, catabolism exceeds anabolism and a net loss occurs. For example, with muscle inactivity and immobilization, muscle protein degradation exceeds protein synthesis and muscle atrophy (decreases in muscle mass) occurs.[7]

Anabolism includes the chemical reactions that cause different molecules to combine to larger, more complex ones. The net result of anabolism is the creation of new cellular material, such as cytoskeletal proteins, structural proteins, contractile proteins, and enzymes. Typically, in anabolism, small precursor molecules are assembled into larger organic molecules. This always requires the input of energy (often as ATP) because anabolism is necessary for growth, maintenance, and tissue repair. Catabolism includes the chemical reactions that denature complex molecules into simpler ones for energy production. This process usually occurs with the release of energy (usually as ATP), for recycling of cellular components or for their excretion. If energy is produced, it is typically either used immediately to perform cellular work (e.g., muscle contraction) or stored as glycogen in skeletal muscle and/or liver, or fat in skeletal muscle and/or adipose tissue. By reducing the rate of catabolism, anabolism is increased, resulting in faster recovery from exercise, stress, injury, and a higher level of performance and an increased growth rate. Both anabolism and catabolism are necessary for survival and good health, and understanding these processes can help one make good decisions about exercise and diet. From this perspective, it should be somewhat clear that one's diet should be adequate in regard to total calories along with an appropriate ratio of macronutrients that correspond to the type of exercise, along with the volume and intensity, in which one is engaged. Simply being in a hypocaloric state, regardless of the macronutrient ratio, can instigate catabolic mechanisms thereby decreasing the anabolism/catabolism ratio. Therefore, to help ensure that protein synthesis exceeds degradation, a person should be aware of their nutritional and dietary needs relative to their exercise-training regimen. Some nutritional supplements may help to augment protein synthetic mechanisms or also blunt protein proteolytic mechanisms. However, these will be of benefit only if a proper nutritional approach is routinely practiced.

**FIGURE 5.12.** An illustration of the general components involved in cellular anabolism and catabolism.

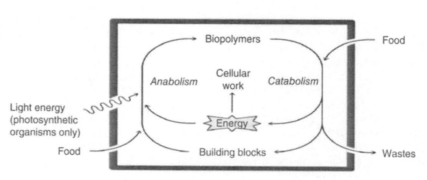

# HORMONAL CONTROL OF CELLULAR FUNCTION

The endocrine system is involved in maintaining the normal functional cellular environment through the release of hormones. Hormones are cell-signaling substances secreted from various tissues within the body (usually categorized as endocrine glands) that exert a physiologic response on appropriate target tissues. Hormones regulate mechanisms controlling growth, development, and reproduction, and augment the body's capacity for handling physical and psychologic stress. Hormones differ in how they affect their target cells, and are classified as amine, peptide, or steroid. Amine hormones are derived from amino acids, whereas peptide hormones are structured by peptide bonds between multiple amino acids. Amine and peptide hormones are soluble and are transported in blood plasma in solution. The water-soluble characteristics of amine and peptide hormones make them easily removed from the circulation but allow only a short time (minutes) to exert their function. Steroid hormones are not water soluble and therefore must be bound to plasma proteins to be transported through cell membranes where they are then able to bind to their intracellular receptors for translocation to the nucleus for DNA binding to their appropriate hormone response element.

The major function of hormones is to alter the rates of cellular reactions assisted with their specific target cells. This is typically accomplished by altering the rate of intracellular protein synthesis, changing the rate of enzyme activity, modifying plasma membrane transport, and by inducing secretory activity. Hormones are able to reach virtually all tissues because they travel in the blood. However, the ability for a target tissue to respond to a hormone depends on the presence of specific membrane-bound or intracellular receptors. Amine and peptide hormones exert their action on target cells by binding to specific receptors on the membrane of the target tissue. In response to the hormone binding to its receptor, an enzymatic reaction by way of enzymes such as adenyl cyclase or tyrosine kinase will produce a second messenger molecule typically known as cyclic adenosine monophosphate (cyclic AMP), which initiates a signal transduction cascade of covalent modification then inevitably stimulates a cellular response. Control of hormone secretion must be rapid in order to meet the demands of changing bodily functions. Hormone secretion is usually pulsatile in nature and constant hormone release rarely exists. The predominant hormonal control mechanism is feedback regulation, discussed above (Figure 5.2).

Testosterone, growth hormone (GH), and insulin-like growth factor (IGF)-1 are sensitive to mechanical overload and the levels of each increase in response to resistance training. These hormones have specific receptors responsible for cell signaling located at the cell membrane or within the cell. Testosterone is produced in the testes (women's ovaries produce small amounts of testosterone). There are androgen receptors located within muscle cells and androgen response elements within muscle-specific genes that these receptors bind and facilitate gene transcription. Resistance training also increases testosterone production. There are data showing testosterone to increase after sequential bouts of heavy resistance exercise in males that corresponded in concomitant increases in the up-regulation of the gene and protein expression for the intracellular androgen receptor in skeletal muscle.[10] Testosterone works in opposition to cortisol; therefore, the challenge is to maximize the hypertrophic effects of testosterone while minimizing the atrophic effects of cortisol. Therefore, one would desire an elevated testosterone/cortisol ratio. Most IGF-1 is derived from the liver, and there exists a feedback mechanism by which IGF-1 feedback to the hypothalamus and pituitary regulates GH secretion. However, IGF-1 is synthesized in skeletal muscle independent of GH release upon mechanical overload, and IGF-1 receptors are increased in response to resistance training. A variant of IGF-1 called mechano-growth factor (MGF) is expressed in muscle and is thought to act in an autocrine/paracrine manner to cause muscle hypertrophy. GH is a peptide hormone synthesized by the anterior pituitary gland and is released after acute bouts of high-intensity resistance training. GH facilitates the transport of amino acids into cells and the subsequent synthesis of protein. This exerts a stimulatory effect on IGF-1 and affects carbohydrate and fat metabolism. It stimulates glucose uptake in muscle and fat, and mobilizes free fatty acids from adipose tissue.

Cortisol is a catabolic hormone that reduces body protein stores in all tissues except the liver. The body reacts to high-intensity resistance training as it would to any stressor by increasing the secretion of cortisol from the adrenal gland. Cortisol helps maintain blood glucose levels by breaking down muscle protein into amino acids by way of the ubiquitin system, which the liver then converts to glucose by gluconeogenesis. It has been shown that eccentric exercise increases cortisol secretion, and decreases myofibrillar protein content, which is likely linked to the associated increases in the expression of the ubiquitin pathway.[11] Insulin opposes cortisol, but high stress activity can promote cortisol domination over insulin. When elevated in the blood, cortisol enters the muscle cells where it binds with its glucocorticoid receptor; this hormone receptor complex then binds on ubiquitin pathway-related genes and accelerates proteolysis.[11] It has also been shown that elevated cortisol and a glucocorticoid receptor-mediated mechanism are associated with an up-regulation expression in myostatin during heavy resistance training.[9] Cortisol can inhibit GH levels by stimulating the release of somatostatin (a GH antagonist). It may also reduce the expression of IGF-1.

## SUMMARY

The basis for improvements in exercise performance typically revolves around the systemic processes, that is, what happens at the molecular level, that govern our body's ability to adapt to various methods of training and nutritional intervention. It is a well-known and accepted fact that many of these processes of adaptation are governed by regulatory signals centered at the molecular level; however, at present, many of these signals are not well elucidated. For instance, these signals are many times responsible for regulating the activity of protein synthesis. Furthermore, protein synthesis is, in many ways, completely dependent on the expression patterns of various genes which, when up-regulated, are responsible for initiating the cascade of events leading to the synthesis of a respective protein. Involved in this cascade are the events of transcription, translation, and posttranslation modification. Each of these three events contains multiple regulatory steps that can be highly sensitive to an individual's exercise training and nutritional status. To maintain a physiological balance favoring exercise adaptation, an individual must attempt to keep themselves in an overall anabolic state conducive to adaptation. This involves a person's nutritional status and dietary habits which can oftentimes have a significant role in regulating the molecular regulatory mechanisms that seem to govern many of the processes of physiologic adaptation to exercise.

## PRACTICAL IMPLICATIONS

Both acute and chronic exercise induces a myriad of molecular responses that regulate physiologic adaptations on multiple physiologic levels. Additionally, both endurance and resistance exercise result in the integration of a numerous amount of biochemical and physiologic mechanisms that regulate the cardiorespiratory, neuromuscular, and neuroendocrine systems, to also instigate exercise-induced adaptations. These system adaptations occur as a result of changes on the tissue and cellular level, and adaptations on the cellular level in turn depend on qualitative and quantitative shifts in gene expression. Furthermore, the appropriately governed cells respond to the stimulus of repeated exercise bouts by changing their patterns of gene expression. The molecular regulatory network in which many of these exercise-induced adaptations are established is based on nutritional issues, particularly those dealing with macronutrient metabolism. Carbohydrate and fat are essential because they provide oxidative power in providing a critical link to the synthesis of ATP energy substrate whereas dietary protein is critical in providing the necessary amino acids for protein synthesis.

## GLOSSARY OF TERMS

*Anabolism*: The building up of complex molecules.

*Catabolism*: The breakdown of complex molecules.

*DNA polymerase*: An enzyme that binds to DNA and assists in replication.

*Endocrine system*: A system of various organs and glands that have the ability to secrete hormones into the blood.

*Genome*: All of the genes contained within DNA.

*Hormone*: Cell-signaling substances secreted from various tissues within the body (usually categorized as endocrine glands) that exert a physiologic response on appropriate target tissues.

*Myogenic regulatory factors*: A group of DNA binding proteins in skeletal muscle that serves as transcription factors by regulating the expression of various genes.

*Oligomeric proteins*: Proteins with multiple polypeptide chains.

*Polypeptide*: A linear chain of amino acids attached by a peptide bond that constitutes a protein's primary structure.

*Promoter*: A short nucleotide sequence within a gene that serves as the starting point for transcription.

*Proteome*: The complement of all the expressed proteins of an individual.

*Quaternary structure*: A protein composed of four subunits of tertiary structure.

*RNA polymerase*: An enzyme that binds to the promoter sequence on the DNA and assists in transcription.

*Signal transduction pathway*: An intracellular pathway in which various proteins are intermittently activated and deactivated by the levels of their phosphorylation in order to elicit a cellular response, oftentimes resulting in gene expression.

*Tertiary structure*: The complete three-dimensional structure of the polypeptide units of a given protein.

*Transcription*: The process in which DNA codes for mRNA (messenger RNA) and produces a template for translation.

*Translation*: The process in which the 20 different amino acids (9 essential and 11 nonessential) are used to synthesize proteins from the mRNA template.

## QUESTIONS

1. During DNA replication, a new DNA strand is synthesized using one strand as a template by which of the following enzymes?
   a. RNA polymerase
   b. Phosphorylase
   c. Tyrosine kinase
   d. DNA polymerase

2. What enzyme has a role in assisting transcription once transcription factors bind to the gene's promoter?
   a. Creatine kinase
   b. DNA polymerase
   c. RNA polymerase
   d. Lactate dehydrogenase

3. Which of the following are characteristics of mRNA?
   a. Synthesized from a DNA template strand by the enzyme RNA polymerase
   b. Relies on elongation factors for transcription
   c. Is a double stranded, α-helical molecule
   d. Undergoes DNA replication

4. Which of the following steps are not involved in the process of translation?
   a. Initiation
   b. Elongation

c. Extension
d. Termination

5. Which of the following are true of translation?
   a. Amino acids are used to create a polypeptide
   b. Proteins are not degraded by protease enzymes
   c. Myogenic regulatory factors cause termination
   d. Exercise cannot facilitate increases in protein synthesis

6. A short nucleotide sequence within a gene that serves as the starting point for transcription is the:
   a. mRNA
   b. Promoter
   c. Transcription factor
   d. Ribosome

7. A linear chain of amino acids attached by a peptide bond that constitutes a protein's primary structure is:
   a. mRNA
   b. Polypeptide
   c. Transcription factor
   d. β-Pleated sheet

8. A system of various organs and glands that have the ability to secrete hormones into the blood is known as the:
   a. Cardiovascular system
   b. Neuromuscular system
   c. Endocrine system
   d. Pulmonary system

9. The tertiary structure of a protein is defined as:
   a. A sequence of amino acids attached by a peptide bond
   b. An arrangement of protein into either an α-helix or β-pleated sheet
   c. The complete three-dimensional structure of the polypeptide
   d. A protein composed of four subunits of tertiary structure

10. The folding of many newly synthesized proteins in the cell depends on the assistance from a set of proteins known as:
    a. DNA binding proteins
    b. RNA polymerase
    c. Molecular chaperones
    d. Kinase enzymes

11. The process in which DNA codes for mRNA and produces a template for translation is known as:
    a. Transcription
    b. Replication
    c. Translation
    d. Posttranslational modification

12. The process in which both essential and nonessential amino acids are used to synthesize proteins from the mRNA template is known as:
    a. Transcription
    b. Replication
    c. Translation
    d. Posttranslational modification

13. What kind of enzymes are a class of membrane-bound receptor proteins with the ability to phosphorylate other proteins?
    a. Phosphatases
    b. Phosphorylases
    c. Polymerases
    d. Kinases

14. Once polypeptides are synthesized, the processing in the primary structure many will need to undergo to assume a shape that will allow for a fully active protein is known as:
    a. Transcription
    b. Replication
    c. Translation
    d. Posttranslational modification

15. Which of the following hormones are anabolic with regards to skeletal muscle?
    a. Insulin
    b. Testosterone
    c. Growth hormone
    d. All of the above

16. Which of the following contain proteases and are responsible for the non-selective degradation of many macromolecules, including proteins, and mostly degrade soluble and extracellular proteins?
    a. Peroxisomes
    b. Mitochondria
    c. Lysosomes
    d. Creatine kinase

17. Which of the following is a calcium-dependent protease, primarily degrades cytoskeletal but not myofibrillar proteins, and is mostly involved in limited proteolysis of some specific target proteins?
    a. Lysosome
    b. Calpain
    c. Cathepsin
    d. Ubiquitin

18. Which proteolytic system involves the selective breakdown of abnormal and short-lived regulatory proteins but seems to be the primary system for degradation of the majority of myofibrillar proteins?
    a. Ubiquitin system
    b. Lysosome system
    c. Calcium-dependent calpain system
    d. Protease system

19. The process in which chemical reactions cause different molecules to combine to larger, more complex ones resulting in the creation of new cellular material, such as cytoskeletal proteins, structural proteins, contractile proteins, and enzymes is known as:
    a. Proteolysis
    b. Catabolism
    c. Anabolism
    d. Muscle atrophy

20. The process in which chemical reactions denature complex molecules into simpler ones for energy production and usually occurs with the release of energy for recycling of cellular components or for their excretion is known as:
    a. Protein synthesis
    b. Catabolism
    c. Anabolism
    d. Muscle hypertrophy

21. Which of the following types of molecules have cell-signaling functions, are secreted from endocrine glands that exert a physiologic response on appropriate target tissues, and regulate mechanisms controlling growth, development, and the body's capacity for handling physical and psychologic stress?
    a. Hormones
    b. Nucleic acids
    c. Kinase enzymes
    d. Carbohydrates

22. During the elongation phase of translation, which of the following prevent inappropriate association or aggregation of exposed hydrophobic surfaces and direct their substrates into productive folding, transport, or degradation pathways?
    a. RNA polymerase
    b. Myogenic regulatory factors
    c. DNA binding proteins
    d. Molecular chaperones

23. The principle that the flow of genetic information travels from DNA to RNA and finally to the translation of proteins is referred to as:
    a. A signal transduction pathway
    b. The central dogma of molecular biology
    c. The ligand-receptor complex
    d. An intracellular degradation pathway

24. Which of the following terms describe a control process in which gene expression can be regulated?
    a. Large ribosomal subunit
    b. Feedback
    c. Elongation factor
    d. 20S proteasome

25. The protein, oftentimes a hormone, that binds with its associated membrane or intracellular receptor in order to initiate a physiologic response is referred to as a:
    a. Ribosome
    b. Transcription factor
    c. Elongation factor
    d. Ligand

26. An enzyme known to have a role in the removal of phosphate groups from molecules involved in signal transduction pathways is referred to as a:
    a. Phosphorylase
    b. Phosphatase
    c. Kinase
    d. Ligase

27. Which of the following is not considered an intracellular degradation pathway?
    a. Lysosomal
    b. Calcium-dependent calpain
    c. Ubiquitin
    d. Covalent modification

28. Which of the following is not considered a steroid hormone?
    a. Insulin
    b. Testosterone
    c. Cortisol
    d. Estrogen

29. In regard to skeletal muscle, if the rate of protein synthesis exceeded the rate of protein degradation, then the net result would favor:
    a. Muscle atrophy
    b. Muscle hypertrophy
    c. DNA replication
    d. Muscle proteolysis

30. In regard to skeletal muscle, if the rate of protein degradation exceeded the rate of protein synthesis, then the net result would favor:
    a. Muscle atrophy
    b. Muscle hypertrophy
    c. DNA replication
    d. Muscle strength

# REFERENCES

1. Willoughby DS, Pelsue S. Effects of high-intensity strength training on steady-state myosin heavy chain isoform mRNA expression. J Exerc Physiol 2000;3(4):13–25.
2. Willoughby DS, Nelson M. Myosin heavy chain mRNA expression after a single session of heavy resistance exercise. Med Sci Sports Exerc 2002;34(8):1262–1269.
3. Willoughby DS, Rosene J. Effects of oral creatine and resistance training on myosin heavy chain expression. Med Sci Sports Exerc 2001;33(10):1674–1681.
4. Willoughby DS, Rosene JM. Effects of oral creatine and resistance training on myogenic regulatory factor expression. Med Sci Sports Exerc 2003;35(6):923–929.
5. Willoughby DS, Rosene J, Myers J. Ubiquitin and HSP-72 expression and apoptosis after a single session of eccentric exercise. J Exerc Physiol 2003;6(2):88–95.
6. Willoughby DS, Priest J, Nelson M. Expression of the stress proteins, ubiquitin and HSP-72, and myofibrillar protein content after 12 weeks of leg cycling in persons with spinal cord injury. Arch Phys Med Rehabil 2002;83(5):649–654.
7. Willoughby DS, Sultemeire S, Brown M. Human muscle disuse atrophy after 28 days of immobilization in a lower-limb walking boot: a case study. J Exerc Physiol 2003; 6(2):96–104.
8. Willoughby DS, Priest J, Jennings R. Myosin heavy chain isoform and ubiquitin protease mRNA expression after passive leg cycling in persons with spinal cord injury. Arch Phys Med Rehabil 2000;81(2):157–163.
9. Willoughby DS. Effects of heavy resistance training on myostatin mRNA and protein expression. Med Sci Sports Exerc 2004;36(4):574–582.
10. Willoughby DS, Taylor L. Effects of sequential bouts of resistance exercise on androgen receptor expression. Med Sci Sports Exerc 2004;36(9):1499–1506.
11. Willoughby DS, Taylor M, Taylor L. Glucocorticoid receptor and ubiquitin expression after repeated eccentric exercise. Med Sci Sports Exerc 2003;35(12):2023–2031.

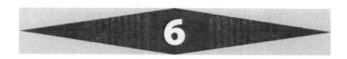

# Aspects of Overtraining

## Mike Greenwood

## OBJECTIVES

On the completion of this chapter you will be able to:

1. Differentiate between overreaching and overtraining.
2. Describe the physiologic signs and symptoms of overtraining.
3. Explain the differences between parasympathetic and sympathetic overtraining.
4. Understand the physiologic and psychologic consequences of overtraining.
5. Illustrate the major factors that make up the central fatigue hypothesis.
6. Describe the major components of a needs analysis.
7. Understand the basic components of a periodized training program.
8. Explain the role of glutamine, protein, vitamin C, zinc, and Echinacea as tools for avoiding overtraining.
9. Illustrate the role of sound nutrition in the prevention of overtraining.
10. Conceptualize the role of nutrient timing in the prevention of overtraining.
11. Understand the importance of maintaining appropriate hydration.
12. Describe the dietary carbohydrate, protein, and fat needs of athletes.

## ABSTRACT

The road to a safe, effective, and enjoyable fitness and athletic lifestyle should be considered an ultramarathon and not a 100-meter sprint. The often quoted phrase that "Rome was not built in one day" really holds credence here because of the number of annual exercisers that initiate an exercise protocol only to quit within a few weeks because they did not attain the desired results in "their" specified time frame. Because of inappropriate dietary habits and or training protocols that lead to overreaching (short-term) and overtraining (long-term), decrements of physiologic and psychologic outcomes occur in many exercisers (Kreider et al. In: Kreider et al., eds. Overtraining in Sport. Champaign, IL: Human Kinetics Publishers; 1998:vii–ix). Whereas intense training is necessary to optimize performance, intense training over prolonged periods can hinder performance. The truth of the matter is, although it may take a person 30 or 40 years to display their current physical fitness state, it is human nature to want to immediately become, although unrealistic, the next Mr. or Ms. Olympia overnight. Yes, an effective athletic or fitness lifestyle becomes a journey and not a weekend vacation that involves the development of knowledge, patience, proper nutritional practices, variety, commitment and tenacity,

From: *Essentials of Sports Nutrition and Supplements*
Edited by J. Antonio, D. Kalman, J. R. Stout, M. Greenwood, D. S. Willoughby, and G. G. Haff © Humana Press, a part of Springer Science+Business Media, Totowa, NJ

not to mention hard work, in order for a person to reach and maintain their optimal athletic/exercise/fitness goals. Although research supports a plethora of reasons why people abandon exercise protocols (Weinberg and Gould. Foundations of Sport and Exercise Psychology. Champaign, IL: Human Kinetics Publishers; 1999:371–395), the scientific literature has varied on the precise reasons why and how the processes of overreaching/overtraining occur and can be reduced or eliminated. With these elements in mind, the purpose of this chapter is to present the following information: 1) physiologic and psychologic effects of overtraining related to sport and exercise, 2) valid fitness and health assessment guidelines to limit aspects of overtraining, 3) strength and conditioning periodization design to reduce occurrences of overtraining, and 4) scientific-based nutritional strategies to promote and prevent overtraining with exercise and sport populations.

*Key Words:* **overtraining, overreaching, central fatigue, delayed onset muscle soreness [DOMS], periodization**

## OVERREACHING AND OVERTRAINING IN SPORT AND EXERCISE

Although most scientific experts agree that the overreaching and overtraining phenomenon exists, the confusion in the literature regarding this topic is centered on the variety of terms and stages used to describe or define this process. The issue of overreaching and overtraining is further complicated with numerous physiologic and psychologic explanations of why and how this phenomenon occurs as well as how this process affects every individual differently. Although terms such as overworked, overstressed, and burnout have been used to describe this process, for the purposes of this chapter an established definition of overreaching and overtraining is presented to evaluate this phenomenon relative to sport and exercise participants.

In their "Overtraining in Sport" text, the authors define overreaching as "an accumulation of training and/or non-training stress resulting in short term decrements in performance capacity with or without related physiological and psychological signs and symptoms of overtraining in which restoration of performance capacity may take from several days to a few weeks."[1] Sometimes, because of a variety of physiologic and psychologic factors that are not completely understood, a state of overreaching may easily lead to a longer, more permanent state of overtraining. Whereas performance standard decrements have been noted as the "gold standard" measure of the overtraining syndrome,[2] there is some degree of variation concerning the duration of substandard performance that would qualify as overtraining.[3] Therefore, a more serious scenario to consider is the "accumulation of training or non-training stress resulting in long term decrements in performance capacity with or without related physiological and psychological signs and symptoms of overtraining in which restoration of performance capacity may take several weeks or months."[1] It is also important to note that the overtraining phenomenon has been explained as a process that occurs in four progressive stages (Table 6.1).[4]

## PHYSIOLOGIC SYMPATHETIC AND PARASYMPATHETIC OVERTRAINING

Although the definitions of overreaching and overtraining provide a foundational base to understand this phenomenon, they do not paint a complete picture for comprehending this entire process. Specifically, in the literature, overtraining has been segmented into the distinct categories of sympathetic and parasympathetic paradigms.[5,6] Sympathetic overtraining has been predominately affiliated with aspects of anaerobic exercise such as power and strength parameters of resistance training. However, parasympathetic overtraining is typically compared with aerobic activities such as long endurance

**TABLE 6.1. Theoretical development of anaerobic overtraining.**

| Stages of overtraining | Neural | Skeletal muscle | Metabolic | Cardiovascular | Immune | Endocrine | Psychologic |
|---|---|---|---|---|---|---|---|
| 1st (no effect on performance) | Altered neuron function | | | | | | |
| 2nd (probably no effect on performance) | Altered motor unit recruitment | | | | | Altered sympathetic activity and hypothalamic control | |
| 3rd (probably decreased performance) | Decreased motor coordination | Altered excitation-contraction coupling | Decreased muscle glycogen | Increased resting heart rate and blood pressure | Altered immune function | Altered hormonal concentration | Mood disturbances |
| 4th (decreased performance) | | Decreased force production | Decreased glycolytic capacity | | Sickness and infection | | Emotional and sleep disturbances |

*Source:* Kraemer.[4] Originally published in Kreider R, Fry AC, O'Toole M. Overtraining in Sport. Champaign, IL: Human Kinetics; 1998. Reprinted with permission.

exercise. It should be noted that the majority of research dedicated to this topic has been primarily centered on parasympathetic overtraining (aerobic) participants because many scientific experts believe that sympathetic (anaerobic) overtraining markers are much more difficult to accomplish via resistance training protocols compared with endurance exercise training regimens.[1] However, a variety of sympathetic and parasympathetic markers have been cited in the research literature that include but are not limited to physiologic aspects such as altered exercise performance, biochemical and immunologic signs and symptoms of overtraining. (Tables 6.2 and 6.3).[4,7] Performance decrements can occur as a result of large increases in training volume/intensity/frequency, lack of rest/recovery days, limited nutritional intake, the central fatigue hypothesis (discussed below), and not acknowledging possible overtraining markers that are brought on by varying exercise protocols.[8]

**TABLE 6.2. The major signs and symptoms of overtraining described in the literature.**

**Physiologic/performance**
Decreased performance
Inability to meet previously attained performance standards or criteria
Recovery prolonged
Reduced toleration of loading
Decreased muscular strength
Decreased maximum work capacity
Loss of coordination
Decreased efficiency/decreased amplitude of movement
Reappearance of mistakes already corrected
Reduced capacity of differentiation and correcting technical faults
Increased difference between lying and standing heart rate
Abnormal T wave pattern in electrocardiogram
Heart discomfort on slight exertion
Changes in blood pressure
Changes in heart rate at rest, exercise, and recovery
Increased frequency of respiration
Perfuse respiration
Decreased body fat
Increased oxygen consumption at submaximal workloads
Increased ventilation and heart rate at submaximal workloads
Shift of the lactate curve toward the $x$-axis
Decreased evening postworkout weight
Elevated basal metabolic rate
Chronic fatigue
Insomnia with and without night sweats
Thirst

*(Continued)*

**TABLE 6.2.** *Continued*

Anorexia nervosa
Loss of appetite
Bulimia
Amenorrhea/oligomenorrhea
Headaches
Nausea
Increased aches and pains
Gastrointestinal disturbances
Muscle soreness/tenderness
Tendonostic complaints
Periosteal complaints
Muscle damage
Elevated C-reactive protein
Rhabdomyolysis

**Psychologic/information processing**
Feelings of depression
General apathy
Decreased self-esteem/worsening feelings of self
Emotional instability
Difficulty in concentrating at work and training
Sensitive to environmental and emotional stress
Fear of competition
Changes in personality
Decreased ability to narrow concentration
Increased internal and external distractibility
Decreased capacity to deal with large amounts of information
Gives up when the going gets tough

**Immunologic**
Increased susceptibility to and severity of illness/colds/allergies
Flu-like illnesses
Unconfirmed glandular fever
Minor scratches heal slowly
Swelling of the lymph glands
One-day colds
Decreased functional activity of neutrophils
Decreased total lymphocyte counts
Reduced response to mitogens
Increased blood eosinophil count
Decreased proportion of null (non-T, non-B lymphocytes)
Bacterial infection
Reactivation of herpes viral infection
Significant variations in CD4:CD8 lymphocytes

**Biochemical**
Negative nitrogen balance
Hypothalamic dysfunction
Flat glucose tolerance curves
Depressed muscle glycogen concentration
Decreased bone mineral content
Delayed menarche
Decreased hemoglobin
Decreased serum iron
Decreased serum ferritin
Lowered total iron-binding capacity
Mineral depletion (Zn, Co, Al, Mn, Se, Cu, etc.)
Increased urea concentrations
Elevated cortisol levels
Elevated ketosteroids in urine
Low free testosterone
Increased serum hormone binding globulin
Decreased ratio of free testosterone to cortisol of more than 30%
Increased uric acid production

*Source:* Fry et al.[7] Reprinted with permission granted from Adis Press International.

**TABLE 6.3.** Signs and symptoms of anaerobic and aerobic overtraining.

| *Markers of anaerobic overtraining* | | *Markers of aerobic overtraining* |
| --- | --- | --- |
| • Psychologic effects: decreased desire to train, decreased joy from training<br>• Acute epinephrine and norepinephrine increases beyond normal exercise-induced levels (sympathetic overtraining system)<br>• Performance decrements, although these occur too late to be a good predictor Unfortunately, because of the limited markers available for anaerobic overtraining, many athletes and coaches monitor the markers of aerobic overtraining whereas typically do not monitor anaerobic overtraining. | • Decreased performance<br>• Decreased percentage of body fat<br>• Decreased maximal oxygen uptake<br>• Altered blood pressure<br>• Increased muscle soreness<br>• Decreased muscle glycogen<br>• Altered resting heart rate<br>• Increased submaximal exercise heart rate<br>• Decreased lactate<br>• Increased creatine kinase | • Altered cortisol concentration<br>• Decreased total testosterone concentration<br>• Decreased ratio of total testosterone to cortisol<br>• Decreased ratio of free testosterone to cortisol<br>• Decreased ratio of total testosterone to sex hormone-binding globulin<br>• Decreased sympathetic tone (decreased nocturnal and resting catecholamines)<br>• Increased sympathetic stress response |

*Source:* Kraemer.[4] Reprinted with permission.

## PSYCHOLOGIC MARKERS OF OVERTRAINING

The majority of psychologic research investigating overtraining paradigms has sought to determine how mood state and personality factors relate to this process.[2] Psychologic researchers have suggested that the overtraining phenomenon causes negative mood states and negatively alters the dynamic mental health model.[3] Of the mood states investigated, fatigue and vigor are considered the most sensitive psychologic overtraining markers, whereas depression and anger provide valuable insight regarding the onset of psychologic overtraining that can lead to performance decrements and mood disturbance.[3] The profile of mood states is a common measure used to evaluate the category of psychologic overtraining (Table 6.1).

As mentioned above, the underlying cause for all overtraining markers is not well understood. Recently reviewed research in this area has focused on the potential mechanisms for the overtraining phenomenon. Explanations deemed plausible include: 1) increased serotonin levels caused by training-induced alterations in nutrient metabolism, 2) inadequate carbohydrate intake, 3) the combined effect of exercise and life stress causing the exerciser to reach the exercise exhaustive stage of the general adaptation syndrome, 4) chronic changes to the neuroendocrine environment (i.e., sympathetic-adrenal medullary or hypothalamic-pituitary-adrenocortical axis), 5) increased incidence of infection or other maladaptive immune response, and 6) disturbance of mood state or onset of depression.[9] Complicating the matter further, the underlying etiology of overtraining for endurance athletes may be different for individuals who engage primarily in intense, anaerobic exercise (Table 6.1).[9]

## CENTRAL FATIGUE HYPOTHESIS

Researchers once believed that fatigue displayed from intense prolonged exercise was primarily caused by peripheral muscle glycogen depletion and possible hypoglycemia.[10-12] Although this was once an accepted explanation for the occurrence of exercise fatigue, additional research findings suggest the "central fatigue hypothesis" as a possible explanation for the onset of this dilemma. As noted earlier in this chapter, limited nutritional intake can lead to performance decrements and as a result exercise-induced fluctuations in the central nervous system or more precisely the central fatigue hypothesis.[12-17]

Central fatigue hypothesis is a theory that suggests that changes in the central nervous system brought on by exercise may result in fatigue after extensive exercise. Various researchers have theorized that during exercise, along with the decline of muscle glycogen fuel, there is an increased oxidation of fat and the branched-chain amino acids (BCAAs) leucine, isoleucine, and valine are used as fuel substrates.[12-17] This results in a decreased availability in the blood of BCAAs, which increases levels of free fatty acids (FFAs). The increase of FFA levels in the blood is accompanied by a release of the amino acid tryptophan from albumin. The release of tryptophan from albumin serves to increase the level of free tryptophan in the blood resulting in a steady increase in the ratio of free tryptophan to BCAA as one continues to exercise.

Exercise-induced imbalances in the ratio of free tryptophan to BCAA have been implicated as a possible cause of central fatigue, both physiologic and psychologic. Although additional research is warranted in this area, the entry of tryptophan into the brain increases as the ratio of free tryptophan to BCAA increases. It has been reported that increased concentrations of tryptophan in the brain promotes the formation of the neurotransmitter 5-hydroxytryptamine, frequently referred to as serotonin. Theoretically, chronic elevations in serotonin levels may be one explanation for the occurrence of various signs and symptoms of overtraining. Increased levels of serotonin in the brain and peripheral tissues have been reported to induce sleep, depress motor neuron excitability, influence autonomic and endocrine function, and suppress appetite in animal and human studies.[13] It should be noted that other researchers believe that heightened levels of free tryptophan and BCAA increase a person's pain threshold levels during exercise which in turn may disguise select markers of fatigue. This disguised pain may make the athlete more susceptible to detrimental levels of injury and negatively affect their health-risk profile.[18] Therefore, it is important that extreme caution be taken in evaluating the overtraining syndrome because confounding markers exist and select individuals show no signs of this process other than decrements in exercise capacity.[19] Finally, nutritional strategy research should continue to be conducted to enhance the possibility of reducing aspects associated with the central fatigue hypothesis thereby promoting safety and performance outcomes.

## VALUE OF ASSESSMENT CONSIDERATIONS TO LIMIT OVERTRAINING

Before initiating any exercise regimen, it is imperative to determine current physical fitness level, previous/current health status, psychologic status, and nutritional intake. It is extremely vital for athletes and exercise participants to consider their exercise history and health history before creating their blueprint to Caesar's Palace.[20] This baseline information (i.e., exercise experience, hereditary conditions, and previous injuries) becomes valuable in shaping one's exercise program.[20] A more in-depth query may be to determine current functioning fitness level in relation to the noted fitness parameters of flexibility, muscular strength/endurance, cardiorespiratory function, and body composition. Just as an auto mechanic typically runs a battery of tests on one's car to determine where precise problems are located, one should be evaluated by a certified personal trainer, certified strength and conditioning specialist, and in some instances a physician (based on age and/or health history) to determine current level of functioning on the fitness parameters and a variety of health status issues noted earlier in this section.[20] The certified personal trainer or strength and conditioning specialist should be able to administer a variety of valid tests and procedures to assess flexibility, body composition, cardiorespiratory function, speed/agility, and muscular strength, power, and endurance. Once the results from the respective assessment procedures have been collected and analyzed, an exercise recipe (prescription) can be used based on current fitness status. It should be noted that many exercise participants discontinue their fitness programs early on because of injuries derived from limited or inaccurate fitness assessment results. It is critical that a qualified expert (i.e., exercise physiologist, certified exercise specialist, and physician) administer fitness/ health assessments and interpret the results in effort to prescribe the most accurate, safe, and functional exercise training program.

The National Strength and Conditioning Association refer to this process as performing a "needs analysis."[21] What this means, basically, is to design strength and conditioning programs that are sport/activity specific. In other words, the type of training and conditioning that is prescribed is specific to the demands of a given sport (i.e., baseball versus track and field). In addition, prescribing sport-specific training should also be different within a given sport (i.e., quarterbacks versus defensive backs). It is still vital to accrue information about health and exercise history of the athlete. However, the athlete goes through a series of assessments to measure their functional athletic ability and fitness levels but the test results are used to prescribe strength training and conditioning methods based on sport-specific movements. For example, the game of basketball requires a variety of movements (i.e., lateral, vertical, linear) whereas running the 100-meter sprint in track primarily requires linear action. Some sports require more power and explosion in a variety of directions and therefore require specialized training methods such as plyometrics, power lifting, speed development, and agility training. The key aspect to remember is that with proper assessment of the athlete and the specific demands of a given sport, a functional strength and conditioning program can be developed and implemented. It is also imperative to conduct periodic assessments (not just baseline and posttest assessments) to determine if the athlete's strength and conditioning program needs any adjustment based on the progression that has been documented. If one only conducts assessments at the beginning and end of a periodization strategy, it becomes too late to help athletes adjust training programs to reach their optimal individual potentials. Strength and conditioning assessments should be periodic, not just before and after, for optimal potentials and to avoid the overtraining syndrome.

In addition to physiologic and psychologic baseline assessments, it is imperative for a registered dietitian or sports nutritionist to perform and collect dietary records to determine an individual's nutritional status. Categories such as caloric and macronutrient needs, meal ingestion timing, and hydration guidelines are a few vital strategies to address the overtraining phenomena not to mention reaching optimal performance and exercise/fitness outcomes. These specific nutritional strategies and more are discussed in length in various sections below.

## CONCEPT OF PERIODIZATION TO REDUCE OVERTRAINING

Before discussing the valuable issue of exercise program design, it is necessary to first define the concept of periodization in relation to all fitness components. Note that for the purpose of general discussion, only "classic" or "traditional" periodization is discussed. Obviously, additional models of periodization exist (i.e., fitness/fatigue theory, undulating model, repeated mesocycle model), and for complete information on these topics the reader is referred to a valuable discussion provided by Plisk and Stone, published in 2003.[22]

In the United States in the 1960s, periodization became a catch phrase and promoted an "exercise system" that if designed correctly helped to prevent "overtraining" while optimizing peak performance through progressive training cycles.[23] Periodization gained its popularity and application from a physiologic theory called the "general adaptation syndrome" or GAS. GAS refers to the body's ability to adapt to a variety of physiologic stresses associated with exercise programs (i.e., strength training, interval training, and aerobic exercise) that occur in one of three phases. Phase I, or what is frequently termed the "shock or alarm" phase, occurs in the initial phases of the exercise program (first 3–4 weeks depending on the fitness level of the exercise participant) which is primarily a neurologic adaptation to the stress being placed on the body. During phase II, or the "super compensation stage," the human body progressively adapts to exercise stress in the form of various physiologic adjustments (i.e., biochemical, skeletal, muscular, connective tissue, cardiorespiratory). This progressive adaptation continues until the individual reaches their desired exercise/fitness goals or when the optimal performance is paramount during competition. In phase III of GAS, which is to be avoided through proper design, the individual enters into the dreaded "overtraining" phenomena primarily associated with physiologic and psychologic staleness or exhaustion, and hence a decrement of performance occurs. This phase is also referred to as the maladaptation stage. Thus, if one supports the notion of exercise training progression, by manipulating GAS, a systematic plan of periodization can be created to enhance performance and prevent overtraining. This innovative systematic progressive training plan has been labeled "periodization cycles." The initial stage of periodization is frequently referred to as the macrocycle. The macrocycle constitutes the overall training period and plan such as preparing for an athletic competition 1 year in advance. During that year of training, an athlete goes through a series of progressive mesocycles, which can last from weeks to months depending on the program goals and the athlete's progress in reaching optimal performance levels before the competition while also avoiding the "overtraining" phenomena. The mesocycle can be divided into smaller segments (microcylces) which can be periods of 1 week to concentrate on or isolate sport-specific training considerations in the periodization scheme.

Although a variety of periodization schemes can be used, a traditional or classic periodization design for an athlete would/could begin with a series of mesocycles starting with a "transition I phase" which includes active rest with little or no formal training. This transition periodization phase would be considered a detraining phase as opposed to training or nontraining phase with low-volume, nonspecific resistance training and conditioning. The transition phase can be followed with the preparatory period that includes the progressive phases of hypertrophy, strength, and power. After the power phase is complete, athletes and exercise participants move into the maintenance phase. In the maintenance phase, the challenge is to maintain some semblance of the physiologic adaptations (i.e., strength, power, speed, flexibility, aerobic function) that were developed over the course of the annual mesocycles to that point. Although competitive schedules vary from sport to sport, it is vital to select training days when hard, medium, light schedules can be used to avoid overtraining and injuries. It is also vital to note that transition phases have recently been included after each phase of the periodization cycle to promote recovery and limit markers of overtraining. For complete information regarding time by number of weeks, intensity, frequency, and volume of each of the previously mentioned training cycles, please refer to Wathen et al.[23]

Another important aspect of reaching optimal training and sport/exercise performance is the restoration/recovery of training/competition attained by adequate rest/recovery—specifically, adequate sleep. A suggestion of 8–10 hours a day is recommended for individuals involved with intense training and competition to reduce various markers of overtraining. Great caution should be taken to ensure that adequate recovery time is obtained to promote optimal performance results and avoid the negative markers of physiologic, psychologic, environmental (i.e., employment, school, family issues) overtraining, or inadequate nutritional strategies. Specific nutritional strategies used to inhibit overtraining are discussed in detail in the next section.

Since the inception of periodization, various professional sports and fitness experts have learned that in addition to helping athletes reach peak performance at the precise time and avoid overtraining, properly designed periodization exercise programs are not only safe and progressive but individualized and sport/activity specific. In other words, any exercise program protocol can be specifically tailored to meet the fitness/health needs of any person in any situation. This has become increasingly evident with the general fitness population, specialized athletes, and individuals functioning in clinical health environments. The main goal in properly designed periodization schemes is to develop the highest levels of strength and power that is required for an individual athlete/person in their given sport/activity which ultimately promotes optimal performance peaking by avoiding overtraining.

## KEY NUTRITIONAL CONSIDERATIONS FOR ENHANCEMENT OF IMMUNE FUNCTION AND DELAYING CENTRAL FATIGUE

Earlier in this chapter, the central fatigue hypothesis was addressed in relation to the model's effects on markers of overtraining as well as how vital nutrients are involved in this theory. In this section, various nutrients are discussed (i.e., glutamine, protein, vitamin C, zinc, and Echinacea) that have been scientifically shown to enhance immune function and assist in delaying central fatigue.

## The Immune System

The issue of immune suppression is one concern of the overtraining syndrome especially regarding specific markers of anaerobic and aerobic training protocols. There is evidence that moderate levels of training and exercise actually improve immune function whereas exercise protocols that are intense and prolonged inhibit immune status for up to 6 hours after the training or competitive event.[24–26] It is during this 6-hour time period that the athlete or exercise participant is most susceptible in acquiring a variety of immune infections from attacks on the lymphocytes. Although this dilemma can occur in anaerobic and aerobic protocols, it has been primarily noted in research settings with individuals training and competing in endurance activities.[26] Unfortunately, these overtrained individuals become much more susceptible to upper respiratory tract infections (URTIs), which often result in colds or ear infections for extended periods of time.[26,27] When evaluating these factors, it becomes evident that athletes and exercise participants who overtrain for extended periods of time ignite health-risk issues of immune system function. Because of suppressed immune system issues resulting from the overtraining phenomena, it is imperative to investigate and discuss viable nutritional strategies that can assist in reducing central fatigue.

## Glutamine

Glutamine is one of the most abundant "conditional" amino acids in the body that has been shown to be a vital metabolic fuel during exercise for a variety of components of the immune system. Glutamine also has an important role in the enhancement of protein and glycogen synthesis.[28] This is specifically evident with lymphocyte function because below-normal glutamine levels after intense exercise over long periods of time can contribute to immune suppression in overtrained athletes and exercise participants. The reduction of blood glutamine levels (hypoglutamina) from intense prolonged training can last up to 6 hours after training which is why it becomes imperative to replace glutamine levels before, during, or after training in order to enhance recovery and reduce the probability of reaching the overtraining phenomena.[29] Chronically low glutamine levels make it more difficult for the body to respond to attacks on the immune system thereby hindering health profiles and performance outcomes.[27,30–32]

## Protein

A second nutrient that has been effective in bolstering immune system function is protein.[26,33,34] Protein contributes greatly to the nutritional needs of athletes and exercise participants in a variety of ways, and it has been shown to be an effective strategy to enhance energy balance during intense training thereby promoting a healthier immune system while contributing to optimal performance outcomes. Increased protein supplementation has also improved immune function status for clinical patients with protein deficiencies.[34] Other benefits of quality protein ingestion will be discussed later in this chapter, but from the existing research, it is apparent that maintaining a positive protein energy balance contributes to a healthier immune function.

## Vitamin C

The next nutrient that may influence immune status from intense exercise protocols is vitamin C.[35] Vitamin C is considered an antioxidant that assists in iron absorption, and its increased consumption has been shown to reduce endurance athletes' susceptibility to URTIs.[36] In a recent study evaluating responses of neutrophils and lymphocytes during high-intensity physical activity in volunteer athletes, increased vitamin C supplementation positively influenced immune status.[37] Additionally, the researchers noted immune function improvements in athletes who increased their vitamin C intake during a period of strenuous exercise.[38] These researchers also revealed that immune function was not altered with the moderate exercise group. Therefore, vitamin C ingestion enhances immune function and reduces URTIs in athletes participating in intense exercise protocols.

## Zinc

Zinc is considered to be a constituent of enzymes that readily assist in the digestive process. Furthermore, zinc is an essential trace element that constitutes many of the enzymes required for normal metabolism. Similar to vitamin C, zinc supplementation (25–100 mg/d) has been shown to reduce various cold symptoms and therefore helps to limit URTIs.[39–41] Recently, zinc supplementation has been shown to enhance the immune status of hospitalized elderly, and liver plasticity in the elderly.[42,43] Although more extensive research is needed in this area, it may be beneficial to use zinc ingestion strategies to enhance the immune status of individuals under strenuous training protocols because these athletes have been shown to experience zinc deficiencies.[44]

## Echinacea

Finally, Echinacea is a very popular supplement that has been labeled the "immune herb." Similar to the effects of an antibiotic, Echinacea has been used with various animal populations and humans to diminish the onset symptoms of colds and help eliminate URTIs, therefore enhancing immune status.[45–47] Whereas current research shows justification for Echinacea supplementation to enhance immune status, to date, this author is not aware of any studies investigating the effects of Echinacea on immune function with athletic or exercise populations. Obviously, continued research is needed in this area.

## EAT TO COMPETE: DIETARY NECESSITIES TO CONTROL OVERTRAINING AND PROMOTE RECOVERY

### Setting the Dietary Stage

As mentioned previously, signs and symptoms associated with the overtraining phenomenon have been linked to a number of aspects including chronic energy consumption deficits.[1,8,28] To establish a solid nutritional foundation, to adequately set the stage for reaching optimal training/performance outcomes, and to control the elements of overtraining, one need not look any further than a properly designed dietary plan. Although this may seem to be an easy goal to accomplish, the commitment, time, and costs often associated with a quality dietary strategy can make it a difficult task to accomplish. It is widely accepted that athletes in high-intensity training and competition often do not ingest the right types or amounts of macronutrients to offset their energy expenditure. Although nutritional supplementation is a viable alternative for athletes to consume and meet their dietary needs, it cannot completely replace a quality, nutrient-dense diet. It is referred to as nutritional supplementation because it is a complement to a properly designed nutrient-dense diet, not a replacement. In this section, nutritional necessities surrounding an "eat to compete" philosophy are addressed in relation to strategies to control overtraining and promote recovery for athletic and exercise populations.

### Determining Energy Requirements

The most critical aspect of establishing a properly implemented dietary strategy to accomplish optimal performance outcomes is to ensure that exercise participants meet quality caloric needs to balance specific energy expenditure.[1,8,28] When considering this nutritional approach, it is always important to include and calculate individual differences regarding select exercise training intensities. Although recommended daily allowance guidelines have been established regarding daily dietary consumption for general populations, these suggested initiatives may be insufficient for athletic populations involved with intense training protocols because of the greater caloric requirements. For example, daily caloric intake needs for untrained individuals are based on the number of kilocalories per kilogram of body weight per day which usually averages between 1900 to 3000 kcal daily.[11,48] Without question, when adding various factors of exercise into the equation, the frequency, duration, and intensity demands of the training protocol requires increased nutritional intake to maintain an effective energy balance. Individuals involved in low-intensity exercise lasting 30–40 minutes a day that is performed 3 times per week typically require 1800–2400 kcal per day because of minimal physical exertion and energy expenditure.[28,49] Athletes undertaking moderate exercise protocols defined as 5–6 times a week for 2–3 hours a day or intense training 5–6 days a week, 3–6 hours a day obviously have greater dietary needs (2500–8000 kcal/d depending on body weight) compared with individuals involved in light exercise protocols.[1,16] When attempting to accurately evaluate the caloric values needed for individuals involved in the various levels of exercise training, it becomes evident that athletes have a difficult time maintaining ingestion of enough calories with simply a well-balanced diet. Because of the enormous energy expenditure for high-volume intensity training, the combination of nutritional supplementation with a quality nutritional dietary profile makes it much more probable that athletes will consume enough to meet caloric needs. The proper replacement of caloric needs based on energy expenditure not only helps control the possibility of overtraining markers but most definitely heightens the recovery process needed for future optimal training bouts. Although a balanced energy status is vital for all athletes in formalized training, it is even more imperative for larger athletes who must consume huge amounts of quality calories to offset the energy expenditures acquired from high-volume and intensity training. Obviously, the ramifications of inappropriate dietary strategies can be tremendous weight loss and susceptibility to the various signs and symptoms of physiologic and psychologic overtraining. Furthermore, there is scientific evidence that the athlete who undertakes intense training has a greater preponderance to a suppressed appetite, which increases the possibility of health risks and ultimately performance decrements.[14] A great strategic plan is to develop a multidisciplinary team approach that combines athletic coaches, athletic trainers, strength and conditioning coaches, parents, and physicians to closely monitor and evaluate the athlete's nutrient-dense dietary status in effort to maintain body weight, enhance performance, and avoid aspects of the overtraining phenomenon. Besides caloric ingestion concerns for larger athletes, there are other athletic groups that require close monitoring in relation to meeting caloric energy demands. Specifically, female gymnasts and distance runners can be highly susceptible to eating disorders, which jeopardize their ability to meet specific energy caloric needs. This can also occur with athletes who participate in sports such as boxing and wrestling and select unsafe dietary strategies in order to make a particular weight class for competition.

## Nutritional Timing and Refueling

Earlier in the chapter, the issue of rest and recovery, specifically adequate sleep patterns, for athletes involved with intense training and competition was addressed. Recently, sports nutritionists and researchers have placed emphasis on the tremendous value of the timing of adequate dietary ingestion to promote viable recovery strategies. Understanding the value of select but quality nutritional timing is critical for athletes to not only increase strength and muscle mass but to avoid the detrimental aspects of overtraining and central fatigue.

Sports nutritionists and researchers in the Exercise and Sport Nutrition Laboratory at Baylor University have suggested the following guidelines for nutritional timing for athletic populations. To enhance the digestive process, athletes are encouraged to eat a full meal complete with high-energy carbohydrates 4–6 hours before practice or competition. For example, this could include the ingestion of a high-carbohydrate breakfast for afternoon training sessions and a carbohydrate snack for events before noon. Thirty to 60 minutes before practice or competition, athletes should consume a combination carbohydrate (30–50 g) protein (5–10 g) snack or shake to help provide needed energy and reduce catabolism. Ready-to-drink products and bars are convenient options for pretraining and precompetition events because they can help control markers of overtraining. One concern associated with posttraining and competition dietary ingestion is that some athletes simply are not hungry after the intense event. However, this is one of the most critical times to replenish dietary energy balance to offset the tremendous energy expenditure. A viable recommendation is to ingest a postworkout snack of a light carbohydrate/protein (50–100 g of carbohydrates and 30–40 g of protein) within 30–60 minutes after the event; then the athlete should consume a complete dietary meal within the 2-hour supported nutritional recovery window. The postworkout/competition meal should be high in carbohydrates and protein because this is the period when the body is most receptive to energy replenishment which helps sustain the valuable energy balance and assists in avoiding the overtraining syndrome. The general dietary suggested guidelines for athletes during heavy training periods include 55%–65% calories from carbohydrates, 15% from protein, and less than 30% from fat. Sport nutritional specialists recommend that athletes involved in heavy, intense training eat as many as 4–6 meals daily. However, it is recommended that power or strength athletes not consume as many carbohydrates as suggested in these guidelines.

In a recent book entitled "Nutrient Timing," the author's further drive home the importance of proper dietary ingestion based on a finely tuned nutritional schedule.[50] This exceptionally written and scientifically based reading promotes the importance of a "nutritional timing system" that is composed of three vital phases: 1) energy, 2) anabolic, and 3) growth. Whereas the majority of nutritional research has been centered on what to eat, this cutting-edge contribution places tremendous emphasis on what and when to eat. Following the concepts of this book will not only allow the athlete to reach optimal potentials but also help to control detrimental markers of overtraining.

## Proper Hydration: Water—The Fluid of Life

Frequently referred to as the fluid of life necessary for survival, water serves numerous extracellular and intracellular functions in the body such as a variety of vital metabolic functions, interacting with other nutrients such as protein to assist with organ and joint lubrication, while also acting as a much-needed solvent that assists in transporting molecules throughout the body. Without question, water is the most important ergogenic nutritional aid for athletes as a normal balance of water is maintained to avoid dehydration and accomplish optimal training and performance outcomes. The athlete's need for water balance is based on the type of foods ingested, the intensity of the activity, the ambient temperature, individual sweat rates, and the chronologic age of the athlete or exercise participant. Therefore, the regulation of water balance should be based on more than the amount of water lost. A key strategy to promote adequate water balance is to drink plenty of water (4–6 cups or 32–48 ounces) before the training event begins. Two common mistakes in hydration practices is the athlete waiting until the sensation of thirst begins, and trying to rehydrate during training when dehydration has already occurred. It has been noted that a decrement in athletic performance will occur when 2% of body weight is lost through perspiration.[28] The athlete's normal sweat rate can be anywhere from 0.5 to 2.0 L per hour and therefore replenishment should be 6–8 ounces of water every 5–15 minutes to reduce elements of dehydration and heat illness. Another promoted recommendation is for the athlete to consume 3 cups of water for every pound lost during training. Sports nutritionists suggest that if the athlete loses 2–3 pounds during training/competition, not enough water was consumed. Common strategies to enhance water balance to optimize performance and maintain exercise capacity include weighing before and after training, properly hydrating before, during, and after training (a common mistake is to wait until thirsty to drink), consuming larger quantities of water during higher ambient temperatures, and avoiding excessive weight loss techniques that increase health risk. A major goal should be to regain any weight loss and maintain that weight before the next exercise or competitive bout. Finally, adding salt to one's diet can be an effective fluid retention strategy.

## Glucose Electrolyte Solution

Ingesting glucose electrolyte solution (GES) drinks during extensive training protocols is an accepted technique to reduce muscle glycogen utilization and to contribute to positive hydration status.[28] In addition, there is evidence that GES ingestion may enhance exercise endurance capacity, delay central fatigue markers by increasing the ratio of free tryptophan to BCAAs, and reduce exercise intensity effects by improving immune function.[51,52] Although additional research is needed in this area, current research promotes GES products for athletes and exercisers participating in intense, prolonged endurance training, especially in excessive heat and humidity. Finally, it is recommended that during intense exercise lasting more than 1 hour, the athlete should ingest 3 cups of GES for every pound lost during training every 5–15 minutes.[28]

## Carbohydrate Intake

A common macronutrient strategy used to optimize performance and prevent overtraining is complex carbohydrate ingestion. In order to help maintain necessary muscle glycogen levels to reduce fatigue, the proper amounts of carbohydrate ingestion should be based on the intensity of the activity and duration of the training period. As mentioned above, the percentage of all dietary macronutrient consumption differs based on low, moderate, and high exercise intensities as well as caloric energy replacement needs. A before-, during-, and after-exercise carbohydrate ingestion philosophy should be used to ensure adequate glycogen levels. One effective approach is to carbohydrate load a few days before competitive events (200–300 more grams than usual), high carbohydrate meals and snacks before competition, and carbohydrate ingestion during and after the event. Whereas specific carbohydrate recommendations were made previously, guidelines during intense training were not. Therefore, to assist in maintaining carbohydrate levels, athletes should ingest 8–10 g of carbohydrates during intense training periods.[12,49] This can be accomplished by ingesting complex carbohydrates with a low to moderate glycemic index such as fruits, grains, and starches.[28] Because this can become a vast quantity of carbohydrates to consume on a daily basis, a nutrient-dense diet can be complemented with a variety of high carbohydrate supplements. Remember, a higher carbohydrate diet applies to athletes involved with moderate- to high-intensity training for long periods of time. Following these dietary strategies will limit the dreaded overtraining syndrome and optimize training.

## Protein Intake

Adequate protein requirements for athletes has been a very controversial topic in sport nutrition research and the nutrition industry. Similar to carbohydrate needs, protein requirements of athletes are greater than those for nontraining individuals. To increase protein synthesis, hasten recovery time, and maintain nitrogen balance, 1.5–2.0 g/kg/d protein is recommended for athletes in high-intensity training.[53-57] If these protein values are not maintained, the athlete becomes susceptible to overtraining thereby hindering optimal performance. Specific protein percentages for athletes training at low-, moderate-, and high-intensity levels vary, and were provided previously in this chapter. The quality of protein consumed is as important as the amount. Some protein sources, such as whey and casein, have been shown to have different digestion rates, which can alter the athlete's recovery time.[34,58-60] High-quality sources of dietary protein are fish, egg white, skim milk, and skinless chicken. Research suggests that the best sources of high-quality protein in nutritional supplements are egg protein, whey, casein, colostrums, and milk proteins.[34,61] It is also important to note that ingesting more protein than recommended will not enhance an athlete's strength or muscle.[8,62]

## Value of Fat

To this point, a constant theme has been higher dietary recommendations for athletes compared with nonathletes. However, fat intake suggestions for athletes have been reported as similar or even slightly higher when compared with nonathletes.[27] The level of adequate fat consumption again depends on the athlete's fitness level, program goals, and the specific training demands of their current periodization cycle. Although fat has negative associations for many people, the ingestion of high fat foods has some positive characteristics that promote viable physiologic functions, which inhibit overtraining thus enhancing performance potentials. For example, in comparison to low-fat diets, high-fat diets help maintain testosterone levels, which are often suppressed during high-intensity training.[62–64] Testosterone suppression is a common occurrence without a quality energy balance, especially under the duress of intense training and competition.[65] As mentioned earlier, athletes are typically encouraged to eat a moderate diet of fat, approximately 30% of their overall caloric intake. However, athletes wishing to diminish body composition have been encouraged to ingest 0.5–1.0 g/kg/d of fat.[1,66] Similar to protein selections, the type of dietary fat consumed has an important role in loss and maintenance of desired body fat. Like any dietary strategy, athletes need to be informed about the quality of dietary fat and the correct way to calculate total fat grams.[1,66]

## Amino Acids

There are mixed results in the existing research regarding the possible benefits amino acid ingestion has on overtraining. Specifically, there is research to support positive effects and limited effects of amino acid supplementation regarding physiologic and psychologic responses to training.[15,16,49,53,67,68] There are a number of amino acid options (i.e., BCAAs, glutamine, creatine) that have been examined to determine potential benefits on physiologic and psychologic responses to optimize performance and limit overtraining. As stated before, the strategy of ingesting BCAA supplementation has been theorized to limit the onset of central fatigue. Specifically, BCAA ingestion before and during training not only heightens BCAA levels, but helps control increases of free tryptophan thereby minimizing various effects of physiologic and psychologic responses to exercise stress.[11,14–16,67–70] A few studies also exist that indicate that BCAA ingestion improves exercise capacity.[69] Specifically, positive physiologic and psychologic responses to exercise have been noted by consuming 4–21 g of BCAA a day while training and 2–4 g of BCAA every hour combined with GESs (6–8 ounces) before and during extensive training. Improved training adaptations have also been noted when ingesting BCAA with carbohydrates and or protein supplements before and during moderate to intense training bouts.[52] Although more extensive research is needed in this area, there is evidence that BCAA supplementation can have an important role in enhancing exercise capacity while assisting with overtraining markers.

In addition to the benefits associated with immune function, glutamine has been shown to enhance glycogen and protein synthesis as well as optimize cell hydration.[71] These findings indicate that supplementing 6–10 g of glutamine before and after exercise promotes muscle mass and strength improvements.[62,72] While more data are needed, current research regarding glutamine supplementation suggests a viable alternative for reducing markers of overtraining by enhancing immune function as well as helping improve select strength-training components.

The final amino acid discussed that can theoretically limit the process of overtraining is creatine. Currently there is an abundance of research to support the efficacy of creatine as an ergogenic aid as well as a nutritional supplement recommended by select members of the medical profession. Although anecdotal concerns have been raised about the safety of creatine supplementation, the only clinically supported side effect has been weight gain.[62,73-75] Because creatine supplementation has been shown to actually decrease the incidence of injury with athletes, some experts contend that creatine may assist the athlete in tolerating intense training and therefore avoid deleterious markers of overtraining.[8,76-78] It is important to conduct additional research to evaluate how creatine scientifically impacts this rationale.

## SUMMARY

Although there are mixed reviews surrounding the scientific rationale for the overtraining phenomena, there is a multitude of evidence to support anaerobic and aerobic signs and symptoms of this syndrome. Although physiologic and psychologic overtraining can occur for a number of reasons (i.e., inaccurate assessment procedures, inadequate periodization schemes, and low caloric intake), the most accepted hypothesis is suppressed hypothalamic function that ultimately hinders an athlete's hormonal response to various stress factors. Nutritional supplementation strategies evaluated through scientific methods have been used to effectively address the issue of overtraining. Typically athletes are exposed to markers of overtraining because they do not consume adequate calories to maintain a healthy nutrient balance. Quality protein and carbohydrate strategies have been effectively used to offset excess energy expenditure. Furthermore, numerous nutritional strategies have been investigated regarding their effectiveness in suppressing factors surrounding the central fatigue hypothesis and thereby supporting immune function. When evaluating the effects of adequate dietary habits and nutritional supplementation on overtraining, researchers have postulated that these practical approaches assist athletes in better tolerating intense prolonged exercise or competition. Although additional research is warranted, current data suggest that solid nutritional strategies provide a vital role in addressing issues of overtraining.

## PRACTICAL APPLICATIONS

1. Nutritional supplements are not a complete substitute for a well-balanced, nutrient-dense diet. However, nutritional supplementation strategies, in addition to a nutrient-dense diet, are vital in assisting the athlete in replacing the necessary caloric losses from high-intensity energy expenditure.
2. In addition to a quality nutrient-dense diet, athletes should take a multivitamin daily (with iron for female athletes).
3. Valid baseline physiologic and psychologic assessments provide important evaluation criteria to monitor markers of overtraining of athletes over various training cycles.
4. In combination with adequate caloric intake, properly designed periodization schemes are viable methods for reducing markers of overtraining.
5. Glutamine, protein, vitamin C, zinc, and Echinacea have been shown to prevent URTI and maintain a healthy immune system.
6. Central fatigue can be delayed by ingesting GES drinks before, during, and after exercise.
7. Because matching caloric intake to energy expenditure is critical, athletes engaged in intense training (2–3 h/d) should ingest between 60 and 80 kcal/kg/d. The caloric requirement should be based on the intensity of training and the total energy expenditure.
8. Because it is difficult to consume large quantities of food in one sitting and difficult to maintain a quality energy balance, athletes are encouraged to eat 4–6 meals per day. Ingesting carbohydrate and protein snacks between meals helps offset energy expenditure.
9. Because athletes are susceptible to negative energy balance during intense training periods, dietary options should be composed of the

following combinations: carbohydrate (8–10g/kg/d), high-quality protein (1.5–2.0g/kg/d), and low to moderate fat intake (less than 30% of diet). It is recommended that this intake occur 4–6 hours before training whenever possible. Recommended fat intake for athletes attempting to lose weight is 0.5–1.0g/kg/d.

10. Nutritional timing is imperative as a dietary strategy. To help maintain energy balance and reduce catabolic states, athletes are encouraged to consume the following 30–60 minutes before exercise: 50–100g of carbohydrate and 30–40g of protein.

11. Physiologic and psychologic recovery is greatly enhanced by caloric intake within 2 hours after training. Because some athletes lose their appetites after intense training, a carbohydrate/protein supplement snack is recommended within 30 minutes after the exercise bout followed by a nutrient-dense meal within the critical 2-hour caloric window.

12. A very effective and convenient way to maintain energy balance between meals is to consume carbohydrate/protein supplements composed of vitamins, minerals, and select amino acids.

13. Ingesting water helps reduce concerns of dehydration. The following hydration strategies are recommended: 4–6 cups of water or GES before training begins, 6–8 cups of water or GES every 5–15 minutes during training, replenish lost fluid amounts after training. The athlete's weight should be monitored closely throughout the training period in effort to reduce heat illness. The hydration standard is to drink 3 cups of water or GES for every pound lost.

14. Although the ergogenic value is minimal, ingesting BCAA with a GES before and during training helps control the dreaded aspects of the overtraining syndrome.

15. Athletes should be evaluated throughout the entire training or competitive period to reduce the possibility of overtraining. If markers of overtraining are detected, training cycles should be adjusted and relevant dietary strategies should be initiated.

16. Various contents in nutritional supplements do not meet National Collegiate Athletic Association [NCAA] requirements. Therefore, athletes should consult a nutrition specialist, athletic trainer, strength and conditioning specialist, or other qualified professional to ensure the supplement(s) is not banned by the NCAA.

## ACKNOWLEDGMENTS

I acknowledge the International Society of Sport Nutrition (ISSN) Board of Directors and Advisor Board Members for their professional commitment in promoting Sport Nutrition and for developing the ISSN. My appreciation and thanks also go out to the many people that supported me during my recent recovery period. I have been blessed with the opportunity to continue to serve my students and the profession.

## QUESTIONS

1. The term "overreaching" applies to:
   a. Recovery from fatigue
   b. Performance enhancement
   c. Short-term performance decrements
   d. Long-term performance decrements

2. An accumulation training and or nontraining stress that can last weeks to months is referred to as:
   a. Detraining period
   b. Nontraining period
   c. Overreaching period
   d. Overtraining period

3. The type of overtraining that has been classified as anaerobic exercise is:
   a. Sympathetic
   b. Parasympathetic
   c. Undulating
   d. Classic fatigue

4. A frequently used assessment to evaluate psychologic overtraining is:
   a. Trait anxiety inventory
   b. State anxiety inventory
   c. Test of interpersonal style
   d. Profile of mood states

5. High levels of nutritional expenditure and central nervous system changes from intense exercise have been associated with:
   a. Increases of free fatty acid levels in the blood
   b. The release of free tryptophan levels in the blood
   c. Increasing the ratio of free tryptophan to branched-chain amino acid during exercise
   d. All of the above

6. A common mistake made in avoiding the overtraining phenomenon is:
   a. Inaccurate physiologic assessment
   b. Progressing too slowly in training protocols
   c. Inaccurate or no nutritional evaluation
   d. a and c

7. Which of the following is the second stage of the general adaptation syndrome?
   a. Super-compensation stage
   b. Alarm stage
   c. Shock stage
   d. None of the above

8. The transition I phase used in classic periodization models to limit over-training typically focuses on:
   a. Intense training
   b. Active recovery
   c. Maintaining previous gains
   d. No training whatsoever

9. What is considered the most naturally abundant amino acid(s) in the body?
   a. Creatine
   b. Branched-chain amino acid
   c. Glutamine
   d. All of these are abundant

10. Which of the following nutrients has been scientifically shown to improve immune function?
    a. Zinc
    b. Vitamin C
    c. Echinacea
    d. All the above

11. Which of the following nutrients is considered an antioxidant that assists in iron absorption?
    a. Echinacea
    b. Vitamin C
    c. Glutamine
    d. Creatine

12. Known as the "immune herb," this popular supplement has similar effects as an antibiotic:
    a. Echinacea
    b. Chromium
    c. Magnesium
    d. Selenium

13. This nutrient is considered to be a constituent of enzymes that readily assist in the digestive process while enhancing immune function:
    a. Zinc
    b. Iron
    c. Niacin
    d. Creatine

14. Individuals involved in low-intensity exercise lasting 30–40 minutes a day and performed 3 times a week typically require:
    a. 1200–1500 kcal/d
    b. 1700–2000 kcal/d
    c. 1800–2100 kcal/d
    d. 1800–2400 kcal/d

15. To reduce the possibilities of overtraining, every aspect of training or competition should be monitored by:
    a. The athlete
    b. The athletic training and athletic coaching staff
    c. Sports nutritionist or registered dietitian
    d. All of the above

16. To bolster energy intake and limit catabolism, 30–60 minutes before training or competition athletes should ingest:
    a. 50–60 g of carbohydrate
    b. 10–20 g of fat
    c. 30–40 g of protein
    d. a and c

17. For proper hydration during training, it is recommended that athletes consume:
    a. 3 cups of water for every pound lost
    b. 6–8 ounces of water every 5–15 minutes
    c. Only glucose electrolyte solution in events lasting less than 1 hour
    d. a and b

18. During intense training periods, in addition to their normal caloric intake, it is recommended that athletes ingest:
    a. 2–4 g of carbohydrate
    b. 4–6 g of protein
    c. 8–10 g of carbohydrate
    d. 12–15 g of protein

19. In an effort to hasten recovery and enhance protein synthesis during intense training, which of the following recommendations are suggested to maintain nitrogen balance and limit overtraining?
    a. Protein 1.5–2.0 g/kg/d
    b. Carbohydrate 2–4 g/kg/d
    c. Protein 4–6 g/kg/d
    d. Carbohydrate 4–6 g/kg/d

20. Which amino acid has been theoretically promoted as one of the best ergogenic aids to assist athletes in tolerating intense training, thus limiting various markers of overtraining?
    a. Branched-chain amino acid
    b. Glutamine
    c. Creatine
    d. None of the above

21. Fat intake suggestions for athletes have been reported to be similar or slightly above nonathletic population requirements.
    a. True        b. False

22. Athletes that desire to lose body weight have been encouraged to ingest fat at a rate of 1.5–2.0 g/kg/d.
    a. True        b. False

23. Glutamine has a vital role in the enhancement of protein and glycogen synthesis.
    a. True          b. False

24. Athletes involved in intense training 5–6 days a week 3–6 hours a day should ingest 2500–8000 kcal/d to balance energy expenditure.
    a. True          b. False

25. The general recommended dietary guidelines for athletes during heavy training periods include 55%–65% carbohydrates, 20% protein, and 15% fat.
    a. True          b. False

26. Nutritional timing considers adequate dietary consumption in relation to a finely tuned nutritional timing schedule.
    a. True          b. False

27. Adequate hydration levels assist intracellular functions in the body such as metabolic functions.
    a. True          b. False

28. Adding salt to one's diet can assist in fluid retention.
    a. True          b. False

29. Based on available research, creatine supplementation has been shown to increase the incidence of injuries in athletes.
    a. True          b. False

30. There is evidence that ingestion of glucose electrolyte solution may enhance exercise capacity and delay central fatigue.
    a. True          b. False

# REFERENCES

1. Kreider RB, Fry AC, O'Toole ML. Overtraining in sport: terms, definitions, and prevalence. In: Kreider RB, Fry AC, O'Toole ML, eds. Overtraining in Sport. Champaign, IL: Human Kinetics Publishers; 1998:vii–ix.
2. Urhausen A, Kindermann W. Diagnosis of overtraining—what tools do we have? Sports Med 2002;32:95–102.
3. O'Connor PJ. Overtraining and staleness. In: Morgan WP, ed. Physical Activity and Mental Health. Washington, DC: Taylor & Francis; 1997:145–160.
4. Kraemer WJ. Physiological adaptations to anaerobic and aerobic endurance training programs. In: Baechle TR, Earle RW, eds. Essentials of Strength Training and Conditioning. 2nd ed. Champaign, IL: Human Kinetics Publishers; 2000:161 and 166.
5. Lehmann M, Foster C, Gastmann U, et al. Physiological responses to short- and long-term overtraining in endurance athletes. In: Kreider RB, Fry AC, O'Toole ML, eds. Overtraining in Sport. Champaign, IL: Human Kinetics Publishers; 1998: 29–46.
6. Keizer H. Neuroendocrine considerations. In: Kreider RB, Fry AC, O'Toole ML, eds. Overtraining in Sport. Champaign, IL: Human Kinetics Publishers; 1998:145–168.
7. Fry RW, Morton AR, Keast D. Overtraining in athletes: an update. Sports Med 1991;12:32–65.
8. Kreider RB, Leutoholtz B. Nutritional considerations for preventing overtraining. In: Antonio J, Stout JR, eds. Sports Supplements. Philadelphia: Lippincott Williams & Wilkins; 2001:199–208.
9. Armstrong L, VanNeest J. The unknown mechanism of the overtraining syndrome: clues from depression and psychoneuroimmunology. Sports Med 2002;32:185–209.
10. Berning JR. Energy intake, diet, and muscle wasting. In: Kreider RB, Fry AC, O'Toole ML, eds. Overtraining in Sport. Champaign, IL: Human Kinetics Publishers; 1998: 275–288.
11. Snyder AC. Overtraining and glycogen depletion hypothesis. Med Sci Sports Exerc 1998;30(7):1146–1150.
12. Sherman WM, Jacobs KA, Leenders N. Carbohydrate metabolism during endurance exercise. In: Kreider RB, Fry AC, O'Toole ML, eds. Overtraining in Sport. Champaign, IL: Human Kinetics Publishers; 1998:289–308.

13. Newsholme EA, Parry-Billings M, McAndrew M, et al. Biochemical mechanism to explain some characteristics of overtraining. In: Brouns F, ed. Medical Sports Science, Advances in Nutrition and Top Sport. Basel, Switzerland: S. Karger; 1991: 79–93.

14. Bloomstrand E, Celsing F, Newshome EA. Changes in plasma concentrations of aromatic and branch-chain amino acids during sustained exercise in man and their possible role in fatigue. Acta Physiol Scand 1988;133:115–121.

15. Bloomstrand E, Hassmen P, Ekblom B, et al. Administration of branch-chain amino acids during sustained exercise—effects on performance and on plasma concentration of some amino acids. Eur J Appl Physiol 1991;63:83–88.

16. Bloomstrand E, Hassmen P, Newsholme E. Effect of branch-chain amino acid supplementation on mental performance. Acta Physiol Scand 1991;143:225–226.

17. Davis JM. Carbohydrates, branched-chain amino acids, and endurance: the central fatigue hypothesis. Int J Sport Nutr 1991;5(Suppl):29–38.

18. Segura R, Ventura J. Effect of L-tryptophan supplementation on exercise performance. Int J Sports Med 1988;9:301–305.

19. Rowbottom DG, Keast D, Morton AR. Monitoring and prevention of overreaching and overtraining in endurance athletes. In: Kreider RB, Fry AC, O'Toole ML, eds. Overtraining in Sport. Champaign, IL: Human Kinetics Publishers; 1998:47–68.

20. Franklin BA, Whaley MH, Howley ET, et al. ACSM's Guidelines for Exercise Testing and Prescription. Baltimore: Lippincott Williams & Wilkins; 2000:1–130.

21. Baechle T, Earle R, Wathen D. Resistance training. In: Baechle TR, Earle RW, eds. Essentials of Strength Training and Conditioning. 2nd ed. Champaign, IL: Human Kinetics Publishers; 2000:395–426.

22. Plisk S, Stone MH. Periodization strategies. Strength Cond J 2003;25:19–37.

23. Wathen D, Baechle T, Earle R. Training variation: periodization. In: Baechle TR, Earle RW, eds. Essentials of Strength Training and Conditioning. 2nd ed. Champaign, IL: Human Kinetics Publishers; 2000:513–528.

24. Venkatraman JT, Pendergast DR. Effect of dietary intake on immune function in athletes. Sports Med 2002;32(5):323–337.

25. Nieman DC, Pedersen BK. Exercise and immune function, recent developments. Sports Med 1999;27:72–80.

26. Nieman DC. Effects of athletic endurance training on infection rates and immunity. In: Kreider RB, Fry AC, O'Toole ML, eds. Overtraining in Sport. Champaign, IL: Human Kinetics Publishers; 1998:193–218.

27. Kreider RB. Central fatigue hypothesis and overtraining. In: Kreider RB, Fry AC, O'Toole ML, eds. Overtraining in Sport. Champaign, IL: Human Kinetics Publishers; 1998:309–331.

28. Kreider RB, Almada AL, Antonio J, et al. ISSN exercise and sport nutrition review: research recommendations. Sports Nutr Rev J 2004;1(1):1–44.

29. Kargotich S, Rowbottom DG, Keast D, et al. Plasma glutamine changes after high intensity exercise in elite male swimmers [abstract]. Med Sci Sports Exerc 1996; 28(suppl):133.

30. Castell LM. Can glutamine modify the apparent immunodepression observed after prolonged, exhaustive exercise? Nutrition 2002;18(5):371–375.

31. Newsholme EA, Calder PC. The proposed role of glutamine in some cells of the immune system and speculative consequences for the whole animal. Nutrition 1997;13:728–730.

32. Parry-Billings M, Budgett R, Koutedakis K, et al. Plasma amino acid concentrations in the overtraining syndrome: possible effects on the immune system. Med Sci Sports Exerc 1992;24:1353–1358.

33. Bucci LR, Unlu LM. Proteins and amino acid supplements in exercise and sport. In: Driskell JA, Wolinsky I, eds. Energy-Yielding Macronutrients and Energy Metabolism in Sports Nutrition. Boca Raton, FL: CRC Press; 1999:191–212.

34. Kreider RB, Miriel V, Bertun E. Amino acid supplementation and exercise performance: proposed ergogenic value. Sports Med 1993;16:190–209.

35. Hemila H. Vitamin C and common cold incidence: a review of studies with subjects under heavy physical stress. Int J Sports Med 1996;17:379–383.

36. Peters EM, Goetzsche JM, Grobbelaar B, Noakes TD. Vitamin C supplementation reduces the incidence of postrace symptoms of upper-respiratory-tract infection in ultramarathon runners. Am J Clin Nutr 1993;57:170–174.

37. Tauler P, Aguilo A, Gimeno I, et al. Differential response of lymphocytes and neutrophils to high intensity physical activity and to vitamin C diet supplementation. Free Radic Res 2003;37(9):931–938.

38. Jeurissen A, Bossuyt X, Ceuppens JL, Hespel P. The effects of physical exercise on the immune system. Ned Tijdschr Geneeskd 2003;147(28):1347–1351.

39. Gleeson M, Lancaster G, Bishop N. Nutritional strategies to minimize exercise-induced immunosuppression in athletes. Can J Appl Physiol 2001;26:523–535.

40. Konig D, Weinstock C, Keul J, Northoff H, Berg A. Zinc, iron, and magnesium status in athletes: influence on the regulation of exercise-induced stress and immune function. Exerc Immunol Rev 1998;4:2–21.

41. Prasad AS. Zinc and immunity. Mol Cell Biochem 1998;188(1–2):63–69.

42. Routsias JG, Kosmopoulou A, Makri A, et al. Zinc ion dependent B-cell epitope, associated with primary Sjögren's syndrome, resides within the putative zinc finger domain of Ro60kD autoantigen: physical and immunologic properties. J Med Chem 2004;47(17):4327–4334.

43. Mocchegiani E, Giacconi R, Muti E, et al. Zinc, immune plasticity, aging, and successful aging: role of metallothionein. Ann NY Acad Sci 2004;1019:127–134.

44. Singh A, Failla ML, Deuster PA. Exercise-induced changes in immune function: effects of zinc supplementation. J Appl Physiol 1994;76:2298–2303.

45. Mishima S, Saito K, Maruyama H, et al. Antioxidant and immuno-enhancing effects of *Echinacea purpurea*. Biol Pharm Bull 2004;27(7):1004–1009.

46. Jurkstiene V, Kondrotas AJ, Kevelaitis E. Compensatory reactions of immune system and action of Purple Coneflower (*Echinacea purpurea* (L.) Moench) preparations. Medicina (Kaunas) 2004;40(7):657–662.

47. Brinkeborn RM, Shah DV, Degenring FH. Echinaforce and other echinacea fresh plant preparations in the treatment of the common cold. A randomized, placebo controlled, double-blind clinical trial. Phytomedicine 1999;6:1–6.

48. American College of Sports Medicine. Encyclopedia of Sports Sciences and Medicine. New York: Macmillan Publishing; 1999:1128–1129.

49. Leutholtz B, Kreider RB. Exercise and sport nutrition. In: Temple N, Wilson T, eds. Nutritional Health. Totowa NJ: Humana Press; 2001:207–239.

50. Ivy J, Portman P. The Future of Sports Nutrition: Nutrient Timing. North Bergen, NJ: Basic Health Publications; 2004:7–14.

51. Davis JM, Baily SP, Woods JA, et al. Effects of carbohydrate feedings on plasma free tryptophan and branched-chain amino acids during prolonged cycling. Eur J Appl Physiol 1992;65:513–519.

52. Henson DA, Nieman DC, Blodgett AD, et al. Influence of exercise mode and carbohydrate on the immune response to prolonged exercise. Int J Sport Nutr 1999;9(2):213–228.

53. Lemon PW, Tarnopolsky MA, MacDougall JD, Chesley A, Phillips S, Schwarcz HP. Protein requirements and muscle mass/strength changes during intensive training in novice bodybuilders. J Appl Physiol 1992;73(2):767–775.

54. Tarnopolsky MA, MacDougall JD, Atkinson SA. Influence of protein intake and training status on nitrogen balance and lean body mass. J Appl Physiol 1988;64(1):187–193.

55. Tarnopolsky MA, Atkinson SA, MacDougall JD, Chesley A, Phillips S, Schwarcz HP. Evaluation of protein requirements for trained strength athletes. J Appl Physiol 1992;73(5):1986–1995.

56. Tarnopolsky MA. Protein and physical performance. Curr Opin Clin Nutr Metab Care 1999;2(6):533–537.

57. Kreider RB. Effects of protein and amino acid supplementation on athletic performance. Sportscience 1999. Available at: http://www.sportsci.org/jour/9901/rbk.html:3(1).

58. Boirie Y, Dangin M, Gachon P, Vasson MP, Maubois JL, Beaufrere B. Slow and fast dietary proteins differently modulate postprandial protein accretion. Proc Natl Acad Sci USA 1997;94(26):14930–14935.

59. Boirie Y, Gachon P, Cordat N, Ritz P, Beaufrere B. Differential insulin sensitivities of glucose, amino acid, and albumin metabolism in elderly men and women. J Clin Endocrinol Metab 2001;86(2):638–644.

60. Boirie Y, Gachon P, Corny S, Fauquant J, Maubois JL, Beaufrere B. Acute postprandial changes in leucine metabolism as assessed with an intrinsically labeled milk protein. Am J Physiol 1996;271(6 Pt 1):E1083–1091.

61. Kreider RB, Kleiner SM. Protein supplements for athletes: need vs. convenience. Your Patient Fitness 2000;14(6):12–18.

62. Kreider RB. Dietary supplements and the promotion of muscle growth with resistance exercise. Sports Med 1999;27:97–110.

63. Williams MH. Facts and fallacies of purported ergogenic amino acid supplements. Clin Sports Med 1999;18:633–649.

64. Di Pasquale MG. Proteins and amino acids in exercise and sport. In: Driskell JA, Wolinsky I, eds. Energy-Yielding Macronutrients and Energy Metabolism in Sports Nutrition. Boca Raton, FL: CRC Press; 1999:119–162.

65. Fry AC, Kraemer WJ, Ramsey LT. Pituitary-adrenal-gland responses to high-intensity resistance exercise overtraining. J Appl Physiol 1998;85(6):2352–2359.

66. Miller WC, Koceja DM, Hamilton EJ. A meta-analysis of the past 25 years of weight loss research using diet, exercise or diet plus exercise intervention. Int J Obes Relat Metab Disord 1997;21:941–947.

67. Struder HK, Hollmann W, Platen P, Donike M, Gotzmann A, Weber K. Influence of paroxetine, branched-chain amino acids and tyrosine on neuroendocrine system responses and fatigue in humans. Horm Metab Res 1998;30(4):188–194.

68. Davis JM, Welsh RS, De Volve KL, Alderson NA. Effects of branched-chain amino acids and carbohydrate on fatigue during intermittent, high-intensity running. Int J Sports Med 1999;20(5):309–314.

69. Mittleman KD, Ricci MR, Bailey SP. Branched-chain amino acids prolong exercise during heat stress in men and women. Med Sci Sports Exerc 1998;30(1):83–91.

70. Calders P, Matthys D, Derave W, Pannier JL. Effect of branched-chain amino acids (BCAA), glucose, and glucose plus BCAA on endurance performance in rats. Med Sci Sports Exerc 1999;31(4):583–587.

71. Varnier M, Leese GP, Thompson J, Rennie MJ. Stimulatory effect of glutamine on glycogen accumulation in human skeletal muscle. Am J Physiol 1995;269(2 Pt 1): E309–315.

72. Antonio J, Street C. Glutamine: a potentially useful supplement for athletes. Can J Appl Physiol 1999;24(1):1–14.

73. Williams MH, Kreider R, Branch JD. Creatine: The Power Supplement. Champaign, IL: Human Kinetics Publishers; 1999.

74. Kreider RB. Effects of creatine supplementation on performance and training adaptations. Mol Cell Biochem 2003;244(1–2):89–94.

75. Kreider RB, Melton C, Rasmussen CJ, et al. Long-term creatine supplementation does not significantly affect clinical markers of health in athletes. Mol Cell Biochem 2003;244(1–2):95–104.

76. Greenwood M, Kreider RB, Melton C, et al. Creatine supplementation during college football training does not increase the incidence of cramping or injury. Mol Cell Biochem 2003;244(1–2):83–88.

77. Greenwood M, Kreider R, Greenwood L, Byars A. *Cramping and injury incidence are not increased by creatine supplementation in collegiate football players.* Journal of Athletic Training 2003;38(3):216–219.

78. Greenwood M, Kreider R, Greenwood L, Byars A. *Creatine supplementation does not increase the incidence of injury or cramping in college baseball players.* Journal of Exercise Physiology: Online 2003;6(4):16–23.

**PART II**

# Exercise Principles and Assessment

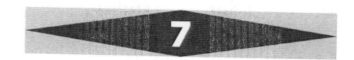

# Principles of Exercise Training

## Steven J. Fleck

## OBJECTIVES

On the completion of this chapter you will be able to:

1. Distinguish between health and fitness benefits of both aerobic and resistance training.
2. Define training volume and intensity for both aerobic and resistance training.
3. Understand the training principles of overload, specificity, and individualization.
4. Explain the possible benefits of both warmup and flexibility training on performance and injury prevention.
5. Design both an aerobic and resistance training session that meets the recommended guidelines for training frequency, duration, and intensity.
6. Learn to implement increases in aerobic and resistance training programs as stress improves.

## ABSTRACT

Virtually all individuals interested in total-body health and fitness should not only follow a sound nutritional program, but should also perform regular physical activity including aerobic or cardiovascular training and weight or resistance training. This is true for adolescents as well as seniors. There are a myriad of health and fitness benefits associated with regular physical activity. Various health and fitness benefits are typically associated with either cardiovascular or resistance training. However, there is much overlap in the benefits of these two training modalities in terms of fitness and health benefits as well as overlap between what is considered a health or a fitness benefit. Health benefits typically associated with aerobic training include reduced blood pressure, improved blood lipid profile, reduced resting heart rate, reduced body fat, and protection from osteoporosis. Health benefits typically associated with resistance training include increased or maintenance of fat-free mass, decreased percent body fat, increased basal metabolic rate, maintenance of activities of daily living in seniors (e.g., rising from a chair, stair climbing), and protection from osteoporosis. Fitness benefits associated with aerobic training include increased maximal oxygen consumption, increased lactate threshold, decreased heart rate during submaximal work, decreased percent body fat, and increased performance in endurance sports and activities. Fitness benefits associated with resistance training include increased strength, increased muscular power, increased fat-free mass, decreased percent body fat, and increased performance in strength/power sports activities. Some of these adaptations, such as improved lipid profile and reduced body fat percentage, are also typical goals of and very

From: *Essentials of Sports Nutrition and Supplements*
Edited by J. Antonio, D. Kalman, J. R. Stout, M. Greenwood, D. S. Willoughby, and G. G. Haff © Humana Press, a part of Springer Science+Business Media, Totowa, NJ

compatible with a healthy nutrition program. In this chapter, basic principles and guidelines for the development of both aerobic and weight training programs for a beginning trainee to a moderately trained individual are described and discussed. These training guidelines and principles are applicable to the vast majority of apparently healthy individuals interested in total-body health and fitness. Programs for athletes, sport-specific programs, cardiovascular rehabilitation programs, and injury rehabilitation programs are only briefly discussed.

*Key Words:* **periodization, specificity, overload, individualization**

## FUNDAMENTAL TRAINING PRINCIPLES

Some fundamental training principles apply to both resistance and aerobic training. These principles must be followed to produce the desired training adaptations or outcomes and to produce continued gains in health and fitness over long training periods.

### Training Variables

Training variables common to both aerobic and resistance training include training volume and intensity. Aerobic training volume is determined by the total distance for which aerobic training was performed (e.g., yards swam, miles ran) or total time for which training was performed (e.g., minutes ran). Resistance training volume is typically determined as the total number of repetitions performed or the total weight lifted (i.e., number of repetitions × weight used). Both of these ways of representing resistance training volume is dependent on total number of exercises performed, number of repetitions performed, and number of sets of each exercise performed. Both aerobic and resistance training volume are dependent on the volume of training performed each training session, training duration per session, and the number of training sessions performed in a specific time (e.g., three sessions per week) or the training frequency.

Resistance training intensity is normally defined as the percentage of the maximal weight it is possible to lift for 1 repetition in a specific exercise. The maximal weight it is possible to lift for 1 repetition in a specific exercise is termed the 1 repetition maximum (RM). Thus, if one is lifting 60 pounds and the 1 RM for the exercise is 100 pounds, training intensity is 60%. Some coaches and strength conditioning professionals also consider whether or not the exercise was performed to "failure" when considering exercise intensity. If an exercise was performed to "failure" it means as many repetitions as possible were performed with the weight being lifted. For most resistance training exercises, this means the concentric phase (lifting phase) of the repetition was not completed in the last repetition attempted. If "failure" occurred during the 11th repetition, 10 complete repetitions were performed. The resistance used when failure occurred during the 11th repetition would be termed a 10 RM. Other RM resistances (e.g., 8 RM, 3 RM) can also be defined as the weight used to perform $x$ repetitions but $x + 1$ repetitions could not be performed. The need to perform sets to absolute failure is unclear because strength gains have been reported with all sets in training being performed to failure, some sets performed to failure, and with no sets performed to absolute failure.[1] However, in programs in which sets were not carried to failure, sets were carried generally close to failure (e.g., could have performed 10 repetitions but performed 8–9 repetitions).

The aerobic training intensity for general health and fitness programs is typically defined as a percentage of maximal heart rate. If an individual with a maximal heart rate of 200 beats per minute is performing aerobic training at a heart rate of 140 beats per minute, they are training at 70% of maximal heart rate. An accurate estimate of maximal heart rate can be obtained by using the equation 208—0.70 (age in years) = maximal heart rate in beats per minute.[2] This and any estimate of maximal heart rate is, however, only an estimate and does have possible large individual variations. Therefore, a training intensity utilizing an estimate of maximal heart rate must be viewed as a guideline because wide individual variation may be present. The equations used to predict maximal heart rate also make it apparent that as aging occurs maximal heart rate decreases and training heart rates at any percentage of maximal heart rate will therefore decrease with aging.

## Overload

Overload refers to the principle that as training and fitness progresses, if further gains in health and fitness are to be achieved, the training must be made more difficult. For aerobic training, overload can be accomplished by training at a higher intensity, or increasing training volume by training more frequently or increasing the duration of each training session. Overload in resistance training is typically accomplished by increasing the resistance being lifted for a specified number of repetitions or increasing training intensity at a certain number of repetitions. Use of RM resistances implies that overload will be applied as strength is gained because as an individual gains strength, the resistance that allows $x$ number of repetitions but not $x + 1$ repetitions will increase. Overload in resistance training can, however, also be accomplished by increasing training volume by either increasing the number of exercises performed per training session, or increasing the number of sets performed of an exercise. No matter how overload is applied, increases in training intensity or volume should progress slowly and cautiously.[3] For example, if training volume is increased, the new higher volume may be performed for one training session with the next training session returning to the original lower training volume. This alternation of the old training session volume and the new higher training session volume can be used for 1–2 weeks of training before all training sessions are performed using the higher training volume.

## Specificity

Specificity means that the physiologic characteristics being trained will be the characteristics that show gains or adaptations. The most basic application of the specificity principle is that aerobic training predominantly leads to adaptations in physiologic characteristics and variables associated with cardiovascular health and endurance. However, strength training predominantly leads to adaptations in physiologic characteristics and variables associated with muscular strength and power. Thus, it is important to include both aerobic and strength training in a conditioning program because although overlap concerning physiologic adaptations exists between aerobic and strength training, both training modalities also result in physiologic adaptations unique to that modality (e.g., weight training increases fat-free mass to a greater extent than aerobic training; aerobic training offers greater adaptations to the lipid profile than strength training) (Figure 7.1).

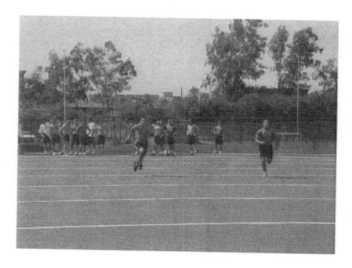

**FIGURE 7.1.** (Photograph courtesy of Athletes' Performance, Tempe AZ.)

Muscle group specificity implies that the muscle(s) trained will be the muscle(s) in which adaptations occur, and is typically thought of in regard to resistance training. For example, if arm curls are performed, then increases in strength and muscle hypertrophy will occur predominantly in the biceps muscle group. However, there is also muscle group specificity with aerobic training. If running or cycling is performed, then increases in endurance and maximal oxygen consumption will occur predominantly when the leg musculature is used during activity. This is in large part because peripheral changes, such as increased aerobic enzyme concentration and increased blood flow, in the musculature being trained occur with little or no change in these same variables in the musculature not trained. However, central adaptations or adaptations to the cardiovascular system, such as decreased resting heart rate, increased blood volume, and positive changes of the blood lipid profile, will occur with any type of aerobic training (e.g., swimming, cycling, running).

## Individualization

Training guidelines and principles can be established. However, a great deal of variation in a specific individual's response and adaptations to a specific training program can be present. All training programs need to be individualized to account for each person's individual response and adaptation to a training program. Individualization takes into account many aspects. For older individuals with a history of knee pain or even artificial joints, some lower body exercises may be contraindicated. Individuals with a history of shoulder pain caused by impingement should have rotator cuff exercises added to their resistance training program. Some individuals, even though their age-predicted maximal heart rate is 188 beats per minute will only have a maximal heart rate of 180 beats per minute, and any aerobic training program based on percentage of maximal heart rate will have to be adjusted accordingly. Individualization is necessary for successful aerobic and resistance training programs.

## Warmup

A warmup before intense aerobic or weight training is usually considered essential for optimum performance; however, there is little scientific evidence supporting a warmup's effectiveness in many situations.[4,5] The effectiveness of a warmup has been attributed to slight increases in body and tissue temperature that decrease muscular stiffness, increase nerve-conduction rate, altered muscular force-velocity relationships, and an increase in aerobic energy availability. Other possible mechanisms proposed for the effectiveness of a warmup include elevated initial oxygen consumption and a psychologic effect increasing preparedness. The majority of studies examining the effects of a warmup are not well controlled and have study-design limitations, such as very small subject numbers. Active warmup, such as performing a period of low-intensity running, tends to result in improvement of short-term (less than 10 seconds) performances.[4,5] However, short-term performance may be impaired if the warmup occurs too close to initiating the performance or is too intense, both of which may not allow sufficient time for recovery of high-energy phosphates before beginning performance. Active warmup also seems to benefit activities ranging in length from 10 seconds to more than 5 minutes.[4,5] Thus, an active warmup may aid performance in both aerobic and weight training programs designed to improve health and fitness. This possible performance improvement is relatively small and probably only of importance to intermediate or higher level fitness enthusiasts.

Typically included as part of a warmup is stretching or flexibility training. Flexibility training does clearly increase joint range of motion. Poor flexibility in some joints has been implicated as contributing to some types of injury, such as the Achilles tendon, plantar fascia, and hamstring tendons, and stretching programs for all the major body joints have been shown to reduce the severity and frequency of some types of injuries.[6] However, some evidence exists that the addition of stretching to a warmup does not significantly affect injury rate.[7]

Although the evidence in support of a warmup increasing performance, and flexibility training reducing injury rate has limitations, it is prudent to include both as part of a total conditioning program. Typically, a warmup consists of approximately 10 minutes of low-intensity aerobic activity followed by a total-body stretching routine. The stretching typically performed is static stretching. Proprioceptive neuromuscular facilitation (PNF) can also be performed. However, this type of stretching does require some minimal training, and for some types of PNF stretching, a partner is required. Static stretches should be held for 10–30 seconds with at least 4 repetitions of each stretch.[6] PNF stretching should include a 6-second contraction followed by a 10- to 30-second assisted stretch for at least 4 repetitions per stretch.[6] The inclusion of stretching as part of a health and fitness conditioning program may be especially important for some population segments, such as seniors for whom decreases in range of motion may impair performance of some activities of daily living. Additionally, severe losses of range of motion may exasperate the injury rate in these populations as well as in younger populations.

# TRAINING FREQUENCY

Frequency normally refers to the number of training sessions per week. During many health and fitness training programs, both aerobic and resistance training are performed 3 days per week. Generally, with a training frequency of 3 days per week, training sessions are separated by at least 1 day. For aerobic training, the optimal frequency for untrained to moderately trained individuals is 3–5 days per week.[6] However, additional fitness benefits may be achieved with training frequencies of 6–7 days per week. However, if the guidelines for training duration and intensity are met, then a training frequency of 3–5 days per week will produce optimal or near optimal aerobic health and fitness gains. It has also been recommended for health gains that some type of physical activity be performed for 30–60 minutes per day. This recommendation is aimed at bringing about health gains and not necessarily fitness gains, and the intensity of the physical activity is generally relatively low. More frequent training sessions above 3–4 sessions per week may be beneficial for weight loss. However, higher training frequencies should not be undertaken until the habit of performing exercise is firmly established and physical condition has improved to a point at which the risk of injury has been reduced.

Resistance training frequency refers to the number of days per week a particular muscle group is trained. It would be possible to utilize a body-part training program (e.g., train chest and arms on Monday, legs on Wednesday, back and abdomen on Friday) having 3 training sessions per week, but only train each muscle group 1 day per week. When considering training frequency for resistance training, the definition of frequency with which a certain muscle group is trained is important. It has been recommended that training frequency for novice and intermediate lifters be 2–3 days per week when using a total-body workout and for advanced lifters 4–5 days per week.[3] However, this recommendation for advanced lifters is based, in part, on not training each muscle group during each training session (i.e., body-part type program). Recent meta-analyses support this recommendation[8,9] and indicate that for untrained and moderately (minimum 1 year of weight training experience) trained individuals the optimal training frequency is 3 days per week per muscle group and for advanced training or training of athletes the optimal frequency is 2 days per week per muscle.

# TRAINING DURATION

The duration of a resistance training session is dependent upon several factors. The factors having the greatest impact on the sessions duration are the number of exercises performed, number of sets performed of each exercise, number of repetitions per set and the rest periods between sets and exercises. Another factor the time to perform each repetition also has an impact, but the impact is smaller than the other factors affecting resistance training duration.

For a total-body fitness and health resistance training session, at least 1 exercise for each major muscle group should be performed. The major muscle groups or body parts are: chest, triceps, biceps, shoulder, upper back, lower back, quadriceps, hamstrings, gluteals, and calf. Using 8–12 exercises, it is possible to have at least 1 exercise for each of the body's major muscle groups or body parts. This range in terms of number of exercises is in part attributable to whether or not single-joint or single–muscle group exercises (e.g., arm curl, triceps extension, knee extension) or multijoint or multi–muscle group exercises (e.g., bench press which trains the chest and triceps, squat which trains quadriceps, hamstrings, gluteals, and to some extent, the calf and lower back) are used in the training session. Both types of exercises have characteristics that make them advantageous in certain training situations. Single-joint exercises isolate a particular muscle group. This makes them ideal for some types of injury rehabilitation (e.g., shoulder rotator cuff) programs or when a certain muscle group limits performance of an activity or sport. Single-joint exercises may also pose a lesser risk of injury because of the reduced level of exercise skill and technique necessary for successful completion of a repetition compared with multijoint exercises. Multijoint exercises produce a greater metabolic load, are more neurally complex, and have generally been regarded as more effective for increasing overall muscular strength because they allow the use of a greater resistance compared with single-joint exercises.[3] Because of this difference in characteristics, generally resistance training programs include a mix of both types of exercises with the multijoint exercises being performed first or early in the training session.

For novice and intermediate trainees, 1–3 sets per exercise using 8–12 repetitions per set has been recommended[3,6] to produce optimal gains in strength and muscle size. This recommendation concerning the number of sets is supported by recent meta-analyses indicating that in untrained and moderately trained individuals, 1 set of an exercise does produce significant strength gains, but further significant strength gains are produced by the performance of 2, 3, and 4 sets of an exercise with the optimal number of sets being 3–4.[9-11]

Rest periods between sets and exercises in part determine how much physical recovery (e.g., lowering blood lactate, replenish intramuscular stores of adenosine triphosphate and phosphocreatine) takes place between sets and exercises during the training session. The length of rest periods affects not only training duration but also perceived difficulty of the training session. For the training of muscular strength 2- to 3-minute rest periods are recommended when using multijoint exercises with heavy resistances and for single-joint exercises the rest periods can be reduced to 1–2 minutes.[3] When muscular hypertrophy is the training outcome being emphasized, shorter rest periods of 1–2 minutes should be used at all times by novice and intermediate lifters.

Speed with which repetitions are performed has a very minor impact on the duration of a resistance training session. It has been recommended that for beginning lifters, slow and moderate repetition velocities be used for both strength and muscle hypertrophy gains.[3] For intermediate lifters, moderate velocities should be used when emphasizing strength gains and slow and moderate velocities used when emphasizing muscle hypertrophy gains. When emphasizing strength and hypertrophy no matter what repetition velocity is used, the resistance should be controlled throughout the full range of motion of exercises.

**TABLE 7.1. Aerobic training guidelines.**

| Volume | Intensity | Type of activity |
|---|---|---|
| 20–60 minutes/session | 55%–90% of heart rate maximum | Large muscle group |
| 3–5 sessions/week | | Rhythmic in nature: running, swimming, walking, aerobic dance, cycling, elliptical trainer |

Research indicates optimal exercise duration for aerobic exercise is 20–60 minutes per training session for novice and moderately trained individuals.[6] There are, however, some major caveats concerning this recommendation. First, this time frame does not include warmup or cool-down time, and second, the exercise intensity during this time frame must meet the minimal exercise intensity (discussed below) for aerobic exercise. Similar gains in measures of health and fitness as a result of aerobic exercise can be obtained with several short-duration sessions adding up to the minimal duration (three 10-minute exercise bouts) or one (20- to 30-minute exercise bout) session of a longer duration (Table 7.1).

## TRAINING INTENSITY

The most common way of determining aerobic training intensity is the percentage of the individual's heart rate maximum (HR max) at which the training is performed. Training intensities ranging from 55% to 90% of HR max do bring about changes in health and fitness variables.[6] The lower intensities of 55%–64% of HR max are generally most applicable to individuals who are just beginning a program or who are quite unfit. Some people can achieve a training effect by performing aerobic training at relatively low intensities of 45% or less of HR max. However, the training effect at these low intensities is generally related to health benefits as opposed to fitness benefits.

Training intensities of resistance training are typically determined as a percent of 1 RM. Recent meta-analyses indicate that for untrained individuals, the optimal mean training intensity for strength gains is 60% of 1 RM and 80% of 1 RM for moderately trained individuals[12] and 85% for trained athletes.[8] This is not to imply that other training intensities cannot or should not be used. Relatively light resistances (12–15 RM) result in only small or nonexistent increases in 1 RM strength, but are effective for increasing absolute local muscular endurance or the ability to perform repeated muscle actions against a relatively light resistance.[13] Conversely, very heavy resistances (1–6 RM) may be most effective to increase maximal (1 RM) strength.[13] So a variety of training intensities may be the optimal training strategy when attempting to increase all of the health and fitness variables associated with resistance training (Table 7.2).

**TABLE 7.2. Resistance training guidelines.**

| Volume | Intensity | Type of activity |
|---|---|---|
| 1–3 sets of each exercise | At or close to repetition maximum resistances | At least 1 exercise for all major muscle groups |
| 8–12 repetitions/set | | |
| 2–3 days/week for total-body program | | Typically 8–12 total exercises |
| 4–5 days/week for body-part program | | Mix of multi- and single-joint exercises |

## TRAINING PROGRESSION

Training progression refers to training variation systematically applied in a planned manner. Training progression relates to the idea of periodization of training. Lack of training variation may result in continued training but with no further gains in fitness[12,14,15] or what is frequently termed "training plateaus." Training variation is not a necessity of training for general health and fitness gains, but may be important to produce optimal long-term fitness gains. Additionally, some training variation may be important for some individuals to keep the training program from becoming psychologically "boring," which may for these individuals help with program compliance.

The use of a percentage of HR max for aerobic training and RM resistances for weight training automatically ensures training progression. As aerobic fitness increases, it will be possible to perform at a higher workload (e.g., run, cycle, or swim faster) at the same percentage of HR max. As strength fitness increases, it will be possible to perform the same number repetitions with a greater resistance (i.e., RM weight increases).

Other common ways to incorporate training variation with aerobic training are to perform training sessions at various training volumes and intensities. The guidelines for aerobic training intensity (55%–90% HR max) and volume (20–60 minutes) offer a wide range of possibilities for training variation. This can mean something as simple as running a different route (e.g., different distance and grade) on various training days. Training variation can also be implemented by performing different types of aerobic training (e.g., cycling, running, walking) on different training days or during different weeks or any other time frame of the training program. This type of variation may be especially applicable if it is necessary to alleviate joint stress and discomfort because each form of aerobic training places different joints under different amounts of compressive forces. Many unfit or overweight individuals may find initially a walking or cycling program most appropriate. When walking or cycling, the compressive forces on the ankle, knee, and hip are relatively low compared with running. This may be advantageous for preventing joint pain. As fitness is gained, progression to a running program may occur.

Many different types of training variation that alter training volume and intensity can be implemented during a resistance training program. Exercises for the same muscle group can be varied (e.g., free weight bench press changed to machine bench press or dumbbell bench press). Rest periods between sets and exercises can be increased or decreased. The number repetitions per set or the number of sets performed can be changed. The two major types of resistance training periodization that have been investigated and shown to produce greater strength, power, and body compositional changes than non-varied training (e.g., only perform training using a constant number of sets and repetitions) are classic strength/power (also termed linear) and undulating (also termed nonlinear). Complete descriptions of these types of periodization and research supporting their efficacy are provided elsewhere.[1,14,16] Briefly, classic periodization is characterized by an initial relatively high volume and low intensity of training, then as the training progresses, training volume decreases and training intensity increases to maximize strength and power or both. The highest training intensity and lowest training volume typically occur before a point in time at which it is desired to maximize strength/power. For athletes, this typically is a major competition. This type of training is typically divided into various training phases each of which varies in length from 3 to 6 weeks (Table 7.3).

Undulating periodization dramatically changes training volume and intensity within 7- to 10-day periods. This type of training typically uses three different training zones that are randomly rotated over a relatively short training period. If training were performed in the typical three session per week pattern with at least 1 day of rest between sessions, resistances of 3–5 RM on Monday, 12–15 RM on Wednesday, and 8–10 on Friday might be used. The same training zones are then performed in the next 7-day period, but perhaps in a different

**TABLE 7.3. Typical classical strength/power resistance training periodization training phases.**

|  | *Hypertrophy* | *Strength* | *Power* | *Peaking* |
|---|---|---|---|---|
| Sets | 3–5 | 3–5 | 3–5 | 1–3 |
| Repetitions/set | 8–12 | 2–6 | 2–3 | 1–3 |
| Intensity | Low | Moderate | High | Very high |
| Volume | High | High | Moderate | Low |

order. In some training programs, this changing pattern of RM resistances is utilized only for the multijoint exercises in the program and single-joint exercises are always performed using 8–10 RM resistances. Obviously, many combinations of resistance training variables can be developed to be used in the training program and the majority of research indicates that training variation during resistance training does produce greater fitness gains than nonvaried resistance training (Figure 7.2).

In summary, a total conditioning program for health and fitness should include a warmup, flexibility training, aerobic training, and strength training to produce all the adaptations related to health and fitness benefits. Health benefits may be gained by training at lower intensities and volumes than are necessary to produce optimal fitness benefits. To produce optimal health and fitness benefits, aerobic and strength training must be performed at the minimal guidelines for each type of training. Some type of training variation for aerobic and weight training is recommended to produce continued long-term gains in fitness and keep the program from becoming psychologically "boring" for some individuals, which may increase their compliance.

## PRACTICAL APPLICATIONS

To produce optimal changes in health and fitness attributable to the performance of aerobic and resistance training, at least the minimal guidelines of each training modality must be met. Health benefits can be gained at lower training volume and intensity. For example, aerobic training health benefits may be produced by performing training at an intensity of 45%–50% of HR max, frequency of 3 times per week, and training duration of 20 minutes. Physical activity performed at very low intensities and consisting of walking or other low-intensity activities (e.g., gardening) for a total duration of 30 minutes per day typically maintains or increases health benefits.

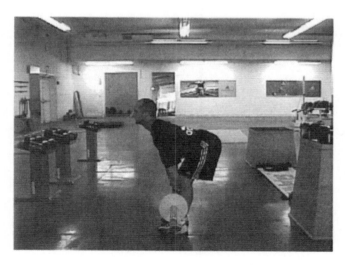

**FIGURE 7.2.** (Photograph courtesy of Athletes' Performance.)

Aerobic training guidelines to produce both health and fitness adaptations are:

- Exercise should be performed using large muscle groups (e.g., running, cycling, swimming, cross country skiing, rowing, elliptical trainer)
- Intensity ranging from 55% to 90% of HR max
- Daily training duration of 20–60 minutes
- Training frequency 3–5 days per week

The equation 208—0.70 (age in years) = heart rate in beats per minute can be used to estimate maximal heart rate for the calculation of aerobic training intensity. However, large individual variation in the actual maximal heart rate can be present. Therefore, training heart rate may have to be adjusted for a particular individual.

Resistance training guidelines to produce both health and fitness adaptations are:

- At least 1 exercise for all of the body's major muscle groups
- Typically 8–12 exercises consisting of both multijoint and single-joint exercises comprise a training session
- 1–3 sets per exercise
- Exercises should be performed close to failure or to failure (i.e., close to or at an RM for the number of repetitions performed)
- When emphasizing strength, rest periods between sets and exercises for untrained and moderately trained individuals should be 2–3 minutes between multi-joint exercises using heavy resistances and 1–2 minutes for single-joint exercises
- When emphasizing muscular hypertrophy, rest periods between sets and exercises for untrained and moderately trained individuals should be 1–2 minutes

All training sessions should be preceded by a warmup. Typically, the warmup consists of low-intensity aerobic training for approximately 10 minutes. After the aerobic training, a total-body stretching routine should be performed before initiation of the actual training included in the session. Static stretching is the most frequently performed type of stretching and should consist of at least 1 stretch for the major muscle groups of the body with each stretch held for 10–30 seconds with at least 4 repetitions of each stretch.

The use of a percentage of HR max for aerobic training and RM resistances for weight training automatically ensures training progression. However, other forms of training variation and progression (e.g., periodization) can also be used to help ensure optimal fitness gains over long training periods.

## QUESTIONS

1. Total resistance training volume depends on:
   a. Number of training sessions per week
   b. Number of repetitions performed per set
   c. Total number of exercises performed per session
   d. All of the above

2. An estimation of maximal heart rate for a 30 year old would be:
   a. 208
   b. 187
   c. 176
   d. 159

3. The recommended training intensity for aerobic training to produce both health and fitness gains is:
   a. 80%–90% of HR max
   b. 65%–80% of HR max

    c. 55%–90% of HR max
    d. 45%–65% of HR max

4. The recommended training duration per session for aerobic training to produce both health and fitness gains is:
    a. 10–30 minutes
    b. 30–40 minutes
    c. 20–60 minutes
    d. 60 minutes or more

5. Meta-analyses indicate that the mean optimal training intensity for moderately trained individuals to experience optimal strength gains is:
    a. 90% of 1 RM
    b. 80% of 1 RM
    c. 60% of 1 RM
    d. 40% of 1 RM

6. Typical health benefits associated with aerobic training include:
    a. Decreased resting blood pressure
    b. Increased muscle hypertrophy
    c. Increased performance in endurance activities
    d. All of the above

7. Effectiveness of a warmup to increase performance has been associated with which of the following?
    a. Increased nerve conduction velocity
    b. Altered muscular force-velocity relationships
    c. Increased aerobic energy availability
    d. All of the above

8. Possible definitions of a repetition maximal (RM) resistance when weight training include:
    a. A set is carried to failure
    b. Resistance used to perform $x$ repetitions but not $x + 1$ repetitions
    c. A set performed using 60% of 1 RM
    d. a and b

9. During resistance training, overload can be applied by:
    a. Use of RM training resistances
    b. Performing more exercises per session
    c. Performing more sets of an exercise
    d. All of the above

10. When training to emphasize muscular hypertrophy gains, resistance training rest periods between sets and exercises should be:
    a. 1/2–1 minute
    b. 1–2 minutes
    c. 3–4 minutes
    d. 4 minutes or more

11. Strength/power (linear) resistance training periodization is characterized by:
    a. Use of 3 training zones that are altered on a training session by training session basis
    b. Performance of only single-joint exercises
    c. Initially training is performed using a relatively high volume and relatively low intensity
    d. a and b

12. Training volume recommendations for a beginning resistance training program include:
    a. 3–5 training sessions per week
    b. 1–3 sets of each exercise per session
    c. 1–6 repetitions per set
    d. All of the above

13. Training volume recommendations for a beginning aerobic training program include:
    a. 1–3 training sessions per week
    b. Training at a heart rate of at least 55% of HR max
    c. 20–60 minutes of training per session
    d. a and b

14. Meta-analyses indicate that for a beginning weight trainer the optimal training frequency is:
    a. 1 time per week
    b. 3 times per week
    c. 4 times per week
    d. 6 times per week

15. Aerobic training volume can be practically defined as:
    a. Distance for which training was performed
    b. Time for which training was performed
    c. Heart rate at which training was performed
    d. a and b

16. If the 1 RM for an exercise is 200 pounds, meta-analyses indicate that for a moderately trained individual the minimal resistance training intensity for this exercise to produce optimal gains in strength is:
    a. 160 pounds
    b. 140 pounds
    c. 120 pounds
    d. 100 pounds

17. Which of the following is true concerning static stretching to produce optimal increases in a joint's range of motion?
    a. Each stretch should be performed at least 6 times per session
    b. Each stretch should be held for 10–30 seconds
    c. Stretching should be performed before the warmup
    d. All of the above

18. If an individual is 40 years old, what is their heart rate at a training intensity of 75% of HR max?
    a. 180 beats per minute
    b. 166 beats per minute
    c. 135 beats per minute
    d. 117 beats per minute

19. For beginning lifters, the recommended repetition velocity to produce strength and muscle hypertrophy gains is:
    a. Slow to moderate
    b. Moderate to fast
    c. Fast to very fast
    d. Only very fast

20. Concerning aerobic training intensity, which of the following is true?
    a. Recommended intensity is 55%–90% of HR max
    b. Intensities of 55%–64% of HR max are applicable to unfit individuals
    c. Intensities of 45% or less of HR max can produce aerobic health gains in some individuals
    d. All of the above

21. Aerobic and resistance training frequency typically refers to the number of training sessions per week.
    a. True          b. False

22. Individualization of aerobic and resistance training needs only to take place with high-level athletes.
    a. True          b. False

23. In a typical warmup, flexibility training should be performed before approximately 10 minutes of aerobic activity.
    a. True          b. False

24. Typically, at least 1 day of rest is allowed between total-body resistance training sessions for beginning and moderately trained individuals.
    a. True        b. False

25. A beginning resistance training session is typically composed of only multijoint exercises.
    a. True        b. False

26. With aging, HR max increases.
    a. True        b. False

27. Health benefits can be achieved with aerobic training without concurrent fitness benefits.
    a. True        b. False

28. Resistance training performed using light resistances (12–15 RM) produces maximal strength gains.
    a. True        b. False

29. An example of a single-joint resistance training exercise is the knee extension.
    a. True        b. False

30. The training guidelines for aerobic and resistance training make it very difficult to have variations in training volume and intensity.
    a. True        b. False

# REFERENCES

1. Fleck SJ, Kraemer WJ. Design Resistance Training Programs. Champagne, IL: Human Kinetics Publishers; 2004.
2. Tanka H, Monohan KG, Seals DS. Age predicted maximal heart rate revisited. J Am College Cardiol 2001;37:153–156.
3. American College of Sports Medicine Position Stand. Progression models in resistance training for healthy adults. Med Sci Sports Exerc 2004;34:364–380.
4. Bishop D. Warm up I potential mechanisms and the effects of passive warm up on exercise performance. Sports Med 2003;33:439–454.
5. Bishop D. Warm up II performance changes following active warm up and how to structure the warm up. Sports Med 2003;33:484–498.
6. American College of Sports Medicine Position Stand. The recommended quantity and quality of exercise for developing and maintaining cardiorespiratory and muscular fitness, and flexibility in healthy adults. Med Sci Sports Exerc 1998;30:975–991.
7. Pope RP, Herbert RD, Kirwan JD, Graham BJ. A randomized trial of preexercise stretching for prevention of lower-limb injury. Med Sci Sports Exerc 2000;32:271–277.
8. Peterson MD, Rhea MR, Alvar BA. Maximizing strength development and athletes: a meta-analysis to determine the dose-response relationship. J Strength Cond Res 2004;18:377–382.
9. Rhea MR, Alvar BA, Burkett LN, Ball SD. A meta-analysis to determine the dose response for strength development. Med Sci Sports Exerc 2003;35:456–464.
10. Rhea MR, Alvar BA, Burkett LN. Single versus multiple sets for strength: a meta-analysis to address the controversy. Res Quart Exerc Sport 2002;73:485–488.
11. Wolfe BL, LeMura LM, Cole PJ. Quantitative analysis of single vs multiple-set programs in resistance training. J Strength Cond Res 2004;18:35–47.
12. Marx JO, Ratamess NA, Nindl BC, et al. Low-volume circuit versus high-volume periodized resistance training in women. Med Sci Sports Exerc 2001;33:635–647.
13. Kraemer WJ, Ratamess NA. Fundamentals of resistance training: progression and exercise prescription. Med Sci Sports Exerc 2004;36:674–688.
14. Fleck SJ. Periodized strength training: a critical review. J Strength Cond Res 1999;13:82–89.
15. Kraemer WJ, Hakkinen K, Triplett-McBride NT, et al. Physiological changes with periodized resistance training in women tennis players. Med Sci Sports Exerc 2003;35:157–168.
16. Fleck SJ. Periodization of strength training. In: Kraemer WJ, Hakkinen KO, eds. Strength Training For Athletes. Oxford: Blackwell Scientific Publications; 2001: 55–68.

# Laboratory and Field Techniques for Measuring Performance

Ronald W. Mendel and Christopher C. Cheatham

## OBJECTIVES

On the completion of this chapter you will be able to:

1. Understand the rationale for implementing testing procedures before, during, and after a training program has been designed.
2. Explain the strengths and weaknesses of laboratory- and field-based testing programs.
3. Conceptualize the importance of measuring aerobic capacity, anaerobic capacity, muscular force, power, and flexibility in a testing program.
4. Describe and differentiate the different methods used to evaluate aerobic power.
5. Explain the contributing factors associated with an individual's $VO_2$ max.
6. Understand the key criteria for determining if a $VO_2$ max has been achieved.
7. Give a rationale for the value of testing the lactate threshold.
8. Explain the different methods for assessing anaerobic power, muscular strength, and flexibility.
9. Diagnose strengths and weaknesses an athlete might have based on the results achieved in a battery of physiologic tests.
10. Calculate power from a vertical jump and maximal strength from a repetition maximum weight

## ABSTRACT

As a scientist, coach, athlete, or other fitness-type professional, knowledge of tests to measure specific physiologic characteristics that may ultimately contribute to performance in a sport or event is imperative. Baseline measurements of these factors influencing performance are critical for many different reasons. First, it is difficult to get to a predetermined end point if the baseline is unknown. Second, these specific physiologic characteristic, once measured, can be evaluated and used as a guide to develop appropriate training strategies for continued improvement. As such, this chapter explores and details the most widely used laboratory and field techniques used to measure human performance. Performance can be thought of as the way an individual or something functions. There are many levels of performance such as poor, average, or elite. Many times, performance is measured by the outcome of the game or event with wins and losses. So what determines an athlete's ability to perform, or more importantly, excel at his or her sport? Of particular interest in this chapter are the physiologic components that comprise a portion of sport performance. Technical skill and tactical awareness are not considered here but are extremely

From: *Essentials of Sports Nutrition and Supplements*
Edited by J. Antonio, D. Kalman, J. R. Stout, M. Greenwood, D. S. Willoughby, and G. G. Haff © Humana Press, a part of Springer Science+Business Media, Totowa, NJ

important to overall sport performance. Certainly, genetic endowment is at the top of the list of physiologic parameters that affect sport performance. As has often been said, we must choose our parents wisely and realize that genetic predisposition to exercise performance is uncontrollable. Along with genetics, the overall health and nutritional status of an athlete can affect their performance. These factors of health and nutritional status are controllable and must be optimized. Another factor and arguably the most recognized influential and controllable component of performance is training. A tremendous amount of scientific study along with trial and error have produced increasingly better performances across the athletic spectrum through the improvement of training programs. A cornerstone to these improved training programs is the ability to monitor an athlete's progress. This monitoring can be achieved by properly selecting and administering specific laboratory and field tests based on sport-specific physiologic demands.

*Key Words:* **testing, assessment, measurements, aerobic power, anaerobic capacity, power, strength, speed**

## RATIONALE FOR TESTING

Regular testing of an athlete, although potentially time consuming and costly, can provide specific and useful information. The first recognized benefit of testing physiologic parameters is general recognition of the athlete's current health and fitness status. With this baseline measure, a regular testing program will provide feedback to the athlete, coach, or scientist. This feedback allows for assessment of the effectiveness of the training program.

Feedback from testing also allows for an objective evaluation of an athlete's strengths and weaknesses for his or her particular sport. As such, the results of the assessment allow for specific exercise prescription of an optimal training program to focus on the athlete's weakness.

As important and effective as testing can be, it is not and should not be considered a training tool. Testing provides objective measures of physiologic components such as aerobic and anaerobic capacity, muscular strength and endurance, as well as measures of flexibility to evaluate potentials needed to perform in competition. Testing does not project or identify winners of a race or competition. If it did, sporting events would be quite boring, not to mention useless. Also, testing cannot determine the genetic limits of an individual to determine the degree of improvement with training. Limitations certainly exist, in that laboratory and even field testing cannot exactly simulate some sports or events. However, some events and sports lend themselves nicely to physiologic testing, but it should always be remembered that many components (skill and psychologic makeup) contribute to an athlete's ability to perform, and physiology is but one component.

## LABORATORY VERSUS FIELD TESTING

Determining whether to use laboratory or field testing poses some interesting challenges and obstacles. Laboratory tests are conducted in highly controlled environments and use standardized protocols, expensive equipment, and qualified personnel. Simulation of the particular sport or event is extremely critical so that appropriate conclusions can be drawn. Conversely, field test measurements are conducted in an ambient environment generally with little equipment while the athlete performs the actual or simulated event or activity. Some activities, such as cycling and running, are easily transferred from the laboratory to the field. For cyclists, physiologic measures such as anaerobic threshold can be measured on a stationary bike in the laboratory whereas time trials can be performed in the field. Other events or sports such as soccer and basketball are more difficult to simulate in the laboratory or even measure in the field. Laboratory testing is oftentimes more reliable (or reproducible) because physiologic characteristics can be more precisely measured, but field tests which simulate actual competition events tend to be more valid (measure what is intended) because of their greater specificity.[1] It should be noted that field tests are not necessarily more valid than laboratory tests in terms of validity coefficients even though they may, in some cases, have more practical application to a particular sport. Environmental conditions also make field testing less reliable because of influences of wind, rain, ground conditions, and temperature. As was also previously mentioned, field tests have equipment limitations. All that being said, field tests should not be ignored or unused. Properly controlled and appropriate field tests should be used in conjunction with measurements obtained in the laboratory setting.

Effective testing measures those variables that are relevant and contribute to the performance outcome. There is no need to test grip strength if vertical jump height is the performance measure of interest because the two are not related. Tests must be valid and reliable to be useful. Effective testing also needs trained test administrators. Test administrators must have the competency to evaluate the tests and procedures to make sure they are appropriate. Valid tests measure what they claim to measure and reliable tests produce consistent and reproducible results.[1] Another consideration of appropriate and effective testing is optimal practical significance. In other words, specificity of testing and training is crucial. Aerobic capacity testing on a treadmill is of no practical use to a cyclist or swimmer because it provides little information on cycling or swimming performance. A final consideration is that standardized testing protocols be used. This consistent administration of testing procedures will allow for proper comparisons between testing trials.

## WHAT IS MEASURED

Physiologic factors most often measured are aerobic capacity, anaerobic capacity, muscular force and power, and flexibility. The importance of these factors vary as widely as the number of events and sports. Some events rely almost completely on sheer strength and/or power, other events are almost completely skill related, and some are a combination of both. Body composition can also be a critical factor in sports performance, particularly in gymnastics and wrestling and other such events. However, body composition is not discussed in this chapter, but can be found in Chapters 9 and 26.

## ASSESSMENT OF MAXIMAL AEROBIC POWER

Maximal aerobic power, also referred to as maximal oxygen uptake, is defined as the maximal amount of oxygen one's body can transport and utilize. Maximal aerobic power, also termed $VO_2$ max, is one of the most frequently measured physiologic variables in exercise physiology laboratories. The term $VO_2$ max represents the maximal volume of oxygen consumed or used per minute using the large muscle groups of the body. $VO_2$ max can be expressed in both absolute $(LO_2 \cdot min^{-1})$ and relative $(mLO_2 \cdot kg^{-1} \cdot min^{-1})$ terms. Absolute $VO_2$ max refers to the actual or total amount of oxygen that is used by the body per minute whereas relative $VO_2$ max refers to the amount of oxygen that is used every minute per kilogram of body weight. It is important to understand the differences between absolute and relative $VO_2$ max and the usefulness of each value. Absolute $VO_2$ max is used as an indicator of the total amount of energy produced by the body. Research has established that for every liter of oxygen consumed, approximately 5 kcal of energy is produced. Therefore, absolute $VO_2$ max can be useful to determine the maximal rate that energy can be produced. Because an individual's $VO_2$ max is partially determined by one's body size (i.e., larger individuals will typically use more oxygen than smaller individuals), it is important to be able to express $VO_2$ max in a manner in which individuals of differing body size can be compared. Therefore, by expressing $VO_2$ max relative to one's body weight, a 50-kg individual can be compared with an 80-kg individual. For example, assume that $VO_2$ max is assessed in a bodybuilder who weighs 100 kg and a marathon runner who weighs 65 kg. It would be expected that the bodybuilder has a higher absolute $VO_2$ max because of the much larger body size. However, one would also expect that the marathon runner has a much higher level of maximal aerobic power than the bodybuilder because of the type of training that the marathon runner participates in. Results from this hypothetical assessment of $VO_2$ max display this relationship. We observe that the bodybuilder has an absolute $VO_2$ max of 4.0 $LO_2 \cdot min^{-1}$ and the marathon runner has an absolute $VO_2$ max of 3.5 $LO_2 \cdot min^{-1}$. Based on this sole piece of information, it may be incorrectly assumed that the bodybuilder displays a greater level of maximal aerobic power. However, when we express $VO_2$ max relative to body weight, it is observed that the bodybuilder has a relative $VO_2$ max of 40 $mLO_2 \cdot kg^{-1} \cdot min^{-1}$ whereas the marathon runner has a relative $VO_2$ max of 54 $mLO_2 \cdot kg^{-1} \cdot min^{-1}$. By expressing $VO_2$ max relative to each individual's body weight, we observe that the marathon runner exhibits a higher level of maximal aerobic power or cardiorespiratory endurance.

## Physiologic Significance of Maximal Oxygen Uptake

$VO_2$ max is an important determinant of performance in events that are of a longer duration and require the production of more energy. These type of events are often labeled as aerobic activities or activities that require more sustained levels of energy production. Some examples include swimming, longer distance running, and cycling. These type of activities require a greater production of adenosine triphosphate (ATP). ATP is the major source of energy for cellular activity or work and is mainly produced by the oxidative metabolic pathways which require oxygen for the synthesis of ATP. Therefore, a greater $VO_2$ max will result in a greater potential for the production of ATP and the maintenance of an adequate energy supply for cellular activity.

There are a variety of body systems that contribute to determining an individual's $VO_2$ max. The determination of $VO_2$ max primarily involves the ability of the respiratory system to oxygenate the blood, the cardiovascular system to transport the oxygenated blood, and the skeletal muscle system to extract and utilize the oxygen from the blood to synthesize ATP. Therefore, an individual's $VO_2$ max is determined by the functioning of these three systems. There has been much scientific debate about the contribution of each of these systems to an individual's $VO_2$ max, or in other words, what system actually is the limiting factor to $VO_2$ max. It is generally assumed that in most individuals the respiratory system functions at an adequate level to fully oxygenate the blood at all levels of exercise intensity. However, some researchers have hypothesized that the respiratory system may be a limiting factor to $VO_2$ max especially in highly endurance-trained athletes.[2] Most researchers believe that the functioning of the cardiovascular system or the musculoskeletal system limits $VO_2$ max. Again though, there is much debate as to which system truly limits $VO_2$ max.[3,4] Those who believe that the cardiovascular system limits performance or $VO_2$ max point to the fact that when an individual reaches his or her maximal ability to deliver oxygen-rich blood (maximal cardiac output), there is no further mechanism to deliver more oxygen-rich blood to the muscles for the production of ATP. Those who believe that the muscular system limits performance or $VO_2$ max point to the fact that at the highest level of exercise intensity an individual can perform at, the muscles are not able to extract or utilize any more oxygen for the production of ATP. The exact mechanisms that determine an individual's $VO_2$ max are still questionable and more research continues to be conducted to answer this question.

It is important to understand that the assessment of $VO_2$ max is not truly an assessment of performance. Rather, it is an assessment of physiologic function that may contribute to an individual's athletic performance. Research has examined the relationship between $VO_2$ max and performance in events typically thought to require a greater level of aerobic metabolism. Although different researchers have reported differing levels of contribution of $VO_2$ max to performance, the consensus is that an individual's $VO_2$ max does significantly contribute to performance in events of longer durations.[5-9]

## Determining Maximal Oxygen Uptake

There are a variety of methods available to assess an individual's VO$_2$ max. VO$_2$ max may be predicted or estimated using nonexercise prediction equations, field tests, and submaximal exercise tests. In addition, VO$_2$ max can be measured in a laboratory using a metabolic measurement system. These various methods to assess VO$_2$ max are discussed below.

### NONEXERCISE PREDICTION EQUATIONS AND FIELD TESTS

VO$_2$ max can be predicted using nonexercise prediction equations. These equations utilize information about an individual's age, gender, body composition, and activity level to predict VO$_2$ max. An example of such an equation is shown below[10]:

$$VO_2 \text{ max } (mLO_2 \cdot kg^{-1} \cdot min^{-1}) = 50.513 + 1.589 \text{ (PA[0–7])} - 0.289 \text{ (years)} \\ - 0.552 \text{ (\%BF)} + 5.863 \text{ (female = 0, male = 1)}$$

where PA represents physical activity and %BF represents percent body fat. The reader is referred to the original citation for the categorical levels of physical activity. As one may expect, using an equation to predict VO$_2$ max is not the most accurate and reliable method to assess VO$_2$ max and is not the most preferable method to use. Field tests may also be used to estimate VO$_2$ max. Field tests are advantageous because they do not require expensive equipment, they are easy to perform, and large groups of individuals may be tested concurrently. Field tests usually utilize the time to complete the test or the heart rate response during a test to predict VO$_2$ max. Examples of field tests include the 1.0 walk[11] and 1.5 mile run[12] tests. The accuracy of these tests depends on an individual's motivation to perform the test and/or the accurate measurement of heart rate. In addition, because these tests do not actually measure oxygen consumption but rather predict VO$_2$ max, their accuracy is quite variable.

### SUBMAXIMAL EXERCISE TESTS

VO$_2$ max can be estimated using submaximal exercise tests. These tests typically measure the heart rate response at submaximal levels of exercise and then use this information to estimate an individual's VO$_2$ max. The heart rate response during exercise can be used to estimate VO$_2$ max because a linear relationship exists between heart rate and exercise intensity and oxygen consumption. The utilization of submaximal exercise tests to estimate VO$_2$ max is based on several assumptions that must be met[13]:

1. A steady-state heart rate is obtained for each submaximal exercise level performed.
2. There is a linear relationship between exercise intensity and heart rate.
3. The prediction of maximal heart rate (220 – age) is accurate.
4. Mechanical efficiency, or the level of oxygen consumption at a given exercise intensity, is uniform from person to person.

One of the most frequently used submaximal exercise tests is the YMCA Cycle Test.[14] This test requires that the subject perform between two and four stages of exercise, each lasting 3 minutes in length while cycling at a pedal rate of 50 revolutions per minute. Heart rate is recorded during the last 15–30 seconds of the second and third minute of each stage of exercise. If the heart rates at the end of the second and third minute differ by more than 6 beats per minute, then the stage of exercise is continued for an additional minute and heart rate is again recorded. The final heart rate for the exercise stage is then recorded and represents the steady-state heart rate for the given stage of exercise.

Each subject begins at an exercise intensity of 150 kg·m·min$^{-1}$ and then the exercise intensity is increased based on the heart rate response for this initial stage of exercise. Figure 8.1 displays the progression of exercise intensity for the YMCA Cycle Test. The goal of the YMCA Cycle Test is to achieve two steady-state heart rates between 110 beats per minute and 85% of the age-predicted maximal heart rate (220 – age).

**FIGURE 8.1.** YMCA Cycle Test protocol. (From Golding et al.[14])

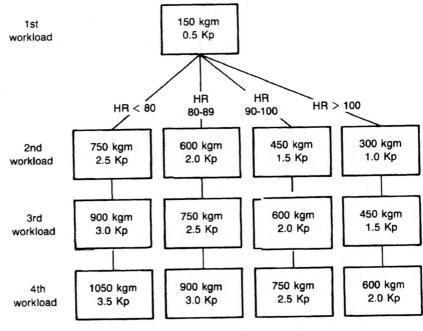

Directions:

1. Set the first workload at 150 kgm/min (0.5 Kp).
2. If the HR in the third min is
   - less than (<) 80, set the second load at 750 kgm (2.5 Kp);
   - 80 to 89, set the second load at 600 kgm (2.0 Kp);
   - 90 to 100, set the second load at 450 kgm (1.5 Kp);
   - greater than (>) 100, set the second load at 300 kgm (1.0 Kp).
3. Set the third and fourth (if required) loads according to the loads in the columns below the second loads.

To estimate VO₂ max, the exercise intensity and the associated steady-state heart rate values are plotted for the two consecutive stages of exercise which met the criteria for the heart rate range of 110 beats per minute to 85% of the age-predicted maximal heart rate. A line is then drawn through these points and this line is extrapolated up to the age-predicted maximal heart rate. A perpendicular line is then drawn down from the point where the extrapolated line meets the age-predicted maximal heart rate line and the VO₂ max is then recorded. Specialized graph paper has been developed to facilitate this calculation and is shown in Figure 8.2.

The benefits of using the YMCA Cycle Test are that the heart rate response for several stages of submaximal exercise intensity are recorded, it requires very little expensive equipment besides a cycle ergometer, and the test is easy to perform for most individuals. However, the accuracy of the estimation of VO₂ max is limited by the accuracy of the 220 – age equation to predict an individual's maximal heart rate.

### Maximal Laboratory Test to Determine Maximal Oxygen Uptake

The most accurate method to assess an individual's VO₂ max is through the use of a graded exercise test in which oxygen consumption is actually measured. This type of test is typically performed in a laboratory or clinical setting because of the use of expensive, specialized equipment and the need for qualified personnel to perform the test. This section describes the general principles of measuring VO₂ max in a laboratory setting, and the equipment and protocols typically used.

The measurement of VO₂ max is based on the Fick equation:

$$VO_2 = Q \times \text{a-v}O_2 \text{ difference}$$

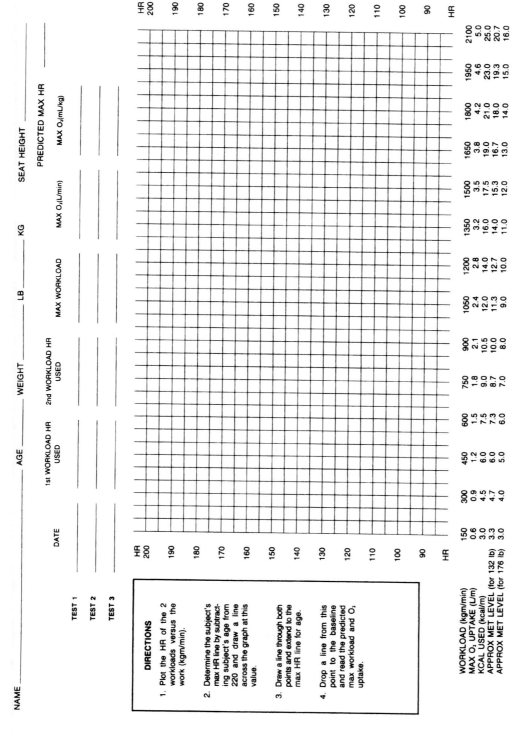

**FIGURE 8.2.** Graph paper to estimate VO$_2$ max from the YMCA Cycle Test. HR = heart rate. (From Golding et al.[14])

where $VO_2$ represents oxygen consumption, Q represents cardiac output, and a-v$O_2$ difference represents the arteriovenous oxygen difference. The measurement of cardiac output and arteriovenous oxygen difference would require invasive techniques such as the catheterization of an artery and a vein. Obviously, this technique is impractical for most purposes and could only be performed in a hospital setting. Therefore, techniques have been established to measure oxygen consumption using measurements that are more easily made in a laboratory setting. Specifically, by measuring ventilation and the difference in oxygen concentration between inspired air and expired air, oxygen consumption can be measured. In a sense then, the measurement of ventilation is comparable to the measurement of cardiac output and the difference in oxygen concentration between inspired and expired air is comparable to the arteriovenous oxygen difference.

## EQUIPMENT

The measurement of $VO_2$ max in a laboratory setting requires equipment that allows for the measurement of ventilation and the concentration of oxygen in expired air. When performing a $VO_2$ max test, the subject typically breathes through a one-way non-rebreathing valve consisting of a rubber mouthpiece and rubber diaphragms. When the subject inspires, the rubber diaphragm on the inspiration side of the mouthpiece opens allowing the subject to breathe in room air while the expiration diaphragm remains closed. Conversely, when the subject expires, the inspiration side of the mouthpiece closes and the expiration diaphragm opens allowing all of the expired air to be directed to the measurement equipment. The subject wears a nose clip so all of the inspired or expired air is directed out of the mouth. Ventilation is measured either on the inspired or expired side of the system using a flowmeter. The expired air is directed to equipment that allows for the measurement of oxygen concentration of the expired air using gas analyzers. By measuring the oxygen concentration of the expired air, and based on the fact that the concentration of inspired room air is 20.93%, the amount of oxygen extracted from the air by the body can be calculated. Thus, by knowing the level of ventilation and the amount of oxygen extracted from the air, oxygen consumption can be calculated. There are several commercially available "metabolic measurement systems" that incorporate a flowmeter, gas analyzers (oxygen and carbon dioxide), and a computer in an integrated package to facilitate the calculations involved in determining oxygen consumption. Before using a metabolic measurement system, it is essential that the system be calibrated to ensure the accurate measurements of ventilation and oxygen and carbon dioxide concentrations in the expired air. The calibration of the flowmeter is performed using a calibration syringe and the oxygen and carbon dioxide analyzers are calibrated using calibration gases of known concentrations.

In addition to the aforementioned equipment, it is also necessary to have an ergometer for the subject to exercise on. Ergometers allow for the precise control of exercise intensity during a graded exercise test. The most common types of ergometers used for graded exercise tests are treadmills and stationary cycle ergometers; however, other types of ergometers may be used such as rowing ergometers and swimming simulators.

Although not necessary for the measurement of $VO_2$ max, heart rate is typically measured during these tests and is usually obtained from an electrocardiograph or a telemetry heart rate monitor. Lastly, it is important to assess the subject's perceptual response to how hard the exercise feels. This measurement is accomplished through the use of the Borg Ratings of Perceived Exertion (RPE) scale (Table 8.1), which requires that the subject point to a number representing how hard the exercise feels.

## PROTOCOLS TO ASSESS MAXIMAL OXYGEN UPTAKE

A true measurement of $VO_2$ max utilizes a graded exercise test. A graded exercise test requires that the subject begin exercising at a low exercise intensity and then the exercise intensity is gradually increased until the person reaches his or her maximal potential. There are a variety of factors to consider when

**TABLE 8.1. Ratings of perceived exertion (RPE) scales.**

| Fifteen category RPE scale | | | Category-ratio RPE scale |
|---|---|---|---|
| 6 | No exertion at all | 0 | Nothing at all |
| 7 | Extremely light | 0.5 | Very, very weak (just noticeable) |
| 8 | | 1 | Very weak |
| 9 | Very light | 2 | Weak (light) |
| 10 | | 3 | Moderate |
| 11 | Light | 4 | Somewhat strong |
| 12 | | 5 | Strong (heavy) |
| 13 | Somewhat hard | 6 | |
| 14 | | 7 | Very strong |
| 15 | Hard (heavy) | 8 | |
| 16 | | 9 | |
| 17 | Very hard | 10 | Very, very strong (almost maximal) |
| 18 | | | |
| 19 | Extremely hard | * | Maximal |
| 20 | Maximal exertion | | |

*Sources:* Borg GV. Psychophysical bases of perceived exertion. Med Sci Sports Exerc 1982;14:377–381; Noble B, Borg GV, Jacobs I, Ceci R, Kaiser P. A category-ratio perceived exertion scale: relationship to blood and muscle lactates and heart rate. Med Sci Sports Exerc 1983;15:523–528.

choosing an appropriate protocol for the graded exercise test. These factors include the mode of exercise, the starting exercise intensity and the rate of progression, and the overall test time.

Most graded exercise tests are performed on a treadmill or a cycle ergometer. However, other modes of exercise may be used as long as the exercise involves the use of a large percentage of the overall muscle mass. The primary consideration to be made when choosing the mode of exercise involves the concept of specificity. When testing athletes, it is best to use a mode of exercise that most closely simulates the type of athletic competition that the athlete performs. For example, when testing a marathon runner, it would make very little sense to use a cycle ergometer instead of a treadmill. Similarly, when testing a competitive cyclist, the results from a graded exercise test using a treadmill would have very little applicability. When testing nonathletes, it is best to choose a mode of exercise that the individual is used to, or determine if there are extenuating circumstances that would make one mode of exercise more safe or appropriate than another. The mode of exercise can also influence the values obtained for an individual's VO$_2$ max. Typically, cycle ergometry protocols result in VO$_2$ max values that are approximately 5%–10% lower than values obtained using treadmill protocols, likely because of the relatively smaller muscle mass involved in cycle ergometry exercise.

When choosing a protocol for a graded exercise test, there are some basic principles that should be followed. The initial exercise intensity should be low enough that this stage of exercise serves as a warmup for the subject. The rate of progression of exercise intensity should be gradual so that local muscular fatigue or the sudden onset of an increase in blood lactic acid concentration does not limit test performance. In addition, the rate of progression of exercise intensity should be at a level that results in an overall test time between 8 and 12 minutes. Lastly, a protocol should be used that is appropriate to the subject [e.g., walking versus running, appropriate treadmill speed (if treadmill is used)]. Although any protocol that meets these aforementioned characteristics will be effective in determining an individual's VO$_2$ max, there are many established protocols that are used in laboratory and clinical settings. The most frequently used treadmill protocols are the Bruce[16] and Balke protocols.[17] These protocols are listed in Table 8.2. There are fewer defined cycle ergometry protocols, but an example of one protocol is listed below:

- 2 minutes of exercise at 40 watts (females) or 60 watts (males)
- 1-minute stages in which the watts are increased 20 watts every minute until volitional exhaustion

TABLE 8.2. Treadmill protocols for maximal graded exercise tests.

| Stage | Time (min) | Speed (mph) | Grade (%) |
|---|---|---|---|
| Bruce protocol for maximal graded exercise test | | | |
| 1 | 0–3 | 1.7 | 10 |
| 2 | 3–6 | 2.5 | 12 |
| 3 | 6–9 | 3.4 | 14 |
| 4 | 9–12 | 4.2 | 16 |
| 5 | 12–15 | 5.0 | 18 |
| 6 | 15–18 | 5.5 | 20 |
| Balke protocol for maximal graded exercise test | | | |
| 1 | 0–1 | 3.3 | 0 |
| 2 | 1–2 | 3.3 | 2 |
| 3 | 2–3 | 3.3 | 3 |
| 4 | 3–4 | 3.3 | 4 |
| 5 | 4–5 | 3.3 | 5 |
| 6 | 5–6 | 3.3 | 6 |
| 7 | 6–7 | 3.3 | 7 |
| 8 | 7–8 | 3.3 | 8 |
| 9 | 8–9 | 3.3 | 9 |
| 10 | 9–10 | 3.3 | 10 |

Sources: Bruce RA. Multistage treadmill test of submaximal and maximal exercise. In: American Heart Association, ed. Exercise Testing and Training of Apparently Healthy Individuals: A Handbook for Physicians. New York: American Heart Association; 1972:32–34; and Balke.[17]

Note: After stage 10, increase grade by 1% every minute while maintaining a speed of 3.3 mph.

In summary, any protocol that meets the aforementioned principles should be effective in determining an individual's $VO_2$ max. However, one must always consider that the protocol be appropriate to the individual being tested and that the individualization of a protocol is sometimes necessary to achieve the proper test characteristics and the goals of the test.

### INTERPRETATION OF MAXIMAL OXYGEN UPTAKE TEST DATA

Interpretation of $VO_2$ max test data is used to: 1) determine if a true maximal effort has been achieved during the test, 2) classify an individual's fitness level, and 3) determine the effectiveness of a training program.

Because a graded exercise test to determine $VO_2$ max requires the motivation of the subject to provide a true maximal effort, objective criteria have been established to confirm that a maximal effort has been achieved. These criteria include[13]:

- A plateau in oxygen consumption. A plateau is defined as an increase in oxygen consumption less than $150 \text{ mL·min}^{-1}$ with an increase in exercise intensity. Although this is the single best indicator of a true maximal effort, it must be used with caution because a plateau is not consistently observed when using many protocols.
- A maximal heart rate within 10 beats per minute of the age-predicted maximal heart rate.
- A respiratory exchange ratio greater than 1.1 or 1.15.
- An RPE greater than 17 (using the Borg 6–20 scale).

To classify an individual's fitness level, one must compare the individual's $VO_2$ max value to population norms. Many studies have established population norms for $VO_2$ max. These tables will typically classify an individual as poor, fair, good, very good, excellent, or provide a percentile ranking. An example of a classification table is provided in Table 8.3.

Lastly, one can use the $VO_2$ max value to determine the effectiveness of a training program. This interpretation requires that the individual be tested before the onset of a training program (pretest) and after the training program (posttest). A comparison of the pre- and posttest $VO_2$ max values can then be used to determine if the training program has resulted in physiologic adaptations influencing $VO_2$ max.

## Specialized Test—The Lactate Threshold

For decades, lactic acid production during exercise has been of interest to scientists because of the relationships among lactic acid, muscle fatigue, and

**TABLE 8.3. Maximal oxygen uptake (VO₂ max) norms for men and women.**

| Percentile | Age | | | | |
|---|---|---|---|---|---|
| | 20–29 | 30–39 | 40–49 | 50–59 | 60+ |
| *Men* | | | | | |
| 90 | 51.4 | 50.4 | 48.2 | 45.3 | 42.5 |
| 80 | 48.2 | 46.8 | 44.1 | 41.0 | 38.1 |
| 70 | 46.8 | 44.6 | 41.8 | 38.5 | 35.3 |
| 60 | 44.2 | 42.4 | 39.9 | 36.7 | 33.6 |
| 50 | 42.5 | 41.0 | 38.1 | 35.2 | 31.8 |
| 40 | 41.0 | 38.9 | 36.7 | 33.8 | 30.2 |
| 30 | 39.5 | 37.4 | 35.1 | 32.3 | 28.7 |
| 20 | 37.1 | 35.4 | 33.0 | 30.2 | 26.5 |
| 10 | 34.5 | 32.5 | 30.9 | 28.0 | 23.1 |
| *Women* | | | | | |
| 90 | 44.2 | 41.0 | 39.5 | 35.2 | 35.2 |
| 80 | 41.0 | 38.6 | 36.3 | 32.3 | 31.2 |
| 70 | 38.1 | 36.7 | 33.8 | 30.9 | 29.4 |
| 60 | 36.7 | 34.6 | 32.3 | 29.4 | 27.2 |
| 50 | 35.2 | 33.8 | 30.9 | 28.2 | 25.8 |
| 40 | 33.8 | 32.3 | 29.5 | 26.9 | 24.5 |
| 30 | 32.3 | 30.5 | 28.3 | 25.5 | 23.8 |
| 20 | 30.6 | 28.7 | 26.5 | 24.3 | 22.8 |
| 10 | 28.4 | 26.5 | 25.1 | 22.3 | 20.8 |

*Sources:* Institute for Aerobics Research, Dallas, TX (1994); American College of Sports Medicine. ACSM's Guidelines for Exercise Testing and Prescription. 6th ed. Philadelphia: Lippincott Williams & Wilkins; 2000.

*Note:* Study population for the data set was predominately white and college educated. A modified Balke treadmill test was used with $\dot{V}O_2$ max estimated from the last grade/speed achieved. The following may be used as descriptors for the percentile rankings: well above average (90), above average (70), average (50), below average (30), and well below average (10).

the disruption of the maintenance of homeostasis within the human body. Lactate threshold is defined as the workload, or exercise intensity, at which lactate begins to accumulate in the blood.[18,19] At lower intensity exercise, blood lactate concentrations remain low because of the low level of lactic acid production as well as an adequate level of removal of lactic acid by the body. However, as exercise intensity increases, lactic acid production increases whereas lactic acid removal from the blood decreases. This combination of effects increases the lactic acid concentration in the blood. In the blood, lactic acid quickly dissociates into a lactate ion and a hydrogen ion. This increase in hydrogen ions may lead to pH disturbances within the body. Thus, the body must buffer the increase in hydrogen ions. This buffering is accomplished though the bicarbonate system. In blood, hydrogen ions originating from lactic acid combine with bicarbonate to eventually produce carbon dioxide and water. This excess carbon dioxide is then expelled from the body via an increase in respiration or ventilation.

The lactate threshold is also frequently referred to as the anaerobic threshold. However, the term anaerobic threshold implies that the increase in lactic acid is solely a result of an increased reliance on anaerobic metabolism. As previously mentioned, the increase in lactic acid may in part be attributable to an increased reliance on anaerobic metabolism, but it may also be attributable to a decrease in the removal of lactic acid from the blood. Therefore, the term lactate threshold is the preferred nomenclature. The term ventilatory threshold is also used to describe the point during exercise at which lactic acid begins to accumulate in the blood as a result of the mechanisms responsible for buffering the increase in hydrogen ions associated with an increase in lactic acid concentrations. Ventilatory threshold is defined as the point during an incremental exercise test at which ventilation increases out of proportion to the increase in oxygen consumption.[20] Again, this increase in ventilation is thought to be the result of the buffering of lactic acid and the subsequent increase in carbon dioxide production which stimulates ventilation.

Because an increase in lactic acid concentration in the body is associated with muscular fatigue, the assessment of the lactate threshold is an important predictor of performance in endurance events such as longer distance running, cycling, and triathlons. In theory, the greater the exercise intensity that the athlete can perform at without a marked increase in blood lactic acid concentration, the greater potential for improved performance. Research has shown a high degree of correlation between the lactate threshold and performance in endurance-type events.[21,22]

The lactate threshold is typically assessed using a graded exercise test similar to that described for the assessment of VO2 max. In addition to the typical physiologic measurements that are made during a VO2 max test, lactate concentration in the blood is measured at the end of each stage of exercise, usually from a venous blood sample or a capillary blood sample obtained from a fingerprick. To determine an individual's lactate threshold, a graph is made plotting the exercise intensity or the rate of oxygen consumption on the x-axis and the lactate concentration on the y-axis. The point at which lactate concentration begins to increase in the blood represents the lactate threshold. Usually the lactate threshold is quantified as the exercise intensity or the percentage of VO2 max at which the lactate concentration begins to increase. Although the protocols used to assess lactate threshold are similar to those described for a VO2 max test, there are many variations that are used by researchers and practitioners that include altering the length of each exercise stage and/or using a discontinuous test with varying rest periods between the stages of exercise.[1] Lastly, more objective methodologies have been developed to aid the researcher or the practitioner in determining the point at which lactic acid concentration begins to increase in the blood.[23,24]

## ASSESSMENT OF ANAEROBIC POWER

Simply stated, anaerobic means without oxygen. Any anaerobic work that is performed occurs without the use of oxygen, metabolically speaking. There are 3 energy systems the body relies on for producing mechanical work. During maximal exercise, each energy system has a definitive timeframe for which each is the dominant energy system (Figure 8.3). The first energy system is the immediate system made up of stored ATP and phosphocreatine. The second energy system is the glycolytic energy system which can be both oxidative (use of oxygen) and nonoxidative depending on the exercise intensity. The third system is oxidation whereby oxygen is the final electron acceptor in the electron transport chain for the formation of ATP, $H_2O$, and $CO_2$.[25]

**FIGURE 8.3.** Three systems of energy transfer. ATP-CP = adenosine triphosphate–creatine phosphate. (From McArdle et al.[25])

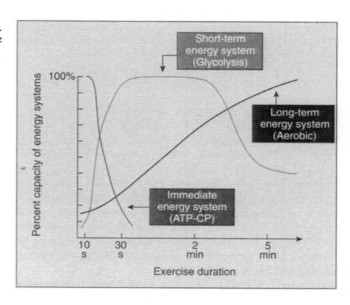

Volumes have been written on each of these energy systems, so this section only provides a brief review as necessary. The immediate energy system is just that, immediate. It is capable of replenishing ATP for only a few seconds during high- or maximal-intensity exercise. To maintain maximal or near-maximal intensity after the initial few seconds, the glycolytic energy system becomes the primary energy system. This system can maximally supply ATP for up to 2 minutes before reliance on those substrates begins to decline. The oxidative system cannot support ATP resynthesis at maximal intensity. Instead, its function is to serve as the primary energy provider in low-power endurance-type activities (submaximal). The oxidative system uses oxygen and, therefore, is not considered in this section of anaerobic (without oxygen) testing.

Anaerobic performance can be further delineated to anaerobic capacity and anaerobic power. Although anaerobic performance is significantly affected by training, it is also partially determined by endogenous ATP and phosphocreatine stores. Glycogen storage is also a significant factor in the ability of the glycolytic system to produce energy. Capacity is measured as the total amount of energy of the system. Power is determined as the maximal amount of energy per unit time.[1] The easiest example to consider is the bench press. Two men may be able to move the absolute same amount of weight on the bench press (200 lbs.). If however, man A is able to move the 200 lbs. from his chest to full extension in 1 second and it takes man B 2 seconds to move the same distance, then man A exhibits more power (200 lbs./1 second).

In general, activities that last less than 10 seconds primarily rely on the immediate energy system. Such activities include 100-m sprint (or distances less than), shot put, American football running plays, running bases in baseball, and a golf swing. The glycolytic system is primarily responsible for activities that last up to 90 seconds and include longer sprints (400 m), ice hockey shift, indoor soccer shift, and 100-m swim.

## Stair-Sprinting Power Test

One of the most well known and frequently used tests to assess anaerobic capacity is the Margaria Staircase Test.[26] This test almost entirely relies on the immediate energy system (stored ATP). It lasts for a time period of less than 3 seconds. The Margaria Staircase Test can be classified as a field test because a laboratory setting is not necessary. However, some specialized equipment is fundamental to this test. The protocol is as follows:

- The subject stands 2 m from the bottom of a set of stairs.
- Timing mats are placed on the 8th and 12th stairs.
- The subject is instructed to run at top speed from the 2-m start point up the stairs, two at a time.

Total power for this test is calculated as:

$$\text{Power (kg·m·s}^{-1}) = \text{wt of subject (kg)} \times \text{vertical distance between mats (m)/time (s)}$$

There are some variations to the Margaria Staircase Test, but the objective of measuring muscular power remains constant. Once such variation is that the subject travels up the stairs three at a time. The protocol for this is similar to the previous:

- The subject begins 6 m from the bottom of a set of stairs.
- Timing mats are placed on the 3rd and 9th stairs.
- The subject is instructed to run at top speed from the 6-m start point up the stairs, three at a time.

## 30-Second Cycle Sprint Test

If there has been one test that has been the most widely used test to assess anaerobic performance, it is the 30-second Wingate Test.[27] Although there are variations relative to the length of this test, the 30-second test predominates. The Wingate Test is performed on a cycle ergometer whereby the subject pedals

**TABLE 8.4. Percentile norms for peak and average power.**

| % Rank | Average power | | Peak power | |
|---|---|---|---|---|
| | Male | Female | Male | Female |
| | watts (W) | | watts (W) | |
| 90 | 662 | 470 | 822 | 560 |
| 80 | 618 | 419 | 777 | 527 |
| 70 | 600 | 410 | 757 | 505 |
| 60 | 577 | 391 | 721 | 480 |
| 50 | 565 | 381 | 689 | 449 |
| 40 | 548 | 367 | 671 | 432 |
| 30 | 530 | 353 | 656 | 399 |
| 20 | 496 | 336 | 618 | 376 |
| 10 | 471 | 306 | 570 | 353 |
| | $W \cdot kg \cdot BW^{-1}$ | | $W \cdot kg \cdot BW^{-1}$ | |
| 90 | 8.24 | 7.31 | 10.89 | 9.02 |
| 80 | 8.01 | 6.95 | 10.39 | 8.83 |
| 70 | 7.91 | 6.77 | 10.20 | 8.56 |
| 60 | 7.59 | 6.59 | 9.80 | 8.14 |
| 50 | 7.44 | 6.39 | 9.22 | 7.65 |
| 40 | 7.14 | 6.15 | 8.92 | 6.96 |
| 30 | 7.00 | 6.03 | 8.53 | 6.86 |
| 20 | 6.59 | 5.71 | 8.24 | 6.57 |
| 10 | 5.98 | 5.25 | 7.06 | 5.98 |

*Source:* Adapted from McArdle WD, Katch FI, Katch VL. Exercise Physiology: Energy, Nutrition and Human Performance. 5th ed. Baltimore: Williams & Wilkins; 2001.

at maximal speed for a period of 30 seconds. After a proper warmup, the protocol is as follows:

- Subject pedals against zero resistance until maximal pedaling rate is achieved.
- Subject then pedals against a resistance that equals 75 g/kg body weight for the duration of the test.
- Subject then pedals against zero resistance for a cool-down period.

Results from this test include mean power, peak power, and fatigue index. Mean power represents the mean output over the 30-second test period and is assumed to represent the capacity of the glycolytic energy system. Peak power represents the highest power output over a 5-second period and is assumed to represent the energy-generating capacity of high-energy phosphates (immediate energy system) and the fatigue index is the difference between the peak power and the lowest 5-second power output divided by the peak power.[28] Norms for the Wingate Test have been established (Table 8.4).[29]

## Vertical Jump

The vertical jump test is another means to assess muscular power, and a very objective measurement for determining the progress of the athlete through his or her training program (see Table 8.5). The vertical jump test is a very simple way of measuring the height an athlete can jump from a two-footed standing position. To begin, the athlete stands next to a wall and fully extends an arm over the head and reaches the highest position with fingers fully extended and palm facing the wall while standing flat-footed. This spot is marked on the wall. Next, the athlete performs a countermovement jump (arms move downward and knees bend into a squat position) and then jumps as high as possible touching the wall at the peak height of the jump. This spot is then marked and the difference between the marks is the vertical jump height. Usually three jumps are performed with a rest of 15–30 seconds between jumps. The highest jump should be recorded. Different types of commercial apparatus are available to assess muscular power via vertical jump height. Leg power can be determined by the following equation:

$$\text{Leg power (kgm/s)} = 2.21 \times \text{wt in kg} \times \sqrt{\text{vertical jump(m)}}$$

**TABLE 8.5.** Classification table for vertical jump height (cm).

| Age | Excellent | Very good | Good | Fair | Needs improvement |
|---|---|---|---|---|---|
| **15–19** | | | | | |
| Male | ≥104 | 88–103 | 73–87 | 61–72 | ≤60 |
| Female | ≥74 | 67–73 | 58–66 | 51–57 | ≤50 |
| **20–29** | | | | | |
| Male | ≥121 | 102–120 | 89–101 | 74–88 | ≤73 |
| Female | ≥78 | 65–77 | 56–64 | 52–55 | ≤51 |
| **30–39** | | | | | |
| Male | ≥120 | 102–119 | 87–101 | 70–86 | ≤69 |
| Female | ≥74 | 64–73 | 56–63 | 51–55 | ≤50 |
| **40–49** | | | | | |
| Male | ≥113 | 96–112 | 81–95 | 73–80 | ≤72 |
| Female | ≥72 | 60–71 | 56–59 | 52–55 | ≤51 |
| **50–59** | | | | | |
| Male | ≥105 | 93–104 | 76–92 | 68–75 | ≤67 |
| Female | ≥71 | 63–70 | 57–62 | 54–56 | ≤53 |
| **60–69** | | | | | |
| Male | ≥98 | 84–97 | 75–83 | 67–74 | ≤66 |
| Female | ≥64 | 56–63 | 53–55 | 49–52 | ≤48 |

*Source:* Adapted from Nieman DC. Exercise Testing and Prescription. 4th ed. Mountain View, CA: Mayfield Publishing; 1999.

## ASSESSMENT OF MUSCULAR STRENGTH

Muscular strength tests are used quite often in fitness testing athletes for a variety of reasons. One main reason is to assess absolute strength and make comparisons between athletes. Also, as has already been mentioned, initial testing allows for a starting point to determine the appropriate program design to attain a specific goal. Periodic testing also allows an objective measure to determine if the training is resulting in the intended outcome. Strength can be used very effectively as an objective measure to determine if an athlete can move more weight. This, however, does not always directly translate to an athlete improving his or her performance unless that performance is based solely on lifting a specified weight such as power-lifting competitions. In today's sports, strength training is used in conjunction with many other performance-related criteria (skill training, tactical training, speed, agility, and coordination) to improve overall performance. There are, however, many different means to measure muscular strength.

### 1 Repetition Maximum

The most widely used field measure for testing strength (the amount of force or weight that a particular muscle or group of muscles can move one time) is the 1 repetition maximum (1 RM). Bench press and squat are the two most frequently used movements for measuring 1 RM. The bench press is used to measure strength of the triceps, pectoralis major, and anterior deltoid. The squat is a measure of strength for the quadriceps and gluteus maximus. The 1-RM tests are truly a mixture of science and art. There should always be a warmup period in which the athlete becomes familiar with the movement and that allows the muscles to be properly prepared. Weight should be continually added to a successful 1 RM until the athlete can no longer lift the weight. A rest period of 1–3 minutes between trials should be allowed. For the bench press test and after a proper warmup, the athlete lies on his or her back on a bench with arms fully extended. Grip on the bar should be approximately shoulder width apart with the palms facing forward. The bar should be lowered until it touches the chest and then pushed back upward until arms are once again fully extended. Breathing during this movement should not be ignored. Inspiration during the eccentric movement (bar moving down to chest) and expiration during the concentric movement (bar moving upward to full arm extension) is the proper technique for breathing during the bench press. The 1-RM bench press can be performed using either free weights or machines. Free weights require the help of a spotter. Machines offer an easier and safer test, but may not allow for exact measuring of muscular strength because of inexact weight selection.

The 1-RM testing can also be estimated as may be warranted with certain populations such as preadolescents. Prediction equations are used to determine the 1 RM from a 7- to 10-RM weight. This means that the athlete can lift a weight no more than 7–10 times. This 7–10 RM represents approximately 68% of a 1 RM.[30] Depending on the training status of the person, one of two equations can be used to estimate the 1 RM[30]:

Trained:     1 RM (kg) = 1.554 (7–10 RM wt in kg) – 5.181

Untrained:   1 RM (kg) = 1.172 (7–10 RM wt in kg) + 7.704

Laboratory testing of muscular strength requires much more expensive equipment and qualified personnel to run the testing. There are some advantages to laboratory testing compared with traditional field testing such as the 1 RM but these advantages do not always overcome the simplicity and ease of field testing. To begin, most, if not all, laboratory testing require some form of equipment. With any type of equipment, it is imperative that it is calibrated on a regular basis. This, in and of itself, increases the time aspect of strength testing when using sophisticated laboratory equipment. Also, each individual piece of equipment may have norms that are only relative to that particular piece of equipment. Therefore, it is a very important consideration when making comparisons of strength using different equipment.

## Isometric Strength Testing

The first type of strength testing is isometric. Isometric means that displacement and velocity are equal to zero with no change in muscle fiber length so no movement occurs. With proper equipment (isometric dynamometers), peak force can be measured but that peak force is only applicable at the specific joint angle at which the test is performed. Some apparatus are designed to allow measurements at different joint angles throughout a range of motion.[1] For example, a traditional biceps curl using a dumbbell is performed by placing a dumbbell in one hand with the arm fully extended hanging down by the athlete's side. The movement calls for the dumbbell to be raised by forearm flexion to the highest point possible and then lowered under control back to the original starting position. The maximal strength (weight) achieved in this movement will occur at the weakest joint angle throughout that entire range of motion. Therefore, in an isometric test, the peak force recorded for a specific joint angle does not necessarily represent the peak force of that muscle or group of muscles. Therefore, isometric testing must be performed through a variety of joint angles. Although isometric exercise can be used to increase strength, it has very little application to sports which tend to be dynamic in nature.

## Isokinetic Strength Testing

Isokinetic testing is another aspect of laboratory testing. Isokinetic means constant velocity.[31] Isokinetic dynamometers are used to control the velocity of movement throughout a range of motion. The apparatus provides resistance so that force is matched to the resistance mechanism not allowing for acceleration to occur. This allows for measurement of work, power, and torque of muscles at a specific and constant velocity. Strength gains can be realized with isokinetic training but direct application to sports is negligible. However, isokinetic exercises can be beneficial to regaining strength after injury, but again it has little application to sports or events that are dynamic or have a need for changing velocities.

## Isotonic Strength Testing

Isotonic testing is yet another type of strength testing in which there is constant tension or force output throughout the range of motion (different joint angles). Classical weightlifting is considered isotonic because the same weight is lifted throughout a range of motion. However, this is often criticized because the actual force applied throughout that range of motion is rarely constant because of changes in acceleration, deceleration, and mechanical advantage of joint angles. Isotonic dynamometers are used to measure acceleration, work, power, and peak velocity at various preset constant loads. This is the most applicable scenario when it comes to strength training for sports performance.

## ASSESSMENT OF FLEXIBILITY

Flexibility refers to the movement of a joint through its full range of motion. Flexibility may contribute to the ability to perform various tasks associated with athletic competition and may also decrease the risk of injury when performing these athletic events. In addition, flexibility is an important component to an individual's health and fitness status because it is associated with the ability to perform various activities of daily living. There are a variety of factors that may influence an individual's level of flexibility. These factors include age, level of physical activity, and the tightness of muscles, ligaments, and tendons.[13,32] Preexercise behaviors such as stretching and adequate warmup will also affect the level of flexibility.[13]

Although there are several frequently used methods to assess an individual's flexibility, there is no single test that serves as an indicator of whole-body flexibility. This is because the measurement of flexibility is specific to the joint being tested. The most frequently used test to assess an individual's level of flexibility is the sit and reach test. There are a variety of sit and reach tests that are used in the assessment of flexibility, specifically the YMCA,[14] the Traditional,[33] and the Wall[34] sit and reach tests.

### Methods to Assess Flexibility

This section describes the most frequently used methods to assess an individual's level of flexibility. Before testing, stretching and a light warmup should be performed to optimize the measurement of flexibility and reduce the chances of injury.

The YMCA Sit and Reach Test is easy to perform and requires no special equipment except for a typical yard/meter stick. The protocol to administer the YMCA Sit and Reach Test follows:

1. A yard/meter stick is placed on the ground and a piece of tape is placed perpendicular to the yard/meter stick and the 15-inch line.
2. The subject sits on the floor (without shoes) with the legs extended and the heels of the feet placed at the taped line approximately 10–12 inches apart.
3. With the hands together and the arms extended, the subject then reaches forward as far as possible along the yard/meter stick without bending the knees and holds this position for a few seconds. It is important that the legs remain extended (i.e., no knee bend), but the tester should not press down on the knees of the subject.
4. The score is recorded as the distance the subject reaches. Three trials are typically performed with the best score of the three trials representing the subject's level of flexibility.

The Traditional Sit and Reach Test utilizes a sit and reach box to determine an individual's level of flexibility. A sit and reach box is a box-like structure with a flat horizontal surface that extends over the box toward the subject and has a measuring scale in centimeters. When using a sit and reach box, the subject's heels are placed against the box and this surface is perpendicular to the 23-cm mark on the measuring scale. Sit and reach boxes are commercially available or are easily constructed. The protocol to administer the Traditional Sit and Reach Test follows:

1. The subject sits on the floor (without shoes) with the legs extended and the feet placed against the sit and reach box. The sit and reach box is either stabilized by the tester or placed against a wall to ensure that the box does not move.

2. With the hands together and the arms extended, the subject then reaches forward four times without bending the knees. The first three movements may be submaximal, but the fourth measurement should be maximal and the final position should be held for a few seconds. It is important that the legs remain extended (i.e., no knee bend). The tester may apply slight downward pressure on the knees, but the tester should not exert maximal pressure on the knees.
3. The score is recorded as the distance the subject reaches on the fourth attempt. Three trials are typically performed with the best score of the three trials representing the subject's level of flexibility.

The Wall Sit and Reach Test is very similar to the Traditional Sit and Reach Test with the exception that there is a preliminary measurement that accounts for individual differences in limb length. The protocol to administer the Wall Sit and Reach Test is identical to the Traditional Sit and Reach Test except for the following additions/modifications:

1. The subject sits on the floor (without shoes) with the head, back, and hips against a wall.
2. With the hands together and arms extended, the subject reaches forward as far as possible while keeping the head, back, and hips along the wall. The shoulders may be rolled forward. The tester then records the measurement and this score represents the "starting point."
3. The subject then performs the sit and reach test using the same procedures described for the Traditional Sit and Reach Test.
4. The final score is calculated as the maximal distance reached minus the starting point.

There are a variety of other methods to assess an individual's flexibility that include assessments of specific joints.[35] In addition, devices such as a goniometer (a device to measure the range of motion in degrees) and the Leighton Flexometer are useful because they can be used to test the range of motion of specific joints of the body.

## Interpretation of Flexibility Test Data

The sit and reach tests are frequently used to assess an individual's flexibility because these protocols are thought to assess the flexibility of the hamstrings and lower back, which is associated with low-back function. However, various research studies have questioned the validity of these tests in measuring flexibility in relation to low-back function.[36] Regardless, these tests are still the most typical tests performed. Tables 8.6, 8.7, and 8.8 provide population norms for the YMCA, Traditional, and Wall Sit and Reach Tests, respectively.

TABLE 8.6. Population norms for the YMCA Sit and Reach Test (in).

| | Age (years) | | | | | | | | | | | |
| | 18–25 | | 26–35 | | 36–45 | | 46–55 | | 56–65 | | >65 | |
| | Gender | | | | | | | | | | | |
| Percentile | M | F | M | F | M | F | M | F | M | F | M | F |
|---|---|---|---|---|---|---|---|---|---|---|---|---|
| 90 | 22 | 24 | 21 | 23 | 21 | 22 | 19 | 21 | 17 | 20 | 17 | 20 |
| 80 | 20 | 22 | 19 | 21 | 19 | 21 | 17 | 20 | 15 | 19 | 15 | 18 |
| 70 | 19 | 21 | 17 | 20 | 17 | 19 | 15 | 18 | 13 | 17 | 13 | 17 |
| 60 | 18 | 20 | 17 | 20 | 16 | 18 | 14 | 17 | 13 | 16 | 12 | 17 |
| 50 | 17 | 19 | 15 | 19 | 15 | 17 | 13 | 16 | 11 | 15 | 10 | 15 |
| 40 | 15 | 18 | 14 | 17 | 13 | 16 | 11 | 14 | 9 | 14 | 9 | 14 |
| 30 | 14 | 17 | 13 | 16 | 13 | 15 | 10 | 14 | 9 | 13 | 8 | 13 |
| 20 | 13 | 16 | 11 | 15 | 11 | 14 | 9 | 12 | 7 | 11 | 7 | 11 |
| 10 | 11 | 14 | 9 | 13 | 7 | 12 | 6 | 10 | 5 | 9 | 4 | 9 |

*Sources:* Based on data from Golding et al.[14] Adapted from American College of Sports Medicine. ACSM's Guidelines for Exercise Testing and Prescription. 6th ed. Philadelphia: Lippincott Williams & Wilkins; 2000.

*Note:* Data are in inches.

**TABLE 8.7. Population norms for the Traditional Sit and Reach Test (cm).**

| | Age (years) | | | | | | | | | |
| | 20–29 | | 30–39 | | 40–49 | | 50–59 | | 60–69 | |
| | Gender | | | | | | | | | |
| Percentile | M | F | M | F | M | F | M | F | M | F |
|---|---|---|---|---|---|---|---|---|---|---|
| 90 | 42 | 43 | 40 | 42 | 37 | 40 | 38 | 40 | 35 | 37 |
| 80 | 38 | 40 | 37 | 39 | 34 | 37 | 32 | 37 | 30 | 34 |
| 70 | 36 | 38 | 34 | 37 | 30 | 35 | 29 | 35 | 26 | 31 |
| 60 | 33 | 36 | 32 | 35 | 28 | 33 | 27 | 32 | 24 | 30 |
| 50 | 31 | 34 | 29 | 33 | 25 | 31 | 25 | 30 | 22 | 28 |
| 40 | 29 | 32 | 27 | 31 | 23 | 29 | 22 | 29 | 18 | 26 |
| 30 | 26 | 29 | 24 | 28 | 20 | 26 | 18 | 26 | 16 | 24 |
| 20 | 23 | 26 | 21 | 25 | 16 | 24 | 15 | 23 | 14 | 23 |
| 10 | 18 | 22 | 17 | 21 | 12 | 19 | 12 | 19 | 11 | 18 |

*Sources:* Based on data from The Canada Fitness Survey, 1981. Canadian Standardized Test of Fitness (CSTF) Operations Manual. 3rd ed. Adapted from American College of Sports Medicine. ACSM's Guidelines for Exercise Testing and Prescription. 6th ed. Philadelphia: Lippincott Williams & Wilkins; 2000.

*Note:* Data are in centimeters.

## OTHER CONSIDERATIONS

Testing order and proper (standardized) warmup are probably the most often overlooked aspects of physiologic testing in both laboratory and field testing. Clearly, a proper warmup should always be performed before testing. Warmup is necessary to prepare the body and all relevant physiologic systems for work. Unfortunately, there are few, if any, standardized warmups found in the literature. Many scientists and their respective laboratories have developed their own standardized warmups so useful comparisons can be made. Therefore, it is our recommendation to develop your own standardized warmup based on sound scientific principles for the physiologic components covered in this chapter.

**TABLE 8.8. Population norms for the Wall Sit and Reach Test (in).**

| | Age (years) | | | | | |
| | <35 | | 36–49 | | >50 | |
| | Gender | | | | | |
| Percentile | M | F | M | F | M | F |
|---|---|---|---|---|---|---|
| 99 | 24.7 | 19.8 | 18.9 | 19.8 | 16.2 | 17.2 |
| 95 | 19.5 | 18.7 | 18.2 | 19.2 | 15.8 | 15.7 |
| 90 | 17.9 | 17.9 | 16.1 | 17.4 | 15.0 | 15.0 |
| 80 | 17.0 | 16.7 | 14.6 | 16.2 | 13.3 | 14.2 |
| 70 | 15.8 | 16.2 | 13.9 | 15.2 | 12.3 | 13.6 |
| 60 | 15.0 | 15.8 | 13.4 | 14.5 | 11.5 | 12.3 |
| 50 | 14.4 | 14.8 | 12.6 | 13.5 | 10.2 | 11.1 |
| 40 | 13.5 | 14.5 | 11.6 | 12.8 | 9.7 | 10.1 |
| 30 | 13.0 | 13.7 | 10.8 | 12.2 | 9.3 | 9.2 |
| 20 | 11.6 | 12.6 | 9.9 | 11.0 | 8.8 | 8.3 |
| 10 | 9.2 | 10.1 | 8.3 | 9.7 | 7.8 | 7.5 |
| 5 | 7.9 | 8.1 | 7.0 | 8.5 | 7.2 | 3.7 |
| 1 | 7.0 | 2.6 | 5.1 | 2.0 | 4.0 | 1.5 |

*Sources:* Hoeger WWK. Principles and Laboratories for Physical Fitness and Wellness. Englewood, CO: Morton Publishing; 1991. Adapted from Adams GM. Exercise Physiology Laboratory Manual. 3rd ed. Boston: WCB McGraw-Hill; 1998:257.

*Note:* Data are in inches.

Testing order is another issue that needs to be addressed so that useful comparisons of research can be made. Another consideration to determine sequence of testing is determining what battery of tests will be conducted and the time-frame allowable for testing. It is generally accepted that nonfatiguing tests should be administered first. These tests would include such things as height, weight, blood pressure, flexibility, body composition, and anaerobic power tests such as vertical jump. Maximum power and strength testing should be performed next. Such tests would include the 1-RM bench press. After an appropriate recovery period, at least 5–10 minutes, muscular endurance tests can be performance such as reps to failure. Fatigable anaerobic tests such as the Margaria Stairstep Test or the Wingate cycle test should then follow. It is important that a considerable rest period lasting at least 1 hour be given if an aerobic capacity test must be performed on the same day. Preferably, however, aerobic tests should be conducted on a separate day for the fatigable anaerobic tests.

## QUESTIONS

1. Which of the following would be an assessment of performance in a marathon runner?
   a. Maximal aerobic power
   b. Maximal anaerobic power
   c. Flexibility
   d. Time to complete the marathon event
   e. None of the above are correct
   f. All of the above are correct

2. Physiologic/performance testing of athletes is beneficial for all of the following reasons except:
   a. Determine current health and fitness status
   b. Determine strengths and weaknesses relating to performance in a specific event
   c. Project the likely winner of an athletic competition
   d. Assess the effectiveness of a training program
   e. All of the above
   f. None of the above

3. Tom, a track and field athlete, had his flexibility assessed on 3 consecutive days. The results of these three tests varied by upwards of 20%. Assuming Tom's flexibility has not changed over the 3 days of testing, one might conclude that the test used to assess flexibility has a low degree of:
   a. Validity
   b. Reliability
   c. Reproducibility
   d. a and b are correct
   e. b and c are correct
   f. All of the above are correct

4. In relation to an individual's $VO_2$ max, this body system is primarily responsible for the transport of oxygen-rich blood to the muscles of the body:
   a. Respiratory system
   b. Endocrine system
   c. Sympathetic nervous system
   d. Cardiovascular system
   e. All of the above are correct
   f. None of the above are correct

5. An athlete, who weighs 70 kg, has an absolute $VO_2$ max of 4.2 $LO_2 \cdot min^{-1}$. What is his $VO_2$ max in relative terms?
   a. $60\,mLO_2 \cdot kg^{-1} \cdot min^{-1}$
   b. $42\,mLO_2 \cdot kg^{-1} \cdot min^{-1}$
   c. $55\,mLO_2 \cdot kg^{-1} \cdot min^{-1}$
   d. $0.06\,mLO_2 \cdot kg^{-1} \cdot min^{-1}$
   e. $82\,mLO_2 \cdot kg^{-1} \cdot min^{-1}$
   f. None of the above are correct

6. Submaximal exercise tests are able to predict $VO_2$ max because of what assumptions:
    a. A linear relationship exists among heart rate, $VO_2$, and exercise intensity
    b. That the maximum heart rate at a given age is uniform
    c. That the mechanical efficiency ($VO_2$ at a given workload) is the same for everyone
    d. That the heart rate at a given submaximal exercise intensity is the same for everyone
    e. a, b, c
    f. a, b, d
    g. All of the above

7. Grace, who is 27 years of age, is completing a YMCA Cycle Test. The goal of the test is to complete two stages of exercise with heart rates between:
    a. 110–150 bpm
    b. 120–150 bpm
    c. 60–193 bpm
    d. 110–164 bpm
    e. 120–150 bpm
    f. None of the above

8. Janet recently completed the YMCA Cycle Test. Her data are listed below. What is Janet's estimated absolute $VO_2$ max?

    Age = 21 years, body weight = 60 kg

    | | | |
    |---|---|---|
    | Workload 1: | 150 kg·m·min$^{-1}$ | heart rate = 98 |
    | Workload 2: | 450 kg·m·min$^{-1}$ | heart rate = 130 |
    | Workload 3: | 600 kg·m·min$^{-1}$ | heart rate = 148 |

    a. 2.3 LO$_2$·min$^{-1}$
    b. 1.5 LO$_2$·min$^{-1}$
    c. 2.9 LO$_2$·min$^{-1}$
    d. 3.5 LO$_2$·min$^{-1}$
    e. 4.2 LO$_2$·min$^{-1}$
    f. None of the above are correct

9. All of the following are the criteria for a "true" maximal effort on a graded exercise test, except for:
    a. Plateau in oxygen uptake
    b. Maximum heart rate within ± 10 beats of age-predicted maximum
    c. Respiratory Exchange Ratio <1.05
    d. Ratings of perceived exertion >17
    e. All of the above are criteria

10. This component of a "Metabolic Measurement System" measures the amount of air an individual inspires or expires:
    a. Oxygen analyzer
    b. Carbon dioxide analyzer
    c. One-way non-rebreathing valve
    d. Flowmeter
    e. None of the above are correct

11. The lactate threshold is defined as:
    a. The workload, or exercise intensity, at which lactate begins to decrease in the blood
    b. The workload, or exercise intensity, at which lactate begins to accumulate in the blood
    c. The workload, or exercise intensity, at which lactate concentration in the blood remains constant
    d. The workload, or exercise intensity, at which ventilation begins to decrease
    e. None of the above are correct

12. The initial energy source for mechanical work comes from:
    a. Stored adenosine triphosphate
    b. Phosphocreatine

c. The breakdown of glucose

d. The breakdown of free fatty acids

e. a and b are correct

f. c and d are correct

g. All of the above are correct

13. An athlete, who weighs 165 lbs., performed the Margaria Staircase Test. The vertical distance between the timing mats was 110 cm and the time recorded between the timing mats was 0.5 seconds. The calculated power for this athlete is:

a. $165 \, kg \cdot m \cdot s^{-1}$

b. $220 \, kg \cdot m \cdot s^{-1}$

c. $363 \, kg \cdot m \cdot s^{-1}$

d. $16,500 \, kg \cdot m \cdot s^{-1}$

e. None of the above are correct

14. For the Wingate Test, the recommended resistance to be used for an 80-kg individual is:

a. 4000 g

b. 4.0 kg

c. 6.0 kg

d. 3.0 kg

e. 3500 g

f. None of the above are correct

15. An untrained individual has an 8 RM of 45 kg. This individual's predicted 1 RM is:

a. 64.7 kg

b. 60.4 kg

c. 150 lbs.

d. 180 lbs.

e. None of the above are correct

16. This type of assessment measures muscle strength at a constant velocity:

a. Isometric testing

b. Isotonic testing

c. Isokinetic testing

d. All of the above are correct

e. None of the above are correct

17. This type of assessment of muscular strength provides a constant tension or force output throughout the entire range of motion:

a. Isometric testing

b. Isotonic testing

c. Isokinetic testing

d. All of the above are correct

e. None of the above are correct

18. A 40-year-old woman performed the YMCA Sit and Reach Test and obtained a score of 18 inches. The percentile ranking for this individual is:

a. 80th percentile

b. 30th percentile

c. 60th percentile

d. 45th percentile

e. None of the above are correct

19. A 22-year-old male athlete performed the Wall Sit and Reach Test and was able to reach 20 inches. His final score for the test was 17.5 inches. What was his "starting point" score?

a. 5.0 inches

b. 2.5 inches

c. 3.5 inches

d. 10 cm

e. None of the above are correct

20. An athlete is undergoing a battery of tests which include a 1-RM bench press test, an assessment of body composition, and a Wingate Test. These tests should be performed in what order:
    a. 1-RM bench press, body composition, Wingate Test
    b. Wingate Test, 1-RM bench press, body composition
    c. Body composition, Wingate Test, 1-RM bench press
    d. Body composition, 1-RM bench press, Wingate Test
    e. The order of the testing is nonconsequential

# REFERENCES

1. MacDougall JD, Wenger HA, Green HJ, Canadian Association of Sport Sciences. Physiological Testing of the High-Performance Athlete. 2nd ed. Champaign, IL: Human Kinetics Publishers; 1991.
2. Dempsey JA, Wolffe JB. Memorial lecture. Is the lung built for exercise? Med Sci Sports Exerc 1986;18:143–155.
3. Bassett DR Jr, Howley ET. Limiting factors for maximum oxygen uptake and determinants of endurance performance. Med Sci Sports Exerc 2000;32:70–84.
4. Saltin B, Strange S. Maximal oxygen uptake: "old" and "new" arguments for a cardiovascular limitation. Med Sci Sports Exerc 1992;24:30–37.
5. Taylor HL, Buskirk E, Henschel A. Maximal oxygen intake as an objective measure of cardio-respiratory performance. J Appl Physiol 1955;8:73–80.
6. Cooper KH. Testing and developing cardiovascular fitness within the United States Air Force. J Occup Med 1968;10:636–639.
7. Mayhew JL, Andrew J. Assessment of running performance in college males from aerobic capacity percentage utilization coefficients. J Sports Med Phys Fitness 1975; 15:342–346.
8. Getchell LH, Kirkendall D, Robbins G. Prediction of maximal oxygen uptake in young adult women joggers. Res Q 1977;48:61–67.
9. Kumagai S, Tanaka K, Matsuura Y, Matsuzaka A, Hirakoba K, Asano K. Relationships of the anaerobic threshold with the 5 km, 10 km, and 10 mile races. Eur J Appl Physiol Occup Physiol 1982;49:13–23.
10. Jackson AS, Blair SN, Mahar MT, Wier LT, Ross RM, Stuteville JE. Prediction of functional aerobic capacity without exercise testing. Med Sci Sports Exerc 1990; 22:863–870.
11. Kline GM, Porcari JP, Hintermeister R, et al. Estimation of VO2max from a one-mile track walk, gender, age, and body weight. Med Sci Sports Exerc 1987;19:253–259.
12. Cooper KH. The Aerobics Way: New Data on the World's Most Popular Exercise Program. New York: M. Evans; distributed in U.S. by JB Lippincott; 1977.
13. American College of Sports Medicine, Whaley MH, Brubaker PH, Otto RM, Armstrong LE. ACSM's Guidelines for Exercise Testing and Prescription. 7th ed. Baltimore: Lippincott Williams & Wilkins; 2005.
14. Golding LA, Myers CR, Sinning WE. Y's Way to Physical Fitness: The Complete Guide to Fitness Testing and Instruction. 3rd ed. Champaign, IL: Human Kinetics Publishers; 1989.
15. Astrand PO, Ryhming I. A nomogram for calculation of aerobic capacity (physical fitness) from pulse rate during sub-maximal work. J Appl Physiol 1954;7:218–221.
16. Bruce RA, Kusumi F, Hosmer D. Maximal oxygen intake and nomographic assessment of functional aerobic impairment in cardiovascular disease. Am Heart J 1973;85:546–562.
17. Balke B. Advanced Exercise Procedures for Evaluation of the Cardiovascular System. Milton, WI: Burdick; 1970.
18. Brooks GA. Anaerobic threshold: review of the concept and directions for future research. Med Sci Sports Exerc 1985;17:22–34.
19. Davis JA. Anaerobic threshold: review of the concept and directions for future research. Med Sci Sports Exerc 1985;17:6–21.
20. Wasserman K, Whipp BJ, Koyl SN, Beaver WL. Anaerobic threshold and respiratory gas exchange during exercise. J Appl Physiol 1973;35:236–243.
21. Farrell PA, Wilmore JH, Coyle EF, Billing JE, Costill DL. Plasma lactate accumulation and distance running performance. Med Sci Sports 1979;11:338–344.
22. Sjodin B, Jacobs I. Onset of blood lactate accumulation and marathon running performance. Int J Sports Med 1981;2:23–26.
23. Wasserman K, McIlroy MB. Detecting the threshold of anaerobic metabolism in cardiac patients during exercise. Am J Cardiol 1964;14:844–852.
24. Wasserman K. Determinants and detection of anaerobic threshold and consequences of exercise above it. Circulation 1987;76:VI29–39.

25. McArdle WD, Katch FI, Katch VL. Exercise Physiology: Energy, Nutrition, and Human Performance. 4th ed. Baltimore: Williams & Wilkins; 1996.
26. Margaria R, Aghemo P, Rovelli E. Measurement of muscular power (anaerobic) in man. J Appl Physiol 1966;21:1662–1664.
27. Nelson RC, Morehouse CA. Biomechanics IV; proceedings. Baltimore: University Park Press; 1974.
28. Inbar O, Bar-Or O. Anaerobic characteristics in male children and adolescents. Med Sci Sports Exerc 1986;18:264–269.
29. Maud PJ, Shultz BB. Norms for the Wingate anaerobic test with comparison to another similar test. Res Q Exerc Sport 1989;60:144–151.
30. Braith RW, Graves JE, Leggett SH, Pollock ML. Effect of training on the relationship between maximal and submaximal strength. Med Sci Sports Exerc 1993;25:132–138.
31. Hislop HJ, Perrine JJ. The isokinetic concept of exercise. Phys Ther 1967;47:114–117.
32. Hein V, Jurimae T. Measurement and evaluation of trunk forward flexibility. Sports Med Training Rehabil 1996;7:1–6.
33. American Alliance for Health, Physical Education, Recreation and Dance. AAHPERD Health Related Physical Fitness Test. Reston, VA: American Alliance for Health, Physical Education, Recreation and Dance; 1980.
34. Hoeger WWK, Hoeger SA. Lifetime Physical Fitness and Wellness: A Personalized Program. 6th ed. Englewood, CO: Morton Publishing; 2000.
35. Howley ET, Franks BD. Health Fitness Instructor's Handbook. 4th ed. Champaign, IL: Human Kinetics Publishers; 2003.
36. Jackson A, Langford NJ. The criterion-related validity of the sit and reach test: replication and extension of previous findings. Res Q Exerc Sport 1989;60:384–387.

# Methods of Body Composition Assessment

## Joe Weir

## OBJECTIVES

On the completion of this chapter you will be able to:

1. Understand the various levels of body composition assessment.
2. Describe the basic procedures associated with hydrostatic weighing.
3. Demonstrate how to calculate body composition from body density.
4. Discuss the limitations associated with the various methods for assessing body composition.
5. Explain the basic procedures associated with skinfold analysis.
6. Understand the methods associated with air-displacement plethysmography.
7. Describe the factors that can affect the accuracy of the different methods of assessing body composition.
8. Discuss the basic principles behind the use of bioelectrical impedance analysis of body composition.
9. Explain the basic procedures and limitations associated with dual-energy X-ray absorptiometry.
10. Demonstrate the basic calculations associated with the body mass index.
11. Understand the limitations associated with the body mass index.
12. Describe the differences among two-, three-, and four-compartment models for assessing body composition.
13. Illustrate the different combinations of procedures that can be used to make two-, three-, and four-compartment body composition assessment models.

## ABSTRACT

Body composition refers to the physical material that makes up the body. This chapter focuses on body composition assessment in humans. Because of the health effects of excess body fat (e.g., increased risk of Type 2 diabetes, heart disease, cancer) and of being underweight (e.g., anorexia nervosa), and because of the deleterious effects of excess fat on athletic performance, quantifying body composition in terms of percent fat has important uses (e.g., for implementing and monitoring weight loss programs). In addition, quantifying fat-free mass and its components (muscle, bone) is important because of the health implications of sarcopenia and osteopenia/osteoporosis. The characterization of body composition can be divided into two broad divisions: levels and models. Herein, the "levels" of body composition characterization are briefly examined. These include atomic, molecular, cellular, tissue-system, and whole-body levels. Specific techniques of determining body composition such as underwater weighing, skinfold assessments, bioelectrical impedance analysis, and dual-energy

From: *Essentials of Sports Nutrition and Supplements*
Edited by J. Antonio, D. Kalman, J. R. Stout, M. Greenwood, D. S. Willoughby, and G. G. Haff © Humana Press, a part of Springer Science+Business Media, Totowa, NJ

X-ray absorptiometry are then examined. Finally, different "models" of body composition analysis are explained. The different models segregate the body into different compartments, and currently there are two-, three-, and four-component models.

*Key Words:* **body composition, body fat, lean body mass, fat-free mass, DEXA, skinfolds, underwater weighing, BIA**

## BODY COMPOSITION LEVELS

The levels of body composition analysis include the atomic, molecular, cellular, tissue-system, and whole-body levels.[1] Many of these levels of analysis require sophisticated technology that is generally limited to a relatively few laboratories. Therefore, only a cursory description will be provided here.

At the atomic level, the body can be characterized based on the elements that compose it. The bulk of the body is composed of the elements oxygen, carbon, hydrogen, and nitrogen, which account for more than 95% of body mass.[2] Other elements such as sodium, potassium, phosphorus, and calcium contribute the balance of mass. Technology such as neutron activation analysis and whole-body potassium 40 counting are required for an atomic level of analysis.[1,2] Whereas this level of analysis is not practical for application to most settings, research using these techniques is important for validation of body composition models.

The molecular level of analysis segregates the body into water (~60% in males and ~50% in females), lipid, protein, glycogen, and minerals (~5% of body mass).[1,2] These can be further partitioned. For example, lipid includes fats (primarily triglycerides) as well as steroids and phospholipids. Similarly, water can be segregated into extracellular (e.g., plasma, interstitial fluid, gastrointestinal tract) and intracellular compartments.

At the cellular level of analysis, the body is segregated into cells (e.g., adipose cells, muscle cells), extracellular fluid (e.g., interstitial fluid, plasma, lymph), and extracellular solids (e.g., collagen fibers in connective tissue, bone matrix).[1,2] Determination of cellular mass requires techniques such as potassium 40 counting.

The tissue-system level is categorized as adipose tissue (subcutaneous, visceral, and bone marrow), skeletal muscle tissue, visceral organs, brain, and skeletal tissue.[1] Techniques such as computerized tomography and magnetic resonance imaging are used to quantify the amount of these various tissues.

At the level of the whole body, the analysis includes such factors as height, body mass, circumferences, and body density. The techniques of body composition at the whole-body level are used in most applied settings.[1]

## METHODS OF BODY COMPOSITION ASSESSMENT

### Underwater Weighing

Underwater weighing, or hydrostatic weighing, is based on the two-component model of body composition. In the two-component model of body composition, the body is divided into a fat-mass component and a fat-free mass (FFM) component. Fat mass is primarily made up of adipose tissue (both subcutaneous and deep), but other tissues primarily composed of lipid tissues such as myelinated nerve cells are also fat weight. FFM is all the tissue that is left, such as muscle, bone, and most organs. The FFM is composed of four main components: water, protein, bone mineral, and nonbone mineral.[3] Most of the common body composition tools in use for everyday applications [underwater weighing, air-displacement plethysmography (ADP), skinfolds, bioelectrical impedance analysis (BIA)] are based on the two-component model. The concept of density forms the basis of the two-component model. Density is defined as mass divided by volume. The two-component model assumes that fat weight has a density of 0.9 kg/L, whereas FFM has a density of 1.1 kg/L. The closer the body density to 1.1 kg/L, the leaner is the person. The closer the body density is to 0.9 kg/L, the higher is the percentage of body fat of the person.

Underwater weighing, then, attempts to determine the density of the body, and it is sometimes referred to as hydrodensitometry. Underwater weighing determines body density using the Archimedes Principle, which states that an object immersed in a fluid loses an amount of weight equal to the weight of the fluid displaced. Therefore, if one is weighed on land and then weighed underwater, the difference between those two values will equal the weight of the fluid that was displaced. Although physicists will note that mass and weight are not equivalent concepts, as a practical matter, the terms are used interchangeably here. Because we know the density of water is approximately 1.0 kg/L (the exact density varies depending on the temperature of the water), we can solve for the volume of water displaced by rearranging the basic density equation as follows:

$$Volume = mass/density$$

where volume = volume (L) of water displaced, mass = mass (kg) of water displaced, and density = density of water (kg/L). The volume of water that was displaced, as determined by underwater weighing, is equal to the body volume of the person. Because

$$Body\ density = body\ mass/body\ volume$$

and we have determined body volume from underwater weighing, we can solve for body density by simply incorporating the dry land mass of the person in the numerator of the equation, so that

$$body\ volume = [(body\ mass - underwater\ mass)/$$
$$density\ of\ water] - residual\ volume$$

where residual volume = the volume of air in the lungs after a complete exhalation. The actual procedure involves the subject being weighed underwater after completely exhaling as much air from the lungs as possible. This is an uncomfortable process, and some people have difficulty with the procedure. In practice, the subject is seated on a chair attached to a scale or a series of load cells. After becoming completely submerged, the subject must exhale all the air that is possible from the lungs (so that the only air left is residual volume), and sit quite still while the mass measurements are made. Naïve subjects need practice and become more skilled at the maneuver over time, so most tests involve repeated trials until three trials occur that are within 0.1 kg of each other.[4] The largest source of error in the underwater weighing procedure is error in the determination of residual volume.[4] An error of 100 mL in the measurement of residual volume results in an error of about 1% fat.[5] Residual volume can be estimated based on standard open circuit spirometry, but is more accurately assessed using closed-circuit nitrogen washout, helium dilution, or oxygen dilution.

The ultimate goal of the procedure is to calculate a body-fat percentage for the person based on the body-density calculation. There are two main equations that are used to convert body density into percent fat. The Brozek equation[6] is as follows:

$$\%\ fat = (457/body\ density) - 414.2$$

Similarly, the Siri equation is:

$$\%\ fat = (495/body\ density) - 450$$

The two equations differ because of small differences in assumptions regarding the density and temperature of fat. Differences between the two equations for a given body density are shown in Figure 9.1. For most the physiologic range, the equations yield percent fat values that are within 1% fat of each other.

There are two primary concerns of this approach. First is that the two-component model, on which the Siri and Brozek equations are based, makes certain assumptions concerning the density of FFM. The density of individual FFM components are assumed to be as follows: water = 0.9937 kg/L, protein = 1.34 kg/L, bone mineral = 2.982 kg/L, and nonbone mineral = 3.317 kg/L[6] and

**FIGURE 9.1.** Percent fat calculated from body density using the Brozek and Siri equations.

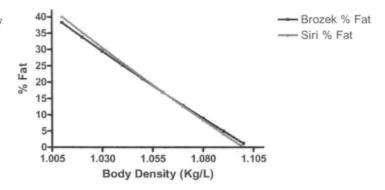

the proportions of water, protein, and minerals are assumed to be 73.8%, 19.4%, and 6.8% respectively.[6] It should also be noted that the density assumptions of the various FFM components are originally based on a very small number of human cadaver dissections.[3,5] Although the average FFM density value of 1.1 kg/L seems to hold in a variety of analyses, the density of FFM can vary across individuals.[7] The density of tissues can vary with age, gender, ethnicity, disease, hydration, etc.[4,5] For example, resistance training resulting in marked muscle hypertrophy tends to decrease the aggregate density of FFM, and standard densitometric calculations can overpredict percentage of fat.[8] Similarly, the density of FFM has been shown to be higher in blacks than whites, so that equations other than the Brozek and Siri equations have been suggested for use with blacks,[9,10] although not all studies support this view.[8] Therefore, even if underwater weighing is performed with perfect technique, the actual percentage of fat is likely to be somewhat different from the value calculated from body density. Ellis[5] notes that "the total cumulative error for body fatness (% fat) is on the order of 3–4% of body weight for the individual."

Second, most facilities do not have the equipment to perform underwater weighing, although most exercise physiology laboratories do perform this measurement. This limits the use of underwater weighing as an easily accessible tool for body composition assessment in most applied settings. Despite these limitations, the use of underwater weighing has served as a standard laboratory procedure for body composition assessment and is still considered by many to be the "gold standard" by which most other field tests of body composition are compared.[5]

## Skinfold Thickness

A popular "field test" for body composition is the measurement of skinfold thickness. Skinfold procedures are designed to predict body density (from underwater weighing) based on the thickness of various skinfold sites throughout the body. Skinfold thickness is primarily determined by the thickness of the subcutaneous fat layer. Precision skinfold calipers are used to manually measure the thickness of the skinfolds at different sites throughout the body. At each site, the skinfold is pinched by hand and pulled away from the underlying muscle and fascia, and the calipers are then placed along the fold and the thickness measured. Because people differ with respect to the distribution of subcutaneous fat throughout the body, skinfold procedures involve the measurement of multiple skinfold sites. Skinfold thickness is measured using calipers, and a strict measurement protocol is required for accurate results (Figure 9.2). Because skinfold equations are usually designed to predict body density, the calculation of % fat requires the implementation of the Brozek or Siri equation (or appropriate population-specific equation) as described above.

It is possible to predict % fat based on skinfold thickness because, on average, people with a thicker subcutaneous fat layer also have a higher % fat. The prediction of body density from skinfold thickness uses a statistical procedure called regression analysis. When researchers develop skinfold prediction equations, a sample of people from the population of interest undergoes

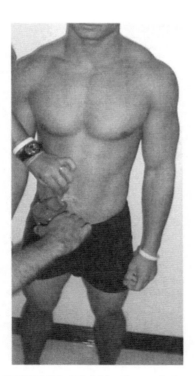

**FIGURE 9.2.** Skinfold caliper technique.

TABLE 9.1. Three-site generalized skinfold equations.

| Title | Equation | $R^2$ | SEE |
|---|---|---|---|
| 3-site equation for men | Body density = 1.1093800 − 0.0008267 (sum of chest, abdomen, and thigh) + 0.0000016 (sum of chest, abdomen, and thigh)$^2$ − 0.0002574 (age in years) | 0.91 | 0.008 |
| 3-site equation for women | Body density = 1.099421 − 0.0009929 (sum of triceps, thigh, and suprailium) + 0.0000023 (sum of triceps, thigh, and suprailium)$^2$ − 0.0001392 (age in years) | 0.84 | 0.009 |

SEE = standard error of estimate.

measurement of both skinfold thickness as well as the criterion (underwater weighing). Regression analysis allows one to generate a regression equation (prediction equation) that describes the relationship between a predictor(s) (e.g., skinfold thickness) and the variable of interest (e.g., body density). The validity of the equation is usually further tested by applying the equation to a separate sample and comparing the results of the prediction to the criterion. This process is referred to as cross-validation.[11]

One limitation of the use of skinfolds is that regression equations are population specific.[12] That is, an equation developed on college-age men would be invalid in predicting values from elderly women. To date, there are more than 100 skinfold regression equations in the scientific literature.[12] Despite this, some generalized regression equations have been developed that are successful in widespread application. The 7-site and 3-site skinfold equations of Jackson and Pollock[13] for males and Jackson et al.[14] for females have been shown to be highly correlated with body density determined from underwater weighing.[13,14] Because the sum of 3 skinfolds is highly correlated with the sum of 7 skinfolds, the extra information provided by the 7-site equations is trivial relative to the 3-site equations.[15,16] The 3-site equations are recommended for field use and are presented in Table 9.1. Note the squared terms for the sum of 3 skinfolds. This indicates that the relationship between skinfold thickness and body density is not linear, but somewhat curvilinear. Also note that these equations include age as well as skinfold thickness, which indicates that age contributes information to the prediction of body density above that provided simply by skinfold thickness. This may be attributable to age-related differences in fat distribution (e.g., increased intraabdominal fat relative to subcutaneous fat with increased age) or FFM characteristics (e.g., bone loss with age).[15] Statistically, the inclusion of age in the equations allows for the use of these equations across an age span, thus yielding "generalized" prediction equations.[13,14] Another limitation of skinfold testing is that the skill of the person performing the skinfold measurements can influence the scores. Training is required to properly administer the skinfold test (e.g., pinch the appropriate amount of tissue at a given site). Differences in technique among different testers can lead to bias in % fat estimates when measures are taken on the subject.

In lieu of the use of generalized equations, population-specific equations can be used. As noted above, there are more than 100 skinfold regression equations.[12] To facilitate use of the appropriate skinfold equation for a specific population, Heyward and Stolarczyk[17] have developed decision trees for equation selection, and the interested reader is invited to examine these in various publications.[17,18]

A variety of factors can affect the accuracy of a prediction equation. Technical errors in the measurement of the skinfolds and of the underwater-weighing procedure add error to the prediction equations. Additional error is introduced because body density and % fat are influenced by more than just subcutaneous fat (e.g., intraabdominal fat is not measured by skinfolds but influences % fat and body density). Therefore, it is important to keep in mind that the predicted body density of an individual from a skinfold equation (and the resulting % fat) likely varies from the value that would be obtained from underwater weighing. The accuracy of a prediction equation is assessed using standard statistics such as $R^2$ and the standard error of estimate (SEE). The $R^2$ value represents the variance in the criterion variable (e.g., body density from underwater weighing) accounted for, or explained by, the predictors (e.g., skinfold thickness). An $R^2$

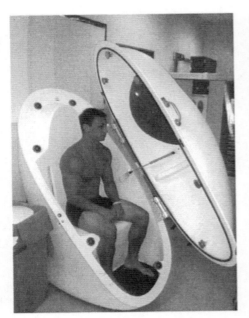

**FIGURE 9.3.** Air-displacement plethysmography.

of 0.85 for a skinfold equation means that 85% of the variance in body density was accounted for by skinfold thickness. The $R^2$ value can vary from 0.0 to 1.0, and the closer the value to 1.0, the better the equation. Whereas the $R^2$ value provides important information regarding the equation, the SEE can be used to gain a sense of the potential errors of prediction for an individual. To illustrate, assume that person's predicted score for % fat was 15%, the mean % fat for the subjects that the equation was developed from was also 15%, and the equation had a SEE of 3% fat. Based on the properties of a normal distribution, we would be approximately 68% confident that this person's true % fat (based on some criterion such as underwater weighing) fell between 12% and 18% (i.e., ±1 SEE), and about 95% confident that this person's true % fat fell between 9% and 21% fat (±2 SEE). This represents a substantial error of prediction for a given individual. Furthermore, the potential errors increase as the difference between the person's % fat and the mean % fat of the sample increase. Assuming there is no systematic bias in an equation, the individual errors tend to cancel and regression equations can give accurate estimates of samples of people. On an individual basis, however, the errors can be quite large and use of these equations to make assessments of individuals should be done with caution.

## Air-Displacement Plethysmography

Although underwater weighing can accurately determine body volume, there are several disadvantages to the use of underwater weighing. First is that underwater weighing requires subjects to be completely immersed in water, and completely exhale. This can be difficult for many people. Second, the equipment needs are not trivial (tank, scales, water, etc.). Recently, a new approach to determine body volume has been developed using air displacement instead of water displacement. The volume of air displaced by the body is equal to body volume in the same way that the volume of water displaced by the body equals body volume.

The ADP measurements are made by examining the pressure differences between a chamber containing the subject and an adjacent chamber after manipulating the volume in the chambers[12] (Figure 9.3). Specifically, because the relationship between pressure and volume is defined as

$$P1/P2 = V2/V1$$

where P1 and P2 represent the pressures in chambers 1 and 2, and V1 and V2 represent the volumes of chambers 1 and 2. By manipulating the volume of each chamber (using an oscillating diaphragm located between the two chambers), and measuring the resulting pressure, the body volume can be determined.[19] As with underwater weighing, the results of ADP are based on the two-component model, and the body volume determined from air displacement is converted to body density and then % fat using the procedures described above (e.g., Brozek or Siri equation). Unlike underwater weighing, subject compliance with the procedure is relatively easy.

To date, the only commercial product available for ADP is the "Bod Pod." The error of the volumetric measures relative to underwater weighing are generally small when evaluated on groups as a whole, although more research is required to improve accuracy.[19] Notably, the validity of ADP for use with children and differences between males and females require further study. For example, Biaggi et al.[20] reported that % fat tended to be underestimated in men and overestimated in women (by about 1%) relative to results from underwater weighing. Furthermore, although differences between ADP and other techniques such as underwater weighing, dual-energy X-ray absorptiometry (DEXA), and higher-order body composition models (see below) seem to be relatively small when looking at groups as a whole, errors for individuals can be potentially large (9%–16% fat).[19] Assuming accurate body-mass measurement, differences between ADP and underwater weighing must be attributed to differences in body-volume calculation. Factors such as breathing pattern during the ADP test, air trapped in hair, and type of clothing can affect ADP values.

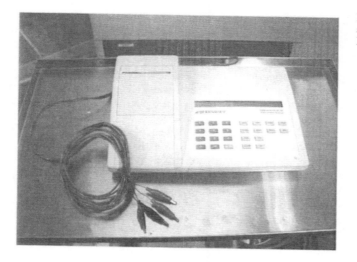

**FIGURE 9.4.** Bioelectrical impedance analysis machine. (Photograph courtesy of Miami Research Associates.)

## Bioelectrical Impedance Analysis

BIA is an easily administered technique that is a part of a family of procedures used to determine total body water (Figure 9.4). Because FFM contains a relatively constant proportion of water (0.732 L of water per kg), one can estimate FFM based on measures of total body water.[12] The most accurate approaches for measuring total body water (e.g., isotope dilution) are limited to research laboratories and therefore have little use in field studies. However, BIA can be used to estimate total body water.[21] The principle is relatively straightforward. The resistance to the flow of an electrical current is high in fat tissue and low in fat-free tissue, because FFM (with the exception of bone) has a high percentage of water and electrolytes. Therefore, the lower the resistance, the higher the total body water and FFM, all else being equal. By injecting a small electrical current through the body and measuring the resistance, one can estimate percent fat. Most BIA systems use tetrapolar electrode lead systems in which two electrodes are placed at the wrist/hand and two at the ankle/foot. One commercial system has incorporated BIA measurement into a device that resembles a bathroom scale, so that as body mass is measured, current is injected through the feet. The typical BIA systems use a single frequency (50 kHz) with a painless current (e.g., 500 μA) level.[18] More recently, the development of multifrequency BIA machines allows for the estimation of body water in both the extracellular and intracellular compartments, which should improve FFM estimates.

As noted above, one can estimate total body water (TBW) with BIA. Because water is approximately equal to 73% of FFM, one can also estimate FFM as[1]:

$$FFM = TBW/0.73$$

Fat mass can then be estimated by simple subtraction of FFM from body mass. In practice, however, regression equations have been developed to predict body density and % fat directly from BIA-based resistance values.[22] Although impedance is a function of both resistance and reactance, resistance values alone can be used instead of impedance because reactance contributes only a small amount to impedance relative to the contribution of resistance to impedance, so resistance can suffice as an estimate of impedance.[5] BIA equations also typically present the resistance information in the denominator of the ratio $ht^2/R$.[5,22] The rationale for this is that the volume of the conductor (total body water or FFM) is proportional to the length of the conductor squared divided by the resistance.[22] In this case, height is used as a proxy for conductor length. As with skinfolds, the validity of the BIA estimates depends on the regression equations used and are typically validated against underwater weighing, or more recently, using higher-order body composition models described in a subsequent section.

Early use of BIA to predict % fat resulted in only modest accuracy when validated against underwater weighing.[23,24] The predictive validity between BIA values and underwater weighing was markedly poorer than that found with skinfold-based predictions,[16,23,25] in some cases performed poorer than simple visual estimation of % fat,[16] and were comparable to those found with simple height- and weight-based assessments [e.g., body mass index (BMI); see below]. Eckerson et al.[26] found that BIA systematically overestimated % fat in lean males. Jackson et al.[23] noted "that wt/ht$^2$ is the major source of variance in BIA prediction models" and indeed most equations still include body mass and ht$^2$/R for prediction so that much of the variance explained by the equations can be attributed to the influence of mass and stature.

That said, improvements in population-specific BIA equations have occurred and BIA has been shown to accurately predict total body water (from which fat-free weight and % fat can be derived) and % fat,[22] and can result in standard error of estimate values markedly smaller than those yielded by equations based only on height and weight.[27] Several authors have noted that population-specific regression equations yield R$^2$ and SEE values comparable to skinfold equations.[18,22] Similar to population-specific skinfold equations, decision trees for choosing BIA equations have been developed.[17,18]

Errors in body composition assessment with BIA can be introduced if proper protocol is not followed.[28] Because BIA is reflective of total body water, all subjects must be properly hydrated. In addition, use of different instruments, loss of instrument calibration, subject body position, body temperature, and improper electrode placement can affect results.[22,29]

As with skinfolds and other regression-based methods, caution must be used when evaluating individuals. Houtkooper et al.[22] have noted that even though BIA techniques result in acceptable R$^2$ and SEE values, the "impedance approach, and most other body composition methods, has limited accuracy for estimating body composition in individuals."

## Dual-Energy X-Ray Absorptiometry

DEXA technology was originally developed to assess the health of the skeletal system as is needed in screening for osteoporosis. The term "dual-energy" derives from the fact that the devices transmit X-ray energy at two distinct energy peaks.[30,31] The basis for the technique is that X-ray energy is more readily absorbed in bone tissue than soft tissue, so the absorption of X-rays (or more precisely, the degree of attenuation of X-rays) should be reflective of bone density and bone mineral content. Fat and muscle also differ from each other in X-ray absorption at the two energy levels,[30] and it soon became apparent that body composition could also be simultaneously assessed with DEXA. These DEXA-based estimates of body composition are essentially a three-component model of body composition: bone mineral content, bone-free FFM, and fat mass (Figure 9.5).[30,32]

Numerous studies have examined the validity of DEXA-based body composition estimates.[30,33] The body composition results are affected by factors such as anterior-posterior thickness of the person, the hydration status of FFM, the specific hardware system used, and the software system.[31–35] A review by Lohman et al.[33] indicates that, using the most recent software, DEXA-based estimates of % fat are within 1%–3% fat of values derived from more sophisticated multicomponent models (see below). Although the validity of DEXA technology is generally good, systematic errors in the analysis of body composition do occur. For example, Van Der Ploeg et al.[36] found that DEXA tends to underestimate fat mass in lean subjects and overestimates fat mass in subjects with higher fat.

Since DEXA's development, differences in hardware and software among DEXA vendors have led to differences in validity estimates,[5] and newer hardware and software systems may further complicate the issue. Earlier technology used a "pencil-beam" X-ray system. Newer technology incorporates "fan-beam" technology which has a wider X-ray swath (shaped like a fan) that decreases scanning time. To date, only a few studies have assessed the validity of the fan-beam system. Recently, Norcross and Van Loan[32] showed good agree-

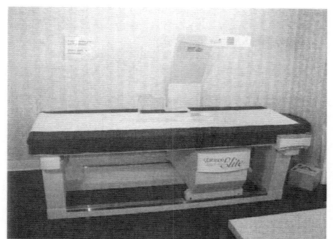

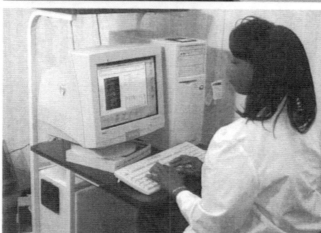

**FIGURE 9.5.** Dual-energy X-ray absorptiometry imaging. (Photographs courtesy of Miami Research Associates.)

ment between body composition values from fan-beam DEXA and hydrodensitometry in healthy adults (18–45 years of age). Soriano et al.[35] showed that % fat values among four different systems (two of each beam type) were highly correlated with each other, but there were small but statistically significant differences in mean % fat estimates between fan- and pencil-beam systems from different vendors and from the same vendors. More validation studies are required, especially for multicomponent models, which are described below.

There are several advantages of DEXA over other methods. Perhaps of most importance is that those tested receive information regarding bone health in addition to body composition. Furthermore, body composition of different segments of the body can be estimated. For example, arm, leg and whole-body muscle mass can be estimated from DEXA.[37] In addition, similar to BIA, the physical demands of the person being tested are minimal (as opposed to underwater weighing) and the procedure is painless and comfortable. The radiation exposure is small (~20% of the background radiation of a typical day).[3] Nonetheless, users of DEXA need to be aware of errors introduced by the use of different machines from different vendors.

## Body Mass Index

BMI is a simple technique that requires only height and mass to determine if a person is "overweight." The idea is that for a given height, there is an acceptable range of body weight, and values above that range reflect a condition of overweight or obesity. The calculation of BMI is:

$$BMI = mass/height^2$$

where mass is in kilograms and height is in meters.[15] The normal range of BMI is 18.5–24.9. People with BMI values below 18.5 are considered underweight, those with values between 25 and 29.9 are considered overweight, and those ≥30 are classified as obese.[38] Because of the simplicity of the measurement, BMI is useful in large epidemiologic studies to estimate population characteristics. However, there are several weaknesses to the use of BMI in the assessment of individuals. First, BMI does not estimate body composition per se. Rather, it attempts to assess whether someone is overweight (based on height). On an individual basis, highly muscular individuals may be classified as overweight even if they have a low % fat. Athletes who compete in strength- and power-based sports often are heavy but relatively lean. For example, McGee and Burkett[39] studied data from the National Football League (NFL) combine before the 2000 NFL draft. Athletes drafted in the first and second rounds had a mean height of 1.88 m and a mass of 112.46 kg. The resulting BMI was 31.8, which falls in the obese category. More recently, Kraemer et al.[40] examined the BMI and body composition (Bod Pod) of an NFL team, and found that the average BMI at each position, including "skill" positions such as running back and wide receiver, fell into the overweight category. However, the % fat values were often quite low. For example, the mean BMI for defensive backs was 26.9 whereas the mean % fat was only 6.3%. Clearly, caution and common sense need to be applied when interpreting BMI data.

## Beyond the Two-Component Model

As noted above, underwater weighing is based on the two-component model in which the body is segregated into fat mass and FFM, with assumed densities of 0.9 kg/L for fat and 1.1 kg/L for FFM. Similarly, techniques such as air displacement and skinfolds that are validated against underwater weighing also depend on these assumptions. However, the densities of the two components are known to be affected by factors such as hydration, age, gender, and race. For example, the 1.1 kg/L density value of FFW assumes fixed proportions and densities of the components of FFM, yet factors such as bone and muscle mass that constitute the FFM component vary from person to person. Furthermore, variations in hydration status of FFM and mineral content of bone can affect the validity of the two-component model.

In theory, measuring the subcomponents of the FFM component should allow for improved accuracy over the two-component model. By combining underwater weighing (for body density) and DEXA (for bone mass), one can create the three-component model mentioned above in regard to the validation of DEXA: bone mass, bone-free FFM, and fat mass. Alternatively, quantification of total body water would remove variability caused by FFM hydration assumptions, and could yield a different three-component model: fat mass, total body water, and dry fat-free solid.[3] This partitioning of the FFM component into either bone and bone-free components, or water and dry fat-free solid, should improve the accuracy of the model because the "noise" created by variability in bone mass (as a component of FFM), or noise created by variability in hydration of FFM, is now accounted for. In practice, because the contribution of water to FFM is much greater than the contribution of bone to FFM, the three-component model using total body water improves accuracy over the two-component model more than the three-component model that accounts for bone.[21]

Similarly, by measuring total body water and bone mineral content, a further partitioning of FFM can occur, resulting in a four-component model of body composition. In the four-component model, underwater weighing is used to determine body density and DEXA is used to quantify bone mass. In addition, total body water is measured using a technique such as isotope dilution. The most frequently used isotope dilution procedure involves oral administration of deuterium oxide ($^2H_2O$). If a known amount of $^2H_2O$ is administered and allowed to evenly disperse in the total body water pool (~3–3.5 hours), then measures of $^2H_2O$ concentration in body fluids such as saliva, urine, or plasma will yield estimates of total body water.[3] The resulting model segregates the body into water, fat, bone mineral mass, and residual. The residual includes factors such as the dry mass of muscle. The improved accuracy of this approach has led many to replace underwater weighing as the "gold standard" for body composition with the four-component model. The increased technical demands of the four-component model make it impractical for routine use. However, research laboratories can now use this model to improve the validity of techniques such as BIA and DEXA.

## SUMMARY

Body composition assessment can be performed at an extremely sophisticated level using techniques such as neutron activation, or can involve simple technology such as height and weight measurements. All approaches have strengths and weaknesses. For advanced techniques, very accurate determinations are possible, but factors such as radiation risk and the fact that very few facilities can perform the tests limit their use to research laboratories. Underwater weighing has been a staple of body composition assessment but is not widely available to the public, and is constrained by the limits of the two-component model and its assumptions regarding the density of FFM. Likewise, DEXA has limited use in determining body composition in large numbers of individuals, and differences in hardware and software add uncertainty to the body composition estimates. Air-displacement technology is still relatively expensive, certain issues regarding validity relative to underwater weighing are still being studied, and similar to underwater weighing ADP depends on the two-component model. Nonetheless, its relative ease of use and potential for testing large numbers of people are encouraging. Techniques such as skinfolds and BIA are effective in evaluating characteristics of groups of people, but large errors can occur on an individual basis even with "good" regression equations. When using these techniques in consultation with individual clients, it is wise to keep these limitations in mind. The advent of combining more than one approach has led to the three- and four-component models. These models will improve the accuracy of future body composition research but are unlikely to be in widespread use for testing individuals.

## PRACTICAL APPLICATIONS

There is no perfect method of body composition assessment. Techniques available for routine use are prone to errors. Sports nutritionists need to be aware of these limitations when consulting with clients regarding body composition scores. Because of these concerns, it may be prudent to minimize emphasis on actual % fat values and simply use the procedures to monitor progress as part of a larger assessment protocol. Furthermore, standardization of procedures and strict adherence to the appropriate protocols need to occur to minimize error.

It is likely that the two most accessible techniques for body composition assessment of individual clients will be skinfolds and BIA. When using skinfolds with a diverse client base, it is recommended that either the 3-site generalized equations of Jackson and Pollock[13] for men or Jackson et al.[14] for women be used, or a population-specific equation be selected as outlined by Heyward and Stolarczyk[17] and Going and Davis.[18] Keep in mind that individual calculated % fat will likely differ from the "true" value, even if the technique is performed well. Clients should be made aware of the likely ranges for their true score about the calculated value. In addition, interpretation of body composition should be made in the larger context of the individual's health and/or athletic goals. In particular, multiple measurements over time are more useful to track changes in body composition than are single-point estimates of % fat. These serial measurements are more reliable if the same tester performs the measurements each time. When using BIA, factors such as hydration, body temperature, and physical activity can negatively influence results. Therefore, care must be taken to standardize the testing and follow the manufacturer's testing instructions as much as possible.

Because of the numerous skinfold and BIA equations that are in the literature, one should critically evaluate the merits of a particular equation. Examination of the data regarding $R^2$ and SEE is informative. In addition, equations that have been adequately cross-validated are less likely to give erroneous data. Because of the improved accuracy of higher-order body composition models, one should give particular attention to equations or procedures that were successfully validated and cross-validated against the four-component model.

## QUESTIONS

1. Body density =
   a. Body volume/body mass
   b. Body mass/body volume
   c. $ht^2/R$
   d. Mass/$ht^2$

2. In the two-component model of body composition, fat-free mass is assumed to have a density of:
   a. 0.9 kg/L
   b. 1.0 kg/L
   c. 1.1 kg/L
   d. 1.2 kg/L

3. In the two-component model of body composition, fat mass is assumed to have a density of:
   a. 0.9 kg/L
   b. 1.0 kg/L
   c. 1.1 kg/L
   d. 1.2 kg/L

4. The primary predictive power of bioelectrical impedance analysis comes from:
   a. Body volume/body mass
   b. Body mass/body volume
   c. $ht^2/R$
   d. Mass/$ht^2$

5. Bioelectrical impedance analysis is mainly a predictor of:
   a. Fat mass
   b. Bone mineral density
   c. Body density
   d. Total body water

6. All of the following are based on the two-component model of body composition except:
   a. Hydrostatic weighing
   b. Dual-energy X-ray absorptiometry
   c. Skinfolds
   d. Air-displacement plethysmography

7. The largest source of error in underwater weighing comes from errors in the measurement of:
   a. Residual lung volume
   b. Intestinal gas volume
   c. Body mass on dry land
   d. Body mass under water

8. When estimating fat-free mass from total body water, it is assumed that fat-free mass is composed of ____ water.
   a. 50%
   b. 60%
   c. 73%
   d. 95%

9. Which of the following procedures is the most physically demanding of the person being tested?
   a. Dual-energy X-ray absorptiometry
   b. Skinfolds
   c. Air-displacement plethysmography
   d. Underwater weighing

10. Which of the following represents a three-component model currently in use?
    a. Water, bone, and protein
    b. Fat mass, protein-free fat-free mass, and bone mineral
    c. Subcutaneous fat, visceral fat, fat-free mass
    d. Fat mass, total body water, dry fat-free solid

11. The most accurate estimates of total body water are based on:
    a. Dual-energy X-ray absorptiometry
    b. Bioelectrical impedance analysis
    c. Isotope dilution
    d. Underwater weighing

12. The atomic level of body composition analysis characterizes the body based on the elements that compose it. Which of the following elements contributes the least to body mass?
    a. Carbon
    b. Hydrogen
    c. Oxygen
    d. Calcium

13. At the molecular level of analysis, which of the following contributes the most body mass?
    a. Water
    b. Protein
    c. Glycogen
    d. Lipid

14. An object's mass on land is found to be 100 kg. The underwater mass is found to be 10 kg. The mass of the water that was displaced by the object while underwater is:
    a. 10 kg
    b. 0.1 kg
    c. 90 kg
    d. 100 kg

15. Which of the following tissues absorbs the most X-ray energy?
    a. Muscle
    b. Fat
    c. Bone
    d. Visceral organs

16. Which of the following techniques would be most influenced by the skill of the person administering the test?
    a. Dual-energy X-ray absorptiometry
    b. Bioelectrical impedance analysis
    c. Skinfolds
    d. Air-displacement plethysmography

17. In the technique of air-displacement plethysmography, which of the following variables is directly measured to determine body volume?
    a. Chamber mass
    b. Chamber pressure
    c. Chamber temperature
    d. Chamber humidity

18. A certain population is determined to have a density of fat-free mass that is lower than is the standard value assumed for the two-component model of body composition. If the Brozek equation is applied to this population, the percent fat scores will tend to be:
    a. Too low
    b. Too high
    c. Just right

19. Which of the following techniques can estimate regional body composition (i.e., in the arms and legs)?
    a. Bioelectrical impedance analysis
    b. Body mass index
    c. Dual-energy X-ray absorptiometry
    d. Underwater weighing

20. Muscular athletes are most likely to be misclassified as being overweight when assessed using:
    a. Bioelectrical impedance analysis
    b. Body mass index
    c. Dual-energy X-ray absorptiometry
    d. Underwater weighing

21. Body mass index is a measure of body composition.
    a. True
    b. False

22. Skinfolds are the most accurate measure of percent body fat.
    a. True
    b. False

23. The Siri and Brozek equations yield similar percent fat values for a given body density.
    a. True
    b. False

24. Air-displacement plethysmography is most similar to underwater weighing.
    a. True
    b. False

25. On average, blacks have a lower bone density than whites.
    a. True
    b. False

26. The Brozek and Siri equations are valid for all populations.
    a. True
    b. False

27. Currently, the best "gold standard" against which to validate body composition procedures is the four-component model.
    a. True
    b. False

28. Use of 7 skinfolds results in much better percent fat prediction equations than the use of 3 skinfold sites.
    a. True
    b. False

29. The X-ray dose from dual-energy X-ray absorptiometry is quite high, so few people should be tested.
    a. True
    b. False

30. Bioelectrical impedance analysis gives highly accurate estimates of body composition in individuals.
    a. True
    b. False

31. Resistance values from bioelectrical impedance analysis are inversely proportional to total body water.
    a. True
    b. False

# REFERENCES

1. Pietrobelli A, Heymsfield SB. Establishing body composition in obesity. J Endocrinol Invest 2002;25:884–892.
2. Heymsfield SB, Wang Z, Baumgartner RN, Ross R. Human body composition: advances in models and methods. Annu Rev Nutr 1997;17:527–558.
3. Withers RT, LaForgia J, Heymsfield SB. Critical appraisal of the estimation of body composition via two-, three-, and four-component models. Am J Hum Biol 1999; 11:175–185.
4. Wagner DR, Heyward VH. Techniques for body composition assessment: a review of laboratory and field methods. Res Quart Exerc Sport 1999;70:135–149.
5. Ellis KJ. Human body composition: in vivo models. Physiol Rev 2000;80:649–680.
6. Brozek J, Grande F, Anderson JT, Keys A. Densitometric analysis of body composition: revision of some quantitative standards. Ann NY Acad Sci 1963;110:1133–1140.
7. Wang Z, Heshka S, Wang J, Wielopolski L, Heymsfield SB. Magnitude and variation of fat-free mass density: a cellular-level body composition modeling study. Am J Physiol 2003;284:E267–E273.
8. Millard-Stafford ML, Collins MA, Modlesky CM, Snow TK, Rosskopf LB. Effect of race and resistance training status on the density of fat-free mass and percent fat estimates. J Appl Physiol 2001;91:1259–1268.
9. Schutte JE, Townsend EJ, Hugg J, Sharp RF, Malina RM, Blomqvist CG. Density of lean body mass is greater in blacks than in whites. J Appl Physiol 1984;56:1647–1649.
10. Wagner DR, Heyward VH. Validity of two-component models for estimating body fat of black men. J Appl Physiol 2001;90:649–656.
11. Guo SS, Chumlea WC, Cockram DB. Use of statistical methods to estimate body composition. Am J Clin Nutr 1996;64(Suppl):428S–435S.
12. Ellis KJ. Selected body composition methods can be used in field studies. J Nutr 2001;131:1589S–1595S.
13. Jackson AS, Pollock ML. Generalized equations for predicting body density of men. Br J Nutr 1978;40:497–504.
14. Jackson AS, Pollock ML, Ward A. Generalized equations for predicting body density of women. Med Sci Sports Exerc 1980;12:175–182.
15. Jackson AS, Pollock ML. Practical assessment of body composition. Phys Sports Med 1985;13:76–90.
16. Eckerson JM, Housh TJ, Johnson GO. The validity of visual estimations of percent body fat in lean males. Med Sci Sports Exerc 1992;24:615–618.
17. Heyward VH, Stolarczyk LM. Applied Body Composition Assessment. Champaign IL: Human Kinetics Publishers; 1996.
18. Going S, Davis R. Body composition. In: Roitman JL, ed. ACSM's Resource Manual for Exercise Testing and Prescription. Philadelphia: Lippincott Williams & Wilkins; 2001:391–400.
19. Fields DA, Goran MJ, McCrory MA. Body composition assessment via air displacement plethysmography in adults and children: a review. Am J Clin Nutr 2002;75:453–467.
20. Biaggi RR, Vollman MW, Nies MA, et al. Comparison of air displacement plethysmography with hydrostatic weighing and bioelectrical impedance analysis for the assessment of body composition in healthy adults. Am J Clin Nutr 1999;69:898–903.
21. Evans EM, Arngrimsson SA, Cureton KJ. Body composition estimates from multicomponent models using BIA to determine body water. Med Sci Sports Exerc 2001;33:839–845.
22. Houtkooper LB, Lohman TG, Going SB, Howell WH. Why bioelectrical impedance analysis should be used for estimating adiposity. Am J Clin Nutr 1996;64(Suppl):436S–448S.
23. Jackson AS, Pollock ML, Graves JE, Mahar MT. Reliability and validity of bioelectrical impedance in determining body composition. J Appl Physiol 1988;64:529–534.
24. Segal KR, Gutin B, Presta E, Wang J, Itallio TB. Estimation of human body composition by electrical impedance methods: a comparative study. J Appl Physiol 1985;58:1565–1571.

25. Eckerson JM, Stout JR, Housh TJ, Johnson GO. Validity of bioelectrical impedance equations for estimating percent fat in males. Med Sci Sports Exerc 1996;28: 523–530.

26. Eckerson JM, Housh TJ, Johnson GO. Validity of bioelectrical impedance equations for estimating fat-free weight in lean males. Med Sci Sports Exerc 1992;24: 1298–1302.

27. Kushner RF, Schooeller DA, Fjeld CR, Danford L. Is the impedance index (ht²/R) significant in predicting total body water? Am J Clin Nutr 1992;56:835–839.

28. NIH. Bioelectrical impedance analysis in body composition measurement: National Institutes of Health Assessment Conference Statement. Am J Clin Nutr 1996; 64(Suppl):524S–532S.

29. Kushner RF, Gudivaka R, Scholler DA. Clinical characteristics influencing bioelectrical impedance analysis measurements. Am J Clin Nutr 1996;64(Suppl):423S–427S.

30. Pietrobelli A, Formica C, Wang Z, Heymsfield SB. Dual-energy X-ray absorptiometry body composition model: review of physical concepts. Am J Physiol 1996;271: E941–E951.

31. Roubenoff R, Kehayias JJ, Dawson-Hughes B, Heymsfield SB. Use of dual-energy X-ray absorptiometry in body composition studies. Not yet a "gold standard." Am J Clin Nutr 1993;58:589–591.

32. Norcross J, Van Loan MD. Validation of fan beam dual energy X ray absorptiometry for body composition assessment in adults aged 18–45 years. Br J Sports Med 2004;38:472–476.

33. Lohman TG, Harris M, Teixeira PJ, Weiss L. Assessing body composition and changes in body composition. Another look at dual-energy X-ray absorptiometry. Ann NY Acad Sci 2000;904:45–54.

34. Modlesky CM, Evans EM, Millard-Stafford ML, Collins MA, Lewis RD, Cureton KJ. Impact of bone mineral estimates on percent fat estimates from a four-component model. Med Sci Sports Exerc 1999;31:1861–1868.

35. Soriano JM, Ioannidou E, Wang J, et al. Pencil-beam vs fan-beam dual-energy X-ray absorptiometry comparisons across four systems. J Clin Densitom 2004;7:281–289.

36. Van Der Ploeg GE, Withers RT, LaForgia J. Percent body fat via DEXA: comparison with a four-compartment model. J Appl Physiol 2003;94:499–506.

37. Kim J, Wang Z, Heymsfield SB, Baumgartner RN, Gallagher D. Total-body skeletal muscle mass: estimation by a new dual-energy X-ray absorptiometry method. Am J Clin Nutr 2002;76:378–383.

38. ACSM. ACSM's Guidelines for Exercise Testing and Prescription. 6th ed. Baltimore: Lippincott Williams & Wilkins; 2000.

39. McGee KJ, Burkett LN. The National Football League combine: a relative predictor of draft status? J Strength Cond Res 2003;17:9–11.

40. Kraemer WJ, Torine JC, Silvestre R, et al. Body size and composition of National Football League players. J Strength Cond Res 2005;19:485–489.

## APPENDIX 9.1: A BRIEF INTERVIEW WITH KRISTIN J. REIMERS, MS, RD

Kristin J. Reimers, MS, RD, is the associate director of The Center for Human Nutrition in Omaha Nebraska. The Center for Human Nutrition is a tax-exempt, nonprofit organization committed to the enhancement of health, performance, and the quality of life through nutrition. Reimers has been with the Center since 1990, and associate director since 1995. Her work focuses primarily on nutrition research and education. She is also an adjunct faculty member in Health, Physical Education and Recreation at the University of Nebraska–Omaha. She holds professional memberships in the American College of Sports Medicine, the American Dietetic Association, the National Strength and Conditioning Association, and the Society for Nutrition Education. Her publications include 14 chapters in textbooks and numerous articles and columns. After receiving a Bachelor of Arts degree from the University of Northern Iowa, Reimers earned a Master of Science degree in human nutrition from the University of Nebraska–Lincoln. She is currently pursuing her doctoral degree in human nutrition.

Q: *In your work as a sports nutritionist, what types of clients do you work with who might need body composition information in the development of their nutritional and exercise program?*
A: Athletes who are contemplating weight loss, for example wrestlers, who are unsure whether they have excess body fat, are one group in whom body composition information is useful in the development of a sport nutrition plan. Body composition assessment is also useful to monitor the progress of an athlete who is gaining weight to determine what proportion is fat and what is lean tissue.

Q: *What type of body composition technology do your clients typically get assessed with?*
A: I usually use calipers to measure skinfold thickness. In my experience, sports nutritionists need to be mobile . . . and work within a budget. That said, I don't think you can beat skinfold measurements.

Q: *How do you use that information (e.g., do you set % fat goals, body mass goals, or anything like that)?*
A: I use body composition measurements in combination with other assessment information I'm gathering. I think percent body fat is quite meaningless in isolation. I am from the school of thought that ideal body composition is quite individualized, and can't be "prescribed" based on group averages. The most useful information is a series of body composition measurements over several years that can be compared with changes in performance and health. For example, let's say a college sophomore soccer player is slower than he or she was as a freshman. There are many variables that may be causing that. If we have serial percent body fat measurements, we can look at those measurements to see if change in body fat is a potential contributing factor.

Q: *Are there any drawbacks to using body comp information?*
Like any technology, body comp information can be overused and abused. It's just one piece of the total assessment for the medical and performance staff working with athletes. Top performance and health, not percent body fat, should be the goal of nutrition interventions.

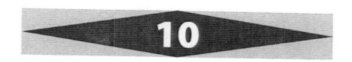

# Nutritional Assessment
# and Counseling of Athletes

## Susan M. Kleiner

## OBJECTIVES

On the completion of this chapter you will be able to:

1. Develop a basic understanding of the relationship between dietary practices and overall health and wellness.
2. Understand the basic components of the 2005 Dietary Guidelines for Americans.
3. Explain the components of an effective nutrition assessment program.
4. Describe the factors that impact an athlete's dietary practices.
5. Integrate the knowledge attained in previous chapters about body composition assessments with the nutritional assessment techniques in order to help athletes with their dietary practices.
6. Determine an athlete's optimal body weight and resting metabolic rate.
7. Explain the limitations of the body mass index as a tool for determining body composition.
8. Discuss the relationship between optimal body fat levels and an athlete's optimal body weight.
9. Develop a basic understanding of the methods for determining caloric needs.
10. Predict an athlete's basal metabolic rate and total caloric need depending on their activity levels.
11. Discuss the relationships among psychosocial factors, dietary practices, and lifestyle.
12. Determine the best method for assessing the dietary practices of athletes.
13. Establish an understanding of how to council athletes about their dietary practices.

## ABSTRACT

Athletes' nutritional needs are based on their age, gender, lifestyle, health status, level of physical activity, physical conditioning, and type of sport. An athlete's diet will affect his/her health and physical performance now, and in the future. According to the National Center for Health Statistics, of the 10 leading causes of death, five of them—coronary heart disease and generalized atherosclerosis, cancer, stroke, diabetes, and diseases of the kidney—have been associated with dietary excesses or imbalances, and another—accidents—is often the result of excessive alcohol intake. Together, these six conditions account for as many as 68% of all United States deaths each year (www.cdc.gov/nchs/fastats/lcod.htm.). By following good nutritional practices, athletes

From: *Essentials of Sports Nutrition and Supplements*
Edited by J. Antonio, D. Kalman, J. R. Stout, M. Greenwood, D. S. Willoughby, and
G. G. Haff © Humana Press, a part of Springer Science+Business Media, Totowa, NJ

**TABLE 10.1. Key messages of the 2005 United States Dietary Guidelines.**[1]

- Consume a variety of foods within and among the basic food groups while staying within energy needs.
- Control calorie intake to manage body weight.
- Be physically active every day.
- Increase daily intake of fruits and vegetables, whole grains, and nonfat or low-fat milk and milk products.
- Choose fats wisely for good health.
- Choose carbohydrates wisely for good health.
- Choose and prepare foods with little salt.
- If you drink alcoholic beverages, do so in moderation.
- Keep food safe to eat.

not only have a better chance of maintaining health and improving their performance, but if they do become injured, an appropriate diet can assist with the process of returning them to the playing field as quickly as possible.

Athletes are prey to nutrition faddism and misinformation. The diets of many athletes are inadequate for a number of reasons: 1) poor information; 2) pressures of time, money, and access; and 3) overly restrictive eating habits and obsessions with body weight and food. Making sure that athletes get appropriate nutrition advice, and then learn to apply the information correctly, is a task that must be approached with care. As a health professional, you have an important role in helping athletes learn appropriate nutrition behaviors. Accomplishing this task requires an understanding of the physiologic, as well as psychosocial influences that affect athletes' dietary practices. Practical skills in counseling and education are needed to motivate athletes to modify their food choices and eating habits. The purpose of this chapter is to introduce you to the basic principles of nutrition assessment, evaluation, and counseling. Then, by giving you the tools to apply these principles and appropriately evaluate dietary information, you can positively influence the nutrition practices of athletes and other active individuals.

*Key Words:* **assessment, diet, dietary guidelines, dietitian, nutrition, counseling**

## REVIEW OF THE LITERATURE

The publication of the 2005 Dietary Guidelines for Americans (see Table 10.1) has given us a dietary model to follow while counseling athletes.[1] Whereas all people have individual nutritional requirements, these guidelines offer general dietary recommendations that can be applied to the majority of people. For some athletes, the guidelines may serve as minimum dietary recommendations. The Dietary Guidelines emphasize the positive, rather than negative, aspects of eating behavior. Instead of stating "avoid" or "do not eat" certain foods, the guidelines suggest that foods be chosen "wisely," based on a basic knowledge of nutrient and energy density. This positive approach is more successful in promoting behavior change.

## BASIC PRINCIPLES OF NUTRITION ASSESSMENT AND SCREENING

An effective nutrition care plan for athletes is based on the four principles of a classical nutrition assessment:

- Anthropometric,
- dietary,
- biochemical, and
- clinical studies

Nutrition and physical performance indicators are integrated to determine the physiologic needs of the athlete and compared with food intake. Additional factors that will affect the athlete's dietary choices, such as level of motivation, social pressures, beliefs, competitive goals, work and school schedules, must be considered before attempting to counsel the athlete about dietary change.[2]

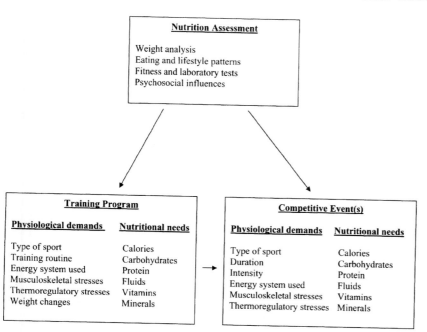

**FIGURE 10.1.** Flowchart for the nutritional assessment of athletes.[2]

A conceptual framework for conducting nutritional assessments of athletes has been described by Storlie[2] (Figure 10.1). Because most athletes have several different diet and training schedules, such as in-season, competitive season, and off-season training regimens, it is important to include the various training modalities in the nutrition assessment protocol. This model promotes a comprehensive approach to nutrition assessment. In practice, circumstances may render some of the data included in the comprehensive model unavailable or irrelevant.

Depending on the individual athlete's situation, different types of data collection techniques may be used. When nutritional assessments are conducted in a primary care setting, or away from a medical facility (e.g., school, athletic facility), we need practical and reliable methods to quickly assess an athlete's nutritional status and to solve common problems. Common nutritional problems should be addressed directly, so that athletes understand the importance of the diagnosis and recommended intervention. A designated professional who has good rapport with the athletes should also perform preventive nutrition assessment and counseling on a regular basis.

When uncommon or more complicated disease-oriented situations are detected (such as hypoglycemia, diabetes, eating disorders), athletes should be referred to specialists. Referrals to specialists such as registered dietitians, psychologists, and specialty physicians with experience in working with athletes can complement the care of the primary physician, coach, or trainer, resulting in improved compliance and outcome.

## Nutrition Assessment Strategy

### WEIGHT ANALYSIS (ANTHROPOMETRIC)

The body weight of an athlete has a crucial role in physical performance, as well as long-term health. The determination of the energy needs of an athlete is based on his/her average daily energy expenditure, as well as whether the athlete needs to lose weight, maintain weight, or gain weight. Because this is generally a primary concern for athletes, it is most productive to begin the nutrition assessment process by addressing and evaluating this issue thoroughly.

The determination of optimal body weight is a somewhat subjective process. Generally, three methods are applied and evaluated in order to determine an athlete's optimal body weight[2]:

- Personal goal weight
- Height/weight formula
- Percent body fat prediction

The athlete's personal goal weight is an indicator of both the athlete's knowledge of his/her own body and at what weight it performs and feels the best, as well as his/her motivation and body image. The collection of anthropometric data such as current weight, height, and percent body fat, offers the tools to predict optimal body weight. These data can then be reviewed and applied to determine how the athlete's present weight deviates from both the predicted weight and the athlete's personal weight goal.

## Weight Assessment Tools

There are a number of sources that thoroughly discuss the various protocols for anthropometric and body composition assessment (see Chapter 9). Because the tools used for the assessment of an athlete's weight must be practical yet reliable, optimal body weight should be determined using both height/weight and percent body fat assessment techniques.

## Field Methods of Body Composition Assessment

Field methods allow for simple techniques to estimate body weight and composition in a non–medical facility setting. Testing them against several other more rigorous assessment methods has validated the techniques. The common field methods utilize anthropometric measures of height, weight, and body mass index (BMI). Measures of skinfold and circumference sites are useful tools to assess body composition and distribution of body fat. Bioelectrical impedance has been validated as a portable tool to assess body composition.

Using BMI to predict optimal body weight for an athlete can be misleading. The predictive formula was developed based on average individuals, not athletes. Athletes tend to be less fat and more muscular than the average individual. A very lean, muscular bodybuilder or strength-training athlete may appear overweight when compared with a BMI standard, yet this athlete is far from overfat. A lean, small-boned endurance athlete may appear underweight according to the BMI standards, yet according to their body structure and the requirements of their sport, their weight is appropriate.

Although BMI is an acceptable starting point, predictive equations of body fat based on skinfold measures and body circumferences are more accurate for assessing the body composition of athletes. One predictive equation based on a population of fit individuals is the "Navy Chart of Percent Body Fat Estimated from Height and Circumference Values."[3] These predictive values are based on different equations and data points for men and women. To collect the pertinent data from an athlete, an accurate height measurement and a tape measure for circumference values are required. (See Tables 10.2 and 10.3.)

Bioelectrical impedance analysis is another acceptable field method for measuring body composition. Numerous tools are available on the market. The reliability of the measurement is greatly dependent on the preparation of the subject and the equations used for translating impedance into a body fat calculation. Equations developed from athletic populations should be used when determining body composition of fit individuals. To obtain the most accurate results from bioelectrical impedance analysis, the following conditions should be met:

- No alcohol 48 hours before the test
- Avoid intense exercise 12 hours before the test
- Avoid eating or drinking (especially caffeinated products) 4 hours before the test
- Come to your consult well hydrated
- Empty bladder 30 minutes before the test
- Avoid all diuretics for 7 days before test (only if medically possible)
- Measure in bare feet
- Illness at the time of measurement may affect individual hydration levels, which may affect results

Guidelines for percent body fat predictors can be found in Tables 10.4 and 10.5. Once an athlete's present body weight and percent body fat are determined, optimal body weight can be calculated from the following formula using the desired percent body fat. Then, considering all three predictors (personal goal, height/weight goal, percent body fat goal), the counselor and the athlete must work toward a realistic goal through negotiation and professional judgment.

Calculation of optimal body weight using desired percent body fat:

Present body weight: 140 pounds
Present percent body fat: 18%
Desired percent body fat: 14%
140 (0.18) = 25.2 pounds fat
140 − 25.2 = 114.8 pounds lean body mass
114.8/0.86 = 133.4 total pounds at 14% body fat

# GUIDELINES FOR ACCEPTABLE PERCENT BODY FAT LEVELS

The process of determining optimal body weight is generally a dynamic one. Body weight goals change with age and with sport. Athletes that participate in several different sports throughout the year may have different weight goals that are sport specific. Body weight goals fluctuate with on-season, competitive-season, and off-season training. Athletes who participate in events with official weight classifications such as wrestling, boxing, and bodybuilding will alter their weight goals frequently and repetitively. Sometimes the competitive goals of the athlete are potentially at odds with health goals. Yet an athlete may be determined to achieve what he or she believes is the competitive edge with rapid weight loss. Because performance is the bottom-line goal of the athlete, counselors must keep this factor in mind when athletes desire to reach an unrealistic weight goal. Research has shown that rapid weight loss in wrestlers trying to compete in lower weight classes adversely affects their performance.[4] Bodybuilders who have been on rigid dietary regimens before competitive events are at risk of metabolic abnormalities that can affect their performance as they enter competition.[5,6] Using this information may be the most helpful way to achieve a negotiated optimal body weight that can meet both performance and health goals. Finally, if the counselor suspects that eating disorders are present, this approach may not be appropriate, and assistance should be sought from an eating disorders specialist.

# DETERMINATION OF CALORIE REQUIREMENTS

After optimal body weight has been determined, approximate energy needs can be calculated. This process requires either an actual measure of total daily energy expenditure or an equation to predict energy expenditure.

## Methods of Determining Energy Expenditure

Until recently, actually measuring energy expenditure required a laboratory setting. Direct calorimetry, which measures the amount of heat given off by the body, is conducted in an air-tight, room-sized chamber. Subjects live in the chamber for a period of time and heat production is assessed by measuring the change in temperature in the water that surrounds the room. Indirect calorimetry estimates the heat released by the body through the measurement of the respiratory oxygen–carbon dioxide exchange ratio over a period of 24 hours. This ratio is called the respiratory exchange ratio (RER) and is a measure of the amount of oxidized carbohydrates and lipids. Respiratory quotient is generally the same as the RER except that the respiratory quotient represents respiratory exchange at the cellular level, and the RER is a measure of expired gases. This ratio can then be used to estimate total energy expenditure. Although there are versions of this equipment that can be worn as portable units, they are still bulky and are used primarily for research purposes.

TABLE 10.2. Percent body fat estimated from height and circumference value (lower abdominal girth – neck girth).

| Circumference Value | 60.0 | 60.5 | 61.0 | 61.5 | 62.0 | 62.5 | 63.0 | 63.5 | 64.0 | 64.5 | 65.0 | 65.5 | 66.0 | 66.5 | 67.0 | 67.5 | 68.0 | 68.5 | 69.0 |
|---|---|---|---|---|---|---|---|---|---|---|---|---|---|---|---|---|---|---|---|
| 11.0 | 3 | 2 | 2 | 2 | 2 | 1 | 1 | 1 | 1 | 1 | 0 | 0 | – | – | – | – | – | – | – |
| 11.5 | 4 | 4 | 4 | 3 | 3 | 3 | 3 | 2 | 2 | 2 | 2 | 2 | 1 | 1 | 1 | 1 | 1 | 0 | 0 |
| 12.0 | 6 | 5 | 5 | 5 | 5 | 4 | 4 | 4 | 4 | 3 | 3 | 3 | 3 | 3 | 2 | 2 | 2 | 2 | 2 |
| 12.5 | 7 | 7 | 6 | 6 | 6 | 6 | 6 | 5 | 5 | 5 | 5 | 4 | 4 | 4 | 4 | 4 | 3 | 3 | 3 |
| 13.0 | 8 | 8 | 8 | 8 | 7 | 7 | 7 | 7 | 6 | 6 | 6 | 6 | 6 | 5 | 5 | 5 | 5 | 5 | 4 |
| 13.5 | 10 | 9 | 9 | 9 | 9 | 8 | 8 | 8 | 8 | 8 | 7 | 7 | 7 | 7 | 6 | 6 | 6 | 6 | 6 |
| 14.0 | 11 | 11 | 10 | 10 | 10 | 10 | 10 | 9 | 9 | 9 | 9 | 8 | 8 | 8 | 8 | 8 | 7 | 7 | 7 |
| 14.5 | 12 | 12 | 12 | 11 | 11 | 11 | 11 | 11 | 10 | 10 | 10 | 10 | 9 | 9 | 9 | 9 | 9 | 8 | 8 |
| 15.0 | 13 | 13 | 13 | 13 | 12 | 12 | 12 | 12 | 12 | 11 | 11 | 11 | 11 | 10 | 10 | 10 | 10 | 10 | 9 |
| 15.5 | 15 | 14 | 14 | 14 | 14 | 13 | 13 | 13 | 13 | 12 | 12 | 12 | 12 | 12 | 11 | 11 | 11 | 11 | 11 |
| 16.0 | 16 | 15 | 15 | 15 | 15 | 15 | 14 | 14 | 14 | 14 | 13 | 13 | 13 | 13 | 12 | 12 | 12 | 12 | 12 |
| 16.5 | 17 | 17 | 16 | 16 | 16 | 16 | 15 | 15 | 15 | 15 | 14 | 14 | 14 | 14 | 14 | 13 | 13 | 13 | 13 |
| 17.0 | 18 | 18 | 17 | 17 | 17 | 17 | 16 | 16 | 16 | 16 | 16 | 15 | 15 | 15 | 15 | 14 | 14 | 14 | 14 |
| 17.5 | 19 | 19 | 19 | 18 | 18 | 18 | 18 | 17 | 17 | 17 | 17 | 16 | 16 | 16 | 16 | 16 | 15 | 15 | 15 |
| 18.0 | 20 | 20 | 20 | 19 | 19 | 19 | 19 | 18 | 18 | 18 | 18 | 17 | 17 | 17 | 17 | 17 | 16 | 16 | 16 |
| 18.5 | 21 | 21 | 21 | 20 | 20 | 20 | 20 | 19 | 19 | 19 | 19 | 18 | 18 | 18 | 18 | 18 | 17 | 17 | 17 |
| 19.0 | 22 | 22 | 22 | 21 | 21 | 21 | 21 | 20 | 20 | 20 | 20 | 19 | 19 | 19 | 19 | 19 | 18 | 18 | 18 |
| 19.5 | 23 | 23 | 23 | 22 | 22 | 22 | 22 | 21 | 21 | 21 | 21 | 20 | 20 | 20 | 20 | 19 | 19 | 19 | 19 |
| 20.0 | 24 | 24 | 23 | 23 | 23 | 23 | 22 | 22 | 22 | 22 | 22 | 21 | 21 | 21 | 21 | 20 | 20 | 20 | 20 |
| 20.5 | 25 | 25 | 24 | 24 | 24 | 24 | 23 | 23 | 23 | 22 | 22 | 22 | 22 | 22 | 22 | 21 | 21 | 21 | 21 |
| 21.0 | 26 | 26 | 25 | 25 | 25 | 25 | 24 | 24 | 24 | 23 | 23 | 23 | 23 | 23 | 22 | 22 | 22 | 22 | 22 |
| 21.5 | 27 | 26 | 26 | 26 | 26 | 25 | 25 | 25 | 25 | 24 | 24 | 24 | 24 | 24 | 23 | 23 | 23 | 23 | 22 |
| 22.0 | 28 | 27 | 27 | 27 | 27 | 26 | 26 | 26 | 26 | 25 | 25 | 25 | 25 | 24 | 24 | 24 | 24 | 24 | 23 |
| 22.5 | 28 | 28 | 28 | 28 | 27 | 27 | 27 | 27 | 26 | 26 | 26 | 26 | 25 | 25 | 25 | 25 | 25 | 24 | 24 |
| 23.0 | 29 | 29 | 29 | 29 | 28 | 28 | 28 | 28 | 27 | 27 | 27 | 27 | 26 | 26 | 26 | 26 | 25 | 25 | 25 |
| 23.5 | 30 | 30 | 30 | 29 | 29 | 29 | 29 | 28 | 28 | 28 | 28 | 27 | 27 | 27 | 27 | 26 | 26 | 26 | 26 |
| 24.0 | 31 | 31 | 30 | 30 | 30 | 30 | 29 | 29 | 29 | 28 | 28 | 28 | 28 | 28 | 27 | 27 | 27 | 27 | 27 |
| 24.5 | 32 | 31 | 31 | 31 | 31 | 30 | 30 | 30 | 30 | 29 | 29 | 29 | 29 | 29 | 28 | 28 | 28 | 28 | 27 |
| 25.0 | 33 | 32 | 32 | 32 | 31 | 31 | 31 | 31 | 30 | 30 | 30 | 30 | 30 | 29 | 29 | 29 | 29 | 28 | 28 |
| 25.5 | 33 | 33 | 33 | 33 | 32 | 32 | 32 | 31 | 31 | 31 | 31 | 31 | 30 | 30 | 30 | 30 | 29 | 29 | 29 |
| 26.0 | 34 | 34 | 34 | 33 | 33 | 33 | 32 | 32 | 32 | 32 | 32 | 31 | 31 | 31 | 31 | 30 | 30 | 30 | 30 |
| 26.5 | 35 | 35 | 34 | 34 | 34 | 33 | 33 | 33 | 33 | 32 | 32 | 32 | 32 | 32 | 31 | 31 | 31 | 31 | 30 |
| 27.0 | 36 | 35 | 35 | 35 | 34 | 34 | 34 | 34 | 33 | 33 | 33 | 33 | 32 | 32 | 32 | 32 | 32 | 31 | 31 |
| 27.5 | 36 | 36 | 36 | 35 | 36 | 35 | 35 | 34 | 34 | 34 | 34 | 33 | 33 | 33 | 33 | 32 | 32 | 32 | 32 |
| 28.0 | 37 | 37 | 36 | 36 | 36 | 36 | 35 | 35 | 35 | 34 | 34 | 34 | 34 | 34 | 33 | 33 | 33 | 33 | 33 |
| 28.5 | 38 | 37 | 37 | 37 | 37 | 36 | 36 | 36 | 36 | 35 | 35 | 35 | 35 | 34 | 34 | 34 | 34 | 33 | 33 |
| 29.0 | 38 | 38 | 38 | 38 | 37 | 37 | 37 | 37 | 36 | 36 | 36 | 36 | 35 | 35 | 35 | 35 | 34 | 34 | 34 |
| 29.5 | 39 | 39 | 39 | 38 | 38 | 38 | 37 | 37 | 37 | 36 | 36 | 36 | 36 | 36 | 35 | 35 | 35 | 35 | 35 |
| 30.0 | 40 | 39 | 39 | 39 | 39 | 38 | 38 | 38 | 38 | 37 | 37 | 37 | 37 | 36 | 36 | 36 | 36 | 35 | 35 |
| 30.5 |  |  | 40 | 40 | 39 | 39 | 39 | 39 | 38 | 38 | 38 | 38 | 37 | 37 | 37 | 37 | 36 | 36 | 36 |
| 31.0 |  |  |  |  | 40 | 40 | 39 | 39 | 39 | 38 | 38 | 38 | 38 | 38 | 37 | 37 | 37 | 37 | 37 |
| 31.5 |  |  |  |  |  |  |  | 40 | 40 | 39 | 39 | 39 | 39 | 38 | 38 | 38 | 38 | 37 | 37 |
| 32.0 |  |  |  |  |  |  |  |  |  |  | 40 | 40 | 39 | 39 | 39 | 38 | 38 | 38 | 38 |
| 32.5 |  |  |  |  |  |  |  |  |  |  |  |  | 40 | 40 | 39 | 39 | 39 | 39 | 38 |
| 33.0 |  |  |  |  |  |  |  |  |  |  |  |  |  |  | 40 | 40 | 39 | 39 | 39 |
| 33.5 |  |  |  |  |  |  |  |  |  |  |  |  |  |  |  |  |  | 40 | 40 |
| 34.0 |  |  |  |  |  |  |  |  |  |  |  |  |  |  |  |  |  |  |  |
| 34.5 |  |  |  |  |  |  |  |  |  |  |  |  |  |  |  |  |  |  |  |
| 35.0 |  |  |  |  |  |  |  |  |  |  |  |  |  |  |  |  |  |  |  |
| 35.5 |  |  |  |  |  |  |  |  |  |  |  |  |  |  |  |  |  |  |  |
| 36.0 |  |  |  |  |  |  |  |  |  |  |  |  |  |  |  |  |  |  |  |
| 36.5 |  |  |  |  |  |  |  |  |  |  |  |  |  |  |  |  |  |  |  |
| 37.0 |  |  |  |  |  |  |  |  |  |  |  |  |  |  |  |  |  |  |  |
| 37.5 |  |  |  |  |  |  |  |  |  |  |  |  |  |  |  |  |  |  |  |

| 69.5 | 70.0 | 70.5 | 71.0 | 71.5 | 72.0 | 72.5 | 73.0 | 73.5 | 74.0 | 74.5 | 75.0 | 75.5 | 76.0 | 76.5 | 77.0 | 77.5 | 78.0 | 78.5 | 79.0 | 79.5 |
|---|---|---|---|---|---|---|---|---|---|---|---|---|---|---|---|---|---|---|---|---|
| – | – | – | – | – | – | – | – | – | – | – | – | – | – | – | – | – | – | – | – | – |
| – | – | – | – | – | – | – | – | – | – | – | – | – | – | – | – | – | – | – | – | – |
| 1 | 1 | 1 | 1 | 1 | 0 | 0 | 0 | – | – | – | – | – | – | – | – | – | – | – | – | 1 |
| 3 | 3 | 2 | 2 | 2 | 2 | 2 | 1 | 1 | 1 | 1 | 1 | 1 | 0 | 0 | – | – | – | – | – | – |
| 4 | 4 | 4 | 4 | 3 | 3 | 3 | 3 | 3 | 2 | 2 | 2 | 2 | 2 | 1 | 1 | 1 | 1 | 1 | 1 | 0 |
| 5 | 5 | 5 | 5 | 5 | 4 | 4 | 4 | 4 | 4 | 4 | 3 | 3 | 3 | 3 | 3 | 2 | 2 | 2 | 2 | 2 |
| 7 | 7 | 6 | 6 | 6 | 6 | 6 | 5 | 5 | 5 | 5 | 5 | 4 | 4 | 4 | 4 | 4 | 3 | 3 | 3 | 3 |
| 8 | 8 | 8 | 7 | 7 | 7 | 7 | 7 | 6 | 6 | 6 | 6 | 6 | 5 | 5 | 5 | 5 | 5 | 5 | 4 | 4 |
| 9 | 9 | 9 | 9 | 8 | 8 | 8 | 8 | 8 | 7 | 7 | 7 | 7 | 7 | 6 | 6 | 6 | 6 | 6 | 6 | 5 |
| 10 | 10 | 10 | 10 | 9 | 9 | 9 | 9 | 9 | 8 | 8 | 8 | 8 | 8 | 7 | 7 | 7 | 7 | 7 | 7 | 6 |
| 11 | 11 | 11 | 11 | 11 | 10 | 10 | 10 | 10 | 10 | 9 | 9 | 9 | 9 | 9 | 8 | 8 | 8 | 8 | 8 | 8 |
| 13 | 12 | 12 | 12 | 12 | 12 | 11 | 11 | 11 | 11 | 11 | 10 | 10 | 10 | 10 | 10 | 9 | 9 | 9 | 9 | 9 |
| 14 | 13 | 13 | 13 | 13 | 13 | 12 | 12 | 12 | 12 | 12 | 11 | 11 | 11 | 11 | 11 | 10 | 10 | 10 | 10 | 10 |
| 15 | 14 | 14 | 14 | 14 | 14 | 13 | 13 | 13 | 13 | 13 | 12 | 12 | 12 | 12 | 12 | 11 | 11 | 11 | 11 | 11 |
| 16 | 15 | 15 | 15 | 15 | 15 | 14 | 14 | 14 | 14 | 14 | 13 | 13 | 13 | 13 | 13 | 12 | 12 | 12 | 12 | 12 |
| 17 | 16 | 16 | 16 | 16 | 16 | 15 | 15 | 15 | 15 | 15 | 14 | 14 | 14 | 14 | 14 | 13 | 13 | 13 | 13 | 13 |
| 18 | 17 | 17 | 17 | 17 | 17 | 16 | 16 | 16 | 16 | 16 | 15 | 15 | 15 | 15 | 15 | 14 | 14 | 14 | 14 | 14 |
| 19 | 18 | 18 | 18 | 18 | 18 | 17 | 17 | 17 | 17 | 17 | 16 | 16 | 16 | 16 | 16 | 15 | 15 | 15 | 15 | 15 |
| 20 | 19 | 19 | 19 | 19 | 18 | 18 | 18 | 18 | 18 | 17 | 17 | 17 | 17 | 17 | 16 | 16 | 16 | 16 | 16 | 16 |
| 20 | 20 | 20 | 20 | 20 | 19 | 19 | 19 | 19 | 19 | 18 | 18 | 18 | 18 | 18 | 17 | 17 | 17 | 17 | 17 | 16 |
| 21 | 21 | 21 | 21 | 20 | 20 | 20 | 20 | 20 | 19 | 19 | 19 | 19 | 19 | 18 | 18 | 18 | 18 | 18 | 18 | 17 |
| 22 | 22 | 22 | 22 | 21 | 21 | 21 | 21 | 21 | 20 | 20 | 20 | 20 | 20 | 19 | 19 | 19 | 19 | 19 | 18 | 18 |
| 23 | 23 | 23 | 22 | 22 | 22 | 22 | 22 | 21 | 21 | 21 | 21 | 21 | 20 | 20 | 20 | 20 | 20 | 19 | 19 | 19 |
| 24 | 24 | 23 | 23 | 23 | 23 | 23 | 22 | 22 | 22 | 22 | 22 | 21 | 21 | 21 | 21 | 21 | 20 | 20 | 20 | 20 |
| 25 | 25 | 24 | 24 | 24 | 24 | 23 | 23 | 23 | 23 | 23 | 22 | 22 | 22 | 22 | 22 | 21 | 21 | 21 | 21 | 21 |
| 26 | 25 | 25 | 25 | 25 | 24 | 24 | 24 | 24 | 24 | 23 | 23 | 23 | 23 | 23 | 22 | 22 | 22 | 22 | 22 | 21 |
| 26 | 26 | 26 | 26 | 25 | 25 | 25 | 25 | 25 | 24 | 24 | 24 | 24 | 24 | 23 | 23 | 23 | 23 | 23 | 22 | 22 |
| 27 | 27 | 27 | 26 | 26 | 26 | 26 | 26 | 25 | 25 | 25 | 25 | 25 | 24 | 24 | 24 | 24 | 24 | 23 | 23 | 23 |
| 28 | 28 | 27 | 27 | 27 | 27 | 27 | 26 | 26 | 26 | 26 | 26 | 25 | 25 | 25 | 25 | 25 | 24 | 24 | 24 | 24 |
| 29 | 28 | 28 | 28 | 28 | 28 | 28 | 27 | 27 | 27 | 27 | 26 | 26 | 26 | 26 | 26 | 25 | 25 | 25 | 25 | 25 |
| 29 | 29 | 29 | 29 | 29 | 28 | 28 | 28 | 28 | 27 | 27 | 27 | 27 | 27 | 26 | 26 | 26 | 26 | 26 | 25 | 25 |
| 30 | 30 | 30 | 29 | 29 | 29 | 29 | 29 | 28 | 28 | 28 | 28 | 28 | 27 | 27 | 27 | 27 | 27 | 26 | 26 | 26 |
| 31 | 31 | 30 | 30 | 30 | 30 | 30 | 29 | 29 | 29 | 29 | 28 | 28 | 28 | 28 | 28 | 27 | 27 | 27 | 27 | 27 |
| 32 | 31 | 31 | 31 | 31 | 30 | 30 | 30 | 30 | 30 | 30 | 29 | 29 | 29 | 29 | 29 | 28 | 28 | 28 | 28 | 27 |
| 32 | 32 | 32 | 32 | 31 | 31 | 31 | 31 | 31 | 30 | 30 | 30 | 30 | 30 | 29 | 29 | 29 | 29 | 28 | 28 | 28 |
| 33 | 33 | 33 | 32 | 32 | 32 | 32 | 31 | 31 | 31 | 31 | 31 | 30 | 30 | 30 | 30 | 30 | 29 | 29 | 29 | 29 |
| 34 | 33 | 33 | 33 | 33 | 33 | 33 | 32 | 32 | 32 | 32 | 31 | 31 | 31 | 31 | 31 | 30 | 30 | 30 | 30 | 29 |
| 34 | 34 | 34 | 34 | 33 | 33 | 33 | 33 | 32 | 32 | 32 | 32 | 32 | 31 | 31 | 31 | 31 | 31 | 30 | 30 | 30 |
| 35 | 35 | 35 | 34 | 34 | 34 | 34 | 33 | 33 | 33 | 33 | 33 | 32 | 32 | 32 | 32 | 32 | 31 | 31 | 31 | 31 |
| 36 | 35 | 35 | 35 | 35 | 35 | 35 | 34 | 34 | 34 | 34 | 33 | 33 | 33 | 33 | 32 | 32 | 32 | 32 | 32 | 31 |
| 36 | 36 | 36 | 36 | 35 | 35 | 35 | 34 | 34 | 34 | 34 | 34 | 33 | 33 | 33 | 33 | 33 | 32 | 32 | 32 | 32 |
| 37 | 37 | 36 | 36 | 36 | 36 | 36 | 35 | 35 | 35 | 35 | 34 | 34 | 34 | 34 | 34 | 33 | 33 | 33 | 33 | 33 |
| 38 | 37 | 37 | 37 | 37 | 36 | 36 | 36 | 36 | 36 | 35 | 35 | 35 | 34 | 34 | 34 | 34 | 34 | 33 | 33 | 33 |
| 38 | 38 | 38 | 37 | 37 | 37 | 37 | 37 | 36 | 36 | 36 | 35 | 35 | 35 | 35 | 35 | 34 | 34 | 34 | 34 | 33 |
| 39 | 39 | 38 | 38 | 38 | 38 | 38 | 37 | 37 | 37 | 37 | 36 | 36 | 36 | 36 | 35 | 35 | 35 | 35 | 35 | 34 |
| 39 | 39 | 39 | 39 | 38 | 38 | 38 | 38 | 38 | 37 | 37 | 37 | 37 | 36 | 36 | 36 | 36 | 36 | 35 | 35 | 35 |
| 40 | 40 | 39 | 39 | 39 | 39 | 39 | 38 | 38 | 38 | 38 | 37 | 37 | 37 | 37 | 37 | 36 | 36 | 36 | 36 | 36 |
|  |  | 40 | 40 | 39 | 39 | 39 | 38 | 38 | 38 | 38 | 38 | 37 | 37 | 37 | 37 | 37 | 36 | 36 | 36 | 36 |
|  |  |  |  | 40 | 40 | 39 | 39 | 39 | 38 | 38 | 38 | 38 | 38 | 37 | 37 | 37 | 37 | 37 | 36 | 36 |
|  |  |  |  |  |  | 40 | 40 | 40 | 39 | 39 | 38 | 38 | 38 | 38 | 38 | 37 | 37 | 37 | 37 | 37 |
|  |  |  |  |  |  |  | 40 | 40 | 39 | 39 | 39 | 39 | 39 | 38 | 38 | 38 | 38 | 38 | 37 | 37 |
|  |  |  |  |  |  |  |  |  | 40 | 40 | 39 | 39 | 39 | 39 | 39 | 38 | 38 | 38 | 38 | 38 |
|  |  |  |  |  |  |  |  |  |  |  | 40 | 40 | 39 | 39 | 39 | 39 | 39 | 38 | 38 | 38 |
|  |  |  |  |  |  |  |  |  |  |  |  |  | 40 | 40 | 39 | 39 | 39 | 39 | 38 | 38 |
|  |  |  |  |  |  |  |  |  |  |  |  |  |  |  | 40 | 40 | 39 | 39 | 39 | 39 |
|  |  |  |  |  |  |  |  |  |  |  |  |  |  |  |  |  | 40 | 40 | 39 | 39 |
|  |  |  |  |  |  |  |  |  |  |  |  |  |  |  |  |  |  |  | 40 | 40 |
|  |  |  |  |  |  |  |  |  |  |  |  |  |  |  |  |  |  |  |  | 40 |

**TABLE 10.3.** Percent body fat estimated from height and circumference value (upper abdominal girth + hip girth − neck girth).

| CV | 58.0 | 58.5 | 59.0 | 59.5 | 60.0 | 60.5 | 61.0 | 61.5 | 62.0 | 62.5 | 63.0 | 63.5 | 64.0 | 64.5 | 65.0 | 65.5 | 66.0 | 66.5 | 67.0 |
|---|---|---|---|---|---|---|---|---|---|---|---|---|---|---|---|---|---|---|---|
| 34.5 | 1 | 0 | – | – | – | – | – | – | – | – | – | – | – | – | – | – | – | – | – |
| 35.0 | 2 | 1 | 1 | 1 | 0 | – | – | – | – | – | – | – | – | – | – | – | – | – | – |
| 35.5 | 3 | 2 | 2 | 2 | 1 | 1 | 0 | 0 | – | – | – | – | – | – | – | – | – | – | – |
| 36.0 | 4 | 3 | 3 | 3 | 2 | 2 | 1 | 1 | 1 | 0 | 0 | – | – | – | – | – | – | – | – |
| 36.5 | 5 | 4 | 4 | 4 | 3 | 3 | 2 | 2 | 2 | 1 | 1 | 1 | 0 | – | – | – | – | – | – |
| 37.0 | 6 | 5 | 5 | 4 | 4 | 4 | 3 | 3 | 3 | 2 | 2 | 2 | 1 | 1 | 1 | 0 | – | – | – |
| 37.5 | 7 | 6 | 6 | 5 | 5 | 5 | 4 | 4 | 4 | 3 | 3 | 3 | 2 | 2 | 2 | 1 | 1 | 1 | 0 |
| 38.0 | 7 | 7 | 7 | 6 | 6 | 6 | 5 | 5 | 5 | 4 | 4 | 3 | 3 | 3 | 2 | 2 | 2 | 1 | 1 |
| 38.5 | 8 | 8 | 8 | 7 | 7 | 7 | 6 | 6 | 5 | 5 | 5 | 4 | 4 | 4 | 3 | 3 | 3 | 2 | 2 |
| 39.0 | 9 | 9 | 9 | 8 | 8 | 7 | 7 | 7 | 6 | 6 | 6 | 5 | 5 | 5 | 4 | 4 | 4 | 3 | 3 |
| 39.5 | 10 | 10 | 9 | 9 | 9 | 8 | 8 | 8 | 7 | 7 | 7 | 6 | 6 | 6 | 5 | 5 | 5 | 4 | 4 |
| 40.0 | 11 | 11 | 10 | 10 | 10 | 9 | 9 | 8 | 8 | 8 | 7 | 7 | 7 | 6 | 6 | 6 | 5 | 5 | 5 |
| 40.5 | 12 | 12 | 11 | 11 | 10 | 10 | 10 | 9 | 9 | 9 | 8 | 8 | 8 | 7 | 7 | 7 | 6 | 6 | 6 |
| 41.0 | 13 | 12 | 12 | 12 | 11 | 11 | 11 | 10 | 10 | 10 | 9 | 9 | 8 | 8 | 8 | 7 | 7 | 7 | 6 |
| 41.5 | 14 | 13 | 13 | 13 | 12 | 12 | 11 | 11 | 11 | 10 | 10 | 10 | 9 | 9 | 9 | 8 | 8 | 8 | 7 |
| 42.0 | 14 | 14 | 14 | 13 | 13 | 13 | 12 | 12 | 12 | 11 | 11 | 10 | 10 | 10 | 9 | 9 | 9 | 8 | 8 |
| 42.5 | 15 | 15 | 15 | 14 | 14 | 13 | 13 | 13 | 12 | 12 | 12 | 11 | 11 | 11 | 10 | 10 | 10 | 9 | 9 |
| 43.0 | 16 | 16 | 15 | 15 | 15 | 14 | 14 | 14 | 13 | 13 | 12 | 12 | 12 | 11 | 11 | 11 | 10 | 10 | 10 |
| 43.5 | 17 | 17 | 16 | 16 | 15 | 15 | 15 | 14 | 14 | 14 | 13 | 13 | 13 | 12 | 12 | 12 | 11 | 11 | 11 |
| 44.0 | 18 | 17 | 17 | 17 | 16 | 16 | 16 | 15 | 15 | 14 | 14 | 13 | 13 | 13 | 13 | 12 | 12 | 12 | 11 |
| 44.5 | 19 | 18 | 18 | 17 | 17 | 17 | 16 | 16 | 16 | 15 | 15 | 14 | 14 | 14 | 14 | 13 | 13 | 13 | 12 |
| 45.0 | 19 | 19 | 19 | 18 | 18 | 17 | 17 | 17 | 16 | 16 | 16 | 15 | 15 | 15 | 14 | 14 | 14 | 13 | 13 |
| 45.5 | 20 | 20 | 19 | 19 | 19 | 18 | 18 | 18 | 17 | 17 | 16 | 16 | 16 | 15 | 15 | 15 | 14 | 14 | 14 |
| 46.0 | 21 | 20 | 20 | 20 | 19 | 19 | 19 | 18 | 18 | 18 | 17 | 17 | 17 | 16 | 16 | 16 | 15 | 15 | 15 |
| 46.5 | 22 | 21 | 21 | 20 | 20 | 20 | 19 | 19 | 19 | 18 | 18 | 18 | 17 | 17 | 17 | 16 | 16 | 16 | 15 |
| 47.0 | 22 | 22 | 22 | 21 | 21 | 20 | 20 | 20 | 19 | 19 | 19 | 18 | 18 | 18 | 17 | 17 | 17 | 16 | 16 |
| 47.5 | 23 | 23 | 22 | 22 | 22 | 21 | 21 | 21 | 20 | 20 | 19 | 19 | 19 | 18 | 18 | 18 | 17 | 17 | 17 |
| 48.0 | 24 | 23 | 23 | 23 | 22 | 22 | 22 | 21 | 21 | 21 | 20 | 20 | 20 | 19 | 19 | 18 | 18 | 18 | 18 |
| 48.5 | 25 | 24 | 24 | 23 | 23 | 23 | 22 | 22 | 22 | 21 | 21 | 21 | 20 | 20 | 20 | 19 | 19 | 19 | 18 |
| 49.0 | 25 | 25 | 25 | 24 | 24 | 23 | 23 | 23 | 22 | 22 | 22 | 21 | 21 | 21 | 20 | 20 | 20 | 19 | 19 |
| 49.5 | 26 | 26 | 25 | 25 | 24 | 24 | 24 | 23 | 23 | 23 | 22 | 22 | 22 | 21 | 21 | 21 | 20 | 20 | 20 |
| 50.0 | 27 | 26 | 26 | 26 | 25 | 25 | 24 | 24 | 24 | 23 | 23 | 23 | 22 | 22 | 22 | 21 | 21 | 21 | 20 |
| 50.5 | 27 | 27 | 27 | 26 | 26 | 26 | 25 | 25 | 24 | 24 | 24 | 23 | 23 | 23 | 22 | 22 | 22 | 21 | 21 |
| 51.0 | 28 | 28 | 27 | 27 | 27 | 26 | 26 | 25 | 25 | 25 | 24 | 24 | 24 | 23 | 23 | 23 | 22 | 22 | 22 |
| 51.5 | 29 | 28 | 28 | 28 | 27 | 27 | 27 | 26 | 26 | 25 | 25 | 25 | 24 | 24 | 24 | 23 | 23 | 23 | 22 |
| 52.0 | 29 | 29 | 29 | 28 | 28 | 28 | 27 | 27 | 27 | 26 | 26 | 25 | 25 | 25 | 24 | 24 | 24 | 23 | 23 |
| 52.5 | 30 | 30 | 29 | 29 | 29 | 28 | 28 | 28 | 27 | 27 | 26 | 26 | 26 | 25 | 25 | 25 | 24 | 24 | 24 |
| 53.0 | 31 | 30 | 30 | 30 | 29 | 29 | 29 | 28 | 28 | 27 | 27 | 27 | 26 | 26 | 26 | 25 | 25 | 25 | 24 |
| 53.5 | 31 | 31 | 31 | 30 | 30 | 30 | 29 | 29 | 28 | 28 | 28 | 27 | 27 | 27 | 26 | 26 | 26 | 25 | 25 |
| 54.0 | 32 | 32 | 31 | 31 | 31 | 30 | 30 | 30 | 29 | 29 | 28 | 28 | 28 | 27 | 27 | 27 | 26 | 26 | 26 |
| 54.5 | 33 | 32 | 32 | 32 | 31 | 31 | 31 | 30 | 30 | 29 | 29 | 29 | 28 | 28 | 28 | 27 | 27 | 27 | 26 |
| 55.0 | 33 | 33 | 33 | 32 | 32 | 32 | 31 | 31 | 30 | 30 | 30 | 29 | 29 | 29 | 28 | 28 | 28 | 27 | 27 |
| 55.5 | 34 | 34 | 33 | 33 | 33 | 32 | 32 | 31 | 31 | 31 | 30 | 30 | 30 | 29 | 29 | 29 | 28 | 28 | 28 |
| 56.0 | 35 | 34 | 34 | 33 | 33 | 33 | 32 | 32 | 32 | 31 | 31 | 31 | 30 | 30 | 30 | 29 | 29 | 29 | 28 |
| 56.5 | 35 | 35 | 34 | 34 | 34 | 33 | 33 | 33 | 32 | 32 | 32 | 31 | 31 | 31 | 30 | 30 | 30 | 29 | 29 |
| 57.0 | 36 | 35 | 35 | 35 | 34 | 34 | 34 | 33 | 33 | 33 | 32 | 32 | 32 | 31 | 31 | 31 | 30 | 30 | 30 |
| 57.5 | 36 | 36 | 36 | 35 | 35 | 35 | 34 | 34 | 34 | 33 | 33 | 32 | 32 | 32 | 31 | 31 | 31 | 30 | 30 |
| 58.0 | 37 | 37 | 36 | 36 | 36 | 35 | 35 | 35 | 34 | 34 | 33 | 33 | 33 | 32 | 32 | 32 | 31 | 31 | 31 |
| 58.5 | 38 | 37 | 37 | 37 | 36 | 36 | 35 | 35 | 35 | 34 | 34 | 34 | 33 | 33 | 33 | 32 | 32 | 32 | 31 |
| 59.0 | 38 | 38 | 38 | 37 | 37 | 36 | 36 | 36 | 35 | 35 | 35 | 34 | 34 | 34 | 33 | 33 | 33 | 32 | 32 |
| 59.5 | 39 | 38 | 38 | 38 | 37 | 37 | 37 | 36 | 36 | 36 | 35 | 35 | 35 | 34 | 34 | 34 | 33 | 33 | 33 |
| 60.0 | 39 | 39 | 39 | 38 | 38 | 38 | 37 | 37 | 37 | 36 | 36 | 35 | 35 | 35 | 34 | 34 | 34 | 33 | 33 |
| 60.5 | 40 | 40 | 39 | 39 | 39 | 38 | 38 | 37 | 37 | 37 | 36 | 36 | 36 | 35 | 35 | 35 | 34 | 34 | 34 |
| 61.0 | 41 | 40 | 40 | 39 | 39 | 39 | 38 | 38 | 38 | 37 | 37 | 37 | 36 | 36 | 36 | 35 | 35 | 35 | 34 |
| 61.5 | 41 | 41 | 40 | 40 | 40 | 39 | 39 | 39 | 38 | 38 | 38 | 37 | 37 | 37 | 36 | 36 | 36 | 35 | 35 |

| 67.5 | 68.0 | 68.5 | 69.0 | 69.5 | 70.0 | 70.5 | 71.0 | 71.5 | 72.0 | 72.5 | 73.0 | 73.5 | 74.0 | 74.5 | 75.0 | 75.5 | 76.0 | 76.5 | 77.0 | 77.5 |
|---|---|---|---|---|---|---|---|---|---|---|---|---|---|---|---|---|---|---|---|---|
| – | – | – | – | – | – | – | – | – | – | – | – | – | – | – | – | – | – | – | – | – |
| – | – | – | – | – | – | – | – | – | – | – | – | – | – | – | – | – | – | – | – | – |
| – | – | – | – | – | – | – | – | – | – | – | – | – | – | – | – | – | – | – | – | – |
| – | – | – | – | – | – | – | – | – | – | – | – | – | – | – | – | – | – | – | – | – |
| – | – | – | – | – | – | – | – | – | – | – | – | – | – | – | – | – | – | – | – | – |
| – | – | – | – | – | – | – | – | – | – | – | – | – | – | – | – | – | – | – | – | – |
| – | – | – | – | – | – | – | – | – | – | – | – | – | – | – | – | – | – | – | – | – |
| 1 | 0 | 0 | – | – | – | – | – | – | – | – | – | – | – | – | – | – | – | – | – | – |
| 2 | 1 | 1 | 1 | 0 | 0 | – | – | – | – | – | – | – | – | – | – | – | – | – | – | – |
| 3 | 2 | 2 | 2 | 1 | 1 | 1 | 0 | 0 | – | – | – | – | – | – | – | – | – | – | – | – |
| 4 | 3 | 3 | 3 | 2 | 2 | 2 | 1 | 1 | 1 | 0 | 0 | – | – | – | – | – | – | – | – | – |
| 4 | 4 | 4 | 3 | 3 | 3 | 3 | 2 | 2 | 2 | 1 | 1 | 1 | 0 | 0 | – | – | – | – | – | – |
| 5 | 5 | 5 | 4 | 4 | 4 | 3 | 3 | 3 | 2 | 2 | 2 | 2 | 1 | 1 | 1 | 0 | 0 | – | – | – |
| 6 | 6 | 5 | 5 | 5 | 5 | 4 | 4 | 4 | 3 | 3 | 3 | 2 | 2 | 2 | 2 | 1 | 1 | 1 | 0 | 0 |
| 7 | 7 | 6 | 6 | 6 | 5 | 5 | 5 | 4 | 4 | 4 | 4 | 3 | 3 | 3 | 2 | 2 | 2 | 2 | 1 | 1 |
| 8 | 8 | 7 | 7 | 7 | 6 | 6 | 6 | 5 | 5 | 5 | 4 | 4 | 4 | 4 | 3 | 3 | 3 | 2 | 2 | 2 |
| 9 | 8 | 8 | 8 | 7 | 7 | 7 | 6 | 6 | 6 | 6 | 5 | 5 | 5 | 4 | 4 | 4 | 3 | 3 | 3 | 3 |
| 9 | 9 | 9 | 9 | 8 | 8 | 8 | 7 | 7 | 7 | 6 | 6 | 6 | 5 | 5 | 5 | 5 | 4 | 4 | 4 | 3 |
| 10 | 10 | 10 | 9 | 9 | 9 | 8 | 8 | 8 | 7 | 7 | 7 | 7 | 6 | 6 | 5 | 5 | 5 | 5 | 5 | 4 |
| 11 | 11 | 10 | 10 | 10 | 9 | 9 | 9 | 9 | 8 | 8 | 8 | 7 | 7 | 6 | 6 | 6 | 6 | 6 | 5 | 5 |
| 12 | 12 | 11 | 11 | 11 | 10 | 10 | 10 | 9 | 9 | 9 | 8 | 8 | 8 | 8 | 7 | 7 | 7 | 6 | 6 | 6 |
| 13 | 12 | 12 | 12 | 11 | 11 | 11 | 10 | 10 | 10 | 10 | 9 | 9 | 9 | 8 | 8 | 8 | 7 | 7 | 7 | 7 |
| 13 | 13 | 13 | 12 | 12 | 12 | 12 | 11 | 11 | 11 | 10 | 10 | 10 | 9 | 9 | 9 | 9 | 8 | 8 | 8 | 7 |
| 14 | 14 | 14 | 13 | 13 | 13 | 12 | 12 | 12 | 11 | 11 | 11 | 10 | 10 | 10 | 10 | 9 | 9 | 9 | 8 | 8 |
| 15 | 15 | 14 | 14 | 14 | 13 | 13 | 13 | 12 | 12 | 12 | 12 | 11 | 11 | 11 | 10 | 10 | 10 | 9 | 9 | 9 |
| 16 | 15 | 15 | 15 | 14 | 14 | 14 | 13 | 13 | 13 | 13 | 12 | 12 | 12 | 11 | 11 | 11 | 11 | 10 | 10 | 10 |
| 16 | 16 | 16 | 15 | 15 | 15 | 15 | 14 | 14 | 14 | 13 | 13 | 13 | 12 | 12 | 12 | 12 | 11 | 11 | 11 | 10 |
| 17 | 17 | 17 | 16 | 16 | 16 | 15 | 15 | 15 | 14 | 14 | 14 | 13 | 13 | 13 | 13 | 12 | 12 | 12 | 11 | 11 |
| 18 | 18 | 17 | 17 | 17 | 16 | 16 | 16 | 15 | 15 | 15 | 15 | 14 | 14 | 14 | 13 | 13 | 13 | 12 | 12 | 12 |
| 19 | 18 | 18 | 18 | 17 | 17 | 17 | 16 | 16 | 16 | 15 | 15 | 15 | 15 | 14 | 14 | 14 | 13 | 13 | 13 | 13 |
| 19 | 19 | 19 | 18 | 18 | 18 | 17 | 17 | 17 | 17 | 16 | 16 | 16 | 15 | 15 | 15 | 14 | 14 | 14 | 14 | 13 |
| 20 | 20 | 19 | 19 | 19 | 18 | 18 | 18 | 18 | 17 | 17 | 17 | 16 | 16 | 16 | 15 | 15 | 15 | 15 | 14 | 14 |
| 21 | 20 | 20 | 20 | 19 | 19 | 19 | 19 | 18 | 18 | 18 | 17 | 17 | 17 | 16 | 16 | 16 | 16 | 15 | 15 | 15 |
| 21 | 21 | 21 | 20 | 20 | 20 | 20 | 19 | 19 | 19 | 18 | 18 | 18 | 17 | 17 | 17 | 17 | 16 | 16 | 16 | 15 |
| 22 | 22 | 21 | 21 | 21 | 20 | 20 | 20 | 19 | 19 | 19 | 18 | 18 | 18 | 17 | 17 | 17 | 17 | 16 | 16 | 16 |
| 23 | 22 | 22 | 22 | 22 | 21 | 21 | 21 | 20 | 20 | 20 | 19 | 19 | 19 | 18 | 18 | 18 | 18 | 17 | 17 | 17 |
| 23 | 23 | 23 | 22 | 22 | 22 | 22 | 21 | 21 | 21 | 20 | 20 | 20 | 19 | 19 | 19 | 19 | 18 | 18 | 18 | 17 |
| 24 | 24 | 23 | 23 | 23 | 23 | 22 | 22 | 22 | 21 | 21 | 21 | 20 | 20 | 20 | 20 | 19 | 19 | 19 | 18 | 18 |
| 25 | 24 | 24 | 24 | 23 | 23 | 23 | 22 | 22 | 22 | 21 | 21 | 21 | 20 | 20 | 20 | 20 | 19 | 19 | 19 | 19 |
| 25 | 25 | 25 | 24 | 24 | 24 | 24 | 23 | 23 | 23 | 22 | 22 | 22 | 21 | 21 | 21 | 21 | 20 | 20 | 20 | 19 |
| 26 | 26 | 25 | 25 | 25 | 24 | 24 | 24 | 23 | 23 | 23 | 22 | 22 | 22 | 21 | 21 | 21 | 21 | 20 | 20 | 20 |
| 27 | 26 | 26 | 26 | 25 | 25 | 25 | 24 | 24 | 24 | 24 | 23 | 23 | 23 | 22 | 22 | 22 | 22 | 21 | 21 | 21 |
| 27 | 27 | 27 | 26 | 26 | 26 | 25 | 25 | 25 | 25 | 24 | 24 | 24 | 23 | 23 | 23 | 22 | 22 | 22 | 22 | 21 |
| 28 | 28 | 27 | 27 | 27 | 26 | 26 | 26 | 25 | 25 | 25 | 25 | 24 | 24 | 24 | 23 | 23 | 23 | 22 | 22 | 22 |
| 29 | 28 | 28 | 28 | 27 | 27 | 27 | 26 | 26 | 26 | 25 | 25 | 25 | 25 | 24 | 24 | 24 | 23 | 23 | 23 | 23 |
| 29 | 29 | 29 | 28 | 28 | 28 | 27 | 27 | 27 | 27 | 26 | 26 | 26 | 25 | 25 | 25 | 25 | 24 | 24 | 24 | 23 |
| 30 | 30 | 29 | 29 | 29 | 28 | 28 | 28 | 28 | 27 | 27 | 27 | 26 | 26 | 26 | 26 | 25 | 25 | 25 | 24 | 24 |
| 30 | 30 | 30 | 29 | 29 | 29 | 29 | 28 | 28 | 28 | 27 | 27 | 27 | 26 | 26 | 26 | 26 | 25 | 25 | 25 | 24 |
| 31 | 31 | 30 | 30 | 30 | 29 | 29 | 29 | 29 | 28 | 28 | 28 | 27 | 27 | 27 | 26 | 26 | 26 | 26 | 25 | 25 |
| 32 | 31 | 31 | 31 | 30 | 30 | 30 | 29 | 29 | 29 | 28 | 28 | 28 | 28 | 27 | 27 | 27 | 26 | 26 | 26 | 26 |
| 32 | 32 | 32 | 31 | 31 | 31 | 30 | 30 | 30 | 29 | 29 | 29 | 28 | 28 | 28 | 28 | 27 | 27 | 27 | 26 | 26 |
| 33 | 32 | 32 | 32 | 32 | 31 | 31 | 31 | 30 | 30 | 30 | 29 | 29 | 29 | 28 | 28 | 28 | 28 | 27 | 27 | 27 |
| 33 | 33 | 33 | 32 | 32 | 32 | 31 | 31 | 31 | 31 | 30 | 30 | 30 | 29 | 29 | 29 | 28 | 28 | 28 | 28 | 27 |
| 34 | 34 | 33 | 33 | 33 | 32 | 32 | 32 | 31 | 31 | 31 | 31 | 30 | 30 | 30 | 29 | 29 | 29 | 28 | 28 | 28 |
| 35 | 34 | 34 | 34 | 33 | 33 | 33 | 32 | 32 | 32 | 31 | 31 | 31 | 31 | 30 | 30 | 30 | 29 | 29 | 29 | 28 |

*(Continued)*

**TABLE 10.3.** Percent body fat estimated from height and circumference value (upper abdominal girth + hip girth − neck girth). *Continued*

| CV | 58.0 | 58.5 | 59.0 | 59.5 | 60.0 | 60.5 | 61.0 | 61.5 | 62.0 | 62.5 | 63.0 | 63.5 | 64.0 | 64.5 | 65.0 | 65.5 | 66.0 | 66.5 | 67.0 |
|---|---|---|---|---|---|---|---|---|---|---|---|---|---|---|---|---|---|---|---|
| 62.0 | 42 | 41 | 41 | 41 | 40 | 40 | 40 | 39 | 39 | 38 | 38 | 38 | 37 | 37 | 37 | 36 | 36 | 36 | 35 |
| 62.5 | 42 | 42 | 42 | 41 | 41 | 40 | 40 | 40 | 39 | 39 | 39 | 38 | 38 | 38 | 37 | 37 | 37 | 36 | 36 |
| 63.0 | 43 | 42 | 42 | 42 | 41 | 41 | 41 | 40 | 40 | 40 | 39 | 39 | 39 | 38 | 38 | 38 | 37 | 37 | 37 |
| 63.5 | 43 | 43 | 43 | 42 | 42 | 42 | 41 | 41 | 40 | 40 | 40 | 39 | 39 | 39 | 38 | 38 | 38 | 37 | 37 |
| 64.0 | 44 | 44 | 43 | 43 | 42 | 42 | 42 | 41 | 41 | 41 | 40 | 40 | 40 | 39 | 39 | 39 | 38 | 38 | 38 |
| 64.5 | 45 | 44 | 44 | 43 | 43 | 43 | 42 | 42 | 42 | 41 | 41 | 41 | 40 | 40 | 40 | 39 | 39 | 39 | 38 |
| 65.0 |  | 45 | 44 | 44 | 44 | 43 | 43 | 42 | 42 | 42 | 41 | 41 | 41 | 40 | 40 | 40 | 39 | 39 | 39 |
| 65.5 |  |  | 45 | 44 | 44 | 44 | 43 | 43 | 43 | 42 | 42 | 42 | 41 | 41 | 41 | 40 | 40 | 40 | 39 |
| 66.0 |  |  |  |  | 45 | 44 | 44 | 44 | 43 | 43 | 43 | 42 | 42 | 41 | 41 | 41 | 40 | 40 | 40 |
| 66.5 |  |  |  |  |  | 45 | 44 | 44 | 44 | 43 | 43 | 43 | 42 | 42 | 42 | 41 | 41 | 41 | 40 |
| 67.0 |  |  |  |  |  |  | 45 | 45 | 44 | 44 | 44 | 43 | 43 | 43 | 42 | 42 | 42 | 41 | 41 |
| 67.5 |  |  |  |  |  |  |  | 45 | 44 | 44 | 44 | 43 | 43 | 43 | 42 | 42 | 42 | 42 | 41 |
| 68.0 |  |  |  |  |  |  |  |  | 45 | 45 | 44 | 44 | 44 | 43 | 43 | 43 | 42 | 42 | 42 |
| 68.5 |  |  |  |  |  |  |  |  |  |  |  | 45 | 44 | 44 | 44 | 43 | 43 | 43 | 42 |
| 69.0 |  |  |  |  |  |  |  |  |  |  |  |  | 45 | 45 | 44 | 44 | 44 | 43 | 43 |
| 69.5 |  |  |  |  |  |  |  |  |  |  |  |  |  |  | 45 | 44 | 44 | 44 | 43 |
| 70.0 |  |  |  |  |  |  |  |  |  |  |  |  |  |  |  | 45 | 45 | 44 | 44 |
| 70.5 |  |  |  |  |  |  |  |  |  |  |  |  |  |  |  |  |  | 45 | 44 |
| 71.0 |  |  |  |  |  |  |  |  |  |  |  |  |  |  |  |  |  |  | 45 |
| 71.5 |  |  |  |  |  |  |  |  |  |  |  |  |  |  |  |  |  |  |  |
| 72.0 |  |  |  |  |  |  |  |  |  |  |  |  |  |  |  |  |  |  |  |
| 72.5 |  |  |  |  |  |  |  |  |  |  |  |  |  |  |  |  |  |  |  |
| 73.0 |  |  |  |  |  |  |  |  |  |  |  |  |  |  |  |  |  |  |  |
| 73.5 |  |  |  |  |  |  |  |  |  |  |  |  |  |  |  |  |  |  |  |
| 74.0 |  |  |  |  |  |  |  |  |  |  |  |  |  |  |  |  |  |  |  |
| 74.5 |  |  |  |  |  |  |  |  |  |  |  |  |  |  |  |  |  |  |  |
| 75.0 |  |  |  |  |  |  |  |  |  |  |  |  |  |  |  |  |  |  |  |
| 75.5 |  |  |  |  |  |  |  |  |  |  |  |  |  |  |  |  |  |  |  |

**TABLE 10.4.** Health standards for percent body fat.

|  | Recommended body fat levels | | | | |
|---|---|---|---|---|---|
|  | *Not recommended* | *Low* | *Mid* | *Upper* | *Obesity* |
| Men |  |  |  |  |  |
|   Young adult | <8 | 8 | 13 | 22 | → |
|   Middle adult | <10 | 10 | 18 | 25 | → |
|   Elderly | <10 | 10 | 16 | 23 | → |
| Women |  |  |  |  |  |
|   Young adult | <20 | 20 | 28 | 35 | → |
|   Middle adult | <25 | 25 | 32 | 38 | → |
|   Elderly | <25 | 25 | 30 | 35 | → |

*Source:* Lohman TG, Houtkooper L, Going SB. Body fat measurement goes high-tech: not all are created equal. ACSM's Health Fit J 1997;7:30–35.

**TABLE 10.5.** New fat fitness standards for percent body fat in active men and women.

|  | Recommended body fat levels | | |
|---|---|---|---|
|  | *Low* | *Mid* | *Upper* |
| Men |  |  |  |
|   Young adult | 5 | 10 | 15 |
|   Middle adult | 7 | 11 | 18 |
|   Elderly | 9 | 12 | 18 |
| Women |  |  |  |
|   Young adult | 16 | 23 | 28 |
|   Middle adult | 20 | 27 | 33 |
|   Elderly | 20 | 27 | 33 |

*Source:* Lohman TG, Houtkooper L, Going SB. Body fat measurement goes high-tech: not all are created equal. ACSM's Health Fit J 1997;7:30–35.

| 67.5 | 68.0 | 68.5 | 69.0 | 69.5 | 70.0 | 70.5 | 71.0 | 71.5 | 72.0 | 72.5 | 73.0 | 73.5 | 74.0 | 74.5 | 75.0 | 75.5 | 76.0 | 76.5 | 77.0 | 77.5 |
|---|---|---|---|---|---|---|---|---|---|---|---|---|---|---|---|---|---|---|---|---|
| 35 | 35 | 34 | 34 | 34 | 34 | 33 | 33 | 33 | 32 | 32 | 32 | 31 | 31 | 31 | 30 | 30 | 30 | 30 | 29 | 29 |
| 36 | 35 | 35 | 35 | 34 | 34 | 34 | 33 | 33 | 33 | 33 | 32 | 32 | 32 | 31 | 31 | 31 | 30 | 30 | 30 | 30 |
| 36 | 36 | 36 | 35 | 35 | 35 | 34 | 34 | 34 | 33 | 33 | 33 | 32 | 32 | 32 | 31 | 31 | 31 | 30 | 30 | 30 |
| 37 | 36 | 36 | 36 | 35 | 35 | 35 | 35 | 34 | 34 | 34 | 33 | 33 | 33 | 32 | 32 | 32 | 32 | 31 | 31 | 31 |
| 37 | 37 | 37 | 36 | 36 | 36 | 35 | 35 | 35 | 35 | 34 | 34 | 34 | 33 | 33 | 33 | 32 | 32 | 32 | 32 | 31 |
| 38 | 38 | 37 | 37 | 37 | 36 | 36 | 36 | 35 | 35 | 35 | 34 | 34 | 34 | 34 | 33 | 33 | 33 | 32 | 32 | 32 |
| 38 | 38 | 38 | 37 | 37 | 37 | 37 | 36 | 36 | 36 | 35 | 35 | 35 | 34 | 34 | 34 | 34 | 33 | 33 | 32 | 32 |
| 39 | 39 | 38 | 38 | 38 | 37 | 37 | 37 | 36 | 36 | 36 | 36 | 35 | 35 | 35 | 34 | 34 | 34 | 33 | 33 | 33 |
| 39 | 39 | 39 | 39 | 38 | 38 | 38 | 37 | 37 | 37 | 36 | 36 | 36 | 35 | 35 | 35 | 35 | 34 | 34 | 34 | 33 |
| 40 | 40 | 39 | 39 | 39 | 38 | 38 | 38 | 37 | 37 | 37 | 37 | 36 | 36 | 36 | 35 | 35 | 35 | 35 | 34 | 34 |
| 41 | 40 | 40 | 40 | 39 | 39 | 39 | 38 | 38 | 38 | 37 | 37 | 37 | 37 | 36 | 36 | 36 | 35 | 35 | 35 | 34 |
| 41 | 41 | 40 | 40 | 40 | 39 | 39 | 39 | 39 | 38 | 38 | 38 | 37 | 37 | 37 | 36 | 36 | 36 | 36 | 35 | 35 |
| 42 | 41 | 41 | 41 | 40 | 40 | 40 | 39 | 39 | 39 | 38 | 38 | 38 | 38 | 37 | 37 | 37 | 36 | 36 | 36 | 36 |
| 42 | 42 | 41 | 41 | 41 | 40 | 40 | 40 | 40 | 39 | 39 | 39 | 38 | 38 | 38 | 37 | 37 | 37 | 37 | 36 | 36 |
| 43 | 42 | 42 | 42 | 41 | 41 | 41 | 40 | 40 | 40 | 39 | 39 | 39 | 39 | 38 | 38 | 38 | 37 | 37 | 37 | 37 |
| 43 | 43 | 42 | 42 | 42 | 42 | 41 | 41 | 41 | 40 | 40 | 40 | 39 | 39 | 39 | 38 | 38 | 38 | 38 | 37 | 37 |
| 44 | 43 | 43 | 43 | 42 | 42 | 42 | 41 | 41 | 41 | 40 | 40 | 40 | 40 | 39 | 39 | 39 | 38 | 38 | 38 | 37 |
| 44 | 44 | 43 | 43 | 43 | 43 | 42 | 42 | 42 | 41 | 41 | 41 | 40 | 40 | 40 | 39 | 39 | 39 | 39 | 38 | 38 |
| 45 | 44 | 44 | 44 | 43 | 43 | 43 | 42 | 42 | 42 | 41 | 41 | 41 | 40 | 40 | 40 | 39 | 39 | 39 | 39 | 38 |
|  | 45 | 44 | 44 | 44 | 43 | 43 | 43 | 43 | 42 | 42 | 42 | 41 | 41 | 41 | 40 | 40 | 40 | 39 | 39 | 39 |
|  |  | 45 | 45 | 44 | 44 | 44 | 43 | 43 | 43 | 42 | 42 | 42 | 42 | 41 | 41 | 41 | 40 | 40 | 40 | 40 |
|  |  |  | 45 | 44 | 44 | 44 | 44 | 43 | 43 | 43 | 43 | 42 | 42 | 42 | 41 | 41 | 41 | 41 | 40 | 40 |
|  |  |  |  | 45 | 44 | 44 | 44 | 44 | 43 | 43 | 43 | 43 | 42 | 42 | 42 | 42 | 41 | 41 | 41 | 41 |
|  |  |  |  |  | 45 | 44 | 44 | 44 | 44 | 43 | 43 | 43 | 43 | 42 | 42 | 42 | 42 | 41 | 41 | 41 |
|  |  |  |  |  |  | 45 | 44 | 44 | 44 | 44 | 43 | 43 | 43 | 43 | 42 | 42 | 42 | 42 | 41 | 41 |
|  |  |  |  |  |  |  | 45 | 44 | 44 | 44 | 44 | 43 | 43 | 43 | 43 | 42 | 42 | 42 | 42 | 41 |
|  |  |  |  |  |  |  |  | 45 | 44 | 44 | 44 | 44 | 43 | 43 | 43 | 43 | 42 | 42 | 42 | 42 |
|  |  |  |  |  |  |  |  |  | 45 | 45 | 44 | 44 | 44 | 43 | 43 | 43 | 43 | 42 | 42 | 42 |
|  |  |  |  |  |  |  |  |  |  | 45 | 45 | 44 | 44 | 44 | 43 | 43 | 43 | 43 | 42 | 42 |
|  |  |  |  |  |  |  |  |  |  |  | 45 | 45 | 44 | 44 | 44 | 44 | 43 | 43 | 43 | 43 |

Current technology has allowed for the invention of mini, portable devices worn by subjects that are able to estimate energy expenditure. These devices use sensors to measure a number of variables. These measured variables may include motion, heat flux, galvanic skin response, skin temperature, and near-body temperature. When combined with other variables such as gender, age, height, and weight, predictive equations can be calculated to estimate energy expenditure. Some of these devices have been validated in peer-reviewed published literature.[7]

Daily energy expenditure can be estimated without the use of equipment. By combining valid historical data on a subject's diet and activity with specific formulas to predict resting metabolic rate (RMR), reliable estimates of daily energy expenditure can be reached. Energy intake from a diet history, energy expenditure from an activity history, and body weight changes over a period of 6–12 months should together represent a picture of predictive energy needs. When accurately collected, these data should correspond to the calculated energy values from the predictive formulas.

A number of predictive formulas for RMR have been developed. Because the data used to develop these formulas are the measured RMR values from a population of individuals, it is essential that the formula chosen to predict RMR be based on a similar population of individuals as the subject in question.

The most frequently used formula to predict RMR is the Harris-Benedict equation, which uses age (years), body mass (kg), and height (cm):

Women: RMR = 655.1 + (9.56 × mass) + (1.85 × height) − (4.68 × age)

Men: RMR = 66.47 + (13.75 × mass) + (5.0 × height) − (6.76 × age)

This equation was published in 1919, and was based on a population of 136 men (mean age 27 ± 9 years; mean weight 64 ± 10 kg) and 103 women (mean age 33.1 ± 14; mean weight 56.5 ± 11.5 kg).[8]

According to Thompson and Manore,[9] among five different RMR predictive equations used on endurance-trained men and women, one most closely predicted the actual measured RMR. This equation was published by Cunningham in 1980 using 223 of the original subjects from the 1919 Harris-Benedict data set. Sixteen males who were trained athletes were removed from the database. Lean body mass (LBM) accounted for 70% of the predictive value of the equation. Cunningham calculated LBM from body mass and age data.[9] The resulting formula is:

$$RMR = 500 + 22 \ (LBM)$$

Once RMR has been estimated, it is multiplied by an activity factor to estimate total energy expenditure. By interviewing the athlete about daily activities, the activity factor can be determined. Information about daily routines (eating, sleeping, shopping, reading, walking, stair climbing) as well as specific sports activities (type of activity, frequency, intensity, and duration) over a week's time are required to achieve accurate results (see Table 10.6).

The final step is to consider whether the athlete wants to gain, maintain, or lose weight. By adding or subtracting calories per day from the calculated energy requirement, athletes will gain or lose weight. A calorie deficit should be designed as a *combination* of reduced nutritional intake and increased energy expenditure through exercise. As with the determination of optimal body weight, energy requirements are dynamic, based on the changing activity levels of athletes throughout their seasons. To maintain weight goals, periodic adjustments in calories must be made to reflect changes in training and competition. Refer to specific chapters for detailed discussions of this topic.

## Eating and Lifestyle Patterns (Dietary)

Evaluating the diet of an athlete consists of understanding what the athlete eats, as well as why, where, when, and how the athlete eats. It includes everything that an athlete consumes, including all dietary supplements and sports nutrition products. The lifestyle routines and stresses that athletes face profoundly affect food selection, food preparation, and eating habits, which ultimately impact health and performance. It is critically important to collect information about the athlete's daily routines, such as training, work or school

TABLE 10.6. Physical activity factors for various levels of activity for adults of average size 19 years and older.

| Activity category | Physical activity factor |
|---|---|
| Sedentary<br>Seated and standing activities, office work, driving, cooking; no vigorous activity | 1.39 |
| Low active<br>In addition to the activities of a sedentary lifestyle, 30 minutes of moderately intensive activity equivalent to walking 2 miles in 30 minutes; most office workers with additional planned exercise routines | 1.49 |
| Active<br>In addition to the activities of a low active lifestyle, an additional 3 hours of activity such as: bicycle 10–12 mph, stair-treadmill, walk 4.5 miles/hour, run 6 miles/hour; individuals with active jobs or with 3 hours of planned vigorous exercise each day | 1.75 |
| Very active<br>Full-time athletes, unskilled laborers, military on active duty, steel workers, etc. | 2.06 |

*Source:* Adapted from Food and Nutrition Board. Dietary Reference Intakes for Energy, Carbohydrate, Fiber, Fat, Protein and Amino Acids (Macronutrients). Washington, DC: The National Academy of Sciences; 2002.

commitments, and travel. With this information in mind, you and the athlete can design a program that fits the athlete's lifestyle, and will really work.

## Dietary Assessment Tools

All dietary assessment tools have strengths and weaknesses, yet the collection of food intake data is critical to the complete nutritional assessment of athletes. The collection of dietary data is also important for the development of an intervention and counseling strategy, as well as a follow-up plan.

The following dietary assessment tools can be applied as they stand, or can be adapted to specific groups by adding or deleting pertinent questions or sections. With athletes in particular, it may be appropriate to always include questions regarding whether the same dietary pattern is followed during in-season, off-season, or competitive-season training schedules. Examples of each tool follow. Because each tool has its strengths and weaknesses, two or more tools may be used to provide more complete and accurate information about the dietary intake of an athlete.

### GENERIC NUTRITION QUESTIONNAIRE

The generic nutrition questionnaire (Figure 10.2) is a universal questionnaire. Counselors can select those questions that are appropriate for each situation then add others to elicit specific information required in their particular setting.

### TWENTY-FOUR-HOUR RECALL

The 24-hour recall (Figure 10.3) is a dietary assessment tool that provides a historical window on food intake during a specific time. It can be used for any age group. The recall is based on the premise that information about foods and beverages that were consumed during the previous 24-hour period represents a broad picture of the athlete's food intake and habits. This assumption is flawed if the previous 24-hour period was not a typical day for the athlete. It is therefore extremely important to determine whether the previous day's food intake was typical of the athlete's diet. The 24-hour recall is best used with a second dietary assessment tool. It can also be useful during follow-up visits to determine whether the athlete is adapting to dietary recommendations.

### FOOD FREQUENCY FORM

The food frequency form (Figure 10.4) is a checklist that elicits data regarding the kinds of food eaten (usually based on food groupings, i.e., dairy, fruit, vegetables, etc.) and the frequency of intake over a period of time. It can help to confirm the adequacy or deficiency of an athlete's diet and is best used with a second dietary assessment tool.

### FOOD DIARY

The food diary (Figure 10.5) is a self-recorded description of intake over a period of days (usually 3–7). Different from a recall, which is a historical record based on the athlete's memory of the past 24 hours, the food diary is recorded by the athlete immediately after he/she eats. The athlete is given instructions on how to complete the diary at the first visit and returns the diary at the follow-up visit.

### FOOD AND ACTIVITY RECORD

The food and activity record (Figure 10.6) describes food intake, activity, and mood. It gives the most comprehensive picture of lifestyle and the impact that the lifestyle has on mood. However, it also takes the most dedication on the part of the client in order to be completed with the detailed accuracy necessary to make the tool most useful. A minimum of 3 and a maximum of 7 days are generally required for a reliable record. Each of these tools may be used as it appears or each may be adapted to specific situations.

Name: _____     Date: _____

**Data**                                                                    **Follow-up**
                                                                            **Required**

   I. Appetite

      a. How would you describe your appetite?

        ( ) Hearty          ( ) Moderate          ( ) Poor

      b. Do you enjoy eating?

        ( ) Yes             ( ) No                ( ) Sometimes

  II. Eating pattern and attitudes about food

      a. Do you eat at approximately the same time every day?

        ( ) Yes             ( ) No                ( ) Sometimes

      b. Do you skip meals?

        ( ) Yes             ( ) No

      If yes, at what times?

      _____

      c. Are there any foods that you do not eat because you don't think
        they are good for you?

        ( ) Yes             ( ) No

      If yes, what?

      _____

      d. Do you usually eat anything between meals?

        ( ) Yes             ( ) No

      If yes, name the two or three snacks (including bedtime snacks) that
      you have most often.

      _____

      _____

      e. During one week, where do you eat most of your food?

        Home _____     School _____

        Work _____     Restaurant _____

        Other _____ (identify)

      f. Are there any foods that you regularly eat because you think that they
        are good for you?

        ( ) Yes             ( ) No

      If yes, what?

      _____

 III. Food choices

      a. Are there any foods you can't eat?

        ( ) Yes             ( ) No

      If yes, what food(s)?

*(continued)*

**FIGURE 10.2.** Generic nutrition questionnaire.

**Data**

What happens when you eat this food?

_____

_____

b. Are you allergic to any foods?

( ) Yes          ( ) No

If yes, what food(s)? _____

What happens when you eat this food?

_____

_____

c. Are there certain foods that you do not eat because you don't like them?

( ) Yes          ( ) No

If yes, what food(s)? _____

d. Are there certain foods that you avoid eating because of your religious beliefs?

( ) Yes          ( ) No

If yes, what food(s)? _____

e. Are there certain foods that you avoid eating because of your ethnic/cultural background?

( ) Yes          ( ) No

If yes, what food(s)? _____

f. Are there certain foods that you eat regularly because of your ethnic/cultural background?

( ) Yes          ( ) No

If yes, what food(s)? _____

g. How is your food usually prepared?

( ) Baked        ( ) Broiled        ( ) Fried

Other _____

h. Do you drink milk?

( ) Yes          ( ) No

If yes:

( ) Whole milk   ( ) Skim milk

( ) Other; specify _____

i. List five of your favorite foods:

_____

j. List five of your least favorite foods:

_____

IV. Weight history

a. Have you ever had any problems with weight?

( ) Yes          ( ) No

b. If yes, what?

(continued)

**FIGURE 10.2.** _Continued_

**Data**

( ) Underweight    ( ) Overweight

( ) Other _____

c. Are you now on a diet to lose weight?

( ) Yes              ( ) No

If yes, what kind? _____

_____

How long? _____
Who recommended it? _____

d. How do you feel about your weight?

( ) Too heavy       ( ) Too thin        ( ) Okay

e. Do you ever vomit to keep your weight down?

( ) Every day       ( ) 3-4 times/week

( ) Every week      ( ) Sometimes       ( ) Never

V.  Supplements and medications

a. Are you now taking any vitamins or mineral supplements?

( ) Yes              ( ) No

If yes, what, now often, and what brand?

_____

b  Do you regularly take any medications prescribed by your doctor?

( ) Yes              ( ) No

If yes, what? _____

c. Do you regularly take any "over-the-counter" medications?

( ) Yes              ( ) No

If yes, what? _____

VI.  Smoking, alcohol, and substance use

a. Do you smoke?

( ) Yes              ( ) No

If yes, what, how many cigarettes per day?

_____

b. Do you drink any alcoholic beverages (liquor, wine, wine coolers, beer)?

( ) Yes              ( ) No

If yes, what do you drink and how often?

_____

_____

c. Do you smoke marijuana?

( ) Yes              ( ) No

If yes, how often? _____

d. How often do you use crack, cocaine, speed, or other street drugs?

( ) Every day       ( ) 3-4 times/week

( ) Every week      ( ) Sometimes       ( ) Never

*(continued)*

**FIGURE 10.2.** *Continued*

**Data**

**Follow-up Required**

VII. Exercise

    a. How often do you exercise?

        ( ) Every day    ( ) 3-4 times/week

        ( ) Every week    ( ) Sometimes    ( ) Never

    b. List kinds of exercise you do most often _____

    c. How often do you get out of breath when you exercise?

        ( ) Every week    ( ) Sometimes    ( ) Never

VIII. Household information

    a. Indicate the person who does the following in your household:

    Plans the meals _____

    Buys the food _____

    Prepares the food _____

    b. How much is spent on food each week for your household?

    $ _____    ( ) Don't know

    For how many people? _____

    c. Are there periods in the month when there isn't enough money for food or you run out of food?

        ( ) Yes    ( ) No

    If yes, when and how long are these periods? _____

    _____

    d. Indicate the types of kitchen equipment you have in your home.

        ( ) Refrigerator    ( ) Working stove

        ( ) Hot plate    ( ) Piped water    ( ) Sink

IX. Food programs

    a. Are you receiving any of the following:

        ( ) Food stamps    ( ) WIC vouchers    ( ) Commodity foods

    b. Does your family use:

        ( ) Food co-ops    ( ) Food shelves

        ( ) Food pantries    ( ) Soup kitchens

        ( ) Free or reduced-price school lunch and/or breakfast

        ( ) Summer feeding program

    c. How many hot meals do you have each week?

        >7        7        6        <6

Modified from Simko, M.D., Cowell, C., and Gilbride, J.A.: *Nutrition assessment: a comprehensive guide for planning intervention*, Rockville, Md, 1984, Aspen Publishers.

**FIGURE 10.2.** *Continued*

Name: _____    Date of Birth: _____
                                                          month / date / year

ID# _____    Sex _____

| Time | Place | Food | Amount | For Practitioner Use |
|------|-------|------|--------|----------------------|
|      |       |      |        | Summary              |
|      |       |      |        |                      |

a.  This is a typical day.   Yes _____   No _____

b.  I take vitamin/mineral supplements.   Yes _____   No _____

    If yes, name the brand _____

c.  I have been on a special diet during the past 3 months.   Yes _____   No _____

    If yes, the kind of special diet _____

Instructions:

1.  Record time of day or night when you ate food or drank beverages (8 AM, 9 PM, etc.).

2.  Indicate the place where you ate (home-kitchen, home-living room, restaurant, etc.).

3.  Describe the specific food eaten or drunk during a 24-hour period, beginning with the first meal or snack (e.g., fried chicken, plain yogurt); use brand names.

4.  Indicate the amount of food or beverage (e.g., ½ cup, 1 slice, 1 chicken leg, etc.).

Modified from Simko, M.D., Cowell, C., and Gilbride, J.A.: *Nutrition assessment: a comprehensive guide for planning intervention*, Rockville, Md, 1984, Aspen Publishers.

**FIGURE 10.3.** Twenty-four-hour recall.

Client's Name: _____     Date: _____

Interviewer: _____

| Food | Don't eat | Do eat | Serving Size | Number of Servings Per Week |
|------|-----------|--------|--------------|------------------------------|
| **I. Animal and vegetable protein foods** | | | | |
| Chicken | | | | |
| Beef, hamburger, veal | | | | |
| Liver, kidney, tongue, etc. | | | | |
| Lamb, goat | | | | |
| Cold cuts, hot dogs | | | | |
| Pork, ham, sausage | | | | |
| Bacon | | | | |
| Fish | | | | |
| Kidney beans, pinto beans, lentils | | | | |
| Soybeans | | | | |
| Tofu | | | | |
| Eggs | | | | |
| Nuts or seeds | | | | |
| Peanut butter | | | | |
| **II. Milk and milk products** | | | | |
| Milk, fluid: Type: _____ | | | | |
| Milk, dry | | | | |
| Milk, evaporated | | | | |
| Condensed milk | | | | |
| Cottage cheese | | | | |
| Cheese (all kinds except cottage) | | | | |
| Yogurt | | | | |
| Pudding and custard flan | | | | |
| Milkshake | | | | |
| Sherbert | | | | |
| Ice cream | | | | |
| Ice milk | | | | |
| | | | | |

*(continued)*

**FIGURE 10.4.** Food Frequency Form.

| Food | Don't eat | Do eat | Serving Size | Servings Per Week |
|---|---|---|---|---|
| **III.  Grain Products** | | | | |
| Whole grain bread | | | | |
| White bread | | | | |
| Rolls, biscuits, muffins | | | | |
| Crackers, pretzels | | | | |
| Pancakes, waffles | | | | |
| Cereals: Brand: _____ | | | | |
| White rice | | | | |
| Brown rice | | | | |
| Noodles, macaroni, grits, hominy | | | | |
| Tortillas (flour) | | | | |
| Tortillas (corn) | | | | |
| Bulgar | | | | |
| Popcorn | | | | |
| Wheat germ | | | | |
| **IV.  Vitamin-C-rich fruits and vegetables** | | | | |
| Tomato, tomato sauce, or tomato juice | | | | |
| Orange or orange juice | | | | |
| Tangerine | | | | |
| Grapefruit or grapefruit juice | | | | |
| Papaya, mango | | | | |
| Strawberries, cantaloupe | | | | |
| White potato, yautia, yams, plantain, yucca | | | | |
| Turnip | | | | |
| Peppers (green, red, chili) | | | | |
| **V.  Leafy green vegetables** | | | | |
| Dark green or red lettuce | | | | |
| Asparagus | | | | |
| Swiss chard | | | | |
| Bok choy | | | | |
| Cabbage | | | | |
| Broccoli | | | | |
| Brussel sprouts | | | | |
| Scallions | | | | |

*(continued)*

**FIGURE 10.4.** *Continued*

| Food | Don't eat | Do eat | Serving Size | Number of Servings Per Week |
|---|---|---|---|---|
| Spinach | | | | |
| Greens (beet, collard, kale, turnip, mustard) | | | | |
| **VI. Other fruits and vegetables** | | | | |
| Carrots | | | | |
| Artichoke | | | | |
| Corn | | | | |
| Sweet potato or yam | | | | |
| Zucchini | | | | |
| Summer squash | | | | |
| Winter squash | | | | |
| Green peas | | | | |
| Green and yellow beans | | | | |
| Beets | | | | |
| Cucumbers or celery | | | | |
| Peach | | | | |
| Apricot | | | | |
| Apple | | | | |
| Banana | | | | |
| Pineapple | | | | |
| Cherries | | | | |
| **VII. Snacks, sweets, and beverages** | | | | |
| Potato chips | | | | |
| French fries | | | | |
| Cakes, pies, cookies | | | | |
| Sweet rolls, doughnuts | | | | |
| Candy | | | | |
| Sugar or honey | | | | |
| Carbonated beverages (sodas) | | | | |
| Coffee: Type: _____ | | | | |
| Tea: Type: _____ | | | | |
| Cocoa | | | | |
| Wine, beer, cocktails | | | | |
| Fruit drink | | | | |
| **VIII. Other foods not listed that you regularly eat** | | | | |
| | | | | |
| | | | | |

Modified from California Dept. of Health, 1975.

**FIGURE 10.4.** *Continued*

Name: _____    Date: _____

Please write down everything you eat for 3 days before your next appointment.

To do this:

1. Write down everything you eat or drink in the order in which it was eaten. Use brand names.
2. Include meals and snacks as well as gum and candy.
3. Write down the amount you eat. Use standard measuring cups and spoons. Record meat portions as ounces.
4. Write down items added to food (sugar on cereal, butter on bread, salad dressing to salad, etc.).
5. Write down the time you eat.
6. Write down how you prepared it (baked, fried, broiled, etc.).
7. Include a list of any vitamin and/or mineral supplements you take. Write down the name of the supplement, the amount of vitamins or minerals it contains, and the amount taken.

Examples:

| Day 1: Time | Food and Preparation | Amount |
|---|---|---|
| 12:30 PM | Peanut butter sandwich | 1 tablespoon peanut butter 2 slices bread, whole wheat |
| | Milk, 2% | 6 ounces |

Make a separate sheet for each day.

Modified from California Dept. of Health, 1975.

**FIGURE 10.5.** Food diary.

---

Date _____    Name _____

| Time | Food (quantity-type) | Activity and Length of Time | Where/ with whom | Mood* | How hungry |
|---|---|---|---|---|---|
| *Examples* | | | | | |
| 9:00 AM | Hershey's chocolate candy bar (1 large) | 15 min. in hall | School, friend | Tired | Very |
| 3:00 PM | Potato chips ½ medium bag | 30 min. watching TV | Home, alone | Bored | A little |
| 5:30 PM | Cola (regular) 1 can | Thirsty | Work, another store clerk | "Down" | Thirsty |
| 7:00 PM | Cookies (3 small chocolate chip) | Late for dinner | Work, alone | Upset | Very |

*Anxious, bored, content, depressed, "down," angry, tired, happy, relaxed, "up," celebrating, other

Modified from J. Endres & R. Rockwell (1985). *Food, Nutrition, and the Young Child.* Columbus, OH: Merrill Publishing Co.

**FIGURE 10.6.** Food and Activity Record.

In addition to these traditional tools, there are nutrition Web sites that offer dietary assessments. Although the databases are not as comprehensive as those developed for professional use, clients can enter their dietary data themselves and receive immediate feedback of fairly reliable, albeit general, nature. The Interactive Healthy Eating Index is a government-sponsored free online dietary assessment tool that includes nutrition messages. Once dietary data are entered, a dietary "score" is given based on recommendations from the Dietary Guidelines for Americans and the Food Guide Pyramid. Up to 20 days of diet records can be entered and scored, to see a picture of eating habits over time (www. forcevbc.com/good/food.htm).

## Fitness and Laboratory Tests (Biochemical/Clinical)

The biochemical and clinical assessment of an athlete through fitness and laboratory tests is an essential component to a complete nutrition assessment. Some practice settings, such as sports medicine clinics or fitness centers, will allow for partial or full access to these types of tests or information. Other settings, such as schools or athletic facilities, may not be equipped for the collection of such complete data. In these instances, contacting a medical practitioner to access information in medical records, such as blood tests, diagnoses, or histories, will assist in the development of a comprehensive nutrition care plan. The counselor and/or medical practitioner, depending on the age, sex, and health status of the athlete, can determine the importance of medical data. A list of suggested physical fitness, laboratory, and clinical tests can be found in Table 10.7.

## Psychosocial Influences

The psychologic and social influences on an athlete can be positive and negative. In either case, these influences affect the eating habits and overall lifestyle of an athlete (see Table 10.8). Nutrition counselors need to be aware of the relevant issues affecting dietary intake, even though a complete psychologic assessment is outside the scope of practice of most individuals acting as nutrition counselors. During the nutrition assessment and counseling process, many psychologic issues may be uncovered. Because most nutrition counselors are

**TABLE 10.7. Physical fitness and laboratory tests.**

| Test/assessment | Relevant information |
|---|---|
| Fitness assessment | Heart rate<br>Blood pressure<br>Aerobic capacity<br>Strength<br>Flexibility<br>Percent body fat |
| Blood tests | Complete blood count<br>Comprehensive metabolic panel<br>Blood lipids<br>Iron status (serum iron,* ferritin†)<br>Food allergy‡ |
| Medical assessment | Current health status<br>Medical history<br>Cardiovascular risk status<br>Orthopedic problems<br>Recent and past injuries<br>Gynecologic problems |

*Source:* Adapted from Storlie,[2] and T. Incledon, personal communication, 2004.

*Note:* Appropriateness of some of these tests will depend on the athlete's age and sex. In many practice settings, some of this information will not be available.

*Serum iron can be evaluated in women.

†Ferritin can be evaluated if anemia is suspected.

‡Tests should be conducted if food allergies are suspected.

TABLE 10.8. Psychosocial influences.[2]

| Dimension | Factors to consider |
|---|---|
| Social influences<br>Family members<br>Friends<br>Teammates<br>Coaches<br>Celebrities | Forms of support<br>Sources of conflict/friction<br>Vicarious interests<br>Expectations/pressures<br>Role modeling |
| Self-concept | Body image<br>Self-efficacy<br>Self-confidence<br>Fears of failure, fears of competition<br>Locus of control |
| Competitive goals and commitment | Realistic aspirations (athletic talent, self-discipline)<br>Priority/importance<br>Competitive anxieties |
| Attitudes and philosophy | Balanced versus imbalanced approach toward life<br>Aspirations (career, school, other areas)<br>Tendency to be driven or single-minded<br>Need for power and control<br>Stress patterns/life satisfaction |

not qualified to accurately assess and treat these issues, referrals to qualified professionals are recommended in order to evaluate and care for potential problems.

Eating behaviors are determined by:

- Biologic factors
- Psychologic factors
- Sociocultural factors[10]

Gut hormones, thermoregulatory mechanisms, and blood glucose levels are biologic factors affected by exercise that influence eating behaviors. Depending on these biologic changes, an athlete's brain will receive messages from the body that it needs to eat and/or drink. But these natural biologic urges can be overcome. Psychologic factors are often more powerful in influencing eating behaviors than biologic factors. These are many and varied, and include emotional conflict, self-image, and attitudes toward nutrition. For example, an athlete may be emotionally torn between an internal noncompetitive spirit and an external motivation to compete in order to make his/her parents proud. This conflict can cause psychologic instability, which will ultimately affect eating behaviors, the most classic of which is either loss of appetite or overeating.

Sociocultural factors also have a strong role in determining eating patterns and behaviors. Peer influence, time constraints, and lack of accurate information, among other factors, have a significant part in forming the eating behaviors of individuals. The dietary choices of athletes who travel on the road together are clearly influenced by the eating establishments made available to them, and the foods that coaches and other teammates select. Nutrition misinformation and the lack of practical and accurate nutrition information is a notorious sociocultural factor that influences the eating patterns of athletes. In fact, Madison Avenue may have a greater influence on the eating patterns of many athletes than bona fide sources of nutrition information.

## NUTRITION COUNSELING STRATEGIES

When a professional nutritionist is not available, the athletic trainer or sports physician usually leads nutrition counseling. However, the intervention is usually the most successful when a team approach that includes all the sports medicine professionals is used. The athletic trainer or sports physician may take the lead role, conducting the counseling sessions and giving direction to the other sports medicine professionals. The coach and physical therapist are usually involved on a more daily basis, observing the athlete and answering questions or referring the athlete back to the athletic trainer or physician for more specific information.

## The Nutrition Care Plan

Developing a practical nutrition care plan requires assessing the athlete's present nutritional status and requirements, taking into consideration biologic, psychologic, and sociocultural determinants of eating behaviors. Most athletes need a normal, well-balanced diet. The design of the diet itself can be based on the United States Dietary Guidelines (Table 10.1) and the athlete's calorie requirements, as discussed above. In specific situations, however, the demands of training and competition may result in increased physiologic demands, which, if not met by diet, may negatively influence performance. (See chapters that follow for specific information.) To appropriately address these circumstances, a specialist with a sophisticated knowledge and understanding of sports nutrition is required, and such a referral should be made to ensure the health and performance of the athlete.

## Counseling Strategies for Lifestyle Change

It should be clear by now that dietary change is really lifestyle change. Altering eating behaviors often requires changing other life habits beyond diet. For instance, an athlete who lacked an appetite after most training sessions and never ate much until the next day learns that eating good carbohydrate sources immediately after training assists with the replenishment of spent glycogen in the muscles, thereby improving endurance for the next day's training session. This athlete has decided to make one dietary change—to consume a good source of carbohydrates shortly after each training session. This singular dietary change might involve:

- Changes in shopping habits, to have an appropriate food on hand after training
- Knowledge acquisition, to learn about good food sources of carbohydrates
- Time management skills, because the athlete never had to stop to eat after training before
- Some experimentation and emotional considerations, because the athlete will have to find foods that are satisfying, as well as convince his/her body that even though there is no hunger, it needs to eat.[11]

Obstacles block the path of many changes, but lifestyle changes seem to be the most difficult to achieve. Athletes are motivated to improve their performance. If they understand that these diet and lifestyle changes will assist with this process, they generally put forth a good effort.

It is crucial for the nutrition counselor to recognize that food is more than just a mode of transportation for nutrients into the body. Food is a very intimate and emotional component of our lives. It is at the center of many religious and cultural celebrations and is often linked to significant family memories, both good and bad. Food has been used for reward and punishment, and may represent a powerful emotional concept to some individuals.[12]

The nutrition counselor must recognize that although an athlete may cognitively understand the benefits of changing eating behaviors, he or she cannot do so until the emotional barriers to that change are overcome. Instead of the counselor designing a strategy for diet and behavior change, the athlete must be involved in the process to set his/her own goals for gradual change. This will help to secure the athlete's commitment and ensure effective and permanent change.[12]

Regular follow-up is essential to successful behavior change. If, by monitoring the athlete's progress, the athlete seems to be having difficulty in adhering to the jointly established plan for change, the counselor should consider involving other health professionals, such as social and psychologic counselors, registered dietitians, and nurse educators.

## SUMMARY

The relationship between diet and exercise is clear, and what, where, and how an athlete eats will affect health and physical performance now and in the future. Athletes obtain nutrition information from many sources. Unfortunately, many of those sources are either incorrect or unscrupulous, and athletes suffer the consequences of nutrition misinformation.

Dietary practices are affected by physiologic and psychosocial influences. Changing dietary behaviors is a complex issue, and often requires lifestyle changes. As authority figures, coaches, trainers, and physicians must be aware of their athletes' nutritional health. With appropriate education, tools, and experience, these individuals may be able to counsel athletes regarding dietary requirements, eating behaviors, and food choices. At the least, they must be able to spot a problem and refer the athlete to an appropriate health care practitioner.

## PRACTICAL APPLICATIONS

The counseling process can be divided into the following 10 strategies.[10]

### Develop a Partnership with the Athlete

Because it is essential that the person undergoing counseling trust the counselor, taking the time to get to know the athlete, as well as for him/her to get to know you, is essential to a successful counseling outcome.

### Educate the Athlete

Accurate information is a powerful tool in behavior modification. Bright, motivated athletes, looking for information, often succumb to false or misleading nutrition information. By giving them accurate information, and not berating them for following poor advice, they often will change their behaviors quite easily.

### Explain Behavior–Health–Performance Relationship

Similar to the previous strategy, giving the athlete more information about how his/her health does matter because it will ultimately affect athletic performance is a powerful technique. Again, never berate an athlete for following incorrect or unscientific information. Educate them about the positive influences of the accurate information.

### Assess Barriers to Behavior Change

Just like one cannot drive a car through a brick wall, athletes cannot make behavior changes with barriers in the way, be they real or imagined. Barriers to behavior change must be discussed at the outset of counseling so that they can be dealt with in a way that either allows the athlete to eliminate them or work around them.

### Obtain Athlete Commitment

The athlete must want to change, and concur with the method of achieving change. Without a commitment from the athlete, it is unlikely that any positive changes will occur. In the eyes of the athlete, it will always be someone else's responsibility (e.g., the nutrition counselor, the coach, the athletic trainer) to effect the behavior change, rather than the athlete's own responsibility.

### Encourage Athlete Participation

By having some control of the process, the athlete becomes involved and committed to the goal. Participating in the design of his or her own nutrition plan places the athlete in a role of responsibility for the outcome of the plan. Most athletes do not want to fail.

## Use a Combination of Strategies

Not all strategies will work for every athlete, but at least one of the strategies should work for any athlete who really wants change. Sometimes the appropriate strategy is not obvious, so trying a variety or combination of strategies might prove to be successful, when a singular approach did not work. As long as an athlete is still interested, keep trying.

## Design a Behavior Modification Plan

Most athletes like to know where they are going and how they are going to get there. A behavior modification plan allows the athlete to design a set of small, short-term goals, as well as larger, long-term goals. This plan allows for the achievement of frequent successes, supporting further positive change. When failures occur, they do not seem so overwhelming, and because the plan is clearly laid out, it is easy to get back to it and continue toward the goal.

## Monitor Progress

As the health professional, it is important for you to monitor the athletes that have been counseled, to make sure that there have been no misunderstandings in the delivery of information between you and your client, and in the planning and execution of their nutrition goals. In addition, it is reassuring to the athlete and the process of change for you to "check up on them" periodically. Monitoring progress is a helpful tool for reinforcing the goals that have been set for behavior change, answering any questions that have arisen, and dealing with any new barriers or situations that might occur during the process.

## Involve Other Health Professionals

Frequently, an athlete will have a problem that cannot be taken care of by a non-nutrition professional. An athlete may also encounter a problem that requires other health care expertise, such as a physician or a psychologist. It is imperative that health care providers understand their own practice limitations, and involve other health professionals when necessary to provide adequate care for the athletes whom they counsel.

# ACKNOWLEDGMENTS

The author thanks Tom Incledon, PhD(c), RD, LD/LN, RPT, NSCA-CPT, CSCS, CFT, (www.thomasincledon.com) for a valuable interview on biochemical assessment.

# QUESTIONS

1. An effective nutrition care plan for athletes is based on these four assessments:
   a. Weight analysis, physical activity, psychosocial influences, and diagnosis studies
   b. Weight analysis, percent body fat, eating and lifestyle patterns, and laboratory studies
   c. Anthropometric, weight analysis, physical activity, and laboratory studies
   d. Weight analysis, eating and lifestyle patterns, fitness and laboratory studies, and psychosocial influences

2. Three methods should be applied and evaluated when determining optimal body weight. These include:
   a. Personal goal weight, team goal weight, percent body fat prediction
   b. Personal goal weight, height/weight formula, percent body fat prediction
   c. Personal goal weight, ideal body weight, height/weight formula
   d. Personal goal weight, team goal weight, height/weight formula

3. According to research conducted by Thompson and Manore, this equation most closely predicted actual resting metabolic rate among male and female athletes:
   a. Harris-Benedict (1919)
   b. Owen (1986)
   c. Cunningham (1980)
   d. Mifflin (1990)

4. The Food Frequency Form is a dietary assessment tool that is:
   a. A checklist that elicits data regarding the kinds and frequency of foods and food groups eaten over a period of time
   b. A historical window on food intake during a specific time
   c. A self-recorded description of actual food intake over a period of days
   d. A generic questionnaire of food intake

5. The 24-hour recall is best used:
   a. With the physical activity factor
   b. With a second dietary assessment tool
   c. When yesterday was not a typical representation of daily food intake
   d. When clients are not sure of what they ate yesterday

6. The Food and Activity Record:
   a. Is flawed if the previous 24-hour period was not a typical food intake day
   b. Is a universal nutrition questionnaire
   c. Can help confirm the adequacy or deficiency of an athlete's diet based on frequency of food group intake
   d. Is the most comprehensive lifestyle assessment tool

7. A standard biochemical assessment consists of:
   a. A lactose intolerance test
   b. Complete blood count and comprehensive metabolic panel
   c. Complete blood count, comprehensive metabolic panel, and blood lipids
   d. Food allergy tests

8. Psychosocial influences on an athlete can be:
   a. Positive
   b. Negative
   c. Positive and negative
   d. None of the above

9. Eating behaviors of athletes are determined by:
   a. Biologic, psychologic, and sociocultural factors
   b. Biologic factors only
   c. Psychologic factors only
   d. Biologic and psychologic factors

10. This key message is missing in the 2005 United States Dietary Guidelines for Americans:
    a. Control calorie intake to manage body weight
    b. Choose and prepare foods with little sugar
    c. Be physically active every day
    d. Choose and prepare foods with little salt

11. A practical tool that a client can use to assess their own general dietary intakes is:
    a. The online Healthy Eating Index
    b. A professional database of tables of food composition

c. A private nutrition counseling session

d. To use a kitchen scale to weigh all foods eaten

12. Of the 10 leading causes of death in the United States, ____ is/are related to diet and account for 68% of all deaths.
    a. One
    b. Ten
    c. Six
    d. Five

13. The diets of many athletes are inadequate because of:
    a. Poor information; working parents; restrictive eating habits
    b. Poor information; pressures of time, money, and access; restrictive eating habits
    c. Restrictive eating habits; poor coaching; influence from others
    d. Pressures of time, money, and access; vending machines in schools; too much sugar in the diet

14. The recommended fit standards for percent body fat in active men and women are ____ the health standards for percent body fat in average individuals.
    a. Greater than
    b. Less than
    c. The same as
    d. As low as you can go compared with

**Select which counseling strategy is being used in the following scenarios.**

15. The coach of the swim team meets individually with each athlete to discuss the diet diary. During this meeting, the coach and the athlete discuss each other's goals: the athlete's personal goals, and the coach's goals for the team. Together they determine how the athlete can best contribute to the team. With these goals in mind, the athlete's diet is discussed and compared with a healthy dietary pattern. This evaluation process leads to dietary goal setting for the athlete.
    a. Develop a partnership with the athlete
    b. Encourage athlete participation
    c. Monitor progress
    d. Involve other health professionals

16. Coach Strong realized that Janet's cross country-running performance was probably suffering because of dehydration when Janet complained that it was too hard to run with water in her stomach, so she skipped most of her fluid stops. The only way to get Janet to change her behavior was to educate her about the importance of fluids and exercise. Then they could begin to talk about how Janet could get used to having fluid in her stomach while she was running, without discomfort.
    a. Develop a partnership with the athlete
    b. Monitor progress
    c. Educate the athlete
    d. Involve other health professionals

17. Once the regular playing season began, Ted was feeling like he was following his diet, but he began to gain weight. He went back to his athletic trainer, and they both realized that even though it was now the regular playing season, Ted wasn't getting as hard a workout on a daily basis as he had been during training camp. So he needed to eat fewer calories to maintain his weight loss. After adjusting Ted's diet plan, his athletic trainer recommended that they meet again every few weeks just to check on Ted's progress, and make sure that nothing else had changed to interfere with their weight loss strategy. At the end of the season, they would have to evaluate how his body weight had changed,

and probably readjust his diet plan again to reflect off-season activity
level.

a. Develop a partnership with the athlete
b. Monitor progress
c. Educate the athlete
d. Involve other health professionals

18. Mark plays high school football in the fall and wrestles in the winter. He
    needs to bulk up for football and get lean for wrestling. Each year,
    Mark stuffs himself to gain weight before football, and then starves
    himself and sweats to lose weight for wrestling. After doing this for 2
    years in a row, Mark's mother interfered, and suggested that he see a reg-
    istered dietitian to help him design a healthier strategy to manage his body
    weight.

    With the registered dietitian, Mark designed a long-term weight-control
    strategy. Instead of trying to gain and lose weight in very short amounts of
    time, Mark set several short-term goals for his body weight over periods of
    several months. He also decided that he wouldn't try to have such a dra-
    matic weight change between wrestling and football. He stated, in fact, that
    he probably performed better in the higher wrestling weight class. He also
    planned to add strength training to his training routine, so that he would
    be gaining muscle before football, and maintaining muscle before wrestling.
    In this way, the management of his body weight wouldn't be as difficult,
    and certainly not as unhealthy.

    a. Obtain athlete's commitment
    b. Assess barriers to behavior change
    c. Monitor progress
    d. Design a behavior modification plan

19. Dave is a diver on his college swim team. He has always watched his
    weight, because he knows that it makes a difference in his performance.
    He recently went to see the team physician because he's had several colds
    back to back, making it hard for him to train.

    During his examination, the physician asked Dave to get on the scale.
    He had lost 15 pounds since last season, placing him in the underweight
    category for his height. When he asked Dave about his diet, Dave was rather
    reluctant to talk about how much he was eating.

    At this point, the physician became concerned that Dave was having
    some abnormal eating behaviors or possibly an eating disorder. The physi-
    cian talked to Dave about the effects of low body weight on health,
    immune function, and ultimately on athletic performance. He told Dave
    that because he was not an expert with diet, but he was concerned that
    Dave's diet might be inadequate, he referred Dave to a team of experts
    with experience in working with athletes, diet, and behavior. The group
    of experts included a registered dietitian, a psychologist, and a physician.
    The team physician assured Dave that he would be in close contact with
    this expert team, so that Dave's athletic goals were not set aside, and he
    could continue to dive for the team as long as he remained healthy and
    able.

    a. Develop a partnership with the athlete
    b. Educate the athlete
    c. Involve other health professionals
    d. Monitor progress

20. Steve, a cyclist, walked into the registered dietitian's office with a grocery
    bag full of the dietary supplements that he'd been taking for the last year.
    He was there to have his diet evaluated, and see if he could improve his
    athletic performance. After describing his diet, he showed the dietitian
    what supplements he used. She asked him how and why he took each sup-
    plement. Steve explained that most of the supplements were recommended
    by a friend who was an Olympic contender, and who had sold Steve the
    supplements.

After analyzing Steve's diet, the dietitian showed him the strong points and weak points of his diet. Basically, he was eating great. His diet wasn't lacking any of the components found in the supplements that he was taking. But Steve was still sure that at least some of those supplements were making a difference.

After the dietitian explained that there may be a few nutrients that are needed in extra amounts by athletes performing high-energy exercise, she and Steve negotiated the supplements that he would continue to take, and those he was willing to give up. They decided that as long as his performance did not diminish, he would stay away from the supplements that he had given up, and that they would discuss whether or not he felt he needed to continue on any supplements at a future meeting. In a way, Steve was partially relieved, because he was spending more than $150.00 a month on the bagful of pills and powders.

a. Obtain athlete commitment
b. Assess barriers to behavior change
c. Educate the athlete
d. Monitor progress

21. The United States Dietary Guidelines are developed without any political influence.
   a. True
   b. False

22. When uncommon or more complicated disease-oriented situations are detected, athletes should be referred to specialists.
   a. True
   b. False

23. The body weight of an athlete does not impact long-term health.
   a. True
   b. False

24. Bioelectrical impedance analysis is a reliable field method to assess body composition immediately after exercise.
   a. True
   b. False

25. Changing dietary behaviors is a complex issue.
   a. True
   b. False

26. A medical assessment is not really necessary for the development of a nutrition care plan.
   a. True
   b. False

27. Psychologic factors can overpower biologic urges in influencing an athlete's eating behaviors.
   a. True
   b. False

28. The dietary choices of athletes are not affected by traveling to games away from home.
   a. True
   b. False

29. It is often necessary to use a combination of counseling strategies to effectively change behavior.
   a. True
   b. False

30. It is usually better to just tell the athlete how to change behaviors, rather than having them involved in the planning.
   a. True
   b. False

## REFERENCES

1. Dietary Guidelines for Americans Advisory Committee. Nutrition and Your Health: The Report of the Dietary Guidelines for Americans, 2005. Washington, DC: Department of Health and Human Services and the Unites States Department of Agriculture. 2005. Available at: www.health.gov/dietaryguidelines.
2. Storlie J. Nutrition assessment of athletes: a model for integrating nutrition and physical performance indicators. Int J Sport Nutr 1991;1:192–204.
3. Adams GM. Exercise Physiology Laboratory Manual. 2nd ed. Dubuque, IA: WCB Brown & Benchmark Publishers; 1994.
4. Tipton CM. Making and maintaining weight for interscholastic wrestling. Sports Sci Exch 1990;3:2.
5. Kleiner SM, Bazzarre TL, Litchford MD. Metabolic profiles, diet, and health practices of championship male and female bodybuilders. J Am Diet Assoc 1990;90(7): 962–967.
6. Kleiner SM, Bazzarre TL, Ainsworth BE. Nutritional status of nationally ranked elite bodybuilders. Int J Sport Nutr 1994;4:54–69.
7. King GA. Comparison of activity monitors to estimate energy cost of treadmill exercise. Med Sci Sports Exerc 2004;36(7):1244–1251.
8. Manore MM, Thompson JL. Sport Nutrition for Health and Performance. Champaign, IL: Human Kinetics Publishers; 2000:152.
9. Thompson JL, Manore MM. Predicted and measured resting metabolic rate of male and female endurance athletes. J Am Diet Assoc 1996;96:30–34.
10. Michener JL. Nutrition counseling. Translating research into practice. Presented at the Opinion Leaders' Symposium for "Rx Nutrition: Good Health in Practice," sponsored by University of Washington School of Medicine. Little Falls, NJ: Health Learning Systems; 1989.
11. Laquatra I, Danish SJ. A primer for nutritional counseling. In: Frankle RT, Yang M-U, eds. Obesity and Weight Control. Rockville, MD: Aspen Publishers; 1988. 205–224
12. Kleiner SM. Nutrition screening and assessment. In: Matzen RN, Lang RS, eds. Clinical Preventive Medicine. St. Louis: Mosby-Year Book; 1993. 441–477

## APPENDIX 10.1: PUBLIC HEALTH OR POLITICAL AGENDA?

### What Are the Dietary Guidelines for Americans?

The Dietary Guidelines for Americans "provide science-based advice to promote health and to reduce risk for major chronic disease through diet and physical activity."[1] By law, the Guidelines are updated every 5 years and the report is issued from the Secretaries of the Department of Health and Human Services and the Department of Agriculture (USDA). Every Federal agency with a food, nutrition, or health program must promote the Dietary Guidelines and apply the key messages in their menu planning and programming. They influence policy, education, and practice across the entire spectrum of Federal agencies. Because these guidelines dictate national food policy and menu planning, farmers, food manufacturers, and many others have much to gain or lose based on the key messages of the guidelines. Food purchases increase or decrease based on the key messages.

### Politics and Public Health

These key messages are the only part of the document that most people will ever read, and they cover all the healthy food and activity advice with which many of us are already familiar. However, if you have ever paid any attention to the Dietary Guidelines in the past, you may notice that a fairly important point is missing from these messages: sugar. In the last five sets of Dietary Guidelines, sugar has been singled out not only in the body of the scientific text, but as a salient point in the key messages. The key messages of the 1980 Dietary Guidelines clearly stated: "Avoid too much sugar." As political pressure from the food industry and their representatives mounted, the 2000 Dietary

Guidelines Committee tried to take a more positive approach and stated: "Choose beverages and foods to moderate your intake of sugar."

According to the Committee, the exclusion of the mention of sugar from the key messages does not mean that the Committee views the topic of sugars to be unimportant. "On the contrary," the Executive Summary states, "the Committee provides a strong rationale for limiting one's intake of added sugars (that is, sugars and syrups that are added to foods during processing or preparation or at the table). The Committee's intent is to make this point clearly under the new topic, 'Choose Carbohydrates Wisely for Good Health,' and also under the first and second topics, which address energy needs and controlling calorie intake, respectively."

And in fact, there is an excellent discussion of the dangers of refined foods and added sugars in the diet in several places in the fine print of the report that most people will never read. So here is some of the fine print:

"Compared with individuals who consume small amounts of foods and beverages that are high in added sugars, those who consume large amounts tend to consume more calories but smaller amounts of micronutrients. Although more research is needed, available prospective studies suggest a positive association between consumption of sugar-sweetened beverages and weight gain. A reduced intake of added sugars (especially sugar-sweetened beverages) may help in achieving recommended intakes of nutrients and in weight control."

That's a bold statement! Why bury it where it will never be put into practice by Federal agencies or the public? The answer likely lies with the other constituency of the USDA: The Sugar Association, the Soft Drink Association, and the National Food Processors Association.

Cheryl Digges, the director of public policy for the Sugar Association, was quoted in the New York Times (August 25, 2004) after the publication of the new Guidelines: "We prefer this way to the way it was in the previous guidelines. We think there is too much emphasis on sugars. Sugars are just a part of the diet." She goes on to say, "There is no negative health impact for sugar; there never has been."

Experts from the World Health Organization (WHO) disagree with the Sugar Association. According to the 2003 recommendations from the WHO, a healthy diet should contain no more than 10% of calories from added sugar. Before the publication of this document, the Sugar Association, backed by the United States Department of Health and Human Services, tried to eliminate the sugar limitation from the WHO recommendations. Fortunately, this attempt was unsuccessful.

Even though the 2005 Dietary Guidelines Committee Report is in more agreement with the WHO recommendations than the stand taken by the Sugar Association, political pressure seems to have hit its target this time. The scientific process has been overrun by special interests, and the lack of clarity in the key messages has unfortunately spoken louder than the written words.

## APPENDIX 10.2: CASE STUDY

At the end of his senior year of college, Tim was drafted to play professional basketball for the NBA. After graduation, Tim weighed 225 pounds and was 6 feet 7 inches tall, with a medium frame size. He felt that he was a little overfat, so before basketball training camp, Tim had been trying to lose weight. His 2-week precamp diet consisted of:

Weekdays:

8:00 am   6 ounces orange juice or 8–12 ounces of cola drink
1:00 pm   Wendy's chicken sandwich, french fries, lemonade
8:00 pm   Sometimes just fruit; sometimes a casserole that included noodles
          or potatoes, and some kind of meat and vegetable

Only breakfast changed on the weekend.

Weekend breakfast:

10:00 am   3 eggs, 3 links sausage, 1 piece of fruit, 6 ounces orange juice

Tim only drinks beverages at meals, never between meals, and rarely while he is in practice or playing. He states that he does not drink much during practice or games because his former coach believed strongly that full bellies inhibited performance on the court. Tim does not drink any alcohol.

When training camp began and Tim moved from his family home to his new city with the team, he lived at a hotel until he knew that he would have a permanent position with the team. Soon into training camp, Tim lost his appetite. After the first week, his performance began to diminish. After the second week of training camp, the coach asked the team physician to take a look at Tim. After stepping on the scale, Tim and the physician learned that Tim had lost 13 pounds since the beginning of training camp 2 weeks before. He now weighed 203 pounds.

Questions for analysis:

1. Tim is suffering from several problems. What is the most likely and serious health concern?
2. What are Tim's other health concerns?
3. What would be your first counseling strategy in approaching this case?
4. What barriers does Tim have to behavior change?

Design a care plan of strategies for Tim that will support his efforts to win a spot on the NBA team in the next few weeks, as well as help him maintain his health now and into the future.

# PART III

# Basic and Applied Nutrition

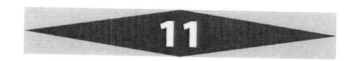

# An Overview of Macronutrients

## Jennifer Hofheins

## OBJECTIVES

On the completion of this chapter you will be able to:

1. Understand the differences among monosaccharides, oligosaccharides, and polysaccharides.
2. Explain the glycemic index and glycemic loads of a variety of carbohydrate sources.
3. Describe the health benefits of having high-fiber content in the diet.
4. Present sources of soluble and insoluble fiber.
5. Give examples of monosaccharides, oligosaccharides, and polysaccharides.
6. Describe the three major forms of fat.
7. Explain what linolenic and linoleic acids are.
8. Discuss what trans fatty acids are and why they are unhealthy.
9. Present the major functions of carbohydrates, fats, and proteins in the body.
10. Describe the different sources of fat in the body and give dietary examples.
11. Differentiate between essential and nonessential amino acids.
12. Understand what is meant by biologic value.
13. Give examples of food combinations that offer complete proteins.
14. Explain the basics of protein metabolism.

## ABSTRACT

Carbohydrate, fat, and protein ultimately provide the energy necessary to maintain body functions at rest and during physical activity. These macronutrients maintain the body's structural and functional integrity. In this chapter, each macronutrient's function, metabolism, and sources in the diet are reviewed. For a more detailed explanation of the roles of these macronutrients, the reader is referred to Chapters 12–14.

*Key Words:* **nutrition, carbohydrate, protein, fat, nutrient, food**

## CARBOHYDRATES

As their name suggests, carbohydrates are carbon-, hydrogen-, and oxygen-based molecules that are abundant in most plant foods, especially fruits and grains. Regardless of the size of the carbohydrate, once it has been ingested, it is metabolized in the mouth, stomach, and intestines to the smallest unit, which is usually glucose.

From: *Essentials of Sports Nutrition and Supplements*
Edited by J. Antonio, D. Kalman, J. R. Stout, M. Greenwood, D. S. Willoughby, and G. G. Haff © Humana Press, a part of Springer Science+Business Media, Totowa, NJ

**TABLE 11.1. Sources of dietary fiber.**

| Insoluble fiber | Soluble fiber |
| --- | --- |
| Wheat | Oats |
| Rye | Legumes |
| Rice | Beans and peas |
| Most whole grains | Fruits |
| Bran | Vegetables |

Dietary carbohydrate exists in three major classes: the monosaccharides, oligosaccharides, and polysaccharides. Monosaccharides are structurally the simplest form of carbohydrate, in that they cannot be hydrolyzed to smaller units by hydrolysis. For this reason, they are sometimes referred to as simple sugars. The most abundant and certainly the most nutritionally important monosaccharide is glucose. Oligosaccharides consist of short-chain monosaccharide units joined together. An example is a disaccharide, which is the most abundant oligosaccharide. Within this group, sucrose, consisting of glucose and fructose, is nutritionally most significant. Polysaccharides are long chains of monosaccharide units that may number from several into the hundreds or thousands. Polysaccharides are often referred to as complex carbohydrates. The two major forms of complex carbohydrates are starch and fiber.

Starch serves as a storage form of carbohydrate in plants and represents the most common form of digestible plant polysaccharide. Starches are digested more slowly than simple sugars and therefore provide less energy in the short term but more energy in the long term. Glycogen is the storage form of carbohydrate in animal tissues, and is found primarily in liver and skeletal muscle (80% stored in skeletal muscle).

Fiber is an indigestible carbohydrate. There are two types of dietary fiber: soluble and insoluble (see Table 11.1). Soluble fiber dissolves in water and forms a gel or paste. This gel forms within the digestive tract and serves to slow the rate at which food passes through the small intestine. This increases the rate of absorption of nutrients from food. Insoluble fiber, or cellulose is the constituent that gives structure to plants. Cellulose provides a number of important benefits including absorbing and removing toxins and contributing to healthy functioning of the digestive tract. It tends to absorb water and increase in bulk, greatly contributing to the volume of feces.

Numerous health benefits have been attributed to fiber in the diet including increased laxation, lower blood glucose levels, and normalization of blood cholesterol levels.[1] Research also shows that certain kinds of fiber bind with cholesterol and prevent it from being absorbed by the body, resulting in decreased risk of cardiovascular disease.[2]

In 2002, the Food and Nutrition Board reported the first recommended intakes for fiber. According to the report, men and women 50 years and younger should ingest at least 38 and 25 g, respectively, of total fiber each day. For men and women older than 50 years, the recommended intakes are at least 30 and 21 g per day, respectively.[1]

## Function

- The primary function of carbohydrate is to provide energy to the cells of the body, particularly the brain.
- Facilitate the body's metabolism of fat.
- Spare muscle protein.

The glycemic index (GI) is a ranking of foods based on their measured blood glucose response compared with a reference food, either white bread or glucose. The GI is calculated by measuring the incremental area under the blood glucose curve after ingestion of a test food providing 50 g of carbohydrate, compared with the area under the blood glucose curve after an equal carbohydrate intake from the reference food. This test is conducted after an overnight fast.[3] A food with a low GI produces a mild, sustained increase in glucose. A food with a high GI produces a larger, more transient glucose spike.

**TABLE 11.2. Glycemic load and glycemic index ranges.**

|        | Glycemic index | Glycemic load |
|--------|----------------|---------------|
| High   | >70            | >20           |
| Medium | 56–69          | 11–19         |
| Low    | <55            | <10           |

*Source:* Adapted from Foster-Powell et al.[5]

Glycemic Load (GL) is another method used to categorize foods by their effect on blood glucose levels. This method provides a better indication of food choices because it takes into account the total carbohydrate rather than a small 50-g portion of food. The GL is calculated by multiplying the GI of a food by the grams of carbohydrate per serving size.[4] The higher the GL, the greater the expected increase in blood glucose.[5] The long-term consumption of a diet with a relatively high GL is associated with an increased risk of Type 2 diabetes and coronary heart disease.[6]

Generally, whole grains have a lower GI than refined grains, high-fiber foods have a lower GI than low-fiber foods, and foods containing high amounts of protein and/or fat have a lower GI than foods with small amounts of protein and fat. This is because fiber, fat, protein, and acidity help blunt the glycemic response. Lowering the GI and GL has been shown to improve blood sugar levels and high blood cholesterol (Tables 11.2 and 11.3).[7]

## Metabolism

The cellular use of carbohydrates depends on their absorption from the gastrointestinal tract into the bloodstream, a process that is usually restricted to monosaccharides. Therefore, polysaccharides and disaccharides must be hydrolyzed to monosaccharide units (simplest form) before absorption can occur. Once this occurs, the monosaccharides are transported into the muscles and other tissues where they are broken down further to generate energy. When glucose is not needed immediately for energy, it is stored in the muscle and liver in long, branched chains called glycogen. The body's capacity for storing glycogen is limited. Once glycogen stores in the muscle and liver are replenished, excess glucose is converted into fat.

## Types/Sources

All living cells contain carbohydrate. Except for lactose and a small amount of glycogen, plants provide the main source of carbohydrate in the human diet (Table 11.4).[8]

**TABLE 11.3. Glycemic index and glycemic load of common foods.**

|                 | Glycemic index | Glycemic load |
|-----------------|----------------|---------------|
| Carrots         | 47             | 3             |
| Green peas      | 48             | 3             |
| Sweet potato    | 61             | 17            |
| Baked potato    | 85             | 26            |
| Orange          | 48             | 5             |
| Apple           | 40             | 6             |
| Banana          | 51             | 13            |
| Skim milk       | 32             | 4             |
| Cranberry juice | 68             | 24            |
| Cola            | 63             | 16            |
| Long-grain rice | 41             | 16            |
| White rice      | 53             | 20            |
| Spaghetti       | 47             | 23            |
| Wheat bread     | 52             | 10            |
| Pancakes        | 102            | 22            |
| Bagel           | 72             | 25            |

*Note:* For a complete list see Foster-Powell.[5]

**TABLE 11.4. Types of carbohydrates.**

| Type of carbohydrate | Common name | Food sources |
|---|---|---|
| Monosaccharides | | |
|   Glucose | Dextrose, blood sugar | Fruits, sweeteners |
|   Fructose | Fruit sugar | Fruits, honey |
|   Galactose | — | Milk products |
| Oligosaccharides and Disaccharides | | |
|   Sucrose (glucose + fructose) | Table sugar | Sugar cane, beet sugar, |
|   Lactose (glucose + galactose) | Milk sugar |   high fructose corn |
|   Maltose (glucose + glucose) | Malt sugar |   syrup, honey, maple |
| | |   syrup, brown sugar |
| | | Milk and milk products |
| | | Germinating seeds, |
| | |   beer, cereal |
| Polysaccharides | | |
|   Starch | Dextrin | Potatoes, corn, wheat, |
|   Fiber indigestible | Cellulose |   rye, and legumes |
|     Soluble | Hemicellulose | Fruits, legumes, oats, |
|     Insoluble | Pectin |   rye, and barley |
| | Gums | Vegetables and wheat |
| | Mucilage |   bran |
| | Psyllium | |
| | Lignin | |

# FAT

Lipid is the collective name given to a wide variety of water-insoluble chemicals, including all fats and oils in the diet and in the body. Fat or lipids are made up of carbon, hydrogen, and oxygen, which is similar to carbohydrates and protein. The ratio of oxygen to carbon and hydrogen is much lower in lipids than carbohydrates and therefore lipids are a more concentrated source of energy.[9]

The type of fat in the diet has an important role in general health and the onset of several chronic diseases. There are three major types of fatty acids. Their molecular bonds and the number of hydrogen atoms they contain distinguish these three types from one another. Fats may be saturated, monounsaturated (possessing one carbon–carbon double bond) or polyunsaturated (having two or more carbon–carbon double bonds).

Humans must ingest two types of polyunsaturated fatty acids, linolenic acid (omega-3 fatty acid) and linoleic acid (omega-6 fatty acid), from the foods they eat, because the body cannot make them. A lack of either one of these essential fatty acids will result in symptoms of deficiency, including scaly skin, dermatitis, and reduced growth. Studies have shown that populations with diets naturally high in alpha-linolenic acid and longer-chain omega-3 fatty acids, common in countries where larger quantities of fatty fish are consumed, have a decreased risk of cardiovascular disease.[1]

Cholesterol is another group of lipids that is required for the formation of many essential substances in the body, including steroid hormones, vitamin D, and bile salts. It is also an integral part of cell membranes and myelin that forms an insulating sheath around nerve fibers. Cholesterol is not a dietary essential because it can be synthesized by the liver. In general, low-density lipoproteins are considered bad cholesterol because they transport cholesterol to cells of the body. In contrast, high-density lipoproteins are considered good cholesterol because they carry cholesterol away from the body cells and back to the liver (for excretion). As future editions of this text will attest, recent research is already changing this simplistic view, however.

The most nutritionally significant lipid/fat is triglycerides, which are formed when three fatty acid molecules combine with glycerol. Triglycerides are the main source of ingested fat and provide the majority of energy derived from dietary lipid. Triglycerides are more properly referred to as triacylglycerols because the part of the triglyceride molecule derived from the fatty acid forms what are known as acyl groups.[9]

Trans fatty acids, which are chemically classified as unsaturated fatty acids, but behave more like saturated fatty acids in the body, are found in partially hydrogenated vegetable oils, such as margarine and shortening, with lower levels found in meats and dairy products. Both types of fat heighten the risk of heart disease in some people by boosting the level of harmful, low-density lipoprotein cholesterol in the bloodstream; this occurs even with very small quantities in the diet. Because there is no intake level of saturated fatty acids, trans fatty acids, or dietary cholesterol at which there are no adverse effects, no upper limit is set for them; instead, the Dietary Reference Intakes recommend keeping intake as low as possible while consuming a nutritionally adequate diet, because many of the foods containing these fats also provide valuable nutrients.[1] Saturated fat and trans fat may promote heart disease, diabetes, certain cancers, and obesity because they raise low-density lipoprotein cholesterol levels, aggravate inflammation in the arteries, elevate triglycerides and lower healthy high-density lipoprotein cholesterol levels.[10]

## Function

Fats serve many functions in the body.

- They are the most energy-dense macronutrient, and they provide many of the body's tissues and organs (including the heart) with most of their energy. Fat is an ideal fuel because it contains almost twice the energy as glucose, weighs less, and is easily transported and stored.
- Cell membranes are partly composed of a specific type of fat called phospholipids.
- Critical for the transmission of nerve signals that generate muscle contraction.
- Serve as a transporter for vitamins A, D, E, and K.
- Provide cushioning for the protection of vital organs and insulation from the thermal stress of cold environments.
- Fat helps delay the onset of hunger pangs, because fat empties more slowly from the stomach. This is one reason why diets containing moderate amounts of fat tend to be more successful than low-fat diets.

## Metabolism

Fat gets metabolized into short-, medium-, or long-chain fatty acids and glycerol. However, because fats are insoluble in water, their digestion requires an aqueous environment. Triglycerides, the storage form of fats, are found in liver, muscles, or adipose tissues for use as energy at a later time. The body can store unlimited amounts of fat.

## Types/Sources

The types and sources of fat are listed in Table 11.5.

**TABLE 11.5. Fat types and their sources.**

| | Type of fat | | | |
|---|---|---|---|---|
| | **Monounsaturated** | **Polyunsaturated** | **Saturated** | **Trans fat** |
| | Sources | | | |
| | Olive, canola, and peanut oils, nuts, and avocados | Omega-3: herring, mackerel, salmon, sardines, and tuna; flax seed, canola oil, and walnuts<br><br>Omega-6: corn, safflower, soy, and sunflower oils; nuts and seeds | Meat, poultry, butter, cheese, cream and whole milk, coconut, palm and palm kernel oils, processed foods, e.g., cookies, crackers, chips, and baked goods | Stick margarine, shortening, packaged cookies, pastries, crackers, candy, fried foods; very small amounts found naturally in meat, poultry, and dairy products |
| Daily amounts | 10%–15% of calories | Up to 10% of calories | Up to 10% of calories | As little as possible |

## PROTEIN

The importance of protein in nutrition and health cannot be overemphasized. Proteins are essential nutritionally because of their constituent amino acids, which the body must have to synthesize its own variety of proteins and nitrogen-containing molecules that make life possible. Proteins are the major structural components of all cells of the body, and amino acids are the basic building blocks of proteins. The building blocks of protein are 20 amino acids that may be consumed from both animal and plant sources. Of these 20 amino acids, 9 are considered to be essential because the carbon skeletons cannot be synthesized by human enzymes. The remaining 11 amino acids are considered nonessential because they can be synthesized endogenously. These nonessential amino acids can be synthesized from one another by the transfer of amino groups to carbon compounds as a result of carbohydrate and lipid metabolism (Table 11.6).

## Function

Proteins have many essential roles in the body.

- Produce antibodies for the immune system.
- Produce enzymes that are required for many chemical reactions in the body (i.e., digestion and absorption, blood coagulation, and contractibility and excitability of muscle tissue).
- Component of structural hormones:
  - Contractile proteins for muscle tissue (i.e., actin and myosin).
  - Fibrous proteins found in connective tissue, skin, hair, and nails (i.e., collagen, elastin, and keratin).
- Component of transport proteins (i.e., albumin, prealbumin, hemoglobin, ceruloplasmin, transferrin, and retinol-binding protein).
- Component of peptide hormones (i.e., insulin, glucagon, parathyroid hormone, thyroid hormone, growth hormone, adrenocorticotropic hormone, and antidiuretic hormone).
- Source of fuel when muscle glycogen levels are low (i.e., during prolonged, intense exercise).

TABLE 11.6. Essential and nonessential amino acids.

| Nine essential amino acids (must be consumed in your diet) | Nonessential amino acids (can be produced by the body) |
| --- | --- |
| Histidine | Alanine |
| Isoleucine* | Arginine |
| Leucine* | Asparagine |
| Lysine | Aspartic acid |
| Methionine | Cysteine |
| Phenylalanine | Glutamic acid |
| Threonine | Glutamine |
| Tryptophan | Glycine |
| Valine* | Proline |
| | Serine |
| | Tyrosine |

*Branched-chain amino acids (BCAAs): leucine, isoleucine, and valine are the three BCAAs that are unique among the essential amino acids in that they can be taken up directly by skeletal muscle instead of having to be metabolized by the liver. They are able to serve as a fairly efficient muscle energy source during exercise. Researchers have shown that supplementation of BCAAs before and after exercise has a beneficial effect for decreasing exercise-induced muscle damage, and promoting muscle-protein synthesis and therefore may be beneficial for athletes.[11]

**TABLE 11.7. Complete protein sources.**

| | |
|---|---|
| Milk and dairy products | Macaroni and cheese |
| Whole egg | Peanuts and sunflower seeds |
| Fish | Yogurt and granola |
| Meat/poultry | Corn and peas or beans |
| Soy | Oatmeal with milk |
| Rice and beans | Lentils and bread |
| Peanut butter on whole wheat bread | Bean and cheese burrito |

## Metabolism

Ingested proteins serve as sources of the essential amino acids and are the primary source of the additional nitrogen needed for the synthesis of the nonessential amino acids and nitrogen-containing compounds.[12] Dietary protein combines with endogenous protein from gastrointestinal secretions in the gut and is digested and absorbed as amino acids.[3] The amino acid then loses its nitrogen molecule in the liver (deamination) to form urea, which is excreted by the body. A new amino acid then becomes synthesized from the deaminated amino acid. The remaining deaminated carbon compound can be used to form carbohydrate or fat, or can be metabolized directly for energy. In muscle, enzymes facilitate nitrogen removal from certain amino acids and subsequently pass it to other compounds in the biochemical reactions of transamination. An amino group shifts from a donor amino acid to an acceptor acid (keto-acid); the acceptor then becomes a new amino acid.

If protein intake is inadequate, then protein synthesis cannot keep up with protein breakdown and body proteins (i.e., muscle tissue) are broken down and used to fulfill the requirements for amino acids. This results in slowing of tissue repair, and a decrease in strength and muscle size, which results in decreased physical performance.[13] It is essential to consume enough protein on a daily basis because unlike carbohydrates and fat, which the body can store as glycogen or triglycerides respectively for later use, amino acids cannot be stored in the body.

## Types/Sources

One of the most common methods of classifying proteins is by their biologic value (BV). The BV of a dietary protein is determined by the amount and proportion of essential amino acids it provides. Protein from animal sources (fish, meats, eggs, dairy products) is considered high BV protein or a complete protein because all nine essential amino acids are present in these proteins. Plant protein sources (grains, seeds, nuts, and legumes) generally do not contain sufficient amounts of one or more of the essential amino acids and are therefore considered intermediate BV protein or partially complete. Plant protein sources (most fruits and vegetables) that are lacking the essential amino acids are considered low BV protein or incomplete proteins. It is very important to combine different sources of protein to ensure adequate consumption of the essential amino acids. Only animal sources (and soy) contain all the essential amino acids, but by combining different plant proteins complete protein foods can be made. Protein quality improves when dairy products are added to a plant food and when plant-based foods, such as wheat and beans, are mixed together (see Table 11.7).

## CONCLUSION

Fats, carbohydrates, and proteins substitute for one another to some extent to meet the body's energy needs. Acceptable ranges of intake for each of these energy sources are set, based on evidence that consumption above or below these ranges may be associated with nutrient inadequacy and increased risk of developing chronic diseases, including coronary heart disease, obesity, diabetes, and/or cancer.

Optimal nutrition includes adequate quality as well as quantity of food and fluids to provide the essential nutrients before, during, and after training or a competition. In subsequent chapters, proper nutrition to maximize athletic performance and recovery are discussed.

## Sidebar 11.1. The Vegetarian Athlete of the Millennium

### By Theresa Romano

The classroom and textbook learning accomplished over the years regarding vegetarian athletes left me with the knowledge that it is difficult for a vegetarian athlete to meet their total caloric needs because of their large intake of fresh vegetables—a low kilocalorie food.

Over the past 10 years of practice, I have found two key issues a vegetarian athlete faces. The first is the basic fundamentals of vegetarianism; the second is macronutrient distribution. Whether working with a vegetarian who is a recreational athlete, a collegiate athlete, or a professional athlete, the focus becomes macronutrient content or lack of one particular macronutrient because of the food selection process. The main issue is no longer hypocaloric intake as a result of high consumption of low-calorie vegetables, but rather composition of total diet.

In our "carb phobic" nation, I find it ironic to meet with vegetarian athletes who are barely meeting the general protein requirements, otherwise known as the recommended daily allowance (RDA) of 8 g/kg of body weight, while practically overdosing on carbohydrates. Keep in mind that an athlete's protein requirements are normally above the RDA to promote muscle growth and repair. Traditionally, vegetarians have had a wealth of knowledge about nutrition. Traditionally, a vegetarian had truly done their homework when it came to what they put into their bodies. I think the tradition has been broken!

For whatever the reason a person chooses to become vegetarian, whether it is religious, ethical, or otherwise, vegetarian athletes of today are not learning the basic fundamentals of what it means to be a good vegetarian. When meeting with a vegetarian client, my first question is, "Are you a GOOD vegetarian or a BAD vegetarian?" This not only serves as an icebreaker, but also gets the client thinking about their food intake and what it means to be a good or a bad vegetarian. Nine times out of ten the athlete sitting with me admits their diet could improve, but they need the tools to do so. Let's review a typical diet of a vegetarian athlete:

| Meal | Food selection |
|---|---|
| Breakfast | 1 Bagel with cream cheese, 16 oz. orange juice |
| Snack | Veggie booty (small snack bag) |
| Lunch | 1 slice of pizza, 20-oz. soda or 20-oz. iced tea |
| Snack | Handful of pretzels |
| Dinner | 2 cups pasta with tomato sauce |
| Snack | "Too late to eat" |

Are you thinking what I am thinking? The above is pretty scary! Clearly, we need improvement here. This population defines vegetarianism solely by not eating animal protein in the form of meat, pork, or poultry. Many vegetarians will consume dairy (in the form of yogurt and cheese) and some will consume eggs. Let's get back to basics!

- A good vegetarian chooses foods that optimize their health, but are in alignment with their beliefs.
- A good vegetarian athlete utilizes protein sources such as beans, lentils, chickpeas, tofu, and soy products. Educate them to use dry beans or beans in a can, not just beans added to soup. Educate clients to cook with tofu and other soy products. Encourage them to get a tofu cookbook. If all else fails, there are great processed soy products on the market.
- When using starchy foods, help clients utilize whole grains, some of which have great amino acid profiles: Legumes come to mind once again, as well as soba noodles (buckwheat), millet, quinoa, brown rice, and whole grain breads. Again, encourage your clients to buy a whole-grains cookbook or you can do the research yourself and provide your clients with recipes that base the meal around these whole grains.

The above diet was deficient in vegetables and fresh fruit. Fit vegetables in any way you can:

- Add them to omelets (eggs or egg substitutes).
- Cut up and use as snacks (cucumber slices, bell peppers, snap peas, string beans).
- Add cubed vegetables to grain dishes, or lettuce and mushroom to tofu sandwiches.

If legumes and tofu are not sufficient and additional protein is needed, use amino acids powders or whey protein in shakes. Remember Little Miss Muffet who ate her "curds and whey"? Advise your vegetarian athletes to do the same!

## Sidebar 11.2. Macronutrient Differences of Athletes

### By Theresa Romano

One of the best ways a coach can learn is by on-the-job training. Combine life experience with cutting-edge information (continuing education) via national and local meetings and you've got the right components to be a success.

As sports nutritionists, we are often thought of as the "fuel coach." Through life experience, I have learned that not all athletes consume the same cookie-cutter macronutrient ratios. Of course, we have our textbook standards for carbohydrate, protein, and fat ingestion, but sometimes you will be required to think outside of the box.

Be proactive in your learning! A great method of gaining understanding of an athlete's diet is to work with as many different athletes as you possibly can. Experience gained from working with male versus female athletes, variety of sports, and levels of competitive sport—whether it be recreational, collegiate, or professional—will be beneficial.

I'm hoping if you are looking to be a sports nutritionist that you lead by example. Assess not only your dietary intake, but also your training program and methods of exercising mental fitness. Are you practicing what you preach? If so, it is time to move on and work with athletes. A great learning experience is working with collegiate athletes. The level of competition is high and the commitment of the athletes and coaching staff is commendable. This forum provides you with gender and sport differentiation. To add to your pool of athletic case studies, you may want to work with people at your local gym. If you are fortunate, you will not only have contact with recreational athletes, but also former athletes, bodybuilders, and/or fitness competitors.

Dietary assessments are excellent tools. They allow you to view the macronutrient content of diets and critically review if changes are necessary based on performance. When I began working with athletes in my junior year of college, I used textbook standards for everyone, with slight variation. While assessing dietary intakes via computer programs for an accurate breakdown of diet, I found athletes consuming a wide variation of nutrients and quickly altered my approach.

Collaborating with the coaching staff provides you with the ability to inquire about the athlete's performance levels. Is your athlete living up to potential? How is their speed and strength? Is their level of training acceptable or below par during workouts? All of these are important questions that lead you to an understanding of whether or not this athlete's diet is working for him or her. See below for a few examples of macronutrient assessments:

| Athlete | Sport | Gender | Total kcals | Macronutrient distribution (carbohydrate, protein, fat) | Changes made based on performance |
|---------|-------|--------|-------------|------------------------------------------|----------------------------------|
| AP | LAX (defense) | Male | 3400 | 40, 30, 30 | 45, 30, 26 |
| SM | Football (O/ST) | Male | 3800 | 52, 30, 18 | No change |
| SG | Football (OLine) | Male | 4400 | 58, 20, 23 | 50, 27, 24 ↓kcals to 2800 |
| AT | Baseball (P) | Male | 2850 | 42, 33, 25 | 50, 30, 20 |
| KE | Bodybuilder | Male | 5200 | 45, 30, 25 | 40, 33, 27 |
| KO | Vball, Sball | Female | 2300 | 50, 18, 32 | 50, 22, 28 ↓kcals to 2100 |
| JO | Track and Field | Female | 1900 | 63, 15, 22 | 60, 18, 22 ↑kcals to 2200 |
| AF | Kickline | Female | 2250 | 65, 15, 20 | 58, 20, 22 |
| JB | Sports model | Female | 1600 | 50, 25, 25 | ↑kcals to 1800, then 2000 |

- First conduct a full assessment with your athlete.
- What is their body composition?
- How much are they training?
- How is their performance?
- Can performance be improved by diet and/or training?
- Make alterations to diet and training to optimize performance as necessary.
  - First tackle caloric intake. Are basic needs being met?
  - Next change macronutrient content if necessary.

We will use the athlete SG for example. The coach reported SG was "slow on his feet." The coaches wanted SG to not only lose 40 pounds, 20 of which he gained in the off-season, but also optimize his playing potential. The coach needed SG leaner and quicker. Coaches were hoping this would improve SG's agility during practice, which would translate to on-the-field play making.

- SG had a hypercaloric intake. We first decreased calories to induce weight loss.
- Macronutrients were then manipulated to help increase lipolysis and retain lean muscle mass.
- SG and coaches were able to see quick results with the above alterations, however you need to adjust as you go along. Do not be afraid to modify a meal plan periodically.

Remember to think outside of the box. Listen to what your athletes are telling you and what the goals of the athlete and the coaches are. Your job is to help athletes and please coaching staff. Results are what are important. Results will always be measured by performance and athletic gains! Therefore, learn from each and every athlete you meet with, and remember to critically assess macronutrient content in relation to performance.

## PRACTICAL APPLICATIONS

### Functions of Carbohydrate

- The primary function of carbohydrate is to provide energy to the cells of the body, particularly the brain.
- Facilitate the body's metabolism of fat.
- Spare muscle protein.

### Functions of Fat

- Fat is an ideal fuel because it contains almost twice the energy as glucose, weighs less, and is easily transported and stored.
- Cell membranes are partly composed of a specific type of fat called phospholipids.
- Critical for the transmission of nerve signals that generate muscle contraction.
- Serve as a transporter for vitamins A, D, E, and K.
- Provide cushioning for the protection of vital organs and insulation from the thermal stress of cold environments.
- Fat helps delay the onset of hunger pangs, because fat empties more slowly from the stomach.

### Functions of Protein

- Produce antibodies for the immune system.
- Produce enzymes that are required for many chemical reactions in the body (i.e., digestion and absorption, blood coagulation, and contractibility and excitability of muscle tissue).
- Component of structural hormones:
  - Contractile proteins for muscle tissue (i.e., actin and myosin).
  - Fibrous proteins found in connective tissue, skin, hair, and nails (i.e., collagen, elastin, and keratin).
- Component of transport proteins (i.e., albumin, prealbumin, hemoglobin, ceruloplasmin, transferrin, and retinol-binding protein).
- Component of peptide hormones (i.e., insulin, glucagon, parathyroid hormone, thyroid hormone, growth hormone, adrenocorticotropic hormone, and antidiuretic hormone).
- Source of fuel when muscle glycogen levels are low (i.e., during prolonged, intense exercise).

## QUESTIONS

1. What is most frequently referred to as complex carbohydrates?
   a. Monosaccharides
   b. Disaccharides
   c. Oligosaccharides
   d. Polysaccharides

2. What serves as a storage form of carbohydrate in animal tissues, and is primarily found in liver and skeletal muscle?
   a. Soluble fiber
   b. Insoluble fiber
   c. Starch
   d. Glycogen

3. Metabolism of carbohydrate begins in the:
   a. Small intestine
   b. Mouth
   c. Stomach
   d. Large intestine

4. What provides the most concentrated source of energy?
   a. Lipid
   b. Carbohydrates
   c. Amino acids
   d. Protein

5. What is not a dietary essential because it can be synthesized by the liver?
   a. Linoleic acid
   b. Triglyceride
   c. Cholesterol
   d. Linolenic acid

6. These are critical for the transmission of nerve signals that generate muscle contraction:
   a. Amino acids
   b. Low-density lipoproteins
   c. High-density lipoproteins
   d. Lipids

7. These are the main source of ingested fats and provide the majority of energy derived from dietary lipid:
   a. Trans fatty acids
   b. Triglycerides
   c. Low-density lipoprotein
   d. High-density lipoprotein

8. These are found in partially hydrogenated vegetable oils, such as margarine and shortening:
   a. Trans fatty acids
   b. Triglycerides
   c. Low-density lipoprotein
   d. High-density lipoprotein

9. This may heighten the risk of heart disease by boosting levels of low-density lipoprotein cholesterol in the bloodstream:
   a. Trans fat
   b. Saturated fat
   c. Triglycerides
   d. Trans fat and saturated fat

10. This helps delay the onset of hunger pangs, because it empties more slowly from the stomach:
   a. Protein
   b. Carbohydrate
   c. Fat
   d. Fiber

11. This serves as a storage form of carbohydrate in plants, and represents the common form of digestible plant polysaccharide:
   a. Soluble fiber
   b. Insoluble fiber
   c. Starch
   d. Glycogen

12. An excellent source of omega-6 fatty acids is:
   a. Salmon
   b. Beef
   c. Flax seed oil
   d. Sunflower seeds

13. Which of the following is false about protein?
   a. Production of enzymes
   b. Component of hormones
   c. Transports vitamins A, D, E, and K
   d. Component of transport proteins

14. Which of the following amino acids are essential in the diet?
    a. Glutamine
    b. Glutamic acid
    c. Tyrosine
    d. Tryptophan

15. During deamination, the amino acid loses its ____ molecule in the liver to form urea, which is then excreted.
    a. Hydrogen
    b. Oxygen
    c. Nitrogen
    d. Ammonia

16. What is the best source of a complete protein (contains all the essential amino acids)?
    a. Granola
    b. Soy
    c. Peanut butter
    d. Oatmeal

17. Protein from fruits and vegetables are considered ____ biologic value protein.
    a. High
    b. Intermediate
    c. Low

18. Protein produces enzymes that are required for:
    a. Digestion
    b. Coagulation of blood
    c. Contraction of muscle
    d. All of the above

19. Protein is used as a source of fuel primarily during:
    a. 100-meter sprint
    b. 90-minute professional soccer game
    c. Backstroke 2 lengths of the pool
    d. A sprint to home base

20. Which macronutrient produces antibodies for the immune system?
    a. Fat
    b. Protein
    c. Carbohydrate

21. Branched-chain amino acids are a fairly efficient source of energy.
    a. True
    b. False

22. Ingesting foods with a high glycemic index and a high glycemic load can improve blood glucose levels.
    a. True
    b. False

23. According to the Food and Nutrition Board (2002), women younger than 50 years of age should ingest at least 25 g of fiber a day.
    a. True
    b. False

24. A good source of soluble fiber is bran.
    a. True
    b. False

25. Protein can be used as a source of fuel during prolonged intense exercise.
    a. True
    b. False

26. The body's capacity for storing glycogen is unlimited.
    a. Tru e
    b. False

27. Plants provide the sole source of carbohydrate in the diet.
    a. True
    b. False

28. A deficiency of essential fatty acids can result in dermatitis and scaly skin.
    a. True
    b. False

29. The ratio of oxygen to carbon and hydrogen is lower in lipids than carbohydrates.
    a. True
    b. False

30. Protein quality improves when dairy products are added to plant food and when plant-based foods are consumed together.
    a. True
    b. False

# REFERENCES

1. Trumbo P, Schlicker S, Yates AA, Poos M; Food and Nutrition Board of the Institute of Medicine, The National Academies. Dietary reference intakes for energy, carbohydrate, fiber, fat, fatty acids, cholesterol, protein and amino acids. J Am Diet Assoc 2002;102(11):1621–1630.
2. Anderson JW, Tietyen-Clark J. Dietary fiber: hyperlipidemia, hypertension, and coronary heart disease. Am J Gastroenterol 1986;81(10):907–919.
3. Rosenbloom C, American Dietetic Association. Sports Cardiovascular and Wellness Dietetic Practice Group. Sports Nutrition: A Guide for the Professional Working with Active People. 3rd ed. Chicago: The American Dietetic Association; 2000:viii, 759.
4. Ludwig DS. The glycemic index: physiological mechanisms relating to obesity, diabetes, and cardiovascular disease. JAMA 2002;287(18):2414–2423.
5. Foster-Powell K, Holt SH, Brand-Miller JC. International table of glycemic index and glycemic load values: 2002. Am J Clin Nutr 2002;76(1):5–56.
6. Liu S, Willett WC, Stampfer MJ, et al. A prospective study of dietary glycemic load, carbohydrate intake, and risk of coronary heart disease in US women. Am J Clin Nutr 2000;71(6):1455–1461.
7. Jenkins DJ, Kendall CW, Augustin LS, et al. Glycemic index: overview of implications in health and disease. Am J Clin Nutr 2002;76(1):266S–273S.
8. McArdle WD, Katch FI, Katch VL. Sports and Exercise Nutrition. Philadelphia: Williams & Wilkins; 1999:xlvii, 750.
9. Guthrie HA, Picciano MF, Scott A. Human Nutrition. St. Louis: Mosby; 1995:xix, 659, [147].
10. Duyff RL, American Dietetic Association. American Dietetic Association Complete Food and Nutrition Guide. 2nd ed. Hoboken, NJ: John Wiley & Sons; 2002:xii, 658.
11. Shimomura Y, Murakami T, Nakai N, Nagasaki M, Harris RA. Exercise promotes BCAA catabolism: effects of BCAA supplementation on skeletal muscle during exercise. J Nutr 2004;134(6 Suppl):1583S–1587S.
12. Gropper SAS, Smith JL, Groff JL. Advanced Nutrition and Human Metabolism. 4th ed. Belmont, CA: Thomson/Wadsworth; 2005:600.
13. Lemon PW, Berardi JM, Noreen EE. The role of protein and amino acid supplements in the athlete's diet: does type or timing of ingestion matter? Curr Sports Med Rep 2002;1(4):214–221.

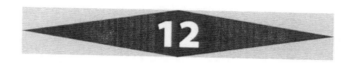

# Protein

## Tim N. Ziegenfuss and Jamie Landis

## OBJECTIVES

On the completion of this chapter you will be able to:

1. Understand the basics functions of proteins in the body.
2. Describe the components of the amino acid pool.
3. Discuss the process by which proteins are digested and absorbed into the body.
4. Differentiate among essential, conditionally essential, and nonessential amino acids.
5. Understand the difference between complete and incomplete protein sources.
6. Discuss the three major methods for quantifying protein quality.
7. Describe the recommended protein needs for various populations.
8. Contrast the effects of increasing protein intake on adaptations that occur in response to a resistance training program.
9. Describe the effects of consuming various types of proteins on muscle proteins synthesis.
10. Understand the importance of protein timing and its relationship to adaptive responses.
11. Discuss the potential hazards of high protein diets and determine if these risks are exaggerated.

## ABSTRACT

Although it has been fairly well established that most athletes ingest sufficient protein in their habitual diet, recent scientific evidence has shown that the type (animal versus vegetable) and timing of protein intake (pre- versus post-exercise) can affect protein kinetics and adaptations to training. This chapter reviews basic protein and amino acid metabolism, discusses methods of measuring protein quality, provides prudent levels of protein intake for various athletic populations, compares different protein types, and discusses what is currently known about timing of protein intake relative to exercise. The chapter concludes by providing practical applications for sports nutritionists that maximize the benefits of protein/amino acid ingestion while balancing the potential adverse effects of excessive protein intake.

*Key Words:* biologic value, protein efficiency ratio, fast protein, slow protein, protein requirements, essential amino acids

From: *Essentials of Sports Nutrition and Supplements*
Edited by J. Antonio, D. Kalman, J. R. Stout, M. Greenwood, D. S. Willoughby, and G. G. Haff © Humana Press, a part of Springer Science+Business Media, Totowa, NJ

**TABLE 12.1. Functional roles of protein.**

| | |
|---|---|
| Energy | After protein undergoes degradation, amino acids can be transaminated or deaminated to form glucose. |
| Growth and maintenance | Proteins are found in many body structures, including skin, hair, nails, tendons, ligaments, muscles, organs, and bones. |
| Hormones | Growth hormone, glucagon, insulin, prolactin, and antidiuretic hormone are some examples of hormones that are classified as proteins. |
| Enzymes | Enzymes are proteins that speed up chemical reactions. Almost all enzymes are proteins or have protein components. |
| Antibodies | Antibodies are proteins produced by β-lymphocytes to fight infections. |
| Acid-base balance | In addition to carrying oxygen, hemoglobin (which is a protein) serves as a blood buffer to help regulate pH within narrow limits. |
| Fluid balance | The blood proteins, albumin and globulin, help draw fluid into the capillary beds, thus preventing edema. |
| Transportation | Hemoglobin carries oxygen, lipoproteins carry fats, and specialized transport proteins carry certain vitamins and minerals. |

## OVERVIEW OF PROTEIN AND AMINO ACID METABOLISM

For more than 150 years, scientists have explored the role of dietary protein in human anatomy and physiology. In sports and exercise nutrition, few topics have received more attention (and heated debate) than protein. In the mid-1800s, von Leibig proposed that protein was the major source of fuel for muscle contraction.[1] By 1925, this was shown to be false and most scientists believed that protein needs were unaffected by exercise.[2] Only in the past 30 years has the middle ground been occupied—that although it is not a major source of energy during most types of exercise, under certain circumstances, dietary protein and/or certain amino acids can have very important roles in muscle metabolism and exercise performance.

There are approximately 50,000 different protein-containing compounds in the body, and 65% of them are found in skeletal muscle. In addition to its role as a macronutrient, protein has vital roles in our health, for example, as components of RNA, DNA, insulin, hemoglobin, epinephrine, and serotonin. Table 12.1 lists some of the general functions of various body proteins.

## PROTEIN BASICS

Along with carbohydrates and fat, protein is one of the three macronutrients. Similar to fat, protein is an essential nutrient, and similar to carbohydrate, protein has an energy density of 4 kcals per gram. Unlike either of the other macronutrients, however, protein contains nitrogen atoms. It is these nitrogen atoms that give the name amino ("nitrogen containing") to the amino acids. Structurally, proteins consist of various combinations of amino acids linked together by peptide bonds. Most body proteins are polypeptides that contain >100 amino acids linked together.

Figure 12.1 provides an overview of whole-body protein metabolism. The liver, skeletal muscles, and blood make up the amino acid pools of the body. These pools are constantly turning over and equilibrating with one another. When entry (of nitrogen) into the amino acid pools equals its rate of excretion, an individual is in a state of nitrogen balance. During periods of fasting and overtraining, nitrogen losses typically outstrip nitrogen intake, and a state of negative nitrogen balance (or more correctly, nitrogen *status*) ensues. During the accretion of lean tissue, the opposite occurs (positive nitrogen status).

## DIGESTION AND ABSORPTION OF PROTEIN AND AMINO ACIDS

Protein digestion begins in the stomach where the proenzyme pepsinogen is converted to the active enzyme pepsin by hydrochloric acid. Pepsin starts cleaving the peptide bonds that link amino acids together, forming smaller peptides and some free amino acids. Once the gastric contents enter the small intestine,

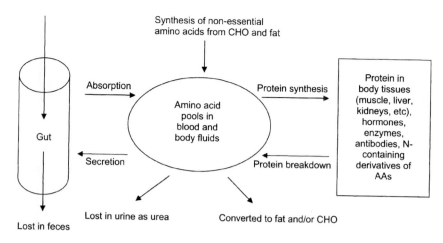

**FIGURE 12.1.** An overview of protein and amino acid metabolism. CHO = cholesterol, AAs = amino acids.

enzymes from the pancreas (trypsin, chymotrypsin, elastase, carboxypeptidase) and the brush border itself (aminopeptidases, intracellular peptidases) complete the cleavage to absorbable amino acids. It should be noted that pepsin, chymotrypsin, and elastase are endopeptidases that hydrolyze peptide bonds *within* chains, whereas aminopeptidases and carboxypeptidases are exopeptidases that act on amino acids at the N or C terminus, respectively. Amino acids are then absorbed from the lumen of the small intestine into the blood by one of six sodium-dependent cotransporters, and/or facilitated diffusion. Amino acids transported into the intestine and kidneys react with glutathione before their release into the cell. Proteins that are not absorbed are acted on by flora of the large intestine and converted largely to methane and hydrogen sulfide. Contrary to popular belief, there is no known maximum amount of protein that can be absorbed in one meal. However, in general, it is known that humans typically absorb approximately 95% of ingested animal proteins, and approximately 85% of ingested plant proteins.[3]

As mentioned above, protein turnover is a dynamic process that involves a constant input of entry into and exit from the amino acid pools. Upon entry into the amino acid pools, amino acids can be used to synthesize proteins and other nitrogen-containing compounds, oxidized for energy, or excreted in the urine (Figure 12.1). Before amino acids can be used for energy, the nitrogen-containing amino group must be removed by one of two mechanisms: 1) transamination, or 2) oxidative deamination. It is thought that all amino acids except lysine and threonine can undergo transamination; however, in exercising humans, transamination of the branched-chain amino acids (BCAAs) (leucine, isoleucine, valine) is particularly important because these amino acids are oxidized in significant amounts in muscle.[4] Transamination occurs when the amino group from one amino acid ($NH_3^+$) is transferred to a carbon skeleton (usually alpha-ketoglutarate), forming a new amino acid (usually glutamate). This reaction requires vitamin B6 as a cofactor and an intracellular enzyme called transaminase. The two most common transaminase reactions are shown in the equations below. Reaction (a) utilizes alanine aminotransferase [ALT, formerly known as serum glutamate-pyruvate transaminase (SGPT)], whereas reaction (b) utilizes aspartate aminotransferase [AST, formerly known as serum glutamate-oxaloacetate transaminase (SGOT)].

(a) pyruvate + glutamate ↔ alanine + alpha-ketoglutarate

(b) oxaloacetate + glutamate ↔ aspartate + alpha-ketoglutarate

It should be noted that these two enzymes are sometimes used as clinical markers of hepatocellular injury. However, because AST and ALT can also be released from skeletal muscle, it is not uncommon to see elevated levels (within 1.5 times the upper limits of normal) in intensely training athletes. This is normal, and does not indicate liver damage.

In oxidative deamination, the amino group is removed, converted to ammonia and urea in the liver, and subsequently removed by the kidneys and

**TABLE 12.2. Amino acids.**

| Essential amino acids | Nonessential amino acids |
|---|---|
| Histidine | Alanine |
| Isoleucine* | Arginine† |
| Leucine* | Asparagine |
| Lysine | Aspartic acid |
| Methionine | Cysteine† |
| Phenylalanine | Glutamic acid |
| Threonine | Glutamine† |
| Tryptophan | Glycine† |
| Valine* | Proline† |
| | Serine |
| | Tyrosine† |

*Branched-chain amino acid.
†Conditionally essential amino acid.

sweat glands. This process is called the urea cycle, and is particularly active during prolonged fasting and high protein diets.[5,6] Besides urea, major excretory products from protein are uric acid and creatinine. Uric acid is derived from the metabolism of nucleic acids, and is typically elevated in a condition known as gout. Creatinine is a waste product formed from creatine. Whereas urea excretion varies directly with protein intake (i.e., as protein intake increases, so does urea excretion), creatinine excretion is relatively constant and is directly related to muscle mass. For this reason, urinary creatinine excretion is sometimes used as an indirect measure of muscle mass.[7]

## FOOD SOURCES OF PROTEIN

Different sources of protein can vary widely in their amino acid profile, digestibility, and nutritional value. A food protein is only considered "complete" if it contains all nine essential amino acids, thus allowing for tissue growth and repair. Examples of complete proteins include animal proteins such as milk, eggs, meat, poultry, and fish. Proteins that lack one or more of the essential amino acids are termed "incomplete," are not capable of causing growth, and instead can lead to protein malnutrition if eaten in isolation (i.e., not combined with other complementary foods). Examples of incomplete proteins include plant proteins such as corn, lentils, beans, and nuts. Soy is one of the few examples of a plant protein that is considered "complete." Table 12.2 lists the various "essential" (must be obtained through the diet), "conditionally essential" (must be obtained from the diet under stressful conditions—such as exercise), and "nonessential" (not necessary in the diet because the body can produce them from other compounds) amino acids.

As general guidelines, one 8-oz. glass of milk provides 8 g of protein, a 1-oz. serving of chicken breast provides 7 g of protein, 1 slice of wheat bread provides 3 g of protein, 1/2 cup of mixed vegetables provides 2 g of protein, and 1 scoop of protein powder (or 1 regular-sized protein bar) provides 20 g of protein. Fruits are essentially devoid of protein. Readers are referred to the Food and Information Center of the United States Department of Agriculture Nutrient Database (www.nal.usda.gov/fnic) for a complete listing of the protein content of foods. For specific examples of dietary menus, readers should seek the advice of a qualified (licensed) dietitian, preferably with a background in sports nutrition and exercise science.

## METHODS OF MEASURING PROTEIN QUALITY

Protein quality refers to the ability of a specific dietary protein to support body growth and maintenance.[8] The three most common methods of determining protein quality are biologic value (BV), protein efficiency ratio (PER), and the Protein Digestibility-Corrected Amino Acid Score (PDCAAS). Table 12.3 compares the BV, PER, and PDCAAS of various foods and protein sources.

**TABLE 12.3. A comparison of protein quality of selected foods and protein sources.**

| Protein | BV | PER | PDCAAS |
|---|---|---|---|
| Hydrolyzed whey | 100 | >3.0 | 1.00 |
| Whey concentrate | 100 | >3.0 | 1.00 |
| Whole egg | 100 | 2.8 | 1.00 |
| Milk | 91 | 2.8 | 1.00 |
| Beef/poultry, fish | 79–83 | 2.0–2.9 | 0.80–0.92 |
| Soy | 74 | 1.8–2.3 | 0.91–1.00 |
| Casein | 71 | 2.9 | 1.00 |

*Source:* Adapted from Kreider and Kleiner.[9]

BV = biologic value, PER = protein efficiency ratio, PDCAAS = Protein Digestibility-Corrected Amino Acid Score.

BV measures the amount of nitrogen retained in comparison to the amount of nitrogen absorbed. Values are derived from humans and laboratory animals to generate BV of different food proteins. Although measuring nitrogen balance in humans is technically challenging, BV is considered a valid method of assessing protein quality in humans.

PER measures the ability of a protein to support the growth of a weaning rat. It is calculated as the ratio of the weight gained to the amount of protein consumed (i.e., PER = g weight gain/g protein consumed). Aside from the known species' differences between humans and rats, PER is not considered the ideal method of assessing protein quality because it does not address the maintenance needs of adults (which are likely to be vastly different from the growth needs of weanlings).

The PDCAAS is a relatively new method of assessing protein quality for children older than 1 year of age and nonpregnant adults. The PDCAAS compares the amino acid profile of a specific dietary protein with the essential (human) amino acid requirements established by the Food and Agriculture Organization. A correction is made for digestibility differences, and the resulting value is adjusted so that a value of unity (1.0) indicates that the protein exceeds the essential amino acid requirements of the body. Although the PDCAAS is an excellent method of assessing protein quality, most food labels (i.e., nutrition facts panels) do not contain the percent daily value for protein because of the costs associated in determining the PDCAAS.

## PROTEIN REQUIREMENTS—HOW MUCH DIETARY PROTEIN DO ACTIVE INDIVIDUALS NEED?

Several different experimental techniques have been used to study protein metabolism and determine protein requirements in humans (e.g., nitrogen balance, isotopic tracers, and arteriovenous measurements of amino acids across a tissue bed). Classically, the recommended daily allowance (RDA) has relied on the nitrogen balance technique, wherein nitrogen intake (from food) is compared with nitrogen output (from urine, sweat, and feces). When nitrogen intake exceeds output, the subject is said to be in positive nitrogen balance (or more correctly, positive nitrogen *status*); when the reverse is true, the subject is in negative nitrogen balance (status). Although nitrogen balance studies are conceptually very easy to understand, they are technically very difficult to perform and have historically overestimated nitrogen retention.[10] For this reason, and because the RDA is based on data from essentially sedentary subjects, some[11-13] but not all[14] researchers have suggested that physically active individuals need more protein than is currently recommended. In addition, it is known that certain factors such as energy intake, exercise intensity, exercise duration, training status, and possibly gender can influence protein needs.[11-19] With this in mind, as well as the acknowledgment that the relationship between protein intake and optimal health/performance is unclear, Table 12.4 lists the current RDA for protein for sedentary adults, along with values we consider prudent for physically active individuals (also note Figures 12.2–12.4).

**TABLE 12.4. Recommended protein intakes.**

| Activity level | Grams of protein/kg body weight/day |
|---|---|
| Sedentary (adult) | 0.8 (0.4 g/lb.) |
| Recreational exerciser (adult) | 1.0–1.4 (0.5–0.7 g/lb.) |
| Resistance-trained (maintenance) | 1.2–1.4 (0.6–0.7 g/lb.) |
| Resistance-trained (gain muscle mass)* | 1.4–1.8 (0.7–0.9 g/lb.) |
| Endurance-trained | 1.2–1.4 (0.6–0.7 g/lb.) |
| Intermittent, high-intensity training | 1.2–1.8 (0.6–0.9 g/lb.) |
| Weight-restricted sports | 1.4–2.0 (0.7–1.0 g/lb.) |

*Source:* Adapted from Williams[20] and refs. 9–19.

*Note:* Growing teens should add ~10% to all values.

*In athletes using anabolic agents (e.g., growth hormone, insulin, testosterone), it is our opinion that a much higher protein intake may be required to maximize gains.

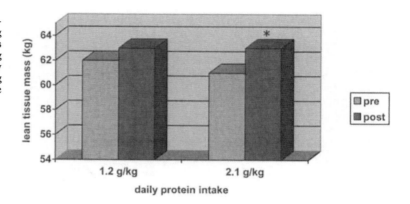

**FIGURE 12.2.** Lean mass changes in experienced weightlifters after 6 weeks of ingesting either 1.2 or 2.1 g of protein/kg per day. In this study, the group that ingested 2.1 g of protein/kg per day increased their lean mass significantly more than the group that ingested 1.2 g of protein/kg per day. (Adapted from Burke et al.[21])

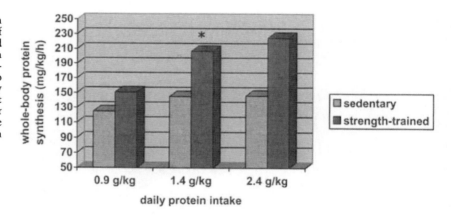

**FIGURE 12.3.** Changes in whole-body protein synthesis in response to different amounts of dietary protein. In this study, strength-trained men who increased their protein intake from 0.9 to 1.4 g/kg body weight per day had significant increases in protein synthesis; however, no additional increase was noted at 2.4 g/kg body weight per day. This study also showed that sedentary men who simply increased their protein intake did not sustain an increase whole-body protein synthesis. (Adapted from Tarnopolsky et al.[22])

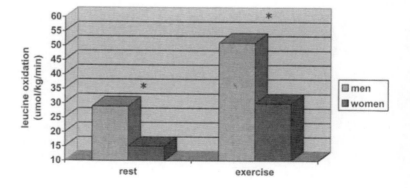

**FIGURE 12.4.** Effect of exercise and gender on leucine oxidation (a marker of protein breakdown) in male and female endurance runners. In this study, exercise significantly increased leucine oxidation, and values for men were significantly greater than women. (Adapted from Phillips et al.[23])

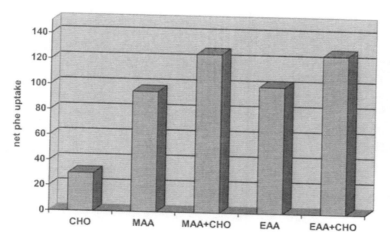

**FIGURE 12.5.** Comparison of net phenylalanine uptake (as a marker of muscle protein synthesis) to the ingestion of carbohydrate (CHO), mixed amino acid (MAA—essential + nonessential), and essential amino acid (EAA) after resistance exercise. CHO = 100 g sucrose; MAA = 6 g ingested at 1 and 2 hours postexercise (12 g total); MAA + CHO = 6 g + 35 g sucrose ingested at 1 and 2 hours postexercise (12 g + 70 g total); EAA = 6 g ingested at 1 and 2 hours postexercise (12 g total); EAA + CHO = 6 g + 35 g sucrose ingested at 1 hours postexercise. (Adapted from Tipton and Wolfe.[13])

In one of the few studies examining potential gender differences in protein metabolism, Phillips et al.[23] reported that nitrogen balance (status) was less, and leucine oxidation was more, in male versus female endurance runners adapted to a protein intake of ~0.8–0.9 g/kg body weight per day (Figure 12.4). Although confirmatory data are necessary, this may indicate that the protein needs of women endurance athletes are less than their male counterparts.

## DOES PROTEIN TYPE MATTER?

In a word, yes. Several studies have shown that diets that include animal proteins are superior in promoting improvements in strength and body composition compared with vegetarian diets,[24] and that milk proteins are superior to hydrolyzed soy proteins.[25] In addition, a series of studies have convincingly established that only the essential amino acids are necessary to stimulate muscle protein synthesis, and the inclusion of nonessential amino acids offers no additional benefit (as reviewed in ref. 13). Figure 12.5 compares the results from various studies to date on net muscle protein balance. It is important to note that in all of these studies, resistance training was used as the mode of exercise. Although it is known that resistance exercise and endurance exercise both increase mixed muscle protein synthesis, the latter does not usually result in muscle hypertrophy because the changes in protein kinetics occur primarily in mitochondrial proteins.

The BCAAs, which are also essential amino acids, are also a popular topic in nutritional research.[26] Whereas most studies to date have examined the potential of BCAA supplementation to improve various types of performance (the results of which have been equivocal), one interesting aspect of BCAAs that has only recently been explored is their potential effect on weight loss. During a moderate protein (1.5 g/kg of body weight per day), lower carbohydrate (100–200 g/day) diet, the increased intake of BCAAs (especially leucine) is thought to have positive effects on muscle protein synthesis, insulin signaling, and sparing of glucose use by stimulation of the glucose-alanine cycle. This leads to more fat loss and a greater sparing of lean tissue compared with an isoenergetic, higher carbohydrate diet.[27] Although exciting, further confirmatory research into the effects of BCAAs on changes in body composition is warranted.

## TIMING OF PROTEIN INTAKE

One relatively new development in the field of sports nutrition is the knowledge that the timing of nutrient ingestion influences the physiologic responses to exercise. Figure 12.6 shows that net muscle protein balance (as reflected by phenylalanine uptake) increases substantially more when a protein + carbohydrate mixture is ingested before an acute bout of resistance exercise compared

**FIGURE 12.6.** Net phenylalanine uptake over 3 hours after the ingestion of 6g of essential amino acids + 35g of sucrose before (PRE) or after (POST) acute resistance exercise. In this study, an approximately fourfold greater increase in net protein synthesis was noted during PRE compared with POST. (Modified from Tipton et al.[38])

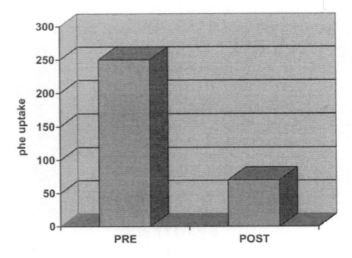

with after exercise. Subsequent studies that have utilized this "nutrient timing" concept have reported greater increases in muscle mass and strength in subjects receiving protein-containing supplements immediately after resistance exercise compared with subjects receiving the same supplement 2 hours after exercise.[28] In a follow-up study from the same laboratory,[29] young men who supplemented with 25g of protein immediately before and after resistance training for 14 weeks had 18%–26% greater gains in muscle hypertrophy than men supplemented with an equal amount of carbohydrate. In women performing 7 days of intense cycling exercise, postexercise macronutrient supplementation reduced the loss of body weight and improved nitrogen status.[30] Some studies show that the combination of protein and carbohydrate can enhance glycogen synthesis compared with ingesting carbohydrate alone[31–33]; however, when carbohydrate intake is very high in the immediate 4 hours after exercise, there seems to be little added benefit[34,35]. It has also been reported that acute administration of a combination of whey protein, amino acids, and carbohydrate causes greater increases in muscle protein synthesis than an isoenergetic amount of carbohydrate.[36] In a recent study of United States marine recruits during basic training,[37] postexercise protein supplementation reduced bacterial/viral infections, decreased medical visits caused by muscle or joint problems, diminished episodes of heat exhaustion, reduced muscle soreness, and improved rifle scores compared with the placebo and control groups. These and other studies highlight that regardless of how much protein an athlete consumes, the timing of the meal relative to exercise as well as the co-ingestion of other nutrients is of critical importance.

## HAZARDS OF "HIGH" PROTEIN INTAKE EXAGGERATED

The purported adverse effects from ingesting excessive protein generally revolve around an increased risk of cardiovascular disease, impaired liver and kidney function, calcium loss, and dehydration. Aside from dehydration, it is our belief that these potential adverse effects have been exaggerated. In their review of the literature, the National Academy of Sciences and the Harvard School of Public Health have concluded that high protein diets do not seem to increase the risk for coronary heart disease (as referenced in 20, 39, and 40).

Relative to organ damage, in contrast to data on subjects with impaired kidney function, no study has ever reported liver or kidney damage in healthy subjects consuming a high protein diet. This includes a recent study of bodybuilders consuming 2.8g of protein/kg body weight per day[41] and studies in rodents fed 80% of their total energy as protein for more than half their lifespan.[42] Thus, unless an individual has known kidney disease or is predisposed to kidney disorders (i.e., kidney stones), there seems to be little reason to consume less protein than is recommended in this chapter.

Regarding high protein diets and calcium loss, it is known that dietary protein increases urine acidity, and that calcium might be drawn from bones to buffer the acid load. However, many early studies reporting this effect were limited by small sample sizes, methodologic errors, and the use of high doses of purified forms of protein.[43] It is now known that the phosphate content of protein foods (and supplements fortified with calcium and phosphorous) negates this effect, and recent studies have generally found a positive relationship between protein intake and bone health. Because inadequate protein intake itself can increase bone loss,[44] athletes should make sure they are obtaining at least the RDA for protein as well as adequate daily amounts of calcium, vitamin D, and phosphorous.

Finally, as the urea cycle processes dietary nitrogen, water is eliminated via the urinary system. If left unchecked, dehydration can result. Because dehydration of as little as 3% can impair performance, athletes ingesting extra protein should weigh themselves regularly to ensure they are properly hydrated.

## Sidebar 12.1. Key Concepts

- Proteins are composed of amino acids, some of which must be obtained through the diet (essential), and others which can be formed from other substrates (nonessential).
- Most athletes already ingest sufficient quantities of protein on a daily basis; however, it is less clear if athletes are consuming protein at the optimal time relative to exercise.
- Amino acid availability is a potent regulator of muscle protein synthesis.
- Only the essential amino acids are necessary to stimulate muscle protein synthesis.
- Carbohydrates alone have a minimal effect on muscle protein synthesis, but carbohydrates + amino acids have a synergistic effect on muscle protein synthesis.

## Sidebar 12.2. How Much Extra Protein Is Required to Build Muscle?

- Skeletal muscle is approximately 72% water, 22% protein, and 6% fat, glycogen, and minerals.
- One pound of muscle tissue contains ~100 g of protein.
- To gain 1 lb. of lean mass per week, an athlete would have to ingest an extra 14 g of protein per day (100 g/7 days).
- Although the calculation is easy, in practice, it is not that simple. Most experts believe that the single most impor-

tant factor in gaining lean mass (along with resistance training, of course) is consuming a hyperenergetic diet.
- Therefore, to ensure the body has sufficient energy for lean mass accretion, consume an additional 200–400 kcal/day (3–5 kcal/kg per day) above maintenance requirements in addition to consuming a little extra protein.

## Sidebar 12.3. Why Is It Difficult to Determine Optimal Protein Requirements?

- Subjects consuming the same absolute amount of protein could consume different amounts and types of amino acids.
- The timing of ingestion relative to exercise (before or after) alters protein kinetics.
- The addition of nonprotein energy (cholesterol or any other insulinogenic compound) can also affect protein kinetics.

## Sidebar 12.4. The Glucose-Alanine Cycle and the Role of Branched-Chain Amino Acids

- During exercise, pyruvate is formed from the breakdown of glycogen and glucose.
- Within the muscle, BCAAs donate their amino group to pyruvate to form alanine.
- Alanine is transported to the liver where it is used to regenerate glucose.

- Glucose can then be transported back to skeletal muscle to be used for energy.
- Thus, BCAAs (especially leucine) help reform glucose—this mechanism whereby glucose homeostasis is maintained during fasting and prolonged exercise is known as the "glucose-alanine" cycle.

## Sidebar 12.5. Fast Versus Slow Proteins, Casein Versus Whey

- Although whey and casein are both high-quality protein sources derived from milk, there are differences in how fast they are digested, influence serum amino acid levels, and affect protein turnover.
- Because it is digested slowly and leads to a relatively sustained increase in amino acids, casein (a "slow" protein) seems to inhibit protein breakdown to a greater degree than whey (a "fast" protein).
- Conversely, whey protein leads to a rapid but short-lived spike in amino acid levels which increases muscle protein synthesis more than casein.[45]

- In the only head-to-head studies conducted to date, casein supplementation resulted in superior gains in strength and muscle mass, along with greater fat loss, compared with whey.[46] In the end, there are good reasons to use both whey and casein in that both contain biologically active peptides that the other lacks.
- One current strategy that some athletes use is to ingest whey protein upon waking and immediately postexercise and casein before bed. During the remainder of the day, protein intake usually comes from a combination of whole food sources.

## Sidebar 12.6. Glutamine—All Show and No Go?

- The most abundant free amino acid in the body, glutamine, has important roles in muscle tissue (as a nitrogen shuttle), the brain (as a component of cerebrospinal fluid), and intestinal mucosa as well as immune cells (as an energy substrate).
- For years, many athletes have used glutamine in the hopes of stimulating muscle growth through direct (anabolic) effects, or by attenuating losses of lean mass via indirect (anticatabolic) actions. Although there is fairly strong theoretical bases for these effects, supporting data in free-living humans is lacking.
- For example, in a recent study of 31 men, subjects who ingested 45 g of glutamine per day for 6 weeks had no greater increase in muscle strength or size than subjects ingesting a placebo.[47]
- In contrast, some, but not all, research supports a beneficial effect of glutamine supplementation on immune function and the prevention of upper respiratory tract infections.[48-50]
- At this time, data linking glutamine supplementation with improvements in immune function, body composition, or athletic performance in humans are weak. That said, because there is no apparent downside to supplementation, athletes engaged in heavy training may find it prudent to ingest 5–10 g of glutamine immediately before and after exercise.

## SUMMARY AND PRACTICAL APPLICATIONS

Although it is not possible to make conclusive recommendations regarding protein intake for optimal performance, the following recommendations are made considering the current body of literature:

- Sound sports nutrition starts with meeting energy needs, fluid requirements, and addressing any micronutrient deficiencies. Do not micromanage— handle the big stuff first.
- Depending on their particular sport and training background, athletes should ingest between 1.0 and 1.8 g of high-quality protein per kilogram of body weight per day (0.5–0.9 g/lb./d). Based on protein kinetic data, pulse feedings are preferable to large boluses, so at least some protein should be included in every meal and snack.
- If an athlete does not eat high-quality proteins, they should consider supplementing with essential amino acids. Although the optimal single dose of essential amino acids is not known, a prudent recommendation is to consume at least 0.1 g/kg body weight several times per day.
- Most athletes should never train fasted or remain fasted in the immediate postexercise period. For athletes attempting to gain (or even maintain) muscle mass, at least 6 g of essential amino acids, with or without 20–30 g of carbohydrate, is a good preworkout strategy. Team sport and endurance athletes should ingest proportionally more carbohydrate to match the energy needs of their event.
- During the 1–3 hours postexercise, athletes should ingest 1–2 mixed meals providing approximately 400–600 kcals (each). For strength/power athletes, a carbohydrate ratio of 2 parts carbohydrates to 1 part protein is recommended. For team sport athletes, a 3 : 1 ratio is recommended. For endurance athletes, a 4 : 1 ratio is recommended. The first postexercise meal should include high glycemic index carbohydrates (dextrose and maltodextrin) and rapidly digesting protein (whey protein concentrates and/or hydrolysates). More energy is necessary for larger athletes and/or for higher volumes of training.
- For athletes consuming protein in excess of 2 g/kg body weight per day, changes in body weight should be carefully monitored to ensure proper hydration.

## QUESTIONS

1. Which of the following is found in protein, as compared with carbohydrate and fat?
   a. Carbon
   b. Hydrogen
   c. Nitrogen
   d. Oxygen

2. Which of the following accounts for the differences among different amino acids?
   a. The amine group
   b. The side chain (R group)
   c. The acid group
   d. a and b

3. How many amino acids are considered to be essential amino acids?
   a. 5
   b. 7
   c. 9
   d. 13

4. A ____ bond is formed between the amine group end of one amino acid and the acid group end of the next amino acid in a protein.
   a. Peptide
   b. Amino acid

c. Denatured
d. Sulfur

5. A major gluconeogenic amino acid is ____.
    a. Creatine
    b. Alanine
    c. Glutamine
    d. Glycine

6. When amino acids are degraded for energy, their amine groups are stripped off and used elsewhere or incorporated by the liver into:
    a. Bile
    b. Urea
    c. Glucose
    d. Urine

7. If amino acids are oversupplied:
    a. The body stores them until they are needed
    b. The body removes and excretes their amine groups
    c. The body converts amino acid residues to glycogen or fat
    d. b and c

8. Which of the following provides amino acids that are best absorbed by the body?
    a. Legumes
    b. Animal proteins
    c. Grains
    d. Vegetables

9. Of the following foods, which has the highest Protein Digestibility-Corrected Amino Acid Score?
    a. Chickpeas
    b. Soybean protein
    c. Kidney beans
    d. Tuna

10. Protein Digestibility-Corrected Amino Acid Score takes into account:
    a. The digestibility of a protein
    b. The proportions of amino acids in a food
    c. How well the protein supports weight gain
    d. a and b

11. The RDA for protein is based solely on:
    a. Height
    b. Body weight
    c. Body size
    d. Sex

12. Which of the following statements is true?
    a. Athletes need more protein than other healthy adults
    b. Athletes should consume protein supplements to build muscle
    c. Dieters need more protein than the RDA to spare lean mass
    d. a and c

13. What is the RDA of protein for a 40-year-old man who is 6′4″ tall and weighs 180 lbs.?
    a. 34 g
    b. 49 g
    c. 65 g

14. Protein contributes an average of about ____% of the total fuel used during rest, and up to ____% during heavy physical activity.
    a. 5, 15
    b. 10, 10
    c. 10, 20
    d. None of these

15. Which of the following athletes would use less protein for fuel during exercise?
    a. Joe, who consumes a protein-rich diet
    b. Charles, who consumes a fat-rich diet
    c. Gary, who consumes a carbohydrate-rich diet
    d. Rick, who consumes a diet rich in branched-chain amino acids

16. What is considered the most naturally abundant amino acid(s) in the body?
    a. Branched-chain amino acids
    b. Creatine
    c. Glutamine
    d. Each of these is equally abundant

17. To stimulate protein synthesis immediately after resistance training:
    a. Acute ingestion of a free amino acid supplement is required
    b. Fasting is recommended
    c. Acute ingestion of intact protein or free essential amino acids is beneficial
    d. Low glycemic index carbohydrate supplementation is required

18. Which of the following results in the greatest stimulation of muscle protein synthesis?
    a. Ingestion of essential and nonessential amino acids immediately postexercise
    b. Ingestion of large quantities of carbohydrate postexercise
    c. Ingestion of carbohydrates and essential amino acids preexercise
    d. None of the above

19. Which of the following ratios of carbohydrate-to-protein is recommended for team sport athletes?
    a. 1 part carbohydrate to 1 part protein
    b. 2 parts carbohydrate to 1 part protein
    c. 3 parts carbohydrate to 1 part protein
    d. 4 parts carbohydrate to 1 part protein

20. Which of the following ratios of carbohydrate-to-protein is recommended for team sport athletes?
    a. 1 part carbohydrate to 1 part protein
    b. 2 parts carbohydrate to 1 part protein
    c. 3 parts carbohydrate to 1 part protein
    d. 4 parts carbohydrate to 1 part protein

21. Inadequate intake of protein leads to bone loss.
    a. True
    b. False

22. Diets containing moderate amounts of protein do not adversely affect liver or kidney function in healthy adults.
    a. True
    b. False

23. Two athletes ingesting the same amount of protein per day may be in markedly different nitrogen states (positive or negative N balance).
    a. True
    b. False

24. The amino acid glycine is an important branched-chain amino acid that has a role in the glucose-alanine cycle.
    a. True
    b. False

25. Glutamine release from muscle increases during exercise.
    a. True
    b. False

26. Although leucine seems to be a key regulator of muscle protein synthesis, not all studies have shown leucine supplementation to be beneficial.
    a. True
    b. False

27. When muscle glycogen levels decrease by more than 40%, protein breakdown increases dramatically.
    a. True
    b. False

28. In terms of training for muscle hypertrophy, total caloric intake is more important than protein intake.
    a. True
    b. False

29. Whey protein seems to be superior to casein for promoting gains in strength and size during chronic resistance training.
    a. True
    b. False

30. Because of nutrient timing, it is possible to ingest more than the RDA for protein yet not be in positive nitrogen balance (status).
    a. True
    b. False

## REFERENCES

1. Cathcart EP. Influence of muscle work on protein metabolism. Physiol Rev 1925; 5:225–243.
2. von Leibig J. Animal Chemistry or Organic Chemistry in Its Application to Physiology [transl. G. Gregory]. London: Taylor & Walton; 1842.
3. Young VR, Pellett PL. Plant proteins in relation to human protein and amino acid nutrition. Am J Clin Nutr 1994;59(5 Suppl):1203S–1212S.
4. Shimomura Y, Murakami T, Nakai N, Nagasaki M, Harris RA. Exercise promotes BCAA catabolism: effects of BCAA supplementation on skeletal muscle during exercise. J Nutr 2004;134:1583S–1587S.
5. Lemon PW, Mullin JP. Effect of initial muscle glycogen levels on protein catabolism during exercise. J Appl Physiol 1980;48(4):624–629.
6. Price GM, Halliday D, Pacy PJ, Quevedo MR, Millward DJ. Nitrogen homeostasis in man: influence of protein intake on the amplitude of diurnal cycling of body nitrogen. Clin Sci (Lond) 1994;86(1):91–102.
7. Heymsfield SB, Arteaga C, McManus C, Smith J, Moffitt S. Measurement of muscle mass in humans: validity of the 24-hour urinary creatinine method. Am J Clin Nutr 1983;37(3):478–494.
8. Schaafsma G. The Protein Digestibility-Corrected Amino Acid Score (PDCAAS)—a concept for describing protein quality in foods and food ingredients: a critical review. J AOAC Int 2005;88(3):988–994.
9. Kreider RB, Kleiner SM. Protein supplements for athletes: need vs. convenience. Your Patient Fitness 2000;14(6):12–18.
10. Fuller MF, Garlick PJ. Human amino acid requirements: can the controversy be resolved? Ann Rev Nutr 1994;14:217–241.
11. Lemon PWR. Dietary protein requirements in athletes. Nutr Biochem 1997;8: 52–60.
12. Lemon PW. Beyond the zone: protein needs of active individuals. J Am Coll Nutr 2000;19(5 Suppl):513S–521S.
13. Tipton KD, Wolfe RR. Protein and amino acids for athletes. J Sports Sci 2004; 22:65–79.
14. Rennie MJ, Tipton KD. Protein and amino acid metabolism during and after exercise and the effects of nutrition. Annu Rev Nutr 2000;20:457–483.
15. Lemon PW. Effect of exercise on protein requirements. J Sports Sci 1991;9 Spec No:53–70.
16. Lemon PW, Proctor DN. Protein intake and athletic performance. Sports Med 1991;12(5):313–325.
17. Rankin JW. Role of protein in exercise. Clin Sports Med 1999;18(3):499–511.
18. Tarnopolsky M. Protein requirements for endurance athletes. Nutrition 2004; 20(7–8):662–668.

19. Lambert CP, Frank LL, Evans WJ. Macronutrient considerations for the sport of bodybuilding. Sports Med 2004;34(5):317–327.

20. Williams MH. Nutrition for Health, Fitness, and Sport. 7th ed. New York: McGraw-Hill; 2005.

21. Burke DG, Chilibeck PD, Davidson KS, Candow DG, Farthing J, Smith-Palmer T. The effect of whey protein supplementation with and without creatine monohydrate combined with resistance training on lean tissue mass and muscle strength. Int J Sport Nutr Exerc Metab 2001;11(3):349–364.

22. Tarnopolsky MA, Atkinson SA, MacDougall JD, Chesley A, Phillips S, Schwarcz H. Evaluation of protein requirements for trained strength athletes. J Appl Physiol 1992;72:1986–1995.

23. Phillips SM, Atkinson SA, Tarnopolsky MA, MacDougall JD. Gender differences in leucine kinetics and nitrogen balance in endurance athletes. J Appl Physiol 1993;75:2134–2141.

24. Campbell WW, Barton ML, Cyr-Campbell D, et al. Effects of an omnivorous diet compared with a lactoovovegetarian diet on resistance-training-induced changes in body composition and skeletal muscle in older men. Am J Clin Nutr 1999;70(6):1032–1039.

25. Phillips SM, Hartman JW, Wilkinson JB. Dietary protein to support anabolism with resistance exercise in young men. J Am Coll Nutr 2005;24(2):134S–139S.

26. Blomstrand E, Saltin B. BCAA intake affects protein metabolism in muscle after but not during exercise in humans. Am J Physiol Endocrinol Metab 2001;281(2):E365–374.

27. Layman DK, Baum JI. Dietary protein impact on glycemic control during weight loss. J Nutr 2004;134(4):968S–973S.

28. Esmarck B, Andersen JL, Olsen S, Richter EA, Mizuno M, Kjaer M. Timing of postexercise protein intake is important for muscle hypertrophy with resistance training in elderly humans. J Physiol 2001;535:301–311.

29. Anderson LL, Tufekovic G, Zebis MK, et al. The effect of resistance training combined with timed ingestion of protein on muscle fiber size and muscle strength. Metabolism 2005;54(2):151–156.

30. Roy BD, Luttmer K, Bosman MJ, Tarnopolsky MA. The influence of post-exercise macronutrient intake on energy balance and protein metabolism in active females participating in endurance training. Int J Sport Nutr Exerc Metab 2002;12(2):172–188.

31. Ivy JL, Goforth HW Jr, Damon BM, McCauley TR, Parsons EC, Price TB. Early post-exercise muscle glycogen recovery is enhanced with carbohydrate-protein supplement. J Appl Physiol 2002;93(4):1337–1344.

32. Zawadzki KM, Yaspelkis BB 3rd, Ivy JL. Carbohydrate-protein complex increases the rate of muscle glycogen storage after exercise. J Appl Physiol 1992;72(5):1854–1859.

33. Williams MB, Raven PB, Fogt DL, Ivy JL. Effects of recovery beverages on glycogen restoration and endurance exercise performance. J Strength Cond Res 2003;17(1):12–19.

34. Carrithers JA, Williamson DL, Gallagher PM, Godard MP, Schulze KE, Trappe SW. Effects of postexercise carbohydrate-protein feedings on muscle glycogen restoration. J Appl Physiol 2000;88(6):1976–1982.

35. Jentjens RL, van Loon LJ, Mann CH, Wagenmakers AJ, Jeukendrup AE. Addition of protein and amino acids to carbohydrates does not enhance postexercise muscle glycogen synthesis. J Appl Physiol 2001;91(2):839–846.

36. Borsheim E, Aarsland A, Wolfe RR. Effect of an amino acid, protein, and carbohydrate mixture on net muscle protein balance after resistance exercise. Int J Sport Nutr Exerc Metab 2004;14(3):255–271.

37. Flakoll PJ, Judy T, Flinn K, Carr C, Flinn S. Postexercise protein supplementation improves health and muscle soreness during basic military training in marine recruits. J Appl Physiol 2004;96:951–956.

38. Tipton KD, Rasmussen BB, Miller SL, et al. Timing of amino acid-carbohydrate ingestion alters anabolic response of muscle to resistance exercise. Am J Physiol 2001;281:E197–E206.

39. Vega-Lopez S, Lichtenstein AH. Dietary protein type and cardiovascular disease risk factors. Prev Cardiol 2005;8(1):31–40.

40. Hu FB, Stampfer MJ, Manson JE, et al. Dietary protein and risk of ischemic heart disease in women. Am J Clin Nutr 1999;70:221–227.

41. Poortmans JR, Dellalieux O. Do regular high protein diets have potential health risks on kidney function in athletes? Int J Sport Exerc Metab 2000;10(1):28–38.

42. Zaragoza R, Renau-Piqueras J, Portoles M, Hernandez-Yago J, Jorda A, Grisolia GS. Rats fed prolonged high protein diets show an increase in nitrogen metabolism and liver megamitochondria. Arch Biochem Biophys 1987;258(2):426–435.

43. Ginty F. Dietary protein and bone health. Proc Nutr Soc 2003;62(4):867–876.

44. New SA. Do vegetarians have normal bone mass? Osteoporos Int 2004;15(9): 679–688.

45. Boirie Y, Dangin M, Gachon P, Vasson MP, Maubois JL, Beaufrere B. Slow and fast dietary proteins differently modulate postprandial protein accretion. Proc Natl Acad Sci USA 1997;94(26):14930–14935.

46. Demling RH, DeSanti L. Effect of hypocaloric diet, increased protein intake and resistance training on lean mass gains and fat mass loss in overweight police officers. Ann Nutr Metab 2000;44(1):21–29.

47. Candow DG, Chilibeck PD, Burke DG, Davison KS, Smith-Palmer T. Effect of glutamine supplementation combined with resistance training in young adults. Eur J Appl Physiol 2001;86(2):142–149.

48. Castell LM. Can glutamine modify the apparent immunodepression observed after prolonged, exhaustive exercise? Nutrition 2002;18(5):371–375.

49. Krzywkowski K, Petersen EW, Ostrowski K, Kristensen JH, Boza J, Pedersen BK. Effect of glutamine supplementation on exercise-induced changes in lymphocyte function. Am J Physiol Cell Physiol 2001;281(4):C1259–1265.

50. Miller AL. Therapeutic considerations of L-glutamine: a review of the literature. Altern Med Rev 1999;4(4):239–248.

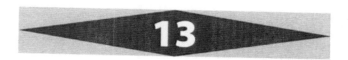

# Fat

## Lonnie Lowery

## OBJECTIVES

On the completion of this chapter you will be able to:

1. Define the major types of fatty acids and relate them to specific food examples.
2. Understand the process by which fat is metabolized.
3. List the steps involved in the metabolism of fatty acids.
4. Describe omega-3, omega-6, and trans fats and their relationship to health and wellness.
5. Discuss the seven potential athletic benefits of manipulating dietary fat content.
6. Explain the relationship between respiratory exchange ratio and respiratory quotient.
7. Discuss the role of fat as a fuel during resting and low-intensity exercise conditions.
8. Understand the effects of high-intensity exercise on fat metabolism.
9. Explain the effect of intensity and duration of exercise on fat metabolism.
10. Understand the effects of increasing exercise intensity on fat metabolism.
11. Explain the two major methods of manipulating dietary fat in an attempt to induce an ergogenic effect.

## ABSTRACT

For decades before the current low-carbohydrate focus pervading public opinion, dietary fat was the primary target of public and academic condemnation. But just as the present trend in macronutrient preference will likely lead to an understanding that the type and not just the amount of carbohydrate matters, so too has awareness grown regarding dietary fat. There are examples. The latest dietary guidelines for Americans has a modified descriptor for total fat intake ("moderate" as opposed to the former "low") and the Harvard School of Public Health has published a radically changed eating pyramid that differs from the longstanding Food Guide Pyramid.[1,2] It flips healthy fat sources such as olive oil and nuts—now near the plentiful bottom—with refined carbohydrates such as white bread and pasta—now limited at the top. More specific to fat type, academicians are discussing saturated fatty acids (not all are equally "bad"), trans fatty acids, monounsaturates, specialty nutraceutical fats, and omega-6 to omega-3 ratio in the diet. It is important for exercise physiology and sports nutrition students to understand the basic chemistry of fat, the metabolism of fat as illustrated by common, whole-body laboratory measurements, and the research regarding biologic systems that are affected by fat. In these ways, one can appreciate the nutritional importance and pharmaceutical-like nature of this macronutrient—and see how it can be applied to athletic endeavors.

From: *Essentials of Sports Nutrition and Supplements*
Edited by J. Antonio, D. Kalman, J. R. Stout, M. Greenwood, D. S. Willoughby, and G. G. Haff © Humana Press, a part of Springer Science+Business Media, Totowa, NJ

**FIGURE 13.1.** A triacylglycerol molecule composed of three fatty acid chains (shown in black) attached to a glycerol "backbone" (shown in light gray).

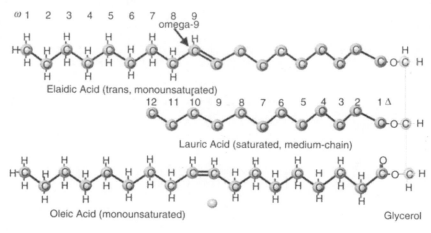

Elaidic Acid (trans, monounsaturated)

Lauric Acid (saturated, medium-chain)

Oleic Acid (monounsaturated)

Glycerol

*Key Words:* **lipids, triglycerides, trans fats, saturated fats, monounsaturated fats, polyunsaturated fats, glycerol, free fatty acids**

## FAT BIOCHEMISTRY: BASIC DEFINITIONS

Before one can make sense of the plethora of fat types and their biologic roles or the research behind the manipulation of fat proportions in the diet, one should start with some definitions.

**Lipids:** A class of compounds consisting of triacylglycerols, sterols, and phospholipids. A full 98% of dietary lipid is constituted of triacylglycerol.

**Triacylglycerol (formerly "triglyceride"):** A glycerol "backbone" molecule with three fatty acids attached (see Figure 13.1). This is the most space- and weight-efficient form of energy storage in the body. One gram of triacylglycerol (TAG) provides 9 kilocalories (kcal) when utilized for energy.[3]

**Glycerol:** A three-carbon molecule that is part of the larger TAG molecule. Glycerol by itself is a three-carbon "sugar" that when released from storage, can be recycled in the liver for the creation of new blood glucose ("gluconeogenesis").

**Fatty acids:** Chains of carbon atoms ("aliphatic chains") of varying lengths that attach to a glycerol molecule to form a TAG. Chains can contain varying numbers and positions of carbon–carbon double bonds, some of which humans cannot make in the body and are thus "essential" in the diet. A fatty acid with no double bonds is called a saturated fatty acid. A chain with one double bond is called a monounsaturated fatty acid. A chain with two or more double bonds comprises a polyunsaturated fatty acid. See Table 13.1 for fat nomenclature of frequently discussed fatty acids.

**TABLE 13.1. Nomenclature of common dietary fatty acids and food sources.**

| Fatty acid (# carbons: # of C=C) | C=C position from methyl (omega) end of chain | C=C position from carboxyl end of chain | Food source |
|---|---|---|---|
| Palmitic acid (168:0) | — | — | Pork fat |
| Stearic acid (18:0) | — | — | Beef fat |
| Oleic acid (18:1) | Omega-9 | cis-9 | Olive oil |
| Trans elaidic acid (18:1) | Omega-9 | trans-9 | Pastries |
| Linoleic acid* (18:2) | Omega-6 | cis-9, cis-12 | Corn oil |
| CLA (18:2) | Varies | cis-9, trans-11 or trans-10, cis-12 | Dairy fat |
| Linolenic acid* (18:3) | Omega-3 | cis-9, cis-12, cis-15 | Flax oil |
| EPA (20:5) | Omega-3 | All cis | Fish oil |
| DHA (22:6) | Omega-3 | All cis | Fish oil |

*Essential fatty acid.

CLA = conjugated linoleic acid, EPA = eicosapentaenoic acid, DHA = docosahexaenoic acid.

## DIETARY FAT

We know that the vast majority of dietary lipid is kilocalorie-dense TAG. With the small exception of a special class called medium-chain TAG (TAG containing fatty acids shorter than 12 carbons in length), these provide a large 9 kcal per gram regardless of type. This is unlike other lipids such as sterols, which do not significantly contribute to kilocalorie intake, and it is more than double the kilocalories provided by carbohydrate and protein at just 4 kcal per gram each.

The digestion, absorption, and storage (or use) of a typical long chain TAG follows the following grossly simplified sequence:

Mouth (lingual lipase) → stomach → duodenum (bile, pancreatic lipase) → ileum → villi → enterocyte → chylomicron packaging → lymphatic system → thoracic duct → large blood vessels → capillaries (lipoprotein lipase) → cells

Once digested fats—packaged into chylomicrons—have reached the cells of their target tissues, they are stored or used depending on one's physiologic state. "Fight or flight" hormones and muscular contractions (up to a point) induce fat breakdown and burning, called lipolysis and oxidation, respectively, whereas "restive–digestive" hormones and relative lack of muscular activity induce fat building/storage, called lipogenesis. Upon reaching the capillary beds of muscle cells (myocytes) or fat cells (adipocytes), circulating chylomicrons interact with the enzyme lipoprotein lipase and release breakdown products of their carried TAG (diacylglycerols and fatty acids) for cellular entry.

## PHARMACOLOGY AND ESSENTIALITY

What makes dietary fats physiologically different than the other major macronutrients? Unlike carbohydrates, which primarily enter cells for storage, fatty acids can become part of the cell membrane. The incorporation of fatty acids into the phospholipid bilayer of the cell membrane leads to membrane fluidity changes and a different prostaglandin cascade that can affect many aspects of physiology, from inflammation to blood clotting to many others (see Sidebar 13.1).[4–6]

The ability of fatty acids to influence physiology in the ways mentioned above can be considered pharmacologic (drug-like) in nature. A primary factor in such pharmacologic effects is the structure of the fatty acids that are enzymatically released (by lipoprotein lipase) from an ingested TAG. Carbon chain length and degree of unsaturation (number of carbon–carbon double bonds along the chain) are important. (See definitions, above.) Furthermore, the position and even the stereochemistry of these carbon–carbon double bonds make critical differences in a fatty acid's pharmacologic effects.

Certain fatty acids are known to be essential because of the inability of humans to synthesize them in the body; thus, these fatty acids must be obtained through the diet from animal and plant species that can synthesize such fats.

## Sidebar 13.1. Potential Athletic Benefits of Manipulating Dietary Fat

- Osteoarthritis and tendonitis improvement (reduced inflammation and breakdown of soft tissues)[5,17–21]
- Muscle recovery[22]
- Reduced catabolic hormone concentrations[23]
- Maintained sex hormone concentrations[24–26]
- Bone preservation[27]
- Resistance to overtraining-induced mental depression[28,29]
- Correction of inadequate energy status (kilocalorie "balance")[30–32]

Humans lack the desaturase enzymes in their tissues to create carbon–carbon double bonds on fatty acids beyond the $C_9$ position.[7] Therefore, the fatty acids essential for humans are linoleic acid (18:2, omega-6) and linolenic acid (18:3, omega-3).

Despite the singular food example of linoleic acid (omega-6) listed in Table 13.1, the typical Western diet has a much larger proportion of these fatty acids—which are known to be proinflammatory—than it does the less common and beneficial omega-3 fatty acids [linolenic acid, eicosapentaenoic acid (EPA), and docosapentaenoic acid (DHA)].[8,9] Unfortunately, the current ratio of omega-6 to omega-3 fatty acids in the diet is closer to 20:1 than the healthful ratio of approximately 7:1 suggested by the Institute of Medicine.[10] These relative amounts are of particular importance because many conditions and diseases of Western society such as obesity, diabetes, and heart disease are now known to be low-grade, systemic inflammatory conditions.[11–13] Thus, public health initiatives should increasingly include education on the health benefits of adding omega-3 fats to the diet, to improve these fatty acid ratios. The American Heart Association is a leading organization in this respect, even recommending intake of EPA/DHA supplements from fish oil for certain populations.[14]

Trans versions of common fatty acids with carbon–carbon double bonds also appear in Table 13.1. Unlike the naturally occurring cis versions, these trans fatty acids are typically the result of food industry alteration. For example, the healthy monounsaturated fatty acid, oleic acid, can be converted under the influence of a catalyst and/or particular commercial cooking procedures to the unhealthy trans fatty acid, elaidic acid. Donuts, French fries, fried chicken, and some partially hydrogenated margarines, are common examples of trans fat-laden foods. Trans fatty acids have been linked to heart disease and inflammation, and are often mentioned as similar to, or even worse than, saturated fatty acids regarding health risks.[15,16] [Special note: conjugated linoleic acid, although technically a trans fatty acid, is sold as a dietary supplement because of its potent health benefits in animal models, making it a highly unusual natural-source trans fat.]

## FAT METABOLISM: REST

Stored cellular fat (as TAG) is the primary fuel source during fasting periods lacking intense physical exertion. Calorimetric research shows that a large percentage (at least 60%) of a human's "fuel mix" at rest—in a fasted state—is from fat usage.[33] Knowing this, one might ask: "Then why don't we all just lounge around in order to get lean?" The answer, of course, is that even a large percentage is unexciting when total caloric expenditure is so low. That is, 60% or even 80% of nothing is still nothing.

But how do we know this percentage at all? It is obtained through laboratory measurements with a device called a metabolic cart (see Figure 13.2). During indirect calorimetry, a type of calorie measurement using gasses rather than direct heat measurements, this large percentage is calculated from the respiratory exchange ratio (RER). This is the ratio of carbon dioxide produced to oxygen consumed, and is a very common—albeit imperfect—laboratory measurement of calorie expenditure and fuel mix. Note the following example:

$$RER = VCO_2/VO_2$$

where V = volume in liters per minute or milliliters per kilogram each minute.

$$RER_{fasted} = (0.220\,L\ CO_2\ \text{exhaled per minute})/$$
$$(0.280\,L\ O_2\ \text{consumed per minute}) = 0.79$$

This RER equates to 70% calorie usage from fat at rest in a fasted state, using a table of known carbohydrate versus fat percentages.[3]

Because fatty acid molecules are "oxygen poor" compared with carbohydrate, much oxygen is consumed in their catabolism ("burning"), thus increasing the denominator of the above equation. A relatively large denominator, of course, results in a lower RER. In our unfed resting example, the denominator

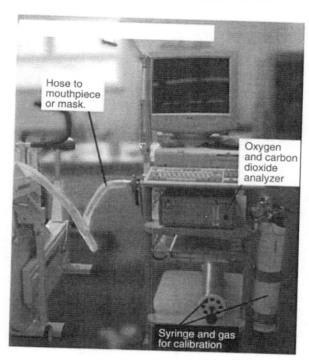

**FIGURE 13.2.** Metabolic cart.

is in fact larger than the numerator, resulting in an RER substantially less than 1.00.

Conversely, in the resting fed state (e.g., after consuming enough carbohydrate), it is possible to watch the RER increase markedly on a metabolic cart, even approaching 1.00. This seems to be attributable to two factors: 1) net fat synthesis rather than breakdown, a state that would result from oxygen liberation as relatively oxygen-rich carbohydrate (glucose) molecules are degraded and reassembled into oxygen-poor fatty acids (called lipogenesis), and 2) production of carbon dioxide during initial glucose breakdown (called glycolysis). These two factors are stimulated by insulin and increase the numerator ($CO_2$) in the RER equation much more than the denominator ($O_2$) as follows:

$$RER_{fed} = (0.305\,L\ CO_2\ \text{exhaled per minute})/$$
$$(0.310\,L\ O_2\ \text{consumed per minute}) = 0.98$$

Bodily fat synthesis (lipogenesis) is not, however, the only way that one's RER can increase dramatically. For somewhat different reasons, very intense exercise can also induce an RER increase, as we will see.

A look at the chemical structure of a fatty acid compared with that of a glucose molecule (the sugar to which ingested carbohydrate degrades in humans) helps a student understand how oxygen usage and carbon dioxide production change on a cellular level (Figure 13.3). At this microscopic level, the RER is

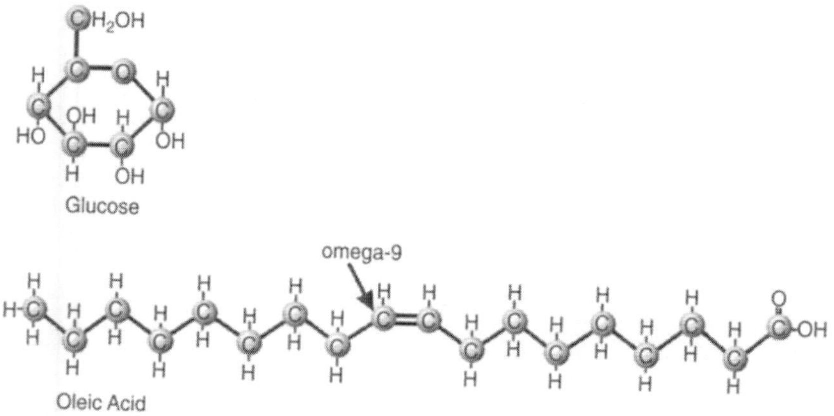

**FIGURE 13.3.** Fatty acid versus glucose comparison (count the oxygen atoms on each).

Glucose

omega-9

Oleic Acid

known as the respiratory quotient, which never actually exceeds 1.00. This limit is sometimes broken on a whole-body systemic level as explained in the next section.

## FAT METABOLISM: EXERCISE

The mobilization and use of stored fatty acids (liberated from stored TAG) change acutely with physical activity. In fact, the physical adaptations of athletes (increased mitochondrial density, increased capillarization, etc.) give them an enhanced capacity to use fat as a fuel. Yet, whether highly trained or sedentary, two phenomena are of note: the effects of exercise duration and the effects of exercise intensity. First, there is a direct relationship between fat use and exercise duration. That is, the longer one exercises at a low–moderate pace, the greater his or her fat breakdown and "burning." Second, and just the opposite, there is an inverse relationship between fat use and exercise intensity. In this latter scenario, the more intensely one exercises, the less stored fat can contribute.

Laboratory measurements such as periodic blood draws and indirect calorimetry during exercise support these two concepts. For example, a student can observe an upward trend in the glycerol content of blood samples taken every 10–20 minutes during exercise. Recall that this glycerol was once the "backbone" of a stored TAG molecule. It has been relieved of its fatty acids, which are increasingly being "burned" (oxidized) in contracting muscles. This same student can also literally watch the RER of the exercising subject slowly decrease on a metabolic cart system as the exercise bout continues. Between these two relatively simple measures, one can witness both TAG breakdown into its component glycerol and fatty acids (lipolysis) and the subsequent oxidation of those liberated fatty acids.

The reverse of these findings generally occurs during highly intense exercise. For example, the RER of a sprinting person meets or exceeds 1.00. Imagine the carbon dioxide numerator (upper number) of our previous equation shooting up dramatically compared with the increase in oxygen use (the denominator). This RER increase with high-intensity exercise signifies a shift from cellular fat metabolism to predominately carbohydrate metabolism, and to the appearance of extra carbon dioxide in the blood from the blood buffer system (bicarbonate, $HCO_3^-$) to counteract the resulting acidity (if the exercise is intense enough). There is no fat catabolism in this case. The abandonment of fat usage is in part attributable to the metabolic demands of the working muscles. Rapidly and strongly contracting muscles require that carbohydrate (primarily glucose stored in the muscle cells as glycogen) be the fuel source.[33,34] This is not only under biochemical control within muscle cells but is related to the fact that intense exercise cannot be prolonged long enough for fat mobilization, transport, uptake, and oxidation to be optimized. Above and beyond this, the glucose breakdown pathway, glycolysis, can ramp up dramatically—even to the point of anaerobic ("without oxygen") metabolism; this is something fatty acids simply cannot do.

Do laboratory practices such as blood sampling for glycerol and RER measures prove that intense exercise is useless in a fat-loss program? Actually, no. Although it is true that intense exercise induces a shift away from fat-specific metabolism (and toward carbohydrate metabolism), other biochemical pathways such as postexercise gluconeogenesis ultimately do result in a replenishment of muscle glycogen and a net loss of body fat. Research comparing brief, intense exercise versus longer, moderate exercise—at least in obese persons—shows that the intensity of the bout matters little regarding whole-body fat loss when total kilocalorie expenditure is controlled.[35] Athletes seem to be little different; a pragmatic look at sprinters reveals extreme leanness despite the acute (bout-specific) biochemistry we have reviewed, which may suggest otherwise at first glance.

Although lower-intensity exercise offers neither cardiovascular conditioning nor body-fat loss that is superior to high-intensity exercise, there is a potential benefit to be considered. The use of less-taxing aerobic exercise, outside of sports-specific training, may be a meaningful way to reduce body fat without degrading overall recovery. Weight-class sports and those sports in which body fat can become a problem (e.g., football linemen) are example targets. By avoiding stress hormone and metabolic thresholds that are known to occur above a moderate intensity (e.g., at the lactate threshold),[36,37] fat-oxidation and caloric expenditure can be achieved with lower-intensity exercise without hindering practice sessions. Indeed, "active recovery" has been shown to actually enhance recuperation such as blood flow to eccentrically damaged muscle, and more acutely, $H^+$ clearance and subsequent work.[38-40] This is of special importance considering that a stale, overtrained state can occur in 30% of team athletes and 48% of individual sport athletes.[41]

## DIETARY FAT MANIPULATION FOR ATHLETIC ENHANCEMENT

Attempts have been made among exercise physiology researchers to use dietary fat as an ergogenic aid. These manipulations have taken two major forms. The first approach is sometimes called fat loading. It involves increasing the amount of fat in the diet (as a percentage of total kilocalorie intake). Providing fat for several days or even immediately before exercise is done in an effort to induce better fat availability and spare glycogen.[42] The second manipulation involves altering the type of fat in the diet rather than the overall amount. This latter approach relies on a more pharmacologic (or at least "functional food") effect as discussed in Sidebar 13.1.

[Note: Both of these fat-related attempts focus on effects that are in addition to maintenance of energy balance and sex hormone concentrations, which are known to be at risk in athletes and are aided by sufficient dietary fat.[24-26,32,43] Such hormonal and energetic support may be of particular interest among the surprising percentage of overtrained athletes.[41,44]]

The first major category of potentially ergogenic fat manipulation essentially involves eating more of it to induce metabolic adaptations. Increasing the amount (proportion) of dietary fat for several days does enhance TAG oxidation and time to exhaustion but conversely seems to make physical effort feel harder. Research shows that despite exhibiting better fat metabolism, subjects' rates of perceived exertion are nonetheless higher after adaptation to a high-fat diet.[45-48] Overall, the scientific literature is mixed regarding this type of ergogenic attempt.[42,46,49-52] Negative findings may be attributable to differences in how ergogenesis is measured (e.g., time to exhaustion versus exercise performances under 1 hour) or perhaps to insufficient carbohydrate intake and subsequent glycogen depletion during days before exercise. Further investigations, such as those that have tried the aforementioned fat loading followed by carbohydrate loading may lead to more consistent results.

The second major category of potentially ergogenic fat manipulation involves altering the type of fat in the diet to achieve ergogenesis via "nutraceutical" means. Acute investigations into performance enhancement such as immediate effects on aerobic capacity or 1 repetition maximums will remain rare, because there is little basis for such a hypothesis. Longer-term nutritional support of athletic recovery or physique enhancement, rather than immediate ergogenesis, seems most promising. For example, Delarue and colleagues[23] found reduced cortisol responses to mental stress in healthy men consuming 7.2 g of fish oils per day. Cortisol is known to be involved in muscle catabolism and intense training,[53] so fish oil supplementation may become beneficial for athletes as well. And although not all researchers agree, muscle-specific recovery may benefit from certain dietary fats. One group of researchers has demonstrated that fish oil in a nutritional supplement can decrease eccentric exercise-induced interleukin (IL)-6 (a proinflammatory cytokine), and C-reactive protein (a marker of inflammation).[22] Others, however, have reported no effects on delayed-onset muscle soreness, hanging arm angle, creatine kinase, cortisol, or IL-6 after 30 days of 1.8 g of fish oil daily.[54] Of the two studies, the former is in better agreement with data on cytokine reductions in other settings,[5,18-20] but time and more athlete-specific research are needed.

The dose and duration of fat administration are of particular interest in dietary fat research. As described, fatty acids integrate with cell membranes and can affect physiologic cascades (prostaglandin and cytokine production); however, this process occurs slowly over a matter of weeks. Slow cell membrane incorporation and fatty acid turnover are demonstrated by the very long "washout" periods for dietary fat which can continue for at least 10–18 weeks.[19,55] Considering the variety of potent biologic effects, this further underscores that duration of dietary fat manipulation must be taken into consideration when determining possible athletic ergogenesis.

A review of all dietary fats and their pharmaceutic properties is beyond the scope of this chapter, but a list of the most promising may be of interest. Common and uncommon dietary fats that may be of benefit to athletes include: oleic acid from olive and canola oils, EPA and DHA from fish oils, linolenic acid from flax and walnuts, gamma-linolenic acid from primrose and borage oils, conjugated linoleic acid from dairy products, medium-chain TAG, structured TAG, and diacylglycerols. These offer health and/or recovery-related benefits via fatty acid structure and length as well as reconfiguration of the natural TAG molecule.

## SUMMARY

Dietary fats are gaining a better reputation among educators and the public, in part because of mounting research that highlights the positive health effects of the various types. Certainly, past research that led to warnings about total fat in the diet, saturated fat, trans fats and even the essential but over-consumed omega-6 fat (linoleic acid found in many vegetable oils) was not wrong. Total fat intake (all types collectively), many saturated fats, and manmade trans fats are still related to certain health consequences. Now, however, it is better understood that not all fats are alike. Much to the contrary—the type of fatty acid and even its arrangement on a TAG molecule are critical in determining its biologic effects.

Dietary fat digestion, absorption, transport, and tissue incorporation are different from the water-soluble macronutrients (carbohydrate and protein). From slowed gastric emptying to lymphatic transport, to cell membrane incorporation and altered prostaglandin function, fats are unique. They are far more than just a rich energy source.

Specific to athletes, moderate amounts of dietary fat, including the less-common healthy varieties, may help support hard training in ways heretofore unrecognized. Possibilities include: antiinflammatory effects (e.g., for tendonitis), preservation of energy balance, bone mass, mental outlook, and sex hormones (e.g., for overtraining syndrome and the "female athlete triad"), reduced cartilage breakdown (e.g., for osteoarthritis), and general whole-body recovery as a result of beneficial effects on catabolic (i.e., muscle wasting) cytokines such as IL-6 and various prostanoids.

Furthermore, exercise duration and intensity greatly affect body-fat biochemistry and thus could be manipulated to improve body composition while enhancing (rather than interfering with) sport-specific training outcomes. As always, exercise specificity remains important and awareness of total training load is necessary. Beyond this, the nutritional, endocrine, and biochemical state of the exerciser should be considered. For example, adding dietary fat to a postworkout nutritional recovery plan, if one wishes, does not seem to interfere with postworkout glycogen recovery and may be included per individual needs.[56]

Regarding ergogenesis, via diet or sports supplements, the scientific literature is still being developed. Research as a whole does not currently support improved exercise performance per se, via either fat loading or via the use of various fat supplements. Further adjustments to the fat-load-followed-by-carb-load concept may lead to a more positive consensus, particularly in certain long-duration events but this is still guesswork. Acute performance benefits from fat supplement ingestion—in either short- or long-duration events—are unlikely, because of the time frames necessary for subcellular changes to occur. Longer-term research with varying doses and in varying species will elucidate the best ways to incorporate these supplements, if at all.

## PRACTICAL APPLICATIONS

1. Healthy athletes should consume 30% of daily caloric requirements from healthy fats while minimizing less healthy fats:
   - Monounsaturate sources such as olive and canola oil (10%–15% of total kilocalories)
   - Omega-6 polyunsaturate sources such as corn oil and safflower oil (6%–7%)
   - Omega-3 polyunsaturate sources such as fish oil, flax oil, walnuts (2%–3%)
   - Saturated fats should be minimized (<10%)
   - Trans fats should be avoided
2. A typical 3000-kcal diet for a college-aged man would thus include 117 g of total fat.
3. If body fat is a concern but so is recovery from sport-specific practice, consider nutrient timing modifications and low- to moderate-intensity aerobic exercise outside of usual sport training.
4. Although they have potent biologic effects that are still being elucidated and exhibit long washout periods (calling for caution), uncommon fats such as fish oils, even in supplemental form, may be advantageous for hard-training athletes. More exercise-specific research is needed.

## ACKNOWLEDGMENTS

Dr. Lowery sincerely thanks his wife, Kelly, for her emotional and editorial support during the writing of this chapter.

## QUESTIONS

1. Which of the following represents an inverse relationship?
   a. Fat breakdown versus exercise duration
   b. Fat breakdown versus exercise intensity
   c. Carbohydrate breakdown versus exercise intensity
   d. None of the above

2. Which is the trans isomer of healthy oleic acid?
   a. Stearic acid
   b. Elaidic acid
   c. Linoleic acid
   d. Linolenic acid

3. How do the less-common fatty acids benefit athletes and health in general?
   a. Altered secretion of cytokines
   b. Altered prostaglandin synthesis
   c. Reduced inflammation
   d. All of the above

4. The favored ratio of omega-6 fatty acids to omega-3 fatty acids is:
   a. 30 : 1 or more
   b. 20 : 1
   c. 15 : 1
   d. 7 : 1 or less

5. Lipolysis means:
   a. Triacylglycerol breakdown
   b. Fatty acid oxidation
   c. Glucose breakdown
   d. Protein breakdown

6. This hormone dramatically slows lipolysis:
   a. Growth hormone
   b. Triiodothyronine
   c. Insulin
   d. Glucagon

7. Which respiratory exchange ratio signifies lipolysis?
   a. 0.99
   b. 0.74
   c. 0.44
   d. None of the above

8. Which respiratory exchange ratio signifies lipogenesis?
   a. 0.99
   b. 0.74
   c. 0.44
   d. None of the above

9. Which respiratory exchange ratio signifies glycolysis during intense exercise?
   a. 0.99
   b. 0.74
   c. 0.44
   d. None of the above

10. Which approach is most likely to benefit hard-training athletes?
    a. Fat loading
    b. Adequate intake of omega-3 fatty acids
    c. Increased intake of omega-6 fatty acids
    d. None of the above

11. This common process underlies many chronic diseases such as diabetes and heart disease and obesity:
    a. Hypermetabolism
    b. Esterification
    c. Inflammation
    d. Hyperandrogenemia

12. The washout period for fish oils is:
    a. 20 minutes or less
    b. 18 days
    c. 4 weeks
    d. 18 weeks or more

13. Eicosapentaenoic acid and docosapentaenoic acid are examples of which type of fatty acid?
    a. Omega-3
    b. Omega-6
    c. Omega-9
    d. Omega-13

14. This hormone inhibits insulin release during exercise, allowing for continued lipolysis even while drinking a mid-workout carbohydrate beverage:
    a. Epinephrine (adrenaline)
    b. Parathyroid hormone
    c. Arginine vasopressin (antidiuretic hormone)
    d. Testosterone

15. Which is the richest source of omega-6 fatty acids?
    a. Fish oil
    b. Corn oil

c. Olive oil

d. Beef fat

16. Which fatty acid is saturated?
    a. Linolenic acid
    b. Stearic acid
    c. Lauric acid
    d. b and c

17. Which has the longest aliphatic (carbon–carbon) chain?
    a. Glycerol
    b. Lauric acid
    c. Stearic acid
    d. Docosahexaenoic acid

18. Athletes possess an improved capacity to "burn" fat because of:
    a. Increased mitochondrial density in cells
    b. Increased capillarization in tissues
    c. Larger cardiac output
    d. All of the above

19. Fats uncommon in the diet such as conjugated linoleic acid in dairy (and supplements) or gamma-linolenic acid from primrose and borage oils are sometimes questioned because of:
    a. Still inconclusive human data
    b. Toxicity in animal studies
    c. No benefits in animal studies
    d. Indigestible qualities

20. Dietary fats and fat supplements are best applied to athletes in what way?
    a. Taken as a preworkout anabolic boost
    b. Taken mid-workout to suppress inflammatory cytokines
    c. Taken for longer-term, chronic recovery and health
    d. Taken as a preworkout fat-loss measure

21. Mild–moderate exercise is vastly superior to intense exercise for body fat control.
    a. True
    b. False

22. All saturated fats are equally detrimental to health.
    a. True
    b. False

23. Stearic acid is an example of a medium-chain triacylglycerol.
    a. True
    b. False

24. The respiratory exchange ratio and respiratory quotient are identical.
    a. True
    b. False

25. A respiratory exchange ratio greater than 1.00 can be achieved because of added $CO_2$ production by the blood buffer system.
    a. True
    b. False

26. Time to exhaustion is the criterion measure for most endurance sports.
    a. True
    b. False

27. Total fat intake is related to diseases such as cancer.
    a. True
    b. False

28. The percentage of fat usage in one's "fuel mix" is the greatest determinant of body-fat reduction.
    a. True
    b. False

29. Healthy fats have fewer kilocalories per gram.
    a. True
    b. False

30. Maintaining fat at 30% (upper end of *Institute of Medicine* recommendations http://www.iom.edu/?id = 4340&redirect = 0) of dietary intake (e.g., about 100 g daily) can help maintain sex hormone concentrations.
    a. True
    b. False

## REFERENCES

1. Gifford K. Dietary fats, eating guides, and public policy: history, critique, and recommendations. Am J Med 2002;113(Suppl 9B):89S–106S.
2. Harvard School of Public Health. Nutrition Book Author Willet Rebuilds USDA Food Pyramid. Harvard Public Health NOW. Roache C, ed. August 4, 2001; Available at: http://www.hsph.harvard.edu/now/aug24/index.
3. Zuntz N. Die bedeutung de verschiendenen nahrstoffe als erzeuger der muskelkraft. Pflugers Arch Physiol 1901;83:557. In: McArdle W, Katch F, Katch V, eds. Exercise Physiology. Philadelphia: Lea & Febiger; 1991:153.
4. Ehringer W, Belcher D, Wassall S, Stillwell W. A comparison of the effects of linolenic (18:3 omega 3) and docosahexaenoic (22:6 omega 3) acids on phospholipid bilayers. Chem Phy Lipids 1990;54(2):79–88.
5. Calder P. Polyunsaturated fatty acids, inflammation, and immunity. Lipids 2001; 36(9):1007–1024.
6. Masley S. Diet therapy for preventing and treating coronary artery disease. Am Fam Physician 1998;57(6):1299–1306.
7. Salway J. Metabolism at a Glance. London: Blackwell Scientific Publications; 1994.
8. Mann NJ, Johnson LG, Warrick GE, Sinclair AJ. The arachidonic acid content of the Australian diet is lower than previously estimated. J Nutr 1995;125(10): 2528–2535.
9. Simopoulos A. The importance of the ratio of omega-6/omega-3 essential fatty acids. Biomed Pharmacother 2002;56(8):365–379.
10. Institute of Medicine. Dietary Reference Intakes for Energy, Carbohydrate, Fiber, Fat, Fatty Acids, Cholesterol, Protein, and Amino Acids. Washington, DC: National Academies Press; 2002:335–432.
11. Schmidt M, Duncan B. Diabesity: an inflammatory metabolic condition. Clin Chem Lab Med 2003;41(9):1120–1130.
12. Wallace J. If heart disease is an inflammatory disease, what about the risk factors? Am Soc Exerc Physiol Natl Mtg, April 2, 2004.
13. Yudkin JS, Kumari M, Humphries SE, Mohamed-Ali V. Inflammation, obesity, stress and coronary heart disease: is interleukin-6 the link? Atherosclerosis 2000;148(2): 209–214.
14. American Heart Association. AHA scientific statement: fish consumption, fish oil, omega-3 fatty acids and cardiovascular disease, #71–0241. *Circulation* 2002;106: 2747–2757.
15. Lichtenstein AH. Dietary trans fatty acid. J Cardiopulm Rehabil 2000;20(3): 143–146.
16. Popkin BM, Siega-Riz AM, Haines PS, Jahns L. Dietary intake of trans fatty acids and systemic inflammation in women. Am J Clin Nutr 2004;79(4):606–612.
17. Browning L. n-3 polyunsaturated fatty acids, inflammation and obesity-related disease. Proc Nutr Soc 2003;62(2):447–453.
18. Endres S. n-3 polyunsaturated fatty acids and human cytokine synthesis. Lipids 1996;31(Suppl):S239–S242.
19. Endres S, Ghorbani R, Kelley V, et al. The effect of dietary supplementation with n-3 polyunsaturated fatty acids on the synthesis of interleukin-1 and tumor necrosis factor by mononuclear cells. N Engl J Med 1989;320(5):265–271.
20. Calder P. n-3 polyunsaturated fatty acids and cytokine production in health and disease. Ann Nutr Metab 1997;41(4):203–234.

21. Curtis C, Hughes C, Flannery C, Little C, Harwood J, Caterson B. n-3 fatty acids specifically modulate catabolic factors involved in articular cartilage degradation. J Biol Chem 2000;275(2):721–724.

22. Phillips T, Childs A, Dreon D, Phinney S, Leeuwenburgh C. A dietary supplement attenuates IL-6 and CRP after eccentric exercise in untrained males. Med Sci Sports Exerc 2003;35(12):2032–2037.

23. Delarue J, Matzinger O, Binnert C, Schneiter P, Chiolero R, Tappy L. Fish oil prevents the adrenal activation elicited by mental stress in healthy men. Diabetes Metab 2003;29(3):289–295.

24. Dorgan J, Judd J, Longcope C, et al. Effects of dietary fat and fiber on plasma and urine androgens and estrogens in men: a controlled feeding study. Am J Clin Nutr 1996;64(6):850–855.

25. Hamalainen E, Adlercreutz H, Puska P, Pietinen P. Decrease of serum total and free testosterone during a low-fat high-fibre diet. J Steroid Biochem 1983;18(3): 369–370.

26. Reed M, Cheng R, Simmonds M, Richmond W, James V. Dietary lipids: an additional regulator of plasma levels of sex hormone binding globulin. J Clin Endocrinol Metab 1987;64(5):1083–1085.

27. Albertazzi P, Coupland K. Polyunsaturated fatty acids. Is there a role in postmenopausal osteoporosis prevention? Maturitas 2002;42(1):13–22.

28. Logan A. Neurobehavioral aspects of omega-3 fatty acids: possible mechanisms and therapeutic value in major depression. Altern Med Rev 2003;8(4):410–425.

29. Su K, Huang S, Chiu C, Shen W. Omega-3 fatty acids in major depressive disorder. A preliminary double-blind, placebo-controlled trial. Eur Neuropsychopharmacol 2003;13(4):267–271.

30. Lowery L. Dietary fat and sports nutrition: a primer. J Sports Sci Med 2004;3(3): 106–117.

31. Hinton P, Sanford T, Davidson M, Yakushko O, Beck N. Nutrient intakes and dietary behaviors of male and female collegiate athletes. Int J Sport Nutr Exerc Metab 2004;14:389–398.

32. Burke L. Energy needs of athletes. Can J Appl Physiol 2001;26(Suppl):S202–S219.

33. Brooks GA. Importance of the 'crossover' concept in exercise metabolism. Clin Exp Pharmacol Physiol 1997;24(11):889–895.

34. Sidossis LS, Gastaldelli A, Klein S, Wolfe RR. Regulation of plasma fatty acid oxidation during low- and high-intensity exercise. *Am J Physiol* 1997;272(6 Pt 1): E1065–E1070.

35. Ballor DL, McCarthy JP, Wilterdink EJ. Exercise intensity does not affect the composition of diet- and exercise-induced body mass loss. Am J Clin Nutr 1990;51(2): 142–146.

36. Yarasheski K. Growth hormone effects on metabolism, body composition, muscle mass, and strength. Exerc Sport Sci Rev 1994;22:285–312.

37. Gabriel H, Schwartz L, Steffens G, Kindermann W. Immunoregulatory hormones, circulating leukocyte and lymphocyte subpopulations before and after endurance exercise at different intensities. Int J Sports Med 1992;13(5):359–366.

38. Tiidus P, Shoemaker J. Effleurage massage, muscle blood flow and long-term post-exercise strength recovery. Int J Sports Med 1995;16(7):478–483.

39. Coffey V, Leveritt M, Gill N. Effect of recovery modality on 4-hour repeated treadmill running performance and changes in physiological variables. J Sci Med Sport 2004;7(1):1–10.

40. Spierer D, Goldsmith R, Baran D, Hryniewicz K, Katz S. Effects of active versus passive recovery on work performed during serial supramaximal exercise tests. Int J Sports Med 2004;25(2):109–114.

41. Kentta G, Hassmen P, Raglin JS. Training practices and overtraining syndrome in Swedish age-group athletes. Int J Sports Med 2001;22(6):460–465.

42. Hargreaves M, Hawley J, Jeukendrup A. Pre-exercise carbohydrate and fat ingestion: effects on metabolism and performance. J Sports Sci 2004;22(1):31–38.

43. Venkatraman J, Leddy J, Pendergast D. Dietary fats and immune status in athletes: clinical implications. Med Sci Sports Exerc 2000;32(7 Suppl):S389–S395.

44. Roberts A, McClure R, Weiner R, Brooks G. Overtraining affects male reproductive status. Fertil Steril 1993;60(4):686–692.

45. Zderic T, Davidson C, Schenk S, Byerley L, Coyle E. High-fat diet elevates resting intramuscular triglyceride concentration and whole body lipolysis during exercise. Am J Physiol Endocrinol Metab 2004;286(2):E217–E225.

46. Fleming J, Sharman M, Avery N, et al. Endurance capacity and high-intensity exercise performance responses to a high fat diet. Int J Sport Nutr Exerc Metab 2003; 13(4):466–478.

47. Stepto N. Effect of short term fat adaptation on high intensity training. Med Sci Sports Exerc 2002;34(3):449–455.

48. Volek J, Sharman M, Love D, et al. Body composition and hormonal responses to a carbohydrate-restricted diet. Metabolism 2002;51(7):864–870.

49. Venkatraman J, Feng X, Pendergast D. Effects of dietary fat and endurance exercise on plasma cortisol, prostaglandin E2, interferon-gamma and lipid peroxides in runners. J Am College Nutr 2001;20(5):529–536.

50. Venkatraman J, Rowland J, Denardin E, Horvath P, Pendergast D. Influence of the level of dietary lipid intake and maximal exercise on the immune status in runners. Med Sci Sports Exerc 1997;29(3):333–344.

51. Horvath P, Eagen C, Fisher N, Leddy J, Pendergast D. The effects of varying dietary fat on performance and metabolism in trained male and female runners. J Am College Nutr 2000;19(1):52–60.

52. Hawley J, Burke L, Angus D, Fallon K, Martin D, Febbraio M. Effect of altering substrate availability on metabolism and performance during intense exercise. Br J Nutr 2000;84(6):829–838.

53. Urhausen A, Gabriel H, Kindermann W. Blood hormones as markers of training stress and overtraining. Sports Med 1995;20(4):251–276.

54. Lenn J, Uhl T, Mattacola C, et al. The effects of fish oil and isoflavones on delayed onset muscle soreness. Med Sci Sports Exerc 2002;34(10):1605–1613.

55. Kremer J, Jubiz W, Michalek A, et al. Fish-oil fatty acid supplementation in active rheumatoid arthritis: a double-blinded, controlled, crossover study. Ann Intern Med 1987;106:497–503.

56. Fox A, Kaufman A, Horowitz J. Adding fat calories to meals after exercise does not alter glucose tolerance. J Appl Physiol 2004;97(1):11–16.

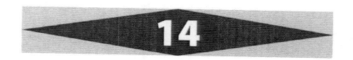

# Carbohydrates

## G. Gregory Haff

## OBJECTIVES

On the completion of this chapter you will be able to:

1. Differentiate among the different types of carbohydrates that are present in the diet.
2. Give examples of the different types of carbohydrates present in the diet.
3. Define the glycemic index and give glycemic index values for selected foods.
4. Define the glycemic load and give glycemic load values for selected foods.
5. Understand the different metabolic pathways associated with the metabolism of carbohydrates.
6. Explain the process by which anaerobic and aerobic exercise bouts are fueled.
7. Discuss why it is important to replenish carbohydrate stores and relate the rate of replenishment to the amount of carbohydrates in the diet.
8. Appreciate the glycogen depletion theory of overtraining.
9. Describe the effects of low carbohydrate diets on anaerobic exercise performance and muscle glycogen stores.
10. Describe the effects of low carbohydrate diets on aerobic exercise performance and muscle glycogen stores.
11. Recommend carbohydrate content needed to meet the exercise demands of athletes who are participating in aerobic and anaerobic training bouts.

## ABSTRACT

One of the fastest growing trends in current dietary concepts is that of the low carbohydrate diet. These diets promise everything from weight loss to improved athletic performance.[2,3] The concept of a low carbohydrate diet is not a new development; in fact, the first notation of a low carbohydrate diet can be traced to the middle of the fifth century. At this time, Stymphalos, a two-time Olympic victor in long-distance running is the first documented case of an athlete using a high-protein, low-carbohydrate diet in an attempt to maximize performance.[4–7] Additionally, the famous Greek wrestler, Milo of Croton, a five-time Olympic champion who competed from 536 to 520 B.C. is reported to have consumed a diet that was low in carbohydrates and high in protein content.[3,8] Currently, many modern athletes are now touting the accolades of the low carbohydrate diet. Proponents of the modern low carbohydrate diet revolution often attack the carbohydrate as being behind the growing obesity trends in the United States[9–12] and promote a reduction in dietary carbohydrate content as a means for enhancing athletic performance.[5,9,13–17] However, many

From: *Essentials of Sports Nutrition and Supplements*
Edited by J. Antonio, D. Kalman, J. R. Stout, M. Greenwood, D. S. Willoughby, and G. G. Haff © Humana Press, a part of Springer Science+Business Media, Totowa, NJ

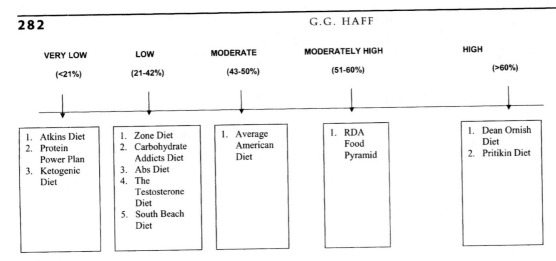

| VERY LOW | LOW | MODERATE | MODERATELY HIGH | HIGH |
|----------|-----|----------|-----------------|------|
| (<21%) | (21-42%) | (43-50%) | (51-60%) | (>60%) |

| | | | | |
|---|---|---|---|---|
| 1. Atkins Diet<br>2. Protein Power Plan<br>3. Ketogenic Diet | 1. Zone Diet<br>2. Carbohydrate Addicts Diet<br>3. Abs Diet<br>4. The Testosterone Diet<br>5. South Beach Diet | 1. Average American Diet | 1. RDA Food Pyramid | 1. Dean Ornish Diet<br>2. Pritikin Diet |

**FIGURE 14.1.** Types of diets. (Modified from Riley,[125] Haff and Whitley.[66])

sports nutritionists and sports scientists have demonstrated the value of carbohydrate in the diet of athletes and continue to promote diets that are rich in carbohydrate content.[2,5,6,18–20] Overall, there seems to be an increased interest in the use of nutrition as a method for improving health, wellness, and sports performance.[5,7,10,11,21–23] With this increased interest, a wide variety of diets have been proposed as methods for dealing with obesity, health wellness, and improving athletic performance (Figure 14.1). Generally, we can classify these diets into categories, which are based on the percentage of dietary carbohydrate supplied by the diet. The categories used to classify these diets range from those that require sparse carbohydrate consumption to those that are rich in carbohydrate content. At present, there is a large debate about the efficacy of the different diets available and their relationship to actual athletic performance. This chapter begins with a detailed discussion that examines the different types of carbohydrates that can be utilized in an athlete's diet. This will include an in-depth look at the concept of the glycemic index and its relationship to the different sources of carbohydrate available in an athletic diet. At this point, how carbohydrates are metabolized are explored in an attempt to clarify why they are important during aerobic and high-intensity exercise such as resistance training. After completing the discussions about the types of carbohydrates and how they are metabolized, the dietary carbohydrate needs of the endurance and strength/power athlete are addressed.

*Key Words:* **carbohydrate, monosaccharides, polysaccharides, glycemic load, glycemic index, glycogen, glycolysis, glycogen depletion, carbohydrate loading**

## CARBOHYDRATES

Carbohydrates, or saccharides, are groups of molecules that are created from carbon, hydrogen, and oxygen atoms. These groups of molecules are generally represented by the simple stoichiometric formula $(CH_2O)_n$, with variations in this basic chemical formula determining the complexity of the carbohydrate molecule. Generally, carbohydrates are divided into three major categories: monosaccharides, oligosaccharides, and polysaccharides. Table 14.1 provides examples of the three major categories of carbohydrates.

**TABLE 14.1.** General classifications and examples of common carbohydrates.

| Monosaccharides | | Oligosaccharides | Polysaccharides | |
|---|---|---|---|---|
| *Pentoses $C_5H_{10}O_5$* | *Hexoses $C_6H_{12}O_6$* | *Disaccharides $C_{12}H_{22}O_{11}$* | *Hexosans $(C_6H_{10}O_6)n^2$* | *Mixed polysaccharides* |
| Ribose | Fructose | Lactose | Cellulose | Pectin |
| Deoxyribose | Galactose | Maltose | Glycogen | Hemicelluloses |
| | Glucose | Sucrose | Starch (amylose and amylopectin) | |

*Source:* Modified from McArdle et al.[50]

**TABLE 14.2. Monosaccharide nomenclature.**

| Name | Number of carbons |
|------|-------------------|
| Trioses | 3 |
| Tetroses | 4 |
| Pentoses | 5 |
| Hexoses | 6 |
| Heptoses | 7 |

*Note:* The term "ose" identifies these as sugars.

## Monosaccharides

Monosaccharides (mono meaning "one" and saccharide meaning "sugar") are the simplest carbohydrate molecules and are often classified as the basic unit of all carbohydrates because they contain only one subunit of sugar. These simple carbohydrate molecules often have a sweet taste and are classified by the number of carbon atoms they have in their structures. Generally, these carbohydrate molecules have between 3 and 7 carbon atoms and are thus termed based upon this number (Table 14.2).[1,12,24–46]

The three most important monosaccharides from a nutritional standpoint are glucose, fructose, and galactose (Figure 14.2). Glucose is the most common mechanism for transport of carbohydrates in the body and is sometimes referred to as blood sugar. It is naturally occurring in food or is the end product of the breakdown of more complex carbohydrates. Additionally, some glucose is synthesized in small amounts in the liver from amino acids, glycerol, pyruvate, and lactate in a process called gluconeogenesis.[16,17,27–29] Overall, glucose is very

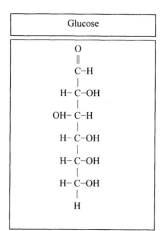

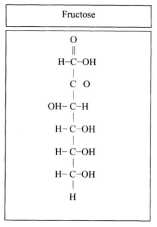

**FIGURE 14.2.** Three most important monosaccharides.

easily broken down by the body and can be 1) used as a fuel substrate to supply energy, 2) stored as muscle or liver glycogen, or 3) converted to triglycerides and stored for later use.

The second monosaccharide of nutritional importance is fructose, or as it is sometimes termed, levulose. Fructose is found in fruits, honey, and high fructose corn syrup. Fructose is generally directly taken from the digestive tract into the blood stream where it eventually is converted into glucose in the liver.[18,19,30] Fructose is considered to be the sweetest of the monosaccharides and high fructose corn syrup is a major component of soft drinks and many other deserts. Recent research has suggested that high fructose corn syrup consumption has increased from 0.8 g·person·day$^{-1}$ in 1970 to 91.6 g·person·day$^{-1}$ in 2000.[20,31] This increase in high fructose corn syrup consumption may be of particular interest because of its relationship to the obesity epidemic currently affecting the United States and many other countries throughout the world.[21,22,31] The consumption of high fructose corn syrup for as little as 3 weeks can result in significant increases in caloric intake and body weight in both genders.[23,32]

The final nutritionally important monosaccharide is galactose. Generally, galactose is not found in any large quantities in nature, but is usually combined with glucose to form the disaccharide lactose or milk sugar. The galactose that is free in nature is absorbed into the body and taken to the liver where it is directly converted to glucose. After galactose is converted to glucose, it is immediately used as a fuel source or is stored as glycogen.

## Oligosaccharides

When monosaccharides are bound together, they can form more complex carbohydrates such as oligosaccharides. Generally, the major oligosaccharide is the disaccharides, or double sugars, as they are sometimes called. Disaccharides are created from the chemical bonding of 2–10 monosaccharides.[1] All disaccharides contain glucose and generally are represented by sucrose, lactose, and maltose.

Sucrose is the most common disaccharide that occurs naturally and is often termed table sugar, beet sugar, or cane sugar. Large quantities of sucrose are found in plants such as sugar cane, sugar beets, and maple syrup. Additionally, fruits and vegetables can contain naturally occurring sucrose. Natural occurring forms of sucrose can be purified and are often sold as brown, white, and powdered sugar in many supermarkets or grocery stores. As with fructose, sucrose consumption may also have a role in contributing to the obesity epidemic. In a recent study, subjects who consumed a sucrose supplement over a 10-week period experienced a 1.6-kg increase in body mass in conjunction with a 1.3-kg increase in body fat.[24,33]

Another common disaccharide is lactose, which is formed from the combination of glucose and galactose. Lactose, or milk sugar, is not found in plants and only exists in milk from lactating animals. In some instances, lactose can be a difficult oligosaccharide to digest resulting in excessive fluid and gas build up in the bowels,[25,34] bloating,[26,35] and cramping.[28,35] Lactose intolerance is considered to be a normal physiologic occurrence[29,34,36] and generally occurs because of a deficiency in the amount of the lactose-digesting enzyme lactase.[35] Deficiencies in lactase are very prevalent in northern Europeans (2%–15%), central Europeans (9%–23%), white Americans (6%–22%), Hispanics (50%–80%), blacks (60%–80%), and Asians (95%–100%).[37] Individuals who have a deficiency in the lactase enzyme need to avoid milk products and be conscious of "hidden" sources of lactose. Trace amounts of lactose may be found in baked goods, cereals, and salad dressings.[35]

The final common disaccharide is maltose, which is created by the combination of two molecules of glucose. Maltose is also sometimes referred to as malt sugar and is produced when seeds sprout. The production of maltose by seeds occurs so that the plant can initiate growth. The sprouting process can be altered with the introduction of heat in a method, which is termed malting. This process is considered the first step in the production of alcoholic beverages such a beer. Malting results in the formation of the enzymes α-amylase and maltase.[38] These enzymes are capable of degrading starch into maltose and other simple sugars. Ultimately, the malt is manipulated into a form, which is termed the wort and is combined with yeast, that initiates the fermentation process. The fermentation process then converts most of the carbohydrates to ethanol and carbon dioxide.[1,38] Very few beverages and food products other than alcohol contain maltose. However, maltose can be produced in the small intestine from the digestion of starches.

## Polysaccharides

Polysaccharides are considered complex carbohydrate molecules. Generally, polysaccharides are linear or complex branching chains that are composed of more than 10 monosaccharides that have been bonded together (Figure 14.3). Polysaccharides that are composed of one type of monosaccharides are termed homopolysaccharides, whereas polysaccharides that contain two or more different types of monosaccharides are termed heteropolysaccharides.[1] Polysaccharides can come from either plant or animal sources.

**FIGURE 14.3.** Types of polysaccharides.

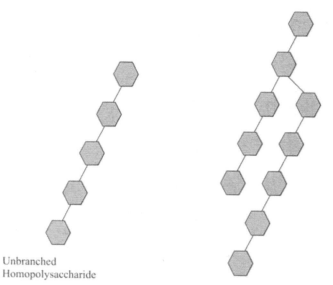

Unbranched
Homopolysaccharide

Branched Homopolysaccharide

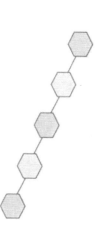

Unbranched Heteropolysaccharide

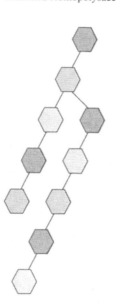

Branched Heteropolysaccharide

## PLANT POLYSACCHARIDES

When examining plant polysaccharides, the two most common forms are starch and fiber. Starch is the storage form of carbohydrates in plants, which exists in two forms: 1) amylose, and 2) amylopectin.[1] Amylose, a linear polymer chain, and amylopectin, a highly branched polymer chain, each can contain several thousand glucose molecules. It seems that the relative proportions of amylose and amylopectin in a plant effect the plants specific characteristics, such as its ability to be digested. Generally, amylose and amylopectin can be found in food sources such as seeds, corn, grains, cereal, potatoes, beans, breads, pastas, and rice.[39] Starches that contain high levels of amylopectin tend to have a high glycemic index (see discussion of the glycemic index in a later section of this chapter), which is represented as a rapid increase in blood glucose.[40,41] The rapid increase of blood glucose associated with amylopectin may partially be explained by the large number of branches found in its structure, which allows many areas for digestive enzymes to break down the starch.

Fiber is considered a nonstarch structural polysaccharide that may be the most abundant organic molecule on earth. The primary components of these nonstarch polysaccharides are cellulose, hemicelluloses, pectins, gums, and mucilages. These structural components are found only in plants and are not digested by the human stomach or small intestine.[39]

## ANIMAL POLYSACCHARIDES

The primary animal polysaccharide is glycogen. Glycogen is a homopolysaccharide that is stored in either the skeletal muscle or the liver and is composed of subunits of glucose. The synthesis of glycogen occurs as a result of adding individual glucose units to an existing glycogen chain. One unique characteristic of a glycogen molecule is that it contains extensively linked branches (Figure 14.4). Generally, branches occur on every 8–12 residues on the glycogen molecule. The branching of the glycogen molecule is particularly important because this type of structure allows for a very rapid breakdown of the molecule to its individual glucose subunits. This rapid degradation of the glycogen molecule, known as glycogenolysis, occurs as a result of many enzymes working on the glycogen molecule at one time.[1] Interestingly, the more extensively

**FIGURE 14.4.** Example of glycogen molecule.

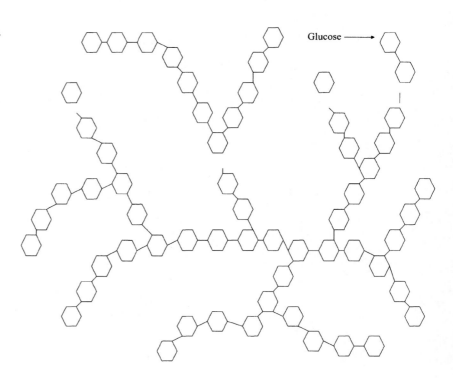

Glucose ⟶

branched the glycogen molecule is, the greater the ability it has to rapidly supply energy.[42]

When looking at the actual storage of glycogen in the body, Felig and Wahren[43] report that a nonobese man weighing 70 kg stores about 350 g of muscle glycogen and 40–50 g of liver glycogen. Because each gram of glycogen or glucose provides approximately 4 calories of energy, the 70-kg man who consumes a normal diet would store about 1600 kcals of energy in the body.[44,45] The amount of carbohydrates stored in the body may be of particular interest during exercise, because the primary supplier of energy during most forms of exercise is carbohydrate, specifically in the form of glycogen.[46] This suggests that glycogen availability may be of particular interest or concern to the competitive athlete.

## Glycemic Index

The glycemic index is an important concept to consider when looking at carbohydrates, because it reflects the metabolic response of the body to a carbohydrate rather than its chemical or structural makeup. Generally, the glycemic index is a ranking system that is used to compare the acute glycemic impact of foods.[47] Foods that are quantified as having a high glycemic index are digested quickly and appear rapidly in the bloodstream as glucose. Conversely, foods that are digested more slowly and appear in the blood stream as glucose at a slower rate are quantified with a lower glycemic index ranking.[47] The glycemic index ranking is based on a standard food such as glucose or white bread, which is given an arbitrary glycemic index ranking of 100.[48] To determine the glycemic index of a carbohydrate, the carbohydrate's 2-hour glucose response curve is compared with 50 g of carbohydrate from a control food such as white bread or glucose.[49] The glycemic index for a particular carbohydrate is primarily impacted by the rate at which the food is digested.[50] The type of carbohydrate,[51] the fiber content, the portion of food, and the fat or protein content of the food[14] all influence the rate of digestion for a particular food.

Recent scientific evidence examining the glycemic response to specific foods suggests that a diet that is centered on low glycemic index carbohydrates might be useful in the prevention of obesity,[50–52] coronary heart disease,[53] colon cancer,[54] and breast cancer.[55] Table 14.3 lists several foods and their glycemic index rankings.

**TABLE 14.3. Glycemic index (GI) and glycemic loads (GL) of various foods using white bread (GI = 100) as a standard.**

| Source | GI | GL | Source | GI | GL |
|---|---|---|---|---|---|
| Bakery products | | | Fruits (continued) | | |
| Angel food cake | 95 | 19 | Peaches | 60 | 5 |
| Croissant | 96 | 17 | Pears | 47 | 4 |
| Doughnut (cake) | 108 | 17 | Pineapples | 94 | 6 |
| Bran muffin | 85 | 15 | Plums | 34 | 3 |
| Scones | 131 | 7 | Watermelon | 103 | 4 |
| Beverages | | | Legumes | | |
| Coca Cola | 76 | 14 | Baked beans | 69 | 7 |
| Gatorade | 111 | 12 | Chickpeas | 47 | 10 |
| Orange juice | 71 | 13 | Kidney beans | 41 | 7 |
| Smoothie, raspberry | 48 | 14 | Lentils | 41 | 5 |
| Breads | | | Pasta and noodles | | |
| Bagel | 103 | 25 | Linguine | 65 | 22 |
| Baguette (French) | 136 | 15 | Macaroni | 67 | 23 |
| Pita bread | 82 | 10 | Spaghetti | 59 | 20 |
| Rye bread | 58 | 5 | | | |
| Breakfast cereals | | | Snack foods | | |
| All bran | 54 | 9 | Corn chips | 103 | 18 |
| Corn Flakes | 130 | 24 | Jelly beans | 112 | 22 |
| Grapenuts | 107 | 16 | M & M (peanut) | 47 | 6 |
| Life | 94 | 14 | Peanuts | 21 | 1 |
| Special K | 98 | 14 | Popcorn | 103 | 8 |
| | | | Potato chips | 77 | 11 |

*(Continued)*

TABLE 14.3. *Continued*

| Source | GI | GL | Source | GI | GL |
|---|---|---|---|---|---|
| Cereal grains and pasta | | | Powerbar (chocolate) | 79 | 24 |
| Barley | 36 | 11 | Pretzels | 119 | 16 |
| Brown rice | 79 | 18 | Skittles | 100 | 32 |
| Cracked wheat | 68 | 12 | Snickers bar | 78 | 19 |
| White rice (long grain) | 80 | 24 | | | |
| | | | Sugars | | |
| Dairy foods | | | Fructose | 27 | 2 |
| Ice cream | 87 | 8 | Glucose | 141 | 10 |
| Ice cream (low fat) | 71 | 3 | Honey | 78 | 10 |
| Milk (full fat) | 38 | 3 | Lactose | 66 | 5 |
| Milk (skim) | 46 | 4 | Maltose | 150 | 11 |
| Yogurt (artificial sweetener) | 20 | 2 | Sucrose | 97 | 7 |
| Fruits | | | Vegetables | | |
| Apples | 52 | 6 | Corn | 78 | 9 |
| Banana | 74 | 12 | Carrots | 131 | 5 |
| Cherries | 32 | 3 | Peas | 68 | 3 |
| Grapefruit | 36 | 3 | Potato (baked) | 121 | 26 |
| Grapes | 62 | 7 | Sweet potato | 87 | 17 |
| Oranges | 60 | 5 | Yam | 53 | 13 |

*Source:* Adapted from Foster-Powell et al.[38]

## Glycemic Load

The glycemic load was first introduced by researches from Harvard University.[56] These researchers have reported that the glycemic load is an independent predictor of an individual's risk for developing Type 2 diabetes[56] and coronary heart disease.[53] The glycemic load is defined as the produce of the glycemic index and the carbohydrate content in a serving of carbohydrate.[56,57] Salmeron et al.[56] suggest that the glycemic load is a variable that represents the quality and quantity of a carbohydrate. The higher the glycemic load for the carbohydrate, the greater the expected increase in blood glucose, which would then result in a significantly greater increase in circulating insulin.[48,57] Diets that get the majority of their carbohydrates from high glycemic load sources are associated with increased risk of Type 2 diabetes and coronary heart disease.[53]

## CARBOHYDRATE METABOLISM

When looking at the ways that carbohydrate can be metabolized there are three basic pathways that can be differentiated. The first two pathways are anaerobic (glycolysis and glycogenolysis) and require no oxygen to produce energy, whereas the third metabolic pathway is termed oxidative metabolism because of its reliance on the availability of oxygen to produce energy.

### Glycolysis and Glycogenolysis

Glycolysis is the metabolic pathway that results in the breakdown of blood glucose to produce adenosine triphosphate (ATP),[1,42] whereas glycogenolysis is the process by which glycogen stores are broken down to produce ATP.[42]

Glycolysis (glykys = sweet and lysis = splitting) is a metabolic process that contains nine enzymatic steps that occur in the cytoplasm of the cells and can be represented with two distinct processes.[58] These two processes are represented by fast and slow glycolysis. Traditionally, fast glycolysis has been termed "anaerobic glycolysis," whereas slow glycolysis is often referred to as "aerobic glycolysis."[42,58] This classic terminology is impractical because glycolysis occurs outside the mitochondria and does not depend on oxygen to produce energy. Because this metabolic pathway does not rely on oxygen, it is termed an anaerobic energy system. When looking closely at fast glycolysis and slow glycolysis it is clear that the two energy pathways are very similar in their enzymatic steps. The primary difference between the two processes is that fast

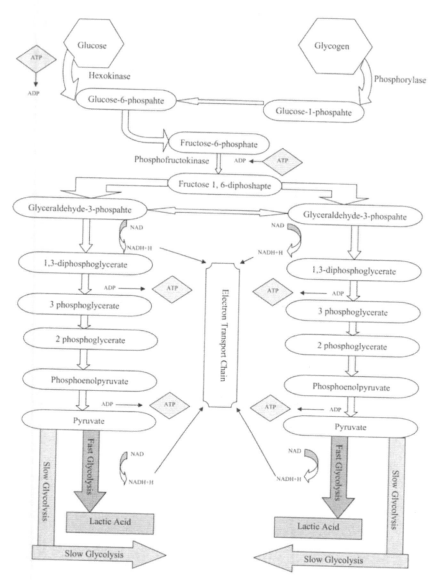

**FIGURE 14.5.** Glycolysis and glycogenolysis.
ATP = Adenosine Triphosphate
ADP = Adenosine Diphosphate
NAD = Nicotinamide adenine dinucleotide
NADH+H = Reduced Nicotinamide adenine dinucleotide

glycolysis results in the production of lactic acid, whereas slow glycolysis results in the formation of pyruvate, which is then shuttled into the mitochondria for use in the oxidative system.[58]

Glycogenolysis is very similar to the process of glycolysis and in some cases is considered to be the same basic pathway of metabolism.[58] The major difference between the metabolism of glucose and glycogen is the entry point into the metabolic pathway. Generally, because of where it enters the metabolic pathway, glycogen metabolism results in a net ATP production of three ATPs whereas the metabolism of glucose (glycolysis) results in the net production of two ATPs. This differentiation in ATP yield occurs because one less ATP is used in the energetic pathway (Figure 14.5). As with glycolysis, the metabolism of glycogen can result in either the formation of lactic acid or the formation of pyruvate, which can be shuttled into the mitochondria where it can be converted into additional energy.

## Oxidative Metabolism (Aerobic Energy System)

Oxidative metabolism occurs in the mitochondria and requires oxygen to produce energy.[1,6,58] Generally, the process of oxidative metabolism primarily utilizes carbohydrates and fats as fuel substrates. Protein, however, does not have a major role in energy supply except in extreme conditions such as starvation, or during long bouts of exercise that last longer than 90 minutes.[59,60]

When looking at the further metabolism of glucose and glycogen, the processes of oxidative metabolism is an extension of the metabolic processes begun during glycolysis and glycogenolysis. If sufficient quantities of oxygen are present, pyruvate, the end product of slow glycolysis, will be transported into the mitochondria where it will enter the Krebs cycle.[58] The Krebs cycle, or the citric acid cycle as it is also known, is a series of reactions that result in the production of two guanine triphosphate molecules, six molecules of nicotinamide adenine dinucleotide (NADH + H), and two molecules of reduced flavin adenine dinucleotide (FADH$_2$) per molecule of glucose or glycogen.[1] Once the NADH + H and FADH$_2$ molecules are generated, they transport hydrogen atoms to the electron transport chain where ATP is produced from the rephosphorylation of adenosine diphosphate or oxidative phosphorylation[6,42] (Figure 14.6).

**FIGURE 14.6.** The Krebs cycle.
FAD = Flavine adenine dinucleotide
FADH$_2$ = Reduced Flavine adenine dinucleotide
NAD = Nicotinamide adenine dinucleotide
NADH + H = Reduced Nicotinamide adenine dinucleotide
GTP = Guanosine triphosphate (energetically equivalent to ATP)

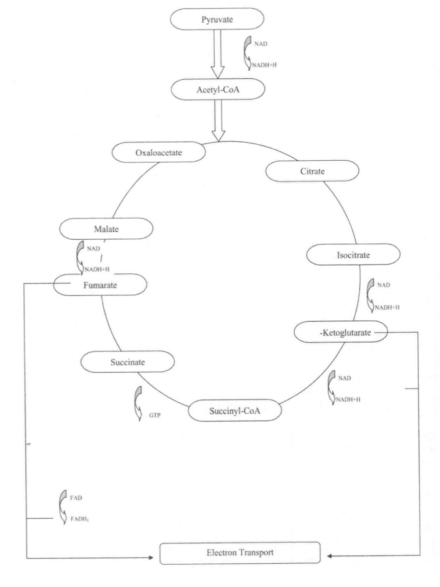

# CARBOHYDRATE METABOLISM AND EXERCISE DURATION AND INTENSITY

The available supply of energy for anaerobic or aerobic exercise is primarily determined by the intensity of the exercise bout and secondarily determined by duration of the exercise bout.[58] Generally, the shorter the duration of the exercise bout, the greater the power output and reliance on anaerobic energy supply.[42] Conversely, the longer the duration of the exercise bout, the lesser the power output and reliance on anaerobic energy supply.[42] Because both glycolysis and glycogenolysis are anaerobic energy systems, it can be concluded that the metabolism of carbohydrates occurs with exercise bouts that are of greater intensity or power outputs. The initial energy supply for short, high-intensity bouts of exercise will be met by the phosphagen system and fast glycolysis. As the duration of the bout increases, the intensity will automatically begin to decline and energy demand will be met by slow glycolysis. If the exercise bout continues, the intensity of the bout will continue to decline as oxidative metabolism begins to be more actively involved in supplying energy[42,61,62] (Table 14.4). As the intensity of exercise declines, a decrease in the metabolism of carbohydrates occurs as an increased metabolism of fats occurs.

## Anaerobic Exercise and Carbohydrate Metabolism

The current body of scientific evidence shows that significant amounts of glycogenolysis can occur in response to acute bouts of anaerobic exercise such as resistance training,[63–66] maximal ergometer sprint activities,[67,68] and maximal sprints.[69,70]

TABLE 14.4. Energy-system relationships during energy supply.

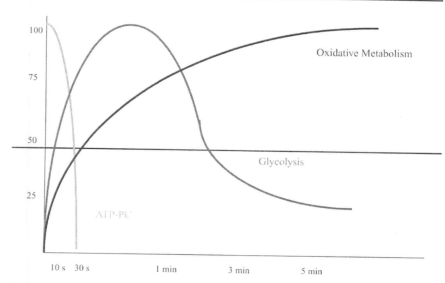

| Contribution | Seconds of exercise | | | | Minutes of exercise | | | | |
|---|---|---|---|---|---|---|---|---|---|
| | 10 | 30 | 60 | 2 | 4 | 10 | 30 | 60 | 120 |
| Anaerobic (%) | 90 | 80 | 70 | 50 | 35 | 15 | 5 | 2 | 1 |
| Aerobic | 10 | 20 | 30 | 50 | 65 | 85 | 95 | 98 | 99 |

*Source:* Modified from refs. 49, 53, 127–129.

ATP-PC = adenosine triphosphate phosphocreatine.

*Note:* Anaerobic mechanisms are the primary energy supply for a short bout of exercise (<60 seconds). Bouts of exercise between 10 seconds to 2 minutes utilize fast and slow glycolysis as the primary energy supplier. Once the bout of exercise crosses over 3 minutes, oxidative mechanisms predominate. Because fast and slow glycolysis only use carbohydrates as fuel sources, athletes who perform bouts of exercise that last less than 2 minutes need carbohydrates to function.

A 20%–50% reduction in muscle glycogen stores has been reported to occur in response to acute bouts of resistance training, even when low total workloads are encountered.[64,65,71–73] This reduction in muscle glycogen may not seem significant when looking at resistance training with few sets or repetitions (low overall workload), but when the athlete is performing multiple sets and repetitions for an overall high total workload, the available muscle glycogen may become a limiting factor that could impact the athlete's ability to handle the prescribed training load.[5,74]

When resistance-training-induced glycogenolysis is examined more closely, a preferential depletion of type II fibers seems to occur.[65,71] Robergs et al.[65] examined the effects of performing 6 sets of 6 repetitions at 35% and 70% of 1 repetition maximum in the leg extension and determined that a significantly greater depletion of type II fibers occurred in response to the bout of exercise. Similarly, Tesch et al.[71] reported that leg extensions performed at 30%, 45%, and 65% of 1 repetition maximum produced a 40%, 40%, and 70% reduction of glycogen in type IIa muscle fibers. Interestingly, only the 65% intensity stimulated a 30% decrease in the muscle glycogen content of type IIab and IIb fibers, whereas the 30% and 45% intensity stimulated no reduction in muscle glycogen in these fibers. Therefore, based on this literature, it seems that high-intensity resistance training stimulates significant reductions in muscle glycogen stores of type II fibers. Although the type II muscle fiber glycogen depletion rates in response to resistance training may seem high, they are not totally unexpected because type II fibers express higher glycolytic and glycogenolytic enzyme activities than type I fibers.[75] Because high-intensity resistance training is reliant on glycolytic and glycogenolytic processes to supply energy, the preferential depletion of type II muscle fibers may pose a significant problem in that compromises in exercise intensity during training as a result of depleted muscle glycogen stores may ultimately lead to impaired performance.[5]

## Aerobic Exercise and Carbohydrate Metabolism

When examining the effects of aerobic exercise on muscle glycogen utilization, it is clear that 1) the intensity of the exercise bout, and 2) the duration of the exercise bout have a role in determining the amount of glycogen used.[76–78]

The rate of glycogenolysis is directly related to the intensity of the aerobic exercise bout,[78–80] which is often quantified as a percentage of the athletes maximal oxygen uptake ($VO_2$ max) (Figure 14.7). When exercising at 20%–30%

**FIGURE 14.7.** The relationship between exercise intensity and glycogenolysis. (Adapted from Costill.[70])

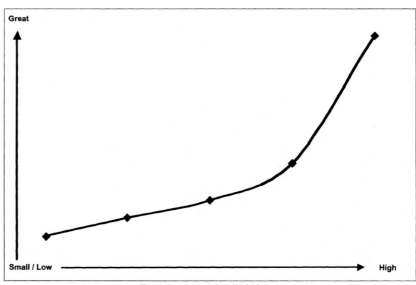

Exercise Intensity (% $VO_{2max}$)

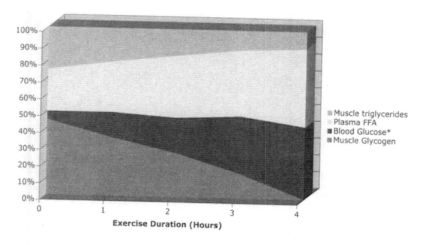

**FIGURE 14.8.** Substrate contribution to exercise over time. *If exercise is extended past 2 hours, exogenous carbohydrate is needed to maintain exercise. FFA = free fatty acid. (Adapted from [73,77,126])

of VO$_2$ max, there is a minimal utilization of muscle glycogen.[77] In fact, when 2 hours of cycling are performed at 30% of VO$_2$ max, muscle glycogen is only depleted by approximately 20% and fat is probably the primary energy supplier.[81] When the intensity of the 2-hour exercise bout is increased to ~75% of VO$_2$ max, muscle glycogen is almost completely depleted.[82,83] Generally, when an exercise bout is undertaken at intensities between 70% to 100% of VO$_2$ max, carbohydrates are considered to be the primary supplier of fuel.[77,81] Conversely, when the intensity of exercise decreases below 60% of VO$_2$ max, the primary fuel supplier during the endurance exercise bout is most likely fat.[79,81] These shifts in fuel suppliers are impacted not only by the intensity, but also the duration of the exercise bout.[77]

During prolonged endurance exercise, the use of muscle glycogen is initially very high, but as the duration of the exercise bout is extended, the reliance on glycogen begins to decline and the utilization of fat as a fuel becomes more prevalent[6,84] (Figure 14.8). This declining reliance on glycogen stores over the duration of an endurance event may partially be explained by the fact that muscle glycogen can be significantly depleted in as little as 1–2 hours of endurance exercise.[78,84–86] It might be expected that substantial decreases in muscle glycogen stores occurs in both type I and type II muscle fibers.[87–89] Interestingly, several researchers suggest that during the initial portion of an endurance event, muscle glycogen is preferentially depleted from type I and type IIa fibers.[85,86] As the duration of the exercise bout progresses, the glycogen stores of the type IIab and type IIb fibers become preferentially depleted.[86] If, however, the intensity of the endurance exercise bout is high (75%–90% VO$_2$ max), the type IIa and IIb fibers will have a greater rate of muscle glycogen depletion than the type I fibers.[77] Costill[77] suggests that the rate of glycogenolysis could be higher during a competitive event when a fast pace is used at the initiation of a race. This practice could increase the possibility of glycogen depletion and premature fatigue.

It seems that glycogen availability is a primary limiting factor in exercise bouts that last longer than 60 minutes. The initial amount of glycogen stored in the muscle is directly proportional to the athlete's ability to sustain exercise for more than 60 minutes at work rates greater than 70% VO$_2$ max.[76] Bergstrom et al.[76] clearly demonstrated that significant reductions in the basal glycogen levels resulted in athletes only being able to sustain a workload of 75% VO$_2$ max for 60 minutes. Conversely, when muscle glycogen stored was increased by 471% with a high carbohydrate diet (35 to 200 mmol glycogen·kg$^{-1}$), the time to exhaustion was increased by 110 minutes. The present scientific knowledge suggests that muscle glycogen content is extremely important for the endurance athlete and that the amount of carbohydrate in the diet can have a deciding role in the outcome of a competitive endurance event. Therefore, it is suggested that endurance athletes take strides to maximize glycogen stores through appropriate carbohydrate replenishment strategies.

# CARBOHYDRATE REPLENISHMENT

## Glycogen Synthesis

Although glycogen synthesis can occur in all animal tissues, the liver and the skeletal muscle are the primary sites in which this process occurs.[1] Generally, glycogen synthesis is stimulated by the enzyme glycogen synthase, which causes the removal of a glucose unit from a donor, specifically UDPglucose (uridine diphosphoglucose). The removed glucose unit is then added to the nonreducing end of the glycogen molecule[1,90] (Figure 14.9). It is important to note that a primer, which contains a glycogen chain of at least 4 glucose units, is required for glycogen synthase to be able to add glucose units. If a totally new glycogen molecule is being synthesized, a core protein termed glycogenin is required.[90–94] Glycogenin is the core primer in which the first 3 glucose units are attached.[1,90–94] Once the glycogen chain contains 4 glucose units then glycogen synthase can actively extend the glycogen chain. The extent to which glycogen is stored has been consistently shown to be directly related to the amount of carbohydrates in the diet.[95,96]

**FIGURE 14.9.** Glycogen synthesis.

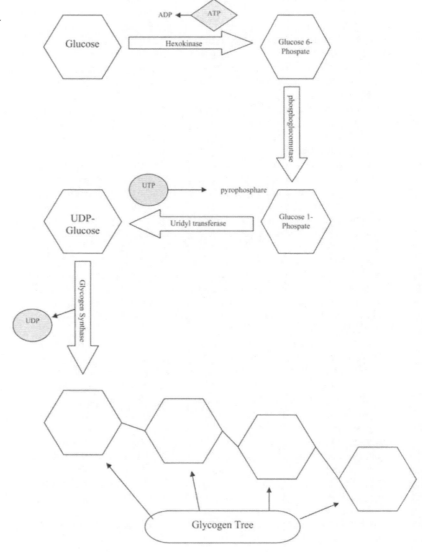

# DIETARY CARBOHYDRATES

When looking at the metabolic processes and their ability to supply energy for athletic performance, it is very clear that carbohydrates are essential components of an athlete's diet.[97] The available scientific literature suggests that dietary carbohydrate content is related to the amount of muscle glycogen that is stored in the body[95,96] and may impact the ability of the athlete to perform either anaerobic[5,98] or aerobic[98,99] exercise. Therefore, it is important for the athlete or coach to be aware of the amounts of carbohydrate in the athlete's diet because this can significantly impact their glycogen stores and ultimately athletic performance.

## Carbohydrates and Muscle Glycogen Stores

In 1981, Costill et al.[95] examined the effect of an isocaloric (~3000 kcal) diet that contained 1) 188 g carbohydrates (CHO)·d$^{-1}$ in two meals (low CHO), 2) a mixed diet containing 375 g CHO·d$^{-1}$ in two meals (mixed CHO), 3) a high carbohydrate diet containing 525 g CHO·d$^{-1}$ spaced out into seven meals (high-7 CHO), or 4) a high carbohydrate diet containing 525 g CHO·d$^{-1}$ in two meals (high-7 CHO). When examining the effects of the different dietary carbohydrate contents, it was clearly demonstrated that the low carbohydrate diet resulted in significantly less glycogen synthesis compared with the high carbohydrate diets. The high-2 CHO diet produced the greatest increases in muscle glycogen stores (Figure 14.10). Overall Costill et al.[95] concluded that the amount of carbohydrate consumed in the diet is directly proportional to the amount of muscle glycogen that is synthesized (r = 0.84).

The daily replenishment of glycogen stores may become even more important when coupling a chronic training regime with a diet that is not adequately supplying dietary carbohydrates.[100] Costill et al.[100] in their classic study examined the effect of multiple days of 2 hours of endurance running on muscle glycogen stores when coupled with a diet that contained ~40% of its calories from carbohydrate. The carbohydrate intake was inadequate and resulted in a progressive decline in resting muscle glycogen over the 3 days of training. Similarly, Sherman et al.[96] compared the effects of a 27% (234 g·d$^{-1}$, 5 g·kg$^{-1}$·d$^{-1}$) carbohydrate diet with that of a 65% (565 g·d$^{-1}$, 5 g·kg$^{-1}$·d$^{-1}$) carbohydrate diet on muscle glycogen stores over a 7-day training week. As expected, the 27% carbohydrate diet was unable to maintain glycogen stores whereas the 65% carbohydrate diet resulted in maintenance of glycogen stores (see Figure 14.11,

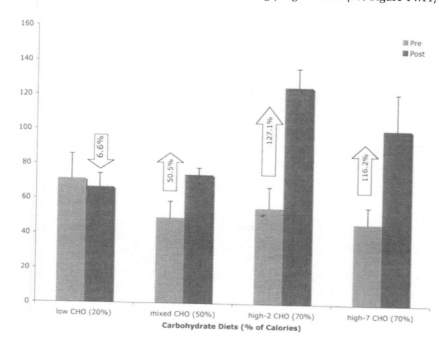

**FIGURE 14.10.** The effect of different carbohydrate (CHO) diets on muscle glycogen. (Adapted from Costill et al.[88])
Low CHO = Low carbohydrate diet
Mixed CHO = Mixed Carbohydrate diet
High-2 CHO = High Carbohydrate diet 2 meals
High-7 CHO = High Carbohydrate diet 7 meals

p. 300). In fact, the cyclists and runners experienced a 30%–36% decrease in muscle glycogen over the 7-day training period when consuming the 27% carbohydrate diet.

It seems that a diet that contains 8 g $CHO \cdot kg^{-1} \cdot d^{-1}$ or more is able to maintain muscle glycogen stores, whereas a diet that contains less than 5 g $CHO \cdot kg^{-1} \cdot d^{-1}$ will result in significant decrements in muscle glycogen.[100-104] The effect of diets that contain inadequate amounts of carbohydrates on muscle glycogen can be magnified when intense training is undertaken over several days.[104] This magnified depletion of muscle glycogen may ultimately result in fatigue during endurance performance[76,82,96] or anaerobic exercise performance[74] that might be interpreted to be a form of overtraining.[105]

## Glycogen Depletion Theory of Overtraining

In 1998, Snyder[105] suggested that low levels of muscle glycogen are associated with exercise-induced muscular fatigue that may be indicative of some form of overtraining. Although the concept of overtraining is a multifaceted problem, the athlete's ability to maintain glycogen stores while training at moderate to high intensities over consecutive days may have a role in the prevention of the occurrence of overtraining. Overtraining syndrome, as it is sometimes termed, can occur when there is an imbalance between exercise training and recovery that is marked by decrements in exercise performance.[106] Overtraining syndrome can be subdivided into two categories: 1) long-term overtraining in which many weeks or months are needed to recover athletic performance, and 2) short-term overtraining or overreaching in which recovery can occur within 14 days.[107]

Snyder[105] based the glycogen depletion hypothesis of overtraining on the fact that 1) moderate- to high-intensity exercise primarily relies on carbohydrates to supply energy,[58] 2) dietary carbohydrate consumption is directly related to the amount of glycogen stored in the body,[76,77,100] 3) successive days of endurance exercise coupled with a moderate to low (42%) carbohydrate diet results in significant decreases in muscle glycogen,[96,100] 4) delayed muscle glycogen resynthesis occurs when the diet is not rich in dietary carbohydrates,[103] and 5) muscle glycogen depletion has been associated with decreases in exercise performance.[83] This line of reasoning suggests that athletes who are performing moderate- to high-intensity exercise over consecutive days will experience decrements in performance, which when coupled with inadequate dietary carbohydrate content, may not replenish muscle glycogen stores and the end result may be expressed as chronic performance decrements. The glycogen depletion theory reveals that it has predominately been based on endurance or aerobic athletes and their performance.

The line of reasoning presented by Snyder[105] may also be extended to the anaerobic athlete. Anaerobic athletes who perform repetitive bouts of exercise also can experience marked decrements in muscle glycogen in response to acute training bouts.[65,108,109] Additionally, suppressed levels of muscle glycogen have been reported to be linked to decreases in isokinetic force production,[110] isometric strength,[111] time to fatigue,[112] and increases in exercise-induced muscle weakness.[105] The fact that inadequate carbohydrate consumption may result in an inability to restore muscle glycogen levels that when coupled with anaerobic interval training may result in decreases in performance, may be indicative of a condition that could contribute to the occurrence of overreaching or overtraining.

## Carbohydrates and the Anaerobic Athlete

Athletes who participate in sports that are predominantly anaerobic tend to have diets that are not rich in carbohydrates.[5,97] Based on current scientific evidence, the consumption of a low carbohydrate diet may be ergolytic and result in decreased training adaptations, or at worst, a decline in anaerobic performance. This response may in part be explained by an inadequate carbohydrate content in the diet coupled with intense training that may require multiple training sessions in 1 day.[5] The carbohydrate intake of anaerobic athletes seems to be between 250–544 g $CHO \cdot d^{-1}$ or 33%–55% of their total caloric

**TABLE 14.5. Energetic breakdown of selected sports and common carbohydrate intakes.**

| Gender | Sport | % Anaerobic | % Aerobic | Total energy intake (kcal) | Dietary carbohydrate content | | |
|---|---|---|---|---|---|---|---|
| | | | | | % | g | g·kg⁻¹ |
| Men | | | | | | | |
| | Soccer | 70 | 30 | 3000–5000 | 42–52 | 390–526 | 4.3–8.3 |
| | Football | 100 | 0 | 2000–11,000 | 44–46 | 366–540 | 4.3–5.2 |
| | Basketball | 90 | 10 | 2000–9000 | 44 | 437–500 | 5.4 |
| | Wrestling | 90 | 10 | 1100–6700 | 52–61 | 329–486 | 4.7–6.7 |
| | Track and field | | | 3500–4700 | 41–55 | 340–429 | 3.7–5.2 |
| | Sprinting | 100 | 0 | 2288–3018 | 50–58 | 283–397 | 4.1–6.1 |
| | Jumping | 100 | 0 | 2585–3141 | 49–59 | 308–410 | 4.2–6.2 |
| | Throwing | 100 | 0 | 2923–4259 | 48–55 | 348–510 | 3.5–4.7 |
| | Body building | 100 | 0 | 2000–5000 | 33–40 | 241–756 | 2.6–8.3 |
| | Weightlifting | 100 | 0 | 2450–4830 | 42–60 | 399–545 | 4.8–7.3 |
| | Distance running | 0–20 | 80–100 | 2500–4000 | 50–58 | 301.6–44 | 5.2–6.1 |
| | Cross-country skiing | 10 | 90 | 3250–4620 | 53–61 | 431–705 | 5.9–9.7 |
| | Triathlon | 0–20 | 80–100 | 2700–4504 | 23–63 | 153–711 | 2.5–8.0 |
| | Swimming | 20–80 | 80–20 | 2797–5152 | 52–54 | 370–696 | 5.2–9.8 |
| Women | | | | | | | |
| | Basketball | 90 | 10 | 1900–3900 | 46 | 229–380 | 3.2 |
| | Volleyball | 85 | 15 | 1100–3200 | 50 | 315 | 4.9 |
| | Track and field | | | 1500–2800 | 46–54 | 244–336 | 4.5–5.1 |
| | Sprinting | 100 | 0 | 1858–2928 | 48–58 | 226–384 | 4.2–7.4 |
| | Jumping | 100 | 0 | 1453–2511 | 48–54 | 184–304 | 3.5–5.5 |
| | Throwing | 100 | 0 | 2052–3182 | 51–57 | 268–404 | 4.0–6.2 |
| | Body building | 100 | 0 | 1000–4000 | 20–65 | 35–425 | 0.7–8.0 |
| | Distance running | 0–20 | 80–100 | 1700–3000 | 56–57 | 222–315 | 4.0–5.7 |
| | Cross-country skiing | 10 | 90 | 2510–3130 | 55–61 | 345–477 | 6.0–8.2 |
| | Triathlon | 0–20 | 80–100 | 1294–3530 | 52–54 | 174–455 | 3.6–6.8 |

Source: Modified from refs. 7–10, 12–15, 17, 19–21, 50, 66, 127–137.

intake (Table 14.5). The carbohydrate content of these athletes is not much different than that seen for the average diet of Americans over the age of 20, in which men consume 304g or 49% of their diet from carbohydrates and women consume 181g or 45% of their diet from carbohydrates.[113] Economos et al.[97] report that anaerobic athletes tend to consume significantly fewer carbohydrates than their aerobic counterparts and tend to consume fewer carbohydrates than recommended to meet the energetic demands of their sports. In fact, the average male athlete who participates in anaerobic training consumes somewhere between 3.3–5.4 g CHO·kg⁻¹·d⁻¹ or 34%–56% carbohydrates per day, whereas their female counterparts consume 2.9–3.4 g CHO·kg⁻¹·d⁻¹ or 46.4%–52.0% carbohydrates per day.[97] Based on these findings, anaerobic or strength-power athletes consume an inadequate amount of carbohydrate in their diet which may ultimately affect athletic performance.[5,97]

# EFFECT OF LOW CARBOHYDRATE DIETS ON HIGH-INTENSITY EXERCISE PERFORMANCE

It seems that high carbohydrate diets (>60%) and moderate carbohydrate diets (43%–50%) produce comparable effects on athletic performance even though high carbohydrate diets result in greater glycogen replenishment.[96,114,115–118] Conversely, it seems that when anaerobic athletes' diets contain <42% carbohydrates, high-intensity anaerobic performance is impaired.[98,115,119] The impairments in athletic performance are most noted in events that last longer than 75 seconds[115,119,120] or require repetitive performances such as interval training.[98] Researchers have suggested that these impairments in performance can be explained by 1) a reduction in muscle glycogen availability,[105] or 2) changes in acid-base status[114] as a result of the low carbohydrate content in the diet.

## Carbohydrate Recommendations for Anaerobic Athletes

Because it is well documented that most anaerobic athletes consume fewer carbohydrates than required to meet the energetic demands of their sports,[97] these athletes need to be educated about the amount of carbohydrates they consume, and need to consume, in their diets.[5,121] The training practices of anaerobic athletes stimulate significant glycogenolysis[63–66,71] that, when coupled with inadequate dietary carbohydrate content,[97] can result in significant performance impairments.[98,121,122]

The current dietary recommendation concerning carbohydrates and anaerobic athletes is to maximize the storage of muscle glycogen, with the expectation of enhanced athletic performance. Burke et al.[123] suggest that athletes should try to maximize the amount of stored glycogen by considering the fuel requirements of their sport and other individual total energy needs. This diet should supply between 6–10g CHO·kg$^{-1}$·d$^{-1}$ or 55%–60% of their total caloric intake when participating in hard training.[97] It is recommended that carbohydrate intake be examined in terms of grams relative to body mass because the utilization of percentage contribution to total dietary caloric intake is not strongly related to the athlete's absolute carbohydrate needs.[97,123] Additionally, Economos et al.[97] recommend that anaerobic athletes consider consuming 45% of their carbohydrate intake from complex or low glycemic index sources and 9%–14% of their carbohydrate intake from simple or moderate to high glycemic index sources. Moderate to high glycemic index sources should be utilized for meals immediately to 4 hours after a training bout. These recovery meals should begin immediately after the cessation of the training bout and contain 1.0–1.5g CHO·kg$^{-1}$·h$^{-1}$ and be consumed over 4 hours at frequent intervals.[97,123]

## Carbohydrates and the Aerobic Athlete

In endurance sports that last longer than 60 minutes, the availability of glycogen has a significant role in the athlete's ability to maintain performance.[76,100] Because a strong relationship between the amount of carbohydrate in the diet and the amount of glycogen stored in the body has been well established in the literature,[100] it is important that the endurance athlete understands that the carbohydrate content of their diet is of particular concern. The carbohydrate intake of aerobic athletes seems to be somewhat better than that of their anaerobic counterparts, but may still fall somewhat short of their energetic needs.[97,123,124] Generally, male endurance athletes tend to consume 5.3–11.5g CHO·kg$^{-1}$·d$^{-1}$ or 44%–65% of their diet from carbohydrates.[97,124] Female endurance athletes tend to consume significantly less carbohydrate in their diets than male endurance athletes. Generally, female endurance athletes consume between 4.4–6.4g CHO·kg$^{-1}$·d$^{-1}$ or 46%–60% of their dietary intake as carbohydrates.[97,124] Similar to the observations made concerning anaerobic athletes, aerobic athletes generally consume inadequate carbohydrate in their diet, which can significantly impact their ability to perform endurance exercise.[97,123]

## Dietary Recommendations for Aerobic Athletes

The carbohydrate consumption of female aerobic athletes has generally been reported to be significantly under the recommended amounts of carbohydrates needed to maximize athletic performance.[97] Conversely, only 14% of male aerobic athletes fall below the carbohydrate demands of their training.[97] Based on these reports, it is important that the aerobic athlete, coach, and sports nutritionist be educated about the carbohydrate needs and dietary practices of aerobic athletes. Inadequate carbohydrate content in the aerobic athlete's diet can result in significant decrements in stored muscle glycogen, especially when coupled with rigorous training,[77,96,100] and can result in significant impairments in aerobic exercise performance.[95,98]

The aerobic athlete should maximize muscle glycogen stores in an attempt to augment endurance performance. To successfully accomplish this goal, the fuel utilization of the sport and the individual's other energy needs should be considered[97,123] (Table 14.6) The general recommendation for carbohydrate intake for the endurance athlete is to consume more than 55% of the caloric intake as carbohydrates or somewhere between 6–10g CHO·kg$^{-1}$·d$^{-1}$.[97] However, Burke et al.[123] suggest that carbohydrate intake should be manipulated based

**TABLE 14.6. Estimates of energy expenditure from selected endurance sports.**

| Endurance activity | Estimated calories | | Carbohydrate (g) | Carbohydrate (g·kg⁻¹) |
| | $kcal·min^{-1}$ | Total kcal | | |
|---|---|---|---|---|
| Running | | | | |
| 2 mile | 20.0 | 216 | 50–55 | 0.71–0.78 |
| 10 km | 17.5 | 700 | 150–170 | 2.14–2.43 |
| Marathon | 15.0 | 2800 | 500–550 | 7.14–7.86 |
| Swimming (front crawl) | | | | |
| 200 m | 25.0 | 50 | 12–15 | 0.17–0.21 |
| 1500 m | 20.0 | 400 | 90–100 | 1.29–1.43 |
| Cycling | | | | |
| 1 hour | 17.0 | 1020 | 230–250 | 3.89–3.57 |

*Source:* Modified from Costill.[70]

on the intensity of the aerobic exercise used by the athlete. When the athlete is training with moderate-duration, low-intensity endurance exercise, the athlete should strive to consume between 5–7 g $CHO·kg^{-1}·d^{-1}$. If the training program is more intense, the carbohydrate needs of the athlete can be met by increasing dietary intake to 7–12 g $CHO·kg^{-1}·d^{-1}$. Finally, when the athlete is undertaking extreme endurance training protocols, which may require the athlete to exercise for 4–6 hours a day or more, they should strive to consume between 10–12 g $CHO·kg^{-1}·d^{-1}$. If the athlete has difficulty consuming this amount of carbohydrate in their diet with food, they should be encouraged to consume carbohydrate liquid supplements that are composed of a 20%–25% carbohydrate solution.[97]

## PRACTICAL APPLICATIONS

From the available scientific literature about dietary carbohydrates and athletic performance it is clear that carbohydrates must make up a substantial portion of the athletic diet, especially when performance is of primary concern. Because strong links have been established among the amount of carbohydrate in the diet, muscle glycogen, and exercise performance, it is essential that athletes, coaches, and sports nutritionists be conscious of the carbohydrate content of the athlete's diet. A minimum of at least 6 g $CHO·kg^{-1}·d^{-1}$ seems to be essential to maintain performance. However, if the athlete is undertaking a particularly intense or period of lengthy training, the amount of carbohydrates in the diet may need to be increased to at least 10 g $CHO·kg^{-1}·d^{-1}$. The carbohydrate choices for most athletes should come from moderate glycemic index sources that are capable of supplying the vast nutrients needed by both the aerobic and anaerobic athlete. High glycemic index carbohydrates may be consumed in the diet if the athlete is unable to meet their carbohydrate needs with other sources. The use of these high glycemic index carbohydrates should be limited to the 1- to 2-hour time period after a training session. This practice will ensure that muscle glycogen stores are maximized in a timely manner.

## Sidebar 14.1. Low Carbohydrate Diets Decrease Anaerobic and Aerobic Exercise Performance Capacity

Recent scientific data suggest that the practice of eating a low carbohydrate diet may reduce body weight but markers of athletic performance may be impaired. Recent research from the Department of Kinesiology at the University of

Connecticut has reported that 6 weeks of a low carbohydrate diet (carbohydrate = 8%, protein = 30%, and fat = 61%) results in significant weight loss when compared with a control diet (carbohydrate = 55%, protein = 16%, and fat =

29%). However, the performance data suggest that the low carbohydrate diet results in significant decreases in anaerobic performance (Figure 14.11). The low carbohydrate diet intervention and training protocol resulted in a 20% decrease in mean power production and a 10% decrease in peak power production. This decrease in anaerobic performance was significantly greater than the decrease in response to a 6-week control diet (mean power = –8% and peak power = –16%). To further their understanding of how low-carbohydrate diets affect athletic performance, the researchers also examined aerobic performance (Figure 14.12). Subjects performed a 45-minute timed cycle ergometer ride to deter-

mine the effects of the low carbohydrate diet on actual endurance performance. The consumption of the low carbohydrate diet for 6 weeks resulted in an 18% decrease in work output, whereas no significant changes were noted for the control diet. These data suggest that athletes who are primarily concerned with athletic performance should avoid low carbohydrate diets because they can stimulate significant decreases in both anaerobic and aerobic exercise performance. Therefore, athletes should choose more traditional moderate to high carbohydrate diets that have the potential to maintain or augment athletic performance when coupled with a sound training program.[98]

**FIGURE 14.11.** The effect of various carbohydrate (CHO) diets on muscle glycogen content. (Adapted from Sherman et al.[89])
CHO = Carbohydrate

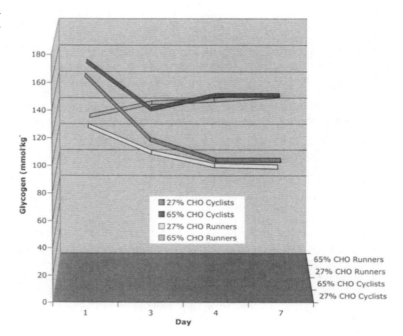

**FIGURE 14.12.** Effect of a 6-week low carbohydrate diet on anaerobic exercise performance.

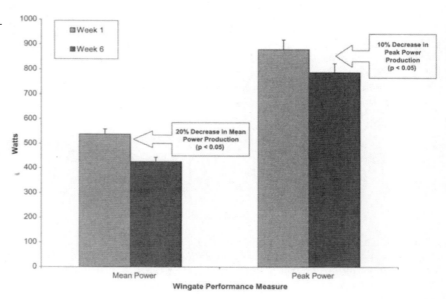

## Sidebar 14.2. Glycogen Loading and Endurance Performance

For many decades, endurance athletes have had the practice of manipulating carbohydrate intake in the diet along with modifying exercise regimes in an attempt to maximize glycogen stores and ultimately improve performance. Hawley et al.[131] suggest that glycogen loading of supercompensation, as it is sometimes termed, can be beneficial for endurance bouts that last longer than 90 minutes. Generally, it has been suggested that a glycogen-loading regime can reduce fatigue during endurance exercise and increase the duration of the exercise bout by 20% while increasing the workload or distance completed by 2%–3%.[131] Therefore, it may be advisable for endurance athletes to use a dietary and exercise strategy designed to maximize glycogen stores.[131,132]

The classic carbohydrate-loading protocol first introduced in the 1960s required athletes to undertake a 3- to 4-day glycogen-depleting regime which contained hard exercise coupled with a low carbohydrate diet followed by a 3- to 4-day repletion phase in which training volume and intensity were decreased whereas carbohydrate consumption was significantly increased.[76] However, this classic glycogen-loading regime has it pitfalls. During the depletion phase, workout quality suffers and many athletes have complained that they do not reach an appropriate physiologic or psychologic peak.

Recently, a modified glycogen-loading regime has been proposed (Table 14.7).[132] This modified method of glycogen requires the athlete to consume a 50% carbohydrate diet for 3 days with a slowly declining amount of exercise. On the fourth day of the protocol, the athlete will consume a 70% carbohydrate diet and the duration of exercise will continue to decline. On the seventh day, the athlete will compete. The modified carbohydrate loading model has been found to be a highly effective mechanism for loading glycogen with less risk of performance decrements than the classic model.[132]

TABLE 14.7. **Comparison of glycogen loading regimes.**

| | Classic model | | Modified model | |
|---|---|---|---|---|
| Day | Exercise time (min) | CHO % | Exercise time (min) | CHO (%) |
| 1 | 90 | 15 | 90 | 50 |
| 2 | 40–60 | 15 | 40–60 | 50 |
| 3 | 40–60 | 15 | 40–60 | 50 |
| 4 | 20–45 | 70 | 20–45 | 70 |
| 5 | 20–45 | 70 | 20–45 | 70 |
| 6 | 0–30 | 70 | 0–30 | 70 |
| 7 | Race | 70 | Race | 70 |

*Source:* Modified from Sherman et al.[119]

CHO = carbohydrate.

## Sidebar 14.3. Postexercise Glycogen Synthesis

The use of carbohydrate supplements to speed the recovery process after an exercise bout has received much attention in the scientific literature.[133–136] Based on this literature, it seems that one of the most important things to consider is the timing of the carbohydrate supplement (Figure 14.13).

When looking at the postexercise time period, the amount of glycogen synthesized is very low when no carbohydrates are consumed.[134,137] When a diet containing high glycemic index carbohydrates is consumed during the first 6 hours after an exercise bout, a greater rate of glycogen synthesis occurs. In fact, it seems that the time period immediately after an exercise bout is a critical time for ingesting carbohydrates.[134] Ivy et al.[134] examined the effects of different postexercise carbohydrate supplementation protocols: 1) a placebo containing no carbohydrates, 2) 1 g glucose·kg$^{-1}$ consumed immediately after and 2 hours after exercise, and 3) 1 g glucose·kg$^{-1}$ consumed only 2 hours after exercise. Muscle biopsies were analyzed immediately after and 4 hours after exercise. The results indicated that the placebo treatment resulted in the lowest rate of glycogen resynthesis (3.2 mmol·kg$^{-1}$·h$^{-1}$), whereas the protocol that required consumption of carbohydrate immediately after and 2 hours after exercise produced the highest rate of resynthesis (6.0 mmol·kg$^{-1}$·h$^{-1}$). Interestingly, if the carbohydrate supplement was only taken 2 hours after exercise, the rate of resynthesis (4.1 mmol·kg$^{-1}$·h$^{-1}$) was lower than the immediately postexercise treatment, but higher than no carbohydrate consumption (Figure 14.3). Based on this study and several others, it seems that 0.7–2.0 g CHO·kg$^{-1}$, at a minimum, should be consumed every 2 hours after exercise to promote glycogen synthesis. If the athlete desires to maximize glycogen synthesis, they should consume carbohydrates immediately after the cessation of the exercise bout.

**FIGURE 14.13.** Effect of different carbohydrate ingestion times on glycogen resynthesis rates.
CHO IP +2P = Carbohydrate consumption immediately post exercise and 2 hours post exercise
CHO 2P = Carbohydrate consumption 2 hours post exercise
No CHO = No carbohydrate consumption

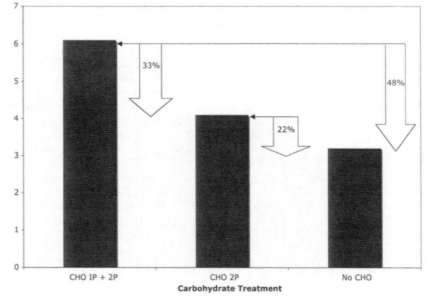

## QUESTIONS

1. The oligosaccharide that is often difficult to digest and results in excess fluid and gas buildup in the bowels is:
   a. Sucrose
   b. Glucose
   c. Lactose
   d. Maltose

2. The monosaccharide that is the most frequently used carbohydrate-transport mechanism is:
   a. Fructose
   b. Galactose
   c. Lactose
   d. Glucose

3. Glucose can be formed in small quantities in the liver from pyruvate, lactate, amino acids, and glycerol in a process called:
   a. Fast glycolysis
   b. Glycogenolysis
   c. Gluconeogenesis
   d. Slow glycolysis

4. The monosaccharide ____ is considered to be the sweetest of all the monosaccharides.
   a. Glucose
   b. Fructose
   c. Galactose
   d. Lactose

5. The oligosaccharide that is most frequently used in the production of alcohol is:
   a. Sucrose
   b. Maltose
   c. Lactose
   d. Glucose

6. Polysaccharides are generally considered complex carbohydrates and contain ____ monosaccharides that have been bound together.
   a. 2
   b. <5
   c. <10
   d. >10

7. Pyruvate is considered the end product of:
   a. Fast glycolysis
   b. Slow glycolysis
   c. Oxidative metabolism
   d. The electron transport chain

8. Glycogen availability is a primary limiting factor in exercise bouts that last:
   a. 15–20 minutes
   b. 30–45 minutes
   c. <15 minutes
   d. >60 minutes

9. Generally, it is recommended that anaerobic athletes consume between ____ g $CHO \cdot kg^{-1} \cdot d^{-1}$.
   a. 3–5
   b. 6–10
   c. 5–7
   d. 10–12

10. If an aerobic athlete is training 5 hours a day, they should strive to consume ____ g $CHO \cdot kg^{-1} \cdot d^{-1}$.
    a. 3–5
    b. 6–10
    c. 5–7
    d. 10–12

11. Running 2 miles results in an estimated caloric expenditure of ____ $kcal \cdot min^{-1}$.
    a. 17
    b. 15
    c. 20
    d. 25

12. Exercise bouts that last longer than 3 minutes will use ____ as their primary energy system.
    a. Oxidative metabolism
    b. Fast glycolysis
    c. Slow glycolysis
    d. Adenosine triphosphate phosphocreatine

13. ____ is considered to be a polysaccharide.
    a. Fructose
    b. Maltose
    c. Starch
    d. Ribose

14. ____ is a monosaccharide that is not found in large quantities in nature.
    a. Galactose
    b. Glucose
    c. Fructose
    d. Maltose

15. Sugar cane contains large quantities of:
    a. Fructose
    b. Sucrose
    c. Lactose
    d. Maltose

16. Approximately ____ of Hispanics are deficient in the enzyme lactase.
    a. 60%–80%
    b. 50%–80%
    c. 2%–15%
    d. 6%–22%

17. Only about ____ of male endurance athletes consume fewer carbohydrates than required by their training.
    a. 28%
    b. 42%
    c. 14%
    d. 7%

18. ____ is an example of a high glycemic food.
    a. Barley
    b. Scones
    c. Yogurt
    d. Plums

19. An example of a very low carbohydrate diet would be the:
    a. Pritikin diet
    b. Average American diet
    c. The testosterone diet
    d. Atkins diet

20. Lactic acid is the end product of:
    a. Fast glycolysis
    b. Slow glycolysis
    c. Oxidative metabolism

21. The effect of increased high fructose corn syrup on the obesity epidemic.
    a. Increase
    b. Decrease
    c. No effect

22. The effect of an acute bout of resistance training on type II muscle fiber glycogen content.
    a. Increase
    b. Decrease
    c. No effect

23. The effect of increasing the intensity of exercise on the rate of glycogenolysis.
    a. Increase
    b. Decrease
    c. No effect

24. The effect of a low carbohydrate diet on the amount of glycogen stored in the body.
    a. Increase
    b. Decrease
    c. No effect

25. The effect of long-duration exercise >60 minutes on the utilization of fat as a fuel.
    a. Increase
    b. Decrease
    c. No effect

26. The effect of consuming a moderate carbohydrate diet (43%–50%) on anaerobic exercise performance.
    a. Increase
    b. Decrease
    c. No effect

27. The effect of a low carbohydrate diet on endurance performance.
    a. Increase
    b. Decrease
    c. No effect

28. The effect of increasing exercise intensity on the rate of glycogenolysis.
    a. Increase
    b. Decrease
    c. No effect

29. The effect of 4 hours of exercise on plasma free fatty acid concentrations.
    a. Increase
    b. Decrease
    c. No effect

30. The effect of a mixed carbohydrate diet (50%) on muscle glycogen stores.
    a. Increase
    b. Decrease
    c. No effect

31. The effect of a 27% carbohydrate diet coupled with 7 days of cycling on muscle glycogen stores.
    a. Increase
    b. Decrease
    c. No effect

32. The effect of a low carbohydrate diet on peak anaerobic power.
    a. Increase
    b. Decrease
    c. No effect

33. The effect of a high glycemic index food on the rate of glucose appearance in the blood stream.
    a. Increase
    b. Decrease
    c. No effect

34. The effect of a diet composed primarily of low glycemic index carbohydrates on the risk of coronary heart disease.
    a. Increase
    b. Decrease
    c. No effect

35. The effect of starvation on the metabolism of protein as a fuel substrate.
    a. Increase
    b. Decrease
    c. No effect

36. Anaerobic athletes tend to consume more carbohydrates than aerobic athletes.
    a. True
    b. False

37. Female athletes tend to consume more carbohydrates than male athletes.
    a. True
    b. False

38. The longer the duration of the exercise bout, the lower the intensity and reliance on carbohydrates as a fuel source.
    a. True
    b. False

39. The greater the intensity of resistance training, the greater the decrease in muscle glycogen.
    a. True
    b. False

40. Type I muscle fibers have higher glycolytic enzyme activity than type II muscle fibers.
   a. True
   b. False

41. Type I muscle fibers are preferentially depleted during endurance exercise bouts.
   a. True
   b. False

42. Glycogen synthesis is stimulated by the enzyme glycogenin.
   a. True
   b. False

43. A minimum of 4 glucose units is needed for glycogen synthase to actively extend the glycogen chain.
   a. True
   b. False

44. Seven days of training coupled with a 27% carbohydrate diet results in a 30%–36% decrease in muscle glycogen.
   a. True
   b. False

45. Overtraining is defined as intense training that the athlete can recover from in as little as 14 days.
   a. True
   b. False

46. Anaerobic athletes generally consume between 33%–55% of their energy needs from carbohydrates.
   a. True
   b. False

47. Carbohydrate content of an athlete's diet should always be calculated on a per kilogram body mass basis.
   a. True
   b. False

48. Impairments in anaerobic performance as a result of a low carbohydrate diet are most noted when the bout of exercise used to test the diet is longer than 75 seconds.
   a. True
   b. False

49. Low carbohydrate diets are effective at reducing body mass.
   a. True
   b. False

50. Monosaccharides contain between 3–12 carbon atoms.
   a. True
   b. False

## REFERENCES

1. Lehninger AL, Nelson DL, Cox MM. Principles of Biochemistry. second ed. New York: Worth Publishers; 1993.
2. Cheuvront SN. The zone diet and athletic performance. Sports Med 1999;27(4): 213–28.
3. Riley RE. Popular weight loss diets. Health and exercise implications. Clin Sports Med 1999;18(3):691–701, ix.
4. Simopoulos AP. Opening address. Nutrition and fitness from the first Olympiad in 776 BC to 393 AD and the concept of positive health. Am J Clin Nutr 1989; 49(5 Suppl):921–6.
5. Haff GG, Whitley A. Low-carbohydrate diets and high-intensity anaerobic exercise. Strength and Cond 2002;24(4):42–53.

6. Mcardle WD, Katch FI, Katch VL. Exercise physiology:energy, nutrition, and human performance. Baltimore, maryland: Lippincott Williams & Wilkins; 2001.

7. Nowak RK, Knudsen KS, Schulz LO. Body composition and nutrient intakes of college men and women basketball players. J Am Diet Assoc 1988;88(5):575–8.

8. Keith RE, Stone MH, Carson RE, Lefavi RG, Fleck SJ. Nutritional status and lipid profiles of trained steroid-using bodybuilders. Int J Sport Nutr 1996;6(3):247–54.

9. Sears B. The Zone: A Dietary Road Map. New York: ReganBooks; 1995.

10. Rico-Sanz J, Frontera WR, Mole PA, Rivera MA, Rivera-Brown A, Meredith CN. Dietary and performance assessment of elite soccer players during a period of intense training. Int J Sport Nutr 1998;8(3):230–40.

11. Rico-Sanz J. Body composition and nutritional assessments in soccer. Int J Sport Nutr 1998;8(2):113–23.

12. Stone MH, Sanborn K, Smith LL, et al. Effects of in-season (5 weeks) creatine and pyruvate supplementation on anaerobic performance and body composition in American football players. Int J Sport Nutr 1999;9(2):146–65.

13. Kleiner SM, Bazzarre TL, Ainsworth BE. Nutritional status of nationally ranked elite bodybuilders. Int J Sport Nutr 1994;4(1):54–69.

14. Volek J. Enhancing exercise performance: nutritional implications. In: Garrett WE, Kirkendall DT, editors. Exercise and sport science. Philadelphia, PA: Lippincott Williams and Wilkins; 2000. p. 980.

15. Marsit JL, Conley MS, Stone MH, et al. Effects of ascorbic acid on serum cortisol and the testosterone:cortisol ratio in junior elite weightlifters. J. Strength Cond. Res. 1998;12(3):179–184.

16. Kirksey B, Stone MH, Warren BJ, et al. The effects of six weeks of creatine monohydrate supplementation on performance measures and body composition in collegiate track and field athletes. Journal of Strength and Conditioning Research 1999;13(2):148–156.

17. Sugiura K, Suzuki I, Kobayashi K. Nutritional intake of elite Japanese track-and-field athletes. Int J Sport Nutr 1999;9(2):202–12.

18. van Erp-Baart AM, Saris WH, Binkhorst RA, Vos JA, Elvers JW. Nationwide survey on nutritional habits in elite athletes. Part I. Energy, carbohydrate, protein, and fat intake. Int J Sports Med 1989;10(Suppl 1):S3–10.

19. Walberg-Rankin J, Edmonds CE, Gwazdauskas FC. Diet and weight changes of female bodybuilders before and after competition. Int J Sport Nutr 1993;3(1):87–102.

20. Peters EM, Goetzsche JM. Dietary practices of South African ultradistance runners. Int J Sport Nutr 1997;7(2):80–103.

21. Fogelholm M, Rehunen S, Gref CG, et al. Dietary intake and thiamin, iron, and zinc status in elite Nordic skiers during different training periods. Int J Sport Nutr 1992;2(4):351–65.

22. Burke LM, Read RS. Diet patterns of elite Australian male triathletes. Phys Sportsmed. 1987;15(2):140–155.

23. Ellsworth NM, Hewitt BF, Haskell WL. Nutrient intake of elite male and female nordic skiers. Phys Sportsmed. 1985;13(2):78–92.

24. Frentsos JA, Baer JT. Increased energy and nutrient intake during training and competition improves elite triathletes' endurance performance. Int J Sport Nutr 1997;7(1):61–71.

25. Nattiv A. Stress fractures and bone health in track and field athletes. J Sci Med Sport 2000;3(3):268–79.

26. Faber M, Spinnler-Benade AJ, Daubitzer A. Dietary intake, anthropometric measurements and plasma lipid levels in throwing field athletes. Int J Sports Med 1990;11(2):140–5.

27. Sumida KD, Donovan CM. Enhanced hepatic gluconeogenic capacity for selected precursors after endurance training. J Appl Physiol 1995;79(6):1883–8.

28. Jonnalagadda SS, Rosenbloom CA, Skinner R. Dietary practices, attitudes, and physiological status of collegiate freshman football players. J Strength Cond Res 2001;15(4):507–13.

29. Krumbach CJ, Ellis DR, Driskell JA. A report of vitamin and mineral supplement use among university athletes in a division I institution. Int J Sport Nutr 1999;9(4):416–25.

30. Jandrain BJ, Pallikarakis N, Normand S, Pirnay F, Lacroix M, Mosora F, et al. Fructose utilization during exercise in men: rapid conversion of ingested fructose to circulating glucose. J Appl Physiol 1993;74(5):2146–54.

31. Bray GA, Nielsen SJ, Popkin BM. Consumption of high-fructose corn syrup in beverages may play a role in the epidemic of obesity. Am J Clin Nutr 2004;79(4):537–43.

32. Tordoff MG, Alleva AM. Effect of drinking soda sweetened with aspartame or high-fructose corn syrup on food intake and body weight. Am J Clin Nutr 1990;51(6):963–9.

33. Raben A, Vasilaras TH, Moller AC, Astrup A. Sucrose compared with artificial sweeteners: different effects on ad libitum food intake and body weight after 10wk of supplementation in overweight subjects. Am J Clin Nutr 2002;76(4): 721–9.

34. Shaw AD, Davies GJ. Lactose intolerance: problems in diagnosis and treatment. J Clin Gastroenterol 1999;28(3):208–16.

35. Swagerty DL, Jr., Walling AD, Klein RM. Lactose intolerance. Am Fam Physician 2002;65(9):1845–50.

36. Vonk RJ, Priebe MG, Koetse HA, et al. Lactose intolerance: analysis of underlying factors. Eur J Clin Invest 2003;33(1):70–5.

37. Sahi T. Hypolactasia and lactase persistence. Historical review and the terminology. Scand J Gastroenterol Suppl 1994;202:1–6.

38. Kleyn J, Hough J. The microbiology of brewing. Annu Rev Microbiol 1971;25: 583–608.

39. Board FaN. Dietary reference intakes for energy, carbohydrate, fiber, fat, fatty acids, cholesterol, protein, and amino acids. Washington, DC: The National Academy Press; 2002.

40. Kabir M, Rizkalla SW, Champ M, et al. Dietary amylose-amylopectin starch content affects glucose and lipid metabolism in adipocytes of normal and diabetic rats. J Nutr 1998;128(1):35–43.

41. Hallfrisch J, Facn, Behall KM. Mechanisms of the effects of grains on insulin and glucose responses. J Am Coll Nutr 2000;19(3 Suppl):320S–325S.

42. Brooks GA, Fahey TD, White TP, Baldwin KM. Exercise physiology: human bioenergetics and its application. 3rd ed. Mountain View, CA: Mayfield Publishing Company; 2000.

43. Felig P, Wahren J. Fuel homeostasis in exercise. N Engl J Med 1975;293(21): 1078–84.

44. Houston ME. Biochemistry Primer for Exercise Science. Champaign, IL: Human Kinetics; 1995.

45. Houston ME. Biochemistry Primer for Exercise Science. 2nd ed. Champagne, IL: Human Kinetics; 2001.

46. Costill DL. Carbohydrate for athletic training and performance. Bol Asoc Med P R 1991;83(8):350–3.

47. Jenkins DJ, Wolever TM, Taylor RH, et al. Glycemic index of foods: a physiological basis for carbohydrate exchange. Am J Clin Nutr 1981;34(3):362–6.

48. Foster-Powell K, Holt SH, Brand-Miller JC. International table of glycemic index and glycemic load values: 2002. Am J Clin Nutr 2002;76(1):5–56.

49. Wolever TM, Jenkins DJ, Jenkins AL, Josse RG. The glycemic index: methodology and clinical implications. Am J Clin Nutr 1991;54(5):846–54.

50. Ludwig DS. Dietary glycemic index and the regulation of body weight. Lipids 2003;38(2):117–21.

51. Ludwig DS, Majzoub JA, Al-Zahrani A, Dallal GE, Blanco I, Roberts SB. High glycemic index foods, overeating, and obesity. Pediatrics 1999;103(3):E26.

52. Ludwig DS. Dietary glycemic index and obesity. J Nutr 2000;130(2S Suppl): 280S–283S.

53. Liu S, Willett WC, Stampfer MJ, et al. A prospective study of dietary glycemic load, carbohydrate intake, and risk of coronary heart disease in US women. Am J Clin Nutr 2000;71(6):1455–61.

54. Franceschi S, Dal Maso L, Augustin L, et al. Dietary glycemic load and colorectal cancer risk. Ann Oncol 2001;12(2):173–8.

55. Augustin LS, Dal Maso L, La Vecchia C, et al. Dietary glycemic index and glycemic load, and breast cancer risk: a case-control study. Ann Oncol 2001;12(11):1533–8.

56. Salmeron J, Ascherio A, Rimm EB, et al. Dietary fiber, glycemic load, and risk of NIDDM in men. Diabetes Care 1997;20(4):545–50.

57. Ludwig DS. Glycemic load comes of age. J Nutr 2003;133(9):2695–6.

58. Conley M. Bioenergetics of Exercise Training. In: Baechle TR, Earle RW, editors. Essentials of Strength Training and Conditioning. 2nd ed. Champaign, IL: Human Kinetics; 2000. p. 73–90.

59. Lemon PW, Mullin JP. Effect of initial muscle glycogen levels on protein catabolism during exercise. J Appl Physiol 1980;48(4):624–9.

60. Millward DJ, Davies CT, Halliday D, Wolman SL, Matthews D, Rennie M. Effect of exercise on protein metabolism in humans as explored with stable isotopes. Fed Proc 1982;41(10):2686–91.

61. Stone MH, O'Bryant HO. Weight Training: A Scientific Approach. Minnesota: Burgess; 1987.

62. Dudley GA, Abraham WM, Terjung RL. Influence of exercise intensity and duration on biochemical adaptations in skeletal muscle. J Appl Physiol 1982;53(4):844–50.

63. Haff GG, Koch AJ, Potteiger JA, et al. Carbohydrate supplementation attenuates muscle glycogen loss during acute bouts of resistance exercise. Int J Sport Nutr Exerc Metab 2000;10(3):326–39.

64. MacDougall JD, Ray S, Sale DG, McCartney N, Lee P, Garner S. Muscle substrate utilization and lactate production during weightlifting. Can J Appl Physiol 1999; 24(3):209–215.

65. Robergs RA, Pearson DR, Costill DL, et al. Muscle glycogenolysis during differing intensities of weight-resistance exercise. J Appl Physiol 1991;70(4):1700–6.

66. Tesch PA, Colliander EB, Kaiser P. Muscle metabolism during intense, heavy-resistance exercise. Eur J Appl Physiol 1986;55(4):362–6.

67. Gaitanos GC, Williams C, Boobis LH, Brooks S. Human muscle metabolism during intermittent maximal exercise. J Appl Physiol 1993;75(2):712–9.

68. Spriet LL, Lindinger MI, McKelvie RS, Heigenhauser GJ, Jones NL. Muscle glycogenolysis and H+ concentration during maximal intermittent cycling. J Appl Physiol 1989;66(1):8–13.

69. Cheetham ME, Boobis LH, Brooks S, Williams C. Human muscle metabolism during sprint running. J Appl Physiol 1986;61(1):54–60.

70. Boobis I, Williams C, Wooton SN. Human muscle metabolism during brief maximal exercise. J Appl Physiol 1983;338:21P–22P.

71. Tesch PA, Ploutz-Snyder LL, Yström L, Castro M, Dudley G. Skeletal muscle glycogen loss evoked by resistance exercise. J Strength Cond Res 1998;12(2):67–73.

72. Tesch PA, Thorsson A, Colliander EB. Effects of eccentric and concentric resistance training on skeletal muscle substrates, enzyme activities and capillary supply. Acta Physiol Scand 1990;140(4):575–80.

73. Haff GG. Carbohydrate supplementation attenuates muscle glycogen loss during acute bouts of resistance training exercise. Unpublished doctoral dissertation, University of Kansas, Lawrence 1999.

74. Haff GG, Lehmkuhl MJ, McCoy LB, Stone MH. Carbohydrate supplementation and resistance training. J Strength Cond Res 2003;17(1):187–96.

75. Gollnick PD, Piehl K, Saltin B. Selective glycogen depletion pattern in human muscle fibres after exercise of varying intensity and at varying pedaling rates. J Physiol Lond 1974;241(1):45–57.

76. Bergstrom J, Hermansen L, Hultman E, Saltin B. Diet, muscle glycogen and physical performance. Acta Physiol Scand 1967;71(2):140–50.

77. Costill DL. Carbohydrates for exercise: dietary demands for optimal performance. Int J Sports Med 1988;9(1):1–18.

78. Blom PC, Vollestad NK, Costill DL. Factors affecting changes in muscle glycogen concentration during and after prolonged exercise. Acta Physiol Scand Suppl 1986;556:67–74.

79. Coyle EF. Physiological determinants of endurance exercise performance. J Sci Med Sport 1999;2(3):181–9.

80. Romijn JA, Coyle EF, Sidossis LS, et al. Regulation of endogenous fat and carbohydrate metabolism in relation to exercise intensity and duration. Am J Physiol 1993;265(3 Pt 1):E380–91.

81. Hultman E. Fuel selection, muscle fibre. Proc Nutr Soc 1995;54(1):107–21.

82. Hermansen L, Hultman E, Saltin B. Muscle glycogen during prolonged severe exercise. Acta Physiol Scand 1967;71(2):129–39.

83. Karlsson J, Saltin B. Diet, muscle glycogen, and endurance performance. J Appl Physiol 1971;31(2):203–6.

84. Coyle EF, Coggan AR, Hemmert MK, Ivy JL. Muscle glycogen utilization during prolonged strenuous exercise when fed carbohydrate. J Appl Physiol 1986;61(1): 165–72.

85. Ball-Burnett M, Green HJ, Houston ME. Energy metabolism in human slow and fast twitch fibres during prolonged cycle exercise. J Physiol 1991;437:257–67.

86. Vollestad NK, Vaage O, Hermansen L. Muscle glycogen depletion patterns in type I and subgroups of type II fibres during prolonged severe exercise in man. Acta Physiol Scand 1984;122(4):433–41.

87. Gollnick PD, Armstrong RB, Saubert CWt, Sembrowich WL, Shepherd RE, Saltin B. Glycogen depletion patterns in human skeletal muscle fibers during prolonged work. Pflugers Arch 1973;344(1):1–12.

88. Essen B. Glycogen depletion of different fibre types in human skeletal muscle during intermittent and continuous exercise. Acta Physiol Scand 1978;103(4):446–55.

89. Vollestad NK, Blom PC. Effect of varying exercise intensity on glycogen depletion in human muscle fibres. Acta Physiol Scand 1985;125(3):395–405.

90. Shearer J, Graham TE. Novel aspects of skeletal muscle glycogen and its regulation during rest and exercise. Exerc Sport Sci Rev 2004;32(3):120–6.

91. Shearer J, Marchand I, Sathasivam P, Tarnopolsky MA, Graham TE. Glycogenin activity in human skeletal muscle is proportional to muscle glycogen concentration. Am J Physiol Endocrinol Metab 2000;278(1):E177–80.

92. Lomako J, Lomako WM, Whelan WJ. The nature of the primer for glycogen synthesis in muscle. FEBS Lett 1990;268(1):8–12.

93. Lomako J, Lomako WM, Whelan WJ. Substrate specificity of the autocatalytic protein that primes glycogen synthesis. FEBS Lett 1990;264(1):13–6.

94. Lomako J, Lomako WM, Whelan WJ. The biogenesis of glycogen: nature of the carbohydrate in the protein primer. Biochem Int 1990;21(2):251–60.

95. Costill DL, Sherman WM, Fink WJ, Maresc C, Witten M, Miller JM. The role of dietary carbohydrates in muscle glycogen resynthesis after strenuous running. Am J Clin Nutr 1981;34(9):1831–6.

96. Sherman WM, Doyle JA, Lamb DR, Strauss RH. Dietary carbohydrate, muscle glycogen, and exercise performance during 7 d of training. Am J Clin Nutr 1993; 57(1):27–31.

97. Economos CD, Bortz SS, Nelson ME. Nutritional practices of elite athletes. Practical recommendations. Sports Med 1993;16(6):381–99.

98. Fleming J, Sharman MJ, Avery NG, et al. Endurance capacity and high-intensity exercise performance responses to a high fat diet. Int J Sport Nutr Exerc Metab 2003;13(4):466–78.

99. Helge JW. Adaptation to a fat-rich diet: effects on endurance performance in humans. Sports Med 2000;30(5):347–57.

100. Costill DL, Bowers R, Branam G, Sparks K. Muscle glycogen utilization during prolonged exercise on successive days. J Appl Physiol 1971;31(6):834–8.

101. Sherman WM, Wimer GS. Insufficient dietary carbohydrate during training: does it impair athletic performance? International journal of sport nutrition 1991;1(1): 28–44.

102. Pascoe DD, Costill DL, Robergs RA, Davis JA, Fink WJ, Pearson DR. Effects of exercise mode on muscle glycogen restorage during repeated days of exercise. Med Sci Sports Exerc 1990;22(5):593–8.

103. Costill DL, Flynn MG, Kirwan JP, et al. Effects of repeated days of intensified training on muscle glycogen and swimming performance. Med Sci Sports Exerc 1988;20(3):249–54.

104. Kirwan JP, Costill DL, Mitchell JB, et al. Carbohydrate balance in competitive runners during successive days of intense training. J Appl Physiol 1988;65(6): 2601–6.

105. Snyder AC. Overtraining and glycogen depletion hypothesis. Med Sci Sports Exerc 1998;30(7):1146–50.

106. O'Toole ML. Overreaching and Overtraining in Endurance Athletes. In: Kreider RB, Fry AC, O'Toole ML, editors. Overtraining in Sport. Champaign, IL: Human Kinetics; 1998. p. 3–18.

107. Kuipers H, Keizer HA. Overtraining in elite athletes. Review and directions for the future. Sports Med 1988;6(2):79–92.

108. McCartney N, Spriet LL, Heigenhauser GJ, Kowalchuk JM, Sutton JR, Jones NL. Muscle power and metabolism in maximal intermittent exercise. J Appl Physiol 1986;60(4):1164–9.

109. Balsom PD, Gaitanos GC, Soderlund K, Ekblom B. High-intensity exercise and muscle glycogen availability in humans. Acta Physiol Scand 1999;165(4):337–45.

110. Jacobs I, Kaiser P, Tesch P. Muscle strength and fatigue after selective glycogen depletion in human skeletal muscle fibers. Eur J Appl Physiol 1981;46(1):47–53.

111. Hepburn D, Maughan RJ. Glycogen availability as a limiting factor in performance of isometric exercise. J. Physiol. 1982;342:52P–53P.

112. Yaspelkis BBd, Patterson JG, Anderla PA, Ding Z, Ivy JL. Carbohydrate supplementation spares muscle glycogen during variable-intensity exercise. J Appl Physiol 1993;75(4):1477–85.

113. Nieman DC, Butler JV, Pollett LM, Dietrich SJ, Lutz RD. Nutrient intake of marathon runners. J Am Diet Assoc 1989;89(9):1273–8.

114. Greenhaff PL, Gleeson M, Maughan RJ. The effects of dietary manipulation on blood acid-base status and the performance of high intensity exercise. Eur J Appl Physiol 1987;56(3):331–7.

115. Jenkins DG, Palmer J, Spillman D. The influence of dietary carbohydrate on performance of supramaximal intermittent exercise. Eur J Appl Physiol 1993;67(4): 309–14.

116. Lamb DR, Rinehardt KF, Bartels RL, Sherman WM, Snook JT. Dietary carbohydrate and intensity of interval swim training. Am J Clin Nutr 1990;52(6):1058–63.

117. Vandenberghe K, Hespel P, Vanden Eynde B, Lysens R, Richter EA. No effect of glycogen level on glycogen metabolism during high intensity exercise. Med Sci Sports Exerc 1995;27(9):1278–83.

118. Wootton SA, Williams C. Influence of carbohydrate status on performance during maximal exercise. Int. J. Sports Med. 1984;5(Supplement):126–127.

119. Maughan RJ, Poole DC. The effects of a glycogen-loading regimen on the capacity to perform anaerobic exercise. Eur J Appl Physiol 1981;46(3):211–9.

120. Pizza FX, Flynn MG, Duscha BD, Holden J, Kubitz ER. A carbohydrate loading regimen improves high intensity, short duration exercise performance. Int J Sport Nutr 1995;5(2):110–6.

121. Haff GG, Kleiner SM, Walberg-Rankin J, Vinci DM, Volek JS. Roundtable Discussion: Low Carbohydrate Diets and Anaerobic Athletes. Strength and Cond J 2001;23(3):42–61.

122. Achten J, Halson SL, Moseley L, Rayson MP, Casey A, Jeukendrup AE. Higher dietary carbohydrate content during intensified running training results in better maintenance of performance and mood state. J Appl Physiol 2004;96(4):1331–40.

123. Burke LM, Kiens B, Ivy JL. Carbohydrates and fat for training and recovery. J Sports Sci 2004;22(1):15–30.

124. Nieman DC. Exercise Testing and Prescription: A Health Related Approach. 4th ed. Mountain View: Mayfield Publsihing; 1999.

125. Faber M, Benade AJ. Mineral and vitamin intake in field athletes (discus-, hammer-, javelin-throwers and shotputters). Int J Sports Med 1991;12(3):324–7.

126. Hickson JF, Jr., Duke MA, Risser WL, Johnson CW, Palmer R, Stockton JE. Nutritional intake from food sources of high school football athletes. J Am Diet Assoc 1987;87(12):1656–9.

127. Burke LM, Gollan RA, Read RS. Dietary intakes and food use of groups of elite Australian male athletes. Int J Sport Nutr 1991;1(4):378–94.

128. Paschoal VC, Amancio OM. Nutritional status of Brazilian elite swimmers. Int J Sport Nutr Exerc Metab 2004;14(1):81–94.

129. Worme JD, Doubt TJ, Singh A, Ryan CJ, Moses FM, Deuster PA. Dietary patterns, gastrointestinal complaints, and nutrition knowledge of recreational triathletes. Am J Clin Nutr 1990;51(4):690–7.

130. Coyle EF. Substrate utilization during exercise in active people. Am J Clin Nutr 1995;61(4 Suppl):968S–979S.

131. Hawley JA, Schabort EJ, Noakes TD, Dennis SC. Carbohydrate-loading and exercise performance. An update. Sports Med 1997;24(2):73–81.

132. Sherman WM, Costill DL, Fink WJ, Miller JM. Effect of exercise-diet manipulation on muscle glycogen and its subsequent utilization during performance. Int J Sports Med 1981;2(2):114–8.

133. Pascoe DD, Costill DL, Fink WJ, Robergs RA, Zachwieja JJ. Glycogen resynthesis in skeletal muscle following resistive exercise. Med Sci Sports Exerc 1993;25(3):349–54.

134. Ivy JL, Katz AL, Cutler CL, Sherman WM, Coyle EF. Muscle glycogen synthesis after exercise: effect of time of carbohydrate ingestion. J Appl Physiol 1988;64(4):1480–5.

135. Ivy JL, Lee MC, Brozinick JT, Jr., Reed MJ. Muscle glycogen storage after different amounts of carbohydrate ingestion. J Appl Physiol 1988;65(5):2018–23.

136. Blom PC, Hostmark AT, Vaage O, Kardel KR, Maehlum S. Effect of different post-exercise sugar diets on the rate of muscle glycogen synthesis. Med Sci Sports Exerc 1987;19(5):491–6.

137. MacDougall JD, Ward GR, Sutton JR. Muscle glycogen repletion after high-intensity intermittent exercise. J Appl Physiol 1977;42(2):129–32.

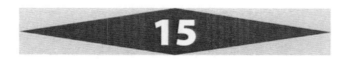

# Vitamins and Minerals

## Darin Van Gammeren

## OBJECTIVES

On the completion of this chapter you will be able to:

1. Explain the difference between fat-soluble and water-soluble vitamins.
2. Differentiate between macronutrients and micronutrients.
3. Give examples of food groups that supply specific vitamins and minerals.
4. Discuss the specific functions in the body of each vitamin and mineral presented.
5. Understand and be able to explain the current body of scientific knowledge regarding the ergogenic properties of each vitamin and mineral.
6. List the different names associated with each vitamin.

## ABSTRACT

The human diet consists of both macro- and micronutrients. Macronutrients include carbohydrates, fats, and proteins, whereas micronutrients consist of vitamins and minerals. (See Table 15.1 for food sources of vitamins and minerals.) As their name implies, the macronutrients comprise most of the required dietary intake whereas the micronutrients are essential in much lower quantities. With the deficiency of micronutrients, athletic performance in addition to normal physiologic function will suffer. However, the very nature of being a micronutrient suggests that excess intake in well-fed athletes will not likely alter performance without an activity-associated increased need. For example, many vitamins and minerals are important in the catabolism of the macronutrients for energy production. Furthermore, many of the micronutrients are involved in endogenous antioxidant defense mechanisms. It has been hypothesized that athletes have an increased requirement for vitamins and minerals because of the increased energy expenditure and excess muscle damage that occurs during training or competition.

During exercise, there is an excess production of various reactive oxygen species and free radicals. Free radicals are reactive molecules that contain one or more unpaired electrons in their outer orbital. Molecules with unpaired electrons are unstable and will oxidize various components of the cell including lipids, proteins, and nucleic acids. The body has multiple antioxidant defense systems to protect itself from these reactive molecules. In addition to endogenous antioxidant enzymes, dietary antioxidants (e.g., vitamin C and E) provide protection against the detrimental effects of reactive oxygen species and free radicals (i.e., oxidative stress).

The following chapter is a review of vitamins and selected minerals. Vitamins are categorized into water-soluble and fat-soluble vitamins. Water-soluble vitamins are found in the fluid portion of the body and do not accumulate to

From: *Essentials of Sports Nutrition and Supplements*
Edited by J. Antonio, D. Kalman, J. R. Stout, M. Greenwood, D. S. Willoughby, and G. G. Haff © Humana Press, a part of Springer Science+Business Media, Totowa, NJ

TABLE 15.1. Food sources of vitamins and minerals.

| Nutrient | Food sources |
| --- | --- |
| Thiamin | Enriched, fortified, or whole-grain products, bread and bread products, cereal |
| Riboflavin | Organ meats, milk, bread products, fortified cereals |
| Niacin | Meat, fish, poultry, enriched and whole-grain breads and bread products, fortified cereals |
| Pantothenic acid | Chicken, beef, potatoes, oats, cereals, tomato products, liver, kidney, yeast, egg yolk, broccoli, whole grains |
| Vitamin B6 | Fortified cereals, organ meats, fortified soy-based meat substitutes |
| Folate | Enriched cereal grains, dark leafy vegetables, enriched and whole-grain breads and bread products, fortified cereals |
| Biotin | Liver and smaller amounts in fruits and meats |
| Vitamin B12 | Fortified cereals, meat, fish, poultry |
| Vitamin C | Citrus fruits, tomatoes, tomato juice, potatoes, brussel sprouts, cauliflower, broccoli, strawberries, cabbage, spinach |
| Vitamin E | Vegetable oils, unprocessed cereal grains, nuts, fruits, vegetables, meats |
| Vitamin A | Liver, dairy products, fish, darkly colored fruits and leafy vegetables |
| Vitamin D | Fatty fish, fortified milk products, fortified cereals |
| Vitamin K | Green vegetables, brussel sprouts, cabbage, plant oils, margarine |
| Calcium | Milk, cheese, yogurt, corn tortillas, broccoli |
| Chromium | Some cereals, meats, poultry, fish, beer |
| Iron | Fruits, vegetables, fortified bread and grain products (nonheme iron sources); meat and poultry (heme iron sources) |
| Magnesium | Green leafy vegetables, unpolished grains, nuts, meat, starches, milk |
| Zinc | Fortified cereals, red meats, certain seafoods |
| Phosphorus | Milk, yogurt, ice cream, cheese, peas, meat, eggs, some cereals and breads |
| Selenium | Organ meats, seafood, plants (depending on soil selenium content) |

a large degree. Fat-soluble vitamins are stored in the lipid portion of the body and, therefore, can accumulate to appreciable amounts. Moreover, almost all of the vitamins and minerals mentioned in this chapter are antioxidants or cofactors involved in the oxidation-reduction balance of the body. Therefore, antioxidant function is a main underlying focal point of this chapter. For each micronutrient, there is a brief description of its physiologic function, in particular its role in maintaining the oxidation-reduction balance of the cell, followed by a review of the scientific literature pertaining to its effect on aerobic, anaerobic, and strength performance.

*Key Words:* **vitamin, mineral, fat-soluble, water-soluble, RDA, overdose, metabolism**

# REVIEW OF LITERATURE

## Water-Soluble Vitamins

### THIAMIN

Thiamin is a B-complex vitamin previously known as vitamin B1. In the body, thiamin can exist as free or phosphorylated thiamin. The phosphorylated forms include thiamin monophosphate, thiamin triphosphate, and thiamin pyrophosphate (TPP). Thiamin triphosphate is found in high concentrations in nerve and muscle cells and can activate ion channels allowing the flow of sodium and calcium. Furthermore, the coenzyme TPP is important in mitochondrial function. Various reactions involved in the Krebs cycle and pentose phosphate pathway require TPP.[1]

Animal research has been conducted on the effects of thiamin and performance. In early studies, repeated bouts (10 days) of swimming exercise were sufficient to deplete thiamin levels whereas one bout of swimming was not.[2] Furthermore, research has determined that trained mice swam 40% longer

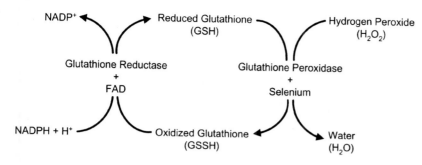

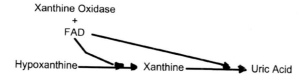

FIGURE 15.1. The glutathione oxidation-reduction (redox) cycle. NADP = nicotinamide adenine dinucleotide phosphate. (Adapted from Higdon.[1])

when given 100 times the minimal daily requirement of thiamin while on a high carbohydrate diet, but no increase in performance was noted with the thiamin supplementation while on a high fat diet.[3] The increase in performance could have been from the high carbohydrate ingestion and not the thiamin.

Research using human subjects has also been used to study the effects of thiamin on performance. Evidence has shown that repeated bouts of eccentric-based exercise decreased blood thiamin levels[4] whereas thiamin supplementation (900 mg/day for 3 days) in highly trained cyclists improved blood lactate levels and heart rate during intense exercise.[5] Nonetheless, thiamin depletion did not alter aerobic performance following 10–12 weeks of treadmill training (60–90 minutes/day).[6] Supplementation of thiamin (1.0 mg/1000 kcal) was also ineffective at altering leg muscle strength, blood lactate, glucose, or pyruvate levels. Finally, short-term, repetitive exercise in moderately trained subjects did not alter thiamin levels.[7]

Theoretically, thiamin supplementation could increase aerobic performance given that it is required for energy production in the Krebs cycle and pentose phosphate pathway. However, because a deficiency in thiamin is uncommon and research has not shown an increase in aerobic or strength performance with thiamin supplementation, excess thiamin intake is not warranted.

## RIBOFLAVIN

Riboflavin is a B-complex vitamin also known as vitamin B2. Riboflavin is primarily a component of the coenzymes flavin adenine dinucleotide (FAD) and flavin mononucleotide, termed flavins. These flavins are critical in the metabolism of all the macronutrients. Furthermore, FAD has a very important antioxidant role. The oxidant, hydrogen peroxide, can be broken down by the antioxidant enzyme glutathione peroxidase in the presence of reduced glutathione (see Figure 15.1). During this reaction, glutathione is oxidized, altering the oxidation-reduction (redox) state of the cell. The FAD-dependent enzyme, glutathione reductase, reduces glutathione maintaining the cellular redox balance. Furthermore, the FAD-dependent enzyme, xanthine oxidase, is used to produce, among other compounds, uric acid (see Figure 15.2). At physiologic concentrations, uric acid contributes to the total antioxidant capacity of the blood plasma more than any other compound including vitamins C and E.[1]

Studies have been performed to ascertain the effects of riboflavin on performance. An early study on 18 male athletes concluded that 45% of the athletes had an inadequate riboflavin status.[8] Nonetheless, more recent studies have shown that athletes have a normal level of riboflavin.[9,10] Furthermore, supplementation of 60 mg/day of riboflavin in male and female elite swimmers for 16–20 days showed no change in their 50-meter freestyle times.[11] A study by van Dokkum and van der Beek[12] also showed no improvement in bicycle ergometry performance with riboflavin supplementation. Overall, riboflavin can function as an antioxidant; however, deficiencies are not common and supplementation does not improve aerobic performance.

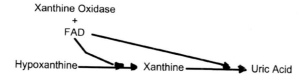

FIGURE 15.2. Flavin adenine dinucleotide (FAD)-dependent xanthine oxidase produces the antioxidant uric acid.

## NIACIN

Niacin is also known as vitamin B3. In the body, niacin is utilized in the forms nicotinic acid, nicotinamide, nicotinamide adenine dinucleotide (NAD), and nicotinamide adenine dinucleotide phosphate (NADP). NAD and NADP are coenzymes that are required by as many as 200 different enzymes. Because these coenzymes are exceptional electron donors, they are essential in the catabolism of all of the macronutrients as well as the synthesis of fatty acids and cholesterol.[1]

Research has been conducted on niacin and performance. One might theorize that supplemental niacin would improve aerobic performance by increasing the availability of NAD and NADP; however, this is not the case.[13] When 10 well-trained runners were given 2 g of nicotinic acid, no changes were noted in their 10-mile run times.[14] Furthermore, nicotinic acid has been administered with and without a carbohydrate supplement.[15] An attenuation in the increase of free fatty acids and an increase in carbohydrate oxidation occurred, but there was no change in performance as measured by the subjects' 3.5-mile cycling time. The attenuated release of free fatty acids and increased carbohydrate oxidation could result in an increase in aerobic performance; however, this has not been scientifically demonstrated.[16]

## PANTOTHENIC ACID

Pantothenic acid is also known as vitamin B5. The major contribution of pantothenic acid to human metabolism is its role as a component of coenzyme A (CoA). CoA is vital in a variety of life-sustaining metabolic reactions including the generation of energy [adenosine triphosphate (ATP)] from macronutrients and the synthesis of essential fats, cholesterol, and acetylcholine.[1]

Research on pantothenic acid and exercise is sparse at best. Supplementation of 2 g/day of pantothenic acid for 2 weeks in cyclists decreased blood lactate and oxygen consumption.[17] However, a study by Nice et al.[18] on 18 athletes from ages 30 to 35 years showed that 1 g/day of pantothenic acid for 2 weeks had no significant effect on performance. The decrease in blood lactate and oxygen consumption would seem to be beneficial, but these effects do not translate to improved aerobic performance.

## VITAMIN B6

Vitamin B6 can be found in the body in the following forms: 1) pyridoxal, 2) pyridoxine, 3) pyridoxamine, and their phosphate derivatives, 4) pyridoxal 5'-phosphate (PLP), 5) pyridoxine 5'-phosphate, and 6) pyridoxamine 5'-phosphate. These permutations of vitamin B6 are important individually and in concert in various metabolic reactions. The most studied form, PLP, is the active coenzyme in the body and is, therefore, very important in human metabolism. For example, PLP is a coenzyme for glycogen phosphorylase, an enzyme that releases muscle glycogen for energy production in the form of glucose. Also, PLP is involved in the conversion of amino acids to glucose (gluconeogenesis). Moreover, PLP is a coenzyme in reactions producing neurotransmitters such as serotonin, dopamine, norepinephrine, and gamma-aminobutyric acid.[1]

Few studies have been conducted on vitamin B6 and performance. Research using rats supplemented with 33 times the amount of vitamin B6 needed for normal maintenance and growth has shown no improvement in skeletal muscle strength.[19] In humans, high carbohydrate diets supplemented with 8–10 g/day of vitamin B6 resulted in an increased use of muscle glycogen and a decrease in free fatty acid levels.[20,21] However, the latest study on vitamin B6 supplementation (20 mg/day) revealed a decrease in plasma free fatty acids but no improvement in endurance.[22] Vitamin B6 supplementation does not seem to improve aerobic performance.

## FOLATE

The B-complex vitamin folate is also known as folic acid. The only function of folate is as a cofactor in the transfer of one-carbon units. By accepting and donat-

**TABLE 15.2. Recommended dietary allowances (RDA)/adequate intakes (AI) of vitamins and selected minerals for young adults.**

| Nutrient | RDA/AI—men | RDA/AI—women | UL |
|---|---|---|---|
| Thiamin (mg/d) | **1.2** | **1.1** | ND |
| Riboflavin (mg/d) | **1.3** | **1.1** | ND |
| Niacin (mg/d) | **16** | **14** | 35 |
| Pantothenic acid (mg/d) | 5 | 5 | ND |
| Vitamin B6 (mg/d) | **1.3** | **1.3** | 100 |
| Folate (µg/d) | **400** | **400** | 1000 |
| Biotin (µg/d) | 30 | 30 | ND |
| Vitamin B12 (µg/d) | **2.4** | **2.4** | ND |
| Vitamin C (mg/d) | **90** | 75 | 2000 |
| Vitamin E (mg/d) | **15** | **15** | 1000 |
| Vitamin A (µg/d) | **900** | **700** | 3000 |
| Vitamin D (µg/d) | 5 | 5 | 50 |
| Vitamin K (µg/d) | 120 | 90 | ND |
| Calcium (mg/d) | 1000 | 1000 | 2500 |
| Chromium (µg/d) | 35 | 25 | ND |
| Iron (mg/d) | **8** | **18** | 45 |
| Magnesium (mg/d) | **400** | **310** | 350 |
| Zinc (mg/d) | **11** | **8** | 40 |
| Phosphorus (mg/d) | **700** | **700** | 4000 |
| Selenium (µg/d) | **55** | **55** | 400 |

*Source:* Adapted from Grandjean.[24]

*Note:* RDA in bold. RDAs are set to meet the needs of 97%–98% of individuals. AIs are believed to meet the requirements of all individuals; however, a lack of data prevents the ability to specify with complete confidence the percent of individuals covered by this intake. Tolerable upper intake levels (ULs) are the maximum amounts that will not likely cause adverse affects. Some levels are not determinable (ND) because of a lack of data on the adverse affects.

ing carbon, folate is important in nucleic acid and amino acid metabolism suggesting that deficiencies in highly trained athletes may affect performance.[1]

To date, only one study has been conducted on folate supplementation and athletic performance in adults.[23] Twenty-three female marathon runners, deficient in folate, were supplemented with 5 mg/day for 10 weeks. Supplementation improved folate levels, but there were no improvements in exercise performance when compared with placebo-supplemented control subjects with normal blood folate levels. With the paucity of data on folate supplementation, conclusions cannot be clearly drawn, but intake of the recommended dietary allowance (RDA) for folate should suffice (see Table 15.2).

### BIOTIN

Biotin, also known as vitamin H, is a B-complex vitamin that cannot be synthesized endogenously and, therefore, must be obtained from the diet (see Table 15.1). Functionally, biotin attaches to four different enzymes. The first enzyme, acetyl-CoA carboxylase, catalyzes the binding of bicarbonate to acetyl-CoA. Acetyl-CoA can form malonyl-CoA which is required for the synthesis of fatty acids. The second enzyme, pyruvate carboxylase, is important in gluconeogenesis. Next, methylcrotonyl-CoA carboxylase is involved in an essential step in leucine metabolism. Finally, propionyl-CoA carboxylase is essential for the metabolism of various amino acids, cholesterol, and odd-chain fatty acids.[1] Studies have not been conducted, to date, on the effects of biotin alone and its effect on exercise performance.

### VITAMIN B12

Vitamin B12 is the largest and most complex vitamin and cannot be synthesized by the body; therefore, individuals must obtain this nutrient in their diet. Vitamin B12 contains cobalt and, therefore, is also called cobalamin. Within the body, vitamin B12 is a constitute of methylcobalamin and 5-deoxyadenosyl

**FIGURE 15.3.** The interaction of vitamin C and vitamin E in scavenging free radicals. (Adapted from Packer and Obermuller-Jevic.[35])

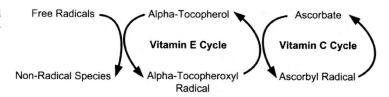

cobalamin. Methylcobalamin is required for methionine synthase activity which converts homocysteine to methionine. 5-Deoxyadenosyl cobalamin is involved in the conversion of L-methylmalonyl-CoA to succinyl-CoA. Succinyl-CoA is important in energy production from fats and proteins.[1]

Only one study has evaluated the effects of vitamin B12 alone on performance.[25] Male students were supplemented with 1 mg of vitamin B12, 3 times per week for 6 weeks in a double-blind, placebo-controlled manner. No effect of supplementation was noted in the maximal oxygen uptake (VO$_2$ max) or strength. In well-nourished individuals, it is unlikely that vitamin B12 supplementation will increase aerobic performance or strength.

### Vitamin C

Vitamin C, or ascorbic acid, is vital for many physiologic functions. Humans cannot synthesize vitamin C and, therefore, must obtain it exogenously. Vitamin C is important in the synthesis of collagen, a component of tendons, ligaments, bones, and blood vessels. Another function of vitamin C is the production of carnitine. Carnitine is a transport molecule for fatty acids into the mitochondria. Once in the mitochondria, fatty acids can be converted into ATP for energy.[1] Finally, vitamin C serves as an antioxidant by scavenging cytotoxic free radicals and recycling the vitamin E radical back to its reduced state (see Figure 15.3).[26]

Because of vitamin C's antioxidant properties, many investigators have studied its effect on reducing free radical mediated muscle damage. In the early 1990s, vitamin C (3 g/day) decreased the delayed onset of muscle soreness (DOMS) in response to 15 minutes of cyclic plantar flexion.[27] Bryer and Goldfarb[28] supplemented subjects with 3 g/day of vitamin C for 2 weeks before eccentric training of the biceps. Supplementation resulted in a decrease in DOMS, creatine kinase, and oxidized proteins during the 4 days after the exercise protocol. In contrast, lower dosages of vitamin C (10 mg/kg) accompanied with N-acetyl-cysteine after eccentric training of the biceps did not reduce DOMS and actually increased muscle damage as indicated by an increase in creatine kinase and lactate dehydrogenase.[29] Similarly, Bryant et al.[30] concluded that vitamin C supplementation may have promoted cellular damage as indicated by an increase of plasma levels of malonaldehyde (MDA). Furthermore, vitamin C did not improve exercise performance during a 30-minute cycle test. Subsequently, Thompson and colleagues[32–34] conducted a series of placebo-controlled experiments to determine the effects vitamin C supplementation (400–1000 mg/day) on muscle soreness and damage after downhill running[31] and intermittent shuttle running. Only one of these studies resulted in a modest benefit of vitamin C with respect to muscle soreness.[34]

Overall, vitamin C supplementation has resulted in improvements in exercise-induced damage. With deficiencies in vitamin C being infrequent, supplementation is rarely thought to improve performance. Nevertheless, the most important consideration with vitamin C is whether or not supplementation above the RDA is warranted. Evidence suggests that supplemental vitamin C may reduce exercise-induced cellular damage; however, when taken in excess, it may act as a prooxidant, actually inducing damage. The author recommends that if supplemental vitamin C is used, it not be taken in excess of the upper limit of the RDA (see Table 15.2).

## Fat-Soluble Vitamins

### Vitamin E

Vitamin E refers to a group of antioxidants including the tocopherols and tocotrienols. Both the tocopherols and tocotrienols have an alpha, beta, gamma, and delta form. In the body, alpha tocopherol is the most active form of vitamin E. Vitamin E serves as a powerful antioxidant by scavenging peroxyl radicals and inhibiting lipid peroxidation in cell membranes (i.e., oxidative damage).[1]

Of all the vitamins and minerals, vitamin E is one of most highly investigated. Studies have shown a beneficial effect of vitamin E supplementation in preventing muscle damage. For example, an early study involving 30 top-class cyclists demonstrated that vitamin E can decrease plasma levels of creatine kinase and malondialdehyde, markers of mechanical and oxidative damage.[36] Furthermore, when 1200 IU of vitamin E were given to 14 male runners in a randomized, placebo-controlled manner, an attenuation in muscle damage was noted.[37] Also, a study by Bryant et al.[30] demonstrated that cyclists given 400 IU/day of vitamin E had a decrease in membrane damage.

In contrast, other studies have shown no benefit of vitamin E supplementation in preventing muscle damage. Healthy men given 1200 IU/day of vitamin E or a placebo for 30 days performed 240 maximal isokinetic eccentric contractions.[38] The results showed no difference in muscle torque, Z-band disruption, creatine kinase, or inflammation. Moreover, 1200 IU/day of vitamin E for 3 weeks had no effect on muscle soreness after 3 resistance-exercise sessions separated by 3 days in previously untrained men.[39]

Whereas investigations of vitamin E supplementation have produced variable results with regard to muscle damage, no study has shown a beneficial effect of vitamin E on performance. Five months of supplementation with vitamin E had no effect on aerobic performance in trained cyclists.[36] Likewise, 1200 IU/day for 4 weeks before and during 6 days of running resulted in no change in $VO_2$ max when compared with a placebo.[37] In a recent study involving seven trained cyclists, vitamin E did not improve cycling performance.[30] Finally, 1200 IU/day of vitamin E for 3 weeks did not improve muscle performance as tested by jump squats, bench throws, and squat endurance.[39] Therefore, vitamin E may attenuate exercise-induced muscle damage, but no evidence exists indicating improved performance with vitamin E supplementation.

## Sidebar 15.1. Vitamin C and E Do Not Improve Performance

A study conducted by Bryant et al.[30] tested the effects of vitamins C and E alone or in combination on cycling performance. Seven young, trained male cyclists were given the following four vitamin supplements in a cross-over design study: 1) placebo, 2) 1 g/day vitamin C, 3) 1 g/day vitamin C and 200 IU/day vitamin E, and 4) 400 IU/day vitamin E. Performance measures included a 60-minute steady-state ride and 30-minute performance ride at 70% of $VO_2$ max. Blood samples were drawn before and after exercise for MDA, a marker of lipid peroxidation, and lactic acid analysis. Pre- and postexercise MDA levels were lower in the vitamin E group as compared with the placebo group. Conversely, vitamin C increased levels of MDA pre- and postexercise. Nonetheless, none of the supplemental regimens improved performance. Therefore, although vitamin E can decrease oxidative damage both before and after exercise, its effects are not ergogenic.

## VITAMIN A

Vitamin A encompasses a group of compounds including the retinoids (i.e., retinol, retinal, and retinoic acid). Of these compounds, retinol can be produced from beta-carotene and other carotenoids. Carotenoids are antioxidants that neutralize free radicals such as singlet oxygen and peroxyl radicals.[1]

Wald et al.[40] supplemented subjects with high doses of vitamin A for 6 weeks and demonstrated no improvement in their ability to perform intense muscular exercise. Mechanistically, vitamin A could improve performance by decreasing oxidative stress; however, because vitamins C and E are more potent antioxidants, vitamin A supplementation is not warranted with respect to redox control.

## VITAMIN D

There are many different forms of vitamin D, but vitamin D3 (cholecalciferol) is the primary form used in the body. Cholesterol can be converted into 7-dehydrocholesterol, a precursor to vitamin D3. Ultraviolet light in sunshine converts 7-dehydrocholesterol to vitamin D3 in skin. With even a minimal exposure to sunlight, there is no need for dietary vitamin D or vitamin D supplementation, and deficiency is virtually nonexistent.[1] Furthermore, no enhancement in physical performance has been noted with vitamin D supplementation.

## VITAMIN K

There are two naturally occurring forms of vitamin K: phylloquinone (vitamin K1) and menaquinone-n (vitamin K2). Plants are capable of making phylloquinone whereas bacteria produce menaquinone-n. The only role of vitamin K is as a coenzyme for vitamin K-dependent carboxylase which is involved in the carboxylation of glutamic acid into gamma carboxyglutamic acid. This reaction is critical for calcium binding to certain proteins.[1] Finally, the mechanistic rationale for vitamin K to improve performance is not readily apparent and therefore no studies have been conducted on its effect on performance to date.

## Minerals

### CALCIUM

Calcium is the most abundant mineral in the body. Calcium concentrations in the body must be closely regulated for normal cellular function. When deficient in the diet, the body will absorb calcium from bone stores to maintain proper blood/cellular calcium concentrations. In light of the critical role of calcium in the maintenance of bone, adequate dietary calcium is essential in protecting the skeleton from degradation. Moreover, calcium is very important in cell signaling. For example, when a nerve conducts an impulse to muscle, the signal will be detected by the ryanodine receptors in the sarcoplasmic reticulum. This will allow calcium ions to be released, stimulating a muscle contraction.[1] Calcium is not an ergogenic aid, but supplementation should be used to prevent osteoporosis if there is a deficiency.

### CHROMIUM

Chromium is an essential mineral and must, therefore, be obtained in the diet. The two common forms include trivalent chromium (III) and hexavalent chromium (VI). Chromium III is the form available in foods and utilized in the body. Chromium is involved in glucose metabolism by enhancing the function of insulin. Insulin is released from the pancreas after the ingestion of food, especially foods high in simple carbohydrates. The binding of insulin to receptors on the surface of cells allows for the uptake of glucose for energy or storage.[1]

In 1989, Evans[41] conducted a two-part study on the effects of 200 μg/day of chromium picolinate (ChrPic). In the first trial, ChrPic significantly increased fat free mass without an increase in fat mass. In the second trial, there was a significant decrease in body fat with ChrPic. Faults of this study were that energy intake and dietary chromium intake were not taken into account. Furthermore, skinfold and limb circumference measurements were used to determine body composition. These measurements are not the ideal way to assess body composition; however, this study sparked a series of experiments on ChrPic supplementation.

Since the Evans study,[41] numerous investigators have tried to replicate the results with no success.[42-47] Using more precise body composition measurements such as hydrostatic weighing[43,44] and dual-energy X-ray absorptiometry,[45] investigators have not shown improvements in body composition with chromium supplementation. Furthermore, none of these studies have shown an increase in strength. Therefore, chromium supplementation is not recommended.

Superoxide ($O_2^-$)
+
Hydrogen Peroxide ($H_2O_2$) $\longrightarrow$
+
Reactive Iron ($Fe^{+2}$)

Oxygen ($O_2$)
+
Hydroxide Anion ($OH^-$)
+
Hydroxyl Radical ($OH\cdot$)

**FIGURE 15.4.** The production of the highly reactive hydroxyl radical via the Haber-Weiss reaction.

## IRON

Iron is a component of hundreds of proteins and enzymes in the body. For example, the heme in hemoglobin and myoglobin contains iron. Hemoglobin is the oxygen transportation molecule found in red blood cells whereas myoglobin is a similar molecule, but it is used in the transport of oxygen within the muscle. Other important heme-containing molecules are cytochromes. Cytochromes are part of the electron transport chain in mitochondria. The cytochromes serve as electron carriers in the production of ATP. Moreover, catalase and peroxidase enzymes contain heme. These molecules can rid the body of excess hydrogen peroxide, a toxic reactive oxygen species. Finally, when free iron is in its ferrous state ($Fe+2$), it can react with hydrogen peroxide and superoxide to form the highly reactive hydroxyl radical (see Figure 15.4).[1]

Anemia, by definition, is a low blood hemoglobin concentration. Of all the single nutrient deficiencies, iron-deficiency anemia is the most common. Iron depletion results in a reduced oxygen transport capacity and a reduction in cellular oxygen capacity. Dietary iron sources include heme and nonheme iron where heme iron is obtained from the hemoglobin and myoglobin found in meat products. Of the two sources of iron, heme iron is more effectively absorbed and the absorption of heme iron is facilitated by animal protein, but inhibited by calcium.[48]

Low iron levels can also alter such processes as the electron transport chain, neurotransmitter synthesis, and protein synthesis. Low hemoglobin and tissue iron can be disadvantageous to exercise performance and athletes may be more susceptible to iron deficiency.[48] It is well known that the iron intake of female athletes is low, making them more prone to iron-deficiency anemia.[49,50] Finally, women may be more susceptible to exercise-induced alterations in iron because of a negative iron balance. It has been determined that an individual's $VO_2$ max is correlated to the blood's oxygen-carrying capacity. However, at lower intensities, tissue iron concentrations are more important because of the importance of iron-dependent oxidative enzymes.[48]

Recent research on iron supplementation has shown positive effects. Twenty iron-depleted, nonanemic, young women received iron for 6 weeks.[51] After the 6-week period, the rate of fatigue during maximal voluntary static contractions of the knee extensors was attenuated with iron supplementation but not the placebo. Furthermore, studies by Brownlie et al.[52,53] have shown improvements in aerobic capacity. Both studies used untrained, iron-depleted, nonanemic women. Subjects were given 100 mg of iron sulfate or a placebo for 6 weeks and the results showed an improvement in $VO_2$ max with iron supplementation. Therefore, in subjects with low iron levels, it is recommend that supplemental iron (not exceeding the upper limit; see Table 15.2) be utilized to improve performance.

## MAGNESIUM

There are approximately 25 g of magnesium in the body of which more than 60% is found in the skeleton and 27% in the muscle. Magnesium is involved in more than 300 essential metabolic reactions. Many of these reactions are involved in the metabolism of carbohydrates, fats, proteins, and nucleic acids. Furthermore, the antioxidant glutathione requires magnesium for its synthesis and the energy-producing molecule, ATP, is usually found in the body as the complex MgATP. Magnesium also has a structural role in bone cells, cell membranes, and chromosomes. Finally, active transport of potassium and calcium across membranes requires magnesium. This ion transport can affect nerve conduction and muscle contraction. Nonetheless, magnesium supplementation and performance has not been investigated.[1]

## ZINC

Zinc is involved in various aspects of cellular metabolism including catalytic, structural, and regulatory roles. More than 100 different enzymes involved in catalytic reactions are zinc dependent. Furthermore, zinc is important in the structure of cell membranes and proteins. Many proteins are stabilized by zinc finger motifs. Also, zinc is important in the structure of the cytosolic antioxidant copper-zinc superoxide dismutase; therefore, a loss of zinc can increase the vulnerability of the cell membrane to oxidative damage. Finally, zinc is involved in cell signaling and, therefore, can release hormones, aid in nerve conduction, and participate in apoptosis (i.e., programmed cell death).[1]

Few studies have been conducted on the supplementation of zinc alone and its effect on performance. In a placebo-controlled, cross-over design study, 16 middle-aged women were supplemented with 135 mg/day of zinc for 14 days.[54] Strength and endurance were evaluated via one-leg isokinetic testing. Zinc increased strength and endurance, but dietary zinc and plasma zinc status were not measured. However, untrained men given various amounts of zinc showed no difference in peak oxygen uptake.[55] Furthermore, rats given 5 or 50 mg/kg of zinc for 3 weeks showed no difference in treadmill running times to exhaustion.[56] Overall, zinc supplementation does not seem to be advantageous.

## Sidebar 15.2. Zinc Magnesium-Aspartate Supplementation

Zinc and magnesium have been touted as an ergogenic aid. It has been reported that athletes may have low zinc and magnesium levels which could decrease their testosterone levels, strength, and muscle mass. Research on the effects of zinc magnesium-aspartate (ZMA) was recently presented at the Experimental Biology Conference in Washington, DC (May 2004).[57,58] In this experiment, 42 resistance-trained males ingested capsules containing 450 mg of magnesium and 30 mg of zinc for 8 weeks. Subjects participated in a standardized weight-training program 4 days per week (two upper- and two lower-body workouts per week) during supplementation. Blood samples were collected at 0, 4, and 8 weeks. No differences in anabolic/catabolic hormones including insulinlike growth factor-1, total testosterone, free testosterone, cortisol, growth hormone, or creatine kinase were noted. However, some markers of catabolism were lower in the ZMA group as compared with a placebo (blood urea nitrogen/creatine ratio and liver enzyme efflux).

Additionally, strength was determined by a 1 repetition maximum strength test for the bench and leg press, whereas muscular endurance was assessed with an 80% 1 repetition maximum endurance test. Also, the Wingate 30-second sprint cycling anaerobic capacity test was performed and body composition was assessed via dual-energy X-ray absorptiometry. No differences in strength, endurance, or body composition parameters existed with ZMA supplementation. These data do not support the use of zinc and magnesium for the enhancement of muscular strength, body composition, or anaerobic performance.

## PHOSPHORUS

Phosphorous is required for every cell in the body to function properly. Most of the phosphorus in the body is in the form of phosphate ($PO_4$), 85% of which is in bone. Phosphorus is a structural component of bone as a calcium phosphate salt called hydroxyapatite. Furthermore, phosphorous is involved in energy production from ATP and creatine phosphate. Although phosphorous is a critical component of all living organisms, phosphorous is not used to improve athletic performance.[1]

## SELENIUM

Selenium-dependent enzymes (selenoproteins) are important in the normal function of the body. To date, 11 selenoproteins have been identified including glutathione peroxidase and thioredoxin reductase. Glutathione peroxidase with glutathione can convert the reactive oxygen species, hydrogen peroxide, into water (see Figure 15.1). Thioredoxin reductase is involved in the regeneration of several antioxidant systems including ascorbate.[1]

Animal studies have shown that selenium-deficient diets decrease the activity of the antioxidant glutathione peroxidase.[59–63] Nonetheless, no study has shown an improvement in performance with selenium supplementation.

## SUMMARY

All of the nutrients discussed in this chapter are, of course, essential for normal, everyday healthy living. All individuals from sedentary to athletic populations need to consume the RDA of all of these nutrients (see Table 15.2). Conversely, none of aforementioned nutrients has been found to enhance performance when taken in excess of the RDA. However, the antioxidant vitamins C and E may enhance recovery after a bout of exercise or strength training by attenuating oxidative stress in the muscle. Furthermore, individuals with a low iron status should consume supplemental iron to ensure proper oxygenation of the working muscle and proper function of the electron transport chain.

## PRACTICAL APPLICATIONS

In a perfect world, everyone would consume a well-balanced diet containing whole grains, fruits, and vegetables, thereby aiding in the assurance of the proper intake of all the micronutrients. Nonetheless, in the real world, people do not have perfect diets. In today's society, the lack of time and the convenience of fast food tempts people to ingest a diet lacking many of the essential vitamins and minerals needed to maintain a healthy lifestyle. If an athlete's diet is less than favorable, it is recommended that they take a high-quality multivitamin as an easy and cost-effective way to ensure the proper intake of all the essential micronutrients. However, first and foremost, it is imperative that athletes strive for a well-balanced diet.

Regarding supplementation with individual vitamins and minerals, there are few data warranting this regimen. Of all the vitamins, only vitamins C and E may enhance recovery after an endurance event or bout of strength training. Deficiencies are rare and supplementation has not been shown to improve performance; nonetheless, as antioxidants, vitamins C and E may decrease oxidant-induced muscle damage. Supplementation not exceeding the upper limit (2000 mg/day for vitamin C and 1000 mg/day for vitamin E including dietary intake) may aid in recovery after prolonged endurance events and strength-training bouts.

Finally, of all the minerals, only iron has been shown to improve performance. Of the single nutrients, iron deficiency is the most common in the world. Furthermore, women, vegetarians, and athletes are all very prone to iron-deficient diets. Moreover, exercise may increase the need for iron by 30%. Athletes at risk should ensure adequate intake of iron and supplement if they are not meeting the recommended dietary intake.

## QUESTIONS

1. Another name for ascorbic acid is:
   a. Vitamin A
   b. Vitamin B12
   c. Vitamin C
   d. Vitamin E

2. Another name for the tocopherols is:
   a. Vitamin A
   b. Vitamin B12
   c. Vitamin C
   d. Vitamin E

3. The most common, single nutrient deficiency is of:
   a. Calcium
   b. Magnesium
   c. Iron
   d. Zinc

4. Which of the following is not considered an antioxidant?
   a. Vitamin A
   b. Vitamin B12
   c. Vitamin C
   d. Vitamin E

5. Adenosine triphosphate is bound to this element in the body:
   a. Iron
   b. Magnesium
   c. Phosphorus
   d. Zinc

6. This vitamin can be obtained from ultraviolet light in the sun:
   a. Vitamin A
   b. Vitamin D
   c. Vitamin E
   d. Vitamin K

7. Which of the following is not a fat-soluble vitamin?
   a. Vitamin A
   b. Vitamin C
   c. Vitamin D
   d. Vitamin E
   e. Vitamin K

8. Which of the following is a powerful scavenger of peroxyl radicals?
   a. Vitamin A
   b. Vitamin C
   c. Vitamin D
   d. Vitamin E

9. Which of the following minerals is important in preventing osteoporosis?
   a. Calcium
   b. Chromium
   c. Magnesium
   d. Zinc

10. This mineral is important in the structure of the cytosolic antioxidant superoxide dismutase.
    a. Chromium
    b. Iron
    c. Magnesium
    d. Zinc

11. This vitamin is a component of flavin adenine dinucleotide and flavin mononucleotide.
    a. Thiamin
    b. Riboflavin
    c. Niacin
    d. Folate

12. This vitamin is a component of adenine dinucleotide and nicotinamide adenine dinucleotide phosphate.
    a. Thiamin
    b. Riboflavin
    c. Niacin
    d. Folate

13. The largest B vitamin is:
    a. Vitamin B6
    b. Biotin

c. Vitamin B12
d. Vitamin C

14. Which vitamin encompasses a group of vitamins known as the retinoids?
    a. Vitamin A
    b. Vitamin D
    c. Vitamin E
    d. Vitamin K

15. This mineral is the most abundant in the body.
    a. Calcium
    b. Iron
    c. Magnesium
    d. Zinc

16. This vitamin aids in the absorption of calcium.
    a. Vitamin A
    b. Vitamin D
    c. Vitamin E
    d. Vitamin K

17. Which of the following vitamins is not toxic?
    a. Vitamin B6
    b. Vitamin A
    c. Vitamin D
    d. Vitamin E

18. Most of this mineral is found in the bones and the teeth.
    a. Calcium
    b. Chromium
    c. Iron
    d. Magnesium

19. Which of the following can serve as an antioxidant?
    a. Biotin
    b. Vitamin C
    c. Vitamin D
    d. Vitamin K

20. Glutathione peroxidase and thioredoxin reductase are dependent on which of the following minerals?
    a. Iron
    b. Magnesium
    c. Zinc
    d. Selenium

21. Pantothenic acid is a component of coenzyme A.
    a. True
    b. False

22. Thiamin is involved in mitochondrial function, Krebs cycle, and the pentose phosphate pathway.
    a. True
    b. False

23. Iron enhances the function of insulin.
    a. True
    b. False

24. A free radical is a molecule with one or more unpaired electrons.
    a. True
    b. False

25. Vitamin B6 has six different forms, one of which is involved in the release of muscle glycogen for energy.
    a. True
    b. False

26. Niacin attaches to four different enzymes.
    a. True
    b. False

27. Selenium is very important in cytochromes involved in the electron transport chain.
    a. True
    b. False

28. Chromium is involved in phosphorylation/dephosphorylation of cells.
    a. True
    b. False

29. Reactive oxygen species must contain oxygen.
    a. True
    b. False

30. Xanthine oxidase is a flavin adenine dinucleotide–dependent enzyme.
    a. True
    b. False

## REFERENCES

1. Higdon J. An Evidence-Based Approach to Vitamins and Minerals. New York: Thieme; 2003.
2. Bialek M, Nijakowski F. Influence of physical effort on the level of thiamin in tissues and blood. Act Physiol Pol 1964;15:192.
3. McNeill AW, Mooney TJ. Relationship among carbohydrate loading, elevated thiamine intake cardiovascular endurance of conditioned mice. J Sports Med Phys Fitness 1983;23:257–262.
4. Nijakowski F. Assay of some vitamins of the B complex group in human blood in relation to muscular effort. Acta Physiol Pol 1966;17:397.
5. Knippel M, Mauri L, Bellushi R, Bana G. The action of thiamin on the production of lactic acid in cyclists. Med Sports 1986;39:11.
6. Keys A, Henschel A, Mickelsen O, Brozek J. The performance of normal young men on controlled thiamin intakes. J Nutr 1943;26:399.
7. Fogelholm M. Micronutrient status in females during a 24-week fitness-type exercise program. Ann Nutr Metab 1992;36:209–218.
8. Haralambie G. Vitamin B2 status in athletes and the influence of riboflavin administration on neuromuscular irritability. Nutr Metab 1976;20:1–8.
9. Guilland JC, Penaranda T, Gallet C, Boggio V, Fuchs F, Klepping J. Vitamin status of young athletes including the effects of supplementation. Med Sci Sports Exerc 1989;21:441–449.
10. Keith R, Alt L. Riboflavin status of female athletes consuming normal diets. Nutr Res 1991;11:727.
11. Tremblay A, Boiland F, Breton M, Bessette H, Roberge A. The effects of a riboflavin supplementation on the nutritional status and performance of elite swimmers. Nutr Res 1984;4:201.
12. van Dokkum W, van der Beek E. Vitamines en prestatievermogen. Voeding 1985; 46:50.
13. Kalman D. Vitamins: are athletes' needs different than the needs of sedentary people? In: Antonio J, Stout J, eds. Sports Supplements. Philadelphia: Lippincott Williams & Wilkins; 2001.
14. Norris B, Schade DS, Eaton RP. Effects of altered free fatty acid mobilization on the metabolic response to exercise. J Clin Endocrinol Metab 1978;46:254–259.
15. Murray R, Bartoli WP, Eddy DE, Horn MK. Physiological and performance responses to nicotinic-acid ingestion during exercise. Med Sci Sports Exerc 1995;27:1057–1062.
16. Lewis R. Riboflavin and niacin. In: Wolinsky I, Driskell J, eds. Sports Nutrition. Vitamins and Trace Elements. Boca Raton, FL: CRC Press; 1997.
17. Litoff D, Scherzer H, Harrison J. Effects of pantothenic acid supplementation on human exercise. Med Sci Sports Exerc 1985;17:287.
18. Nice C, Reeves AG, Brinck-Johnsen T, Noll W. The effects of pantothenic acid on human exercise capacity. J Sports Med Phys Fitness 1984;24:26–29.
19. McMillan J, Keith R, Stone M. The effects of supplemental vitamin B6 and exercise on the contractile properties of rat muscle. Nutr Res 1988;8:73.

20. DeVos A, Leklem J, Campbell D. Carbohydrate loading, vitamin B6 supplementation and fuel metabolism during exercise in man. Med Sci Sports Exerc 1982; 14:137.
21. Manore MM, Leklem JE. Effect of carbohydrate and vitamin B6 on fuel substrates during exercise in women. Med Sci Sports Exerc 1988;20:233–241.
22. Virk RS, Dunton NJ, Young JC, Leklem JE. Effect of vitamin B-6 supplementation on fuels, catecholamines, and amino acids during exercise in men. Med Sci Sports Exerc 1999;31:400–408.
23. Matter M, Stittfall T, Graves J, et al. The effect of iron and folate therapy on maximal exercise performance in female marathon runners with iron and folate deficiency. Clin Sci (Lond) 1987;72:415–422.
24. Grandjean A. Vitamin/mineral supplements and athletics. Strength Cond J 2003; 25:76–78.
25. Tin-May-Tan, Ma-Win-May, Khin-Sann-Aung, Mya-Tu M. The effect of vitamin B12 on physical performance capacity. Br J Nutr 1978;40:269.
26. Powers SK, DeRuisseau KC, Quindry J, Hamilton KL. Dietary antioxidants and exercise. J Sports Sci 2004;22:81–94.
27. Kaminsky M, Boal R. An effect of ascorbic acid on delayed-onset muscle soreness. Pain 1992;50:317–321.
28. Bryer S, Goldfarb A. The effect of vitamin C supplementation on blood glutathione status, DOMS, and creatine kinase. Med Sci Sports Exerc 2001;33:S122.
29. Childs A, Jacobs C, Kaminski T, Halliwell B, Leeuwenburgh C. Supplementation with vitamin C and N-acetyl-cysteine increases oxidative stress in humans after an acute muscle injury induced by eccentric exercise. Free Radic Biol Med 2001; 31:745–753.
30. Bryant RJ, Ryder J, Martino P, Kim J, Craig BW. Effects of vitamin E and C supplementation either alone or in combination on exercise-induced lipid peroxidation in trained cyclists. J Strength Cond Res 2003;17:792–800.
31. Thompson D, Bailey DM, Hill J, Hurst T, Powell JR, Williams C. Prolonged vitamin C supplementation and recovery from eccentric exercise. Eur J Appl Physiol 2004; 92:133–138.
32. Thompson D, Williams C, Garcia-Roves P, McGregor SJ, McArdle F, Jackson MJ. Post-exercise vitamin C supplementation and recovery from demanding exercise. Eur J Appl Physiol 2003;89:393–400.
33. Thompson D, Williams C, Kingsley M, et al. Muscle soreness and damage parameters after prolonged intermittent shuttle-running following acute vitamin C supplementation. Int J Sports Med 2001;22:68–75.
34. Thompson D, Williams C, McGregor SJ, et al. Prolonged vitamin C supplementation and recovery from demanding exercise. Int J Sport Nutr Exerc Metab 2001;11: 466–481.
35. Packer L, Obermuller-Jevic U. Vitamin E: an introduction. In: Packer L, Traber M, Kraemer K, Frei B, eds. The Antioxidant Vitamins C and E. Champaign, IL: AOCS Press; 2002.
36. Rokitzki L, Logemann E, Huber G, Keck E, Keul J. alpha-Tocopherol supplementation in racing cyclists during extreme endurance training. Int J Sport Nutr 1994;4: 253–264.
37. Itoh H, Ohkuwa T, Yamazaki Y, et al. Vitamin E supplementation attenuates leakage of enzymes following 6 successive days of running training. Int J Sports Med 2000;21:369–374.
38. Beaton LJ, Allan DA, Tarnopolsky MA, Tiidus PM, Phillips SM. Contraction-induced muscle damage is unaffected by vitamin E supplementation. Med Sci Sports Exerc 2002;34:798–805.
39. Avery NG, Kaiser JL, Sharman MJ, et al. Effects of vitamin E supplementation on recovery from repeated bouts of resistance exercise. J Strength Cond Res 2003;17: 801–809.
40. Wald G, Brouha L, Johnson R. Experimental human vitamin A deficiency and ability to perform muscular exercise. Am J Physiol 1942;137:551.
41. Evans G. The effect of chromium picolinate on insulin controlled parameters in humans. Int J Biosoc Res 1989;11:163.
42. Hasten DL, Rome EP, Franks BD, Hegsted M. Effects of chromium picolinate on beginning weight training students. Int J Sport Nutr 1992;2:343–350.
43. Clancy SP, Clarkson PM, DeCheke ME, et al. Effects of chromium picolinate supplementation on body composition, strength, and urinary chromium loss in football players. Int J Sport Nutr 1994;4:142–153.
44. Hallmark MA, Reynolds TH, DeSouza CA, Dotson CO, Anderson RA, Rogers MA. Effects of chromium and resistive training on muscle strength and body composition. Med Sci Sports Exerc 1996;28:139–144.

45. Lukaski HC, Bolonchuk WW, Siders WA, Milne DB. Chromium supplementation and resistance training: effects on body composition, strength, and trace element status of men. Am J Clin Nutr 1996;63:954–965.

46. Campbell WW, Polansky MM, Bryden NA, Soares JH Jr, Anderson RA. Exercise training and dietary chromium effects on glycogen, glycogen synthase, phosphorylase and total protein in rats. J Nutr 1989;119:653–660.

47. Campbell WW, Joseph LJ, Anderson RA, Davey SL, Hinton J, Evans WJ. Effects of resistive training and chromium picolinate on body composition and skeletal muscle size in older women. Int J Sport Nutr Exerc Metab 2002;12:125–135.

48. Beard J, Tobin B. Iron status and exercise. Am J Clin Nutr 2000;72:594S–597S.

49. Weaver CM, Rajaram S. Exercise and iron status. J Nutr 1992;122:782–787.

50. Cook JD. The effect of endurance training on iron metabolism. Semin Hematol 1994;31:146–154.

51. Brutsaert TD, Hernandez-Cordero S, Rivera J, Viola T, Hughes G, Haas JD. Iron supplementation improves progressive fatigue resistance during dynamic knee extensor exercise in iron-depleted, nonanemic women. Am J Clin Nutr 2003;77: 441–448.

52. Brownlie T 4th, Utermohlen V, Hinton PS, Haas JD. Tissue iron deficiency without anemia impairs adaptation in endurance capacity after aerobic training in previously untrained women. Am J Clin Nutr 2004;79:437–443.

53. Brownlie T 4th, Utermohlen V, Hinton PS, Giordano C, Haas JD. Marginal iron deficiency without anemia impairs aerobic adaptation among previously untrained women. Am J Clin Nutr 2002;75:734–742.

54. Krotkiewski M, Gudmundsson M, Backstrom P, Mandroukas K. Zinc and muscle strength and endurance. Acta Physiol Scand 1982;116:309–311.

55. Lukaski HC, Bolonchuk WW, Klevay LM, Milne DB, Sandstead HH. Changes in plasma zinc content after exercise in men fed a low-zinc diet. Am J Physiol 1984;247: E88–93.

56. McDonald R, Keen CL. Iron, zinc and magnesium nutrition and athletic performance. Sports Med 1988;5:171–184.

57. Campbell B, Baer J, Thomas A, et al. Effects of zinc magnesium-aspartate (ZMA) supplementation during training on body composition and training adaptations. FASEB J 2004;LB18:A91.

58. Taylor L, Mulligan C, Rohle D, et al. Effects of zinc magnesium-aspartate (ZMA) supplementation during training on markers of anabolism and catabolism. FASEB J 2004;LB18:A91.

59. Hill KE, Burk RF, Lane JM. Effect of selenium depletion and repletion on plasma glutathione and glutathione-dependent enzymes in the rat. J Nutr 1987;117: 99–104.

60. Ji LL, Stratman FW, Lardy HA. Antioxidant enzyme response to selenium deficiency in rat myocardium. J Am Coll Nutr 1992;11:79–86.

61. Ji LL, Stratman FW, Lardy HA. Antioxidant enzyme systems in rat liver and skeletal muscle. Influences of selenium deficiency, chronic training, and acute exercise. Arch Biochem Biophys 1988;263:150–160.

62. Lang JK, Gohil K, Packer L, Burk RF. Selenium deficiency, endurance exercise capacity, and antioxidant status in rats. J Appl Physiol 1987;63:2532–2535.

63. Brady PS, Brady LJ, Ullrey DE. Selenium, vitamin E and the response to swimming stress in the rat. J Nutr 1979;109:1103–1109.

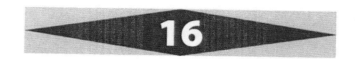

# Nutritional Needs of Endurance Athletes

## Suzanne Girard Eberle

## OBJECTIVES

On the completion of this chapter you will be able to:

1. Discuss the fluid needs and rehydration strategies that are used with endurance athletes.
2. Understand the physiologic ramifications of dehydration and hyponatremia.
3. Explain the macronutrient and micronutrient needs of endurance athletes.
4. Describe the effects of nutrient timing on recovery and performance in endurance athletes.
5. Discuss the ramifications of electrolyte imbalances and how consuming electrolytes can affect recovery and performance.
6. Understand the potential micronutrient needs of endurance athletes and potential food sources that might act as a countermeasure to deficiencies.
7. Outline the proper methods for carbohydrate-loading and explain which athletes this might best benefit.
8. Discuss the pitfalls that can occur when an endurance athlete undertakes a vegetarian dietary regime.
9. Explain the ramifications of a disordered eating pattern coupled with excessive exercise training in endurance athletes.
10. Discuss the three components of the female athlete triad.
11. Outline the warning signs that suggest an athlete is at risk for disordered eating behaviors.
12. Understand the possible factors that might contribute to gastrointestinal distress in endurance athletes.

## ABSTRACT

Endurance athletes, including but not limited to cyclists, runners, triathletes, mountain bikers, and cross-country skiers, have unique and often challenging daily nutritional needs. In fact, the intense and exhaustive endeavors that endurance athletes undertake daily are impossible unless the right foods are eaten in optimal amounts at the correct time. In addition, meeting fluid and fuel needs during exercise—for example, while running a marathon or competing in an Ironman triathlon or multiday adventure race—is another skill the endurance athlete must master.

Nagging injuries, frequent upper respiratory illnesses, and slow recovery from training bouts can all signal that an endurance athlete's nutrition program is out of sync with their training program. Common challenges faced by

From: *Essentials of Sports Nutrition and Supplements*
Edited by J. Antonio, D. Kalman, J. R. Stout, M. Greenwood, D. S. Willoughby, and G. G. Haff © Humana Press, a part of Springer Science+Business Media, Totowa, NJ

endurance athletes include consuming adequate calories, consuming enough of certain key nutrients such as iron, protein, and calcium, and timing food intake around exercise. Endurance athletes who follow a vegetarian eating style as well as those struggling with disordered eating and body image concerns may find it particularly difficult to meet their nutritional needs. This chapter focuses on this specific group of athletes and their nutritional requirements.

*Key Words:* **hydration, fluid replacement, carbohydrate, glycogen, electrolytes, endurance**

## NUTRITIONAL NEEDS AS THEY APPLY TO THE ENDURANCE ATHLETE

Although eating a healthy, well-balanced diet daily does not guarantee success, poor day-to-day eating habits can literally stop an endurance-oriented athlete in their tracks.

## FLUID

Endurance athletes, especially those training multiple times during a 24-hour period, are at particular risk for dehydration, primarily because of increased fluid losses from sweating as a result of prolonged and/or intensive bouts of exercise (especially when exercise is undertaken in extreme conditions such as warm weather, extreme humidity, or at altitude). Being properly hydrated improves endurance, allows the athlete to maintain their desired training intensity, and is vital to protecting against heat illness. Athletes need to know that even minimal dehydration (1%–2% body weight loss) can hinder their performance by reducing blood volume (and consequently the body's ability to maintain a safe core temperature) and reduce the amount of oxygenated blood pumped to working muscles.[1,2]

Endurance athletes will need to monitor their fluid intake throughout the day to minimize acute episodes of dehydration associated with bouts of exercise. For exercise-induced losses, the endurance athlete should weigh in before and after training to determine the amount of fluid lost through sweating. For every pound "lost" after exercise, the athlete needs to drink 20 ounces (2.5 cups) of fluid over the next few hours to meet fluid needs and associated obligatory urine losses that occur during rehydration.[1,2]

Mild dehydration (i.e., <2% body weight loss) is often unavoidable during endurance exercise, particularly during physical endeavors and competitions lasting longer than 3 hours, because the athlete cannot always replenish fluids at a rate that matches the fluid being lost. For example, the capacity of the gastrointestinal (GI) tract, particularly the rate at which ingested fluids empty from the stomach, may become maximized and thus serves to limit the athlete's intake of fluid. If a significant decrease in weight routinely occurs during exercise, however, the athlete needs to do a better job *during* exercise of matching their fluid losses. Gastric emptying rates and tolerance to large volumes of fluids in the stomach vary widely among individuals. During training sessions, endurance athletes are advised to "train" their GI tract "to drink" in an attempt to enhance their ability to tolerate drinking larger volumes of fluid.[3]

In summary, during exercise, endurance athletes will need to closely monitor their fluid intake and be aware of their individual responses. Because fitness levels and sweat rates, and consequently fluid and electrolyte needs, vary widely among athletes, as do the environmental conditions under which endurance athletes train and compete, no "one-size-fits-all" hydration guidelines exist.[1-4] To ensure optimal hydration, endurance athletes must personally establish and monitor their personal fluid needs. Besides dehydration, however, a real and potentially dangerous situation for endurance athletes is overhydration.[1-4] Athletes who *gain* weight during exercise, for example, after running a marathon or participating in a 100-mile bike ride, will need to hydrate less. (See section Electrolytes.) Thus, athletes should not be counseled to "drink as much as possible" during exercise, but more according to thirst,[1-4] with a general recommendation of no more than 400–800 mL per hour.[4]

Chronic dehydration as an athlete trains day after day in hot weather can also affect an athlete's endurance performance. A gradual weight loss, often mistaken as fat loss, accompanied by fatigue or slow recovery and small amounts of dark-colored urine with a strong odor, can indicate a dehydrated state. To combat chronic dehydration, athletes involved in endurance-type activities need to develop a consistent habit of "going out the door" fully hydrated. This is best accomplished by making rehydration a priority after the previous day's exercise, drinking small amounts throughout the day to maximize absorption and by drinking approximately 16 ounces of fluid 2 hours before exercise.[1,2]

## ADEQUATE FUEL (CALORIES) AND MACRONUTRIENTS

To protect their health and lean muscle mass and to maximize performance, serious endurance athletes must consume enough calories on a day-to-day basis to cover the calories expended during exercise (see Table 16.1). As training volume and intensity varies throughout the year, an endurance athlete will need to modify their food intake to match their caloric expenditure. Because carbohydrate is the limiting fuel source during exercise, even for endurance athletes, these individuals will always need to consume enough carbohydrate-rich foods to support their activity level.[5-8] However, because excess body weight is usually a detriment in endurance activities, especially those activities in which the athlete needs to "carry" or propel their own body weight, endurance athletes will need to scale back their total caloric intake during periods of light(er) training or extended rest to maintain a desirable body weight. For example, consuming 5–7 g of carbohydrate/kg should be sufficient in preparation for easy days of moderate-duration, low-intensity training.[8]

Serious-minded endurance athletes have increased protein needs and will benefit from a diet containing adequate amounts of protein-rich foods to meet their performance and recovery demands. Those most likely to consume inadequate amounts of protein are elite athletes with very high training demands as well as those athletes with low or suboptimal energy intakes.[8] Although protein is not a primary energy source during most exercise bouts, an increased breakdown of amino acids (especially leucine, isoleucine, and valine—the branched-chain amino acids) during prolonged exercise has been shown to occur. In well-fed individuals, protein typically supplies about 5% of energy needs at rest and during exercise.[8] This energy contribution from protein may potentially increase up to 10% during the end stages of prolonged exercise.[6]

A recent literature review summarizes that protein needs for endurance athletes vary greatly, with top sport elite athletes requiring the most (up to 1.6 g/kg/day), whereas well-trained endurance athletes (training 4–5 days for longer than 60 minutes) seem to need only a very modest increase in protein (~1.1 g/kg/day, 25%). If energy and carbohydrate intakes are adequate, engaging in low- and moderate-intensity endurance exercise does not seem to increase daily dietary protein requirements.[9] The general recommendation endorsed by most nutrition and exercise science experts is 1.2–1.4 g/kg/day.[5-7]

A very low-fat diet (<20% of total calories consumed) is often the diet of choice among athletes, especially those overfocused on reducing body mass

TABLE 16.1. General estimates for carbohydrate, protein, and fat needs for athletes engaged in moderate or heavy endurance training or competition.[5-9]

| | |
|---|---|
| Carbohydrate | 7–12 g/kg per day |
| | 7 g/kg if training 1 hour per day |
| | 8 g/kg if training 2 hours per day |
| | 10 g/kg if training 3–4 hours per day |
| | 10–12 g/kg if training 4–6 hours per day or more |
| Protein | 1.2–1.4 g/kg per day (elite athletes may need up to 1.6 g/kg per day) |
| Fat | 1 g/kg per day |

and/or body fat below levels associated with performance and long-term health. Endurance athletes may find it difficult, however, to consume adequate calories on a daily diet very low in fat, which can manifest as reduced endurance and suboptimal performances. From a performance standpoint, diets containing less than 15% of energy from fat have not been shown to be any more beneficial than diets containing 20%–25% of energy from fat.[5,10] Adequate intake of key nutrients, such as calcium, zinc, and essential fatty acids, has also been shown to be compromised with a very low intake of fat.[5,10,11]

On the other extreme is "fat-loading," which is an ongoing topic of discussion among researchers.[10,12–15] This potentially performance-enhancing strategy is based on consuming a high-fat diet (studies have examined intakes anywhere from 42% to 70% of total calories) for a period of time (from 5 to 7 days up to 2–4 weeks) followed by a period of high-carbohydrate intake immediately before the event/competition. Although individuals' responses to "fat-loading" seem to vary tremendously, this practice is not recommended at this time because it is unlikely that the majority of endurance athletes would benefit performance or health wise (especially long term because of the associated health risks of a high-fat intake). Some athletes engaged in ultraendurance exercise could potentially see an improvement in performance, because of an increase in fat oxidation and a decreased reliance on muscle glycogen.

## TIMING OF MACRONUTRIENTS

For endurance athletes, consistency in training is often the key to success. In other words, the goal is to minimize time lost to chronic fatigue, illness, and injury. The process of returning to a performance-ready state, known as recovery, hinges on restoring nutrient and fuel stores, repairing damaged muscle fibers, and alleviating mental fatigue. Fueling the body properly for performance and maximizing recovery are especially paramount for those athletes who desire to complete multiple daily workouts or training sessions of prolonged duration, as well as those athletes who must accomplish a high volume of work week after week.

One mistake endurance athletes often make is not fueling properly before training, especially if training occurs in the morning after an 8- to 10-hour fast during sleep. It is recommended that an athlete consume a carbohydrate-rich meal (1.2 g/kg) with a variable content of protein 2–3 hours before an exercise bout. This practice will ensure an increased carbohydrate availability and is warranted if the training bout is to exceed 90 minutes in duration. If the training bout is to be less than 90 minutes, a preexercise carbohydrate snack 15–60 minutes before exercise consisting of 1 g/kg will help to top off glycogen stores and increase carbohydrate availability after an overnight fast (Tables 16.2 and 16.3).

Muscle glycogen depletion is a well-documented detriment to optimal performance during endurance activities and competitions.[5–8] Poor training days can often be linked to poor eating days. Repeated bouts of exercise accompanied by an inadequate intake of carbohydrate will produce a day-to-day decrease in muscle glycogen. Increased muscle soreness (such as "heavy" legs), a lack of usual desire, and physical efforts being perceived as "feeling harder than they should" can all indicate insufficient recovery from previous exercise. Athletes who exercise with low muscle glycogen stores also increase their risk of injury.

Because it takes almost 24 hours to fully replenish muscle glycogen stores, endurance athletes will benefit from consuming a daily diet adequate in carbohydrate to match their activity level, as well as capitalizing on the "carbohydrate window" immediately after exercise. During the first few hours after exercise (especially the initial 15–30 minutes after exercise), muscles convert carbohydrate-rich foods and beverages into glycogen up to 3 times faster than at other times. Endurance athletes can jumpstart the glycogen replenishment process by consuming approximately 1.0–1.5 g of carbohydrate/kg body weight during this time frame.[5–8,16] Consuming a small amount of protein immediately after exercise also seems to be beneficial, by enhancing glycogen repletion, as well as limiting postexercise muscle damage and initiating the muscle repair

**TABLE 16.2.** Carbohydrate and protein recommendations for endurance training and optimal glycogen storage for men (weight 188 lbs./85.5 kgs.).

| When? | Carbs (g) | Type | Protein (g) | Why? |
|---|---|---|---|---|
| Carbohydrate and protein recommendations for "around your endurance training" for men | | | | |
| Preexercise meal (3–5 hours before) | 102 | Polysaccharide (starch maltodextrin) | Varies | To increase carbohydrate availability for prolonged exercise (>90 minutes) |
| Preexercise snack (15–60 minutes before) | 50–85 | Monosaccharide (glucose fructose) | None | To top off glycogen stores/increase carbohydrate availability or after an overnight fast |
| During exercise (per hour) | 30–60+ | Varies but mostly monosaccharide and disaccharide (sucrose) | None | During moderate-intensity or continuous exercise >1 hour in duration |
| Postexercise snack (15–30 minutes after) | 85–130 | Any | 20–30 | For rapid postexercise recovery of muscle glycogen |
| Postexercise meal (2 hours after) | 85–130 | Polysaccharide (starch maltodextrin) | Varies | For continuing postexercise recovery of muscle glycogen |
| Daily carbohydrate recommendations for optimal glycogen storage for men | | | | |
| Daily | 513 | | | Easy training day (<1 hour of activity/ low intensity) |
| Daily | 598–684 | | | Moderate training day (1–3 hours of moderate/high intensity) |
| Daily | 770–855 | | | Hard training day (4–5 hours of moderate/high intensity) |
| Daily | 940+ | | | Extreme training day (>5 hours of moderate/high intensity) |

**TABLE 16.3.** Carbohydrate and protein recommendations for endurance training and optimal glycogen storage for women (weight 128 lbs/58 kgs).

| When? | Carbs (g) | Type | Protein (g) | Why? |
|---|---|---|---|---|
| Carbohydrate and protein recommendations for "around your endurance training" for women | | | | |
| Preexercise meal (3–5 hours before) | 70 | Polysaccharide (starch maltodextrin) | Varies | To increase carbohydrate availability for prolonged exercise (>90 minutes) |
| Preexercise snack (15–60 minutes before) | 25–60 | Monosaccharide (glucose fructose) | None | To top off glycogen stores/increase carbohydrate availability or after an overnight fast |
| During exercise (per hour) | 30–60+ | Varies but mostly monosaccharide and disaccharide (sucrose) | None | During moderate-intensity or continuous exercise >1 hour in duration |
| Postexercise snack (15–30 minutes after) | 58–87 | Any | 15–20 | For rapid postexercise recovery of muscle glycogen |
| Postexercise meal (2 hours after) | 58–87 | Polysaccharide (starch maltodextrin) | varies | For continuing postexercise recovery of muscle glycogen |
| Daily carbohydrate recommendations for optimal glycogen storage for women | | | | |
| Daily | 290–348 | | | Easy training day (<1 hour of activity/low intensity) |
| Daily | 406–469 | | | Moderate training day (1–3 hours of moderate/high intensity) |
| Daily | 522–580 | | | Hard training day (4–5 hours of moderate/high intensity) |
| Daily | 638+ | | | Extreme training day (>5 hours of moderate/high intensity) |

process.[12,16] Endurance athletes should consume the same amount of carbohydrate (usually in the form of a meal) again 2 hours after the completion of exercise to ensure adequate glycogen compensation.

It is well established that endurance athletes engaged in high-intensity, continuous exercise lasting 90 minutes or longer will benefit from consuming supplemental carbohydrate during exercise. General guidelines advise athletes to aim for an intake of approximately 30–60 g of carbohydrate per hour they are engaged in exercise, or approximately 150–300 calories per hour. Relative to body weight, it is recommended that endurance athletes consume 1 g of carbohydrate per kg during each hour of exercise. This rate may need to increase in the later stages of prolonged exercise as the body increasingly draws on blood glucose for fuel. Exact needs vary tremendously among athletes—as well as for the individual athlete on any given day—as a result of fitness levels, preexercise glycogen levels, activity or sport the athlete is engaged in, intensity of the exercise, and the environmental conditions. Therefore, it is necessary to train with different amounts of carbohydrate products to determine the appropriate fuel needs for an individual during exercise.[5-8]

Athletes can best meet their energy needs via carbohydrate-rich sports drink and energy gels and bars specifically designed for use during exercise and/or by eating any "real" carbohydrate-rich beverages and foods that are accessible, practical, palatable, and tolerated.[5-8] Depending on the individual and the physical activity they are involved in (e.g., running versus cycling versus hiking), athletes may also benefit, if tolerated, from consuming small amounts of protein during exercise. Although researchers continue to investigate whether this addition of protein (in conjunction with carbohydrate) actually improves aerobic performance,[17,18] supplemental protein during exercise seems to reduce muscle damage associated with exercise and enhance postexercise protein synthesis. Because of the high caloric needs of athletes engaged in ultraendurance activities, these athletes will often need to consume varying amounts of carbohydrate, protein, and even high-fat food items during training bouts and competitions. Not all athletes can tolerate different substrates during exercise equally, so it is necessary for an individual athlete to experiment by consuming different fuel compositions during exercise.

## ELECTROLYTES

The endurance athlete's performance can be hindered by two fluid and electrolyte-related issues—hyponatremia and/or muscle cramps. Hyponatremia occurs when the concentration of sodium in the blood decreases to a potentially dangerous level, generally accepted as 135 mmol per liter. Feeling weak, lethargic, nauseated, bloated, confused, or developing muscle cramps, a headache, slurred speech, or swollen hands and feet during or after prolonged exercise can be symptoms of hyponatremia. If left untreated, hyponatremia can progress to seizures, coma, permanent brain damage, and even death.[1-4,19,20]

Hyponatremia results from some combination of abnormal water retention and/or sodium loss. Endurance athletes are at an increased risk for hyponatremia because of prolonged or excessive sweating that can set the stage for increased losses of sodium, especially "salty sweaters" who lose abnormally high amounts of sodium in their sweat and those athletes who have high sweat rates. Excessive fluid intake, however, seems to be the primary culprit in most cases of exercise-induced hyponatremia. Ingesting or retaining too much fluid, particularly sodium-free fluids such as plain water, can unavoidably lead to hyponatremia. This can occur even in an otherwise healthy athlete during or after prolonged exercise as urine production decreases and sodium loss (via sweat) increases.[1-4,19-21]

Endurance athletes who have more opportunity to drink, such as triathletes, cyclists, and slower runners, are at increased risk, as are "vigilant" drinkers who are more likely to follow and even overdo hydration advice from coaches and experts. Female athletes, whether attributable to biologic or behavioral factors, seem to be more susceptible to hyponatremia, as are unconditioned individuals. Because sweat losses vary so widely among individuals, the amount of fluid needed to delay dehydration and prevent hyponatremia during prolonged exercise also will vary widely. For intense prolonged exercise lasting longer than 1 hour, athletes should replace both fluid and electrolytes lost in sweat by consuming fluids that contain sodium and/or ingesting salty foods.[1-4,19-21]

The exact cause of muscle cramps remains unknown; however, plausible culprits include muscular fatigue or overexertion, dehydration, and/or an electrolyte imbalance.[22,23] From a nutritional standpoint, athletes tend to suffer muscle cramps more easily when dehydrated, thus starting out well hydrated and monitoring fluid needs during exercise is mandatory. To help assess fluid needs, endurance athletes can monitor their ability to urinate during and after exercise. Consuming a daily diet high in potassium-rich foods (such as legumes, fruits, vegetables, and low-fat dairy foods) and adequate in sodium also may help prevent cramps in susceptible individuals. Although specific electrolyte abnormalities have not been identified with muscle cramps,[23] some experts still believe that for many athletes, sodium depletion is a, if not the, major predisposing factor behind cramping during exercise, particularly in warm weather conditions.[24]

# MICRONUTRIENTS (CALCIUM, IRON, ZINC)

Both iron and zinc are vital for a healthy immune system; plus, adequate iron is needed to build healthy red blood cells and avoid the fatigue associated with iron-deficiency anemia. An iron-poor diet is the primary cause of most iron deficiencies, particularly among active women. Even women making wise food choices, however, can still struggle to meet their daily iron requirement. Female endurance athletes who place a premium on having a lean physique by dieting or restricting calories will find it virtually impossible to consume enough iron. Another at-risk group for developing anemia is vegetarian athletes, male and female, because the iron in plant foods is not as efficiently absorbed as the iron in red meat, poultry, or fish. Athletes who live or train for extended amounts of time at altitude may also fail to fulfill their ongoing iron needs as the body responds by increasing and maintaining more red blood cells.[25]

Iron losses also affect an endurance athlete's ability to maintain a positive iron balance. For women, menstrual blood loss is the second-biggest cause of low iron levels. Additionally, whereas iron losses through sweat and urine are typically negligible, prolonged exercise can boost these looses. The physical jarring of the bladder during prolonged exercise, for example, coupled with dehydration, can cause urinary blood losses (Table 16.4).[25]

Iron can also be lost through GI bleeding that can accompany prolonged exercise, especially for athletes who experience cramping and diarrhea during exercise. The decrease in blood flow and nutrients to the lining of the GI tract, also exacerbated by dehydration, causes cells to die and slough off, resulting in occult, or hidden, blood in bowel movements. Most athletes, however, will not even be aware of this mode of iron loss.[25]

Chronic injury to red blood cells, such as repetitive trauma from hard foot strikes experienced in high-impact sports (such as running), can also contribute to iron depletion. Other theories point to the increase in body temperature associated with exercise or muscle contraction acidosis (a decrease in blood pH) as potentially damaging red blood cells, because swimmers and other athletes in nonimpact sports also experience exercise-induced anemia. Iron supplementation should be done under the guidance of a health professional, with routine monitoring of hemoglobin, hematocrit, and serum ferritin recommended.[25]

**TABLE 16.4. Iron to the rescue.[7]**

| Heme iron (much better absorbed form of iron) | Non-heme iron (poorly absorbed form of iron*) |
|---|---|
| Liver | Iron-fortified breakfast cereal |
| Meat: beef, pork, lamb, veal | Lentils |
| Poultry | Cooked beans: kidney, white, chickpeas, etc. |
| Fish | Baked potato with skin |
| Shellfish (especially oysters) | Whole grain products |
| Egg (whole) | Green leafy vegetables |
| | Dried fruit: apricots, prunes, raisins |
| | Blackstrap molasses |
| | Tofu |
| | *To improve absorption: |
| | 1. Eat with a vitamin C–rich food. |
| | 2. Eat with a food containing heme iron. |
| | 3. Avoid consuming with foods that interfere or block iron absorption, such as coffee, tea, and excessive fiber. |

Zinc is also more efficiently absorbed from animal sources and it helps wounds and injuries heal properly, including the cellular microdamage caused by extensive daily exercise. Endurance athletes who limit or avoid meat, as well as those restricting their calories and/or fat intake, may have difficulty meeting their daily zinc requirement (females 15 mg, males 18 mg). Good dietary sources of zinc include: shellfish, red meat, poultry, fish, dairy foods, legumes, lentils, spinach, soy foods, peanut butter, nuts and seeds, whole grains, and wheat germ.[5-7]

Calcium, a key nutrient necessary for muscle contractions, nerve conduction, and healthy bones, also may be low in the diets of many athletes. Lactose intolerance, perceiving dairy foods as fattening or as potentially causing mucous formation during exercise, may result in an athlete shunning calcium-rich dairy foods. Failure to seek alternate calcium-rich food sources, and/or appropriate supplementation, can leave the athlete short of meeting their daily calcium requirement (males and females aged 19–50/1000 mg, aged 9–18/1200 mg, over age 50/1300 mg). Good dietary sources of calcium include: milk, yogurt, cheese, tofu made with calcium sulfate, canned sardines and salmon (with bones), baked beans, soy nuts, generous portions of dark green leafy vegetables, and calcium-fortified foods such as soy or rice milk, orange juice, and breakfast cereals.[5-7]

## Sidebar 16.1. Racing to the Finish Line—Rehydrating and Fueling While on the Move

Endurance events, such as marathons, triathlons, and adventure races, aren't just about putting one foot in front of the other, keeping one's bike upright and on the road, or who has the best navigational skills—they are eating and drinking contests, too. To excel, endurance athletes need to master the all-important skill of drinking and eating while—literally—on the move. Fluid and caloric needs vary widely because of gender, the particular sport or activity the athlete is engaged in, the intensity and duration of the sport or activity, and, of course, environmental conditions. In some endurance sports, such as marathons and triathlons, fluids and foods will be readily available and easily assessable to athletes during the event. In other cases, such as off-road activities, ultraendurance races, and multiday events, the athlete is often responsible for meeting their own fluid and fuel needs for prolonged portions or even throughout the entire activity.

Logistical planning and practice are paramount, because relying solely on plain water or foods such as many of the popular energy bars that become rock-hard and inedible in the cold, will spell disaster for even the fittest, best-trained endurance athlete.

1. Do your homework before the LONG day: explore various options for carrying a large volume of fluid, such as hydration bladders (backpack style, waist or hip mounted), sports vests or hip belts fitted with flasks or water bottles. On the bike, options include wearing a hydration bladder, or water bottles—standard down tube/top tube combo mount, along with the aero bars or the seat-mounted variety. If the refueling plan calls for extra sports drink powder or foods, plan ahead how these items will be carried or made available.
2. Practice drinking (and if applicable, eating) on the move until it becomes second nature.
3. Experiment with drinks and foods in weather conditions similar to what you expect to encounter during race or event situations.
4. Tolerance to foods and beverages varies immensely during exercise—take personal responsibility to develop an individualized hydration and fueling plan. Develop a plan that takes into account fluid, energy (particularly from carbohydrate sources), and electrolyte (particularly sodium) needs.

## CARBOHYDRATE-LOADING

### Who Should Carbohydrate-Load?

Athletes engaged in high-intensity, continuous-endurance (greater than 90 minutes), and ultraendurance (greater than 4 hours) endeavors or competitive events, such as marathons, triathlons, ultraruns, and century, double-century, and 24-hour cycling events should carbo-load.[5-7]

## Why Carbohydrate-Load?

High-intensity endurance exercise places a greater demand on muscle glycogen stores than nonendurance sports or sports in which intensity is high but only for short periods of time. Normal glycogen stores are inadequate to sustain this type of exercise, so athletes attempt to supersaturate or "load" their muscles with additional glycogen. Carbo-loading can increase glycogen stores by 200%–300%, which can help to delay fatigue related to glycogen depletion ("hitting the wall") and enable an athlete to maintain their desired pace for a greater length of time. Boosted glycogen stores also help to prevent "bonking" or hypoglycemia during exercise.

## What Is the Best Way to Carbohydrate-Load?

The key to successful carbo-loading is to increase one's intake of carbohydrate while simultaneously reducing one's training. At least 3 days (even up to 5 days) of consuming a high-carbohydrate diet (7–10 g/kg/body weight or 70%–85% of energy) is required to attain maximal muscle glycogen stores. Heavy or strenuous training during this time will negate or hold down the amount of muscle glycogen that is stored.

## What Else Is There to Know About Carbohydrate-Loading?

- Research has shown the modified loading protocol described above to be just as effective, with fewer side effects, as the original glycogen loading regimen that included the carbohydrate depletion phase.
- Athletes should expect to "gain" weight with carbohydrate loading, because approximately 3 g of water is stored with every gram of glycogen.
- Athletes may initially experience muscle stiffness and discomfort with elevated muscle glycogen stores (which typically abates once exercise commences).
- (Note: See Sidebar 16.3 for another view on carbohydrate-loading).

# UNIQUE NUTRITIONAL CONCERNS OF ENDURANCE ATHLETES

## Vegetarian Diets

Although a plant-based eating style does not guarantee a physical advantage, a recent review of studies concluded that a vegetarian diet has no detrimental effects on athletic performance, in general, either.[26] Because a vegetarian diet can range from simply eliminating red meat to totally eliminating all animal foods, however, the nutritional adequacy of any athlete's vegetarian diet needs to be assessed on a case-by-case basis. A well-planned vegetarian diet can meet caloric and macro- and micronutrient needs; however, the serious endurance athlete must be committed to putting more thought and planning into their daily food choices.

A potential pitfall of vegetarianism is unbalanced eating whereby animal foods are simply eliminated with little regard given to appropriate substitutes. In this scenario, a vegetarian diet can be extremely unhealthful—high in saturated fat (from full-fat dairy foods such as cheese), refined carbs, sugar, and hydrogenated oils, and low in protein, iron, zinc, and calcium. This puts the athlete at greater risk for iron-deficiency anemia, a weak immune system, nagging injuries, and for females, an out-of-balance menstrual cycle that can contribute to stress fractures as well as the early onset of osteoporosis.[5,26,27]

In some cases, vegetarianism can also be a red flag that a person is restricting food needlessly. Female athletes, especially teens, who struggle with weight and body-image issues may use vegetarianism to justify avoiding certain foods.[5,26,27] For example, they may avoid fat-containing vegetarian fare such as nuts and avocados or they may eliminate meat and dairy foods but then be unwilling to seek out appropriate meat substitutes.

Semi-vegetarians who eat poultry and/or fish can obtain the same range of nutrients as red meat eaters. Those who avoid animal flesh but eat dairy foods and eggs typically meet protein, calcium, and vitamin B12 needs but may have trouble getting enough zinc and iron. Vegans, those who avoid all animal foods, are most at risk for insufficient calories and nutrient deficiencies. Any vegetarian athlete, however, who primarily eats only the starchy side dishes of meat-focused meals, which results in "carbohydrate overload," runs the risk of a diet inadequate in protein, iron, and zinc.[26,28]

Vegetarian athletes can obtain all the essential amino acids needed to form complete proteins by eating a wide variety of plant proteins throughout the day.[28] A potential challenge, particularly for endurance athletes, is to consume enough calories to maintain a healthy weight and fuel the demands of training. Otherwise, the body resorts to using protein for energy rather than building and repairing muscle and other body tissues. Soy foods (e.g., tofu, tempeh, soy milk, and veggies burgers) and legumes (e.g., kidney, pinto, black, and garbanzo beans) offer the highest-quality plant protein and some of each should be consumed daily. Non-vegans can also obtain high-quality protein from eggs and dairy foods.

Vegetarian athletes will need to make a conscious effort to include good meatless sources of iron and zinc daily, especially because animal sources of iron and zinc are better absorbed. Legumes, whole grains, soy foods, and fortified breakfast cereals contribute significant amounts of both. Endurance athletes who opt not to consume dairy foods will need to seek alternative calcium-rich options, such as calcium-fortified orange juice and soy foods made with calcium sulfate. Lastly, vitamin B12 is found almost exclusively in animal foods. Despite being touted as good sources, much of the vitamin B12 in sea vegetables, tempeh, miso, or spirulina is in an inactive form that the body cannot readily use. Options include fortified foods, such as certain brands of soy milk, soy burgers, and cereal, or a multivitamin.

## Disordered Eating, Eating Disorders, and the Female Athlete Triad

Athletes, both male and female, involved in endurance activities and sports are at an increased risk for developing disordered eating habits that can escalate into a full-blown eating disorder, such as anorexia nervosa (self-starvation) or bulimia nervosa (a destructive cycle characterized by binging and purging). An emphasis on leanness, the wearing of tight-fitting or revealing clothing/uniforms, and the erroneous promotion of the myth that "losing weight or weighing less will improve performance" sets the stage for vulnerable endurance athletes of all ages and abilities to struggle with food and weight-related issues. People do recover from eating disorders, however, rarely without professional help. Because early intervention drastically increases the likelihood of a complete recovery, any athlete suffering with food, weight and/or body image issues should immediately be referred to a health professional (medical doctor, registered dietitian, or therapist) who specializes in the treatment of eating disorders.[5–7]

Female endurance athletes also need to be aware of the female athlete triad,[29] a syndrome of medical conditions that occurs in women who exercise. The triad is characterized by three interrelated components: dysfunctional or disordered eating, amenorrhea (the loss of menstrual periods), and osteoporosis. Although bringing a much-needed awareness to this cluster of disorders, the title unfortunately suggests that only female "athletes" or intensely competitive women are at risk. In reality, any physically active female who undereats, overexercises, or both is a prime candidate for experiencing complications associated with the female athlete triad.

Also referred to as the "energy drain scenario," the triad begins when an individual consumes fewer calories than she needs for her activity level. Sometimes female athletes end up in this "energy drain" state because of high-volume training schedules and inadvertently consuming insufficient calories. More often, however, it occurs in physically active girls and women who slip into a pattern of restrictive eating to deliberately lose weight quickly in an attempt to improve their appearance or performance.[30,31]

In response to an inadequate caloric intake, the body attempts to conserve energy by shutting down the reproductive system via the hypothalamic-pituitary-ovarian axis. As the ovaries produce less and less estrogen, menses become irregular and cease altogether, a condition referred to as amenorrhea (three or more consecutive menstrual periods are missed or menstruation fails to begin in an adolescent before the age of 16). Once considered a "normal" part of training or the hallmark of peak fitness, amenorrhea is now viewed as a serious sign that something is amiss in the complex female reproductive system.[29]

With low levels of estrogen that mimic those seen during menopause, the loss of normal bone density accelerates, thereby setting the stage for stress fractures and the early onset of osteoporosis. Amenorrheic women between the ages of 16–30 lose as much as 2%–5% of their bone mass a year, which is particularly troublesome because peak bone mass is reached during this same interval.[31]

The triad has short- and long-term consequences on a female's health and performance. Immediate consequences may include: dehydration, fatigue, loss of concentration and motivation, depression, electrolyte imbalances, moods swings, poor sleep, and sub-par workouts/performances. Depending on the degree and duration of the negative energy state, active females may have delayed puberty and short stature (teens), nutrient deficiencies such as iron-deficiency anemia, loss of lean muscle mass, lingering overuse injuries (e.g., tendonitis) and stress fractures, a full-blown eating disorder (which can be fatal), difficulty conceiving, and the early onset of osteoporosis.[29,32]

Some potential red flags when working with physically active females, of which endurance athletes constitute a high-risk population, include[31]:

- Dysfunctional or disordered eating (e.g., "too busy" or "forgetting" to eat meals, dieting, avoidance of all fat, taking appetite suppressants, self-induced vomiting, laxative use)
- An unbalanced vegetarian eating style (e.g., dislikes legumes and soy foods or resists eating eggs/dairy foods/nuts because of fat content)
- Compulsive or nonpurposeful exercise (e.g., excessive exercise beyond a sensible training program, exercising in secret, exercising with an injury)
- Highly self-critical/low self-esteem/negative body image
- Poor coping skills to deal with emotional/psychologic stress
- Exercise-induced amenorrhea
- Recurrent stress fractures

Oftentimes a gain of 2%–3% of body weight (e.g., approximately 3–5 pounds for a 130-pound woman) will be adequate to restore the body's energy balance and restart the menstrual cycle. Dietary changes alone, however, can rarely totally undo an "energy drain" scenario. Supplementing with 1500 mg of calcium, for example, will simply keep an amenorrheic woman in calcium *balance*—the added calcium does not build bone, because it cannot compensate for a low estrogen level. Other lifestyle factors such as exercise habits (number of rest days and volume/intensity of exercise) and methods to manage stress must be addressed.[29,30]

Because of the impact on bone health, any physically active female (especially a teen) should be advised to seek a thorough medical evaluation if menses become irregular or stop. The use of hormone replacement therapy (e.g., oral contraceptives) to boost low estrogen levels, especially in young females, continues to be debated. It seems that maintenance of bone mineral density can be achieved, but studies to date show limited or no gains in bone mineral density. Body image and disordered-eating issues are often at the root of a female's reluctance to fuel herself properly, hence a multidisciplinary treatment approach (medical doctor, registered dietitian, and therapist) is recommended.[29,31]

# GASTROINTESTINAL ISSUES

Dealing with GI woes, such as nausea, abdominal cramps, vomiting, and diarrhea, particularly if occurring during a competition, are common concerns for endurance athletes. Increased levels of epinephrine associated with intense physical activity, as well as emotional stress, can interfere with the normal functioning of the GI tract. As athletes become dehydrated and blood volume decreases, even less blood flow is available to the GI tract, exasperating the situation. Runners, in particular, seem to be more affected by diarrhea and cramping than other athletes. The repetitive and jarring action of running can actually cause injury to the walls of the colon leading to diarrhea and blood loss. If severe enough or to avoid embarrassment, athletes may resort to limiting or even curtailing their intake of fluid and foods during exercise.[33]

The best defense in preventing abdominal and intestinal problems hinges on the athlete staying well-hydrated and establishing a consistent eating pattern and regular bowel habits. Often, modifying the timing of foods and fluids around exercise can make a substantial difference, such as avoiding gas-forming foods (such as carbonated beverages, legumes, broccoli, and cabbage) and high-fiber foods too close to the time of exercise, artificial sweeteners such as sorbitol and aspartame, caffeine, and any other problem foods identified during training. To minimize GI disturbances during competitions, endurance athletes will need to develop personalized pre-race meals, practice with various drinks and foods during training, and commit to drinking fluids in the early stages of long races/events. The use of antidiarrheal medications during prolonged exercise should be done only with the advice of a health care provider.[5-7,33]

## TRAINING AND COMPETING UNDER EXTREME CONDITIONS—ALTITUDE, HEAT, COLD

Endurance activities and competitions can take athletes anywhere and everywhere—up mountains, through deserts, along backcountry trails, and even across entire countries and continents. Endurance athletes must be prepared to drink and eat in all types of situations and be able to handle whatever Mother Nature dishes out.

The most severe physiologic stress an endurance athlete can face is exercising in the heat. Heat acclimatization is necessary for athletes to obtain optimal performances in the heat, particularly in hot, humid conditions. As an increase in sweat rate accompanies acclimatization, endurance athletes will need to drink more—not less—as they become adjusted to the heat. Consuming adequate sodium, via a daily liberal salt intake, can also help ward off hyponatremia and may help prevent muscle cramps. Endurance athletes will often need to consume salty beverages and foods while performing prolonged exercise (more than 4 hours) under extreme heat conditions.[24,34]

Exercising in the cold for prolonged periods of time presents its own challenges. Frozen fluids and rock-hard, inedible foods can make meeting fluid and fuel a real struggle. Dehydration during cold-weather exercise is not uncommon. Along with sweating (particularly if enhanced as a result of being overdressed), avenues of fluid loss include respiratory water loss and cold-induced diuresis. In addition, fluid is often not available during cold-weather activities because athletes may erroneously give it less thought or struggle with ways to keep it from freezing. Wishing to avoid the logistical problems and discomfort of taking bathroom stops in the cold is another likely reason some athletes avoid or reduce their fluid intake when exercising in the cold.[35]

In cold weather, endurance athletes will need to experiment and devise options for meeting their fluid needs (i.e., insulated hydration bladders), as well as develop a repertoire of food items that remain palatable and edible during cold weather conditions. Energy requirements are typically increased in the cold because the athlete moves over more difficult terrain or carries extra weight as a result of cold-weather clothing and gear. No consensus exists for the most effective diet for prolonged exercising in the cold: a higher-fat diet may improve cold tolerance; however, adequate amounts of carbohydrate must still be consumed to replenish muscle glycogen and prevent excess fatigue. An adequate calorie intake (regardless of the source of these calories) along with good physical conditioning and proper clothing seem to be much more important than the particular percentage of macronutrients consumed.[36]

**TABLE 16.5. Signs of dehydration versus signs of hyponatremia.**

| Dehydration | Hyponatremia |
|---|---|
| Early: headache, fatigue, dizziness, nausea, vomiting, dry mouth and eyes, loss of appetite, flushed skin, heat intolerance/exhaustion, dark-colored urine with a strong odor, irritability, muscle cramps, weight loss during prolonged exercise | Early: feeling bloated, accompanied or followed by nausea and vomiting; visible bloating (i.e., swollen hands and feet, bloated stomach), dizziness, throbbing headache, rapid weight gain during prolonged exercise, cramping |
| More advanced: difficulty swallowing, clumsiness, abnormal chills, shriveled skin, sunken eyes and dim vision, inability to urinate, delirium, heat stroke | More advanced: restlessness/malaise/ apathy, confusion/disorientation, severe fatigue/weakness, respiratory distress, seizure, coma |

*Source:* Adapted from The Right Way to Hydrate for Marathons handout by the American Running Association and the American Medical Athletic Association. Mountain SJ, Sawka MN, Wenger CB. Hyponatremia associated with exercise: rish factors and prognosis. Exerc Sports Sci Rev 29:113–117, 2001.

Exercising at altitude, especially for a prolonged length of time, presents another set of challenges for the endurance athlete. Dehydration and glycogen depletion remain nemeses at high elevations and can be complicated by a limited access to fluids and foods, elevated caloric needs, and/or by a reduced intake caused by acute altitude or mountain sickness. On the whole, digestibility and absorption of macronutrients does not seem to be compromised or contribute to weight loss up to 18,000 feet. At higher, more extreme altitudes, the digestive tract may lose some of its absorptive capacity. The ability to eat, however, can be compromised at much lower elevations.[37–39]

The body's metabolic rate increases upon acute exposure to high altitude (above 9000 feet). Athletes planning extended stays at high altitude will need to be cognizant of working at maintaining their weight or at least minimizing altitude-related weight loss of which a sizable portion is muscle mass. Expending a substantially greater amount of calories performing physical activity at altitude than at sea level, coupled with limited food choices and a lagging appetite (especially with acute mountain sickness), make the daily task of rehydrating and refueling daunting. Athletes should also be aware that at the cellular level, exercising muscles at altitude display an increased reliance on glucose over fat for fuel. Fortunately, carbohydrate-rich foods seem more palatable at altitude than protein and high-fat foods, although athletes can struggle with sport beverages and foods tasting excessively sweet.[37–39]

Lastly, endurance athletes, particularly females, who live and train at moderate altitudes (3000–8000 feet, or 1000–2500 meters) or those planning an extended trip to high altitude, will need to consume plenty of iron-rich foods on a regular basis (see Table 16.5). As the body builds additional red blood cells during acclimatization, extra iron—a key component of hemoglobin—is also required. The need for iron supplementation (beyond the amount in a multivitamin/mineral supplement) should be determined and monitored through routine blood tests, such as hemoglobin, hematocrit, and serum ferritin.[37–39]

## SUMMARY

Endurance athletes face unique nutritional needs and challenges on a daily basis while engaged in prolonged exercise. Serious-minded endurance athletes must undertake certain nutrition-related tasks daily. They must consume adequate calories while maintaining a lean body weight, meet key nutrient needs, such as protein, iron, zinc, and calcium, maintain a favorable fluid and electrolyte balance, fuel properly before and during exercise, and pay close attention to glycogen repletion after exercise. Gender differences, scheduling and time constraints, exercise-associated fatigue, and loss of appetite, as well as a varying fitness levels, changing environmental conditions, and sport-specific situations all serve as challenges when designing an effective nutrition program for endurance athletes. The payoff is enormous, however, as high-performance eating habits improve performances, speed recovery times, and reduce the endurance athlete's risk of injury and illness.

Special nutritional considerations with this population include: hydrating and refueling *during* prolonged exercise, exercise-related GI problems, an increased risk of iron-deficiency anemia, meeting high caloric needs on vegetarian diets, and working with individuals who are at an increased risk for disordered eating habits, eating disorders, and body image issues.

## PRACTICAL APPLICATION: GUIDELINES FOR THE SPORTS NUTRITIONIST

1. Encourage endurance athletes to devote more time and attention to their daily training diet versus just focusing on nutritional needs as an event or competition nears. Remind athletes that appetite is not a reliable indicator of their energy and macronutrient needs. Especially for those who train daily, make certain the athlete is covering the daily basics: hydrated and appropriately fueled before heading out the door, meets fluid, and, if applicable, energy needs, during training situations and is committed to post-exercise nutritional recovery strategies.

2. Determine and discuss potential time and scheduling conflicts to assist athletes with strategies to coordinate eating and exercise. Whereas athletes typically devote ample time and energy to planning and participating in activities of daily life (i.e., work or school) and their training sessions, the logistics of grocery shopping, meal planning, food preparation, and creating actual time to sit down and consume healthy foods are left to chance. Assist athletes in anticipating and effectively dealing with exercise-associated fatigue and loss of appetite.

3. Educate endurance athletes on the signs of both dehydration and hyponatremia. Review guidelines to help prevent dehydration and hyponatremia, especially for athletes new to endurance exercise, those engaged in ultraendurance activities, and for those athletes performing in hot and/or humid environments. Instruct athletes on how to monitor their urine color and volume before, during, and after exercise to asses their fluid balance. Discuss strategies for how the athlete can be certain they consume adequate fluid and sodium—ideally from beverages and foods—before, during, and after prolonged exercise. Be mindful that ultraendurance athletes often take salt or electrolyte tablets during competitions—advise caution, such as taking them with ample fluid to avoid GI problems and experimenting with them in training first under similar conditions.

4. Encourage endurance athletes, particularly females and those living or training for extended amounts of time at altitude, to consume an iron-rich diet daily to help prevent iron-deficiency anemia. Advise athletes that regular blood testing of iron indices should always be undertaken when they consume iron supplements.

5. Assist vegetarian athletes in making daily food choices that supply adequate calories and incorporate alternate sources of key nutrients, such as protein, iron, zinc, calcium, and vitamin B12 that are typically supplied by meat and dairy foods.

6. Work with the athlete to develop individualized sport-specific fluid and fuel plans for use during endurance activities and competitions—based on science and practical factors concerning fluid and food choices, such as accessibility, portability, palatability, and tolerance. Assist athletes in developing a repertoire of "go-to" foods and drinks to rely on, including different flavors to fight "flavor fatigue" that occurs during prolonged exercise. Because many nutritional strategies simply evolve over time through trial and error, remind athletes of their responsibility to implement and practice these strategies during training sessions.

7. Be mindful of the challenges athletes face in meeting their fluid and fuel needs while exercising in extreme conditions. Be certain that recommendations made will work or "hold up" in the anticipated conditions (i.e., heat, cold, at altitude). Be aware that it is not uncommon for athletes to wish to avoid the logistical problems or discomfort associated with making bathroom stops in the cold or while working hard at altitude.

8. Evaluate for, and educate female endurance athletes on, the female athlete triad. Reiterate that nutritional changes alone, such as taking calcium supplements, cannot undo this "energy drain" scenario. Any female with irregular menstrual periods or amenorrhea should be referred to a physician for a thorough medical evaluation. Because disordered eating habits and a distorted body image are often at the root, refer female athletes to medical professionals (i.e., physicians, registered dietitians, therapists) who are experienced in detecting and treating eating disorders.

9. Endurance athletes, particularly but not only females, represent a high-risk group for developing eating disorders. Athletes can suffer significant psychologic and physical consequences long before developing a full-blown eating disorder (and early intervention drives a successful recovery). At the first signs of struggles with food, weight, or a distorted body image, refer the athlete to treatment providers who are familiar with and experienced in treating eating disorders.

## Sidebar 16.2. What Is the Best Sports Drink to Consume During Exercise?

Scientists have consistently documented improved performances among endurance athletes using carbohydrate-containing drinks (4%–6% carbohydrate concentration) during exercise versus water or other placebo beverages.[40] For most athletes, a well-formulated commercial sports drink is the most efficient way to meet carbohydrate, as well as fluid and electrolyte, needs during exercise. The scientific literature also reveals, however, no additional boost in performance when athletes consume sports beverages with higher carbohydrate concentrations (6%–10%).

Although carbohydrate has proven to be the most necessary fuel for endurance athletes, there is recent evidence that the addition of protein may improve performance and enhance recovery. Recent studies suggest that the addition of a small amount of protein (typically 20% of total calories) to a carbohydrate-based sports drink produces the same positive effects or perhaps even a better pay-off than just a carbohydrate drink alone. Using 15 trained male cyclists, Saunders et al.[40] compared a carbohydrate (CHO) beverage with a carbohydrate–protein (CHO + P) beverage (4:1 ratio) in a blinded endurance cycling two-phase trial (two prolonged bouts of cycle ergometry to fatigue with a 12- to 15-hour rest period between rides, first ride at 75% of VO$_2$ peak, second ride at 85% of VO$_2$ peak). During each ride, the cyclists drank 1.8 mL/kg of their randomly assigned beverage every 15 minutes of exercise. The athletes repeated the two performance rides 7–14 days later using the alternate beverage. With the CHO + P drink, the cyclists rode significantly longer before stopped by fatigue (29% longer in the first phase and 40% longer in the second phase). They also seemed to experience less postexercise muscle damage as evidenced by lower post-ride blood creatine phosphokinase values (an indirect assessment of muscle damage).

A limitation of this study is that the beverages were matched for total carbohydrate content but not total calories. However, the authors of this investigation discounted that notion. "Although we cannot entirely discount the potentially beneficial effects of these additional calories in the CHO + P trial, they cannot explain the 318 kcal of additional energy expended during the prolonged performance time (calculated using mean subject values of +24 min at 2.7 L·min$^{-1}$ VO$_2$, and an RER of 0.88). There is general agreement in the literature that the addition of CHO above 6–10% concentration in a sports beverage does not produce additional performance benefits. Thus, if adding protein to a beverage of similar CHO concentration produces performance benefits, it is a practically significant finding. Future studies should examine combinations of isocaloric and isocarbohydrate beverages to elucidate specific mechanisms for these differences in performance."[40]

In the meantime, endurance athletes can determine for themselves what the "best" sports drink is by experimenting with nontraditional CHO + P sports drinks during prolonged exercise.

## Sidebar 16.3. Taking Another Look at Carbohydrate-Loading

Carbo-loading and endurance exercise—can't succeed in the latter if you don't do the former.[41] Or so goes the prevailing science. Some renowned nutrition and exercise science experts decided to give the performance-enhancing benefits of carbohydrate-loading a closer look. They set the stage in the lab by conducting an experiment that closely simulated the demands of a competitive 100-km road cycling race (i.e., time trial with a series of sprints). In other words, a "complete the total distance as fast as you can" trial versus the "time to exhaustion" trials traditionally used in research. They also "blinded" their subjects to whether or not they were actually carbohydrate-loading—

not an easy feat to accomplish and rarely, if ever, done before in research. Each of seven well-trained cyclists completed two experimental rides—carbohydrate-loading for 3 days before one ride (9 g CHO/kg BM/day) and consuming a placebo-controlled moderate-carbohydrate diet (6 g CHO/kg BM/day) for 3 days before the other. All the subjects drank a carbohydrate-based sports drink (1 g CHO/kg BM/hour) during all the rides.

Muscle biopsy results showed that although carbohydrate-loading significantly increased muscle glycogen concentration as expected, the amount of muscle glycogen used during exercise did not differ between the carbohydrate-loaded trials and the placebo trials, nor did the time to complete the time trials differ. In other words, carbohydrate-loading did not significantly improve performance during a 100-km cycling trial (~2.5 hours) during which carbohydrate was consumed! Cyclists, with lower preexercise muscle glycogen stores, who consumed adequate carbohydrate *during* prolonged, intense exercise enhanced their performance (by preventing or offsetting hypoglyce-

mia) just as effectively as those who carbohydrate-loaded before the event.

The researchers suggest the following "food for thought":

- Part or all of the ergogenic effect of carbohydrate-loading recorded in most studies to date could be attributable to a placebo effect (endurance athletes are typically well educated and would expect a performance boost thus introducing a psychologic bias).
- The performance-enhancing effect of carbohydrate-loading is small and in real-life competitions most likely only significant in influencing the finishing order among top elite-level cyclists, not "back-of-the-pack" cyclists.
- Consuming adequate carbohydrate during prolonged exercise (at least non-steady-state events) may be more important than glycogen supersaturation via carbohydrate-loading before exercise.

## QUESTIONS

1. Endurance athletes are at an increased risk for developing iron-deficiency anemia because of:
   a. Injury to red blood cells caused by repetitive trauma from foot strikes
   b. Gastrointestinal bleeding
   c. Living or training for extended amounts of time at altitude
   d. All of the above

2. Athletes at a higher risk for developing hyponatremia during prolonged exercise include:
   a. Female athletes
   b. Elite-level athletes
   c. Those athletes with fewer opportunities to drink during exercise
   d. a and b

3. The potential side effects of carbohydrate-loading include:
   a. Weight gain
   b. Lack of appetite
   c. Muscle discomfort and stiffness
   d. a and c

4. Endurance athletes pursuing a vegetarian eating style may need to pay particular attention to consuming enough:
   a. Iron and zinc
   b. Total calories
   c. Vitamin B12
   d. All of the above

5. Recurrent stress fractures in a female endurance athlete can be a warning sign of:
   a. A calcium deficiency
   b. An energy imbalance
   c. A vitamin D deficiency
   d. Lactose intolerance

6. Treatment for the female athlete triad consists of:
   a. Supplementing with 1500 mg of calcium daily
   b. Referring the individual to qualified health professionals for treatment
   c. Reducing the volume and/or intensity of the athlete's training load
   d. All of the above

7. The most severe physiologic stress an endurance athlete can face is while performing exercise:
   a. In the heat
   b. In extreme cold
   c. At altitude
   d. During gale-force winds

8. To enhance recovery after daily bouts of training, endurance athletes should:
   a. Drink 2 cups of water for every pound of body weight lost during exercise
   b. Consume carbohydrate-rich beverages or food within the first 30 minutes
   c. Speed absorption by drinking their calories for the next few hours
   d. Stretch and nap briefly before they eat

9. To combat muscle cramps during prolonged exercise, athletes should:
   a. Take potassium supplements during the event
   b. Use the salt shaker liberally in the days before the event
   c. Drink fluids containing sodium during exercise
   d. b and c

10. Good vegetarian sources of dietary zinc include:
    a. Most fruit
    b. Legumes and lentils
    c. Red meat and shellfish
    d. Bright or darkly colored vegetables

11. Endurance athletes can best improve their performance during prolonged exercise lasting 4 hours or longer by:
    a. Fat-loading before the event
    b. Consuming carbohydrate-rich fluids and/or foods at regular intervals throughout the event
    c. Taking salt tablets or eating salty foods during exercise
    d. Carbohydrate-loading before the event

12. Signs of chronic dehydration include:
    a. Rapid, otherwise unexplainable weight loss
    b. Small amounts of dark-colored urine with a strong odor
    c. Stress fractures
    d. All of the above

13. To perform best under extreme conditions, such as cold or altitude, endurance athletes should focus on:
    a. Consuming only carbohydrate-rich fluids and foods
    b. Increasing their protein intake to cover increased losses caused by muscle damage
    c. Consuming enough calories to meet their energy needs
    d. Consuming carbohydrate and protein in a 4:1 ratio

14. Endurance athletes are at high risk for developing a full-blown eating disorder because of:
    a. Unrealistic expectations about altering body size and shape
    b. Being involved in sports that favor or emphasize leanness
    c. Belief that losing weight will result in an improved performance
    d. All of the above

15. To determine how much fluid is lost during prolonged exercise, an endurance athlete must:
    a. Visit an accredited laboratory and have their sweat rate tested
    b. Compare their preexercise and postexercise body weights
    c. Record their fluid intake during exercise and collect their urine
    d. Weigh themselves periodically during exercise

16. The healthiest way for endurance athletes to maintain an optimal body weight during periods of light activity or rest is to:
    a. Reduce their fat intake to as little as possible
    b. Increase their protein intake to protect their muscle mass
    c. Reduce their carbohydrate intake to match their decreased energy needs
    d. Cut out carbohydrate-rich foods such as pasta, rice, and bread

17. To effectively carbohydrate-load before prolonged exercise, athletes must:
    a. Eat only carbohydrate-rich foods and drinks the day before and the morning of
    b. Reduce their training
    c. Eat a carbohydrate-rich diet for 3 days leading into the event/race
    d. b and c

18. The most important nutritional strategy an athlete can follow to boost their performance during endurance exercise is:
    a. Take an iron supplement daily
    b. Carbohydrate-load before prolonged events/competitions
    c. Consume carbohydrate during moderate-intensity exercise lasting 90 minutes or longer
    d. Drink a sports drink containing vitamins and minerals during exercise

19. Scientists have consistently documented improved performances during exercise among endurance athletes using carbohydrate-containing drinks:
    a. With a 4%–6% carbohydrate concentration
    b. That also contain a small amount of protein
    c. With a 6%–10% carbohydrate concentration
    d. With added vitamins and minerals

20. During the initial recovery phase after prolonged exercise, an endurance athlete should concentrate on:
    a. Drinking 20 ounces of water for every pound of body weight lost
    b. Fluid and carbohydrate needs
    c. Fluid, carbohydrate, and electrolyte needs
    d. Fluid, carbohydrate, and protein needs

21. Hyponatremia in endurance athletes primarily occurs because of extensive losses of sodium chloride through heavy or prolonged sweating.
    a. True
    b. False

22. The female athlete triad is composed of three interrelated medical conditions: eating disorders, amenorrhea, and osteoporosis.
    a. True
    b. False

23. Athletes who live and train at moderate altitude will benefit from consuming an iron-rich diet on a regular basis.
    a. True
    b. False

24. A common mistake endurance athletes often make is failing to experiment with foods and drinks under environmental conditions similar to what they expect to encounter on race day.
    a. True
    b. False

25. Dehydration is often the underlying cause of gastrointestinal problems, such as abdominal cramps and diarrhea, during prolonged exercise.
    a. True
    b. False

26. One of the prime advantages of becoming acclimatized to exercising in the heat is that an athlete will need to consume less fluid during exercise.
    a. True
    b. False

27. A vegetarian athlete engaged in endurance activities can easily meet their nutritional needs by eating extra portions of carbohydrate-rich foods, such as vegetables and whole grains.
   a. True
   b. False

28. Endurance athletes who eliminate dairy foods from their daily diet can simply meet their nutritional needs by taking calcium supplements and eating calcium-fortified foods, such as orange juice.
   a. True
   b. False

29. An athlete can expect to "gain weight" as they carbohydrate-load because approximately 3 g of water is stored with every gram of carbohydrate stored as muscle glycogen.
   a. True
   b. False

30. A female athlete can correct for all the detrimental effects of the female athlete triad by taking calcium supplements and starting hormone replace therapy, such as oral contraceptives.
   a. True
   b. False

## REFERENCES

1. American College of Sports Medicine. Position stand on exercise and fluid replacement. Med Sci Sports Exerc 1996;28:i–vii.
2. National Athletic Training Association. Fluid replacement for athletes. J Ath Train 2000;35:212–224.
3. Rehrer NJ. Fluid and electrolyte balance in ultra-endurance sport. Sports Med 2001;31(10):701–715.
4. Noakes T. Fluid replacement during marathon running. Clin J Sport Med 2003;13(5):309–318.
5. American College of Sports Medicine, American Dietetic Association, Dietitians of Canada. Joint position stand on nutrition and athletic performance. J Am Diet Assoc 2000;100:1543–1556.
6. Berning JR, Nelson Steen S. Nutrition for Sport and Exercise. Maryland: Aspen Publishers; 1998.
7. Burke L, Deakin V. Clinical Sports Nutrition. Sydney: McGraw-Hill; 1994.
8. Burke LM, Kiens B, Ivy JL. Carbohydrates and fat for training and recovery. J Sport Sci 2004;22:15–30.
9. Tarnopolsky M. Protein requirements for endurance athletes. Nutrition 2004;20:662–668.
10. Horvath PJ, Eagen CK, Ryer-Calvin SD, Pendergast DR. The effects of varying dietary fat on the nutrient intake in male and female runners. J Am Coll Nutr 2000;19(1):42–51.
11. Lowery LM. Dietary fat and sports nutrition: a primer. J Sport Sci Med 2004;3:106–117.
12. Lambert EV, Goedecke JH. The role of dietary macronutrients in optimizing endurance performance. Curr Sport Med Rep 2003;2(4):194–201.
13. Rowlands DS, Hopkins WG. Effects of high-fat and high-carbohydrate diets on metabolism and performance in cycling. Metabolism 2002;51(6):678–690.
14. Lambert EV, Goedecke JH, Zyle C, et al. High-fat diet versus habitual diet prior to carbohydrate loading: effects of exercise metabolism and cycling performance. Int J Sport Nutr Exerc Metab 2001;11(2):209–225.
15. Helge JW. Adaptation to a fat-rich diet: effects on endurance performance in humans. Sports Med 2000;30(5)347–357.
16. Ivy J. Regulation of muscle glycogen repletion, muscle protein synthesis and repair following exercise. J Sports Sci Med 2004;3:131–138.
17. Romano BC, Todd MK, Saunders MJ. Effect of 4:1 ratio of carbohydrate/protein beverage on endurance performance, muscle damage and recovery. Med Sci Sports Exerc 2004;36(5):S126.
18. Ivy JL, Res PT, Sprague RC, Widzer MO. Effect of a carbohydrate-protein supplement on endurance performance during exercise of varying intensity. Int J Sport Nutr Exerc Metab 2003;13:382–395.

19. Hsieh M. Recommendations for treatment of hyponatremia at endurance events. Sports Med 2004;34:231–238.

20. Speedy DB, Noakes TD, Rogeres IR, et al. Hyponatremia in ultradistance triathletes. Med Sci Sports Exerc 1999;31(6):809–815.

21. von Dullivard SP, Braun WR, Markofski M, Beneke R, Leithauser R. Fluids and hydration in prolonged endurance performance. Nutrition 2004;20:651–656.

22. Stamford B. Muscle cramps: untying the knots. Phys Sportmed 1993;21:115–116.

23. Noakes TD. Fluid and electrolyte disturbances in the heat. Int J Sports Med 1998;19: S146–149.

24. Eichner ER. Treatment of suspected heat illness. Int J Sports Med 1998;(19): S150–153.

25. Chatard JC, Mujika I, Guy C, Lacour JR. Anaemia and iron deficiency in athletes: practical recommendations for treatment. Sports Med 1999;27(4):229–240.

26. Nieman DC. Physical fitness and vegetarian diets: is there a relation? Am J Clin Nutr 1999;70:S570–575.

27. Loosli AR, Rudd JS. Meatless diets in female athletes: a red flag. Phys Sports Med 1998;26:45–50.

28. American Dietetic Association. Position stand on vegetarian diets. J Am Diet Assoc 1997;97:1317–1321.

29. American College of Sports Medicine. Position stand on the female athlete triad. Med Sci Sports Exerc 1997;29(5):i–ix.

30. Dueck CA, Matt KS, Manore MM, Skinner JS. Treatment of athletic amenorrhea with a diet and training intervention program. Int J Sport Nutr 1996;6:24–40.

31. Joy E, Clark N, Ireland ML, Nattiv A, Varechok S. Team management of the female athlete triad. Phys Sports Med 1997;25:95–110.

32. Benson JE, Englebert-Fenton KA, Eisenman PA. Nutritional aspects of amenorrhea in the female athlete triad. Int J Sport Nutr 1996;6:134–145.

33. Putukian M, Potera C. Don't miss gastrointestinal disorders in athletes. Phys Sportsmed 1997;25:80–94.

34. Murray R. Fluid needs in hot and cold environments. Int J Sport Nutr 1995;5; S62–73.

35. Shephard R. Metabolic adaptations to exercise in the cold. Sports Med 1993;16: 266–289.

36. Askew EW. Nutrition for a cold environment. Phys Sportsmed 1989;17:89.

37. Kayser B. Nutrition and high altitude exposure. Int J Sports Med 1992;13:S129–132.

38. Kayser B. Nutrition and energetics of exercise at altitude. Sports Med 1994;17: 309–323.

39. Lickteig JA. Exercise at high altitudes. In: Rosenbloom C, ed. Sports Nutrition: A Guide for the Professional Working with Active People. Chicago: The American Dietetic Association; 1993:485–492.

40. Saunders MJ, Kane M, Todd MK. Effects of a carbohydrate-protein beverage on cycling endurance and muscle damage. Med Sci Sports Exerc 2004;36:1233–1238.

41. Burke LM, Hawley JA, Schabort EJ, Gibson AC, Mujika I, Noakes TD. Carbohydrate loading failed to improve 100-km cycling performance in a placebo-controlled trial. J Appl Physiol 2000;88:1284–1290.

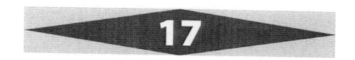

# Nutritional Needs of Strength/Power Athletes

Jim Stoppani, Timothy P. Scheett, and Michael R. McGuigan

## OBJECTIVES

On the completion of this chapter you will be able to:

1. Discuss the different components of the basal metabolic rate.
2. Calculate an individual's basal metabolic rate and account for physical activity.
3. Explain the different methods for determining basal metabolic or resting metabolic rate.
4. Determine the amount of calories needed to add to a diet to gain weight or determine the amount of calories needed to lose weight.
5. Discuss the macronutrient ratios needed by strength/power athletes.
6. Address the issues associated with protein needs of strength/power athletes.
7. Understand the different types of protein supplements and dietary protein that can be used in a healthy diet.
8. Explain the importance of fat in the diet and delineate between the different types.
9. Describe why carbohydrates are important to the strength/power athlete.
10. Address the carbohydrate needs of different types of strength/power athletes.
11. Discuss the different vitamins and minerals that might be needed by strength/power athletes.
12. Understand the ramifications of poor hydration and describe how to rehydrate athletes.
13. Comprehend that water is essential for optimal performance and understand that fluids can be gained from food sources.

## ABSTRACT

Proper dietary guidelines for strength/power athletes have long been lacking. The failure of coaches and the strength/power athletes themselves to recognize the importance of diet is attributable to several reasons. First, strength/power athletes tend to be larger and are required to be larger in lean and overall body mass. Because their goals tend to be gain mass or maintain mass, often the only guideline they are given is simply to eat. Another reason is the type of activity these athletes typically perform. Because they compete in activities that require short bursts of power, the traditional thought was that diet would offer little advantage to their performance. However, as a result of the continuing advances made in the field of sport nutrition, it is now recognized that proper diet enhances all athletes' performance, regardless of body size or type of activity

From: *Essentials of Sports Nutrition and Supplements*
Edited by J. Antonio, D. Kalman, J. R. Stout, M. Greenwood, D. S. Willoughby, and G. G. Haff © Humana Press, a part of Springer Science+Business Media, Totowa, NJ

performed. Sound dietary practices for strength/power athletes are as critical as proper training practices. Because these athletes typically must build and maintain excessive body mass (particularly lean mass), as well as extreme power and strength, a well-designed diet that meets energy intake needs, includes correct macronutrient breakdown, provides adequate fluids and micronutrients, and incorporates proper timing of nutrient intake is a must. Research studies support the concept that athletes who follow a proper dietary strategy experience enhanced training adaptations, whereas those who do not may actually impede training adaptations. This chapter focuses on the proper dietary guidelines for strength/power athletes to follow for optimizing training adaptations and performance.

*Key Words:* **muscle mass, strength, power, protein, dietary energy, calories, muscle hypertrophy, lean body mass**

## ENERGY REQUIREMENTS OF STRENGTH/POWER ATHLETES

The first component to consider regarding the diet of the strength/power athlete is the daily energy requirement. To maintain muscle mass and body weight, as well as to optimize performance and decrease the likelihood of overtraining, the athlete must consume enough calories each day to at least offset their caloric expenditure.[1]

The daily energy requirement of the strength/power athlete is determined by 3 factors: the basal metabolic rate (BMR), physical activity, and the thermic effect of food. BMR is the minimum amount of energy needed to sustain life, often termed the "metabolic cost of living." BMR accounts for about 60%–70% of the total amount of calories the human body uses daily and is determined principally by gender, body size, body composition, and age.[2] Specifically, BMR accounts for the calories expended by the body's organs, tissues, and physiologic systems such as the heart, lungs, liver, kidneys, brain, and muscle mass. It does not include the calories required by the digestive system to digest and absorb nutrients. Physical activity is the most variable component of total energy expenditure. This portion of the athlete's caloric requirement is based on his or her workout frequency, intensity and duration, as well as the amount of physical activity present in a typical day (such as walking and work-related labor). The thermic effect of food makes up the smallest component, and it refers to the amount of calories required to digest and absorb the foods that are consumed.

### Calculating Energy Requirements

There are numerous ways to determine an athlete's daily calorie needs. The more accurate methods typically involve difficult procedures as well as expensive equipment such as doubly labeled water or indirect calorimetry with the use of a metabolic cart. To measure BMR with indirect calorimetry, the metabolic cart measures how much oxygen the athlete's body consumes. By knowing the rate of oxygen consumption (in milliliters per minute), you can accurately calculate energy expenditure. A true BMR must be measured when the individual has been in a postabsorptive state for 12 hours, is completely at rest with absolute minimal muscle movement, and is in a thermoneutral environment that produces the slightest external excitement.[3] The term "BMR" can only be used when a person's metabolic rate is determined when these specified conditions are met. Because it is rare to measure an athlete's metabolic rate under such specific conditions, the term "resting metabolic rate" (RMR) is often used in place of BMR. Regardless, few people have access to a metabolic cart or the time to measure every athlete's BMR/RMR using a metabolic cart, let alone the ability to use tracer methodology. Because of this, several equations have been developed to estimate an individual's RMR based on gender, age, height, and body weight.

The most frequently used RMR equations are the Harris-Benedict equations,[4] given below. There are two different equations, one for males and one for females, because males have a higher metabolic rate (approximately 5%–10% higher) than women as a result of their greater muscle mass. Body size is an important determinant of BMR/RMR and is factored into the Harris-Benedict equations with weight and height. A larger individual will generally have a higher metabolic rate than a smaller individual with comparable body composition. The age of the athlete is also an important factor in determining RMR and is factored into the Harris-Benedict equations. Generally speaking, the older the adult athlete is, the lower the metabolic rate because of age-related decline in muscle mass.

Males: BMR (calories/day) = 66.5 + (13.75 × weight in kg)
+ (5.003 × height in cm) − (6.775 × age in years)

Females: BMR (calories/day) = 655.1 + (9.5663 × weight in kg)
+ (1.85 × height in cm) − (4.676 × age in years)

To determine weight in kilograms, divide weight in pounds by 2.2; to determine height in centimeters, multiply height in inches by 2.54.

Another frequently used system for determining RMR is the one developed by the Food and Agriculture Organization/World Health Organization/United Nations University (FAO/WHO/UNU),[5] given below. Unlike the Harris-Benedict equations, this system does not require the individual's height to determine metabolic rate. It also involves less mathematics. However, the drawback may be some loss of accuracy because fewer individual variables are used to determine the metabolic rate.

| Age (years) | Males | Females |
|---|---|---|
| 10–18 | (17.686 × weight in kg) + 658.2 | (13.38 × weight in kg) + 692.6 |
| 18–30 | (15.057 × weight in kg) + 692.2 | (14.818 × weight in kg) + 486.6 |
| 30–60 | (11.472 × weight in kg) + 873.1 | (8.126 × weight in kg) + 845.6 |
| Over 60 | (11.71 × weight in kg) + 587.7 | (9.082 × weight in kg) + 658.5 |

Whether you use the FAO/WHO/UNU, the Harris-Benedict equations, or indirect calorimetry to determine the athlete's RMR, you will need to enter a factor that represents their average daily physical activity level (PAL) to determine their daily energy expenditure and thus their minimal daily calorie requirements. To do this, you multiply the RMR by a PAL factor that is most appropriate for them. Use the PAL factors found in Table 17.1 to estimate the athlete's minimal daily calorie requirements.

For example, to determine the minimal daily calorie requirements with the Harris-Benedict equation for a 27-year-old athlete who weighs 200 pounds, stands 6 feet tall and trains intensely more than 2 hours per day:
First convert weight and height into SI units.

Weight: 200/2.2 = 91 kg

Height: 72 inches × 2.54 = 183 cm

Next, plug the numbers into the Harris-Benedict equation.

BMR (calories/day) = 66.5 + (13.75 × 91) + (5.003 × 183) − (6.775 × 27)

BMR (calories/day) = 66.5 + 1251.25 + 915.55 − 182.93

BMR = 2050 calories/day

Now multiply the BMR by the appropriate PAL from Table 17.1.

**TABLE 17.1. Physical activity level factors.**

| Activity factor | Activity level |
|---|---|
| 1.53 | Sedentary or light activity |
| 1.76 | Active or moderately active |
| 2.25 | Vigorous active |

Use the most appropriate physical activity level (PAL) factor from the table to determine daily energy expenditure. Multiply the resting metabolic rate by the PAL factor that best suits the athlete. Most athletes who are training and/or competing will have a PAL of 2.25.

$$\text{Minimal daily calorie requirement} = 2050 \times 2.25$$

$$\text{Minimal daily calorie requirement} = 4613$$

## Body Weight Goals

Once you have determined how many calories the athlete needs daily, you must prescribe them a calorie plan that fits their body weight goals. If the athlete is required to simply maintain their body mass, then the estimated RMR multiplied by the appropriate PAL factor should provide sufficient calories for the athlete. However, if the athlete needs to gain or lose body mass, then modifications need to be made to his or her daily calorie plan.

For an athlete to increase or decrease body weight, he or she needs to increase or decrease energy balance, respectively. One pound of body fat equals about 3500 calories.[6,7] Therefore, for weight loss, the athlete should have a weekly caloric intake that is 3500 calories below his or her weekly energy requirements. This will allow him or her to safely lose about 1 pound of fat per week. Daily, the athlete should consume about 500 calories less than his or her daily energy requirements. That means the 200-pound athlete described above would follow a dietary program that averaged about 4113 calories per day.

For weight gain, the opposite is true, and the athlete should consume more calories than his or her energy requirements. Because 1 pound of muscle is about 2500 calories, the strength/power athlete who wants to put on muscle should consume about 300–500 calories beyond their daily energy requirements.[6] For example, the athlete above would need to consume 4913–5113 calories per day. Consuming this many calories can be a difficult task for some athletes. For athletes who cannot consume enough calories for proper weight gain through whole foods, the use of energy/protein powders and bars may be helpful. These dietary supplements are effective tools to help them take in enough calories and macronutrients to put them in a positive energy balance for the day.

Regardless of the exact energy requirements of any athlete, they should follow a daily diet plan that encourages frequent food consumption. It is recommended that the strength/power athlete eat about 4–6 meals per day, with snacks between those meals as necessary to meet their energy needs. This strategy supports lean weight gain by helping to maintain an anabolic environment and supports fat loss by maintaining the metabolic rate and preventing large insulin spikes when not needed.

## Macronutrient Needs

Once energy requirements for the athlete have been established, the issue of macronutrient intake is next to consider. All three macronutrients—protein, carbohydrate, and fat—have key roles in the strength/power athlete's performance. Most strength/power athletes should get 12%–15% of their calories from protein, 55%–60% of their calories from carbohydrates, and 30% of their calories from fat, with less than 10% of that being saturated fats.[1]

## Sidebar 17.1. Ratio Rule

Although the general rule for most strength/power athletes is to shoot for 12%–15% of their calories from protein, 55%–60% of their calories from carbohydrates, and 30% of their calories from fat,[1] it is important to remember that individual differences will influence the ratio of macronutrients for each athlete. The standard ratios given here will provide enough protein to support the normal regenerative processes and promote muscle growth and strength gains; adequate carbohydrates to stock glycogen stores for athletic performance; and fat to maintain a positive energy balance, replenish intramuscular triglyceride stores, and support anabolic hormone production. However, not all sports that strength/power athletes compete in place the same metabolic demands on the athlete's body. Because of the energy continuum that takes place during exercise, activities lasting less than 30 seconds of continual exercise depend little on stored glycogen levels and rely mainly on muscle stores of adenosine triphosphate (ATP) and phosphocreatine. Activities lasting longer than 30 seconds, and those that have multiple intermittent periods of activity, progressively rely more on muscle glycogen levels as the time of exercise increases. This means that strength/power athletes competing and/or training in events that last longer than 30 seconds—such as strongmen, bodybuilders, and football players—will require greater carbohydrate intake. These athletes should take in at least the recommended 55%–60% carbohydrate diet as long as they continue to get 1.5–2.0 g/kg/day of protein and adequate healthy fats. However, athletes who perform activities lasting less than 30 seconds—such as power lifters, shot putters, and sprinters can go with far fewer carbohydrates and higher protein and fat intake to maintain energy balance. Because their sports rely mainly on stored muscle ATP and phosphocreatine with less reliance on muscle glycogen, replenishing glycogen stores via high carbohydrate intake is not necessary to maintain their performance levels. In fact, Day et al.[8] found that low muscle glycogen levels did not impact leg muscle endurance strength.

## PROTEIN INTAKE FOR STRENGTH/POWER ATHLETES

One of the most frequently asked questions by strength/power athletes and their coaches is how much protein is required for increasing muscular size, strength, and power. Muscle-fiber hypertrophy is a result of an increased net protein balance combined with regular resistance training.[9] There are many studies that indicate that intake of protein is advantageous for athletes when muscle hypertrophy is required.[10–12]

Proteins are formed by amino acids, and they serve as the major structural component of tissues such as skeletal muscle as well as being used to produce substances such as hormones (i.e., growth hormone and insulin). Skeletal muscle consists predominantly of water and protein; therefore, to increase muscular size, adequate intakes of amino acids are required. Mixed muscle protein synthesis rate is increased in humans after an acute bout of resistance training.[13] This increase in protein synthesis surpasses the increase in degradation rate and persists for up to 48 hours after an acute exercise bout.[14] There is also evidence that protein intake and hyperaminoacidemia during rest increases protein synthesis,[15,16] and net protein balance remains negative after training if individuals fail to ingest sufficient protein.[14,15] Important questions with protein intake seem to be the amount of protein and the type of protein (i.e., quality) that needs to be consumed to optimize strength and muscle mass gains.

### Enough Is Enough

The amount of protein required by strength/power athletes is a source of much debate by sports nutritionists. Until recently, it was widely suggested that athletes only required the recommended daily intake of 0.8–1.0 g/kg/day. However, there has been a significant body of research recently to suggest that these athletes require greater amounts of protein (i.e., 1.5–2.0 g/kg/day) to maintain positive protein balance.[11,12] This protein intake is equivalent to consuming 3–11 servings of chicken or fish per day for a 50- to 150-kg (110- to 330-pound) athlete.[1] This intake is relatively easy for lighter athletes to achieve, but it can be more difficult for larger athletes. Another important consideration is the total energy intake, which is also a critical factor for athletes who are looking to increase muscle mass.[17] After the strength/power athlete's caloric needs are determined, the total daily protein intake should make up about 12%–15% of the total daily energy intake.[1]

It is perhaps too simplistic to simply state a specific intake amount, given the wide disparity of research findings on protein intake. In addition to the amount of protein consumed, perhaps even more critical is the timing of ingestion of the protein in relation to the exercise bout and the specific type of protein.[18,19] The optimal composition and amount of nutrient ingestion to maximally stimulate muscle-protein synthesis after resistance exercise are currently not known. It does seem that strength/power athletes require more protein than sedentary people,[1] and there are a number of different protein choices available to the strength/power athlete.

## Protein Choices for Strength/Power Athletes

There are a number of different food sources available that can supply protein to the strength/power athlete. In addition, there are also large numbers of protein supplements that are marketed specifically toward this athletic population. However, it is important to note that not all proteins are the same. Proteins differ in terms of their source, the amino acid profile, and the methods of processing. Therefore, the nutritional value of the ingested protein is important, in addition to the composition of the amino acids and the timing of ingestion. Clearly, more research is required to determine specific guidelines in elite strength/power athletes in terms of quantity and quality of protein intake.

The quality of the protein source is an important factor. A number of different methods are used to determine the quality of protein. These include protein-efficiency ratio, biologic value, net protein utilization, and protein digestibility corrected amino acid score.[20] The quality of protein in a food is determined by its essential amino acid content.[21] Some foods contain all of the essential amino acids and in amounts sufficient to maintain protein synthesis, whereas others are lacking in at least one amino acid. The former are called complete protein foods and include such foods as dairy products, eggs, meat, and fish, whereas the latter are called incomplete and include grains, vegetables, and fruits. Because intake of saturated fats and cholesterol is of some concern with complete proteins, athletes can emphasize lean meats, chicken or turkey without the skin, and lowfat dairy products. With a proper combination of sources, vegetable proteins such as nuts and legumes may provide similar benefits to animal sources.

Protein supplements offer a quick and convenient way for strength/power athletes to increase their intake of protein. It should be noted that increasing protein intake above the level necessary to meet protein needs does not result in increased gains in strength, power, or hypertrophy. The best sources of high-quality protein found in supplements are reported to be whey, casein, milk, and egg proteins.[1] Whey protein, especially whey protein isolates or hydrolyzed whey peptides, is widely promoted to strength athletes as being perhaps the best protein, based on its high bioavailability and its content of several critical amino acids (i.e., glutamine, leucine, isoleucine, and valine). Casein is the major component of protein found in dairy products and, like whey, it is a complete protein.

The speed of absorption of dietary amino acids varies according to the type of ingested dietary protein. Research has shown that dietary amino acid absorption is faster with whey protein than with casein.[22] The results of this study indicate that amino acids derived from casein are slowly released from the gut and that slow and fast proteins differently modulate postprandial changes of whole-body protein synthesis, breakdown, and deposition. Overall, results suggest that, in young adults, "slow" proteins (e.g., casein) fare better than "fast" proteins (e.g., whey) with respect to postprandial protein gain. However, other researchers have shown that acute ingestion of both whey and casein after exercise resulted in similar increases in muscle protein net balance, resulting in net muscle protein synthesis despite different patterns of blood amino acid responses.[23] This suggests that the consumption of complete proteins after exercise may be an effective strategy to increase muscle size and strength.

A recent study by Phillips and colleagues[9] examined how the source of protein (i.e., milk versus soy) acutely affected the processes of protein synthesis and protein breakdown after resistance exercise. The findings revealed that even when balanced quantities of total protein and energy were consumed, milk proteins were more effective in stimulating amino acid uptake and net protein deposition in skeletal muscle after resistance exercise than were hydrolyzed soy proteins. There was also a tendency ($p = 0.11$) for greater gains in lean body mass and greater muscle fiber hypertrophy with consumption of milk in the subjects who completed 12 weeks of resistance training. This was also seen in a study with adolescent boys after 12 weeks of progressive resistance training, with greater increases in lean body mass in the subjects who supplemented their diet with milk.[24] However, more recent research has shown no such detriment from soy protein. One study reported that 25 g of soy protein concentrate, soy protein isolate, a soy/whey blend, or whey protein isolate consumed by male subjects after workouts and once more during the day led to similar gains in lean body mass after 12 weeks, and that there was no difference in their individual effect on testosterone or estrogen levels.[25]

The majority of studies investigating the use of protein supplements have been relatively short-term and with small numbers of subjects. Long-term, controlled studies with elite strength/power athletes are required to fully elucidate the effects of increased protein intake and protein quality on strength, power, and muscle hypertrophy. As well, studies specifically using strength/power athletes as subjects may be better able to definitively determine the specific composition and amount of dietary protein needed to optimize gains in muscle strength, power and/or hypertrophy. For now, it appears that the best strategy is to ensure that the strength/power athlete is consuming approximately 1.5–2.0 g of protein per kilogram per day, with the total daily protein intake making up about 12%–15% of the total daily energy intake. In addition, timing seems to be an important factor in muscle hypertrophy. Therefore, not only should emphasis be placed on total daily protein intake for the strength/power athlete, but also on protein timing. Consuming some form of protein immediately before and after the workout is critical for the athlete to gain lean muscle mass.

# CARBOHYDRATE INTAKE FOR STRENGTH/POWER ATHLETES

It is widely recognized that optimum carbohydrate stores in the form of muscle and liver glycogen are required for optimal athletic performance. However, the optimal intake of carbohydrates for strength/power athletes has not been clearly defined. There is little doubt that the macronutrient content of meals after a resistance exercise workout can have a strong influence on the metabolic and hormonal postexercise environment.[26,27] Different macronutrient consumption does influence insulin, testosterone, growth hormone, glucose, and triacylglycerol concentrations after resistance exercise.[26,28,29] It has been shown that muscle glycogen is an important energy substrate during resistance-training activity.[30,31] There is also some evidence that strength and power performance is also enhanced by carbohydrate supplementation during exercise.[32] Thus, it would seem plausible that reduced muscle glycogen would impair strength and power performance. Therefore, the amount and type of carbohydrate consumed is an important consideration for the strength/power athlete.

## Fueling Up

Glycogen is the major substrate used for high-intensity exercise, including resistance training.[33] Several studies have shown muscle glycogen to be reduced by 30%–40% after resistance exercise.[30,31,34] Tesch et al.[31] reported a 26% reduction in muscle glycogen levels after resistance-training activity. Robergs et al.[30] demonstrated that performing multiple sets of leg extensions with 70% and 35% of 1 repetition maximum resulted in 39% and 38% decreases in glycogen, respectively. This decrease in muscle glycogen seems to be particularly marked in the type II fibers.[35] Specific type II muscle fiber glycogen depletion may limit performance during high-volume and/or -intensity workouts, such as resistance training. This could also be an important consideration when multiple workouts or training sessions are performed in a single day and could lead to decreases in strength and power performance. Resistance-training programs that use higher repetition loads (8–15 repetitions), such as those used by bodybuilders and during hypertrophy phases by athletes, could potentially have greater effects on muscle glycogen stores.

Athletes should aim to achieve carbohydrate intakes to meet the fuel requirements of their training program and to optimize restoration of muscle glycogen stores between workouts. The first important consideration is the quantity of nutrient intake. In other words, how much carbohydrate should be consumed? The daily maintenance of glycogen stores is directly related to the amount used during exercise and normal daily activity and the subsequent ingestion of carbohydrates used to replenish the stores. In the case of carbohydrate, strength/power athletes should consume approximately 55%–60% of total energy intake in the form of carbohydrate.[36] This will equate to approximately 5–6 g/kg/day for most athletes. This level of carbohydrate intake seems to be important to maintain the intensity of resistance-training workouts. However, these guidelines should take into account individual total energy needs, specific training needs, and training performance. Potentially, if there is inadequate carbohydrate intake between endurance and/or high-repetition, strength-training sessions, the quality of strength training could be less than optimal. This may then result in less than optimal strength and power development over the course of a training program.

## Carbohydrate Choices for Strength/Power Athletes

As with other macronutrients, an important question is what kind of carbohydrates should be consumed by the athlete (e.g., high-versus low-glycemic carbohydrates). The glycemic index provides a method to rank carbohydrate foods according to the blood-glucose response after their intake. Carbohydrate foods can be divided into those that have a high glycemic index (i.e., white bread, potatoes, sports drinks) or a low glycemic index (i.e., oatmeal, whole grain bread, lentils). Some sports nutritionists recommend manipulating the glycemic index of foods to enhance carbohydrate availability and athletic performance.

In general, before exercise and at times other than postexercise, carbohydrates for strength/power athletes should come from complex carbohydrates that are predominantly low-glycemic sources such as fruits, vegetables, and whole grains. It is better for the athlete to choose nutrient-rich carbohydrate foods and to add other foods to recovery meals and snacks to provide a good source of protein and other nutrients. Because glycogen storage is influenced both by insulin and a rapid supply of glucose substrate, it is logical that carbohydrate sources with a moderate to high glycemic index could enhance postexercise refueling in the strength/power athlete. Carbohydrate foods with a moderate to high glycemic index provide a readily available source of carbohydrate for muscle glycogen synthesis, and should be the major carbohydrate choice in posttraining recovery meals.

It seems that the use of carbohydrate supplementation can potentially enhance muscular strength,[37] although this has not been shown in all studies.[38] This could particularly be the case for lifters who are using high-volume resistance-training programs such as those used by bodybuilders.[32] Compared with placebo, carbohydrate intake (1 g glucose·kg⁻¹ body mass) immediately and 1 hour after a bout of resistance exercise resulted in higher plasma glucose and insulin, decreased myofibrillar protein breakdown and urea nitrogen excretion, and slightly increased fractional muscle protein synthetic rate.[34] An enhanced postexercise insulin response could therefore be of potential benefit to the strength/power athlete, because it may attenuate muscle protein degradation and increase protein synthesis.

Research suggests that providing protein and carbohydrate postexercise enhances accretion of whole body and leg protein.[39] The addition of protein to the carbohydrate seems to have the advantage of limiting postexercise muscle damage and promoting protein accretion.[40] An important question is whether these repeated metabolic alterations are of sufficient magnitude to alter long-term adaptations to resistance training. No studies have systematically addressed the quantity, type, and timing of carbohydrate intake and linked acute physiologic responses to chronic adaptations in strength/power athletes. However, in addition to protein, the strength/power athlete should derive approximately 55%–60% of their total daily energy intake from carbohydrates. The majority of these carbohydrates should be low to moderate on the glycemic index, whereas immediately postexercise the sources should be moderate to high glycemic carbohydrates.

# FAT INTAKE FOR STRENGTH/POWER ATHLETES

Dietary fat intake for strength/power athletes should be fairly similar to that recommended for nonathletes in order to promote general health. However, because strength/power athletes must maintain a positive energy balance, replenish intramuscular triglyceride stores, and support anabolic hormone production, these athletes can tolerate slightly higher dietary fat intake, particularly essential fatty acids, than the general population.[41] Fat is an essential macronutrient that aids in the digestion and absorption of fat-soluble nutrients such as vitamins A, D, E, and K, and beneficial carotenoids, such as lycopene, lutein, and zeaxanthin found in fruits and vegetables.

## Fattening Up

Generally, it is recommended that strength/power athletes receive approximately 30% of their daily caloric intake from fat, with about 10% or fewer of their calories coming from saturated fats. Unlike the general population—who are recommended to limit saturated fat intake—the strength/power athlete should consume some saturated fat in his or her diet. This recommendation is linked with the discovery that higher-fat diets seem to maintain circulating testosterone concentrations better than low-fat diets.[42,43] Maintaining optimal testosterone levels is important for this type of athlete for obvious reasons, such as building muscle mass and strength. It also is important to help combat the suppression of testosterone that can occur during overtraining.[44] In fact, cholesterol may also be important for muscle growth and strength. Riechman and colleagues[45] discovered that in older adults (aged 60–69) following a 12-week weight-training program, subjects who consumed a lower cholesterol diet (<3.5 mg/kg lean mass/day) did not increase their lean mass and experienced strength gains of only 36%. However, in subjects who followed a diet that was higher in cholesterol (>5.7 mg/kg lean mass/day), lean mass was increased by 2.1 kg, and strength increased by 86%. Furthermore, in subjects whose blood cholesterol was <178 mg/dL, lean mass increased by only 0.3 kg and strength by 37%. Yet, subjects with blood cholesterol >238 mg/dL increased their lean mass by 2.3 kg and strength by 70%. Although the exact mechanism for these results is presently uncertain, it may be attributable to the fact that cholesterol is important for testosterone production as well as maintaining the integrity of cell membranes.

Although conventional wisdom has been to limit fat intake, research supports the notion that diets containing higher total and saturated fat are no longer considered detrimental to health. Researchers of The Malmo Diet and Cancer Study[46] reported that individuals receiving more than 30% of their total daily energy from fat and more than 10% from saturated fat did not have increased mortality.

The majority of the strength/power athlete's dietary fat should come from monounsaturated and polyunsaturated fats. About 10%–15% of their daily calories should come from monounsaturated fats and another 10%–15% from polyunsaturated fats. These healthy fats can help fend off diseases and potentially promote athletic performance. Mono- and polyunsaturated fats help to lower total blood cholesterol and triglycerides and increase high density lipoprotein cholesterol levels in the blood.[47,48] These fats, particularly the omega-3 polyunsaturated fats, also help prevent chronic inflammatory-related diseases such as cardiovascular disease.[49,50] In addition, they may improve insulin sensitivity and blood pressure, reducing the risk of diabetes and hypertension.[51–53] More important to the athlete, mono- and polyunsaturated fats are more readily burned for fuel than trans and saturated fats are.[54,55] Diets rich in polyunsaturated fats may help spare muscle glycogen and potentially increase the time it takes to reach muscle exhaustion.[56] In addition, research suggests that omega-3 polyunsaturated fats may actually help to prevent certain cancers and muscle and bone loss during times of inactivity.[57,58]

The strength/power athlete should avoid trans fats whenever possible. Trans fats promote heart disease, diabetes, certain cancers, and obesity.[59–62] They also increase low density lipoprotein cholesterol levels, C-reactive protein, and triglycerides.[60,63,64] In addition, trans fats lower high density lipoprotein cholesterol levels and may encourage muscle breakdown.[63-65]

## Fat Choices

The strength/power athlete should be able to get plenty of these fats in his or her diet by consuming the proper foods. For monounsaturated fats, good choices include olive, canola, and peanut oils; nuts and avocados. Good sources of polyunsaturated fats include corn, safflower, sesame, canola, soy, and sunflower oils; nuts and seeds. The best sources of omega-3 polyunsaturated fatty acids come from cold-water fish such as herring, mackerel, salmon, sardines, and tuna; flaxseed and walnuts. To ensure that he or she receives some saturated fats, the strength/power athlete should eat some beef, poultry, and dairy products, as well as coconut, palm, and palm kernel oils. To avoid trans fats, these athletes should be encouraged to avoid processed foods such as packaged cookies, crackers, pastries, and other baked goods; chips and other snack foods; candy, fried fast food, margarine, and shortening.

## VITAMINS AND MINERALS FOR STRENGTH/POWER ATHLETES

There is limited research supporting the beneficial effects of vitamin and mineral supplements for strength/power athletes. Both fat-soluble (A, D, E, and K) and water-soluble (B and C) vitamins are vital organic compounds that are required for a number of metabolic processes. The metabolic function of vitamins has led to suggestions that additional intake of these vitamins may help athletes tolerate training more effectively. For example, antioxidants are a group of compounds that "combat" free radicals. Several different substances are grouped together and categorized as antioxidants. Some of the most well known include β-carotene (closely related to vitamin A), vitamin C, and vitamin E. In addition, several minerals, such as copper, magnesium, selenium, and zinc also function in an antioxidant role. Many athletes use antioxidants because of their proposed positive health-related aspects and the potential they possess for enhancing recovery from exercise training and/or athletic performance.

McBride et al.[66] investigated whether vitamin E supplementation would have any effect on free-radical formation or variables associated with muscle membrane disruption. The vitamin E–supplemented group elicited a significant decrease in creatine kinase activity at 24 and 48 hours postexercise, compared with the placebo group. These findings suggest that vitamin E supplementation may decrease the muscle membrane disruption that occurs during resistance training. Another recent study investigated the effects of vitamin E supplementation on recovery responses to repeated bouts of resistance exercise.[67] In this study, additional intake of vitamin E was not effective at attenuating performance decrements, muscle soreness, or markers of damage or oxidative stress after repeated bouts of resistance exercise.

The B vitamins (e.g., thiamin, niacin, and riboflavin) are water-soluble and therefore need to be consumed on a daily basis. As a group, B vitamins have a variety of roles in energy metabolism, but dietary availability does not seem to affect exercise capacity when athletes have adequate intakes.

Minerals, which are inorganic compounds such as iron, zinc, magnesium, and calcium, are also used as supplements by some strength/power athletes. For example, chromium, a mineral involved in energy metabolism, has been proposed to enhance the effects of insulin acting as an anabolic agent. However, a study by Campbell et al.[68] found that supplementation with chromium did not enhance muscle size, strength or power development, or lean body mass in older men during a 12-week resistance-training program. In fact, most well-controlled research trials have shown no benefit of chromium supplementation for resistance exercise,[1] and this has been confirmed by a recent meta-analysis.[69]

Calcium is an important mineral for muscle contraction and bone structure. Research also suggests that there is a strong relationship between calcium intake and fat loss.[1] Work by Zemel and colleagues[70] has demonstrated that increasing dietary calcium can increase weight and fat loss secondary to caloric restriction. Calcium seems to modulate 1,25-dihydroxyvitamin D, which serves to regulate intracellular levels of calcium in adipocytes. Vitamin D promotes bone growth, and supplementation along with calcium may be of benefit for athletes at risk of developing osteoporosis.[71]

Optimal immune function requires adequate dietary supply of vitamins and minerals. Studies have indicated that supplementation with zinc can minimize exercise-induced immune responses in athletes,[72] because of zinc's role in immunity. Magnesium is a mineral that activates enzymes involved in protein synthesis. Zinc magnesium-aspartate (ZMA) is a formulation that contains zinc monomethionine aspartate plus magnesium aspartate and vitamin B6. This has been proposed as an effective supplement for improving quality of sleep, recovery, and protein anabolism at night. One study has shown that ingestion of ZMA increased insulin-like growth factor 1 and testosterone levels in football players who were deficient and resulted in greater increases in strength.[73] These findings need to be confirmed with further research, because a more recent study by Wilborn et al.[74] reported conflicting results. They concluded that ZMA seems to have limited value on body composition, hormonal profiles, and performance in experienced weightlifters with normal zinc and magnesium status.

As with any aspect of nutrition, it is critical to determine the dietary sources of vitamins and minerals, in addition to amounts contained in supplements. There may be cases in which athletes are not receiving sufficient amounts of particular vitamins and minerals, and therefore supplementation should be considered. Numerous reports have shown that in individuals lacking sufficient levels of a specific vitamin or mineral, supplementation has increased markers of health as well as athletic performance. Additionally, there is very little research to support the use of vitamin and mineral supplementation in megadoses in attempts to increase athletic performance. However, with this in mind, there is reason to believe that strength/power athletes may benefit from supplementation with certain minerals that are involved in muscle contraction and repair of muscle during recovery from training. One simple recommendation is that athletes consume a low-dose, one-a-day multivitamin during periods of heavy training. In fact, the American Health Association recently recommended that Americans consume a low-dose, one-per-day multivitamin supplement to promote better health.[1]

## HYDRATION AND STRENGTH

"The most important nutritional ergogenic aid for athletes is water."[1] Strength/ power athletes place a formidable demand on their musculature to produce energy during each rep of every workout. In terms of energy metabolism, the body is only 40% efficient in turning fuel energy into usable energy. The remaining 60% of the original fuel energy is lost as heat. The body, utilizing the circulatory system, transfers this heat byproduct from the exercising muscle to the skin (e.g., increased skin blood flow and redness of skin during exercise). Because of this increased load placed on the muscles during repeated contractions, any alteration in fluid status will lead to complications with achieving optimal performance.

Research has shown that sweat-induced body weight losses as small as 2% can elicit significant negative consequences on exercise performance. A 2% loss in body weight equates to a 4-pound loss for a 200-pound athlete. It is not uncommon for a 200-pound football player to lose as much as 6–8 pounds (3%–4% of his body weight) after a single 2-hour early-season practice. Schoffstall et al.[75] reported that sweat-induced body weight reductions of as little as 1.5% led to significant decreases in muscular strength. Thus, the optimal solution to the problems associated with the sweat-induced body weight loss (i.e., decreased strength, power, performance, increased body temperature, and likelihood of muscle cramps) is to prevent the body weight losses rather than trying to replace what was lost after the fact.

In addition to the decreases in strength, power, and performance, sweat-induced body weight losses greater than 4% are not recommended for the additional reason that these losses cause an increase in the resulting physiologic strain (e.g., increased core temperature, heart rate, and perceived effort) placed on the body. Researchers at the United States Army Institute of Environmental Medicine have reported that the body's core temperature, heart rate, and rating of perceived exertion remain at their lowest when the volume of fluid ingested matches as closely as possible to the rate that sweat is lost.[76] Furthermore, acute sweat-induced body weight losses of more than 4% may lead to a heat illness (i.e., heat exhaustion or heat stroke) or possibly death.[77]

Proper hydration is a distinct concern for athletes who participate in sports that require multiple practices or competitions in a single day (e.g., volleyball, basketball, swimming, and bodybuilding), and of even more concern are those athletes who have multiple practices in hot and/or humid conditions (e.g., football, baseball, softball, soccer, lacrosse, track, and tennis). Individuals who begin a second practice in an already dehydrated state will experience further reductions in strength, power, and performance and are at an increased risk of heat illness.[78] Maintaining adequate hydration during and after a single practice takes conscious effort on the part of the athlete and training staff, but maintaining adequate hydration during and after multiple practices takes an even greater substantial effort. Still, maintaining proper hydration is the most efficient and straightforward way to maintain the ability to produce muscular strength and power throughout training, practice, and/or competition.

## Drinking Enough

Based on training status, fitness level, body size, intensity, and heat acclimatization status, athletes typically have sweat rates that range anywhere from 0.5 to 2.0 L per hour. Sweat losses of this magnitude will require an athlete to ingest 0.5–2 L per hour of fluid to maintain optimal fluid balance and/or prevent dehydration, prevent the associated body weight loss, and the subsequent decrease in performance.

To achieve optimal performance during competition or a training session, the best recommendation is to try to prevent a dehydrated state from occurring. It is advisable to tell people to begin their exercise bout in a fully hydrated state. This can be accomplished by consuming at least 34 ounces (1 L) of fluid the day before exercise[79] or alternatively 14–20 ounces (400–600 mL) of fluid 2 hours before beginning exercise and ingesting adequate fluids throughout the exercise bout.[76]

To prevent a sweat-induced body weight loss of only 4 pounds during exercise, our 200-pound athlete would need to consume 61 ounces (1.8 L) of fluid, which equates to ~15 mL of fluid every minute for 2 hours. However, to prevent a 6- to 8-pound loss, the athlete would need to consume 92–122 ounces (2.7–3.6 L) of fluid or 22.5–30 mL/min. Because it would be near impossible, if not just completely impractical, to ingest 15 mL of fluid every minute, this fluid intake recommendation equates to consuming 5–8 ounces (150–225 mL) of fluid every 10–15 minutes. (For the severe sweat-induced, body weight–loss example of 8–10 pounds, fluid consumption would need to be on the order of 8–10 ounces (225–300 mL) every 10–15 minutes.) Of course, these amounts are general recommendations and will need to be adjusted accordingly based on fitness level, intensity (i.e., sweat rate), mode, and/or duration of exercise, as well as individual body size.

Strength/power athletes engaged in intense training or competition in the heat need to give particular attention to their fluid-replenishment protocol. Exercise in any environment (hot and/or humid) that triggers a greater sweat rate requires the athlete to consume even more fluids. In terms of duration, water has been shown to be a sufficient fluid for maintaining hydration levels during exercise sessions that last less than 90 minutes. However, during exercise sessions that last more than 90 minutes, it is advisable to consume some sort of carbohydrate beverage such as those that are commercially available.[76] The carbohydrate contained in the beverage will provide a fuel source to the exercising muscle (e.g., during the 45 minutes of cardiorespiratory exercise often performed after the 90 minutes of resistance training), while the fluid will eventually replace that which was lost to sweat. The addition of electrolytes to a hydration beverage is usually not required because the dietary intake of most strength/power athletes is sufficient enough to provide all of the essential electrolytes that were lost through the sweat and urine; however, during the first few days of training in hot and/or humid conditions or when an individual's caloric intake is less than his or her caloric expenditure, the use of supplemental electrolytes may be warranted.[76]

In terms of knowing when to drink, athletes should be instructed not to wait until they are thirsty to consume fluids. The stimulus to drink for most individuals does not occur (i.e., you do not become thirsty) until blood osmolality (i.e., concentration of particles in the blood) exceeds 295 mosmol/kg. At this level of osmolality, the body is already in a dehydrated state. Thus, it is a good idea to schedule water breaks during the workout and/or instruct athletes to consume a particular amount of fluid during training, practices, and competition. (Furthermore, fluid should *never* be restricted or withheld as a form of punishment.)

During training in hot and/or humid conditions, it is a good idea for athletes to get in the habit of weighing themselves before and after training/practice sessions to make sure they are consuming adequate fluid. A general rule is to consume 24 ounces (710 mL) of fluids for each pound of body weight lost in order to ensure proper rehydration. Athletes should also get in the habit of consuming fluids during practice in the same manner as they will during competition. This will allow the athletes to gauge how the fluids will feel and subsequently affect them during competition. Furthermore, palatability of fluids has been given much consideration. Fluids that taste good are often consumed in much greater quantity than those with an unpleasant or no flavor.[80] Thus, some athletes may want to experiment with different types of fluids during practice to learn which type they prefer to provide them optimal hydration and performance.

## Fluid Is Fluid

We have all heard for as long as we have been alive that we need to consume eight 8-ounce glasses (64 ounces; 1.9 L) of water a day. However, a recent finding of the Institute of Medicine panel of United States and Canadian scientists concluded that men require an average of 16 8-ounce glasses (128 ounces; 3.8 L), and women need 11 8-ounce glasses (88 ounces; 2.6 L) of water a day.[81] This does not mean that this amount of fluid needs to be consumed simply as liquid. All the fluids an individual consumes throughout the day are included in the 3.8 L—including soft drinks, juice, tea, coffee, milk, and, of course, the fluid found in foods. In fact, Grandjean et al.[82] reported that including plain drinking water in the diet, as compared with excluding it, did not affect hydration levels.

Individuals require fluids of these magnitudes because fluid is lost throughout the normal course of a day. The body loses fluid from the kidneys in the form of urine (1500 mL/day), from the skin in the form of sweat evaporation (500 mL/day), from the lungs in the form of moisture in the breath (300 mL/day), and from the gastrointestinal tract (200 mL/day).

We support these recommendations as well as recommend leaning toward the higher values of fluid intake (up to 1 gallon for some individuals) for other reasons beyond hydration and performance. Water, for example, has no calories, yet makes you feel full. This means that dieters fare better the more water they drink. There also is the volumizing effect of supplements such as creatine, which require extra water. But there is a downside. Those individuals who consume large amounts of plain water may be at risk of a condition called hyponatremia (i.e., low sodium). Consuming extreme quantities of water, although rare, has also led to water intoxication and even death in some individuals. Hyponatremia exerts negative consequences on the body in terms of electrolyte imbalances and, if severe enough, cardiac arrhythmias. Electrolyte imbalances result in improper muscle contractions and is a leading theory behind the occurrence of muscle cramps.

Athletes should not worry if they feel they cannot handle taking in these amounts of fluids on a daily basis. Most foods contain a rather high percentage

**TABLE 17.2. Water content of foods.**

| Food | Water content |
|---|---|
| Cucumber (1 large) | 296 mL or 10 ounces |
| Watermelon (1 wedge) | 260 mL or 9 ounces |
| Asian pear (1 large) | 237 mL or 8 ounces |
| Chicken noodle soup (1 cup) | 237 mL or 8 ounces |
| Corn (1 cup) | 213 mL or 7 ounces |
| Salad (1.5 cups) | 213 mL or 7 ounces |
| Lowfat yogurt (1 cup) | 189 mL or 6 ounces |
| Lowfat cottage cheese (1 cup) | 189 mL or 6 ounces |
| Baked beans (1 cup) | 189 mL or 6 ounces |
| Baked potato (1 medium) | 142 mL or 5 ounces |
| Brown rice (1 cup) | 142 mL or 5 ounces |
| Grapes (1 cup) | 142 mL or 5 ounces |
| Apple (1 medium) | 118 mL or 4 ounces |
| Oatmeal (1 cup) | 118 mL or 4 ounces |
| Orange (1 medium) | 118 mL or 4 ounces |

of fluid (Tables 17.2 and 17.3). The fluid consumed through eating foods counts toward the total daily fluid requirements. For example, a large cucumber contains ~10 ounces of water, whereas a medium salad contains ~7 ounces of water and even a medium baked potato contains ~5 ounces of water. Some relatively "dry" foods are in fact a good source of fluid. These particular foods (e.g., beans, grains, and pasta) act like sponges as they cook. A cup of red kidney beans is 77% water, whereas 1 cup of brown rice actually supplies more than 1/2 cup of water. Surprisingly, baked goods are also part liquid—the more moist the food, the more fluid it contains. One slice of whole wheat bread is about 33% water and a tortilla somewhat more. A roasted chicken breast is 65% water, baked salmon totals 62%, and cheeses such as blue and cheddar are about 40% water.

## Drink Up

In January of 2001, the American College of Sports Medicine, American Dietetic Association, and the Dietitians of Canada published the "Joint Position Statement: nutrition and athletic performance."[83] In the statement, the authors concluded in part that "Athletes should be well-hydrated before beginning to exercise; athletes should also drink enough fluid during and after exercise to balance fluid losses. Consumption of sport drinks containing carbohydrates and electrolytes during exercise will provide fuel for the muscles, help maintain blood glucose and the thirst mechanism, and decrease the risk of dehydration or hyponatremia."

The best method to ensure that an individual is well hydrated before training, practice, and/or competition is to regularly consume fluids and foods that are high in water content. Total daily fluid intake should be on the order of 3800 mL for men and 2600 mL for women. It is best to ingest fluid throughout exercise to continually replace fluid losses during exercise. Weighing before and after an exercise bout will allow for the determination of the specific amount of fluid that needs to be consumed to fully rehydrate.

Practice and training sessions are the preferred time for athletes to try different ingestion protocols, volumes or types of fluids that will be ingested during competition. This will allow the athletes to learn which type of fluid they prefer and will provide them the optimal hydration and performance.

Exercise in any environment (hot and/or humid) will increase an individual's sweat rate as their fitness level and acclimatization status increase. Both of these training adaptations require the athlete to consume additional fluids. During exercise bouts less than 90 minutes, water has been shown to be a satisfactory fluid choice for maintaining hydration levels; whereas, during exercise

**TABLE 17.3. Percent water in foods.**

| Food | Percent water | Food | Percent water |
|------|---------------|------|---------------|
| Almonds | 7 | Okra, boiled | 91 |
| Apples | 85 | Olives | 80 |
| Apricots | 85 | Onions | 89 |
| Bananas | 76 | Oranges | 86 |
| Bean sprouts | 92 | Papayas, raw | 89 |
| Beef, raw hamburger | 54 | Parsley, raw | 86 |
| Bread, whole wheat | 35 | Peaches, raw | 90 |
| Broccoli | 91 | Peanuts, shelled | Trace |
| Butter | 20 | Peanut butter | Trace |
| Cabbage, raw | 92 | Pears, raw | 82 |
| Cantaloupe | 91 | Peas, raw | 81 |
| Carrots, raw | 88 | Pecans | 7 |
| Cauliflower, raw | 91 | Peppers, green | 94 |
| Celery | 94 | Pickles, dill | 93 |
| Cheese, American | 37 | Pineapple, raw | 85 |
| Cherries, raw | 80 | Plums, raw | 87 |
| Chicken, broiled | 71 | Pork chops, broiled | 45 |
| Coconut, dried | 7 | Potatoes, raw | 85 |
| Collards, boiled | 91 | Pumpkin, canned | 90 |
| Corn, sweet, fresh | 74 | Radishes, raw | 95 |
| Cucumbers, raw | 96 | Raspberries | 81 |
| Eggs, raw whole | 74 | Rutabagas, boiled | 90 |
| Eggplant, raw | 92 | Sauerkraut, canned | 93 |
| Fruit cocktail | 80 | Spinach, raw | 92 |
| Grapefruit, raw | 88 | Squash, boiled | 96 |
| Grapes | 82 | Strawberries, raw | 90 |
| Ham, smoked, cooked | 54 | Swiss chard | 94 |
| Honey | 15 | Tomatoes, raw | 93 |
| Jams/preserves | 30 | Turkey, roasted | 62 |
| Kale | 87 | Veal, broiled | 60 |
| Lettuce, head | 96 | Walnuts | 4 |
| Macaroni/spaghetti, cooked | 72 | Watercress, raw | 90 |
| Margarine | 20 | Watermelon | 93 |
| Molasses | 25 | | |

sessions lasting more than 90 minutes, experts recommend that a carbohydrate beverage, such as those that are commercially available, be consumed.[76] The carbohydrate source in the beverage will provide fuel to the exercising muscle while the fluid will replace the fluid that was lost during exercise.

Whereas fluid ingestion before and during exercise needs to focus on consuming optimal nutrients (e.g., water, carbohydrates, electrolytes) to maintain fluid levels, postexercise nutrition should be focused toward restoring electrolytes and water, replenishing glycogen stores, and rebuilding/repairing skeletal muscle.

## SUMMARY

Teaching strength/power athletes sound dietary practices is critical for them to gain and maintain muscle mass and perform at the top of their game. Diets designed for these athletes must meet their energy-intake needs, follow proper macronutrient breakdown, provide adequate micronutrients, and offer ample fluids. In general, energy needs should be calculated for each individual athlete through laboratory testing or estimated using a reliable RMR equation. After total daily energy requirements have been determined, the diet should be created taking proper macronutrient amounts into consideration. Diets for strength/power athletes should provide approximately 12%–15% of calories from protein, 55%–60% of calories from carbohydrates, and about 30% from fat. Last but not least, nutrition programs designed for strength/power athletes should also focus on the proper timing of nutrients. Research has demonstrated that the timing of meal consumption, with exercise being the critical time point, may have a role in optimizing performance, training adaptations, and even preventing overtraining. This topic is discussed thoroughly in Chapter 28.

## QUESTIONS

1. The amount of protein required by strength/power athletes is:
   a. <0.8 g per kg body weight
   b. 0.8–1.0 g per kg body weight
   c. 1.5–2.0 g per kg body weight
   d. >2.0 g per kg body weight

2. The quality of protein in a food is determined by:
   a. The number of grams of protein
   b. Its essential amino acid content
   c. Its nonessential amino acid content
   d. Its glycemic index

3. Whey protein is considered to be an excellent source of protein because:
   a. Its high bioavailability
   b. Its content of several critical amino acids such as glutamine, leucine, isoleucine, and valine
   c. Absorption is faster with whey protein than with casein
   d. All of the above

4. Which of the following are important to consider when considering protein intake?
   a. Timing of the intake
   b. Quality of the intake
   c. Quantity of the intake
   d. All of the above

5. Before exercise and at times other than postexercise, the strength/power athlete should consume what type of carbohydrate?
   a. Simple carbohydrates
   b. High glycemic index carbohydrates
   c. Limited intake of carbohydrates is optimal
   d. Low glycemic index carbohydrates

6. Immediately postexercise, the sources of carbohydrate should consist of:
   a. Complex carbohydrates
   b. Moderate to high glycemic index carbohydrates
   c. Limited intake of carbohydrates is optimal and consume only protein
   d. Low glycemic index carbohydrates

7. In the case of carbohydrate, strength/power athletes should consume approximately:
   a. 55%–60%
   b. 10%–20%
   c. 30%
   d. 40%–45%

8. Research suggests that the ingestion of protein and carbohydrate should occur:
   a. Immediately before the workout
   b. Immediately after the workout
   c. 2 hours after the workout
   d. a and b are both correct

9. The glycemic index provides a method to rank carbohydrate foods according to:
   a. Total grams of carbohydrate
   b. Blood glucose response after their intake
   c. Blood free fatty acid response after their intake
   d. The percentage of the food containing glucose

10. Which of the following is not a fat-soluble vitamin?
    a. A
    b. C
    c. D
    d. E

11. During resistance exercise which macronutrient is the preferred fuel substrate?
    a. Fat
    b. Protein
    c. Carbohydrate
    d. Water

12. Which of the following is a true statement? In relation to recovery from resistance training:
    a. Carbohydrates are more important than protein
    b. Protein is more important than carbohydrates
    c. Lipids are more important than both protein and carbohydrates
    d. It is important to consume a combination of protein and carbohydrates

13. Which of the following is the most correct statement? Diets designed for strength/power athletes must:
    a. Meet individual energy-intake needs
    b. Follow proper macronutrient breakdown
    c. Provide adequate micronutrients
    d. Offer ample fluids
    e. All of the above

14. Which of the following is not correct? Strength/power athletes need to consume enough calories each day to at least offset their caloric expenditure in order to:
    a. Maintain muscle mass
    b. Lose body weight
    c. Optimize performance
    d. Decrease the likelihood of overtraining

15. Which of the following does not contribute to the daily energy requirement of the strength/power athlete?
    a. Basal metabolic rate
    b. Physical activity
    c. Macronutrient quality
    d. Thermic effect of food

16. Mixed muscle protein synthesis rate is ____ in humans after an acute bout of resistance training.
    a. Decreased
    b. Increased
    c. Not changed

17. Research has shown that dietary amino acid absorption is ____ with whey protein than with casein protein.
    a. Faster
    b. Not changed
    c. Slower

18. When choosing protein sources for strength/power athletes, which of the following is an important consideration?
    a. Total daily protein intake
    b. Protein timing

c. Protein quality

d. All the above

19. To ensure optimal gains in lean muscle mass, a proper protein source should be consumed immediately ____ the athlete's workout.

a. After

b. Before

c. Before and after

d. During

20. Research has shown that sweat-induced body weight losses as small as ____ can elicit significant negative consequences on exercise performance.

a. 1%

b. 2%

c. 4%

d. 10%

21. Glycogen is the major substrate used for resistance exercise.

a. True

b. False

22. Resistance-training programs that use higher repetition loads, such as those used by bodybuilders and during hypertrophy phases by athletes, would have greater effects on muscle glycogen stores.

a. True

b. False

23. Research suggests that there is a strong relationship between calcium intake and fat loss.

a. True

b. False

24. A one-a-day vitamin/mineral supplementation has been shown to be effective for strength/power athletes.

a. True

b. False

25. All sources of protein provide equal quality protein.

a. True

b. False

26. Strength/power athletes can only get their daily requirement of water by consuming fluids.

a. True

b. False

27. Vitamins function as antioxidants whereas minerals do not.

a. True

b. False

28. Because 60% of the energy the body generates is lost as heat, fluid intake is important for athletes because it helps cool the body.

a. True

b. False

29. To achieve optimal performance during competition or a training session, the best recommendation is to try to prevent a dehydrated state from occurring.

a. True

b. False

30. Weighing before and after an exercise bout will allow for the determination of the specific amount of fluid that needs to be consumed to fully rehydrate.

a. True

b. False

# REFERENCES

1. Kreider RB, Almada AL, Antonio J, et al. ISSN Exercise & Sport Nutrition Review: research & recommendations. Sports Nutr Rev J 2004;1:1–44.
2. Wilmore JH, Costill DL. Metabolism, energy, and the basic energy systems. In: Physiology of Sport and Exercise. 3rd ed. Champaign, IL: Human Kinetics Publishers; 2001:139.
3. Elia M, Stratton R, Stubbs J. Techniques for the study of energy balance in man. Proc Nutr Soc 2003;62:529–537.
4. Harris J, Benedict F. A Biometric Study of Basal Metabolism in Man. Washington, DC: Carnegie Institute of Washington; 1919.
5. Food and Agriculture Organization/World Health Organization/United Nations University Expert Consultation on Human Energy Requirements. Food and Nutrition Technical Report Series no. 1. Rome: FAO; 2001.
6. Kleiner SM. Power Eating. 2nd ed. Champaign, IL: Human Kinetics Publishers; 2001.
7. Lutz CA, Przytulski KR. Nutrition and Diet Therapy. 2nd ed. Philadelphia: F.A. Davis; 1997.
8. Day SM, Brown LE, Beam W, Fortuna J. The effect of pre-exercise carbohydrate status on acute strength. J Strength Cond Res 2005;19:e12.
9. Phillips SM, Hartman JW, Wilkinson SB. Dietary protein to support anabolism with resistance exercise in young men. J Am Coll Nutr 2005;24:134S–139S.
10. Andersen LL, Tufekovic G, Zebis M, et al. The effect of resistance training combined with timed ingestion of protein on muscle fiber size and muscle strength. Metabolism 2005;54:151–156.
11. Lemon PW, Tarnopolsky MA, MacDougall JD, Atkinson SA. Protein requirements and muscle mass/strength changes during intensive training in novice bodybuilders. J Appl Physiol 1992;73:767–775.
12. Tarnopolsky MA, Atkinson SA, MacDougall JD, Chesley A, Phillips S, Schwarcz HP. Evaluation of protein requirements for trained strength athletes. J Appl Physiol 1992;73:1986–1995.
13. Chesley A, MacDougall JD, Tarnopolsky MA, Atkinson SA, Smith K. Changes in human muscle protein synthesis after resistance exercise. J Appl Physiol 1992;73:1383–1388.
14. Phillips SM, Tipton KD, Aarsland A, Wolf SE, Wolfe RR. Mixed muscle protein synthesis and breakdown after resistance exercise in humans. Am J Physiol 1997;273:E99–107.
15. Biolo G, Maggi SP, Williams BD, Tipton KD, Wolfe RR. Increased rates of muscle protein turnover and amino acid transport after resistance exercise in humans. Am J Physiol Endocrinol Metab 1995;268:E514–520.
16. Smith K, Reynolds N, Downie S, Patel A, Rennie MJ. Effects of flooding amino acids on incorporation of labeled amino acids into human muscle protein. Am J Physiol 1998;275:E73–78.
17. Lemon PW. Effects of exercise on dietary protein requirements. Int J Sport Nutr 1998;8:426–447.
18. Esmarck B, Andersen JL, Olsen S, Richter EA, Mizuno M, Kjaer M. Timing of postexercise protein intake is important for muscle hypertrophy with resistance training in elderly humans. J Physiol 2001;535:301–311.
19. Tipton KD, Rasmussen BB, Miller SL, et al. Timing of amino acid-carbohydrate ingestion alters anabolic response of muscle to resistance exercise. Am J Physiol Endocrinol Metab 2001;281:E197–206.
20. Hoffman JR, Falvo MJ. Protein—which is best? J Sports Sci Med 2004;3:118–130.
21. Henley EC, Kuster, JM. Protein quality evaluation by protein digestibility-corrected amino acid scoring. Food Technol 1994;48:74–77.
22. Boirie Y, Dangin M, Gachon P, Vasson MP, Maubois JL, Beaufrere B. Slow and fast dietary proteins differently modulate postprandial protein accretion. Proc Natl Acad Sci USA 1997;94:14930–14935.
23. Tipton KD, Elliott TA, Cree MG, Wolf SE, Sanford AP, Wolfe RR. Ingestion of casein and whey proteins result in muscle anabolism after resistance exercise. Med Sci Sports Exerc 2004;36:2073–2081.
24. Volek JS, Gómez AL, Scheett TP, et al. Increasing fluid milk favorably affects bone mineral density responses to resistance training in adolescent boys. J Am Diet Assoc 2003;103:1353–1356.
25. Rubin S, Kalman D, Martinez M, Krieger DR. A randomized double-blind clinical pilot trial evaluating the effect of protein source when combined with resistance training on body composition and sex hormones in adult males. FASEB J 2005;19:LB250.

26. Volek JS, Kraemer WJ, Bush JA, Incledon T, Boetes M. Testosterone and cortisol in relationship to dietary nutrients and resistance exercise. J Appl Physiol 1997;82:49–54.

27. Bosher KJ, Potteiger JA, Gennings C, Luebbers PE, Shannon KA, Shannon RM. Effects of different macronutrient consumption following a resistance-training session on fat and carbohydrate metabolism. J Strength Cond Res 2004;18:212–219.

28. Chandler RM, Byrne HK, Patterson JG, Ivy JL. Dietary supplements affect the anabolic hormones after weight-training exercise. J Appl Physiol 1994;76:839–845.

29. Volek JS. Influence of nutrition on responses to resistance training. Med Sci Sports Exerc 2004;36:689–696.

30. Robergs RA, Pearson DR, Costill DL, et al. Muscle glycogenolysis during different intensities of weight-resistance exercise. J Appl Physiol 1991;70:1700–1706.

31. Tesch PA, Colliander EB, Kaiser P. Muscle metabolism during intense, heavy-resistance exercise. Eur J Appl Physiol Occup Physiol 1986;55:362–366.

32. Haff GG, Lehmkuhl MJ, McCoy LB, Stone MH. Carbohydrate supplementation and resistance training. J Strength Cond Res 2004;17:186–196.

33. MacDougall JD, Ray S, Sale DG, McCartney N, Lee P, Garner S. Muscle substrate utilization and lactate production. Can J Appl Physiol 1999;24:209–215.

34. Roy BD, Tarnopolsky MA. Influence of different macronutrient intakes on muscle glycogen resynthesis after resistance exercise. J Appl Physiol 1998;72:1854–1859.

35. Tesch PA, Yström L, Ploutz-Snyder LL, Castro M, Dudley GA. Skeletal muscle glycogen loss evoked by resistance exercise. J Strength Cond Res 1998;12:67–73.

36. Lambert CP, Frank LL, Evans WJ. Macronutrient considerations for the sport of bodybuilding. Sports Med 2004;34:317–327.

37. Leveritt M, Abernethy PJ. Effects of carbohydrate restriction on strength performance. J Strength Cond Res 1999;13:52–57.

38. Williams AG, van den Oord M, Sharma A, Jones DA. Is glucose/amino acid supplementation after exercise an aid to strength training? Br J Sports Med 2001;35:109–113.

39. Levenhagen DK, Gresham JD, Carlson MG, Maron DJ, Borel MJ, Flakoll PJ. Post-exercise nutrient intake timing in humans is critical to recovery of leg glucose and protein homeostasis. Am J Physiol Endocrinol Metab 2001;280:E982–993.

40. Ivy JL. Regulation of muscle glycogen repletion, muscle protein synthesis and repair following exercise. J Sports Sci Med 2004;3:131–138.

41. Venkatraman JT, Leddy J, Pendergast D. Dietary fats and immune status in athletes: clinical implications. Med Sci Sports Exerc 2000;32(Suppl):S389–395.

42. Hamalainen EK, Adlercreutz H, Puska P, Pietinen P. Decrease of serum total and free testosterone during a low-fat high-fibre diet. J Steroid Biochem 1983;18:369–370.

43. Reed MJ, Cheng RW, Simmonds M, Richmond W, James VH. Dietary lipids: an additional regulator of plasma levels of sex hormone binding globulin. J Clin Endocrinol Metab 1987;64:1083–1085.

44. Fry AC, Kraemer WJ, Ramsey LT. Pituitary-adrenal-gonadal responses to high-intensity resistance exercise overtraining. J Appl Physiol 1998;85:2352–2359.

45. Riechman SE, Andrews RD, MacLean DA. Dietary and blood cholesterol and statins increase hypertrophy with resistance training. FASEB J 2005;19:902–911.

46. Leosdottir M, Nilsson PM, Nilsson JA, Mansson H, Berglund G. Dietary fat intake and early mortality patterns—data from The Malmo Diet and Cancer Study. J Int Med 2005;258:153–165.

47. Colussi GL, Baroselli S, Sechi L. Omega-3 polyunsaturated fatty acids decrease plasma lipoprotein(a) levels in hypertensive subjects. Clin Nutr 2004;23:1246–1247.

48. Sacks FM, Katan M. Randomized clinical trials on the effects of dietary fat and carbohydrate on plasma lipoproteins and cardiovascular disease. Am J Med 2002;113(Suppl 9B):13S–24S.

49. Pischon T, Hankinson SE, Hotamisligil GS, Rifai N, Willett WC, Rimm EB. Habitual dietary intake of n-3 and n-6 fatty acids in relation to inflammatory markers among US men and women. Circulation 2003;108:155–160.

50. Thies F, Garry JM, Yaqoob P, et al. Association of n-3 polyunsaturated fatty acids with stability of atherosclerotic plaques: a randomised controlled trial. Lancet 2003;361:477–485.

51. Harding AH, Williams DE, Hennings SH, Mitchell J, Wareham NJ. Is the association between dietary fat intake and insulin resistance modified by physical activity? Metabolism 2001;50:1186–1192.

52. Lancaster KJ. Dietary treatment of blood pressure in kidney disease. Adv Chronic Kidney Dis 2004;11:217–221.

53. Minami A, Ishimura N, Sakamoto S, et al. Effect of eicosapentaenoic acid ethyl ester v. oleic acid-rich safflower oil on insulin resistance in type 2 diabetic model rats with hypertriacylglycerolaemia. Br J Nutr 2002;87:157–162.

54. Ide T, Hong DD, Ranasinghe P, Takahashi Y, Kushiro M, Sugano M. Interaction of dietary fat types and sesamin on hepatic fatty acid oxidation in rats. Biochem Biophy Acta 2004;1682:80–91.

55. Piers LS, Walker KZ, Stoney RM, Soares MJ, O'Dea K. Substitution of saturated with monounsaturated fat in a 4-week diet affects body weight and composition of overweight and obese men. Br J Nutr 2003;90:717–727.

56. D'Alessandro ME, Lombardo YB, Chicco A. Effect of dietary fish oil on insulin sensitivity and metabolic fate of glucose in the skeletal muscle of normal rats. Ann Nutr Metab 2002;46:114–120.

57. Watkins BA, Reinwald S, Li Y, Seifert MF. Protective actions of soy isoflavones and n-3 PUFAs on bone mass in ovariectomized rats. J Nutr Biochem 2005;16: 479–488.

58. Fearon KC, Von Meyenfeldt MF, Moses AG, et al. Effect of a protein and energy dense n-3 fatty acid enriched oral supplement on loss of weight and lean tissue in cancer cachexia: a randomised double blind trial. Gut 2003;52:1479–1486.

59. King IB, Kristal AR, Schaffer S, Thornquist M, Goodman GE. Serum trans-fatty acids are associated with risk of prostate cancer in beta-carotene and retinol efficacy trial. Cancer Epidemiol Biomarkers Prev 2005;14:988–992.

60. Lopez-Garcia E, Schulze MB, Meigs JB, et al. Consumption of trans fatty acids is related to plasma biomarkers of inflammation and endothelial dysfunction. J Nutr 2005;135:562–566.

61. Mozaffarian D, Rimm EB, King IB, Lawler RL, McDonald GB, Levy WC. Trans fatty acids and systemic inflammation in heart failure. Am J Clin Nutr 2004;80:1521–1525.

62. Saravanan N, Haseeb A, Ehtesham NZ, Ghafoorunissa. Differential effects of dietary saturated and trans-fatty acids on expression of genes associated with insulin sensitivity in rat adipose tissue. Eur J Endocrinol 2005;153:159–165.

63. Lichtenstein AH, Erkkilä AT, Lamarche B, Schwab US, Jalbert SM, Ausman LM. Influence of hydrogenated fat and butter on CVD risk factors: remnant-like particles, glucose and insulin, blood pressure and C-reactive protein. Atherosclerosis 2003; 171:97–107.

64. Matthan NR, Welty FK, Barrett PH, et al. Dietary hydrogenated fat increases high-density lipoprotein apoA-I catabolism and decreases low-density lipoprotein apoB-100 catabolism in hypercholesterolemic women. Arterioscler Thromb Vasc Biol 2004;24:1092–1097.

65. Hubbard R, Westengard J, Sanchez A, Horning M, Barth J. Apparent skeletal muscle loss related to dietary trans fatty acids in a mixed group of omnivores and vegetarians. Nutr Res 2003;23:651–658.

66. McBride JM, Kraemer WJ, Triplett-McBride T, Sebastianelli W. Effect of resistance exercise on free radical production. Med Sci Sports Exerc 1998;30:67–72.

67. Avery NG, Kaiser JL, Sharman MJ, et al. Effects of vitamin E supplementation on recovery from repeated bouts of resistance exercise. J Strength Cond Res 2003; 17:801–809.

68. Campbell WW, Joseph LJ, Davey SL, Cyr-Campbell D, Anderson RA, Evans WJ. Effects of resistance training and chromium picolinate on body composition and skeletal muscle in older men. J Appl Physiol 1999;86:29–39.

69. Nissen SL, Sharp RL. Effect of dietary supplements on lean mass and strength gains with resistance exercise: a meta-analysis. J Appl Physiol 2003;94:651–659.

70. Zemel MB, Thompson W, Milstead A, Morris K, Campbell P. Calcium and dairy acceleration of weight and fat loss during energy restriction in obese adults. Obes Res 2004;12:582–590.

71. Reid IR. Therapy of osteoporosis: calcium, vitamin D, and exercise. Am J Med Sci 1996;312:278–286.

72. Singh A, Failla ML, Deuster PA. Exercise-induced changes in immune function: effects of zinc supplementation. J Appl Physiol 1994;76:2298–2303.

73. Brilla LR, Conte V. Effects of a novel zinc-magnesium formulation on hormones and strength. J Exerc Physiol Online 2000;3:26–36.

74. Wilborn CD, Kerksick CM, Campbell BI, et al. Effects of ZMA supplementation on the relationship of zinc and magnesium to body composition, strength, sprint performance, and metabolic and hormonal profiles. Sports Nutr Rev J 2004;1: S13.

75. Schoffstall JE, Branch JD, Leutholtz BC, Swain DE. Effects of dehydration and rehydration on the one-repetition maximum bench press of weight-trained males. J Strength Cond Res 2001;15:102–108.

76. Latzka WA, Montain SJ. Water and electrolyte requirements for exercise. Clin Sports Med 1999;18:513–524.

77. Maughan RJ, Noakes TD. Fluid replacement and exercise stress. A brief review of studies on fluid replacement and some guidelines for the athlete. Sports Med 1991; 12:16–31.

78. Godek SF, Godek JJ, Bartolozzi AR. Hydration status in college football players during consecutive days of twice-a-day preseason practices. Am J Sports Med 2005;33:843–851.

79. Scheett TP, Liparulo T, Webster MJ, Diotti K, Kraemer WJ, Dooly CR. Voluntary fluid ingestion ameliorated hypohydration and 24-h ad libitum food and fluid replenishment attenuated dehydration. Med Sci Sports Exerc 2003;35(Suppl I): S311.

80. Minehan MR, Riley MD, Burke LM. Effect of flavor and awareness of kilojoule content of drinks on preference and fluid balance in team sports. Int J Sports Nutr Exerc Metab 2002;12:81–92.

81. Institute of Medicine of the National Academies. Dietary Reference Intakes: Water, Potassium, Sodium, Chloride, and Sulfate. Technical Report. Appel L, Chair; February 11, 2004.

82. Grandjean AC, Reimers KJ, Haven MC, Curtis GL. The effect on hydration of two diets, one with and one without plain water. J Am Coll Nutr 2003;22:165–173.

83. American College of Sports Medicine, American Dietetic Association, and Dietitians of Canada. Joint Position Statement: nutrition and athletic performance. Med Sci Sports Exerc 2000;32:2130–2145.

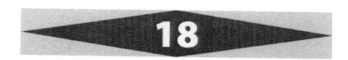

# A Different Look at the Food Guide Pyramid

## Alan E. Shugarman

## OBJECTIVES

On the completion of this chapter you will be able to:

1. Understand the evolution of dietary recommendations.
2. Differentiate between the traditional Food Guide Pyramid and the My Pyramid recommendations.
3. Explain in detail the different components that make up the My Pyramid recommendations.
4. Discuss how the My Pyramid recommendations can be adjusted to address the nutritional needs of athletes.
5. Understand some of the limitations of the My Pyramid recommendations.
6. Describe how the My Pyramid recommendations can be modified to better depict the appropriate dietary recommendations.
7. Discuss how lobbyists, such as the Beef Cattle Lobby, have potentially influenced the recommendations.
8. Give examples of how an individual can meet the My Pyramid recommendations.

## ABSTRACT

The United States Department of Agriculture (USDA) has long been dispensing advice to Americans regarding nutritional intake. Dating back to the early 20th century, the progression of recommendations can be traced to some of the original information provided by the USDA called "Food for Young Children," an attempt to improve the nutritional practices of what parents fed to their children. Throughout the decades, the USDA reviewed the stacks of continuing development on nutritional research to mold and develop recommendations for the citizens of the United States. This chapter focuses on the evolution of dietary guidelines promulgated by the USDA and other agencies. The current "Pyramid" is discussed and critiqued.

*Key Words:* **Food Guide Pyramid, pyramid, diet, dietary guidelines**

## HISTORY OF UNITED STATES DEPARTMENT OF AGRICULTURE FOOD RECOMMENDATIONS

One of the original documents released by the United States Department of Agriculture (USDA) was the National Food Guide published in the 1940s, during World War II (Figure 18.1). The focus at the time was on seven different

From: *Essentials of Sports Nutrition and Supplements*
Edited by J. Antonio, D. Kalman, J. R. Stout, M. Greenwood, D. S. Willoughby, and
G. G. Haff © Humana Press, a part of Springer Science+Business Media, Totowa, NJ

**FIGURE 18.1.** 1946 National Food Guide (also known as "The Basic Seven").

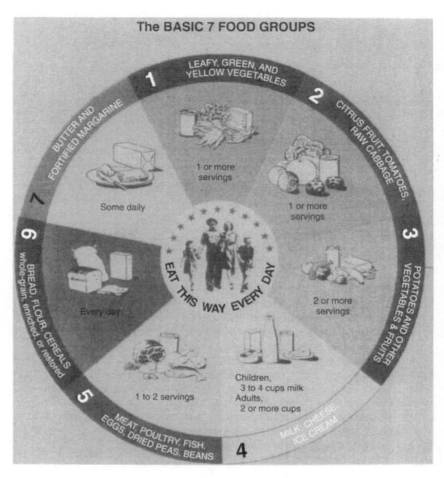

**FIGURE 18.2.** 1956 Food for Fitness (also known as "The Basic Four").

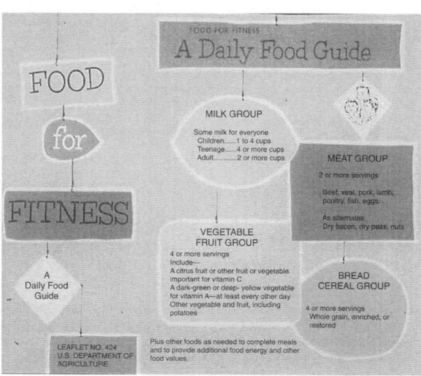

groups of foods to be consumed on a daily basis. Several of the seven groups would now be considered overlapping groups, but back then it seemed to make sense. For example, the Butter and Fortified Margarine Group and the Milk, Cheese, and Ice Cream Group would all be part of what fall under a single Dairy category, but back in the 1940s the USDA had the groups separate. The main focus of the National Food Guide was to promote eating foods that provided the vitamins and minerals needed to prevent deficiencies.

In the 1950s–1980s, the National Food Guide was whittled down to four food groups in an effort to simplify the recommendations. In 1956, the USDA published the "Food for Fitness" guide showing four condensed food groups (Figure 18.2). This condensed food grouping became known as "The Basic Four" representing: Milk, Meat, Vegetable and Fruit, and Breads and Cereals. This concept of The Basic Four continued into and through the 1980s with one small modification in the 1970s when the USDA added a cautionary section on fats, sweets, and alcohol. The USDA made the adjustment to The Basic Four amid growing concern for dietary changes that began to take place as more processed foods entered the food supply in the 1960s and 1970s. This modification of The Basic Four became known as "The Hassle-Free Daily Food Guide," incorporating The Basic Four along with the section cautioning about fats, sweets, and alcohol (Figure 18.3).

The figures depict some of the pamphlets and documents published by the USDA before the first major change in dietary recommendations in 1992 when the original Food Guide Pyramid was introduced.

In 1992, the USDA developed the Food Guide Pyramid amid much revision and debate regarding the failures of the old system of four food groups (Figure 18.4). The Food Guide Pyramid represented what registered dietitians, nutritionists, researchers, and experts thought would be an easily understandable format for teaching and educating the consumer about what to eat, how often, and how much. The Food Guide Pyramid focused heavily on carbohydrates, which was an outcropping of the large amount of research done on high-carbohydrate, low-fat diets in the 1970s and 1980s. Unfortunately, the Food Guide Pyramid did not address individual differences in dietary needs based upon individuality. Rather, the Food Guide Pyramid focused on a high-carbohydrate, low-fat diet for everyone, only varying in the amount of food or calories each person would eat. People are very different and one dietary plan does not

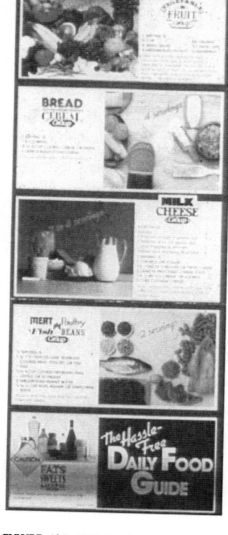

FIGURE 18.3. 1979 Hassle-Free Guide to a Better Diet.

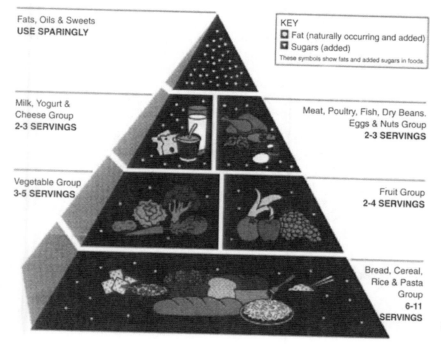

FIGURE 18.4. 1992 Food Guide Pyramid.

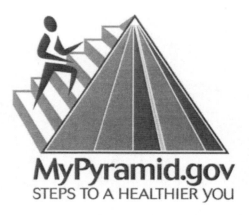

**FIGURE 18.5.** 2005 My Pyramid.

work for everyone. There are differences in how each person processes certain types of macronutrients, how much exercise they perform, and what types of foods they enjoy consuming based on ethnicity, religion, or personal beliefs.

After 12 years the USDA, using the 2005 Dietary Guidelines for Americans and the Dietary Reference Intakes from the National Academy of Sciences, released the latest pyramid dubbed "My Pyramid" (Figure 18.5). The My Pyramid format literally turned the old 1992 Food Guide Pyramid on its side, seeking to incorporate more than just dietary recommendations in this new version. The recommendations conveyed in My Pyramid fall into four categories: Variety, Proportionality, Moderation, and Activity.

## VARIETY

Back when there were four food groups, we were told to simply get a balance of foods from each group on a daily basis. With the advent of the Food Guide Pyramid in 1992, the idea of four food groups went out the window and so did the idea that we should get a balance of foods from each group. Instead, the first pyramid tried to convey importance by promoting foods that should be consumed more often at the wide bottom of the pyramid, in this case grains, breads, and cereals. Alternately, the further up the old pyramid you went, the narrower it got and the less of those foods you were suppose to eat such as dairy, meats, fats, and oils. Of course, we also went from four food groups to five food groups plus oils, making six groups. Each food group is represented by a different color: orange represents grains; green is associated with vegetables; red represents fruits; yellow represents oils; blue represents milk (dairy); and purple represents the meat and beans group.

My Pyramid takes the 1992 Food Guide Pyramid and literally turns it on its ear, meaning My Pyramid is a whole new approach to eating in that each food group goes from the bottom of the pyramid to the top, indicating that you can eat something from each of the six food groups. This change is fundamental in that it represents the fact that you can eat some amount of food from each of the six food groups. Therefore, no foods are particularly excluded from consumption; rather, some groups are minimized or limited in the amount you should consume daily. In this way, My Pyramid is more user friendly and fits more easily within the consumption patterns of the average American diet.

## MODERATION AND PROPORTION

The My Pyramid graphic is very different from the old Food Guide Pyramid. The first thing you notice is that there are six different colors going from top to bottom, only varying in width. It is the width of each color that represents the proportion in which you want to consume that particular item. The My Pyramid shows five food groups along with oils, which is not considered a food group; rather, it is a category found in several food groups. The width of the groups from largest to smallest is as follows: Grains, Milk, Vegetables, Fruits, and Meats & Beans. The smallest color band, yellow, represents the Oils section. The top part of the 1992 Food Guide Pyramid was representative of fats, oils, and sweets, and this theme is carried over to My Pyramid. As each color narrows toward the top of the My Pyramid graphic, it represents that fewer foods should be chosen from this area. Foods toward the top are those that are more highly processed, contain more refined sugar, and are higher in saturated fat and oils and therefore should be eaten in moderation and with less frequency. The wide bottom of each color band represents food choices that are in their natural form and therefore are more nutrient dense without added sugars and fats.

## ACTIVITY

The other major difference in My Pyramid is the stairs and the little figure going up them. This represents activity, a totally new area that was not present in the original 1992 Food Guide Pyramid. The importance of physical activity is added to the My Pyramid because of the overwhelming amount of evidence that diet and exercise are inseparable when it comes to improving and maintaining health and longevity.[1] The stick figure climbing the stairs represents the need for daily physical activity. The steps on the side also convey that you must take steps to improve your physical health and nutritional intake. The My Pyramid slogan is "Steps To A Healthier You" which indicates the gradual nature of the process of improving diet and getting physical exercise. Even though exercise is not nutrition, and never has been a part of any previous food group or pyramid, the authors of My Pyramid recognize the importance and incorporate daily physical exercise as part of a healthy lifestyle.

## GRAIN GROUP

As with the Food Guide Pyramid, My Pyramid features high consumption of the Grain Group. Previously represented by the entire bottom of the Food Guide Pyramid, the orange-colored Grain Group is the widest section of the pyramid indicating its emphasis and higher recommended consumptive level compared with the other groups. The Grain Group includes foods made from wheat, rice, oats, cornmeal, barley, and other grains. Things such as bread, pasta, oatmeal, breakfast cereal, tortillas, and grits are part of this group. The creators of My Pyramid emphasize that at least half of all items consumed daily from the Grain Group should be from whole grain sources. The idea here is for Americans to consume fewer refined and processed grain products, which tend to contain more sugars as opposed to complex carbohydrates (starches and fiber) found in whole grains. The greater the processing of a grain, the more the carbohydrates within the grain tend to be broken down to form simple carbohydrates (sugars). More sugars generally means higher circulating insulin levels and a greater likelihood for the deposition of fat.[2-5] Recommendations are to choose bakery items that are not heavily sweetened with sugars such as sucrose, fructose, or corn syrups.

Make half your grains whole

- Eat at least 3 oz. of whole grain cereals, breads, crackers, rice, or pasta every day
- 1 oz. is about 1 slice of bread, about 1 cup of breakfast cereal, or 1/2 cup of cooked rice, cereal, or pasta
- Choose unsweetened grain products as often as possible

## VEGETABLE GROUP

The Vegetable Group is more heavily emphasized on My Pyramid than on the previous Food Guide Pyramid. Scientific evidence shows that consuming more vegetables will improve nutrient intake and deliver countless health benefits.[6-13] Specifically, My Pyramid recommends eating more dark green and orange-colored vegetables along with greater amounts of dry beans and peas. In the Food Guide Pyramid, dry beans and peas were part of the Meat Group, whereas My Pyramid actually places these foods under both the Vegetable Group and the Meat & Bean Group. Although confusing, the most likely reason for this cross-over is that beans can provide a source of protein as well as being a vegetable. Therefore, the authors put these foods in two groups on My Pyramid. The emphasis in the Vegetable Group is on dark green and orange-colored vegetables, such as broccoli, spinach, carrots, and yams as opposed to starchy vegetables such as potatoes and corn. The Vegetable Group also emphasizes the consumption of more dry beans and peas because of their nutrient value as well as additional protein and high fiber content.

Vary your veggies

- Eat more dark green veggies such as broccoli, spinach, and other dark leafy greens
- Eat more orange vegetables such as carrots and sweet potatoes
- Eat more dry beans and peas such as pinto beans, kidney beans, and lentils

## MILK GROUP

The Milk Group rivals the Grain Group for the most prominent part of My Pyramid. The greatest nutritional source of calcium in the diet comes from dairy-based products. My Pyramid emphasizes the consumption of low-fat or fat-free choices for adults when choosing dairy foods. The Milk Group also contributes high-quality protein along with valuable vitamins and minerals to the diet.[14,15] For those who are lactose intolerant, My Pyramid recommends consuming lactose-free dairy products along with other calcium-fortified foods to assure that the consumer gets adequate calcium on a regular basis. Milk, yogurt, and cheeses are the most frequently consumed dairy products, but My Pyramid also points out that sweetened dairy products should be consumed in moderation because of the extra nonnutrient calories from sugary sweeteners. These additional calories from sweeteners are discussed in the Discretionary Calorie section below.

Get your calcium-rich foods

- Go low fat or fat free when you choose milk, yogurt, and other milk products
- If you don't or can't consume milk, choose lactose-free products or other calcium sources such as fortified foods and beverages
- Choose unsweetened dairy products more often

## FRUIT GROUP

The Fruit Group sits in the middle of the My Pyramid with a slightly lower emphasis compared with the Grain Group. The Fruit Group focuses on consuming a variety of whole fruits whereas minimizing the consumption of fruit juices. The My Pyramid recommendation is a focus on 100% real unsweetened fruit juice, but reminds the consumer that the majority of fruit should come from whole, chopped, or pureed fruit from fresh, frozen, or dried sources. Variety is also a key with the idea that you get a variety of nutrients from the various fruits you consume.

Focus on fruits

- Eat a variety of fruit
- Choose fresh, frozen, canned, or dried fruit
- Go easy on fruit juices

## MEAT & BEAN GROUP

The Meat & Bean Group is the second-smallest portion of the My Pyramid groups. This group mainly focuses on delivering lean sources of protein to the consumer. The recommendations of this group emphasize the selection of low-fat meats, fish, as well as beans, nuts, and seeds. The cooking methods of choice are baked, broiled, or grilled as opposed to frying in an effort to minimize added fats and oils. Along with the Milk Group, the Meat & Bean Group is going to deliver the majority of high-quality complete protein to the consumer.[16,17] It is important to choose lean cuts of meat (beef, pork, lamb, etc.) because although high in protein, high-fat meats can add considerable calories and cholesterol to the diet. Choosing a combination of meat, poultry, fish, beans, nuts, and seeds will provide a variety of nutrients along with healthy fats, fiber, and high-quality protein.

Go lean with protein

- Choose low-fat or lean meats and poultry
- Bake it, broil it, or grill it
- Vary your protein routine—choose more fish, beans, peas, nuts, and seeds

## OILS

Although not an actual food group, the section of the My Pyramid that deals with oils is given special attention because oil and fat come from various animal and vegetable sources. The oils recommended as part of a healthy diet are liquid at room temperature and consist mostly of monounsaturated and polyunsaturated fats. These oils contain fats that are healthier than saturated fats, which are most often solid at room temperature.[18-24] Some foods are also high in healthy oils, such as nuts, olives, some fish, and avocados. Mayonnaise and some tub or liquid margarines are also high in oils, but be sure to watch out for trans fats, an unhealthy type of fat found in oils that have been processed via hydrogenation in order to make them more solid and therefore like a "saturated fat" at room temperature.[25-31] All labels are going to divulge trans fats by 2006.

## DISCRETIONARY CALORIES

This part of My Pyramid is completely new. The idea behind Discretionary Calories is to focus people on consuming nutrient-dense foods to deliver nutrition while not over-delivering calories. The more active you are, the more calories you need to consume in order to provide energy to maintain your body. Discretionary Calories are represented by the difference between the amount of calories you need to consume to maintain your body plus those calories you use during physical activity. If you consume foods high in nutrients and low in added sugars and fats, you can achieve your nutrient needs while still having the extra calories required for your energy needs. In other words, you can meet your nutrient needs while still having extra calories available, allowing you to consume more food that is lower in nutrient density. With these Discretionary Calories, you can eat more foods from a particular group or add in some higher sugar and fat items to your diet. Most people have very small amounts of Discretionary Calories available to them, in the range of 100–300 calories per day. Unfortunately, many people choose foods that are not nutrient dense and therefore use up their Discretionary Calories in the first meal of the day.

## PHYSICAL ACTIVITY

This section makes its debut as part of My Pyramid. Research clearly shows that physical activity has immense benefits on health and quality of life.[32-39] The My Pyramid graphic prominently displays a set of stairs going up the left side of the pyramid with a stick figure walking up. This graphic representation of the act of walking up the steps is designed to show consumers the importance of exercise along with making gradual stepwise improvements in diet and physical activity. The focus of the Physical Activity is to get a total of at least 30 minutes per day of moderate to vigorous exercise. This might not be one bout of exercise. On the contrary, the 30 minutes might come over the course of the day with walking upstairs instead of taking the elevator. Taking a brisk walk while pushing a baby stroller, or digging a posthole in your yard. There are a number of physical activities that can be combined to get the recommended 30 minutes of moderate to vigorous physical activity per day.

## Sidebar 18.1. Adjustments for Athletes

My Pyramid is not aimed at providing nutritional information to maximize physical performance; rather, it is designed to provide minimum nutrition to the average American. Although My Pyramid does indicate the need for physical activity, it certainly does not take into account the nutritional needs of a serious athlete. Adjustments in macronutrient ratios and calorie consumption are needed to achieve extraordinary results whether in athletic performance or physical appearance. The five color-coded groups would need to be restructured and modified in order to accommodate the serious athlete.

The Carbohydrate Group should be adjusted to focus almost exclusively on whole grains such as oatmeal, whole wheat, and barley. The exceptions would be endurance athletes and those preparing for a competition. In this case, the utilization of certain amounts of starchy carbohydrates and sugars is warranted in order to supply and replenish glycogen stores completely and rapidly. Sugars would have a minimal role and would be left off the menu as a source of carbohydrates unless certain glycogen replenishment practices are in place for ultraendurance athletes.

The Vegetable and Fruit Groups would be equal in size and fall slightly behind the Grain Group in prominence. It is necessary for athletes to consume large amounts of fruits and vegetable for the tremendous vitamin and mineral content along with the phytochemicals and antioxidants that help athletes recover and protect against future illness and cellular damage from oxidation.[40-49]

Beans and Nuts would be in a separate group since they have tremendous value to athletes. Beans are a fantastic source of low-glycemic carbohydrates that can provide long-lasting energy without insulin spikes. Beans are also a good source of protein and fiber. Nuts too are a good source of protein and they also offer healthy essential fats. Essential fats are found in every cell of the body and adequate essential fats have a role in reducing inflammation and improving muscular recovery.[50-59]

The Meat Group would be segmented into sources of protein that are the most beneficial for athletes and overall health. Fish and poultry would rank higher than beef and pork. Certain fish contain valuable omega-3 fatty acids whereas the chicken and turkey breast are extremely low-fat sources of high-quality protein. These sources of protein are more heart and cardiovascular healthy meats than beef or pork.

There is no mention of water in My Pyramid. The human body is more than 70% water, so water should not be overlooked as part of a healthy nutrition and exercise plan. Athletes need to focus on water consumption even more than the rest of the population. Dehydration that causes as little as a 2% loss in body fluids decreases endurance performance by as much as 7%.[60-68] Dehydrated exercisers fatigue almost 25% sooner than those who stay hydrated before and during workouts. The average person does not drink the recommended 8–10 8-ounce cups of water per day. The athletic and regular version of My Pyramid should have a section on water and hydration.

These changes are just the tip of the "Pyramid" as it were. The changes needed to make My Pyramid appropriate for athletes go far beyond the few points mentioned above. It would be best to simply rebuild a new program specific for athletes rather than attempt to modify what is a flawed model to begin with, even for average Americans, much less athletes.

## MY PYRAMID PROBLEMS

This latest installment of nutritional advice from the USDA is a big improvement over past efforts even as it falls short in many ways. My Pyramid is the culmination of work by the USDA in concert with the National Academy of Sciences to incorporate the nutrition research completed over the past 12–13 years which has been largely compiled into the 2005 Dietary Guidelines for Americans.[69] Although this version of the pyramid is better than the original, it is by no means ideal, nor is it comprehensive it its advice for the public. My Pyramid lacks information and many valuable concepts that have been shown to improve health and well being. Now that we have explored the basic framework of My Pyramid, let's take a look at some of the possible shortcomings of this latest education campaign by the U.S. government.

### What's in a Shape?

The original Food Guide Pyramid from 1992 was literally a stroke of genius in its design. With one glance, the average American could see what foods to eat more often at the bottom of the pyramid and those to consume less often at the top. My Pyramid starts out as the original Food Guide Pyramid tipped on its side. However, this is where the problems begin.

## Colors = Food Groups?

The pyramid shape remains, but the details have changed drastically and not necessarily for the better. The color stripes representing the food groups stretch from top to bottom with each color representing a different food group. The problem is that the image that the government has put out has no writing on it whatsoever to tell anyone what food group each color represents. This seems to be a major error because it requires people to go to the Web or read a government-published brochure (if they can find one), or third-party literature to find out what each color represents. Millions of Americans don't have access or knowledge of the Web or won't find a brochure and therefore will likely understand little of the new My Pyramid image as to how they should be eating, not even what food each color represents. Why not at least list the group name on each color band to provide some connection between the colors and foods (Figure 18.6)? This way, Americans could at least realize what foods they should consider consuming based on the width of the color band. The inability to tell what each color represents makes My Pyramid useless at first glance on a food package. This would seem to be a major step backward in advising the American public on how to eat.

An example of My Pyramid not thoroughly translating the information from the Dietary Guidelines for Americans, published in January of 2005, can be seen in the lack of information it conveys. According to the Guidelines, Americans should eat foods with little to no trans and saturated fats, choosing foods low in overall fat.[69] The smallest color band on My Pyramid represents oils and fats. The authors seem to think that the narrowness of the band somehow conveys the message about eating low fat and avoiding saturated and trans fats. This simply does not translate and it all starts from that fact that by looking at the My Pyramid image, you can't even tell which band represents oils and fats, much less what it is trying to recommend.

## Serving-Size Omission

The lack of information goes a step further in that not only are the colors devoid of explaining the food groups they represent, they also provide no information on how many servings you should be eating from each group. My Pyramid takes the stance that because this pyramid is suppose to be more individualized, they did not want to show serving sizes for each color on the image. The rationale for this is that small people and large people should be consuming different amounts of food from each group. So instead of providing at least a base level of intake, My Pyramid shows no food group information or serving-size recommendations. The authors were concerned that showing servings on the groups would go against their desire to personalize My Pyramid, a main focus of this revision of the pyramid. In omitting the servings, My Pyramid misses an opportunity to convey basic information about servings relative to each color food group.

One way to address the issue of serving size would be to show servings based on a 1000-calorie consumption level, an admittedly low level of energy consumption. The concept here would be to provide a base level from which people could easily multiply to create servings of 1500 calories, 2000 calories, or any other amount through simple mathematics of addition and/or multiplication. Although not everyone would be able to do the simple math, it would at least offer some basic information. The 2000-calorie diet is ingrained in most consumers' minds from the Nutrition Labeling and Education Act Nutrition Fact panels found on nearly all food labels. By building on the concept of servings through calorie level, My Pyramid could have provided valuable information at a very basic level. Unfortunately, My Pyramid has no basic information to help consumers. Remember, the My Pyramid image is going to finds its way onto millions of labels and the lack of basic information means the image may not convey much of anything to Americans that have not done research into what the image and colors mean.

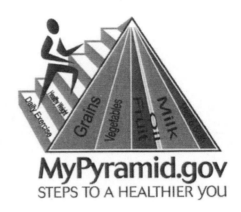

**FIGURE 18.6.** Suggested additions to My Pyramid.

## No Exercise Recommendations

The other part of the image that stands out is the stairs on the left side with the stick figure walking up the side. This was supposed to show the importance of exercise as part of the recommendations for healthy Americans. There are literally stacks of research that show the link between daily physical activity and overall health.[8,22,33,42,70–102] The decision not to write anything on the pyramid hurts its effectiveness in the physical activity area too. A simple line indicating that people should get a minimum of 30 minutes of daily exercise at a target heart rate of at least 65% of predicted maximum would have made a world of difference to this new pyramid image for Americans to pattern their health objective after. Alas, no such information is offered on the image that will be plastered on millions of labels and printed material. If you go to the Web site, you get a decent description of exercise guidelines, but again it is a limited access situation to this simple and invaluable bit of information.

## My Pyramid, No Weighting

The My Pyramid image completely ignores the issue of weight control. Thousands of pages of research are available on the benefits of maintaining a healthy weight.[103–118] The stick figure chugging up the side of the pyramid indicates nothing about weight control. When you consider that even being slightly overweight contributes to preventable diseases such as diabetes, heart disease, and cancer, it is difficult to understand why the authors simply seem to ignore the issue of healthy weight maintenance. Again, a small amount of text discussing the importance of weight could have made a difference. Simply stating that in conjunction with physical activity it is important to maintain appropriate body weight would have provided some information to millions of obese Americans.

## Pyramid Destruction

The pyramid shape is a great concept at the basic level. In execution, My Pyramid seems to forget the concept of the pyramid and its simplicity in conveying information quickly to millions of Americans. By attempting to further personalize the pyramid, it castrated the information at the base level, rendering the pyramid impotent for anyone that has not researched the meaning of the colors and the stick figure and stairs. Additionally, My Pyramid completely ignores the issue of ideal body weight for health maintenance. By simply adding in the names of what each color strip represents and providing a daily serving indication of some kind (be it based on a 1000-kcal diet or another concept), My Pyramid could have provided immediate information that could be used to easily calculate various levels of servings based on caloric intake levels. Also, the addition of words to the side staircase could have served to convey to Americans that daily exercise and maintaining a healthy body weight are critical to overall health and disease prevention. Simple additions to the My Pyramid image could have made a world of difference to all Americans, not just those that cannot or will not read the mypyramid.gov Web site, brochures, or third-party literature.

## Food Group Fiasco

The original Food Guide Pyramid was a giant leap forward in its ability to quickly convey information on food groups and consumption levels. Unfortunately, the old pyramid did not adequately distinguish among such basics as types of carbohydrates, proteins, and fats. My Pyramid is not much better at conveying accurate scientific nutrition information to the American consumer. One major area of debate is within the food groupings.

## Grains Gone Wrong

The most prominent group in My Pyramid is the Grain Group. Dominating the left side of My Pyramid, grains are meant to be consumed in greater quantity in comparison to the other five food groups. The big push behind the Grain Group is to make half of your Grains "whole." Unfortunately, this also means you can make half of your grains from starches and sugars. This is extremely irresponsible as a recommendation in light of the mountains of scientific evidence showing the connection between high starch and sugar consumption and obesity rates and subsequent diabetes and heart disease.[119-133] Starches act effectively similar to sugar in the body by increasing insulin levels, which can have a negative effect on fat storage and cholesterol levels. The authors also continue the practice of using the term "Complex Carbs" as preferred selections in this group. The term "Complex Carbs" is woefully inadequate because it is unlikely that most Americans have a clear understanding of the term, believing that pasta and rice are examples of preferred grain foods when in fact these foods are starches that spike insulin levels significantly. The concept of My Pyramid and the recommendations it conveys should not be based on making the American diet "better," rather it would have been an opportunity to convey what is "ideal" or "optimal." By recommending consumers *avoid* starches and sugar and instead consume unprocessed whole grains that are high in fiber and healthy fats, the government could have contributed toward improving the insulin control of millions of Americans. By controlling insulin levels more effectively, obesity rates would likely decrease along with diseases such as diabetes and cardiovascular disease, which are related to overconsumption of high-glycemic carbohydrates. The recommendations of My Pyramid for the Grain Group fall short of the science as well as what would be ideal.

## Veggie Versus Dairies

The second-largest group on the pyramid seems to be a tie between the Vegetable and Milk Groups (see Sidebar 18.2). The Vegetable Group is filled with efficient foods that are nutrient dense and calorie conscious. Vegetables are quite accurately a "super food" with few exceptions. Starchy vegetables such as potatoes and corn are not as phytonutrient packed as the dark green and orange vegetables. Instead, starchy vegetables have greater impact on insulin levels and My Pyramid does not discuss this issue whatsoever. By not indicating that consumers should choose dark green and orange vegetables more often than starchy vegetables, consumers are misled into believing that a potato is equivalent to broccoli or spinach, and such is a huge mistake when considering the effects of insulin spikes on incidence of obesity, Type 2 diabetes, cholesterol levels, and cardiovascular disease.[134-136] Without going to the My Pyramid Web site, consumers would have no idea of the multitude of health benefits associated with the consumption of higher levels of nonstarchy vegetables. This is another missed opportunity to clearly indicate to Americans that they should focus on consuming dark green and orange vegetables as often as possible and limit the consumption of starchy carbohydrates.

## Sidebar 18.2. The Politics of Food

It is an interesting decision on the part of the authors because one might argue that the nutrient value of the Fruit Group is more valuable than that of the Milk Group, while having fewer negative effects on the body. Consider that fruits can largely be consumed by all Americans, whereas lactose intolerance might prevent millions of Americans from consuming dairy products. The fact that the National Dairy Council is a very powerful lobbying group certainly did not hurt the fact that the Milk Group has greater prominence in My Pyramid than the Fruit Group, which does not have as large a lobbying force on its side (United Fresh Fruit and Vegetable Association). In fact, most people probably have never heard of the United Fresh Fruit and Vegetable Association, but most have probably heard of the National Dairy Council ("Got Milk").

The political pressure surrounding the My Pyramid project should not be overlooked. Other organizations such as the National Cattlemen's Beef Association, American Meat Institute, Wheat Foods Council, and even the Soft Drink Association seem to have an effect on the final My Pyramid product. Although the government should be presenting information to Americans based only on the science, it would seem that the power of the National Dairy Council has effectively pushed their agenda on the authors of My Pyramid. Consider that obesity is one of the biggest problems in the United States, yet My Pyramid recommends the equivalent of three 8-ounce cups of fat-free or low-fat milk for men and women, easily adding about 300 calories to the daily intake of people who may need to achieve and maintain a healthy weight. This amount of extra calories can be extremely detrimental to those people attempting to lose weight. Worse, the rationale for the prominence of the Milk Group is that it provides valuable calcium for the prevention of osteoporosis. Although some data support the effectiveness of dairy calcium for improving bone mineral content, the data are far from conclusive.[137-140] Consider that supplemental sources of calcium (calcium carbonate and calcium citrate) might do as good a job as consuming milk products without the extra 300 calories. The other major nutrients from milk, vitamin D and potassium can be obtained from the sun, many fruits and vegetables, and more calorie-conservative, nutrient-dense foods. If obesity were not such a tremendous problem in the United States, the issue of the Milk Group being larger than the Fruit Group might be less offensive scientifically and ethically, but such is not the case.

## Milk This

The Milk Group is next, although its position may not be warranted (see Sidebar 18.2) when you consider the benefits of the Fruit Group. Milk essentially stands for dairy products produced from milk. My Pyramid focuses on the delivery of calcium, vitamin D, and potassium from milk-based products to build strong bones and teeth. Although calcium has major roles within the body, including muscular contraction (skeletal and heart muscle), the overemphasis of this group by its prominence in My Pyramid is disturbing on several levels. Although there has been much research on dairy products, calcium, osteoporosis, and even weight loss, the information is often equivocal.[141-145] Dairy products are high in protein and calcium; they are also low in fiber, high in lactose, and can contain large amounts of fat, much of which is saturated. One of the biggest pushes by the National Dairy Council is the "Got Milk" campaign. A very successful celebrity-laden campaign that has lasted for more than a decade, the "Got Milk" campaign has now branched off and there is a new campaign focused on weight loss and the consumption of dairy calcium. Unfortunately, the data on weight loss and dairy calcium consumption are far from conclusive, but no one in the United States government is stopping the National Dairy Council from making these largely unsubstantiated claims about milk products. The fact that this is allowed to continue should prove the power of one of the food industries' largest and best financed lobbying organizations in the National Dairy Council. The authors of My Pyramid could not have been looking solely at the scientific data when they made the recommendations and set the size of the Milk Group. This is the most obvious case within My Pyramid that the true scientific data available to the authors were not followed. There is no scientific sense to recommending the Milk Group over the Fruit Group, yet that is exactly what the authors of My Pyramid did, regardless of the nutrient value or caloric compromise it created.

## Fruit Fantastic

The Fruit Group is next in size and therefore importance, based on the width of the color swath in My Pyramid. This group along with the Vegetable Group should have been heavily emphasized in My Pyramid based on the mountain of evidence that supports the many health benefits of consuming fresh fruits and vegetables.[12,146-159] It is interesting that the authors chose to heavily recommend whole grains, giving that group top billing whereas whole vegetables and fruits fall farther down the priority list and after the Milk Group. Whole fruits are nutrient-dense sources of generally high-fiber, calorie-conscious nutrition. The Web site for My Pyramid unfortunately equates whole fruit with 100% fruit juices. This is another big mistake on the part of the authors. Fruit juices are used by registered dietitians in hospitals to specifically add weight back to patients that are underweight because of illness or injury. Why then, in an obesity-prone society such as the United States, do the authors of My Pyramid recommend whole fruits in the same way they do fruit juices? It is unconscionable for the authors to have compared the benefits of calorie-conscious, nutrient-dense whole fruits with the more calorie-dense, easily consumed fruit juices knowing full well of the obesity epidemic in America. The authors also do not strongly differentiate between sugary-syrup-laden canned fruit and fresh, frozen, or pureed whole fruit, a much better choice. Of course there is no differentiation within the Fruit Group to indicate that berries, citrus, melons, and other fruits are extremely different in nutrient content and therefore nutritional value. This is another shortcoming of My Pyramid. Consider the comparison of a whole medium apple, which contains pectin fiber, vitamins, minerals, and phytochemicals including quercetin, catechin, phloridzin, and chlorogenic acid, all of which are strong antioxidants, versus canned fruit cocktail. The benefits of consuming an apple far outweigh the sugary consumption of canned fruit cocktail, yet they are given equal value in the eyes of the My Pyramid authors. My Pyramid does not offer ideal nutritional advice; rather it offers minimum nutritional information. There is also a lack of consideration for the effects of fruit juices on blood sugar and insulin spikes. It is difficult to eat five whole apples, but easy to drink the juice of those same apples. Fruit and vegetable consumption is self-limiting because of the natural bulk of the fiber and structure of the fruit, making it difficult to overconsume and take in too many calories; however, the same cannot be said for fruit juices, be they 100% fruit or not. The authors of My Pyramid made a mistake in not placing more emphasis on the fruit group and specifically focusing on whole fruits as opposed to suggesting fruit juices are equivalent.

## Meat Mismanagement

The Meat & Bean Group is next on the priority of size of color band. The errors from the first pyramid are carried forward into My Pyramid for this group. More than likely, the strong beef cattle lobbyists have a role in the prominence of beef in comparison to fish, poultry, and beans for sources of protein, the true focus of this group. Beef is notoriously high in saturated fat and is known to increase the risk for heart disease and stroke, yet My Pyramid makes no distinction between healthy protein sources such as heart-healthy fish that contain beneficial essential fats, and the saturated fat found in beef and pork. The fact that soy and other beans are lumped into this category is also confusing and unwarranted. In fact, a review of the Web site seems to show that My Pyramid has beans in two groups—the Vegetable Group and the Meat & Bean Group. Which group do beans fall under? Beans might actually deserve their own separate group because they are unique in that they contain many of the benefits of vegetables as well as deliver higher amounts of protein than most other vegetables but have no cholesterol (only animal products contain cholesterol). Beans are also extremely high in valuable fiber, both soluble and insoluble, which has tremendous health benefits on cholesterol levels, gastrointestinal health, and possibly cancer rates.[160–165] My Pyramid makes no distinction between heart-healthy sources of lean protein and those sources that are higher in saturated fat and cholesterol. The lack of separation of this group into at least two if not three groups shows a fundamental flaw in how the U.S. government recommends that consumers get adequate protein. Essentially, My Pyramid favors sources of protein that are higher in fat and cholesterol over splitting the groups to recommend consumers focus on beans, seeds, fish, and poultry while limiting intake of high-fat meat from beef and pork. Because the Meat & Bean Group represents the most protein-dense group on the pyramid, it should be given more specific attention than the authors apparently provided.

## Oil Spill

The last and smallest color on My Pyramid is the Oils Group. Not truly a food group as we would traditionally think, this group is made up of oils and fats from various animal and plant sources. More appropriately, this group should be called the Fat & Oil Group because it includes fats that are solid at room temperature such as butter, lard, and shortening. The authors make a huge mistake in not clearly explaining essential fatty acids to consumers. The multitude of research studies on the benefits of consuming specifically omega-3 fatty acids from fish is completely overlooked in both the Meat & Bean Group as well as the Oils Group.[166–181] In fact, the authors recommend vegetable oils that are high in omega-6 fatty acids which can contribute to greater levels of inflammation, and when out of balance with omega-3s, increase cardiovascular risk factors. Certainly, eating mono- and polyunsaturated fats is better than consuming saturated and trans fats, but the recommendations fall very short of being ideal for health, and in fact don't emphasize strongly enough that butter, margarine, mayonnaise, and other high-fat products are not healthy and should be avoided. My Pyramid does correct part of the problem of "Fat is Bad" that was conveyed in the original Food Guide Pyramid, but does not go far enough in differentiating the good fats from the bad, leaving consumers with the idea that it is acceptable to consume fats and oils that simply are not healthy to consume on a daily basis.

## SIMPLE ADDITION

Some very minor changes could be made to My Pyramid to address some of the issues raised in this text. Adding in group names would make the chart more meaningful to someone who has not seen the My Pyramid Web site. Showing that daily physical activity is necessary along with maintaining a healthy weight is critical for achieving optimal health. These simple changes would make much difference in quickly conveying some of the most important messages for Americans about nutrition, exercise, and the maintenance of health.

## SUMMARY

The authors of My Pyramid failed to adequately convey the breadth and depth of nutrition knowledge available in 2005. It seems that strong lobbying forces had major roles in shaping what should be a purely science- and health-based endeavor. There is also evidence that the authors did not adequately follow the Dietary Guidelines for Americans published in January 2005, which was intended to be one of the guiding documents for the development of the updated pyramid. The new My Pyramid image may actually be a step back in its ability to quickly convey to consumers how they should be eating. The fact that in order to fully understand what My Pyramid is conveying, extensive knowledge of the Web is needed; therefore, many of the people who need the information most (the poor, uneducated, and underserved) will not gain access. The information on the Web site is not user friendly or easy to understand. The confusing nature of the site makes the situation that much worse. Above all, a great opportunity to educate consumers on the latest nutritional information was lost. With the current obesity rates reaching epidemic proportions, and the diseases of over-consumption running rampant, it is difficult to understand why the results of the 2005 My Pyramid project fall so desperately short of achieving some very basic goals of educating the average American. Over time, we will discover whether the shortcomings of My Pyramid have large or negligible effects on the health of Americans. Unfortunately, in the time it takes to discover the results, the outcome could be disastrous to our medical system. In the end, we may all pay physically and financially for the weaknesses of the 2005 My Pyramid.

## QUESTIONS

1. What government organization started publishing dietary recommendations in the 1940s?
    a. National Dairy Council
    b. Government Food Agency

    c. United States Department of Agriculture
    d. Food and Drug Administration

2. In what year was the original Food Guide Pyramid published?
    a. 1984
    b. 1976
    c. 2005
    d. 1992

3. Of these four choices, which is *not* part of the original Food Guide Pyramid?
    a. Milk, Yogurt, & Cheese Group
    b. Vegetable Group
    c. Exercise & Weight Management Group
    d. Fats, Oils, & Sweets Group

4. The recommendations conveyed in My Pyramid fall into four categories. Which of these is incorrect?
    a. Activity
    b. Consistency
    c. Moderation
    d. Variety

5. How many colors represent food groups on the My Pyramid Image?
    a. 5
    b. 7
    c. 4
    d. 9

6. What does the color yellow represent in My Pyramid?
    a. Grains
    b. Oils
    c. Vegetables
    d. Dairy

7. What does the color purple represent on My Pyramid?
    a. Fruit Group
    b. Grain Group
    c. Meat & Bean Group
    d. Milk Group

8. How much grains does My Pyramid suggest should come from whole grain sources?
    a. 60%
    b. 30%
    c. 50%
    d. 100%

9. What items in the Vegetable Group are the same as those in the Meat & Bean Group?
    a. Potatoes
    b. Pheasant
    c. Corn
    d. Beans

10. Changes to My Pyramid, if you are an athlete, include all of the following except:
    a. Drink more water
    b. Eat more fruits
    c. Eat more vegetables
    d. Eat less whole grains

11. What does the color green represent on My Pyramid?
    a. Milk Group
    b. Vegetable Group
    c. Meat & Bean Group
    d. Oil Group

12. The stick figure on the side of My Pyramid is suppose to represent what?
   a. The importance of walking up stairs instead of taking the elevator
   b. The fact that walking stairs is healthy
   c. The importance of daily activity
   d. The importance of taking gradual steps to improve your health through nutrition and exercise

13. What does the color blue represent on My Pyramid?
   a. Milk Group
   b. Vegetable Group
   c. Meat & Bean Group
   d. Sweets Group

14. What is meant by the term "proportion" in relation to My Pyramid?
   a. How much from each color group you want to consume
   b. Your body should be proportionate, not too thin, not to fat
   c. How big your meals should be
   d. The size of the stick person on the side of the pyramid

15. Which of the following does not represent My Pyramid recommendations for getting calcium-rich foods?
   a. Go low fat or fat free when you choose milk, yogurt, and other milk products
   b. Eat at least five dairy-rich foods per day
   c. If you don't or can't consume milk, choose lactose-free products or other calcium sources such as fortified foods and beverages
   d. Choose unsweetened dairy products more often

16. Which of the following are not part of the recommendation in My Pyramid for consuming fruits?
   a. Eat a variety of fruit
   b. Drink a lot of fruit juices
   c. Choose fresh, frozen, canned, or dried fruit
   d. Go easy on fruit juices

17. Which of the following vegetables is not considered starchy?
   a. Potato
   b. Corn
   c. Broccoli

18. Which of these is not mentioned as a lobbying group?
   a. National Cattlemen's Beef Association
   b. Americans For Healthy Food
   c. Wheat Foods Council
   d. Soft Drink Association

19. What does the color red represent in My Pyramid?
   a. Fruit Group
   b. Grain Group
   c. Meat & Bean Group
   d. Milk Group

20. Which of the following is not mentioned as a key problem with My Pyramid?
   a. Strong lobbying forces had major roles in shaping My Pyramid
   b. The Dietary Guidelines for Americans published in January 2005 were followed closely
   c. To fully understand My Pyramid you must visit the MyPyramid.gov Web site
   d. The colors on My Pyramid make perfect sense

21. The authors of My Pyramid follow the Dietary Guidelines for Americans 2005 to the letter.
   a. True
   b. False

22. By looking at My Pyramid, you can immediately adjust your diet to achieve specific goals.
    a. True
    b. False

23. Discretionary Calories are represented by the difference between the amount of calories you need to consume to maintain your body plus those calories you use during physical activity.
    a. True
    b. False

24. The MyPyramid.gov Web site is the main source of information for consumers wanting to know more about My Pyramid.
    a. True
    b. False

25. The Milk Group has valid reason to be placed ahead of the Fruit Group in My Pyramid.
    a. True
    b. False

26. A potato and broccoli are both considered vegetables in My Pyramid.
    a. True
    b. False

27. Beans are found in two groups on My Pyramid, the Meat Group and the Vegetable Group.
    a. True
    b. False

28. My Pyramid clearly shows the importance of maintaining a healthy weight by looking at this diagram:
    a. True
    b. False

29. All meats provide equivalent nutritional value.
    a. True
    b. False

30. Oil is considered a food group in My Pyramid.
    a. True
    b. False

31. My Pyramid will quickly become a valuable and effective tool for educating the consumers of America about nutrition with little confusion.
    a. True
    b. False

32. Simply adding some name tags to the color groups would have helped improve the My Pyramid diagram.
    a. True
    b. False

33. By going to the My Pyramid Web site, you can easily learn everything you want to know about My Pyramid and your particular dietary needs.
    a. True
    b. False

34. Glycemic index is discussed on mypyramid.com Web site as a way to choose vegetables.
    a. True
    b. False

35. My Pyramid was designed as a way to personalize the dietary recommendations.
    a. True
    b. False

# REFERENCES

1. Nutrition and fitness: Diet, genes, physical activity and health. Proceedings of the 4th International Conference on Nutrition and Fitness. Athens, Greece, May 25–29, 2000. World Rev Nutr Diet 2001;89:XI–XXIV, 1–191.
2. Havel PJ. Dietary fructose: implications for dysregulation of energy homeostasis and lipid/carbohydrate metabolism. Nutr Rev 2005;63:133–157.
3. Timlin MT, Barrows BR, Parks EJ. Increased dietary substrate delivery alters hepatic fatty acid recycling in healthy men. Diabetes 2005;54:2694–2701.
4. Timlin MT, Parks EJ. Temporal pattern of de novo lipogenesis in the postprandial state in healthy men. Am J Clin Nutr 2005;81:35–42.
5. Uauy R, Diaz E. Consequences of food energy excess and positive energy balance. Public Health Nutr 2005;8:1077–1099.
6. Engels HJ, Gretebeck RJ, Gretebeck KA, Jimenez L. Promoting healthful diets and exercise: efficacy of a 12-week after-school program in urban African Americans. J Am Diet Assoc 2005;105:455–459.
7. Finley JW. Proposed criteria for assessing the efficacy of cancer reduction by plant foods enriched in carotenoids, glucosinolates, polyphenols and selenocompounds. Ann Bot (Lond) 2005;95:1075–1096.
8. Hung HC, Joshipura KJ, Jiang R, et al. Fruit and vegetable intake and risk of major chronic disease. J Natl Cancer Inst 2004;96:1577–1584.
9. Keck AS, Finley JW. Cruciferous vegetables: cancer protective mechanisms of glucosinolate hydrolysis products and selenium. Integr Cancer Ther 2004;3:5–12.
10. Maclellan DL, Gottschall-Pass K, Larsen R. Fruit and vegetable consumption: benefits and barriers. Can J Diet Pract Res 2004;65:101–105.
11. Ninfali P, Mea G, Giorgini S, Rocchi M, Bacchiocca M. Antioxidant capacity of vegetables, spices and dressings relevant to nutrition. Br J Nutr 2005;93:257–266.
12. Paisley J, Skrzypczyk S. Qualitative investigation of differences in benefits and challenges of eating fruits versus vegetables as perceived by Canadian women. J Nutr Educ Behav 2005;37:77–82.
13. Peltzer K, Promtussananon S. Knowledge, barriers, and benefits of fruit and vegetable consumption and lay conceptions of nutrition among rural and semi-urban Black South Africans. Psychol Rep 2004;94:976–982.
14. Ranganathan R, Nicklas TA, Yang SJ, Berenson GS. The nutritional impact of dairy product consumption on dietary intakes of adults (1995–1996): the Bogalusa Heart Study. J Am Diet Assoc 2005;105:1391–1400.
15. Weinberg LG, Berner LA, Groves JE. Nutrient contributions of dairy foods in the United States, Continuing Survey of Food Intakes by Individuals, 1994–1996, 1998. J Am Diet Assoc 2004;104:895–902.
16. Murphy SP, Allen LH. Nutritional importance of animal source foods. J Nutr 2003;133:3932S–3935S.
17. Nicklas TA, Farris RP, Myers L, Berenson GS. Impact of meat consumption on nutritional quality and cardiovascular risk factors in young adults: the Bogalusa Heart Study. J Am Diet Assoc 1995;95:887–892.
18. MacDonald-Wicks LK, Garg ML. Incorporation of n-3 fatty acids into plasma and liver lipids of rats: importance of background dietary fat. Lipids 2004;39:545–551.
19. Wahrburg U. What are the health effects of fat? Eur J Nutr 2004;43(Suppl 1):I/6–11.
20. Ervin RB, Wright JD, Wang CY, Kennedy-Stephenson J. Dietary intake of fats and fatty acids for the United States population: 1999–2000. Adv Data 2004:1–6.
21. Hulbert AJ, Turner N, Storlien LH, Else PL. Dietary fats and membrane function: implications for metabolism and disease. Biol Rev Camb Philos Soc 2005;80:155–169.
22. Konig D, Vaisanen SB, Bouchard C, et al. Cardiorespiratory fitness modifies the association between dietary fat intake and plasma fatty acids. Eur J Clin Nutr 2003;57:810–815.
23. Kromhout D. Diet and cardiovascular diseases. J Nutr Health Aging 2001;5:144–149.
24. Trichopoulou A, Lagiou P. Worldwide patterns of dietary lipids intake and health implications. Am J Clin Nutr 1997;66:961S–964S.
25. Lopez-Garcia E, Schulze MB, Meigs JB, et al. Consumption of trans fatty acids is related to plasma biomarkers of inflammation and endothelial dysfunction. J Nutr 2005;135:562–566.
26. Steinhart H, Rickert R, Winkler K. Trans fatty acids (TFA): analysis, occurrence, intake and clinical relevance. Eur J Med Res 2003;8:358–362.

27. Sundram K, French MA, Clandinin MT. Exchanging partially hydrogenated fat for palmitic acid in the diet increases LDL-cholesterol and endogenous cholesterol synthesis in normocholesterolemic women. Eur J Nutr 2003;42:188–194.
28. Tsai CJ, Leitzmann MF, Willett WC, Giovannucci EL. Long-term intake of trans-fatty acids and risk of gallstone disease in men. Arch Intern Med 2005;165:1011–1015.
29. Upritchard JE, Zeelenberg MJ, Huizinga H, Verschuren PM, Trautwein EA. Modern fat technology: what is the potential for heart health? Proc Nutr Soc 2005;64:379–386.
30. Wolfram G. Dietary fatty acids and coronary heart disease. Eur J Med Res 2003;8:321–324.
31. Wu D. Modulation of immune and inflammatory responses by dietary lipids. Curr Opin Lipidol 2004;15:43–47.
32. Blaber AY. Exercise: who needs it? Br J Nurs 2005;14:973–975.
33. Brukner PD, Brown WJ. Is exercise good for you? Med J Aust 2005;183:538–541.
34. Cukras Z, Jegier A. [Physical activity and bone mineral density—current knowledge level]. Pol Arch Med Wewn 2005;113:164–171.
35. Jamsa T, Vainionpaa A, Korpelainen R, Vihriala E, Leppaluoto J. Effect of daily physical activity on proximal femur. Clin Biomech (Bristol, Avon) 2006;21(1):1–7.
36. Jankauskiene R, Kardelis K. Body image and weight reduction attempts among adolescent girls involved in physical activity. Medicina (Kaunas) 2005;41:796–801.
37. Liebman M. Promoting healthy weight: lessons learned from WIN the Rockies and other key studies. J Nutr Educ Behav 2005;37(Suppl 2):95–100.
38. Ross KM, Teasdale TA. Prescribing physical activity for older adults. J Okla State Med Assoc 2005;98:443–446.
39. Zahran HS, Kobau R, Moriarty DG, Zack MM, Holt J, Donehoo R. Health-related quality of life surveillance—United States, 1993–2002. MMWR Surveill Summ 2005;54:1–35.
40. Anlasik T, Sies H, Griffiths HR, Mecocci P, Stahl W, Polidori MC. Dietary habits are major determinants of the plasma antioxidant status in healthy elderly subjects. Br J Nutr 2005;94:639–642.
41. Gil L, Lewis L, Martinez G, et al. Effect of increase of dietary micronutrient intake on oxidative stress indicators in HIV/AIDS patients. Int J Vitam Nutr Res 2005;75:19–27.
42. Hassimotto NM, Genovese MI, Lajolo FM. Antioxidant activity of dietary fruits, vegetables, and commercial frozen fruit pulps. J Agric Food Chem 2005;53:2928–2935.
43. Krajcovicova-Kudlackova M, Dusinska M, Valachovicova M, Blazicek P, Paukova V. Products of DNA, protein and lipid oxidative damage in relation to vitamin C plasma concentration. Physiol Res 2006;55(2):227–231.
44. Norman HA, Go VL, Butrum RR. Review of the International Research Conference on Food, Nutrition, and Cancer, 2004. J Nutr 2004;134:3391S–3393S.
45. Serafini M, Del Rio D, Crozier A, Benzie IF. Effect of changes in fruit and vegetable intake on plasma antioxidant defenses in humans. Am J Clin Nutr 2005;81:531–532; author reply 532–534.
46. Takahashi R, Ohmori R, Kiyose C, Momiyama Y, Ohsuzu F, Kondo K. Antioxidant activities of black and yellow soybeans against low density lipoprotein oxidation. J Agric Food Chem 2005;53:4578–4582.
47. Thompson HJ, Heimendinger J, Gillette C, et al. In vivo investigation of changes in biomarkers of oxidative stress induced by plant food rich diets. J Agric Food Chem 2005;53:6126–6132.
48. Waldmann A, Koschizke JW, Leitzmann C, Hahn A. Dietary intakes and blood concentrations of antioxidant vitamins in German vegans. Int J Vitam Nutr Res 2005;75:28–36.
49. Wirth MP, Hakenberg OW. [Prevention of prostate cancer]. Dtsch Med Wochenschr 2005;130:2002–2004.
50. Cleland LG, James MJ, Keen H, Danda D, Caughey G, Proudman SM. Fish oil—an example of an anti-inflammatory food. Asia Pac J Clin Nutr 2005;14:S66–71.
51. de La Puerta Vazquez R, Martinez-Dominguez E, Sanchez Perona J, Ruiz-Gutierrez V. Effects of different dietary oils on inflammatory mediator generation and fatty acid composition in rat neutrophils. Metabolism 2004;53:59–65.
52. Grimble RF, Tappia PS. Modulation of pro-inflammatory cytokine biology by unsaturated fatty acids. Z Ernahrungswiss 1998;37(Suppl 1):57–65.
53. Harbige LS. Fatty acids, the immune response, and autoimmunity: a question of n-6 essentiality and the balance between n-6 and n-3. Lipids 2003;38:323–341.
54. Khor GL. Dietary fat quality: a nutritional epidemiologist's view. Asia Pac J Clin Nutr 2004;13:S22.

55. Maple C, McLaren M, Bancroft A, Ho M, Belch JJ. Dietary supplementation with omega 3 and omega 6 fatty acids reduces induced white blood cell aggregation in healthy volunteers. Prostaglandins Leukot Essent Fatty Acids 1998;58:365–368.

56. Murakami A, Nishizawa T, Egawa K, et al. New class of linoleic acid metabolites biosynthesized by corn and rice lipoxygenases: suppression of proinflammatory mediator expression via attenuation of MAPK- and Akt-, but not PPARgamma-, dependent pathways in stimulated macrophages. Biochem Pharmacol 2005;70:1330–1342.

57. Philpott M, Ferguson LR. Immunonutrition and cancer. Mutat Res 2004;551:29–42.

58. Serhan CN. Novel omega-3-derived local mediators in anti-inflammation and resolution. Pharmacol Ther 2005;105:7–21.

59. Tapiero H, Ba GN, Couvreur P, Tew KD. Polyunsaturated fatty acids (PUFA) and eicosanoids in human health and pathologies. Biomed Pharmacother 2002;56:215–222.

60. Coyle EF. Fluid and fuel intake during exercise. J Sports Sci 2004;22:39–55.

61. Galloway SD. Dehydration, rehydration, and exercise in the heat: rehydration strategies for athletic competition. Can J Appl Physiol 1999;24:188–200.

62. Latzka WA, Montain SJ. Water and electrolyte requirements for exercise. Clin Sports Med 1999;18:513–524.

63. Oppliger RA, Bartok C. Hydration testing of athletes. Sports Med 2002;32:959–971.

64. Rehrer NJ. Fluid and electrolyte balance in ultra-endurance sport. Sports Med 2001;31:701–715.

65. Schoffstall JE, Branch JD, Leutholtz BC, Swain DE. Effects of dehydration and rehydration on the one-repetition maximum bench press of weight-trained males. J Strength Cond Res 2001;15:102–108.

66. Von Duvillard SP, Braun WA, Markofski M, Beneke R, Leithauser R. Fluids and hydration in prolonged endurance performance. Nutrition 2004;20:651–656.

67. Watson G, Judelson DA, Armstrong LE, Yeargin SW, Casa DJ, Maresh CM. Influence of diuretic-induced dehydration on competitive sprint and power performance. Med Sci Sports Exerc 2005;37:1168–1174.

68. Yoshida T, Takanishi T, Nakai S, Yorimoto A, Morimoto T. The critical level of water deficit causing a decrease in human exercise performance: a practical field study. Eur J Appl Physiol 2002;87:529–534.

69. Dietary Guidelines for Americans 2005. In: King JC, Caballero B, Clydesdale FM, et al., eds. Washington, DC: Services USDoHaH, Agriculture USDo; 2005:1–70.

70. Pritchett AM, Foreyt JP, Mann DL. Treatment of the metabolic syndrome: the impact of lifestyle modification. Curr Atheroscler Rep 2005;7:95–102.

71. Nowicka P. Dietitians and exercise professionals in a childhood obesity treatment team. Acta Paediatr Suppl 2005;94:23–29.

72. Nemet D, Barkan S, Epstein Y, Friedland O, Kowen G, Eliakim A. Short- and long-term beneficial effects of a combined dietary-behavioral-physical activity intervention for the treatment of childhood obesity. Pediatrics 2005;115:e443–449.

73. Mendiola AH. Reviewer's comment regarding: "Long-term effects of supervised physical training in secondary prevention of low back pain" (by I. Maul et al.). Eur Spine J 2005;14:612.

74. Kasapis C, Thompson PD. The effects of physical activity on serum C-reactive protein and inflammatory markers: a systematic review. J Am Coll Cardiol 2005;45:1563–1569.

75. Duncan GE, Anton SD, Sydeman SJ, et al. Prescribing exercise at varied levels of intensity and frequency: a randomized trial. Arch Intern Med 2005;165:2362–2369.

76. Bruce B, Fries JF, Lubeck DP. Aerobic exercise and its impact on musculoskeletal pain in older adults: a 14 year prospective, longitudinal study. Arthritis Res Ther 2005;7:R1263–1270.

77. Brownson RC, Boehmer TK, Luke DA. Declining rates of physical activity in the United States: what are the contributors? Annu Rev Public Health 2005;26:421–443.

78. Ball GD, Marshall JD, McCargar LJ. Physical activity, aerobic fitness, self-perception, and dietary intake in at risk of overweight and normal weight children. Can J Diet Pract Res 2005;66:162–169.

79. Andersen LL, Tufekovic G, Zebis MK, et al. The effect of resistance training combined with timed ingestion of protein on muscle fiber size and muscle strength. Metabolism 2005;54:151–156.

80. Volianitis S, Yoshiga CC, Nissen P, Secher NH. Effect of fitness on arm vascular and metabolic responses to upper body exercise. Am J Physiol Heart Circ Physiol 2004;286:H1736–741.

81. Singh MA. Exercise and aging. Clin Geriatr Med 2004;20:201–221.

82. Kouidi E, Grekas D, Deligiannis A, Tourkantonis A. Outcomes of long-term exercise training in dialysis patients: comparison of two training programs. Clin Nephrol 2004;61(Suppl 1):S31–38.

83. Hills AP, Byrne NM. Physical activity in the management of obesity. Clin Dermatol 2004;22:315–318.

84. Flakoll PJ, Judy T, Flinn K, Carr C, Flinn S. Postexercise protein supplementation improves health and muscle soreness during basic military training in Marine recruits. J Appl Physiol 2004;96:951–956.

85. Clement JM, Schmidt CA, Bernaix LW, Covington NK, Carr TR. Obesity and physical activity in college women: implications for clinical practice. J Am Acad Nurse Pract 2004;16:291–299.

86. Blair SN, LaMonte MJ, Nichaman MZ. The evolution of physical activity recommendations: how much is enough? Am J Clin Nutr 2004;79:913S–920S.

87. Santa-Clara H, Fernhall B, Baptista F, Mendes M, Bettencourt Sardinha L. Effect of a one-year combined exercise training program on body composition in men with coronary artery disease. Metabolism 2003;52:1413–1417.

88. Persky AM, Eddington ND, Derendorf H. A review of the effects of chronic exercise and physical fitness level on resting pharmacokinetics. Int J Clin Pharmacol Ther 2003;41:504–516.

89. Karper WB, Stasik SC. A successful, long-term exercise program for women with fibromyalgia syndrome and chronic fatigue and immune dysfunction syndrome. Clin Nurse Spec 2003;17:243–248.

90. Fattirolli F, Cellai T, Burgisser C. [Physical activity and cardiovascular health a close link]. Monaldi Arch Chest Dis 2003;60:73–78.

91. van der Bij AK, Laurant MG, Wensing M. Effectiveness of physical activity interventions for older adults: a review. Am J Prev Med 2002;22:120–133.

92. Singh MA. Exercise to prevent and treat functional disability. Clin Geriatr Med 2002;18:431–462, vi–vii.

93. Mullooly C. Cardiovascular fitness and type 2 diabetes. Curr Diab Rep 2002;2: 441–447.

94. Lowther M, Mutrie N, Scott EM. Promoting physical activity in a socially and economically deprived community: a 12 month randomized control trial of fitness assessment and exercise consultation. J Sports Sci 2002;20:577–588.

95. Hernelahti M, Kujala UM, Kaprio J, Sarna S. Long-term vigorous training in young adulthood and later physical activity as predictors of hypertension in middle-aged and older men. Int J Sports Med 2002;23:178–182.

96. Spirduso WW, Cronin DL. Exercise dose-response effects on quality of life and independent living in older adults. Med Sci Sports Exerc 2001;33:S598–608; discussion S609–610.

97. Scheen AJ, Rorive M, Letiexhe M. [Physical exercise for preventing obesity, promoting weight loss and maintaining weight management]. Rev Med Liege 2001;56: 244–247.

98. New SA. Exercise, bone and nutrition. Proc Nutr Soc 2001;60:265–274.

99. Huuskonen J, Vaisanen SB, Kroger H, Jurvelin JS, Alhava E, Rauramaa R. Regular physical exercise and bone mineral density: a four-year controlled randomized trial in middle-aged men. The DNASCO study. Osteoporos Int 2001;12:349–355.

100. Cox KL, Burke V, Morton AR, Gillam HF, Beilin LJ, Puddey IB. Long-term effects of exercise on blood pressure and lipids in healthy women aged 40–65 years: The Sedentary Women Exercise Adherence Trial (SWEAT). J Hypertens 2001;19: 1733–1743.

101. Messier SP, Royer TD, Craven TE, O'Toole ML, Burns R, Ettinger WH Jr. Long-term exercise and its effect on balance in older, osteoarthritic adults: results from the Fitness, Arthritis, and Seniors Trial (FAST). J Am Geriatr Soc 2000;48: 131–138.

102. Pasman WJ, Saris WH, Muls E, Vansant G, Westerterp-Plantenga MS. Effect of exercise training on long-term weight maintenance in weight-reduced men. Metabolism 1999;48:15–21.

103. Wing RR, Phelan S. Long-term weight loss maintenance. Am J Clin Nutr 2005; 82:222S–225S.

104. Williamson DA, Stewart TM. Behavior and lifestyle: approaches to treatment of obesity. J La State Med Soc 2005;157(Spec No 1):S50–55.

105. Truesdale KP, Stevens J, Cai J. The effect of weight history on glucose and lipids: the Atherosclerosis Risk in Communities Study. Am J Epidemiol 2005;161: 1133–1143.

106. Riebe D, Blissmer B, Greene G, et al. Long-term maintenance of exercise and healthy eating behaviors in overweight adults. Prev Med 2005;40:769–778.

107. Reas DL, Grilo CM, Masheb RM, Wilson GT. Body checking and avoidance in overweight patients with binge eating disorder. Int J Eat Disord 2005;37: 342–346.

108. Raynor HA, Jeffery RW, Phelan S, Hill JO, Wing RR. Amount of food group variety consumed in the diet and long-term weight loss maintenance. Obes Res 2005;13: 883–890.

109. Mathys M. Pharmacologic agents for the treatment of obesity. Clin Geriatr Med 2005;21:735–746, vii.

110. Littman AJ, Kristal AR, White E. Effects of physical activity intensity, frequency, and activity type on 10-y weight change in middle-aged men and women. Int J Obes (Lond) 2005;29:524–533.

111. Lejeune MP, Kovacs EM, Westerterp-Plantenga MS. Additional protein intake limits weight regain after weight loss in humans. Br J Nutr 2005;93:281–289.

112. LeCheminant JD, Jacobsen DJ, Hall MA, Donnelly JE. A comparison of meal replacements and medication in weight maintenance after weight loss. J Am Coll Nutr 2005;24:347–353.

113. Kiehn JM, Ghormley CO, Williams EB. Physician-assisted weight loss and maintenance in the elderly. Clin Geriatr Med 2005;21:713–723, vi.

114. Jakicic JM, Otto AD. Physical activity considerations for the treatment and prevention of obesity. Am J Clin Nutr 2005;82:226S–229S.

115. Hessert MJ, Gugliucci MR, Pierce HR. Functional fitness: maintaining or improving function for elders with chronic diseases. Fam Med 2005;37:472–476.

116. Hart KE, Warriner EM. Weight loss and biomedical health improvement on a very low calorie diet: the moderating role of history of weight cycling. Behav Med 2005;30:161–170.

117. Westerterp-Plantenga MS, Lejeune MP, Nijs I, van Ooijen M, Kovacs EM. High protein intake sustains weight maintenance after body weight loss in humans. Int J Obes Relat Metab Disord 2004;28:57–64.

118. Wallner SJ, Luschnigg N, Schnedl WJ, et al. Body fat distribution of overweight females with a history of weight cycling. Int J Obes Relat Metab Disord 2004;28: 1143–1148.

119. Bessesen DH. The role of carbohydrates in insulin resistance. J Nutr 2001;131: 2782S–2786S.

120. Hallfrisch J, Facn, Behall KM. Mechanisms of the effects of grains on insulin and glucose responses. J Am Coll Nutr 2000;19:320S–325S.

121. Heilbronn LK, Noakes M, Clifton PM. Effect of energy restriction, weight loss, and diet composition on plasma lipids and glucose in patients with type 2 diabetes. Diabetes Care 1999;22:889–895.

122. Kang J, Robertson RJ, Hagberg JM, et al. Effect of exercise intensity on glucose and insulin metabolism in obese individuals and obese NIDDM patients. Diabetes Care 1996;19:341–349.

123. Wallberg-Henriksson H. Exercise and diabetes mellitus. Exerc Sport Sci Rev 1992;20:339–368.

124. Wolfram G. [Is sugar involved in the development of cardiovascular diseases?]. Z Ernahrungswiss 1990;29(Suppl 1):35–38.

125. Fernandez Soto ML, Gonzalez Jimenez A, Lopez-Cozar LN, Lobon Hernandez JA, Aguirre Zamorano MA, Escobar-Jimenez F. [Diet and non-insulin-dependent diabetes mellitus: historic and current perspectives]. Rev Clin Esp 1990;186: 131–133.

126. Bantle JP. The dietary treatment of diabetes mellitus. Med Clin North Am 1988;72:1285–1299.

127. Zimmet PZ, King HO, Bjorntorp SP. Obesity, hypertension, carbohydrate disorders and the risk of chronic diseases. Is there any epidemiological evidence for integrated prevention programmes? Med J Aust 1986;145:256–259, 262.

128. Nuttall FQ, Gannon MC. Sucrose and disease. Diabetes Care 1981;4:305–310.

129. Lee VA. The nutrition significance of sucrose consumption, 1970–1980. Crit Rev Food Sci Nutr 1981;14:1–47.

130. Keen H, Thomas BJ, Jarrett RJ, Fuller JH. Nutrient intake, adiposity, and diabetes. Br Med J 1979;1:655–658.

131. Yudkin J. Dietary factors in arteriosclerosis: sucrose. Lipids 1978;13:370–372.

132. von Knorre G, Bode H. [Obesity and diabetes-morbidity—a prospective 5-year study]. Z Gesamte Inn Med 1976;31:6–9.

133. Walker AR. Whither sugar consumption? S Afr Med J 1973;47:404.

134. Kabir M, Rizkalla SW, Quignard-Boulange A, et al. A high glycemic index starch diet affects lipid storage-related enzymes in normal and to a lesser extent in diabetic rats. J Nutr 1998;128:1878–1883.

135. Vaaler S, Hanssen KF, Aagenaes O. The effect of cooking upon the blood glucose response to ingested carrots and potatoes. Diabetes Care 1984;7:221–223.

136. Bantle JP, Laine DC, Castle GW, Thomas JW, Hoogwerf BJ, Goetz FC. Postprandial glucose and insulin responses to meals containing different carbohydrates in normal and diabetic subjects. N Engl J Med 1983;309:7–12.

137. Bacciottini L, Tanini A, Falchetti A, et al. Calcium bioavailability from a calcium-rich mineral water, with some observations on method. J Clin Gastroenterol 2004;38:761–766.

138. Bhanugopan MS, Rankin A, Hyde ML, Fraser DR, McNeil DM. Improving bone health to optimise calcium metabolism in the dairy cow. Asia Pac J Clin Nutr 2004;13:S54.

139. Pointillart A, Coxam V, Seve B, Colin C, Lacroix CH, Gueguen L. Availability of calcium from skim milk, calcium sulfate and calcium carbonate for bone mineralization in pigs. Reprod Nutr Dev 2000;40:49–61.

140. Aptel I, Cance-Rouzaud A, Grandjean H. Association between calcium ingested from drinking water and femoral bone density in elderly women: evidence from the EPIDOS cohort. J Bone Miner Res 1999;14:829–833.

141. Bawa S. The role of the consumption of beverages in the obesity epidemic. J R Soc Health 2005;125:124–128.

142. Lelovics Z. Relation between calcium and magnesium intake and obesity. Asia Pac J Clin Nutr 2004;13:S144.

143. Zemel MB, Miller SL. Dietary calcium and dairy modulation of adiposity and obesity risk. Nutr Rev 2004;62:125–131.

144. Nicklas TA. Calcium intake trends and health consequences from childhood through adulthood. J Am Coll Nutr 2003;22:340–356.

145. Zemel MB, Shi H, Greer B, Dirienzo D, Zemel PC. Regulation of adiposity by dietary calcium. FASEB J 2000;14:1132–1138.

146. Lea EJ, Crawford D, Worsley A. Consumers' readiness to eat a plant-based diet. Eur J Clin Nutr 2006;60(3):342–351.

147. Reedy J, Haines PS, Campbell MK. Differences in fruit and vegetable intake among categories of dietary supplement users. J Am Diet Assoc 2005;105:1749–1756.

148. Daviglus ML, Liu K, Pirzada A, et al. Relationship of fruit and vegetable consumption in middle-aged men to medicare expenditures in older age: the Chicago Western Electric Study. J Am Diet Assoc 2005;105:1735–1744.

149. Holick CN, De Vivo I, Feskanich D, Giovannucci E, Stampfer M, Michaud DS. Intake of fruits and vegetables, carotenoids, folate, and vitamins A, C, E and risk of bladder cancer among women (United States). Cancer Causes Control 2005;16:1135–1145.

150. Kearney M, Bradbury C, Ellahi B, Hodgson M, Thurston M. Mainstreaming prevention: prescribing fruit and vegetables as a brief intervention in primary care. Public Health 2005;119:981–986.

151. Koebnick C, Garcia AL, Dagnelie PC, et al. Long-term consumption of a raw food diet is associated with favorable serum LDL cholesterol and triglycerides but also with elevated plasma homocysteine and low serum HDL cholesterol in humans. J Nutr 2005;135:2372–2378.

152. Klepp KI, Perez-Rodrigo C, De Bourdeaudhuij I, et al. Promoting fruit and vegetable consumption among European schoolchildren: rationale, conceptualization and design of the pro children project. Ann Nutr Metab 2005;49:212–220.

153. Molaison EF, Connell CL, Stuff JE, Yadrick MK, Bogle M. Influences on fruit and vegetable consumption by low-income black American adolescents. J Nutr Educ Behav 2005;37:246–251.

154. Scalbert A, Manach C, Morand C, Remesy C, Jimenez L. Dietary polyphenols and the prevention of diseases. Crit Rev Food Sci Nutr 2005;45:287–306.

155. Lin J, Zhang SM, Cook NR, et al. Dietary intakes of fruit, vegetables, and fiber, and risk of colorectal cancer in a prospective cohort of women (United States). Cancer Causes Control 2005;16:225–233.

156. Friel S, Newell J, Kelleher C. Who eats four or more servings of fruit and vegetables per day? Multivariate classification tree analysis of data from the 1998 Survey of Lifestyle, Attitudes and Nutrition in the Republic of Ireland. Public Health Nutr 2005;8:159–169.

157. Kang JH, Ascherio A, Grodstein F. Fruit and vegetable consumption and cognitive decline in aging women. Ann Neurol 2005;57:713–720.

158. Wilson DB, Smith BN, Speizer IS, et al. Differences in food intake and exercise by smoking status in adolescents. Prev Med 2005;40:872–879.

159. Vastag B. Recent studies show limited association of fruit and vegetable consumption and cancer risk. J Natl Cancer Inst 2005;97:474–476.

160. Ricketts ML, Moore DD, Banz WJ, Mezei O, Shay NF. Molecular mechanisms of action of the soy isoflavones includes activation of promiscuous nuclear receptors. A review. J Nutr Biochem 2005;16:321–330.

161. Meyer BJ, Larkin TA, Owen AJ, Astheimer LB, Tapsell LC, Howe PR. Limited lipid-lowering effects of regular consumption of whole soybean foods. Ann Nutr Metab 2004;48:67–78.

162. Rizkalla SW, Bellisle F, Slama G. Health benefits of low glycaemic index foods, such as pulses, in diabetic patients and healthy individuals. Br J Nutr 2002;88(Suppl 3): S255–262.

163. Anderson JW, Smith BM, Washnock CS. Cardiovascular and renal benefits of dry bean and soybean intake. Am J Clin Nutr 1999;70:464S–474S.

164. Campbell TC, Parpia B, Chen J. Diet, lifestyle, and the etiology of coronary artery disease: the Cornell China study. Am J Cardiol 1998;82:18T–21T.

165. Anderson JW, Smith BM, Gustafson NJ. Health benefits and practical aspects of high-fiber diets. Am J Clin Nutr 1994;59:1242S–1247S.

166. Doyle PT, Dunshea FR, McIntosh GH. Enhancing health active compounds in milk through cow management. Asia Pac J Clin Nutr 2005;14(Suppl):S13.

167. Buckley JD, Burgess S, Murphy KJ, Howe PR. Effects of omega-3 polyunsaturated fatty acids on cardiovascular risk, exercise performance and recovery in Australian Football League (AFL) players. Asia Pac J Clin Nutr 2005;14(Suppl):S57.

168. Nichols PD, Mansour P, Robert S, et al. Alternate sources of long-chain omega-3 oils. Asia Pac J Clin Nutr 2005;14(Suppl):S112.

169. Harper CR, Jacobson TA. Usefulness of omega-3 fatty acids and the prevention of coronary heart disease. Am J Cardiol 2005;96:1521–1529.

170. Shahidi F, Miraliakbari H. Omega-3 fatty acids in health and disease: part 2—health effects of omega-3 fatty acids in autoimmune diseases, mental health, and gene expression. J Med Food 2005;8:133–148.

171. Harris WS. Extending the cardiovascular benefits of omega-3 fatty acids. Curr Atheroscler Rep 2005;7:375–380.

172. Weinstock-Guttman B, Baier M, Park Y, et al. Low fat dietary intervention with omega-3 fatty acid supplementation in multiple sclerosis patients. Prostaglandins Leukot Essent Fatty Acids 2005;73:397–404.

173. Patch CS, Tapsell LC, Williams PG. Attitudes and intentions toward purchasing novel foods enriched with omega-3 fatty acids. J Nutr Educ Behav 2005;37: 235–241.

174. Stern AH. Balancing the risks and benefits of fish consumption. Ann Intern Med 2005;142:949.

175. Williams LK. Balancing the risks and benefits of fish consumption. Ann Intern Med 2005;142:946–949.

176. Calder PC. n-3 fatty acids, inflammation, and immunity—relevance to postsurgical and critically ill patients. Lipids 2004;39:1147–1161.

177. Oh R. Practical applications of fish oil (omega-3 fatty acids) in primary care. J Am Board Fam Pract 2005;18:28–36.

178. Folsom AR, Demissie Z. Fish intake, marine omega-3 fatty acids, and mortality in a cohort of postmenopausal women. Am J Epidemiol 2004;160:1005–1010.

179. Mori TA, Beilin LJ. Omega-3 fatty acids and inflammation. Curr Atheroscler Rep 2004;6:461–467.

180. Mori TA. Effect of fish and fish oil-derived omega-3 fatty acids on lipid oxidation. Redox Rep 2004;9:193–197.

181. Ruxton C. Health benefits of omega-3 fatty acids. Nurs Stand 2004;18:38–42.

# Special Needs of Youth, Women, and the Elderly

## Marie Spano

## OBJECTIVES

On the completion of this chapter you will be able to:

1. Understand the nutritional issues that relate to the healthy maturation and sports participation in young athletes.
2. Discuss the primary fueling issues as they relate to the specific needs of the young athlete.
3. Explain the precursors for the development of disordered eating and eating disorders in young athletes.
4. Target sports that classically have been linked to athletes with eating disorders.
5. Apply the macro- and micronutrient guidelines to a youth population.
6. Discuss the issues of dehydration and how proper hydration affects sports performance.
7. Understand the specific dietary issues that may be related to female athletes.
8. Explain the ramifications of eating disorders and the interaction of the components of the female athlete triad.
9. Differentiate the nutritional needs of the elderly from those of younger adults.
10. Target the specific micro- and macronutrient needs of the elderly.
11. Discuss why hydration is an important consideration for the elderly individual.

## ABSTRACT

In the past several years, the number of children, women, and elderly participating in sports has increased because of increased availability of competitive leagues and events, the advent of Title 9, and research exposing the benefits of exercise for the elderly. Sport is beneficial for myriad reasons and participants take up athletic endeavors for a variety of these reasons, some being very competitive, others just enjoying being able to "play." To help the pursuit of exercise and sport to be enjoyable, it is important to keep the athlete healthy, well nourished, and hydrated. Sports nutrition as a field has come a long way although research is still limited on children and the elderly, especially for those who are maintaining very strenuous training schedules. This chapter presents several nutritional needs of youth, women, and the elderly that may provide some of the missing links to better athletic performance and, more importantly, better overall health.

*Key Words:* youth, elderly, special needs, vitamins, minerals, children, female, women

From: *Essentials of Sports Nutrition and Supplements*
Edited by J. Antonio, D. Kalman, J. R. Stout, M. Greenwood, D. S. Willoughby, and G. G. Haff © Humana Press, a part of Springer Science+Business Media, Totowa, NJ

Although general sports nutrition guidelines regarding macronutrient composition, meal timing, and recovery nutrition are applicable to all athletes, there are special needs for subgroups of athletes including youth, women, and the elderly. This chapter does not cover all of the nutritional requirements for these subgroups but instead focuses on particular needs that may separate each subgroup from the athletic population as a whole. However, many of the special nutrition issues overlap among the youth, women, and the elderly.

## YOUTH*

According to the National Sporting Goods Association, there was an 11.2% increase in youth (ages 7–11) organized sports participation from 1993 to 2003.[1] With athletic involvement in this age group, as well as younger children and teenagers, hopefully continuing to increase in coming years, the importance of nutrition in these populations cannot be understated. Although nutrition in athletic performance has been studied extensively, there is a paucity of research on the nutritional needs of young athletes, especially those in their elementary and middle school years, making it difficult to develop specific recommendations for these populations. However, there are a few special nutritional needs of young athletes that have been identified. One issue of paramount importance in this age group is their ability to meet their caloric and macronutrient needs to support growth and development as well as their athletic training demands.[2] A second related issue is the risk of eating disorders in preteen and teenage athletes.[3] Third, although micronutrient needs are not different in young athletes in comparison to their nonactive peers, adequate calcium intake is vital because they are in their peak bone accretion years[4] and adequate iron intake is also important because of the prevalence of iron deficiency in the pediatric athlete.[5] And finally, parents and coaches should be cognizant of an increased risk for dehydration and heat illness in young athletes.[6]

### Proper Fueling

Children have additional challenges to meeting their nutritional needs because they depend on their parents, coaches, and the school cafeteria workers to shop for or prepare many, if not all, of their meals. For the young athlete, satisfying their energy and macronutrient needs is critical not only so they meet the training demands of their sport and reach their athletic goals, but more importantly, to support growth and development,[7] ensure rapid recovery from injuries, and for females, start menstruation and maintain regular menstrual cycles when they reach puberty.[6,8] Energy needs for adolescent athletes are dependent on the following variables: growth rate, age, gender, size, weight, and physical activity levels,[2] and therefore it is difficult to determine caloric needs based solely on age, gender, and athletic endeavor (Figure 19.1).

In 2002, the Institute of Medicine produced the latest Dietary Reference Intakes (DRIs) for energy and macronutrients (Table 19.1). An Estimated Energy Requirement is given for the average daily energy intake predicted to maintain energy balance and support growth in a healthy child of a defined age, gender, weight, height, and the "active" physical activity level.[9] These recommendations provide a good reference to start with in estimating a child's caloric needs, although it is important to add calories if training demands are especially intense.

How do parents and coaches determine if a child is meeting their daily caloric needs? The pediatric growth charts can be used as a tool to help track and evaluate a child's growth. Developed by the National Center for Health Statistics from national data collected through the National Health and Nutrition Examination Survey (NHANES), the pediatric growth charts have been

---

*The term youth has been used to describe a variety of age ranges from the young child on through the teenage years. For the purpose of this chapter, it will describe all of those ages unless otherwise noted. Children and adolescents may be interchanged with "youth."

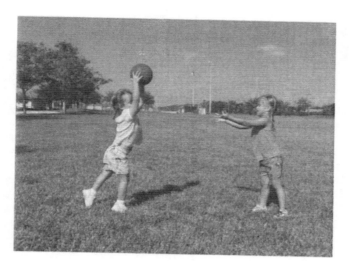

**FIGURE 19.1.** For children to get "exercise," it is not necessary that they engage in an organized sport. Unstructured "play" is often the best way to promote activity.

used by health professionals since 1977 to help determine the adequacy of growth in children. There are several charts as children are grouped by age and sex.[9] They can be found at: http://www.cdc.gov/nchs/about/major/nhanes/growthcharts/clinical_charts.htm. Although one single point on the growth chart does not lend much information, a child's growth plotted over a period of time can help delineate their growth pattern. In the time period from age 2 years until puberty starts, growth should be fairly constant.[7]

As an additional reference, Kuczmarski et al. (2000)[10] established an analytic growth chart data set by combining national health examination surveys collected from 1963 to 1994 with five supplementary data sources. Other ways to examine whether or not a child is meeting their energy needs is to consider if they get tired easily or seem to be worn out by their practice sessions (and they are not overtraining or lacking sleep).

## Disordered Eating and Eating Disorders

During childhood, calorie needs increase throughout growth until they reach their peak during puberty when growth spikes upward. As the energy needs of adolescents increase during the early teenage years, many kids also start to diet,[8] creating a situation of potential impaired athletic performance[2] and interference with growth, bone development, and the onset of puberty.[3,8] In addition, caloric deprivation can increase the athlete's chances for injury, illness, and nutritional deficiencies[11] and put the athlete at risk for the development of a full-blown eating disorder.[12]

Unfortunately, many athletes restrict their calorie intake in an effort to improve performance and/or meet the body image demands of their sport.[12] Several sports are known for the importance they place on body weight and/or body image. These include but are not limited to gymnastics,[7,13] dancing,[7] figure skating,[14] diving,[14] ballet,[14] wrestling,[7] and long-distance running.[15] In Minnesota, researchers distributed a self-administered questionnaire to examine the factors associated with eating disorders in adolescent girls (grades 7, 9, and 11) participating in sports. Of the 5163 girls who answered the questionnaire,

**TABLE 19.1.** Dietary Reference Intakes for energy by life-stage group.

| Life-stage group (years) | Active PAL EER (kcal/day) | |
|---|---|---|
| | *Male* | *Female* |
| 1–2 | 1046 | 992 |
| 3–8 | 1742 | 1642 |
| 9–13 | 2279 | 2071 (to 11 years) |
| 14–18 | 3152 | 2368 (to 16 years) |

*Source:* Food and Nutrition Board, Institute of Medicine.[25]

PAL = physical activity level, EER = estimated energy requirement.

there was a 51% increase in eating disorder symptoms in girls participating in weight-conscious versus non–weight-conscious sports.[16]

In males, wrestling receives the most attention as a weight-conscious sport. Kiningham and Gorenflo[17] utilized surveys to investigate the weight-loss practices of 2532 Michigan high school wrestlers of all skill levels and weight classes. Seventy-two percent of wrestlers practiced at least one harmful weight-loss method (such as fasting, dehydration, laxative use, vomiting) each week during the season, 52% used at least two methods per week, and 12% used five or more harmful weight-loss methods every week during season. Other studies on high school wrestlers confirm that "making weight"—even if it means resorting to unhealthy practices—is necessary to compete in a certain weight class.[18] Unfortunately, in-season weight loss that is so common among these athletes may lead to decreases in both strength and power as a result of fat-free mass loss.[19]

Most studies on eating disorders in females have examined teenage girls who have completed puberty, or women—typically elite athletes. However, it is difficult to quantify the percentage of young athletes with eating disorders, especially because there are very few studies on younger teens and children. A joint study between the National College Athletic Association and the Eating Disorders Program at Laureate Psychiatric Clinic and Hospital in Tulsa, Oklahoma surveyed 1445 student athletes from 11 Division 1 schools to determine the prevalence of eating disorders in this population. Using the DSM-IV criteria (Diagnostic and Statistical Manual of Mental Disorders, 4th edition, published by the American Psychiatric Association, Washington, DC), the 133-question survey revealed that 1.1% of the females and no males were considered bulimic; 9.2% of the females and 0.01% of the males were considered to have clinically significant problems with bulimia; 2.85% of the females and 0% of the males had a clinically significant problem with anorexia nervosa; 10.85% of females and 13.02% of the males were weekly binge eaters; 5.52% of the females and 2.04% of the males reported purging behavior (vomiting, laxatives, diuretics) on a weekly or greater basis.[20]

Review papers on eating disorders in female athletes have estimated the prevalence to be much higher than this.[21] However, by utilizing the Eating Attitudes Test (EAT-26) and the Eating Disorder Inventory Body Dissatisfaction Subscale (EDI-BD), Beals and Manore[22] looked at the prevalence of eating disorders in 425 female collegiate athletes from seven different universities throughout the United States. Whereas only 3.3% of athletes met the diagnostic criteria for anorexia and 2.3% met it for bulimia, using the EAT-26, 15.2% qualified for at-risk behavior and 32.4% qualified for such behavior under the EDI-BD. Overall, 31% of athletes not using oral contraceptives reported menstrual irregularity with the athletes considered at risk for an eating disorder having a significantly greater prevalence of such irregularity.

All of these studies indicate that the prevalence of disordered eating is much higher than that of eating disorders and that some sports have a greater incidence of both because of the emphasis they place on body size.

The following behaviors characterize disordered eating and eating disorders: food restriction; binge eating and/or purging; using laxatives, diuretics, or diet pills; and compulsive exercise.[23] Symptoms may include but are not limited to: dizziness, syncope, weakness, fatigue, hair loss, lanugo, dry skin, constipation, bloating, abdominal pain, menstrual irregularities, and cold intolerance.[3] The DSM-IV is used to diagnose anorexia and bulimia.[24]

For tips on preventing eating disorders, please see Sidebar 19.3.

## Macronutrients

The macronutrient needs for child athletes are higher than their sedentary counterparts mainly because of the increased energy demands of their sports. However, the macronutrient makeup of their diet is basically the same with the possible exception of protein.

The Institute of Medicine's 2002 DRIs include a recommended dietary allowance (RDA) for both carbohydrates and protein (Table 19.2). The RDAs provide an average daily intake that will meet the nutrient requirements of

**TABLE 19.2. Dietary Reference Intakes for carbohydrate and protein.**

| Life-stage group | Carbohydrate (g/d) | Protein (g/d) |
|---|---|---|
| Children (years) | | |
| 1–3 | 130 | 13 |
| 4–8 | 130 | 19 |
| Males | | |
| 9–13 | 130 | 34 |
| 14–18 | 130 | 52 |
| Females | | |
| 9–13 | 130 | 34 |
| 14–18 | 130 | 46 |

*Source:* Food and Nutrition Board, Institute of Medicine.[99]

the majority (97%–98%) of healthy individuals in each age and gender group[25] and they provide a margin of safety.[26] However, an Acceptable Macronutrient Distribution Ranges (AMDR) is given for fat intake. An AMDR is defined as "a range of intakes for a particular energy source that is associated with reduced risk of chronic disease while providing adequate intakes of essential nutrients."[25]

Relative to body weight, children need more protein and a greater percentage of essential amino acids than adults because of physical growth.[26] Although the DRIs provide for this, studies on adult athletes verify an increased protein need and therefore an estimate of 1.5 g/kg/day might be more indicative of the protein needs of child athletes.[26] It is also important to remember that the DRIs are not for very active children who will need more calories overall and, consequently, more carbohydrates, protein, and fat to meet the increased calorie needs.

## Micronutrients

Typically, higher micronutrient needs can be met through an increased intake of nutrient-dense foods[26-28] and it is therefore prudent to encourage young athletes to choose such foods. Supplementation with vitamins and minerals does not enhance sports performance unless a nutrient deficiency exists[26,27] and mega doses of vitamins and minerals are not recommended in this population. A daily multivitamin mineral supplement that meets the recommended dietary intake values should be adequate to meet a young athlete's needs.[12] There are, however, two minerals of concern in this population: calcium[29] and iron.[30]

During childhood and adolescent growth, bone formation exceeds resorption in the bone remodeling process and peak bone mineral density (BMD) is achieved by the end of puberty.[31,32] Peak BMD is essential to the prevention of future bone loss[33] and osteoporosis.[31,34] Among the multitude of factors responsible for bone mineral accretion, adequate calcium intake, especially during childhood, is critical.[35] Athletes who restrict their energy intake may be at particular risk for suboptimal calcium intake.[7] Ninety-four adolescent girls (mean age 11.9) were randomly assigned in a double-blind, placebo-controlled trial examining the effect of 18 months of calcium supplementation (500 mg/day of calcium citrate malate) on bone density and bone mass. After 18 weeks, the calcium-supplemented group (whose overall calcium intake averaged 354 mg/day more than the control group) had significantly greater increases in lumbar spine BMD and bone mineral content (BMC) and total BMD as well as urinary calcium excretion.[36] Many other studies confirm an increase in BMD, BMC, and bone mass with calcium supplementation either through increased intake of dairy products or actual calcium supplements.[37-40]

Although calcium is important for bone mass development in all children, for athletes, inadequate calcium intake and low BMD have also been associated with both shin splits and stress fractures.[41] Bone remodeling is a constant process that is adjusted to accommodate new mechanical stresses upon the skeleton. When calcium intake is inadequate, low blood calcium levels signal bone-resorbing osteoclasts to remove calcium from the bone matrix to help

TABLE 19.3. Acceptable macronutrient distribution ranges.

| Macronutrient | Range (percent of energy) | |
|---|---|---|
| | Children (1–3 years) | Children (4–18 years) |
| Fat | 30–40 | 25–35 |
| Carbohydrate | 45–64 | 45–65 |
| Protein | 5–20 | 10–30 |

Source: National Academy of Sciences.[99]

maintain a normal blood calcium concentration. If calcium intake continues to be inadequate, bone will become more porous and brittle. When calcium intake increases, bone-building osteoblasts will rebuild the bone matrix.[42]

Calcium intake is listed as Adequate Intake (AI) reference value. AI is used when sufficient data to establish an RDA are lacking. AIs are set at a value intended to meet or exceed the amount necessary to maintain nutritional adequacy of the particular nutrient.[29]

According to NHANES, 1999–2000, mean calcium intakes were 853 ± 26.6 mg for children younger than 6 years of age and 889 ± 31.2 mg in children 6–11 years of age,[43] indicating that many children do not meet the AI set for calcium (Table 19.3).

As a component of both hemoglobin and myoglobin, iron carries oxygen in the blood and muscles.[44] Iron-deficiency anemia (normal hemoglobin concentrations but ferritin levels) can hamper athletic performance and it is possible that nonanemic iron deficiency also impairs performance.[45,46]

A few studies show a high percentage of iron deficiency in adolescent athletes, typically in teenage girls. Rowland and Kelleher[47] assessed iron status in 30 male and female high school swimmers in the beginning and at the end of their swim season. Whereas none of the boys were iron deficient, the girls averaged a daily intake of 43% of the RDA for iron and 46.7% of the girls were iron deficient (serum ferritin level less than 12 μg/L).

In a similar study on 50 high school male and female cross-country runners, 3% of males and 40% of females were iron deficient at the beginning of the 11-week season, and at the end of the season, 17% of males and 45% of females were iron deficient; however, no runners were anemic at the beginning or end of the season.[5]

Given that many adolescents may be iron deficient, it is important to examine if iron supplementation will improve performance. Utilizing a randomized, double-blind, placebo-controlled intervention trial, Hinton et al.[46] assigned 42 physically active but untrained women with iron deficiency (serum ferritin <16 μg/L) to the iron supplement (50 mg ferrous sulfate containing 10 mg elemental iron) or placebo group. Pills were taken twice a day for 6 weeks and aerobic training with a cycle ergometer started 2 weeks into the supplementation period and continued 5 times a week for 25 minutes per session (heart rate was kept at a 75% maximum or above) the following 4 weeks. There were no baseline differences in iron measures or time to finish on a 15-km time trial. After 6 weeks, the treatment group showed significant increases in serum ferritin, serum iron, and transferrin saturation in comparison to the placebo group and although both groups decreased their 15-km time, the supplemented group exhibited a significantly greater decrease in 15-km time in comparison to the placebo group.

When assessing adolescents for nonanemic iron deficiency, it is important to assess not just hemoglobin and hematocrit values but also total iron binding capacity, serum ferritin, and transferrin.

## Hydration

Dehydration can lead to decreases in both strength and endurance during exercise resulting in impaired performance.[48–50] In addition, dehydration can increase core body temperature leading to heat illness.[51] Some studies examining how children respond to heat during exercise indicate that young athletes may have an increased risk for heat-related illness (heat cramps, heat exhaustion, and heat stroke) in comparison to adults[52] because they have: 1) lower sweating rates than adults, which decreases their ability to dissipate heat,[53-56] and 2) greater surface area relative to their body mass causing them to gain more heat from the environment.[54-56]

However, not all studies point toward an impaired thermoregulation in children and there seems to be differences among boys and girls in their physiologic responses. Shibasaki et al.[53] compared thermoregulatory responses in seven prepubertal boys (aged 10–11 years) with 11 young men cycling at an intensity of approximately 40% maximal oxygen uptake in a warm environment (86°F, 45% relative humidity). Researchers concluded that the young boys compensated for significantly lower total body sweating and localized sweat rates through significantly greater cutaneous blood flow measured in the chest and back by laser Doppler flowmetry. Therefore, there was no age-related difference in thermoregulation. No age-related differences in rectal temperature or heart rate were noted either. Drinkwater et al.[54] compared the differences between five prepubertal girls with five college-aged women, matched for aerobic power, as they walked on a treadmill in varying degrees of heat and relative humidity. The investigators found that at all temperatures, the prepubertal girls had higher heart rates and significantly higher rectal temperatures. At and above temperatures of 95°F with a relative humidity of 65%, the prepubertal girls could not tolerate the heat as well and thus exercise time until discomfort was much lower than in the college-aged women.

Signs of dehydration and heat illness include excessive sweating, dry skin, tachycardia, dizziness, cramps, stumbling, and apathy.[57] Dehydration and subsequent heat illness in children can be prevented by encouraging children to drink even if they do not feel thirsty,[58] offer sports drinks containing 6%–8% carbohydrate and minor amounts of sodium to stimulate athletes to drink more,[59,60] acclimate athletes to heat,[61] and provide intermittent breaks to children during sporting events, especially during hot, humid days.[62]

Further recommendations put forth by the American Academy of Pediatrics for the prevention of heat illness in children can be found under Practical Guidelines at the end of this chapter.

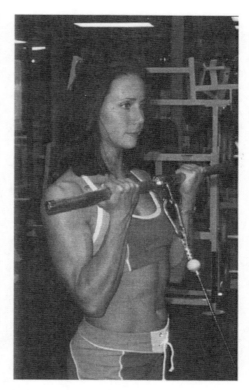

**FIGURE 19.2.** Weight training is an excellent exercise choice for improving bone mineral density in women.

## WOMEN

Athletic women have increased energy, water, and micronutrient needs. An increase in caloric intake should help the athletic woman to meet such needs. However, two micronutrients that athletic women should be especially cognizant of are iron and calcium because many women consume marginal intakes of these minerals.[63] A third nutrition-related concern for women is that of the female athlete triad: disordered eating, amenorrhea, and osteoporosis.[64]

## Calcium

As noted in the section on youth, calcium intake during childhood is significantly related to BMD.[35] Calcium intake in premenopausal women helps maintain BMD serving to prevent stress fractures,[65] osteopenia, and osteoporosis[66] (see Figure 19.2). In 1998, it was estimated that more than 25 million U.S. adults had osteoporosis or an increased risk for developing this disease.[66] Additionally, according to the NHANES, 1999–2000, the mean intake of calcium in all females from 12 years of age to over 60 was less than the AI, sometimes several hundred milligrams less (see Table 19.4).[67] From the risk of injury to the potential threat of osteopenia and osteoporosis, it is essential that athletic women consume the AI of calcium for their respective age group.

Several studies have correlated low BMD with an increased incidence of stress fractures. Lauder et al.[65] examined the association between BMD and the probability of stress fractures in premenopausal women. Twenty-seven active

TABLE 19.4. Dietary Reference Intakes (DRIs): Recommended Intakes for Individuals, Food and Nutrition Board, Institute of Medicine, National Academies of Science.

| Life-stage group (years) | Calcium (mg/d) | Iron (mg/d) |
|---|---|---|
| Children | | |
| 1–3 | 500 | 7 |
| 4–8 | 800 | 10 |
| Males | | |
| 9–13 | 1300 | 8 |
| Females | | |
| 9–13 | 1300 | 8 |

Sources: Food and Nutrition Board, Institute of Medicine.[29,30]

duty Army women with documented stress fractures within the 2 years before the study were compared with 158 female controls. Although there were no significant differences in dual-energy X-ray absorptiometry–measured BMD of the femoral neck and posteroanterior lumbar spine (L2–L4) between groups, low femoral neck BMD was significantly associated with an increased risk for stress fractures. In a similar study comparing 25 women with stress fractures to sex, age, weight, height, and exercise history matched controls, Myburgh et al.[68] found that the athletes with stress fractures had significantly lower BMD of the spine (p = 0.02), femoral neck (p = 0.005), Ward's triangle (p = 0.01), and greater trochanter (p = 0.01) than controls as measured. Significantly more athletes with fractures also exhibited menstrual irregularity (amenorrhea or oligomenorrhea) (p < 0.005). Whereas energy intake as assessed by 7-day diet records was similar between groups, the athletes with fractures had lower calcium intakes (p = 0.02) although both groups of athletes consumed less than the AI for calcium.

## Iron

According to the NHANES, 1999–2000, the mean iron intake for females from 14 to 39 years of age was below the RDA for their respective age groups. It is quite possible that the mean for females younger than 14 and older than the age of 39 was also less than the RDA although this is difficult to elucidate from the given data tables because the NHANES data group women in different age brackets than the DRI tables (Table 19.5).[67]

Similar to the studies on adolescents that reveal a large percentage of the girls are iron deficient or anemic, the same is true for women over the age of 18 before they reach menopause. Low intake of dietary sources of iron, especially heme iron found in meat, is one of the most common contributors to these problems although menstruation-related blood loss may also contribute.

Malczewska et al.[69] examined the causes of iron deficiency in 126 female endurance athletes and 52 control subjects (aged 16–20 years). The mean iron intake for this age group was 14.6 mg with 26% of athletes and 50% of controls

TABLE 19.5. Comparison of the Adequate Intake (AI) for calcium and National Health and Nutrition Examination Survey (NHANES) 1999–2000 calcium intake data.

| Life-stage group, females (years) | AI for calcium (mg/d) | Age group (years) | NHANES (mg/d) |
|---|---|---|---|
| 9–13 | 1300 | | |
| 14–18 | 1300 | 12–19 | 793 ± 26.5 |
| 19–30 | 1000 | 20–39 | 797 ± 32.4 |
| 31–50 | 1000 | 40–59 | 744 ± 28.7 |
| 51–70 | 1200 | ≥60 | 660 ± 21.3 |
| >70 | 1200 | | |

Sources: Food and Nutrition Board, Institute of Medicine.[29] U.S. Department of Health and Human Services.[68]

testing positive for latent iron deficiency without anemia (the second of three stages of iron deficiency). Risser et al.[70] evaluated iron deficiency and its effects on perceived performance in 100 female intercollegiate athletes in a variety of sports in comparison to 66 control subjects. Before supplementation with iron, 31% of the athletes and 45.5% of controls were iron deficient (ferritin less than $12 \, ng \cdot mL^{-1}$; transferrin saturation less than 16%, or both). Significantly more iron-deficient athletes considered their performance to be worse than athletes who were not iron deficient ($p < 0.05$).

## Eating Disorders and The Female Athlete Triad

As noted in the section on children, females are especially at risk for eating disorders, and women with menstrual irregularities, as frequently seen in athletes with eating disorders, are more likely to have lower BMD and BMC values. In a study comparing runners with oligomenorrhea and amenorrhea (n = 13) to eumenorrheic runners (n = 15) and controls (n = 54), all with similar body height, weight, body mass index, and percent body fat, those with menstrual irregularities measured significantly lower on BMD values for the total body, femoral neck, lumbar spine, lower leg, and arms. In addition, past and present menstrual dysfunction severity was linearly associated with declining BMD values in all sites except the lower leg.[71]

This link among disordered eating, amenorrhea, and osteoporosis has been termed the female athlete triad because all three of these frequently occur together. The triad is most often seen in athletes who participate in sports that emphasize leanness, and although it is often through deliberate caloric imbalance that these problems occur, it can also be seen in women who are training at high intensities and very unaware of their high caloric needs. Although the DSM-IV is used to diagnose anorexia and bulimia, most athletes with the female athlete triad do not meet the criteria for a full-blown eating disorder. Factors contributing to the triad are listed in Sidebar 19.1.

## Sidebar 19.1. Factors that Contribute to Eating Disorders in Women

*Jessica Setnick, Understanding Nutrition*

Although sports participation may increase self-esteem for many women, female athletes are still at risk of developing disordered eating, eating disorders, and the female athlete triad. Contributing factors include:

- Nutrition myths and misconceptions promoted by inexperienced coaching or training staff or spread among teammates, such as "Don't eat carbohydrate after 6 pm or you'll get fat";
- Sports that traditionally encourage a specific body size and shape, such as ice dancing, figure skating, cheerleading, drill team, diving, horseback riding, and gymnastics;
- Sport-related weight requirements, including weight classes, weigh-ins, and team-wide body composition testing;
- Training or competition schedules that leave little time for eating adequately;
- Sport-specific misconceptions, such as "The leaner you are the faster you can run";
- Extreme thinking and the determination to pursue it, such as "If low fat is good for you, then no fat is better";

- General misconceptions about the human body, such as "If you still have your period, you're not training hard enough";
- Increasing portrayal of female athletes as sex symbols, with the associated pressure to meet unreasonable body shape ideals;
- A devastating or career-ending injury that is not grieved adequately or addressed appropriately by the athlete's support system.

Not all of these factors can be controlled or eliminated, and not all female athletes will develop eating disorders. Even when training at extreme levels, some female athletes can maintain menstruation and bone health by eating adequate calories to cover the energy cost of their sport.

Anyone working with female athletes should be aware of the risk factors and warning signs of eating disorders in order to promote appropriate eating and attitudes, to prevent as much disordered eating as possible, and to intervene when necessary.

Treatment of the female athlete triad includes a decrease in training intensity until regular menstruation resumes, increasing caloric intake as well as the intake of calcium and vitamin D if necessary, and assessing the athlete for BMD and BMC.[72]

# ELDERLY

According to physical activity prevalence estimates from the 2000 National Health Interview Survey, 13.1% of women and 18.2% of men over the age of 65 are very physically active during usual daily activities and regularly engaged in leisure-time physical activity. Another 18.5% of women and 18.4% of men in this age category fit into the medium–high physical activity level indicating that they are either moderately active during daily tasks and regularly engage in leisure-time activity or are very physically active during leisure tasks and engage in some leisure-time activity.[73] These encouraging statistics indicate that a number of elderly U.S. adults are physically active. In addition, these statistics bring light to the importance of sports nutrition or proper fueling for physical activity in this growing population.

Although many of the nutrition-related issues in the elderly are a function of aging and not the result of athletic demands of those who exercise or compete in sports, these age-related issues can impact the athletic performance and well being of the older individual. It is especially important that active older adults adequately fuel themselves so they do not fatigue during exercise and to help them continue to maintain and build muscle mass. Other important nutritional needs for the exercising elderly include vitamin D and calcium intake and adequate hydration.

## Calorie and Macronutrient Needs

Calorie needs are generally considered to be age-dependent with a decrease later on in life. However, a decline in physical activity[74] and subsequent decrease in lean body mass[75] may be to blame and therefore decreases in lean body mass can be offset if older adults engage in resistance-training exercise.[76] Because many elderly individuals have decreases in muscle mass with aging,[77] it is vital that they consume adequate calories and protein to maintain, and continue to build, muscle mass. There are no studies that estimate the caloric needs of the athletic elderly; however, it has been suggested that the Harris-Benedict equation be used with an activity factor added[78] and that resistance exercise training, in particular, does not dramatically increase the caloric needs of the elderly.[79]

There has been some controversy regarding the adequacy of the RDA for protein in elderly individuals, mainly because of short-term nitrogen balance studies or studies in sedentary older adults.[80] To examine whether this RDA is adequate for resistance-trained adults, Campbell et al.[81] studied 12 men and 17 women consuming the RDA of 0.8 g protein kg$^{-1}$ day$^{-1}$ for 14 weeks. Subjects were then divided into groups performing whole-body resistance training, lower-body resistance training, or no training (sedentary group). Results showed muscle strength increases in those muscle groups being trained, no changes in whole-body muscle mass, protein-mineral mass, and whole-body protein metabolism suggesting adequacy of protein intake. Even if the RDA of 0.8 g/kg is adequate for resistance-trained individuals, it is important to be aware of the decreased caloric consumption in many elderly individuals which may contribute to a decrease in protein intake.

## Micronutrient Requirements

Adequate intake of both vitamin D and calcium are of utmost importance for elderly athletes. In the elderly, calcium intake is vital for the prevention of bone loss because, at this time, bone resorption exceeds formation.[34] Data from

**TABLE 19.6. Comparison of the recommended dietary allowance (RDA) for iron and National Health and Nutrition Examination Survey (NHANES) 1999–2000 iron intake data.**

| Life-stage group, females (years) | RDA for iron (mg/d) | Age group (years) | NHANES (mg/d) |
|---|---|---|---|
| 9–13 | 8 | | |
| 14–18 | 15 | 12–19 | 13.4 ± 0.44 |
| 19–30 | 18 | 20–39 | 13.7 ± 0.47 |
| 31–50 | 18 | 40–59 | 13.6 ± 0.50 |
| 51–70 | 8 | ≥60 | 12.8 ± 0.41 |
| >70 | 8 | | |

*Sources:* Food and Nutrition Board, Institute of Medicine.[30] U.S. Department of Health and Human Services.[68]

NHANES, 1999–2000, indicate that the calcium intake for men was 797 ± 27.0 and for women 660 ± 21.3, both of which are well below the AI for calcium (Table 19.6).

Among other functions, vitamin D promotes calcium absorption and bone mineralization[82] and recent research indicates that it may have a role in muscle strength.[83] Vitamin D deficiency can lead to osteomalacia (softening of the bones) in adults[84] and has been associated with an increase in hip fractures in older Americans.[85,86] Elderly individuals have a higher risk for developing a vitamin D deficiency because of decreased synthesis[87,88] and a decrease in conversion of vitamin D to its active form by the kidneys.[87]

Making matters worse, more than 50% of older women consume below the AI for vitamin D.[89] Moore et al.[90] examined the mean intake of vitamin D in the United States from the NHANES III (1988–1994)[89] and the Continuing Survey of Food Intakes by Individuals 1994–1996, 1998.[91] According to these data, fewer than 10% of adults 51–70 years of age and fewer than 2% of adults over age 70 met the RDA for vitamin D through food alone. Even with supplementation, up to 90% of individuals 51 years of age and older still did not meet the RDA for vitamin D.[89]

The DRIs for vitamin D can be found in Table 19.7. The recommended intake for vitamin D is listed as an AI reference value. An AI is used when there is a lack of sufficient data to establish an RDA. AIs are set at a value intended to meet or exceed the amount necessary to maintain nutritional adequacy of a particular nutrient. The AI for vitamin D is the daily intake necessary to help maintain bone health and calcium metabolism.[43]

## Hydration

Monitoring of proper hydration in the elderly is absolutely vital because of age-related changes in thirst mechanisms and thermoregulation. The elderly are prone to dehydration as a result of a decreased thirst sensation in response to decreases in blood volume, a reduction in renal water conservation capacity, and disturbances in sodium and water balance.[92] Exercise in a warm environment seems to increase the risk of dehydration.[92] Because of dehydration, the elderly are also at risk for hypernatremia (see Sidebar 19.2).

**TABLE 19.7. Dietary Reference Intakes for calcium and vitamin D.**

| Age (years) | Calcium (mg/d) Men and women | Vitamin D* Men (µg/d) | Vitamin D* Women (µg/d) |
|---|---|---|---|
| 51–70 | 1200 | 10 (= 400 IU) | 10 (= 400 IU) |
| ≥71 | 1200 | 15 (= 600 IU) | 15 (= 600 IU) |

*Source:* Food and Nutrition Board, Institute of Medicine.[29]

*Adequate Intake is given for vitamin D; for calcium, recommended dietary allowance is provided.

## Sidebar 19.2. Hypernatremia in the Elderly

*Mona R. Treadwell*

Part of the normal aging process includes changes in fluid and electrolyte homeostasis. This puts the elderly at risk for both dehydration and hypernatremia. Hypernatremia is defined as an increase in plasma sodium concentrations greater than 145 mEq/L, caused by excessive loss of water and electrolytes resulting from polyuria, diarrhea, excessive sweating, or inadequate water intake. For many elderly individuals, age-related decreased thirst may be the primary cause.[92] Thirst tends to diminish with age, and urinary concentration and excretion ability are decreased.[93] Other diseases such as hypertension and cardiovascular disease as well as the use of prescription medications may further exacerbate fluid homeostasis.[94]

Older men and women have altered physiologic control systems associated with thirst, which result from 1) a higher baseline osmolality indicating a higher operating point for thirst sensation, and 2) diminished thirst in response to the unloading and loading of pressure receptors responsible for stimulating thirst.[1] These possible physiologic changes combined with reduced water-conservation capacity, may predispose the elderly to dangerous dehydration when illness increases water losses[95] or the athlete is exercising in hot, humid weather.[96]

Hormonal changes associated with aging, the occurrence of other medical conditions, and the use of medications increase the likelihood of conditions such as hypernatremia.[94] It is important that older men and women drink fluids, preferably on a schedule as opposed to ad lib, when exercising. During exercise, the elderly should drink approximately 6–12 ounces of fluid every 15–20 minutes (if well tolerated).[96] Some low-sodium supplements are given to decrease chances for dehydration, however excess fluids and low-sodium diets may be dangerous to individuals susceptible to overhydration and the ability to excrete excess fluids and retain fluids.[2] Awareness of the homeostatic changes with age and the relationship with disease and medications (especially diuretics) will lead to better management of fluid disorders in the elderly population.[3]

Symptoms of hypernatremia vary depending on the cause. However, when the blood sodium concentration is extremely high, brain cells are affected. Muscle twitching, fatigue, and confusion are likely to set in. In severe cases, coma and death may result. Hypernatremia can be treated through the replacement of lost fluids. In severe cases, fluids may need to be replaced intravenously and blood sodium levels are closely monitored.[97]

Although the extent of hypernatremia in the elderly has not been established, it seems that when there are palatable fluid choices and no illness, the elderly have no problem maintaining fluid balance during sedentary conditions. However, if there is an illness present, access to fluid is restricted, or the elderly are exercising for prolonged periods in hot weather, they may develop undetected dehydration and potentially hypernatremia because of a diminished thirst perception.[2]

## SUMMARY

It is critical that active youth and elderly meet their nutrition needs, not only to ensure they meet their training and performance goals but, more importantly, to ensure there are no nutritional shortfalls that may impact their health. The most critical aspect of sports nutrition for youth is ensuring they meet their macronutrient and calorie needs to support growth and development as well as the added demands of their sport. Parents should also be cognizant of the signs for eating disorders in this group while also being cognizant of young athlete's calcium, iron and fluid intake. The sports nutrition needs of elderly athletes, like those of youth, are tied to their age-related needs and issues. The top issues to watch for in this group include total calorie intake, fluid intake and calcium and vitamin D. This chapter has presented several nutritional needs of youth, women, and the elderly that may provide some of the missing links to better athletic performance and, more importantly, better overall health.

## PRACTICAL APPLICATIONS

### All Athletes

#### HYDRATION

1. Have athletes weigh themselves before and after exercise. Weight loss signifies that the athlete is dehydrated. He/she should immediately take in water

or sports beverages to make up for the dehydration and increase fluid intake during subsequent training sessions and games.

2. Check urine. If urine is dark and scant, then the athlete is probably dehydrated.

3. Encourage athletes to use salt to their own discretion (unless otherwise recommended by their personal clinician) and utilize sports drinks during continuous activity lasting longer than 45 minutes.

4. Be very cognizant of fluid intake in the elderly because of their risk for dehydration and hypernatremia.

## Women and Children

1. Encourage women and children to eat a wide variety of nutrient-dense foods, consume at least 3 servings of dairy daily, and eat iron-rich foods, especially heme iron-rich red meat and dark turkey meat. Other foods rich in iron (although nonheme iron is not absorbed as well) include breakfast cereals, green leafy vegetables, and fortified energy bars.

2. Be very aware of the potential for eating disorders, especially in sports that emphasize leanness. If you suspect disordered eating, seek references such as www.anad.org for help and suggestions on how to approach the person.

3. Test athletes who have disordered eating, the female athlete triad, anorexia, or bulimia for their BMD and BMC. It is important to take steps early to prevent osteoporosis.

## Children

### HYDRATION

Recommendations put forth by the Committee on Sports Medicine and Fitness of the American Academy of Pediatrics for the prevention of heat illness in children are as follows[62]:

1. Children need time to become acclimated to a warmer climate by gradually increasing their level of exposure and of exercise.

2. The duration of exercise and rest periods should be adjusted according to the humidity, air temperature, and degree of sun exposure experienced by the players.

3. Children should be well hydrated before starting prolonged physical activity.

4. They should drink liquids periodically during activities even if they do not feel thirsty: 5 ounces of cold water or a flavored salted beverage such as a sports drink each 20 minutes for a child weighing 40 pounds; 9 ounces every 20 minutes for an adolescent weighing 132 pounds.

5. Clothing should be light-colored, lightweight, and limited to one layer of absorbent fabric to facilitate the evaporation of sweat. If clothes become wet, they should be changed for dry ones.

### ADDITIONAL NUTRITION RECOMMENDATIONS FOR CHILDREN

1. During prolonged, intense exercise, children should consume easily digestible carbohydrate in the form of a sports drink or food between exercise bouts to keep their energy up.

2. Growth charts can be used to plot a child's growth pattern over time thereby helping determine if a child is meeting their nutritional needs. Parents and coaches should also utilize this if a child gets fatigued easily.

## Elderly

1. Ensure that the elderly have access to healthy, nutritious foods because they might not always want to cook, especially if they live alone.

2. Encourage the elderly to take up resistance training; they can still build muscle mass.

## Sidebar 19.3. Steps to Prevent Eating Disorders in Children

*Jessica Setnick, Understanding Nutrition*

1. Don't make disparaging comments on weight, body shapes, or what you or someone else is eating.
2. Throw away your bathroom scale and only weigh children at their medical check-ups.
3. Guide children to follow their own body's signals for when, what, and how much to eat. Teach them to say, "No, thanks" to food that is offered when they're not hungry.
4. When a child or teen announces a decision to change their eating, always ask why. Listen for any ulterior motive that is not food-related, such as "So I'll have more friends" or "So people will like me better."
5. When a child you know is feeling down or disappointed, encourage healthy methods of expression, such as talking, writing, or art, rather than eating or dieting.
6. Seek professional help for any child or teen who seems to be struggling with their weight, shape, or eating. If needed, seek help for yourself in order to be a better role model.

3. Watch for the symptoms of dehydration and hypernatremia in the elderly. Always encourage rest breaks and fluid consumption.
4. To meet nutritional needs, it is vital that the older athlete consume nutrient-dense foods and care for any medical or dental problems that may interfere with their ability to eat a nutritious diet.

## QUESTIONS

1. Dieting can:
   a. Interfere with growth in children
   b. Increase the chance for illness
   c. Make it difficult for the athlete to meet their micronutrient needs
   d. None of the above
   e. All of the above

2. Peak bone mineral density is achieved
   a. By the end of puberty
   b. In middle age
   c. By age 30

3. Symptoms of eating disorders include all of the following except:
   a. Syncope
   b. Lanugo
   c. Hair loss
   d. Flaky skin
   e. Constipation
   f. All are symptoms of an eating disorder

4. Which macronutrient might be needed in greater amounts in younger athletes in comparison to their sedentary peers?
   a. Protein
   b. Fat
   c. Carbohydrate
   d. All of the above

5. Factors that contribute to the female athlete triad include:
   a. Poor coaching
   b. Parents who encourage children who are mildly overweight to lose weight
   c. The belief that if you are menstruating you aren't training enough
   d. None of the above

6. Children are at a greater risk for heat-related illness because they:
   a. Have a smaller body surface area than adults
   b. Have higher sweating rates than adults

   c. Typically exert themselves more than adults
   d. Lower sweating rates than adults

7. Signs of heat illness include all of the following except:
   a. Excessive sweating
   b. Dry skin
   c. Tachycardia
   d. Dizziness
   e. All of the above are signs of heat illness

8. The recommended dietary allowances
   a. Are used when there are not enough data to establish a recommended dietary intake
   b. Provide a range of intakes for a particular energy source that is associated with a reduction in chronic disease risk
   c. Provide the bare minimum each specific age group needs to maintain adequate health
   d. Provide an average daily intake that will meet the nutrient requirements of the majority (97%–98%) of healthy individuals in each age and gender group provided

9. The following things can be done to help prevent eating disorders except:
   a. Don't make disparaging comments about weight
   b. Throw away your bathroom scale
   c. Never make children "clean their plate"
   d. Be aware of non–food-related reasons given for a change in eating
   e. All of the above help prevent eating disorders

10. According to the National Health and Nutrition Examination Survey (NHANES), 1999–2000:
   a. Most children do not consume enough protein
   b. The majority of women do not eat enough calories
   c. Many children do not meet the Adequate Intake for calcium
   d. Many elderly do not meet the recommended dietary allowances for iron

11. An Acceptable Macronutrient Distribution Range is given for:
   a. Fat intake
   b. Iron intake
   c. Vitamin D intake
   d. Protein

12. Much of the data on nutrient intake comes from:
   a. The Youth Behavioral Risk Factor Surveillance System
   b. The National Health and Nutrition Examination Surveys
   c. The National Dietary Assessment Surveys
   d. None of the above

13. The female athlete triad includes all of the following except:
   a. Low calcium intake
   b. Amenorrhea
   c. Disordered eating
   d. Osteoporosis

14. Treatment for those with the female athlete triad includes:
   a. Decrease in training
   b. Increase in calcium intake
   c. Increase in vitamin D intake
   d. Increase in iron intake

15. Which of the following statements are not true?
   a. The elderly are at risk for both hyponatremia and dehydration.
   b. According to government data, many elderly consume less than the Adequate Intake for calcium.
   c. Children are at risk for dehydration.
   d. According to government data, most elderly consume less than the recommended dietary allowances for vitamins.

16. Age-related changes include all of the following except:
    a. Decreased urinary concentration
    b. The elderly should be cautious when exercising in hot, humid weather
    c. The elderly have a reduced water-conservation capacity
    d. The elderly experience increased sweat losses

17. Which of the following is true?
    a. Most of the nutrition requirements for the elderly are related to strength training.
    b. The nutrition requirements for the athletic elderly are not different than their sedentary peers.
    c. Most of the nutrition requirements for the elderly are attributable to age-related changes.
    d. The elderly have all of the same special requirements as premenopausal women.

18. Symptoms of hypernatremia include all of the following except:
    a. Muscle twitching
    b. Fatigue
    c. Confusion
    d. Profuse sweating

19. Which of the following is true?
    a. Exercising in a warm environment helps stimulate thirst in the elderly.
    b. The elderly need to constantly replenish with sports drinks.
    c. Exercise can be especially dangerous for the elderly so care must be taken.
    d. Decreases in blood volume stimulate thirst.

20. Iron
    a. Is a part of myoglobin
    b. Is often deficient in the elderly
    c. Is critical for the metabolism of carbohydrates
    d. Acts as an enzyme in several metabolic reactions

21. Adequacy of a child's growth can be determined by checking it on a growth chart every once in a while.
    a. True
    b. False

22. Although mostly females have eating disorders, the prevalence of disordered eating behaviors among men in very weight-conscious sports is probably fairly high.
    a. True
    b. False

23. Hemoglobin and hematocrit can be used to assess nonanemic iron deficiency.
    a. True
    b. False

24. Most women who have the female athlete triad have anorexia or bulimia.
    a. True
    b. False

25. Boys are at greater risk for dehydration than girls are.
    a. True
    b. False

26. Bone-resorbing osteoclasts remove calcium from the bone matrix.
    a. True
    b. False

27. The elderly have a decreased thirst mechanism.
    a. True
    b. False

28. Many women consume less than the recommended dietary allowances for iron and Adequate Intake for calcium.
   a. True
   b. False

29. The elderly who participate in strength training need substantially more calories than their peers.
   a. True
   b. False

30. Encouraging a child to express themselves by talking, writing, or art when they are feeling down or disappointed, can help with the prevention of an eating disorder.
   a. True
   b. False

# REFERENCES

1. National Sporting Goods Association. 2003 Youth Participation in Selected Sports with Comparisons to 1993. Available at: http://www.nsga.org/public/pages/index.cfm?pageid=158. Accessed September 2004.
2. Unnithan VB, Goulopoulou S. Nutrition for the pediatric athlete. Curr Sports Med Rep 2004;3(4):206–211.
3. American Academy of Pediatrics, Committee on Adolescence. Identifying and treating eating disorders. Pediatrics 2003;111(1):204–211.
4. Schettler AE, Gustafson EM. Osteoporosis prevention starts in adolescence. J Am Acad Nurse Pract 2004;16(7):274–282.
5. Rowland TW, Black SA, Kelleher JF. Iron deficiency in adolescent endurance athletes. J Adolesc Health Care 1987;8(4):322–326.
6. Bar-Or O. Nutritional considerations for the child athlete. Can J Appl Physiol 2001;6(Suppl):S186–S191.
7. Rogol AD, Clark PA, Roemmich JN. Growth and pubertal development in children and adolescents: effects of diet and physical activity. Am J Clin Nutr 2000;72(Suppl):521S–528S.
8. Wahl R. Nutrition in the adolescent. Pediatr Ann 1999;28(2):107–111.
9. Centers for Disease Control. 2000 CDC Growth Charts: United States, May 2004, CDC, National Center for Health Statistics, Health and Nutrition Examination Survey. Available at: http://www.cdc.gov/growthcharts/.
10. Kuczmarski RJ, Ogden CL, Grummer-Strawn LM, et al. CDC growth charts: United States. Adv Data 2000;314:1–27.
11. Exercise and B vitamins. In: Nutrition in Exercise and Sport. 3rd ed. Boca Raton, FL: CRC Press; 1998:179–186.
12. Harvey JS. Nutritional management of the adolescent athlete. Clin Sports Med 1984;3(3):671–679.
13. Lopez-Varela S, Montero A, Chandra RK, Marcos A. Nutritional status of young female elite athletes. Int J Vitam Nutr Res 2000;70(4):185–190.
14. Garner DM, Rosen LW, Barry D. Eating disorders among athletes. Research and recommendations. Child Adolesc Psychiatr Clin North Am 1998;7(4):839–857.
15. West RV. The female athlete: the triad of disordered eating, amenorrhoea and osteoporosis. Sports Med 1998;26(2):63–71.
16. Sherwood NE, Neumark-Sztainer D, Story M, Beuhring T, Resnick MD. Weight-related sports involvement in girls: who is at risk for disordered eating? Am J Health Promot 2002;16(6):341–344.
17. Kiningham RB, Gorenflo DW. Weight loss methods of high school wrestlers. Med Sci Sports Exerc 2001;33(5):810–813.
18. Marquart LF, Sobal J. Weight loss beliefs, practices and support systems for high school wrestlers. J Adolesc Health 1994;15(5):410–415.
19. Roemmich JN, Sinning WE. Weight loss and wrestling training: effects on nutrition, growth, maturation, body composition, and strength. J Appl Physiol 1997;82(6):1751–1759.
20. Johnson C, Powers PS, Dick R. Athletes and eating disorders: the National Collegiate Athletic Association study. Int J Eat Disord 1999;26(2):179–188.
21. West RV. The female athlete. Sports Med 1998;26(2):63–71.
22. Beals KA, Manore MM. Disorders of the female athlete triad among collegiate athletes. Int J Sport Nutr Exerc Metab 2002;12(3):281–293.

23. Johnson MD. Disordered eating in active and athletic women. Clin Sports Med 1994;13:355–369.

24. American Psychiatric Association. Diagnostic and Statistical Manual for Mental Disorders. 4th ed. Washington DC: APA Press; 1994.

25. Food and Nutrition Board, Institute of Medicine. Dietary Reference Intakes for Energy, Carbohydrate, Fiber, Fat, Fatty Acids, Cholesterol, Protein, and Amino Acids (Macronutrients). Washington, DC: The National Academies Press; 2002. Available at: http://books.nap.edu/books/0309085373/html/R1.html#pagetop.

26. Narins DM, Belkengren RP, Sapala S. Nutrition and the growing athlete. Pediatr Nurs 1983;9(3):163–168.

27. Sports Medicine: Health Care for Young Athletes. Elk Grove Village, IL: American Academy of Pediatrics; 1991.

28. Petrie HJ, Stover EA, Horswill CA. Nutritional concerns for the child and adolescent competitor. Nutrition 2004;20(7–8):620–631.

29. Food and Nutrition Board, Institute of Medicine. Dietary Reference Intakes for Calcium, Phosphorus, Magnesium, Vitamin D, and Fluoride. Washington, DC: The National Academies Press; 1997.

30. Food and Nutrition Board, Institute of Medicine. Dietary Reference Intakes for Vitamin A, Vitamin K, Arsenic, Boron, Chromium, Copper, Iodine, Iron, Manganese, Molybdenum, Nickel, Silicon, Vanadium, and Zinc. Washington, DC: The National Academies Press; 2001.

31. Bailey DA, Faulkner RA, McKay HA, Drinkwater RL. Bone mineral acquisition during the adolescent growth spurt. J Bone Miner Res 1996;11:S465.

32. Martin AD, Bailey DA, McKay HA. Bone mineral and calcium accretion during growth. J Bone Miner Res 1996;11:S467.

33. NIH Consensus Development Panel on Optimal Calcium Intake. Optimal calcium intake. J Am Med Assoc 1994;272:1942–1948.

34. Hansen MA, Overgraad K, Riis BJ, Christiansen C. Role of peak bone mass and bone loss in postmenopausal osteoporosis: 12-year study. Br Med J 1991;303:961–964.

35. Mikhail BI. Reduction of risk factors for osteoporosis among adolescents and young adults. Issues Compr Pediatr Nurs 1992;15(4):271–280.

36. Lloyd T, Andon MB, Rollings N, et al. Calcium supplementation and bone mineral density in adolescent girls. JAMA 1993;270(7):841–844.

37. Stear SJ, Prentice A, Jones SC, Cole TJ. Effect of a calcium and exercise intervention on the bone mineral status of 16–18-y-old adolescent girls. Am J Clin Nutr 2003;77(4):985–992.

38. Johnston CC Jr, Miller JZ, Slemenda CW, et al. Calcium supplementation and increases in bone mineral density in children. N Engl J Med 1992;327(2):82–87.

39. Bonjour JP, Chevalley T, Ammann P, Slosman D, Rizzoli R. Gain in bone mineral mass in prepubertal girls 3.5 years after discontinuation of calcium supplementation: a follow-up study. Lancet 2001;358(9289):1208–1212.

40. Cadogan J, Eastell R, Jones N, Barker ME. Milk intake and bone mineral acquisition in adolescent girls: randomised, controlled intervention trial. BMJ 1997;315(7118):1255–1260.

41. Myburgh K, Grobler N, Noakes TD. Factors associated with shin soreness in athletes. Phys Sportsmed 1988;16(4):129–134.

42. Dvorak MM, Riccardi D. Ca2+ as an extracellular signal in bone. Cell Calcium 2004;35(3):249–255.

43. U.S. Department of Health and Human Services. Dietary Intake of Selected Minerals for the United States Population: 1999–2000. Hyattsville, MD: Department of Health and Human Services; Publication No. (PHS) 2004-125004-0304 (4/04).

44. Krause MV, Mahan LK. Minerals. In: Mahan K, Escott-Stump S, eds. Food, Nutrition and Diet Therapy. 11th ed. Philadelphia: WB Saunders; 2003.

45. Brownlie T 4th, Utermohlen V, Hinton PS, Giordano C, Haas JD. Marginal iron deficiency without anemia impairs aerobic adaptation among previously untrained women. Am J Clin Nutr 2002;75(4):734–742.

46. Hinton PS, Giordano C, Brownlie T, Haas JD. Iron supplementation improves endurance after training in iron-depleted, nonanemic women. J Appl Physiol 2000;88(3):1103–1111.

47. Rowland TW, Kelleher JF. Iron deficiency in athletes. Insights from high school swimmers. Am J Dis Child 1989;143(2):197–200.

48. Schoffstall JE, Branch JD, Leutholtz BC, Swain DE. Effects of dehydration and rehydration on the one-repetition maximum bench press of weight-trained males. J Strength Cond Res 2001;15(1):102–108.

49. Bigard AX, Sanchez H, Claveyrolas G, Martin S, Thimonier B, Arnaud MJ. Effects of dehydration and rehydration on EMG changes during fatiguing contractions. Med Sci Sports Exerc 2001;33(10):1694–1700.

50. Walsh RM, Noakes TD, Hawley JA, Dennis SC. Impaired high-intensity cycling performance time at low levels of dehydration. Int J Sports Med 1994;15(7): 392–398.

51. Greenleaf JE, Castle BL. Exercise temperature regulation in man during hypohydration and hyperhydration. J Appl Physiol 1971;30:847–853.

52. Wexler RK. Evaluation and treatment of heat-related illness. Am Fam Physician 2002;65(11):2307–2314.

53. Shibasaki M, Inoue Y, Kondo N, Iwata A. Thermoregulatory responses of prepubertal boys and young men during moderate exercise. Eur J Appl Physiol Occup Physiol 1997;75(3):212–218.

54. Drinkwater BL, Kupprat IC, Denton JE, Crist JL, Horvath SM. Response of prepubertal girls and college women to work in the heat. J Appl Physiol 1977;43:1046–1053.

55. Temperature regulation during exercise in children and adolescents. In: Perspectives in Exercise Sciences and Sports Medicine, II. Youth, Exercise and Sport. Indianapolis: Benchmark Press; 1989:335–367.

56. Delamarche P, Bittel J, Lacour JR, Flandrois R. Thermoregulation at rest and during exercise in prepubertal boys. Eur J Appl Physiol Occup Physiol 1990;60(6): 436–440.

57. Brandt D. Dehydration: examining the examinations—look to signs rather than symptoms when evaluating a child's status. Am J Nurs 2004;104(9):21.

58. Pediatric Nutrition Handbook. 3rd ed. Elk Grove Village, IL: American Academy of Pediatrics; 1991.

59. Passe DH, Horn M, Murray R. Impact of beverage acceptability on fluid intake during exercise. Appetite 2000;35(3):219–229.

60. Passe DH, Horn M, Stofan J, Murray R. Palatability and voluntary intake of sports beverages, diluted orange juice, and water during exercise. Int J Sport Nutr Exerc Metab 2004;14(3):272–284.

61. Costill DL. Heat acclimation: preparing for exercise in hot weather. Sports Med Digest 1989;11(7):3.

62. American Academy of Pediatrics, Committee on Sports Medicine and Fitness. Climatic heat stress and the exercising child and adolescent. Pediatrics 2000;106(1): 158–159.

63. Steinbaugh M. Nutritional needs of female athletes. Clin Sports Med 1984;3(3): 649–670.

64. Manore MM. Nutritional needs of the female athlete. Clin Sports Med 1999;18(3) 549–563.

65. Lauder TD, Dixit S, Pezzin LE, Williams MV, Campbell CS, Davis GD. The relation between stress fractures and bone mineral density: evidence from active-duty Army women. Arch Phys Med Rehabil 2000;81(1):73–79.

66. Reid IR. The roles of calcium and vitamin D in the prevention of osteoporosis. Endocrinol Metab Clin North Am 1998;27:389–398.

67. U.S. Department of Health and Human Services. Dietary Intake of Selected Minerals for the United States Population: 1999–2000. Advance Data from Vital Health Statistics. Washington, DC: Department of Health and Human Services; No. 341, April 27, 2004.

68. Myburgh KH, Hutchins J, Fataar AB, Hough SF, Noakes TD. Low bone density is an etiologic factor for stress fractures in athletes. Ann Intern Med 1990;113(10): 754–759.

69. Malczewska J, Raczynski G, Stupnicki R. Iron status in female endurance athletes and in non-athletes. Int J Sport Nutr Exerc Metab 2000;10(3):260–276.

70. Risser WL, Lee EJ, Poindexter HB, et al. Iron deficiency in female athletes: its prevalence and impact on performance. Med Sci Sports Exerc 1988;20(2):116–121.

71. Tomten SE, Falch JA, Birkeland KI, Hemmersbach P, Hostmark AT. Bone mineral density and menstrual irregularities. A comparative study on cortical and trabecular bone structures in runners with alleged normal eating behavior. Int J Sports Med 1998;19(2):92–97.

72. Gordon N. A review of the female athlete triad (amenorrhea, osteoporosis and disordered eating). Int J Adolesc Med Health 2002;14(1):9–17.

73. Barnes PM, Schoenborn CA. U.S. Department of Health and Human Services. Advance Data from Vital Health Statistics: Physical Activity Among Adults: United States, 2000. Hyattsville, MD: Department of Health and Human Services; Publication No. (PHS) 2003–1250 03–0234; 2003:1–24.

74. Poehlman ET, McAuliffe TL, VanHouten DR. Influence of age and endurance training on resting metabolic rate in women. Med Sci Sports Exerc 1992;24:59–65.

75. Exton-Smith AN. Physiological aspects of aging: relationship to nutrition. Am J Clin Nutr 1980;33:2088–2092.

76. Frontera WR, Meredith CN, O'Reilly KP. Strength conditioning in older men: skeletal muscle hypertrophy and improved function. J Appl Physiol 1988;64:1038–1044.

77. Zheng JJ, Rosenberg IH. What is the nutritional status of the elderly? Geriatrics 1989;44:57–64.

78. Rock CL. Nutrition of the older athlete. Clin Sports Med 1991;10(2):445–456.

79. Campbell WW, Kruskall LJ, Evans WJ. Lower body versus whole body resistive exercise training and energy requirements of older men and women. Metabolism 2002;51(8):989–997.

80. Campbell WW, Trappe TA, Wolfe RR, Evans WJ. The recommended dietary allowance for protein may not be adequate for older people to maintain skeletal muscle. Gerontol A Biol Sci Med Sci 2001;56(6):M373–380.

81. Campbell WW, Trappe TA, Jozsi AC, Kruskall LJ, Wolfe RR, Evans WJ. Dietary protein adequacy and lower body versus whole body resistive training in older humans. J Physiol 2002;542(Pt 2):631–642.

82. Institute of Medicine, Food and Nutrition Board. Dietary Reference Intakes: Calcium, Phosphorus, Magnesium, Vitamin D and Fluoride. Washington, DC: National Academy Press; 1999.

83. Bischoff-Ferrari HA, Dietrich T, Orav EJ, et al. Higher 25-hydroxyvitamin D concentrations are associated with better lower-extremity function in both active and inactive persons aged >60y. Am J Clin Nutr 2004;80(3):752–758.

84. Favus MJ, Christakos S. Primer on the metabolic bone diseases and disorders of mineral metabolism. In: Endocrinology. 3rd ed. Philadelphia: WB Saunders; 1995:1204–1227.

85. Dawson-Hughes B, Harris SS, Krall EA, Dallal GE, Falconer G, Green CL. Rates of bone loss in postmenopausal women randomly assigned to one of two dosages of vitamin D. Am J Clin Nutr 1995;61:1140–1145.

86. LeBoff MS, Kohlmeier L, Hurwitz S, Franklin J, Wright J, Glowacki J. Occult vitamin D deficiency in postmenopausal US women with acute hip fracture. J Am Med Assoc 1999;251:1505–1511.

87. MacLaughin J, Holick MF. Aging decreases capacity of human skin to produce vitamin D3. J Clin Invest 1985;76:1536–1538.

88. Need AG, Morris HA, Horowitz M, Nordin C. Effects of skin thickness, age, body fat, and sunlight on serum 25-hydroxyvitamin D. Am J Clin Nutr 1993;58:882–885.

89. National Center for Health Statistics. Third National Health and Nutrition Examination Survey, 1988–94, Reference Manuals and Reports [http://www.cdc.gov/nchs/about/major/nhanes/datalink.htm#NHANESIII]. Hyattsville, MD: Centers for Disease Control and Prevention; 1996.

90. Moore C, Murphy MM, Keast DR, Holick MF. Vitamin D intake in the United States. J Am Diet Assoc 2004;104:980–983.

91. United States Department of Agriculture, Agricultural Research Service, Food Surveys Research Group. Data [CD-ROM] and documentation for the 1994–96, 1998 Continuing Survey of Food Intakes by Individuals (CSFII). Springfield, VA: National Technical Information Service; Accession No. PB2000-500027; 2000.

92. Kenney WL, Chiu P. Influence of age on thirst and fluid intake. Med Sci Sports Exerc 2001;33(9):1524–1532.

93. Miller M. Hormonal aspects of fluid and sodium balance in the elderly. Endocrinol Metab Clin North Am 1995;24:233–253.

94. Naitoh M, Burrell LM. Thirst in elderly subjects. J Nutr Health Aging 1998;2:172–177.

95. Rolls BJ, Phillips PA. Aging and disturbances of thirst and fluid balance. Nutr Rev 1990;48(3):137–144.

96. Campbell WW. Nutritional considerations for the older athlete. Nutrition 2004;20(7–8):603–608.

97. Hoffman R, Heidrick E, Benz E, Myers J, Shattil SJ, Willerson JT, Cohn JN. Hematology: Basic Principles and Practice. New York: Churchill Livingstone; 2004.

# PART IV

# Supplements

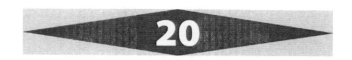

# Sports Applications of Creatine

## Richard B. Kreider

## OBJECTIVES

On the completion of this chapter you will be able to:

1. Understand the biochemical basis for the role of creatine in the body.
2. Recognize the dietary sources of creatine and how different dietary regimes will enhance creatine content of muscle.
3. Differentiate among the different supplementation regimes presented in the literature.
4. Understand the effects of various creatine supplementation regimes on muscular stores of creatine and phosphocreatine.
5. Explain the different theoretical rationales for why creatine supplementation might be an effective ergogenic aid.
6. Describe the ergogenic benefits most noted in the scientific literature.
7. Examine the potential clinical or therapeutic uses of creatine supplements.
8. Discuss the ethical issues involved in creatine supplementation.
9. Understand the best practices used for creatine supplementation: loading, maintenance, dosage, timing, and type of creatine supplements.
10. Discuss the differences between the lay media's reports on creatine safety and the data presented in the scientific literature.

## ABSTRACT

Creatine remains one of the most extensively studied nutritional ergogenic aids available for athletes. Hundreds of studies have reported that increasing muscle creatine stores through creatine supplementation can augment muscle creatine content, improve exercise and training adaptations, and/or provide some therapeutic benefit to some clinical populations. Consequently, creatine represents one of the most effective and popular nutritional ergogenic aids available for athletes. The future of creatine research is very promising. Researchers are attempting to determine ways to maximize creatine storage in the muscle, which types of exercise may obtain the greatest benefit from creatine supplementation, the potential medical uses of creatine, and the long-term safety and efficacy of creatine supplementation. Among these, the most promising area of research is determining the potential medical uses of creatine, particularly in patients with creatine synthesis deficiencies and neuromuscular diseases. Nevertheless, in regard to athletes, creatine has continually proved itself to be one of the most effective and safe nutritional supplements to increase strength, muscle mass, and performance. This is despite oftentimes inaccurate and misleading information that has been written about creatine in the popular media over the last several years.

From: *Essentials of Sports Nutrition and Supplements*
Edited by J. Antonio, D. Kalman, J. R. Stout, M. Greenwood, D. S. Willoughby, and
G. G. Haff © Humana Press, a part of Springer Science+Business Media, Totowa, NJ

*Key Words:* creatine, phosphagen, creatine phosphate, amino acid, hydration, ergogenic aid

During brief explosive exercise lasting 0–15 seconds, the energy supplied to rephosphorylate adenosine diphosphate to adenosine triphosphate (ATP) is dependent to a large degree on the amount of phosphocreatine (PCr) stored in the muscle.[1,2] As PCr stores become depleted during explosive exercise, energy availability deteriorates because of the inability to resynthesize ATP at the rate required.[1,2] Consequently, the ability to maintain maximal-effort exercise declines. Because the availability of PCr in the muscle may significantly influence the amount of energy generated during brief periods of high-intensity exercise, it has been hypothesized that increasing muscle creatine content via creatine supplementation may increase the availability of PCr and allow for an accelerated rate of resynthesis of ATP during and following high-intensity, short-duration exercises.[1–7] Theoretically, creatine supplementation during training may lead to greater training adaptations because of an enhanced quality and volume of work performed. The purpose of this chapter is to overview the available literature regarding the effects of creatine supplementation on muscle bioenergetics and training adaptations, potential medical uses of creatine, and medical safety of creatine. Additionally, a number of common questions about creatine supplementation are answered.

## REVIEW OF LITERATURE

### Background

Creatine is a naturally occurring amino acid–like compound that is found primarily in the muscle (95%). There is also a small amount of creatine in the brain and testes (5%).[3,8] About two thirds of creatine found in the muscle is stored as PCr whereas the remaining amount of creatine is stored as free creatine.[8] The total creatine pool (PCr + free creatine) in the muscle averages about 120 g for a 70-kg individual. However, the body has the capacity to store up to 160 g of creatine under certain conditions.[8] The body breaks down about 1%–2% of the creatine pool per day (about 2 g) into creatinine in the muscle. The creatinine is then excreted in urine.[9] The body can replenish depleted creatine in two ways. First, about half of the daily creatine need can be obtained from the normal diet by eating foods that contain creatine. For example, there is about 1–2 g of creatine in a pound of uncooked beef and salmon.[3] The remaining amount of creatine is synthesized from the amino acids glycine, arginine, and methionine (Figure 20.1).[10,11] Normal dietary intake of creatine from food and creatine synthesis typically maintains creatine levels at about 120 g for a normal-size individual (Table 20.1).[10,11] Vegetarians have been reported to have

**FIGURE 20.1.** Biochemical pathway for creatine synthesis.

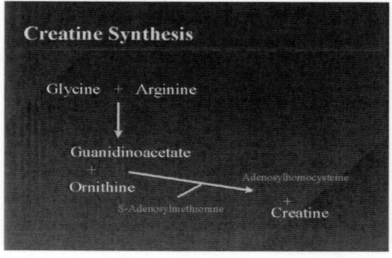

**TABLE 20.1.** Creatine content in selected foods.

| | Creatine content | |
|---|---|---|
| Food | g/lb. | g/kg |
| Shrimp | Trace | Trace |
| Cod | 1.4 | 3 |
| Tuna | 1.8 | 4 |
| Salmon | 2 | 4.5 |
| Herring | 3–4.5 | 6.5–10 |
| Beef | 2 | 4.5 |
| Pork | 2.3 | 5 |
| Cranberries | 0.01 | 0.02 |
| Milk | 0.05 | 0.1 |

*Source:* Adapted from Balsom et al.[3]

lower than normal muscle creatine stores.[12] Additionally, some people have been found to have creatine synthesis deficiencies and therefore must depend on dietary creatine intake to maintain normal muscle concentrations.[13,14]

Most research on creatine has evaluated the effects of creatine supplementation on the content of high-energy phosphates within muscle and its role on exercise capacity and recovery during sprint exercise dependent on the phosphagen energy system.[11,15] However, recent attention has also been given to the role of creatine supplementation on creatine kinases (CK) in muscle as well as the transfer of high-energy phosphates within the cell via what has been called the creatine phosphate shuttle (Figure 20.2).[16–18] CK is an important cellular enzyme that facilitates energy transduction in muscle cells by catalyzing the reversible transfer of a phosphate moiety between ATP and PCr.[19] There are several isoforms of CK that work simultaneously to form a rapid interconversion of PCr and ATP. In this regard, CK is composed of two subunit types including M (muscle) and B (brain) with three isoenzymes, MM-CK, MB-CK, and BB-CK. In addition, a fourth CK isoenzyme (Mi-CK) is located on the outer side of the inner mitochondrial membrane.[19–21] CK activity is greatest in skeletal muscle and CK in the muscle exists almost exclusively in the MM form. MM-CK (also referred to as myofibrillar CK) is bound to the myofibrils and localized to the A bands as well as being distributed across the entire filament. MM-CK generates ATP from adenosine diphosphate. Mi-CK is found on the

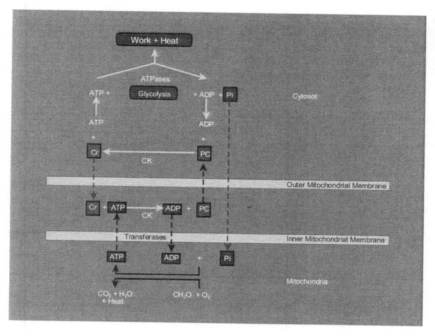

**FIGURE 20.2.** Basic diagram of the creatine phosphate shuttle. ATP = adenosine triphosphate, ATPase = adenosine triphosphatase, ADP = adenosine diphosphate, Cr = creatinine, PC = phosphocreatine, CK = creatine kinase.

outer surface of the inner mitochondrial membrane and is functionally coupled to oxidative phosphorylation. Mi-CK, at the site of oxidative mitochondrial ATP generation, catalyses the phosphorylation of creatine to PCr.[19-21] Fast-twitch fibers have greater CK activity, containing large amounts of MM-CK, than slow-twitch oxidative fibers, but the latter have a higher percentage of Mi-CK.[19-22] Recent studies suggest that dietary and muscle availability of creatine may influence CK activity in various populations.[18,23-29]

From an ergogenic viewpoint, resynthesis of PCr could be the critical factor during sustained very high-intensity exercise. Although the mechanisms are not clearly understood, a creatine phosphate shuttle may be the functional mechanism.[21,30] In addition to its role as an energy buffer, it has been proposed that the CK-PCr system functions in energy transport on the basis of the functional and physical association of CK isoenzymes with subcellular sites of ATP production and hydrolysis. In the creatine phosphate shuttle concept, PCr and Cr act as shuttle molecules between these sites.[22] One proposed shuttle is believed to be functionally coupled to glycolysis,[22] but others believe that the rapid resynthesis of PCr is likely to be oxidative in origin.[19,31,32] Mi-CK promotes the formation of PCr from creatine and from ATP formed via oxidative metabolism in the mitochondria.[21] van Deursen and others[22] note that PCr is presumed to diffuse from the mitochondria to the myofibrillar M band, where it locally serves to replenish ATP with MM-CK as catalyzing agent. Finally, Cr diffuses back to sites of ATP synthesis for rephosphorylation. The potential role of modulating CK activity and the shuttling of adenine nucleotides for synthesis and use has prompted a significant amount of research evaluating the potential clinical uses of creatine as described below. Additionally, because creatine seems to have a role in shuttling of ATP from the mitochondria to the cytosol, it may also be involved in enhancing high-intensity aerobic exercise capacity.[18,21]

## Supplementation Protocols

The most common way described in the scientific literature to increase muscle creatine stores is to "load" creatine by taking 0.3 g/kg/day of creatine monohydrate for 5–7 days (e.g., 5 g taken 4 times per day).[11,33] Studies show that this protocol can increase muscle creatine and PCr by 10%–40%.[33] Studies indicate that, once muscle creatine stores are saturated, you only need to take 3–5 g of creatine monohydrate per day to maintain elevated creatine stores. More recent studies indicate that it may only take 2–3 days to maximize creatine stores, particularly if creatine is ingested with carbohydrate and/or protein.[5,34,35] An alternative supplementation protocol is to ingest 3 g/day of creatine monohydrate for 28 days.[8] Studies show that this method can increase muscle concentrations of creatine as effectively as creatine loading techniques. However, this method would only result in a gradual increase in muscle creatine content compared with the more rapid loading method. Willoughby and Rosene[36] reported that 6 g/day of creatine during 12 weeks of training was sufficient to promote positive changes in strength and muscle mass. Some athletes also cycle on and off creatine by taking loading doses of creatine monohydrate for 3–5 days every 3–4 weeks during training.[11,33] Theoretically, because it takes 4–6 weeks for elevated creatine stores to return to baseline, this protocol would be effective in increasing and maintaining elevated creatine stores over time.[11]

## Sidebar 20.1. Creatine Supplementation Protocols

- Loading/maintenance protocol
  - Ingest 0.3 g/kg/day (15–25 g/day) for 5–7 days
  - Ingest 3–5 g/day to maintain
- High-dose protocol
  - Ingest 15–25 g/day (0.3 g/kg/day) during training
- Low-dose protocol
  - Ingest 3–6 g/day during training
- Cycling protocol
  - Load/maintain during training and reduce/abstain between training periods

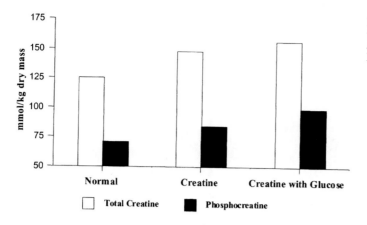

**FIGURE 20.3.** Average change in concentrations of muscle creatine and phosphocreatine after creatine supplementation with or without large amounts of added glucose.

## Effects of Creatine Supplementation on Muscle Creatine Stores

Numerous studies indicate that dietary supplementation of creatine monohydrate increases muscle creatine and PCr content by 10%–40% (Figure 20.3).[8,33] In simple terms, one can think of the normal creatine content of the muscle (about 120 g) as being a gas tank that is normally about three-fourths full. Creatine supplementation typically allows an individual to fill up their creatine storage tank up to 150–160 g (i.e., 20%–30%). It should be noted that the amount of creatine retained in the muscle after creatine supplementation depends on the amount of creatine in the muscle before supplementation. Individuals with low creatine content in muscle before supplementation may increase creatine stores by 20%–40% whereas individuals with relatively high creatine levels before supplementation may only experience a 10%–20% increase in muscle creatine content. Performance changes in response to creatine supplementation have been correlated with the magnitude of increase in muscle creatine levels.[37,38] Once creatine levels are elevated and an individual stops taking creatine, studies indicate it may take 4–6 weeks before creatine levels return to baseline.[39] There is no evidence that muscle creatine levels decrease below baseline after cessation of creatine supplementation which might suggest a long-term suppression of endogenous creatine synthesis.[33,40]

## Theoretical Benefits of Creatine Supplementation

Increasing muscle availability of creatine and PCr can affect exercise and training adaptations in several ways (Table 20.2). First, increasing the availability of PCr in the muscle may help maintain availability of energy during high-intensity exercise such as sprinting and intense weightlifting. Second, increasing the availability of PCr may help speed recovery between sprints and/or bouts of intense exercise. These adaptations would allow an athlete to do more work over a series of sprints and/or sets of exercise, theoretically leading to greater gains in strength, muscle mass, and/or performance over time. For this reason, creatine supplementation has primarily been recommended as an ergogenic aid for power/strength athletes. However, recent research indicates that endurance athletes may also benefit from creatine supplementation. In this regard, studies indicate creatine loading before carbohydrate loading promotes greater glycogen retention.[41] Additionally, studies indicate that ingesting creatine with carbohydrate during carbohydrate loading promotes greater creatine and glycogen retention.[35,42–44] Theoretically, this may improve glycogen availability for endurance athletes. Creatine has also been shown to improve repetitive sprint performance. Because endurance athletes use interval training techniques in an attempt to improve speed and anaerobic threshold, creatine supplementation during training may improve interval training adaptations leading to improved performance. Finally, studies also indicate that creatine supplementation can help maintain body weight and muscle mass during training.[15,39,45–48] Because many endurance athletes have difficulty maintaining body mass during training, creatine supplementation may help maintain optimal body composition.

TABLE 20.2. Examples of sports performance theoretically enhanced by creatine supplementation.

Increased PCr
    Track sprints: 100, 200 meters
    Swim sprints: 50 meters
    Pursuit cycling

Increased PCr resynthesis
    Basketball
    Field hockey
    Football (American)
    Ice hockey
    Lacrosse
    Volleyball

Reduced muscle acidosis
    Downhill skiing
    Rowing
    Swim events: 100, 200 meters
    Track events: 400, 800 meters

Oxidative metabolism
    Basketball
    Soccer
    Team handball
    Tennis
    Volleyball
    Interval training in endurance athletes

Enhanced training
    Most sports

Increased body mass/muscle mass
    American, Australian football
    Bodybuilding
    Heavyweight wrestling
    Power lifting
    Rugby
    Track/field events (shot put, javelin, discus)
    Weightlifting

*Source:* Williams MH, Kreider R, Branch JD. Creatine: the power supplement. Champaign, IL: Human Kinetics Publishers; 1999.
PCr = phosphocreatine.

## Sidebar 20.2. Potential Ergogenic Benefits of Creatine Supplementation

- Increased muscle mass and strength
- Increased single and repetitive sprint performance
- Enhanced glycogen synthesis
- Possible enhancement of aerobic capacity via greater shuttling of ATP from mitochondria and buffering of acidity

- Increased work capacity
- Enhanced recovery
- Greater training tolerance

### Effects of Creatine on Exercise Performance or Training Adaptations

As of this writing, there have been about 1000 articles published in the peer-reviewed scientific literature on creatine supplementation. Slightly more than half of these studies have evaluated the effects of creatine supplementation on exercise performance. The majority of these studies (about 70%) indicate that creatine supplementation promotes a statistically significant improvement in exercise capacity.[15] This means that 95 times out of 100, if you take creatine as described in the study, you will experience an improvement in exercise performance. The average gain in performance from these studies typically ranges between 10% to 15%. For example, short-term creatine supplementation has been reported to improve maximal power/strength (5%–15%), work performed during sets of maximal-effort muscle contractions (5%–15%), single-effort sprint performance (1%–5%), and work performed during repetitive sprint performance (5%–15%).[15] Long-term creatine supplementation seems to enhance the quality of training generally leading to 5%–15% greater gains in strength and performance.[15] Nearly all studies indicate that creatine supplementation increases body mass by about 1–2 kg in the first week of loading.[15] In training studies, subjects taking creatine typically gain about twice as much body mass and/or fat-free mass (FFM) (i.e., an extra 2–4 pounds of muscle mass during 4–12 weeks of training) than subjects taking a placebo. No study has reported that creatine supplementation significantly impairs exercise capacity. Although not all studies report significant results, the preponderance of scientific evidence indicates that creatine supplementation seems to be an effective nutritional ergogenic aid for a variety of exercise tasks in a number of athletic and clinical populations.[11,15] The following highlights some of the recent research that has evaluated the effects of short- and long-term creatine supplementation on exercise performance and/or training adaptations.

## SHORT-TERM SUPPLEMENTATION

Numerous studies have been conducted to evaluate the effects of short-term creatine supplementation (3–7 days) on exercise performance. For example, Volek and colleagues[49] reported that creatine supplementation (25 g/day for 7 days) resulted in a significant increases in the amount of work performed during 5 sets of bench press and jump squats in comparison to a placebo group. Tarnopolsky and MacLennan[50] reported creatine supplementation (20 g/day × 4 days) increased peak cycling power, dorsiflexion maximal voluntary contractions torque, and lactate in men and women with no apparent gender effects. Moreover, Wiroth and colleagues[51] reported that creatine supplementation (15 g/day × 5 days) significantly improved maximal power and work performed during 5 × 10-s cycling sprints with 60-s rest recovery in younger and older subjects.

Creatine supplementation has also been shown to improve exercise performance during various sports activities. For example, Skare and associates[52] reported that creatine supplementation (20 g/day) decreased 100-m sprint times and reduced the total time of 6 × 60-m sprints in a group of well-trained adolescent competitive runners. Mujika and colleagues[53] reported that creatine supplementation (20 g/day × 6 days) improved repeated sprint performance (6 × 15-m sprints with 30-s recovery) and limited the decay in jumping ability in 17 highly trained soccer players. Similarly, Ostojic[54] reported that creatine supplementation (30 g/day for 7 days) improved soccer-specific skill performance in young soccer players. Theodorou et al.[55] reported that creatine supplementation (25 g/day × 4 days) significantly improved mean interval performance times in 22 elite swimmers. Mero and colleagues[56] reported that supplementation of creatine (20 g/day) for 6 days combined with sodium bicarbonate (0.3 g/kg) ingestion 2 hours before exercise significantly improved 2 × 100-m swim performance. Finally, Preen and associates[57] evaluated the effects of ingesting creatine (20 g/day × 5 days) on resting and postexercise creatine and PCr content as well as performance of an 80-minute intermittent sprint test (10 sets of 5–6 × 6-s sprints with varying recovery intervals). The authors reported that creatine increased resting and postexercise creatine and PCr content, mean work performed, and total work performed during 6 × 6-s sets with 54-s and 84-s recovery. In addition, work performed during 5 × 6-s sprints with 24-s recovery tended to be greater. Collectively, these findings and many others indicate that creatine supplementation can significantly improve performance of athletes in a variety of sport-related field activities.

## LONG-TERM SUPPLEMENTATION

Theoretically, increasing the ability to perform high-intensity exercise may lead to greater training adaptations over time. Consequently, a number of studies have evaluated the effects of creatine supplementation on training adaptations. For example, Vandenberghe et al.[39] reported that in comparison to a placebo group, creatine supplementation (20 g/day × 4 days; 5 g/day × 65 days) during 10-weeks of training in women increased total creatine and PCr content, maximal strength (20%–25%), maximal intermittent exercise capacity of the arm flexors (10%–25%), and FFM by 60%. In addition, the researchers reported that creatine supplementation during 10 weeks of detraining helped maintain training adaptations to a greater degree. Noonan and collaborators[58] reported that creatine supplementation (20 g/day × 5 days; 0.1 or 0.3 g/kg/day of FFM × 51 d) in conjunction with resistance and speed/agility training significantly improved 40-yard-dash time and bench press strength in 39 college athletes. Kreider and associates[47] reported that creatine supplementation (15.75 g/day × 28 days) during off-season college football training promoted greater gains in FFM and repetitive sprint performance in comparison to subjects ingesting a placebo. Likewise, Stone et al.[46] reported that 5 weeks of creatine ingestion (~10 or 20 g/day with and without pyruvate) promoted significantly greater increases in body mass, FFM, 1 repetition maximum (RM) bench press, combined 1 RM squat and bench press, vertical jump power output, and peak rate of force development during in-season training in 42 Division IAA college football players.

Volek and coworkers[45] reported that 12 weeks of creatine supplementation (25 g/day × 7 days; 5 g/day × 77 days) during periodized resistance training increased muscle total creatine and PCr, FFM, type I, IIa, and IIb muscle fiber diameter, bench press and squat 1 RM, and lifting volume (weeks 5–8) in 19 resistance-trained athletes. Kirksey and colleagues[59] found that creatine supplementation (0.3 g/kg/day × 42 days) during off-season training promoted greater gains in vertical jump height and power, sprint cycling performance, and FFM in 36 Division IAA male and female track and field athletes. Moreover, Jones and collaborators[60] reported that creatine (20 g/day × 5 days; 5 g/day × 10 weeks) promoted greater gains in sprint performance (5 × 15 s with 15-s recovery) and average on-ice sprint performance (6 × 80-m sprints) in 16 elite ice-hockey players. Interestingly, Jowko et al.[61] reported that creatine supplementation (20 g/day × 7 days; 10 g/day × 14 days) significantly increased FFM and cumulative strength gains during training in 40 subjects initiating training. Additional gains were observed when 3 g/day of calcium beta-hydroxy-beta-methylbutyrate (HMB) was coingested with creatine. Finally, Willougby and Rosene[36] reported that in comparison to controls, creatine supplementation (6 g/day × 12 weeks) during resistance training (6–8 repetitions at 85%–90%); 3 × weeks (three times per week) significantly increased total body mass, FFM, and thigh volume, 1 RM strength, myofibrillar protein content, type I, IIa, and IIx myosin heavy chain mRNA expression, and myosin heavy chain protein expression. In a subsequent article, Willoughby and Rosene[24] reported that Cr supplementation (6 g/day × 12 weeks) increased M-CK mRNA expression apparently as a result of increases in the expression of myogenin and MRF-4. The researchers concluded that increases in myogenin and MRF-4 mRNA and protein may have a role in increasing myosin heavy chain expression. These data indicate that creatine supplementation can directly influence muscle protein synthesis. Collectively, these studies and others provide strong evidence that creatine supplementation during intense resistance training leads to greater gains in strength and muscle mass.

## Potential Therapeutic Uses of Creatine

Creatine and creatine phosphate are involved in numerous metabolic processes. Creatine synthesis deficiencies and/or abnormal availability of creatine and PCr have been reported to cause a number of medical problems. For this reason, the potential medical uses of creatine have been investigated since the mid 1970s. Initially, research focused on the role of creatine and/or creatine phosphate in reducing heart arrhythmias and/or improving heart function during ischemia events (i.e., lack of oxygen).[11] Initial studies also evaluated the effects of treating various medical populations who had creatine deficiencies (gyrate atrophy,[62-65] infants and children with low levels of PCr in the brain,[66–68] etc). Interest in the potential medical uses of creatine has increased over the last 10 years. Researchers have been particularly interested in determining whether creatine supplementation may reduce rates of atrophy and/or muscle wasting; speed the rate of recovery from musculoskeletal and/or spinal cord injuries; and improve strength and muscle endurance in patients with various neuromuscular diseases.[11,33] For example, researchers have been evaluating whether creatine supplementation may improve clinical outcomes in patients with brain and/or spinal cord injuries,[69–73] muscular dystrophy,[28,74,75] myopathies,[26,76–79] Huntington's disease,[29,80–82] amyotrophic lateral sclerosis or Lou Gehrig's disease,[83–86] arthritis,[87] diabetes,[88] high cholesterol and triglyceride levels,[47,89] and elevated homocysteine levels.[90–93] Other studies have reported that creatine supplementation during training reduces injury rates in athletes[94–98] and/or allows athletes to tolerate intensified training to a greater degree.[99] Although more research is needed, some promising results have been reported in a number of clinically related studies suggesting that creatine may have therapeutic benefit in certain patient populations.

# COMMON QUESTIONS ABOUT CREATINE

## Are There Any Side Effects of Creatine?

The only clinically significant side effect that has been consistently reported in the scientific and medical literature from creatine supplementation has been weight gain.[11,33,100] However, there have been a number of anecdotally reported side effects reported in the popular literature such as gastrointestinal distress, muscle cramping, dehydration, and increased risk to musculoskeletal injury (i.e., muscle strains/pulls). Additionally, there has also been concern that short- and/or long-term creatine supplementation may increase renal stress and/or adversely affect the muscles, liver, or other organs of the body. One research group suggested that creatine supplementation may increase anterior compartment pressure in the leg thereby increasing an individual's risk of developing anterior compartment syndrome.[101,102] Over the last few years, a number of studies have attempted to assess the medical safety of creatine. These studies indicate that creatine is not associated with any of these anecdotally reported problems, and that creatine does not increase the likelihood of developing anterior compartment syndrome.[95,103–111] In fact, there is recent evidence that creatine may lessen heat stress and reduce the susceptibility to musculoskeletal injuries among athletes engaged in training.[95,110,111] Although people who take creatine may experience some of these problems, the incidence of occurrence in creatine users does not seem to be greater than in subjects who take placebos, and in some cases has been reported to be less.[104]

## What Is the Best Form of Creatine to Take?

Nearly all studies on creatine supplementation have evaluated pharmacologic-grade creatine monohydrate in powder form or have used oral or intravenous PCr formulations (a more expensive form of creatine). However, because creatine has become a popular supplement, there are a number of different forms of creatine that have been marketed (e.g., creatine candy/bars, liquid creatine, creatine gum, creatine citrate, and effervescent creatine). Many of these forms of creatine claim to be better than creatine monohydrate. However, no data indicate that any of these forms of creatine increases creatine uptake to the muscle better than creatine monohydrate. In fact, a recent study indicates that liquid creatine has no effect on muscle creatine stores.[112] A few published studies have compared the ergogenic value of several of these types of supplements to creatine monohydrate. However, results have generally indicated that although some of these supplements (i.e., creatine candy, creatine gum, and effervescent creatine) can improve exercise capacity, they do not seem to work any better than creatine monohydrate.[47,112-115] Consequently, the only potential benefits that one may derive from many of these different forms of creatine would seemingly be convenience, supplement variety, and/or taste preferences. The greatest disadvantage, however, is that many of these supplements are more expensive than creatine monohydrate. There is absolutely no evidence that you can take less of these types of supplements (e.g., liquid creatine or effervescent creatine) and get the same benefits than ingesting higher amounts of creatine monohydrate supplementation because of less degradation in the stomach, greater intestinal absorption, faster absorption in the blood, and/or greater muscle uptake. Finally, there are three primary sources for creatine (i.e., Germany, United States, and China). Independent testing has revealed that Chinese sources of creatine may have less purity and/or contain higher amounts of contaminants such as dicyandiamide, dihydrotriazine, and/or creatinine (converted form of creatine).[116,117] The best raw sources of creatine monohydrate seem to be from Germany (e.g., Degussa's CreaPure) or the United States (e.g., Ferro Pfansteihl). Care should be taken to only purchase high-quality creatine monohydrate that is produced in inspected facilities that adhere to Food and Drug Administration good manufacturing practice guidelines.

## Should Athletes Load or Not Load?

Research has shown that the most rapid way to increase muscle creatine stores is to follow the loading method described above. Most of the creatine is taken up by muscle during the first 2–3 days of the loading period. Although there is one study that suggests that taking lower doses of creatine over time (3 g/day for 28 days) increased muscle creatine content,[8] it is less clear whether this low-dose protocol enhances exercise capacity. There are only a few well-controlled studies that reported that low-dose creatine supplementation (5–6 g/day of creatine for 10–12 weeks) promoted greater gains in strength and muscle mass during training.[24,36,118] However, several other studies found no effect of low-dose (2–3 g/day), long-term creatine supplementation on exercise capacity. Consequently, it seems that the most effective way to increase creatine stores is to follow the creatine loading technique for at least 3 days followed by ingestion of 3–5 g/day thereafter to maintain creatine stores.

## Should Athletes Take Creatine Alone or with Other Nutrients?

There has been considerable interest in finding ways to enhance muscle uptake of creatine. Many commercially available supplements boast of new, improved transport systems that optimize creatine storage via greater intestinal and/or muscle uptake. The question then arises whether coingesting creatine with other nutrients enhances creatine uptake and/or effectiveness. Before this question is answered, it is important that you know some of the creatine basics. First, research since the early 1900s has indicated that orally ingested creatine monohydrate is absorbed intact through the intestine into the blood.[1,119-123] The creatine is then either taken up by the muscle or excreted as creatine in the urine. Creatine is not degraded into creatinine in the stomach and intestinal absorption is not a limiting factor to muscle uptake of creatine.[124] In fact, one of the ways that muscle creatine storage can be measured is by subtracting urine creatine output from oral creatine intake.[9,113,125] If a significant amount of creatine was digested or degraded to creatinine in the stomach (its only known byproduct), these measurements would be invalid. Second, creatine uptake into the muscle has been reported to be sodium dependent and mediated by insulin.[42,43,126-129] This means that ingesting creatine with large amounts of glucose (e.g., 80–100 g) or carbohydrate/protein (e.g., 50–80 g of carbohydrate with 30–50 g of protein), which is known to increase blood insulin levels, may be an effective way to enhance creatine uptake.[34,112,113,130,131] There is also evidence that coingesting creatine with D-pinitol may augment creatine uptake into muscle.[113] Consequently, it is recommended that athletes take creatine with a high-carbohydrate drink (e.g., juice or concentrated carbohydrate solution) or with a carbohydrate/protein supplement in order to increase insulin and promote creatine uptake.

## When Is the Best Time to Take Creatine?

Research indicates that intense exercise increases anabolic hormone release. Additionally, ingesting carbohydrate and protein or essential amino acids after intense exercise may accelerate glycogen resynthesis as well as promote protein synthesis.[132–136] The primary mechanism seems to be related to a carbohydrate- and protein-stimulated increase in insulin as well as stimulation of protein synthesis by essential amino acids.[132,133,135,136] Because insulin levels enhance creatine uptake, ingestion of creatine after exercise with a carbohydrate and/or protein supplement may be an effective way to increase and/or maintain muscle creatine stores.

## Should Athletes Cycle On and Off Creatine?

There is no evidence that cycling on and off creatine is more or less effective than loading and maintaining creatine. However, the greatest benefits of creatine supplementation seem to be to enhance training adaptations.[15,99] Therefore, if an athlete wants to cycle creatine, it would seemingly be more effective to take creatine when they are involved in heavy training and not take it between training phases.

## Does Caffeine or Acidity Affect Creatine?

Athletes often ask whether creatine can be taken with caffeine or whether mixing creatine with acidic drinks will degrade creatine. There are several studies that indicate that coingesting creatine with large amounts of caffeine may negate some of the performance-enhancing effects of creatine supplementation.[137–140] For this reason, many have warned not to take creatine with caffeine. However, many of the initial studies on creatine mixed creatine in hot coffee or tea to help dissolve the creatine. Additionally, these studies indicated that caffeine did not affect muscle uptake of creatine. Consequently, it is my view that this concern is somewhat overstated. Some have also warned that mixing creatine in acidic solutions (e.g., juices) may degrade creatine to creatinine. Yet, the acid level (pH) of coffee (about 4.5), grape juice (about 3), and orange juice (about 2.8) is less acidic than gastrointestinal secretions (about 1) and the acid in the stomach (about 1.5). It is well established that creatine is not degraded through the normal digestive process.[9] Moreover, a number of creatine studies instructed the subjects to mix creatine with juice and reported ergogenic benefit. Therefore, it is unlikely that mixing creatine in fruit juice would degrade creatine unless you let it sit for several days.

## Do Men and Women Respond Differently to Creatine Supplementation?

About a third of the studies on creatine have evaluated its use in women and/or mixed cohorts of men and women. Several initial short-term studies conducted on female athletes revealed limited ergogenic value. This led some researchers to question whether women respond to creatine differently than men. However, a number of recent well-controlled short- and long-term studies in women have reported ergogenic benefits.[50] In our research, we have found that women typically observe ergogenic benefit after short-term supplementation. However, gains in body mass and FFM are generally are not as rapid as men. Nevertheless, women do gain strength and muscle mass over time during training. Survey research has indicated that men tend to be more interested in creatine supplementation than women.[96,141–143] The primary reason why women are less interested in creatine supplementation seems to be attributable to a fear of excessive gains in weight and/or muscularity.[96,141–143]

## Weight Gain Derived from Creatine Ingestion: Is It Water or Muscle?

As stated above, creatine supplementation typically promotes gains in body mass and/or FFM. Some have suggested that because the gains are fairly rapid, that the gains observed must be attributable to fluid retention. Although it is generally accepted that the initial weight gain may promote some water retention, a number of recent studies do not support this concept. In this regard, most studies that have evaluated the effects of creatine supplementation on fluid retention and body composition indicate that although total body water increases, the increase seems to be proportional to the weight gained. In this regard, muscle is about 73% water. Therefore, if someone gained 10 pounds of muscle, 7.3 pounds of the weight gain would be water and the percentage of total body water would not be changed. Numerous studies report that long-term creatine increases FFM without an increase in the percent of total body water. Additionally, several studies have found that these gains were accompanied by increased muscle fiber diameter (hypertrophy) and gains in strength.[24,36,45] Consequently, it seems that the weight gain associated with long-term creatine supplementation is muscle mass.

## Should Children or Teenagers Take Creatine?

No study has indicated that creatine supplementation could be harmful for children or adolescent athletes. In fact, long-term creatine supplementation (e.g., 4–8 g/day for up to 3 years) has been used as an adjunctive therapy for a number of creatine synthesis deficiencies and neuromuscular disorders in children. However, it should be noted that much less is known about the effects of creatine supplementation in younger individuals. Consequently, it is my view that adolescent athletes should *only* consider taking creatine *if* the following conditions hold true:

1. The athlete is past puberty and is involved in serious/competitive training that may benefit from creatine supplementation;
2. The athlete is eating a well-balanced, performance-enhancing diet;
3. The athlete and his/her parents understand the potential benefits and side effects of creatine supplementation;
4. The athlete's parents approve that their child takes creatine;
5. That creatine supplementation can be supervised by the athlete's parents, trainers, coaches, and/or physician;
6. That quality supplements are used; and
7. The athlete does not exceed recommended dosages.

If these conditions are met, then I personally do not see a reason why high school athletes should not be able to take creatine. Doing so may actually provide a safe nutritional alternative to anabolic steroids or other potentially ineffective or dangerous supplements or drugs. If these conditions are not met, then I do not believe that creatine supplementation would be appropriate unless prescribed by their physician. To me, this is no different than teaching young athletes proper training and dietary strategies to optimize performance. Creatine is not a panacea or short cut to athletic success. It can, however, offer some benefits to optimize training of athletes involved in intense exercise in a similar manner that ingesting a high-carbohydrate diet, sports drinks, and/or carbohydrate loading can optimize performance of an endurance athlete.

## Is Long-Term Creatine Supplementation Safe?

Athletes have been using creatine as a nutritional supplement since the mid-1960s. Widespread use as a dietary supplement began in the early 1990s. No clinically significant and reproducible side effects directly attributable to creatine supplementation have been reported in the scientific literature. Nevertheless, there are some concerns about the long-term side effects of creatine supplementation. Over the last few years, a number of researchers have begun to report long-term safety data on creatine supplementation. So far, no long-term side effects have been observed in athletes (up to 5 years), infants with creatine synthesis deficiency (up to 3 years), or in patient populations (up to 5 years).[11,104,105,108,109] One cohort of patients taking 1.5–3 g/day of creatine has been monitored since 1981 with no significant side effects.[62,63] Conversely, research has demonstrated a number of potentially helpful clinical uses of creatine in heart patients, infants and patients with creatine synthesis efficiency, patients with orthopedic injury, and patients with various neuromuscular diseases. Consequently, all available evidence suggests that creatine supplementation is safe when taken within recommended guidelines.

## Is Creatine Supplementation Ethical?

Several athletic governing bodies and special interest groups have questioned whether it is ethical for athletes to take creatine as a method of enhancing performance. Their rationale is that because studies indicate that creatine can improve performance and it would be difficult to ingest enough food in the diet to creatine load, that it is unethical to do so. Others argue that if you allow athletes to take creatine, they may be more predisposed to try other dangerous supplements and/or drugs. Still others have attempted to lump creatine in with anabolic steroids and/or banned stimulants and have called for a ban on the use of creatine among athletes. Finally, fresh off of the ban of dietary supplements containing ephedra, some have called for a ban on the sale of creatine citing safety concerns. Creatine supplementation is not currently banned by any athletic organization although the National Collegiate Athletic Association does not allow institutions to provide creatine or other "muscle-building" supplements to their athletes (e.g., protein, amino acids, and HMB). Moreover, although some countries limit how much creatine can be provided per serving in nutritional supplements, I am not aware of any country that has banned the sale of creatine. The International Olympic Committee considered these arguments and ruled that because creatine is readily found in meat and fish, there was no need to ban creatine. Frankly, I don't see creatine loading any different than carbohydrate loading. Many athletes ingest high-calorie concentrated carbohydrate drinks in an effort to increase muscle glycogen stores and/or supplement their diet. If carbohydrate loading is not a banned practice, then creatine loading should not be banned. This is particularly true when one considers that creatine supplementation has been reported to decrease the incidence of musculoskeletal injuries,[94,95,105,144] heat stress,[94,110,111] provide neuroprotective effects,[25,69,70,72,81] and/or expedite rehabilitation from injury.[73,84,145] It could be argued that not allowing athletes to take creatine may actually increase the risk of athletic competition.

## SUMMARY AND CONCLUSIONS

Creatine remains one of the most extensively studied nutritional ergogenic aids available for athletes. Hundreds of studies have reported that increasing muscle creatine stores through creatine supplementation can augment muscle creatine content, improve exercise and training adaptations, and/or provide some therapeutic benefit to some clinical populations. Consequently, creatine represents one of the most effective and popular nutritional ergogenic aids available for athletes. The future of creatine research is very promising. Researchers are attempting to determine ways to maximize creatine storage in the muscle, which types of exercise may obtain the greatest benefit from creatine supplementation, the potential medical uses of creatine, and the long-term safety and efficacy of creatine supplementation. Among these, the most promising area of research is determining the potential medical uses of creatine, particularly in patients with creatine synthesis deficiencies and neuromuscular diseases. Nevertheless, in regard to athletes, creatine has continually proved itself to be one of the most effective and safe nutritional supplements to increase strength, muscle mass, and performance. This is despite oftentimes inaccurate and misleading information that has been written about creatine in the popular media over the last several years.

## Sidebar 20.3. Should Athletes Take Creatine?

After extensively evaluating the literature, Williams et al.[11] concluded the following in their book *Creatine: The Power Supplement* (available at http://www.humankinetics.com):

- Individuals contemplating creatine supplementation should do so after being informed of potential benefits and risks so that they may make an informed decision.
- Adolescent athletes involved in serious training should consider creatine supplementation only with approval/ supervision of parents, trainers, coaches, and/or appropriate health professionals.

- If you plan to take creatine, purchase quality supplements from reputable vendors.
- Athletic administrators in organized sports who desire to establish policies on creatine supplementation for teams should base such policies on the scientific literature. Any formal administration policy should be supervised by a qualified health professional.
- Although more research is needed, available studies indicate that creatine supplementation seems to pose no health risk when taken at recommended doses and may provide therapeutic benefit for various medical populations.

## PRACTICAL APPLICATIONS

A significant body of research indicates that creatine supplementation during training can help optimize muscle creatine stores, increase high-intensity intermittent work output, and promote greater gains in strength and muscle mass. Additionally, creatine supplementation may provide some therapeutic benefit for a number of clinical populations. Available research indicates that short- and long-term creatine supplementation is safe and may lessen the incidence of injury in athletes. Creatine supplementation may be particularly beneficial for individuals attempting to increase strength and muscle mass, those involved in intermittent high-intensity exercise such as track and field (60–200 m), football, basketball, volleyball, swimming, and baseball. However, recent studies also indicate that athletes involved in more prolonged athletic events such as soccer may also benefit from creatine supplementation. Also, creatine loading with carbohydrate loading may help maximize glycogen retention. Therefore, because most endurance athletes incorporate interval training in their workouts and are interested in maximizing glycogen availability before events, there may also be some indirect benefit for endurance athletes. Creatine remains one of the most extensively studied and most consistently found nutrients to possess ergogenic value for a variety of athletes. Consequently, creatine monohydrate will no doubt remain a key nutrient in the nutritional arsenal of competitive athletes and clinical populations who may benefit from creatine supplementation.

## QUESTIONS

1. The *primary* energy system used during explosive, maximal exercise of short duration (e.g., 1 repetition maximum lift, 1- to 5-s sprint) is?
   a. ATP–PCr/phosphagen system
   b. Anaerobic glycolysis (lactic acid system)
   c. Aerobic glycolysis
   d. Oxidation of fats and proteins

2. Which of the following statements is *false* concerning the ATP-PCr energy system?
   a. ATP is stored in the muscle at a lesser concentration than PCr.
   b. The ATP-PCr system represents the most rapidly available source of usable energy for the muscle.

  c. The ATP-PCr system does not depend on transporting oxygen to the working muscles to produce energy.
  d. The ATP-PCr system requires a long series of chemical reactions in order to provide energy for muscular contraction.

3. What is the normal concentration of creatine in muscle?
  a. 80 mmol/kg dry mass
  b. 120 mmol/kg dry mass
  c. 160 mmol/kg dry mass
  d. 200 mmol/kg dry mass

4. Creatine supplementation has been reported to increase creatine and PCr content by ____?
  a. 5%–10%
  b. 10%–40%
  c. 30%–60%
  d. 50%–80%

5. Increasing total muscle creatine content has been suggested to provide ergogenic benefit to which of the following energy systems?
  a. ATP–PCr/phosphagen system
  b. Glycolysis
  c. Oxidative phosphorylation
  d. All of the above

6. Which of the following is not a theoretical benefit of creatine supplementation?
  a. Increased single and repetitive sprint performance, muscle mass, and strength during training
  b. Possible enhancement of aerobic capacity via greater shuttling of ATP from mitochondria and buffering of acidity
  c. Increased fat oxidation
  d. Greater training tolerance

7. Which of the following would be the best dietary source of creatine?
  a. Herring
  b. Tuna
  c. Beef
  d. Shrimp

8. Which of the following sports/activities would likely benefit the least from creatine supplementation?
  a. Football
  b. Marathon
  c. Weightlifting
  d. Basketball

9. Creatine supplementation has been studied as a potential therapeutic agent in all of the following diseases except?
  a. Myopathies
  b. Muscular dystrophy
  c. Brain and spinal cord injuries
  d. Hypertension

10. Which of the following is the most common side effect from creatine supplementation reported in the scientific literature?
  a. Muscle cramping
  b. Dehydration
  c. Weight gain
  d. Muscle pulls/tears

11. The creatine transporter mechanism has been reported to be influenced by which of the following?
  a. Amount of creatine ingested
  b. Sodium
  c. Glucose

    d. Insulin
    e. All of the above

12. Creatine may influence oxidative metabolism and recovery via which of the following pathways?
    a. Creatine phosphate shuttle
    b. Glucose-pentose pathway
    c. Adenine nucleotide de novo synthesis pathway
    d. Cytosolic glycolysis

13. Which of the following would be the best marker of adenine nucleotide degradation?
    a. Lactate
    b. Ammonia
    c. Glucose
    d. Ribose
    e. None of the above

14. Which of the following enzymes is most involved in creatine metabolism?
    a. Phosphofructokinase
    b. Citrate synthase
    c. Creatine kinase
    d. Creatinine dehydrogenase

15. Which of the following forms of creatine has been reported to be the most effective form to increase muscle creatine and PCr content?
    a. Serum/liquid creatine
    b. Creatine citrate
    c. Cyclocreatine
    d. Creatine monohydrate

16. Coingestion of creatine with all of the following nutrients has been reported to enhance creatine storage except.
    a. D-Pinitol
    b. HMB (beta-hydroxy-beta-methylbutyrate)
    c. Glucose
    d. Carbohydrate/protein

17. It takes approximately ____ week(s) after creatine loading in order for creatine stores to return to baseline levels.
    a. 1
    b. 2
    c. 4
    d. 8

18. Which of the following has been reported to inhibit the performance-enhancing effects of creatine?
    a. Protein
    b. Arginine
    c. Caffeine
    d. Branched-chain amino acid

19. How long would it take for muscle creatine stores to become fully saturated after a low-dose supplementation protocol (e.g., 2–3 g/day)?
    a. 3 days
    b. 7 days
    c. 1–2 weeks
    d. 3–4 weeks

20. Which of the following organizations ban the use of creatine among their athletes?
    a. Major League Baseball
    b. National Football League
    c. National Collegiate Athletic Association
    d. International Olympic Committee
    e. None of the above

21. The most effective way to increase muscle creatine stores is to ingest 2–3 g of creatine per day for 1 week.
    a. True
    b. False

22. Creatine loading typically increases total creatine and PCr content by 10%–40%.
    a. True
    b. False

23. Vegetarians generally have lower muscle creatine content and may experience large increases in creatine content in the muscle in response to creatine supplementation.
    a. True
    b. False

24. Creatine supplementation during training has been reported to increase strength, repetitive sprint performance, and muscle mass.
    a. True
    b. False

25. The weight gain associated with creatine supplementation is attributable to an increase in total-body and intramuscular water content.
    a. True
    b. False

26. The primary side effects described in the scientific and medical literature from creatine supplementation are dehydration, muscle cramping, and musculoskeletal injury.
    a. True
    b. False

27. Creatine supplementation is contraindicated in individuals with neuromuscular disease or injury because of neurotoxic effects on nerve transmission and brain function.
    a. True
    b. False

28. The normal daily turnover of creatine is 1%–2% (about 2 g).
    a. True
    b. False

29. Daily creatine needs in the body are met from dietary intake of foods containing creatine (e.g., fish, meat) and endogenous creatine synthesis from glycine, arginine, and methionine.
    a. True
    b. False

30. Long-term creatine supplementation results in irreversible suppression of endogenous creatine synthesis leading to a number of creatine deficiency disorders.
    a. True
    b. False

# REFERENCES

1. Chanutin A. The fate of creatine when administered to man. J Biol Chem 1926;67: 29–34.
2. Hultman E, Bergstrom J, Spreit L, Soderlund K. Energy metabolism and fatigue. In: Taylor A, Gollnick PD, Green H, eds. Biochemistry of Exercise VII. Champaign, IL: Human Kinetics Publishers; 1990:73–92.
3. Balsom PD, Soderlund K, Ekblom B. Creatine in humans with special reference to creatine supplementation. Sports Med 1994;18:268–280.
4. Greenhaff P. The nutritional biochemistry of creatine. J Nutr Biochem 1997;11: 610–618.

5. Greenhaff PL. Muscle creatine loading in humans: procedures and functional and metabolic effects. Sixth International Conference on Guanidino Compounds in Biology and Medicine. Cincinnati, OH, 2001.

6. Greenhaff P, Casey A, Green AL. Creatine supplementation revisited: an update. Insider 1996;4:1–2.

7. Harris RC, Soderlund K, Hultman E. Elevation of creatine in resting and exercised muscle of normal subjects by creatine supplementation. Clin Sci (Colch) 1992;83:367–374.

8. Hultman E, Soderlund K, Timmons JA, Cederblad G, Greenhaff PL. Muscle creatine loading in men. J Appl Physiol 1996;81:232–237.

9. Burke DG, Smith-Palmer T, Holt LE, Head B, Chilibeck PD. The effect of 7 days of creatine supplementation on 24-hour urinary creatine excretion. J Strength Cond Res 2001;15:59–62.

10. Williams MH, Branch JD. Creatine supplementation and exercise performance: an update. J Am Coll Nutr 1998;17:216–234.

11. Williams MH, Kreider R, Branch JD. Creatine: the power supplement. Champaign, IL: Human Kinetics Publishers; 1999.

12. Burke DG, Chilibeck PD, Parise G, Candow DG, Mahoney D, Tarnopolsky M. Effect of creatine and weight training on muscle creatine and performance in vegetarians. Med Sci Sports Exerc 2003;35:1946–1955.

13. DeGrauw TJ, Cecil KC, Salomons GS, et al. The clinical syndrome of creatine transporter deficiency. Abstracts of 6th International Conference on Guanidino Compounds in Biology and Medicine, 2001.

14. Stockler S, Hanefeld F. Guanidinoacetate methyltransferase deficiency: a newly recognized inborn error of creatine biosynthesis. Wien Klin Wochenschr 1997;109:86–88.

15. Kreider RB. Effects of creatine supplementation on performance and training adaptations. Mol Cell Biochem 2003;244:89–94.

16. Wallimann T, Dolder M, Neumann D, Schlattner U. Compartmentation, structure, and function of creatine kinases: a rationale for creatine action. Abstracts of 6th International Conference on Guanidino Compounds in Biology and Medicine, 2001.

17. Bessman S, Savabi F. The role of phosphocreatine energy shuttle in exercise and muscle hypertrophy. In: Conway MA, Clark JF, eds. Creatine and Creatine Phosphate: Scientific and Clinical Perspectives. San Diego: Academic Press; 1988:185–198.

18. Wallimann T, Dolder M, Schlattner U, et al. Some new aspects of creatine kinase (CK): compartmentation, structure, function and regulation for cellular and mitochondrial bioenergetics and physiology. Biofactors 1998;8:229–234.

19. Clark JF, Field ML, Ventura-Clapier R. An introduction to the cellular creatine kinase system in contractile tissue. In: Conway MA, Clark JF, eds. Creatine and Creatine Phosphate: Scientific and Clinical Perspectives. San Diego: Academic Press; 1996:51–64.

20. Clark JF. Creatine and phosphocreatine: a review of their use in exercise and sport. J Athl Train 1997;32:45–50.

21. Ma TM, Friedman DL, Roberts R. Creatine phosphate shuttle pathway in tissues with dynamic energy demand. In: Conway MA, Clark JF, eds. Creatine and Creatine Phosphate: Scientific and Clinical Perspectives. San Diego: Academic Press; 1996:17–32.

22. van Deursen J, Heerschap A, Oerlemans F, et al. Skeletal muscles of mice deficient in muscle creatine kinase lack burst activity. Cell 1993;74:621–631.

23. Askenasy N, Koretsky AP. Differential effects of creatine kinase isoenzymes and substrates on regeneration in livers of transgenic mice. Am J Physiol 1997;273:C741–746.

24. Willoughby DS, Rosene JM. Effects of oral creatine and resistance training on myogenic regulatory factor expression. Med Sci Sports Exerc 2003;35:923–929.

25. Wyss M, Schulze A. Health implications of creatine: can oral creatine supplementation protect against neurological and atherosclerotic disease? Neuroscience 2002;112:243–260.

26. Tarnopolsky MA, Parshad A, Walzel B, Schlattner U, Wallimann T. Creatine transporter and mitochondrial creatine kinase protein content in myopathies. Muscle Nerve 2001;24:682–688.

27. Hespel P, Eijnde BO, Derave W, Richter EA. Creatine supplementation: exploring the role of the creatine kinase/phosphocreatine system in human muscle. Can J Appl Physiol 2001;26:S79–102.

28. Felber S, Skladal D, Wyss M, Kremser C, Koller A, Sperl W. Oral creatine supplementation in Duchenne muscular dystrophy: a clinical and 31P magnetic resonance spectroscopy study. Neurol Res 2000;22:145–150.

29. Matthews RT, Yang L, Jenkins BG, et al. Neuroprotective effects of creatine and cyclocreatine in animal models of Huntington's disease. J Neurosci 1998;18: 156–163.
30. Newsholme E, Beis I. Old and new ideas on the roles of phosphagens and the kinases. In: Conway MA, Clark JF, eds. Creatine and Creatine Phosphate: Scientific and Clinical Perspectives. San Diego: Academic Press; 1996:3–15.
31. Blei ML, Conley KE, Kushmerick MJ. Separate measures of ATP utilization and recovery in human skeletal muscle. J Physiol 1993;465:203–222.
32. Radda GK. Control of energy metabolism during energy metabolism. Diabetes 1996;45:S88–S92.
33. Kreider RB, Leutholtz BC, Greenwood M. Creatine. In: Wolinsky I, Driskell J, eds. Nutritional Ergogenic Aids. Boca Raton, FL: CRC Press LLC; 2004:81–104.
34. Steenge GR, Simpson EJ, Greenhaff PL. Protein- and carbohydrate-induced augmentation of whole body creatine retention in humans. J Appl Physiol 2000;89: 1165–1171.
35. Green AL, Hultman E, Macdonald IA, Sewell DA, Greenhaff PL. Carbohydrate ingestion augments skeletal muscle creatine accumulation during creatine supplementation in humans. Am J Physiol 1996;271:E821–826.
36. Willoughby DS, Rosene J. Effects of oral creatine and resistance training on myosin heavy chain expression. Med Sci Sports Exerc 2001;33:1674–1681.
37. Greenhaff PL, Casey A, Short AH, Harris R, Soderlund K, Hultman E. Influence of oral creatine supplementation of muscle torque during repeated bouts of maximal voluntary exercise in man. Clin Sci (Colch) 1993;84:565–571.
38. Greenhaff PL, Bodin K, Soderlund K, Hultman E. Effect of oral creatine supplementation on skeletal muscle phosphocreatine resynthesis. Am J Physiol 1994;266: E725–730.
39. Vandenberghe K, Goris M, Van Hecke P, Van Leemputte M, Vangerven L, Hespel P. Long-term creatine intake is beneficial to muscle performance during resistance training. J Appl Physiol 1997;83:2055–2063.
40. Kreider R, Greenwood M, Melton C, et al. Long-term creatine supplementation during training/competition does not increase perceptions of fatigue or adversely affect health status. Med Sci Sport Exerc 2002;34:S146.
41. Nelson AG, Arnall DA, Kokkonen J, Day R, Evans J. Muscle glycogen supercompensation is enhanced by prior creatine supplementation. Med Sci Sports Exerc 2001;33:1096–1100.
42. van Loon LJ, Murphy R, Oosterlaar AM, et al. Creatine supplementation increases glycogen storage but not GLUT-4 expression in human skeletal muscle. Clin Sci (Lond) 2004;106:99–106.
43. Op 't Eijnde B, Richter EA, Henquin JC, Kiens B, Hespel P. Effect of creatine supplementation on creatine and glycogen content in rat skeletal muscle. Acta Physiol Scand 2001;171:169–176.
44. Kehnder M, Rico-Sanz J, Kuhne G, Dambach M, Buchli R, Boutellier U. Muscle phosphocreatine and glycogen concentrations in humans after creatine and glucose polymer supplementation measured noninvasively by 31P and 13C-MRS. Med Sci Sports Exerc 1998;30:S264.
45. Volek JS, Duncan ND, Mazzetti SA, et al. Performance and muscle fiber adaptations to creatine supplementation and heavy resistance training. Med Sci Sports Exerc 1999;31:1147–1156.
46. Stone MH, Sanborn K, Smith LL, et al. Effects of in-season (5 weeks) creatine and pyruvate supplementation on anaerobic performance and body composition in American football players. Int J Sport Nutr 1999;9:146–165.
47. Kreider RB, Ferreira M, Wilson M, et al. Effects of creatine supplementation on body composition, strength, and sprint performance. Med Sci Sports Exerc 1998;30: 73–82.
48. Earnest CP, Snell P, Rodriguez R, Almada A, Mitchell TL. The effect of creatine monohydrate ingestion on anaerobic power indices, muscular strength and body composition. Acta Physiol Scand 1995;153:207–209.
49. Volek JS, Kraemer WJ, Bush JA, et al. Creatine supplementation enhances muscular performance during high-intensity resistance exercise. J Am Diet Assoc 1997;97: 765–770.
50. Tarnopolsky MA, MacLennan DP. Creatine monohydrate supplementation enhances high-intensity exercise performance in males and females. Int J Sport Nutr Exerc Metab 2000;10:452–463.
51. Wiroth JB, Bermon S, Andrei S, Dalloz E, Hebuterne X, Dolisi C. Effects of oral creatine supplementation on maximal pedalling performance in older adults. Eur J Appl Physiol 2001;84:533–539.
52. Skare OC, Skadberg, Wisnes AR. Creatine supplementation improves sprint performance in male sprinters. Scand J Med Sci Sports 2001;11:96–102.

53. Mujika I, Padilla S, Ibanez J, Izquierdo M, Gorostiaga E. Creatine supplementation and sprint performance in soccer players. Med Sci Sports Exerc 2000;32:518–525.

54. Ostojic SM. Creatine supplementation in young soccer players. Int J Sport Nutr Exerc Metab 2004;14:95–103.

55. Theodorou AS, Cooke CB, King RF, et al. The effect of longer-term creatine supplementation on elite swimming performance after an acute creatine loading. J Sports Sci 1999;17:853–859.

56. Mero AA, Keskinen KL, Malvela MT, Sallinen JM. Combined creatine and sodium bicarbonate supplementation enhances interval swimming. J Strength Cond Res 2004;18:306–310.

57. Preen D, Dawson B, Goodman C, Lawrence S, Beilby J, Ching S. Effect of creatine loading on long-term sprint exercise performance and metabolism. Med Sci Sports Exerc 2001;33:814–821.

58. Noonan D, Berg K, Latin RW, Wagner JC, Reimers K. Effects of varying dosages of oral creatine relative to fat free body mass on strength and body composition. J Strength Cond Res 1998;12:104–108.

59. Kirksey KB, Stone MH, Warren BJ, et al. The effects of 6 weeks of creatine monohydrate supplementation on performance measures and body composition in collegiate track and field athletes. J Strength Cond Res 1999;13:148–156.

60. Jones AM, Atter T, Georg KP. Oral creatine supplementation improves multiple sprint performance in elite ice-hockey players. J Sports Med Phys Fitness 1999; 39:189–196.

61. Jowko E, Ostaszewski P, Jank M, et al. Creatine and beta-hydroxy-beta-methylbutyrate (HMB) additively increase lean body mass and muscle strength during a weight-training program. Nutrition 2001;17:558–566.

62. Sipila I, Rapola J, Simell O, Vannas A. Supplementary creatine as a treatment for gyrate atrophy of the choroid and retina. N Engl J Med 1981;304:867–870.

63. Vannas-Sulonen K, Sipila I, Vannas A, Simell O, Rapola J. Gyrate atrophy of the choroid and retina. A five-year follow-up of creatine supplementation. Ophthalmology 1985;92:1719–1727.

64. Heinanen K, Nanto-Salonen K, Komu M, et al. Creatine corrects muscle 31P spectrum in gyrate atrophy with hyperornithinaemia. Eur J Clin Invest 1999;29:1060–1065.

65. Nanto-Salonen K, Komu M, Lundbom N, et al. Reduced brain creatine in gyrate atrophy of the choroid and retina with hyperornithinemia. Neurology 1999;53:303–307.

66. Ensenauer R, Thiel T, Schwab KO, et al. Guanidinoacetate methyltransferase deficiency: differences of creatine uptake in human brain and muscle. Mol Genet Metab 2004;82:208–213.

67. Schulze A, Ebinger F, Rating D, Mayatepek E. Improving treatment of guanidinoacetate methyltransferase deficiency: reduction of guanidinoacetic acid in body fluids by arginine restriction and ornithine supplementation. Mol Genet Metab 2001;74:413–419.

68. Ganesan V, Johnson A, Connelly A, Eckhardt S, Surtees RA. Guanidinoacetate methyltransferase deficiency: new clinical features. Pediatr Neurol 1997;17:155–157.

69. Zhu S, Li M, Figueroa BE, et al. Prophylactic creatine administration mediates neuroprotection in cerebral ischemia in mice. J Neurosci 2004;24:5909–5912.

70. Hausmann ON, Fouad K, Wallimann T, Schwab ME. Protective effects of oral creatine supplementation on spinal cord injury in rats. Spinal Cord 2002;40:449–456.

71. Brustovetsky N, Brustovetsky T, Dubinsky JM. On the mechanisms of neuroprotection by creatine and phosphocreatine. J Neurochem 2001;76:425–434.

72. Sullivan PG, Geiger JD, Mattson MP, Scheff SW. Dietary supplement creatine protects against traumatic brain injury. Ann Neurol 2000;48:723–729.

73. Jacobs PL, Mahoney ET, Cohn KA, Sheradsky LF, Green BA. Oral creatine supplementation enhances upper extremity work capacity in persons with cervical-level spinal cord injury. Arch Phys Med Rehabil 2002;83:19–23.

74. Tarnopolsky MA. Potential use of creatine monohydrate in muscular dystrophy and neurometabolic disorders. Abstracts of 6th International Conference on Guanidino Compounds in Biology and Medicine, 2001.

75. Tarnopolsky MA, Parise G. Direct measurement of high-energy phosphate compounds in patients with neuromuscular disease. Muscle Nerve 1999;22:1228–1233.

76. Zange J, Kornblum C, Muller K, et al. Creatine supplementation results in elevated phosphocreatine/adenosine triphosphate (ATP) ratios in the calf muscle of athletes but not in patients with myopathies. Ann Neurol 2002;52:126; discussion 126–127.

77. Koumis T, Nathan JP, Rosenberg JM, Cicero LA. Strategies for the prevention and treatment of statin-induced myopathy: is there a role for ubiquinone supplementation? Am J Health Syst Pharm 2004;61:515–519.

78. Borchert A, Wilichowski E, Hanefeld F. Supplementation with creatine monohydrate in children with mitochondrial encephalomyopathies. Muscle Nerve 1999;22: 1299–1300.

79. Tarnopolsky MA, Roy BD, MacDonald JR. A randomized, controlled trial of creatine monohydrate in patients with mitochondrial cytopathies. Muscle Nerve 1997;20: 1502–1509.

80. Andreassen OA, Dedeoglu A, Ferrante RJ, et al. Creatine increases survival and delays motor symptoms in a transgenic animal model of Huntington's disease. Neurobiol Dis 2001;8:479–491.

81. Ferrante RJ, Andreassen OA, Jenkins BG, et al. Neuroprotective effects of creatine in a transgenic mouse model of Huntington's disease. J Neurosci 2000;20:4389–4397.

82. Verbessem P, Lemiere J, Eijnde BO, et al. Creatine supplementation in Huntington's disease: a placebo-controlled pilot trial. Neurology 2003;61:925–930.

83. Andreassen OA, Jenkins BG, Dedeoglu A, et al. Increases in cortical glutamate concentrations in transgenic amyotrophic lateral sclerosis mice are attenuated by creatine supplementation. J Neurochem 2001;77:383–390.

84. Tarnopolsky MA. Potential benefits of creatine monohydrate supplementation in the elderly. Curr Opin Clin Nutr Metab Care 2000;3:497–502.

85. Drory VE, Gross D. No effect of creatine on respiratory distress in amyotrophic lateral sclerosis. Amyotroph Lateral Scler Other Motor Neuron Disord 2002;3: 43–46.

86. Mazzini L, Balzarini C, Colombo R, et al. Effects of creatine supplementation on exercise performance and muscular strength in amyotrophic lateral sclerosis: preliminary results. J Neurol Sci 2001;191:139–144.

87. Willer B, Stucki G, Hoppeler H, Bruhlmann P, Krahenbuhl S. Effects of creatine supplementation on muscle weakness in patients with rheumatoid arthritis. Rheumatology (Oxford) 2000;39:293–298.

88. Op 't Eijnde B, Urso B, Richter EA, Greenhaff PL, Hespel P. Effect of oral creatine supplementation on human muscle GLUT4 protein content after immobilization. Diabetes 2001;50:18–23.

89. Earnest CP, Almada A, Mitchell TL. High-performance capillary electrophoresis-pure creatine monohydrate reduced blood lipids in men and women. Clin Sci 1996;91:113–118.

90. Jacobs RL, Stead LM, Ratnam S, Brosnan ME. Regulation of homocysteine metabolism—effects of insulin, glucagon and creatine. FASEB J 2001;15.

91. Steenge GR, Verhoef P, Greenhaff PL. The effect of creatine and resistance training on plasma homocysteine concentration in healthy volunteers. Arch Intern Med 2001;161:1455–1456.

92. McCarty MF. Supplemental creatine may decrease serum homocysteine and abolish the homocysteine "gender gap" by suppressing endogenous creatine synthesis. Med Hypotheses 2001;56:5–7.

93. Taes YE, Delanghe JR, De Vriese AS, Rombaut R, Van Camp J, Lameire NH. Creatine supplementation decreases homocysteine in an animal model of uremia. Kidney Int 2003;64:1331–1337.

94. Greenwood M, Kreider RB, Melton C, et al. Creatine supplementation during college football training does not increase the incidence of cramping or injury. Mol Cell Biochem 2003;244:83–88.

95. Greenwood M, Kreider RB, Greenwood L, Byars A. Cramping and injury incidence in collegiate football players are reduced by creatine supplementation. J Athl Train 2003;38:216–219.

96. Greenwood M, Farris J, Kreider R, Greenwood L, Byars A. Creatine supplementation patterns and perceived effects in select division I collegiate athletes. Clin J Sport Med 2000;10:191–194.

97. Greenwood M, Kreider R, Greenwood L, Byars A. Creatine supplementation does not increase the incidence of injury or cramping in college baseball players. J Exerc Physiol Online 2003;6:16–22.

98. Ortega Gallo PA, Dimeo F, Batista J, et al. Creatine supplementation in soccer players, effects in body composition and incidence of sport-related injuries. Med Sci Sports Exerc 2000;32:S134.

99. Volek JS, Ratamess NA, Rubin MR, et al. The effects of creatine supplementation on muscular performance and body composition responses to short-term resistance training overreaching. Eur J Appl Physiol 2004;91:628–637.

100. Kreider R, Rasmussen C, Melton C, et al. Long-term creatine supplementation does not adversely affect clinical markers of health. Med Sci Sports Exerc 2000;32: S134.

101. Schroeder C, Potteiger J, Randall J, et al. The effects of creatine dietary supplementation on anterior compartment pressure in the lower leg during rest and following exercise. Clin J Sport Med 2001;11:87–95.

102. Carper MJ, Potteiger JA, Randall JC, Jacobsen DJ, Hulver MW, Thyfault JP. Lower leg anterior compartment pressure response prior to, during, and following chronic creatine supplementation. Med Sci Sports Exerc 2001;33.

103. Yoshizumi WM, Tsourounis C. Effects of creatine supplementation on renal function. J Herb Pharmcother 2004;4:1–7.

104. Kreider RB, Melton C, Rasmussen CJ, et al. Long-term creatine supplementation does not significantly affect clinical markers of health in athletes. Mol Cell Biochem 2003;244:95–104.

105. Schilling BK, Stone MH, Utter A, et al. Creatine supplementation and health variables: a retrospective study. Med Sci Sports Exerc 2001;33:183–188.

106. Earnest CP, Almada A, Mitchell TL. Influence of chronic creatine supplementation on hepatorenal function. FASEB J 1996;10:A790.

107. Poortmans JR, Auquier H, Renaut V, Durussel A, Saugy M, Brisson GR. Effect of short-term creatine supplementation on renal responses in men. Eur J Appl Physiol Occup Physiol 1997;76:566–567.

108. Poortmans JR, Francaux M. Long-term oral creatine supplementation does not impair renal function in healthy athletes. Med Sci Sports Exerc 1999;31:1108–1110.

109. Robinson TM, Sewell DA, Casey A, Steenge G, Greenhaff PL. Dietary creatine supplementation does not affect some haematological indices, or indices of muscle damage and hepatic and renal function. Br J Sports Med 2000;34:284–288.

110. Kilduff LP, Georgiades E, James N, et al. The effects of creatine supplementation on cardiovascular, metabolic, and thermoregulatory responses during exercise in the heat in endurance-trained humans. Int J Sport Nutr Exerc Metab 2004;14:443–460.

111. Volek JS, Mazzetti SA, Farquhar WB, Barnes BR, Gomez AL, Kraemer WJ. Physiological responses to short-term exercise in the heat after creatine loading. Med Sci Sports Exerc 2001;33:1101–1108.

112. Kreider RB, Willoughby DS, Greenwood M, Parise G, Payne E, Tarnopolsky MA. Effects of serum creatine supplementation on muscle creatine content. J Exerc Physiol Online 2003;6:24–33.

113. Greenwood M, Kreider RB, Rasmussen C, Almada AL, Earnest CP. D-Pinitol augments whole body creatine retention in man. J Exerc Physiol Online 2001;4:41–47.

114. Gill ND, Hall RD, Blazevich AJ. Creatine serum is not as effective as creatine powder for improving cycle sprint performance in competitive male team-sport athletes. J Strength Cond Res 2004;18:272–275.

115. Michaelis J, Vukovich MD. Effect of two different forms of creatine supplementation on muscular strength and power. Med Sci Sports Exerc 1998;30:S272.

116. Benzi G. Is there a rationale for the use of creatine either as nutritional supplementation or drug administration in humans participating in a sport? Pharmacol Res 2000;41:255–264.

117. Persky AM, Brazeau GA. Clinical pharmacology of the dietary supplement creatine monohydrate. Pharmacol Rev 2001;53:161–176.

118. Pearson DR, Hamby DG, Russel W, Harris T. Long-term effects of creatine monohydrate on strength and power. J Strength Cond Res 1999;13:187–192.

119. Cathcart EP. The influence of carbohydrates and fats on protein metabolism. J Physiol 1909;39:311–330.

120. Mendel LB, Rose WC. Experimental studies on creatine and creatinine: the role of the carbohydrates in creatine-creatinine metabolism. J Biol Chem 1911;10:213–253.

121. Benedict SR, Osterberg E. Studies in creatine and creatinine metabolism: III. On the origin of creatine. J Biol Chem 1914;18:195–214.

122. Chanutin A. A study of the effect of creatine on growth and its distribution in the tissues of normal rats. J Biol Chem 1927;75:549–557.

123. Chanutin A. A study of the effect of feeding creatine on growth and its distribution in the liver and muscle of normal mice. J Biol Chem 1928;78:167–180.

124. Schedel JM, Tanaka H, Kiyonaga A, Shindo M, Schutz Y. Acute creatine ingestion in human: consequences on serum creatine and creatinine concentrations. Life Sci 1999;65:2463–2470.

125. Havenetidis K, Bourdas D. Creatine supplementation: effects on urinary excretion and anaerobic performance. J Sports Med Phys Fitness 2003;43:347–355.

126. Haughland RB, Chang DT. Insulin effects on creatine transport in skeletal muscle. Proc Soc Exp Biol Med 1975;148:1–4.

127. Salomons GS, van Dooren SJ, Verhoeven NM, et al. X-linked creatine transporter defect: an overview. J Inherit Metab Dis 2003;26:309–318.

128. Queiroz MS, Berkich DA, Shao Y, Lanoue K, Ismail-Beigi F. Thyroid hormone regulation of cardiac creatine content: role of Na+/creatine transporter expression. FASEB J 2001;15.

129. Young JC, Young RE, Young CJ. The effect of creatine supplementation on glucose transport in rat skeletal muscle. FASEB J 2000;14.

130. Green AL, Simpson EJ, Littlewood JJ, Macdonald IA, Greenhaff P. Carbohydrate ingestion augments creatine retention during creatine feeding in humans. Acta Physiol Scand 1996;158:195–202.

131. Green AL, Hultman E, Macdonald IA, Sewell DA, Greenhaff P. Carbohydrate feeding augments skeletal muscle creatine accumulation during creatine supplementation in humans. Am J Physiol 1996;271:E821–E826.

132. Borsheim E, Aarsland A, Wolfe RR. Effect of an amino acid, protein, and carbohydrate mixture on net muscle protein balance after resistance exercise. Int J Sport Nutr Exerc Metab 2004;14:255–271.

133. Borsheim E, Cree MG, Tipton KD, Elliott TA, Aarsland A, Wolfe RR. Effect of carbohydrate intake on net muscle protein synthesis during recovery from resistance exercise. J Appl Physiol 2004;96:674–678.

134. Miller SL, Tipton KD, Chinkes DL, Wolf SE, Wolfe RR. Independent and combined effects of amino acids and glucose after resistance exercise. Med Sci Sports Exerc 2003;35:449–455.

135. Bohe J, Low A, Wolfe RR, Rennie MJ. Human muscle protein synthesis is modulated by extracellular, not intramuscular amino acid availability: a dose-response study. J Physiol 2003;552:315–324.

136. Wolfe RR. Regulation of muscle protein by amino acids. J Nutr 2002;132:3219S–3224S.

137. Doherty M, Smith PM, Davison RC, Hughes MG. Caffeine is ergogenic after supplementation of oral creatine monohydrate. Med Sci Sports Exerc 2002;34:1785–1792.

138. Vandenberghe K, Van Hecke P, Van Leemputte M, Vanstapel F, Hespel P. Inhibition of muscle phosphocreatine resynthesis by caffeine after creatine loading. Med Sci Sports Exerc 1997;29:S249.

139. Vandenberghe K, Gillis N, Van Leemputte M, Van Hecke P, Vanstapel F, Hespel P. Caffeine counteracts the ergogenic action of muscle creatine loading. J Appl Physiol 1996;80:452–457.

140. Hespel P, Op't Eijnde B, Van Leemputte M. Opposite actions of caffeine and creatine on muscle relaxation time in humans. J Appl Physiol 2002;92:513–518.

141. Ray TR, Eck JC, Covington LA, Murphy RB, Williams R, Knudtson J. Use of oral creatine as an ergogenic aid for increased sports performance: perceptions of adolescent athletes. South Med J 2001;94:608–612.

142. Smith J, Dahm DL. Creatine use among a select population of high school athletes. Mayo Clin Proc 2000;75:1257–1263.

143. Sheppard HL, Raichada SM, Kouri KM, Stenson-Bar-Maor L, Branch JD. Use of creatine and other supplements by members of civilian and military health clubs: a cross-sectional survey. Int J Sport Nutr Exerc Metab 2000;10:245–259.

144. Tyler TF, Nicholas SJ, Hershman EB, Glace BW, Mullaney MJ, McHugh MP. The effect of creatine supplementation on strength recovery after anterior cruciate ligament (ACL) reconstruction: a randomized, placebo-controlled, double-blind trial. Am J Sports Med 2004;32:383–388.

145. Hespel P, Op't Eijnde B, Van Leemputte M, et al. Oral creatine supplementation facilitates the rehabilitation of disuse atrophy and alters the expression of muscle myogenic factors in humans. J Physiol 2001;536:625–633.

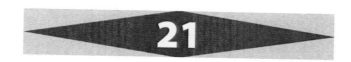

# Weight Loss Ingredients

## Christopher R. Mohr

## OBJECTIVES

On the completion of this chapter you will be able to:

1. Understand why weight loss ingredients are so popular.
2. Explain the current obesity trends in the United States.
3. Discuss the origin and theoretical mechanisms of function for a series of weight loss ingredients.
4. Differentiate between the proposed and actual scientifically proven effects of a variety of weight loss ingredients.
5. Understand the potential ramifications of using weight loss ingredients.

## ABSTRACT

Dietary supplements are and always will be immensely popular. Fat loss supplements are particularly popular as America is currently facing an obesity epidemic. Therefore, dietary supplements intended to enhance weight loss will continue to come and go over the years. Unfortunately, after reading this chapter, it should be apparent that few scientific data support many of the fat loss supplements available. The ephedra-containing supplements were effective for fat loss, but supplements with ephedra have been banned because it was surrounded by controversy as a result of some health concerns reported by consumers. Ironically, pure ephedrine can still be purchased.

*Key Words:* **body mass, obesity, thermogenesis, lipolysis, appetite**

Obesity is an epidemic and a significant public health problem.[1] The prevalence of overweight and obesity has increased substantially to 64.5%.[1] Overweight is classified as having a body mass index of $25–29.9\,kg\cdot m^2$ and obesity is classified by a body mass index of $\geq 30.0\,kg\cdot m^2$. Overweight and obesity are precursors to numerous major health problems including, but not limited to, cardiovascular disease, non–insulin-dependent diabetes mellitus, hypertension, sleep apnea, dyslipidemia, osteoarthritis, and many cancers.[2]

Obesity is a complex disease that encompasses a number of physiologic and psychologic aspects. Therefore, it is recommended that individuals who are overweight or obese decrease their body weight by making healthy lifestyle changes through a decrease in energy intake and increase in energy expenditure. Successful weight loss not only entails dietary and activity modifications, but also behavioral changes, and as a very last resort, sometimes pharmacologic or surgical treatments as well.

From: *Essentials of Sports Nutrition and Supplements*
Edited by J. Antonio, D. Kalman, J. R. Stout, M. Greenwood, D. S. Willoughby, and G. G. Haff © Humana Press, a part of Springer Science+Business Media, Totowa, NJ

Furthermore, individuals often turn to dietary supplements to enhance their fat loss goals. Because of this, in 2002, according to the Federal Trade Commission, consumers spent approximately $35 billion on weight loss products (e.g., books, dietary supplements, and weight loss franchises). This chapter discusses a number of the current dietary supplements in vogue and reviews the research associated with each. Just because they are easily accessible in health food stores and vitamin shops does not necessarily ensure they are safe or efficacious; understanding the research associated with each is crucial.

## REVIEW OF THE LITERATURE

### Citrus aurantium

*Citrus aurantium* has taken over for ephedrine and is in a majority of fat loss supplements available. Although its inclusion in "ephedrine-free" products is common, there is surprisingly little research to support or refute its purported claims. One recent review was published about *C. aurantium* as a specific ingredient,[3] but at this time only one study[4] has specifically measured the effects of synephrine on fat loss. However, the product used in this study included other ingredients as well, making it difficult to assess the specific effects of synephrine on fat metabolism.

*C. aurantium*, also known as bitter or Seville orange, is a small citrus tree; its most active components are synephrine and octopamine, both of which are derived from inedible portions of immature fruits.[3] *C. aurantium* also contains small amounts of alkaloids such as hordenine, m-methyltyramine, and tyramine.[5] Structurally, both active components (synephrine and octopamine) are similar to ephedrine[3] and are frequently referred to as ephedrine's "chemical cousins." Of these two components, synephrine is typically in much higher concentrations than octopamine in fat loss supplements because of its known stimulation β receptors and particularly the β-3 receptors.

The β-3 receptors seem to be responsible for lipolytic and thermogenic effects, whereas the β-1 and β-2 receptors cause a relaxation of smooth muscle and stimulation of cardiac muscle. Not surprisingly, it would be ideal to stimulate the β-3 receptor and minimize the stimulation of β-1 and β-2 receptors, when looking for fat loss.

In vitro research demonstrates that synephrine does just this; it works specifically on β-3 receptors, with limited action on the other two.[5] However, although synephrine's activation of the β-1 and β-2 receptors is limited, there is still concern regarding the effects on the cardiovascular system because of the limited available evidence on *C. aurantium* in general.[6]

This primary outcome of the aforementioned study by Colker et al.[4] was to assess if a product that included synephrine enhanced weight loss; however, the researchers also considered some cardiovascular system outcome measurements. The product in this study contained 975 mg of *C. aurantium* extract (6% synephrine compounds), 528 mg of caffeine, and 900 mg of St. John's wort (3% hypericum). The subjects took the product for 6 weeks and the researchers measured fat loss, weight, metabolic rate, blood lipids, blood pressure, and mood. The researchers reported a 1.4-kg weight loss in the supplement group versus a 0.9-kg loss in the placebo group. Although these results were statistically significant, the groups were not compared against one another, but rather only versus the baseline values of their respective groups. Therefore, it is difficult to draw a logical conclusion with regard to this product's efficacy for weight loss. There was also a higher percentage of fat lost in the supplemented group versus the placebo; however, this too was compared with the baseline value, rather than the other group. Furthermore, there was a significant increase in metabolic rate, which is not surprising considering that the product contains the same amount of caffeine as approximately 4 cups of coffee. Although measuring metabolic rate does show a bit more promise, it would be interesting if this effect would be reduced over time as the body grew accustomed to the dosages used. No significant changes were seen in any of the other outcome measures and no side effects were reported. This is the only full-length, peer-reviewed published literature to date using

*C. aurantium* as a weight loss aid in humans; therefore, it is impossible to draw a sound conclusion because this study provides very weak evidence in favor of *C. aurantium*.

## Green Tea

Green tea extract has also recently seen a surge in popularity; it is hard not to find it on the ingredient list of fat loss supplements. Even green tea as a beverage has surged in popularity as it is the most widely consumed beverage in the world, second only to water.[7] The particular extract in green tea that is of importance is epigallocatechin-3-gallate (EGCG), which is one of four catechins found in green tea.[8] Among the four, EGCG has shown promise as an adjunct to an effective diet and exercise regimen.[8] However, it is not only the EGCG that seems to be relevant in green tea, but also the naturally occurring caffeine.[9] There is approximately 10–80 mg of caffeine/cup[10] and EGCG and caffeine are synergistic in the process of increasing thermogenesis.

Here is how it works: the catecholamines norepinephrine and epinephrine act as regulators of glycogen catabolism and liploysis.[9] They are released in response to fright, exercise, stress, cold, etc.; they are part of a coordinated response to prepare an individual for emergencies and are often referred to as the "fight or flight" reactions.[11] A release in catecholamines results in an increase in heart rate[11] and, subsequently, thermogenesis; but this is a transient process, which is where EGCG comes into play.[9]

The catecholamine norepinephrine is quickly hydrolyzed by a specific enzyme, catechol *O*-methyltransferase.[12] However, it has been shown in vitro that green tea extract inhibits this enzyme,[9] thereby allowing norepinephrine to be up-regulated. This can be important because norepinephrine normally binds to the receptor and activates the enzyme adenylate cyclase. When activated, this enzyme converts adenosine triphosphate (ATP) into cyclic adenosine monophosphate (cAMP). cAMP activates hormone sensitive lipase (HSL), but is rapidly degraded to 5-adenosine monophosphate (5-AMP) via another enzyme, phosphodiesterase (PDE).[13] Because HSL is important in breaking down triglyceride molecules, it would be ideal for cAMP to be preferentially shuttled to HSL, rather than being hydrolyzed. Subsequently, green tea catecholamines allow the first part of this reaction to occur and prolong the thermogenic process.[9] However, this process will ultimately come to an end as well; cAMP is also quickly hydrolyzed to 5-AMP rather than continuing on its path to activating HSL.[13] Here is where caffeine comes into play. It is well established that caffeine can inhibit PDE and allow cAMP to continue its job as a "second messenger" allowing for the enzyme HSL to break down triglycerides and prolong the thermogenic process.[9,14]

A study published in 1999 demonstrated that green tea does in fact increase metabolic rate.[9] In this particular study, researchers gave subjects one of three supplements: green tea extract (providing a total of 270 mg of EGCG plus 150 mg of caffeine per day), 150 mg of caffeine per day, or a placebo. The caffeine-only group was used to determine if the EGCG had any additive effect to the known ergogenic benefits of caffeine. After the short, 24-hour study, researchers noted a significant increase in resting metabolic rate (4%) in the EGCG + caffeine group versus the caffeine or placebo groups. Although this did not correlate to a decrease in body weight, it was only a 1-day study. Therefore, longer-term research is necessary to determine if the body would grow accustomed to this stimulant, or if this increase in metabolic rate would continue for the duration of supplementation, which could obviously enhance weight loss.

There have been several other papers and abstracts published using products that contain green tea, but they are typically combined with other ingredients, making it difficult to tease out the effects of green tea.[15,16]

At this time, it seems that green tea extract is safe, but again, longer studies need to be conducted to truly assess the efficacy of this supplement on weight management. Keep in mind that 1 cup of brewed green tea supplies approximately 50–100 mg of EGCG. However, this value is dependent on temperature of the water, type of leaf, season of cultivation, etc. Nonetheless, because there is also research to support the notion that tea consumption as a beverage is correlated to lower bodyweight,[17] coupled with the known health benefits of green tea,[10,18–20] if there are no known contraindications, such as use of coumadin,[21,22] regular consumption is a wise idea.

## Caffeine

Caffeine is often the cornerstone of many fat loss supplements because of its well-documented effects on thermogenesis and lipolysis.[23–27] However, it is not necessarily considered as a stand-alone product intended to enhance fat loss; rather, it is included with other ingredients with the intention of producing a synergistic effect.

Caffeine exerts its effects in a number of ways. To reiterate the aforementioned section on caffeine, it effects lipolysis by inhibiting a specific enzyme necessary to allow HSL to continue on its thermogenic pathway of breaking down triglycerides.[9] In addition, it also seems to stimulate energy expenditure vis a vis increased sympathetic nervous system,[27] and has been suggested to enhance lipolysis.[28] However, results from in vitro studies demonstrate that caffeine also works synergistically with adrenaline to enhance lipolysis.[14] Therefore, the metabolic effects of caffeine seem to come from other mechanisms as well and not solely the interaction with the sympathetic nervous system.

A recent study sought to ascertain where the lipolytic effect of caffeine is derived from: lipid oxidation or via the sympathetic nervous system.[27] This may provide information for supplement manufacturers to design products around the functioning of caffeine, when considering what ingredients would work synergistically to enhance fat loss. There were eight male volunteers in this study who were given either caffeine or placebo; heart rate, energy expenditure, substrate utilization, and free fatty acid turnover were all measured. The results from this study demonstrated that caffeine ingestion increased energy expenditure (~13%), lipid turnover, and oxidation. However, this study and others show that caffeine has a much greater effect on lipolysis than on energy expenditure, which the authors note as a "pharmacologic model of stimulated lipolyis."[27] They also note that from this study, it is apparent that caffeine exerts its effects through both sympathetic and nonsympathetic components.

It is important to note that high doses of caffeine can also have some negative side effects. Studies have demonstrated that caffeine may elevate blood pressure and heart rate,[29] as well as result in diuresis, with one study suggesting that high doses of caffeine may elicit loose bowels or diarhea.[30] A regular cup of coffee contains approximately 100 mg of caffeine (which will vary with bean type, length of brewing, etc.), so caution is advised when taking doses of caffeine that are much higher than this.

## Conjugated Linoleic Acid

Conjugated linoleic acid (CLA) is one of many supplements on the market touted to reduce body fat, decrease weight, and possess antiatherogenic and antidiabetic effects in animals.[31] This led to a widespread use of CLA in the United States as well as Europe, especially among obese individuals.

CLA is a supplement that has been proposed to increase metabolic rate, increase fat utilization, and thus, with these combined, result in weight loss. CLA is a group of positional and geometric isomers[32]; that is, they are positioned differently as if putting them in front of a mirror, of a fatty acid known as linoleic acid.[33] Linoleic acid, as well as linolenic acid, are fatty acids both required by our bodies. CLA is found primarily in dairy products (not in skimmed dairy products) and meat, specifically, beef and lamb.[34] The typical dietary intake is around 212 mg/day for men and 151 mg/day for women.[34,35]

The predominant isomer that is found in cattle and other ruminant animals is "Cis-9, Trans-11-CLA" (this simply refers to the chemistry of the CLA), which seems to be the most biologically active form.[36] Researchers often call this type of CLA "Rumenic Acid" because it is the "natural" form from ruminant animals. Commercial CLA preparations are those found in supplements, and are often in a 1:1 ratio of the Cis-9, Trans-11-CLA and Trans-10, Cis-12-CLA.

CLA has been studied for various effects on health including: effects on the immune system,[37,38] cancer prevention,[39] blood lipid and glucose levels,[40,41] and body composition/weight loss.[41-45]

The research on CLA and body composition in animals has been extremely positive. For example, it has resulted in leaner pigs, mice, rats, and cows. However, these positive results have not been so consistent with humans. Most researchers have reported no change in body composition with CLA supplementation in humans. Furthermore, CLA may potentially have negative effects on blood lipid levels and glucose levels,[40] although these results have been mixed as well.

A recent meta-analysis published in the *American Journal of Clinical Nutrition* reviewed the few human studies available on CLA.[32] This meta-analysis only included studies that were published as full-length articles. It was noted that the dosages in the studies reviewed ranged from as low as 1.4 g/day (approximately 6 times that of "normal" dietary intake for men) up to 6.8 g/day (approximately 30 times that of the normal dietary intake for men). Of the eight studies considering weight loss as an outcome reviewed in this meta-analysis, none found a significant reduction in body weight and only two showed a significant, but small decrease in body fat. The authors drew the conclusion that "the results of the studies in humans indicate that the effect of CLA on body fat is considerably less than that anticipated from mice studies . . ."

It is important to note, however, that because there are various isomers of CLA, some speculate there may be a difference among the available isomers, contributing to the lack of consistency in results. For example, although the CLA contained naturally in the diet is primarily the cis-9 trans-11 isomer, the majority of studies have instead utilized the trans-10, cis-12 isomer, potentially resulting in mechanistic differences.

Therefore, because of this potential variation among CLA isomers, a group recently published their work comparing two different isomers on body fat mass in overweight humans.[42] This particular 24-week study included 88 overweight, but otherwise healthy men and women. Subjects were randomly split into 5 groups and were randomly assigned to either 3 g high oleic acid sunflower oil (placebo), 1.5 or 3 g cis-9, trans-11 CLA and 1.5 g or 3 g of trans-10, cis-12 CLA. Body fat mass and lean body mass were assessed at baseline and again at the end of the 24 weeks. Dietary intake was also collected to ensure there were no significant differences among groups. At the end of the study, the authors noted there were no significant differences among any of the groups for fat loss, body weight loss, or dietary intake. The authors suggest several potential differences when comparing their research to others; they suggest their study may have been too short or the doses of CLA too low to observe changes. These facts alone demonstrate the need for more research.

Another noticeable difference when comparing the animal data and human data is the doses are inconsistent. If considering the dose of CLA as a percentage of total energy, animal studies that have demonstrated a positive effect from CLA have provided approximately 0.70 g/kg body mass, whereas human studies (such as that described above) provide approximately 0.04 g/kg.[42] For humans to take the same dose of CLA as used in the animal studies, they would need to consume more than 50 g of CLA/day (which would of course vary according to body weight). This dose is not cost-effective and may in fact have negative effects in humans because of the prooxidant effect of CLA that has been suggested.[40]

Although the data in mice seem promising, the existing data in humans suggest that more research is required in humans in which energy intake, energy expenditure, overall nutrient intake, CLA type, and CLA amount are all better controlled. This will allow researchers to truly identify if CLA has a consistent role in decreasing body weight in humans.

Gaullier et al.[46] recently published a study looking at the effectiveness of CLA on body mass, body fat, and various lipid values. This study was the first to show long-term safety and efficacy of CLA in healthy, overweight individuals with no change in lifestyle. Subjects supplemented with either 4.5 g of CLA (in either free fatty acid form or triacylglycerol) or 4.5 g of placebo (olive oil) given in 6 soft gels per day. Because of the different types of isomers identified, this study used equal amounts of c9, t11 and t10, c12 isomers. Results indicated significant reductions in body fat, body weight, and increases in lean body mass through the 12 months. Earlier studies suggested diverse results in total cholesterol and high density lipoprotein. However, this study demonstrated no adverse effects on lipid profiles, which in turn, was predicted to have no increased risk of cardiovascular disease with long-term (10 years) CLA supplementation.

Even though Gaullier et al. had positive results with CLA, and the studies summarized by Wang and Jones[47] showed decreases in body fat and weight only in overweight or obese populations, there is very little research showing a benefit in nonobese, healthy individuals.

## Chitosan

Whereas some dietary supplements are purported to increase metabolic rate or enhance fat metabolism, others, such as Chitosan, are supposed to decrease the amount of fat absorbed and digested.[48] Chitosan is essentially an *N*-deacetylated form of chitin that is extracted from the shells of crustaceans.[48] In the simplest terms, it is a type of positively charged fiber; the goal with use of this product is that it will bind to the negatively charged fat in the intestine and excrete it, similar to the pharmaceutic agent, Orlistat.[49,50] However, although in theory this sounds promising, the results of the studies that have been published are equivocal.

A recent study published by Mhurchu et al.,[48] suggested that treatment with chitosan did not result in a clinically significant change in body weight compared with placebo. This 24-week, double-blind, placebo-controlled, randomized trial was completed on 164 male and female subjects. At baseline and every 4 weeks thereafter, until the end point, subjects completed the following assessments: weight, waist circumference, blood pressure, capsule count, and adverse events. Furthermore, at baseline, 12 weeks, and 24 weeks, blood samples were taken to gather information on serum lipids; it seems logical that if chitosan does in fact decrease fat absorption, there would be a positive effect on lipid levels too.

At the end of 24 weeks, the researchers found no significant changes among any of the outcome variables measured. Those in the chitosan group lost just over 0.5 kg more than the 24-week study period; however, this is not statistically or clinically significant. This study also combined lifestyle and dietary advice throughout the program to all subjects and concluded that "it therefore seems appropriate to focus public attention on the proven effective means of weight loss such as improved nutrition and increased physical activity."

There are some safety concerns with chitosan as well. Although supplementing with chitosan does not seem to be effective at enhancing weight loss, research has suggested that use of this supplement does in fact enhance fat absorption and elimination. Because of this, one common side effect is diarrhea. Moreover, there is concern that some minerals and fat-soluble vitamins would be excreted as well.[51]

## Chromium

Chromium is an essential trace mineral widely used in fat loss supplements. In fact, according to a report in 1999, approximately 10 million Americans took chromium supplements and spent about $150 million per year on the ingredient, making chromium the second largest selling mineral after calcium.[52] This is despite the fact that many well-conducted studies using chromium have not supported its claims as a weight loss agent.

Chromium is sometimes referred to as glucose tolerance factor (GTF), although technically it is the active component of the complex. GTF is actually a complex of molecules found in the body that enhances the effectiveness of insulin. Chromium can be obtained through a varied diet; some of the better sources of the mineral are meats, liver, brewer's yeast, and some grains.[53] The role of chromium and insulin was discovered more than 30 years ago, when researchers realized that chromium-deficient humans on total parenteral nutrition also exhibited signs of insulin resistance and hypercholesterolemia; these signs were reversed with chromium supplementation.[54] Subsequently, researchers have speculated that chromium supplementation might be an effective treatment for diabetes and hypercholesterolemia, with more recent claims suggesting that chromium will enhance body fat loss and lean body mass gains, because of its connection with insulin.

The initial thoughts of how chromium acts in the body is related primarily to enhancing the cell's sensitivity to insulin,[55] thereby increasing the muscle cells' uptake of amino acids, and subsequently improving lean body mass.[56,57] This increase would then result in an increased resting metabolic rate, and incidentally, body fat loss.

One study published considered many of the aforementioned parameters regarding chromium supplementation.[58] This 12-week, double-blind, placebo-controlled study tested the effects of 400 μg/day of chromium picolinate supplementation on body composition, resting metabolic rate, and strength along with several other biochemical parameters. Thirty-seven subjects completed the study, in which each participated in a supervised exercise program, to increase compliance among subjects. All subjects also completed diet records to reduce the confounding factor of energy changes or difference throughout the 12-week protocol. The results at the end of the study showed that supplementing with 400 μg/day chromium picolinate for 12 weeks had no significant effects on any of the outcome parameters measured: body composition, resting metabolic rate, or strength.

Other studies found similar results when assessing the effects of chromium, body composition, and strength gains.[59–62] Yet, this has not swayed eager consumers from trying to find the magic bullet when it comes to weight loss; a majority of the well-controlled studies using chromium supplementation as a means for weight loss show it is ineffective. The more exciting area of research with this mineral is its potential connection to those with diabetes, but even here it seems that the true benefit may be realized in an individual who is chromium deficient, not in someone who is not.

## Sidebar 21.1. "If It Saves Just One Life"—The Fallacy of Absolute Safety

### Jose Antonio

How often have you heard the argument which basically is as follows: "If doing ____ (you fill in the blank) saves just one life, then it's worth doing"? As seductive as it sounds at face value, this argument is at best intellectually vapid and at worst misguided and harmful. The Food and Drug Administration's (FDA) ban on ephedra in 2004 is a perfect illustration of this fallacy. The media coverage of this event frequently referred to a number of adverse events regarding ephedra consumption. However, notions of absolute safety are nothing less than absurd. Whether something is useful or useless, good or harmful, is often related to manner of consumption and dose consumed. To take into perspective, according to the *Nutrition Business Journal*, approximately 9–12 million people consumed an estimated 12–17 billion doses of ephedra-containing supplements annually (before the FDA ban which has since been struck down by a Utah court ruling).[63] However, according to the RAND report, 5 deaths, 5 heart attacks, 11 cerebrovascular accidents, 4 seizures, and 8 psychiatric episodes over a prolonged period of time (8–12 years) are believed to possibly be related to ephedra supplementation. Note that demonstrating causality is virtually impossible.

Clearly, if the argument of "if it saves just one life" is taken to heart, then a ban of ephedra may seem plausible. However, how would one reconcile this with the beneficial effect of ephedra consumption as it applies to weight loss? Would not the human lives and medical costs saved fighting the epidemic of obesity in this country outweigh the potential risks? Should the consumer decide this? The Federal government?

For the sake of comparison, the Centers for Disease Control report that each year more than 400,000 Americans die from cigarette smoking causes (more than 1100 per day).[64] Reports in the medical literature also indicate that more than 100,000 Americans die annually after use of over-the-counter (OTC) or prescription medications (280 per day).[65,66] In 1994 alone, it was estimated that there were 2.2 million severe adverse drug reactions treated in hospitals in response to taking prescription medications that resulted in more than 106,000 fatalities. Moreover, according to the government's Drug Abuse Warning Network (DAWN), in 1999 alone there were 641 deaths linked to diphenhydramine (Benadryl), 477 deaths linked to the antidepressant Elavil, 427 deaths linked to acetaminophen (Tylenol), 305 deaths linked to Prozac, and 104 deaths linked to aspirin.[67]

Certainly, the aforementioned OTC drugs should not be banned; in fact, when you weigh the benefits versus the risks, it is clear that millions of individuals benefit from these drugs. However, are there any positive health benefits from cigarette smoking?

And again, for the sake of comparison, let's look at the fatality rate for a popular winter sport—snowmobiling. Of the nearly half of the 200 people killed on snowmobiles in

Wisconsin over the last decade, most had been drinking.[68] In the state of Michigan, there were 48 deaths from snowmobile accidents during the 1995–96 snow season.[69] Compare that to the 5 total deaths that were attributed to ephedra. Should the state(s) or Federal government seek the ban of a sport that clearly is more dangerous than consuming ephedra?

Clearly not. As with all behaviors, there are risks and trade-offs. Whether one examines relative or absolute risk, it is evident that ephedra, when used properly, is not dangerous.

## Coleus forskohlii

*Coleus forskohlii* is an herb that has been used since ancient times to treat heart and respiratory disorders; more recently, it has been added to weight loss products as well. Herbal product manufacturers are now producing *C. forskohlii* extracts with elevated levels of the constituent forskolin.

Although no full-length manuscripts have been published measuring the effects of this herb on fat loss, there is currently one published abstract. The logic behind its inclusion is apparent when considering its mechanism. *C. forskohlii* stimulates the enzyme adenylate cyclase, which in turn catalyzes the conversion of ATP to cAMP,[70] which, as described earlier in the chapter, increases the effects of HSL to break down triglycerides.

The one small study completed to date provided six overweight women with 250 mg of *C. forskohlii*, standardized to provide 10% (25 mg) of forskolin twice daily for 12 weeks.[70] At the end of the study, the authors found no statistical difference in body weight or body fat, over the 12-week period. This is only one small study; however, at this time, it is the only published evidence regarding this particular supplement.

Consequently, it is safe to say that although the use of *C. forskohlii* seems useful on paper, this conclusion cannot be drawn without more evidence to support or refute the statement. Moreover, there is concern regarding its safety and efficacy because forskolin may worsen cardiovascular conditions, by causing vasodilation and lowering blood pressure.[71]

## Hydroxycitric Acid

Hydroxycitric acid (HCA) is produced from the rind of the fruit of *Garcinia cambogia*, which is native to India and popular as a food additive in Asian cultures.[72] In America, HCA has grown in popularity and its inclusion in weight loss aids is common. However, this popularity has not resulted in many well-controlled human research studies assessing the claims; most of the supportive literature is in rodents.

Early research has shown that administration of HCA inhibits the extramitochondrial enzyme ATP citrate-lyase, which catalyzes the cleavage of citrate to acetyl-coenzyme A and oxaloacetate.[72,73] This is a crucial step in lipogenesis, which would lead one to believe that administration of HCA would enhance fat loss.

van Loon et al.[72] published a small study measuring the acute effects of HCA on substrate oxidation in humans in 2000. This study was designed to determine if HCA would enhance fat oxidation during bicycling; this is important because increased fat oxidation is one of the purported mechanisms of HCA and, if true, one that could increase fat loss. Ten cyclists participated in this pilot study; subjects were provided with a flavored beverage that contained 0.5 g/kg body weight of HCA, resulting in a total of 18 ± 0.4 g HCA over the entire HCA trial. At the end of the trial, it was determined that HCA concentrations were increased higher than would be expected with the doses used in previous studies and what is included in most weight loss products; no other human trials have measured plasma HCA, however, but this study alleviated concern that HCA may not be absorbed. Although plasma HCA levels were increased, this did not translate to increased fat or carbohydrate oxidation rates, suggesting that this mechanism of action does not contribute to weight loss. There is still thought that HCA may inhibit dietary intake as another mechanism, thereby enhancing weight loss.

Therefore, Leonhardt and Langhans[74] investigated the effect of HCA on feeding behavior, body weight regain, and metabolism after weight loss in male rats. This 22-day feeding study fed ad libitum diets to two groups of rats. The rats were first all fed 10 g of a standard rodent diet for 10 days intended to cause weight loss. The rats were then divided into two groups and matched for weight loss and body weight. They were then fed one of two diets (one provided only 1% fat and the other provided 12% fat) and within each group, one group of rats was supplemented with 3 g/100 g HCA, whereas the other solely fed the rodent diet. The results showed that HCA did cause a reduction of body weight regain in both groups. Similarly, for the rats consuming the 12% fat diet (but not the 1% diet) there was a significant long-term suppressive effect on food intake, suggesting that the increased fat content was necessary for this change. Unfortunately, although these results show promise, it is difficult to extrapolate them to humans because the dose of HCA provided would be extremely high in humans, and this is not cost-effective.

The small amount of data available using HCA as a weight loss aid in humans does not provide solid evidence that it is effective. Although the rodent data seem promising, the doses used have been much higher than those used in human studies and the human studies have not solely considered HCA but rather as a component of a proprietary formula. This makes it impossible to tease out the individual effects of each component.

## Summary

Dietary supplements are and always will be immensely popular (Table 21.1). Fat loss supplements are particularly popular because America is currently facing an obesity epidemic. Therefore, dietary supplements intended to enhance weight loss will continue to come and go over the years. Unfortunately, after reading this chapter, it should be apparent that few scientific data support many of the fat loss supplements available. The ephedra-containing supplements were effective for fat loss, but supplements with ephedra have been banned because it was surrounded by controversy as a result of some health concerns reported by consumers. Ironically, pure ephedrine can still be purchased.

**TABLE 21.1. Fat loss supplements and their purported mechanisms.**

| Ingredient | Purported mechanism |
| --- | --- |
| *Citrus aurantium* | Acts primarily on β-3 receptors, which are responsible for lipolytic and thermogenic effects |
| Green tea (EGCG) | EGCG may prolong thermogenesis by inhibiting enzymes necessary in this reaction |
| Caffeine | Enhances lipolysis and thermogenesis by inhibiting enzymes that are otherwise hydrolyzed to halt the process |
| Conjugated linoleic acid | May increase metabolic rate and increase fat utilization |
| Chitosan | Will bind to negatively charged fat in the intestine for excretion |
| Chromium | May enhance the cell's sensitivity to insulin, thereby increasing cellular uptake of amino acids and enhancing lean body mass and subsequently increasing metabolic rate |
| Hydroxycitric acid | Inhibits ATP citrate-lyase, which catalyzes another reaction that would otherwise slow lipogenesis, thereby prolonging this "fat burning" |

EGCG = epigallocatechin-3-gallate, ATP = adenosine triphosphate.

## Sidebar 21.2. Ephedra

### Eric S. Rawson

On April 12, 2004, subsequent to numerous reports of adverse events,[75–79] the FDA banned the sale of the ephedrine-containing herb ephedra. Ephedrine is a sympathomimetic drug and central nervous system stimulant that is structurally related to amphetamines.[80] Ephedrine has been used for weight loss[81] because of its thermogenic and anorectic properties,[82,83] and to increase alertness and improve sports performance because it is a central nervous system stimulant.[84–89] Whereas ephedrine is a synthetic drug, ephedra is an herb (e.g., ma huang, ephedra sinica) that contains a mixture of alkaloids that includes ephedrine, pseudoephedrine, norephedrine, and methylephedrine.[90,91]

### Quality Control

The ephedrine content of ephedra plants varies based on species, where the plant is grown, the type of growing conditions, and the time of harvest,[92] which makes standardization of ephedra in dietary supplements difficult. Not surprisingly, the absolute ephedrine alkaloid content and the ratio of ephedrine alkaloids varies markedly both within and between lots of the same dietary supplements.[91] Gurley et al.[90] assessed the content of ephedra alkaloids in 20 ephedra-containing supplements and reported a 0.0–18.5 mg of total alkaloid content per dosage unit. Lot-to-lot variations in one product for ephedrine, pseudoephedrine, and methylephedrine exceeded 180%, 250%, and 1000%, respectively. The large variability in ephedra alkaloid content makes studying the therapeutic and adverse effects of ephedra supplements complicated.

### Weight Loss

The effectiveness of ephedrine as a weight loss agent is enhanced by caffeine and aspirin.[93,94] Ephedrine stimulates the release of norepinephrine, which stimulates the release of adenosine. Adenosine is a prejunctional inhibitor of norepinephrine, but caffeine blunts the effects of adenosine and in turn potentiates the release of norepinephrine. Additionally, norepinephrine stimulates the synthesis of prostaglandins, which also act as prejunctional inhibitors. Aspirin inhibits the synthesis of prostaglandins and can prevent norepinephrine release.[93] In hope of potentiating the thermogenic effect of ephedra, many ephedra products contained herbal sources of caffeine (e.g., guarana, kola nut) and salicin (e.g., white willow bark) which is converted to the prostaglandin inhibitor salicylic acid in the body. Although ephedrine was marketed primarily as a "thermogenic" supplement that induced weight loss through increased metabolic rate, this marketing strategy was somewhat misleading. It is estimated that 75% of weight loss from ephedrine/caffeine combinations is attributable to an anorectic effect and only 25% is attributable to a thermogenic effect.[82,83]

A recent meta-analysis reported that ephedrine, ephedrine plus caffeine, ephedra, and ephedra plus caffeine (from herbal sources) promote weight loss.[79] However, these differences are small when compared with a placebo (0.9 kg per month > placebo). Reportedly, weight loss in excess of placebo was 7.9 kg greater for those receiving phentermine, 4.3 kg greater for those receiving sibutramine, and 3.4 kg greater for those receiving orlistat.[95] Thus, ephedrine is only modestly effective as a weight loss agent compared with prescription drugs. As an example, Astrup et al.[81] examined the effects of a 24-week diet plus either an ephedrine/caffeine combination (20 mg/200 mg), ephedrine (20 mg), caffeine (200 mg), or placebo ingested 3 times a day. Weight loss was significantly greater in the ephedrine/caffeine group (ephedrine/caffeine 16.6 kg versus placebo 13.2 kg), and weight loss in both the ephedrine and the caffeine-alone groups was similar to the placebo group. Although the ephedrine/caffeine combination resulted in a statistically greater weight loss, Astrup and colleagues[81,96] commented that the additional weight loss attributed to ephedrine (1.7 kg) seemed "clinically irrelevant" compared with the weight loss achieved through diet, nutritional education, frequent monitoring, and behavior therapy (13 kg).

Boozer et al.[97,98] reported that an herbal ephedra/caffeine supplement plus diet and exercise decreased body mass and body fat more than a placebo plus diet and exercise. However, the difference between herbal and placebo treatments was small after 8 weeks (ephedra/caffeine versus placebo: body mass −4.0 versus −0.8 kg; body fat percent—2.1 versus 0.2% fat)[98] and 6 months of supplementation (ephedra/caffeine versus placebo: body mass −5.3 versus—2.6 kg; body fat −4.3 versus −2.7 kg).[97] No studies have assessed the effects of ephedrine/ephedra on long-term weight loss maintenance. Therefore, it is unknown if the weight-reducing effects of ephedrine/caffeine and ephedra/caffeine combinations are more likely to be sustained when compared with weight loss without the use of these drugs.

*Adverse Effects*

Haller and Benowitz[76] conducted an independent review of reports of adverse events related to the use of ephedra-containing supplements. One hundred forty case reports were reviewed and 31% of cases were considered to be definitely or probably related to the use of supplements containing ephedra alkaloids, and 31% were judged to be possibly related. Of the adverse events that were considered related to the use of supplements containing ephedra, there were 17 reports of hypertension, 13 reports of palpitations, tachycardia, or both, 10 cases of stroke, and 7 cases of seizures. Ten deaths and 13 events that produced permanent disability were related to ephedra. In a similar analysis, Samenuk et al.[78] examined 926 cases of possible ephedra toxicity. The authors concluded that 1) ephedra use is temporally related to stroke, myocardial infarction, and sudden death; 2) underlying heart or vascular disease is not a prerequisite for ephedra-related adverse events; and 3) the cardiovascular

toxic effects associated with ephedra were not limited to massive doses. Bent et al.[75] reported that 64% of all adverse reactions to herbs in the United States were accounted for by ephedra products, despite that fact that these products represented only 0.82% of herbal product sales.

However, some researchers remain less convinced of the dangers of ephedra. Kreider[99] reported that in 1999 there were 641 deaths linked to the OTC drugs diphenhydramine (Benadryl), 427 deaths linked to acetaminophen (Tylenol), and 104 deaths linked to aspirin. In comparison, five deaths occurred over several years that were believed to be associated with ephedra ingestion.[99] Nonetheless, the FDA removed ephedra from the market in 2004.

*Conclusion*

Although the removal of herbal ephedra from the market in the United States is seen by some as a solution, ephedrine is readily available through the Internet. Furthermore, the removal of ephedra from the market in the United States left a gap in weight loss supplements that was rapidly filled by products with little research to support their safety or efficacy. One such product is synephrine which is found in *C. aurantium* (bitter orange, sour orange, Seville orange) and is often included in ephedra-free products.[100] Few data are available regarding the safety[101] and efficacy of synephrine,[4] but one case study has already associated synephrine with myocardial infarction.[103] It is likely that nutritional supplements such as ephedra and *C. aurantium* will continue to be marketed as long as people are interested in using supplements to lose weight.

One year after ephedra was banned, a United States District Court in Utah determined that the FDA did not prove by a preponderance of evidence that a 10 mg or less dose of ephedra alkaloids presents a "significant or unreasonable risk of injury." Consequently, supplement manufacturers may be able to sell ephedra supplements without enforcement action taken against them, as long as the daily dose is less than 10 mg. Thus, it seems that ephedra was not gone for long, and certainly was not forgotten.

# PRACTICAL APPLICATIONS

Americans have seen a surge in obesity rates, causing an epidemic that is soon to surpass smoking as the most preventable cause of death. A successful weight loss program encompasses many components: changes in energy intake and energy expenditure, as well as behavioral strategies. Individuals are also bombarded daily with infomercials, fad diets, and charlatans who pass themselves off as authorities. Consequently, the health and nutrition professional must keep abreast of the latest trends, which will ultimately help their clients.

Dietary supplements are one popular trend; some do show promise, but most are not backed by science. Therefore, it is up to professionals to inform clients of the current research or lack thereof. Rather than quickly drawing conclusions about the efficacy of dietary supplements without delving into the available research, it is recommended that professionals do everything in their power to educate clients; provide both the pros and cons of the supplements in question, and, unless it has the potential to cause harm, allow the client to use the sound information provided to make a decision.

An effective weight loss program should encompass trained professionals from a variety of backgrounds: nutrition, exercise physiology, and psychology.

All weight loss efforts should focus on dietary and exercise habits, while providing the necessary behavior model to tell clients not only how to do the right thing, but why they should do the right thing. A client can be well informed on what to do (decrease energy intake and increase energy expenditure), but if they are unaware of how to make these changes, the efforts of the health professional are futile.

The key with any long-term program is to get to the root of the situation, rather than only cutting down the weeds; solely using dietary supplements for weight loss is akin to cutting down the weeds. A sound program of moderate energy reduction and increased exercise are most important when trying to decrease body weight and body fat.

## QUESTIONS

1. Using the body mass index as a marker, overweight is classified as:
   a. $15.0$–$19.9\,kg\cdot m^2$
   b. $20.0$–$24.9\,kg\cdot m^2$
   c. $25.0$–$29.9\,kg\cdot m^2$
   d. $30.0$–$34.9\,kg\cdot m^2$

2. Using the body mass index as a marker, obese is classified as:
   a. $20.0$–$24.9\,kg\cdot m^2$
   b. $25.0$–$29.9\,kg\cdot m^2$
   c. $\geq 30.0\,kg\cdot m^2$
   d. None of the above

3. Several diseases are secondary to obesity, including:
   a. Cardiovascular disease
   b. Osteoarthritis
   c. Diabetes
   d. All of the above
   e. None of the above

4. Health professionals should recommend a comprehensive weight loss regimen including a (an):
   a. Modest reduction in energy only
   b. Increase in energy expenditure only
   c. Modest reduction in energy, an increase in energy expenditure with behavioral modifications
   d. Only taking dietary supplements

5. *Citrus aurantium* is purported to enhance weight loss because:
   a. It increases thermogenesis through the β-3 receptors
   b. It acts on all three β receptors
   c. It causes a reduction in appetite
   d. It binds fat inside the body and excretes it

6. The β-1 and β-2 receptors are primarily responsible for:
   a. Causing a relaxation of smooth muscle and stimulation of cardiac muscle
   b. Increasing thermogenesis and lipolysis
   c. Insulin release from the pancreas
   d. Decreasing appetite

7. The β-3 receptors seem to be responsible for:
   a. Causing a relaxation of smooth muscle and stimulation of cardiac muscle
   b. Increasing thermogenesis and lipolysis
   c. Insulin release from the pancreas
   d. Decreasing appetite

8. In terms of weight loss, the crucial components of green tea extract are:
   a. Caffeine
   b. Epigallocatechin-3-gallate (EGCG)
   c. Ephedrine

d. a and b
e. b and c

9. EGCG may be effective for enhancing fat loss because it:
   a. Inhibits an enzyme that would otherwise be quickly hydrolyzed and is an important part of increasing thermogenesis
   b. Suppresses appetite
   c. Blocks fat absorption in the intestine
   e. Increases the heart rate

10. Caffeine is an important component of green tea because it:
    a. Inhibits an enzyme that would otherwise be quickly hydrolyzed and is an important part of increasing thermogenesis
    b. Suppresses appetite
    c. Blocks fat absorption in the intestine
    d. Works synergistically with EGCG to prolong the thermogenic process

11. CLA is an all-inclusive term for:
    a. A group of proteins that enhance thermogenesis
    b. Trans fats
    c. An amino acid found only in ruminant meats
    d. A group of positional and geometric isomers of a fatty acid known as linoleic acid

12. The primary source(s) of CLA in the diet is:
    a. Whole milk
    b. Beef
    c. Lamb
    d. Green leafy vegetables
    e. All of the above
    f. a, b, and c

13. Chitosan is extracted from:
    a. Whole fat dairy products
    b. Shells of crustaceans
    c. Red meat
    d. None of the above

14. The purported mechanism of chitosan is to:
    a. Bind to the negatively charged fat in the intestine and excrete it
    b. Increase thermogenesis by increasing the heart rate and catecholamine excretion in the brain
    c. Enhance the use of fatty acids for energy
    d. Block cortisol levels

15. Regular use of chitosan may have side effects, including:
    a. Giving a person the "jitters"
    b. Binding and excreting fat-soluble vitamins
    c. Diarrhea
    d. All of the above
    e. b and c

16. Chromium is the second largest selling mineral to:
    a. Selenium
    b. Zinc
    c. Calcium
    e. Iron

17. Some of the best food sources of chromium are:
    a. Brewer's yeast
    b. Grains
    c. Meat
    d. Liver
    e. All of the above

18. *Coleus forskohlii* is an herb that has traditionally been used to treat:
    a. Heart disorders
    b. Respiratory disorders
    c. Overweight and obesity
    d. a and c
    e. a and b

19. The purported mechanism for hydroxycitric acid is:
    a. Absorb fat in the intestine and excrete it
    b. Increase thermogenesis
    c. Suppress appetite
    d. Inhibit an enzyme that may enhance lipolysis

20. Dietary supplements purported to enhance weight loss typically utilize these mechanisms:
    a. Increase thermogenesis
    b. Block fat absorption
    c. Suppress appetite
    d. All of the above

21. Overweight and obese are interchangeable terms.
    a. True
    b. False

22. All fat loss supplements are safe and efficacious because they are sold over the counter.
    a. True
    b. False

23. *Citrus aurantium* is a well-researched supplement with a tremendous amount of safety and efficacy data to support it.
    a. True
    b. False

24. The benefits of green tea can be found in a dietary supplement or by drinking the beverage itself.
    a. True
    b. False

25. The typical nonvegetarian American diet contains CLA.
    a. True
    b. False

26. Americans consume doses of CLA that are equivalent to those used in most studies.
    a. True
    b. False

27. *Coleus forskohlii* has been around since ancient times, ensuring its safety and efficacy through the numerous studies published on the ingredient.
    a. True
    b. False

28. Dietary supplements should always be a component of a sound weight loss regimen.
    a. True
    b. False

29. A modest energy reduction and increase in energy expenditure is a safe bet for a sound weight reduction program.
    a. True
    b. False

30. Dietary supplements that are sold over the counter are all safe and effective
    a. True
    b. False

# REFERENCES

1. Flegal KM, Carroll MD, Ogden CL, Johnson CL. Prevalence and trends in obesity among US adults, 1999–2000. JAMA 2002;288(14):1723–1727.
2. Kopelman PG. Obesity as a medical problem. Nature 2000:635–643.
3. Fugh-Berman A, Myers A. *Citrus aurantium*, an ingredient of dietary supplements marketed for weight loss: current status of clinical and basic research. Exp Biol Med (Maywood) 2004:698–704.
4. Colker CM, Kalman DS, Torina GC, Perlis T, Street C. Effects of *Citrus aurantium* extract, caffeine, and St. John's wort on body fat loss, lipid levels, and mood states in overweight healthy adults. Curr Ther Res 1999:145–153.
5. Pellati F, Benvenuti S, Melegari M, Firenzuoli F. Determination of adrenergic agonists from extracts and herbal products of *Citrus aurantium* L. var. amara by LC. J Pharm Biomed Anal 2002:1113–1119.
6. D'Andrea G, Terrazzino S, Fortin D, Farruggio A, Rinaldi L, Leon A, eds. HPLC electrochemical detection of trace amines in human plasma and platelets and expression of mRNA transcripts of trace amine receptors in circulating leukocytes. Neurosci Lett 2003;346(1–2):89–92.
7. Chantre P, Lairon D. Recent findings of green tea extract AR25 (Exolise) and its activity for the treatment of obesity. Phytomedicine 2002:3–8.
8. Kao YH, Hiipakka RA, Liao S. Modulation of endocrine systems and food intake by green tea epigallocatechin gallate. Endocrinology 2000:980–987.
9. Dulloo AG, Duret C, Rohrer D, et al. Efficacy of a green tea extract rich in catechin polyphenols and caffeine in increasing 24-h energy expenditure and fat oxidation in humans. Am J Clin Nutr 1999:1040–1045.
10. Kaegi E. Unconventional therapies for cancer: 2. Green tea. The Task Force on Alternative Therapies of the Canadian Breast Cancer Research Initiative. CMAJ 1998:1033–1035.
11. Powers SH, Howley ET. Exercise Physiology: Theory and Application to Fitness and Performance. Hormonal Responses to Exercise. Boston: McGraw Hill; 2001: 66–97.
12. Durand J, Giacobino JP, Girardier L. Catechol-O-methyl transferase activity in whole brown adipose tissue of rat in vitro. Experientia Suppl 1978:45–53.
13. Houston ME. Biochemistry Primer for Exercise Science. 2nd ed. Champaign, IL: Human Kinetics Publishers; 2001:113–140.
14. Butcher RW, Baird CE, Sutherland EW. Effects of lipolytic and antilipolytic substances on adenosine 3′,5′-monophosphate levels in isolated fat cells. J Biol Chem 1968:1705–1712.
15. Kalman DS, Rubin S, Martinez T, Schwartz H. Efficacy of a commercial green tea extract/caffeine based product to increase basal metabolism in healthy adults. NIH/NIDDK: The Interaction of Physical Activity and Nutrition: Biological Remodeling and Plasticity Conference, 2002.
16. Kalman DS, RS, Schwartz H. An acute clinical trial to evaluate the safety of a popular commercial weight loss supplement when used with exercise. Experimental Biology Conference, 2003, San Diego CA.
17. Wu CH, Lu FH, Chang CS, Chang TC, Wang RH, Chang CJ. Relationship among habitual tea consumption, percent body fat, and body fat distribution. Obes Res 2003:1088–1095.
18. Mitscher LA, ML, Jung M, Shankel D, et al. Chemoprotection: a review of the potential therapeutic antioxidant properties of green tea (*Camellia sinensis*) and certain of its constituents. Med Res Rev 1997:327–365.
19. Bushman JL. Green tea and cancer in humans: a review of the literature. Nutr Cancer 1998:151–159.
20. Siddiqui IA, Afaq F, Adhami VM, Ahmad N, Mukhtar H. Antioxidants of the beverage tea in promotion of human health. Antioxid Redox Signal 2004:571–582.
21. Taylor JR, Wilt VM. Probable antagonism of warfarin by green tea. Ann Pharmacother 1999:426–428.
22. Booth SL, Madabushi HT, Davidson KW, Sadowski JA. Tea and coffee brews are not dietary sources of vitamin K-1 (phylloquinone). J Am Diet Assoc 1995:82–83.
23. Astrup A, Toubro S, Christensen NJ, Quaade F. Pharmacology of thermogenic drugs. Am J Clin Nutr 1992:246S–248S.
24. Bracco D, Ferrarra JM, Arnaud MJ, Jequier E, Schutz Y. Effects of caffeine on energy metabolism, heart rate, and methylxanthine metabolism in lean and obese women. Am J Physiol 1995:E671–678.
25. Arciero PJ, Gardner AW, Calles-Escandon J, Benowitz NL, Poehlman ET. Effects of caffeine ingestion on NE kinetics, fat oxidation, and energy expenditure in younger and older men. Am J Physiol 1995:E1192–1198.

26. Acheson KJ, Zahorska-Markiewicz B, Pittet P, Anantharaman K, Jequier E. Caffeine and coffee: their influence on metabolic rate and substrate utilization in normal weight and obese individuals. Am J Clin Nutr 1980:989–997.

27. Acheson KJ, Gremaud G, Meirim I, et al. Metabolic effects of caffeine in humans: lipid oxidation or futile cycling? Am J Clin Nutr 2004:40–46.

28. Bellet S, Roman L, DeCastro O, Kim KE, Kershbaum A. Effect of coffee ingestion on catecholamine release. Metabolism 1969:288–291.

29. Debrah K, Haigh R, Sherwin R, Murphy J, Kerr D. Effect of acute and chronic caffeine use on the cerebrovascular, cardiovascular and hormonal responses to orthostasis in healthy volunteers. Clin Sci (Lond) 1995:475–480.

30. Wald A, Back C, Bayless TM. Effect of caffeine on the human small intestine. Gastroenterology 1976:738–742.

31. Park Y, Albright KJ, Storkson JM, Liu W, Cook ME, Pariza MW. Changes in body composition in mice during feeding and withdrawal of conjugated linoleic acid. Lipids 1999;34:243–248.

32. Terpstra AH. Effect of conjugated linoleic acid on body composition and plasma lipids in humans: an overview of the literature. Am J Clin Nutr 2004:352–361.

33. Pariza MW, Ha YL. Conjugated dienoic derivatives of linoleic acid: a new class of anticarcinogens. Med Oncol Tumor Pharmacother 1990:169–171.

34. Ritzenthaler KL, McGuire MK, Falen R, Shultz TD, Dasgupta N, McGuire MA. Estimation of conjugated linoleic acid intake by written dietary assessment methodologies underestimates actual intake evaluated by food duplicate methodology. J Nutr 2001:1548–1554.

35. Terpstra AH. Effect of conjugated linoleic acid on body composition and plasma lipids in humans: an overview of the literature. Am J Clin Nutr 2004:352–361.

36. Pariza MW, Ha YL, Benjamin H, et al. Formation and action of anticarcinogenic fatty acids. Adv Exp Med Biol 1991:269–272.

37. Bontempo V, Sciannimanico D, Pastorelli G, Rossi R, Rosi F, Corino C. Dietary conjugated linoleic acid positively affects immunologic variables in lactating sows and piglets. J Nutr 2004:817–824.

38. Sebedio JL, Gnaedig S, Chardigny JM. Recent advances in conjugated linoleic acid research. Curr Opin Clin Nutr Metab Care 1999:499–506.

39. MacDonald H. Conjugated linoleic acid and disease prevention: a review of current knowledge. J Am Coll Nutr 2000:111S–118S.

40. Riserus U, Smedman A, Basu S, Vessby B. CLA and body weight regulation in humans. Lipids 2003:133–137.

41. Brown JM, McIntosh MK. Conjugated linoleic acid in humans: regulation of adiposity and insulin sensitivity. J Nutr 2003:3041–3046.

42. Malpuech-Brugere C, Verboeket-van de Venne WP, Mensink RP, et al. Effects of two conjugated linoleic acid isomers on body fat mass in overweight humans. Obes Res 2004:591–598.

43. Park Y, Storkson JM, Albright KJ, Liu W, Pariza MW. Evidence that the trans-10,cis-12 isomer of conjugated linoleic acid induces body composition changes in mice. Lipids 1999:235–241.

44. Azain MJ, Hausman DB, Sisk MB, Flatt WP, Jewell DE. Dietary conjugated linoleic acid reduces rat adipose tissue cell size rather than cell number. J Nutr 2000:1548–1554.

45. Gavino VC, Gavino G, Leblanc MJ, Tuchweber B. An isomeric mixture of conjugated linoleic acids but not pure cis-9, trans-11-octadecadienoic acid affects body weight gain and plasma lipids in hamsters. J Nutr 2000:27–29.

46. Gaullier JM, Halse J, Hoye K, et al. Conjugated linoleic acid supplementation for 1 y reduces body fat mass in healthy overweight humans. Am J Clin Nutr 2004;79:1118–1125.

47. Wang Y, Jones PJ. Dietary conjugated linoleic acid and body composition. Am J Clin Nutr 2004;79:1153S–1158S.

48. Mhurchu CN, Poppitt SD, McGill AT, et al. The effect of the dietary supplement, Chitosan, on body weight: a randomised controlled trial in 250 overweight and obese adults. Int J Obes Relat Metab Disord 2004:1149–1156.

49. Kanauchi O, Deuchi K, Imasato Y, Shizukuishi M, Kobayashi E. Mechanism for the inhibition of fat digestion by chitosan and for the synergistic effect of ascorbate. Biosci Biotechnol Biochem 1995:786–790.

50. Deuchi K, Kanauchi O, Imasato Y, Kobayashi E. Effect of the viscosity or deacetylation degree of chitosan on fecal fat excreted from rats fed on a high-fat diet. Biosci Biotechnol Biochem 1995:781–785.

51. Deuchi K, Kanauchi O, Shizukuishi M, Kobayashi E. Continuous and massive intake of chitosan affects mineral and fat-soluble vitamin status in rats fed on a high-fat diet. Biosci Biotechnol Biochem 1995:1211–1216.

52. Hellerstein MK. Is chromium supplementation effective in managing type II diabetes? Nutr Rev 1998:302–306.
53. Guthrie H, Picciano MF. Micronutrient Minerals. In: Human Nutrition. Mosby. St. Louis; 1995:333–380.
54. Jeejeebhoy KN, Chu RC, Marliss EB, Greenberg GR, Bruce-Robertson A. Chromium deficiency, glucose intolerance, and neuropathy reversed by chromium supplementation in a patient receiving long-term total parenteral nutrition. Am J Clin Nutr 1977:531–538.
55. Evans GW, Bowman TD. Chromium picolinate increases membrane fluidity and rate of insulin internalization. J Inorg Biochem 1992:243–250.
56. Vincent JB. The biochemistry of chromium. J Nutr. 2000:Apr;130(4):715–8.
57. Trent LK, Thieding-Cancel D. Effects of chromium picolinate on body composition. J Sports Med Phys Fitness 1995:273–280.
58. Volpe SL, Huang HW, Larpadisorn K, Lesser II. Effect of chromium supplementation and exercise on body composition, resting metabolic rate and selected biochemical parameters in moderately obese women following an exercise program. J Am Coll Nutr 2001:293–306.
59. Clancy SP, Clarkson PM, DeCheke ME, et al. Effects of chromium picolinate supplementation on body composition, strength, and urinary chromium loss in football players. Int J Sport Nutr 1994:142–153.
60. Hallmark MA, Reynolds TH, DeSouza CA, Dotson CO, Anderson RA, Rogers MA. Effects of chromium and resistive training on muscle strength and body composition. Med Sci Sports Exerc 1996:139–144.
61. Lefavi RG, Anderson RA, Keith RE, Wilson GD, McMillan JL, Stone MH. Efficacy of chromium supplementation in athletes: emphasis on anabolism. Int J Sport Nutr 1992:111–122.
62. Lukaski HC, Bolonchuk WW, Siders WA, Milne DB. Chromium supplementation and resistance training: effects on body composition, strength, and trace element status of men. Am J Clin Nutr 1996:954–965.
63. http://www.sfgate.com/cgi-bin/article.cgi?file=/news/archive/2005/04/15/national/a013653D58.DTL.
64. Centers for Disease Control. Cigarette Smoking-Related Mortality. 2001. Available at: http://www.cdc.gov/tobacco/research_data/health_consequences/mortali.htm.
65. Kvasz M, Allen IE, Gordon MJ, et al. Adverse drug reactions in hospitalized patients: a critique of a meta-analysis. MedGenMed 2000;2(2):E3.
66. Lazarou J, Pomeranz BH, Corey PN. Incidence of adverse drug reactions in hospitalized patients: a meta-analysis of prospective studies. JAMA 1998;279(15):1200.
67. Sullum J. What's Wrong With Mahuang? The Weak Case Against Ephedra, in Reason Online. 2003. Available at: http://www.reason.com/links/links030303.shtml.
68. http://newmedia.medill.northwestern.edu/data/snowmobilestory.html.
69. http://www.freep.com/news/mich/snowmo14_20030114.htm.
70. Kreider R, Shonteh H, Magu B, Rasmussen C. Effects of Coleus forskohlii supplementation on body composition and markers of health in sedentary overweight females. FASEB, New Orleans, LA 2002.
71. Baumann G, Felix S, Sattelberger U, Klein G. Cardiovascular effects of forskolin (HL 362) in patients with idiopathic congestive cardiomyopathy—a comparative study with dobutamine and sodium nitroprusside. J Cardiovasc Pharmacol 1990: 93–100.
72. van Loon LJ, van Rooijen JJ, Niesen B, Verhagen H, Saris WH, Wagenmakers AJ. Effects of acute (–)-hydroxycitrate supplementation on substrate metabolism at rest and during exercise in humans. Am J Clin Nutr 2000:1445–1450.
73. Watson JA, Fang M, Lowenstein JM. Tricarballylate and hydroxycitrate: substrate and inhibitor of ATP: citrate oxaloacetate lyase. Arch Biochem Biophys 1969: 209–217.
74. Leonhardt M, Langhans W. Hydroxycitrate has long-term effects on feeding behavior, body weight regain and metabolism after body weight loss in male rats. J Nutr 2002:1977–1982.
75. Bent S, Tiedt TN, Odden MC, Shlipak MG. The relative safety of ephedra compared with other herbal products. Ann Intern Med 2003;138:468–471.
76. Haller CA, Benowitz NL. Adverse cardiovascular and central nervous system events associated with dietary supplements containing ephedra alkaloids. N Engl J Med 2000;343:1833–1838.
77. Rawson ES, Clarkson PM. Ephedrine as an ergogenic aid. In: Bahrke MS, Yesalis CE, eds. Performance-Enhancing Substances in Sport and Exercise. Champaign, IL: Human Kinetics Publishers; 2002:289–298.
78. Samenuk D, Link MS, Homoud MK, et al. Adverse cardiovascular events temporally associated with ma huang, an herbal source of ephedrine. Mayo Clin Proc 2002; 77:12–16.

79. Shekelle PG, Hardy ML, Morton SC, et al. Efficacy and safety of ephedra and ephedrine for weight loss and athletic performance: a meta-analysis. JAMA 2003;289: 1537–1545.

80. Hoffman BB, Lefkowitz RJ. Catecholamines, sympathomimetic drugs, and adrenergic receptor antagonists. In: Hardman JG, Limbird LE, Molinoff PB, Ruddon RW, Gilman AG, eds. Goodman & Gilman's The Pharmacological Basis of Therapeutics. New York: McGraw-Hill; 1996:199–248.

81. Astrup A, Breum L, Toubro S, Hein P, Quaade F. The effect and safety of an ephedrine/caffeine compound compared to ephedrine, caffeine and placebo in obese subjects on an energy restricted diet. A double blind trial. Int J Obes Relat Metab Disord 1992;16:269–277.

82. Astrup A, Toubro S. Thermogenic, metabolic, and cardiovascular responses to ephedrine and caffeine in man. Int J Obes Relat Metab Disord 1993;17(Suppl 1): S41–43.

83. Dulloo AG, Miller DS. The thermogenic properties of ephedrine/methylxanthine mixtures: human studies. Int J Obes 1986;10:467–481.

84. Bell DG, Jacobs I. Combined caffeine and ephedrine ingestion improves run times of Canadian Forces Warrior Test. Aviat Space Environ Med 1999;70:325–329.

85. Bell DG, Jacobs I, Ellerington K. Effect of caffeine and ephedrine ingestion on anaerobic exercise performance. Med Sci Sports Exerc 2001;33:1399–1403.

86. Bell DG, Jacobs I, McLellan TM, Zamecnik J. Reducing the dose of combined caffeine and ephedrine preserves the ergogenic effect. Aviat Space Environ Med 2000; 71:415–419.

87. Bell DG, Jacobs I, Zamecnik J. Effects of caffeine, ephedrine and their combination on time to exhaustion during high-intensity exercise [see comments]. Eur J Appl Physiol 1998;77:427–433.

88. Bell DG, McLellan TM, Sabiston CM. Effect of ingesting caffeine and ephedrine on 10-km run performance. Med Sci Sports Exerc 2002;34:344–349.

89. Jacobs I, Pasternak H, Bell DG. Effects of ephedrine, caffeine, and their combination on muscular endurance. Med Sci Sports Exerc 2003;35:987–994.

90. Gurley BJ, Gardner SF, Hubbard MA. Content versus label claims in ephedra-containing dietary supplements. Am J Health Syst Pharm 2000;57:963–969.

91. Gurley BJ, Wang P, Gardner SF. Ephedrine-type alkaloid content of nutritional supplements containing Ephedra sinica (Ma-huang) as determined by high performance liquid chromatography. J Pharm Sci 1998;87:1547–1553.

92. Sagara K, Oshima T, Misaki T. A simultaneous determination of norephedrine, pseudoephedrine, ephedrine and methylephedrine in Ephedrae Herba and oriental pharmaceutical preparations by ion-pair high-performance liquid chromatography. Chem Pharm Bull (Tokyo) 1983;31:2359–2365.

93. Dulloo AG. Ephedrine, xanthines and prostaglandin-inhibitors: actions and interactions in the stimulation of thermogenesis. Int J Obes Relat Metab Disord 1993; 17(Suppl 1):S35–40.

94. Dulloo AG, Seydoux J, Girardier L. Paraxanthine (metabolite of caffeine) mimics caffeine's interaction with sympathetic control of thermogenesis. Am J Physiol 1994;267:E801–804.

95. Glazer G. Long-term pharmacotherapy of obesity 2000: a review of efficacy and safety. Arch Intern Med 2001;161:1814–1824.

96. Astrup A, Breum L, Toubro S, Hein P, Quaade F. Ephedrine and weight loss. Int J Obes Relat Metab Disord 1992;16:715.

97. Boozer CN, Daly PA, Homel P, et al. Herbal ephedra/caffeine for weight loss: a 6-month randomized safety and efficacy trial. Int J Obes Relat Metab Disord 2002; 26:593–604.

98. Boozer CN, Nasser JA, Heymsfield SB, Wang V, Chen G, Solomon JL. An herbal supplement containing Ma Huang-Guarana for weight loss: a randomized, double-blind trial. Int J Obes Relat Metab Disord 2001;25:316–324.

99. Kreider RB. Ephedra update: AMA and AHA respond. Muscular Dev 2003;40: 122–127.

100. Marcus DM, Grollman AP. Ephedra-free is not danger-free. Science 2003;301:1669–1671; author reply 1669–1671.

101. Penzak SR, Jann MW, Cold JA, Hon YY, Desai HD, Gurley BJ. Seville (sour) orange juice: synephrine content and cardiovascular effects in normotensive adults. J Clin Pharmacol 2001;41:1059–1063.

102. Nykamp DL, Fackih MN, Compton AL. Possible association of acute lateral-wall myocardial infarction and bitter orange supplement. Ann Pharmacother 2004;38: 812–816.

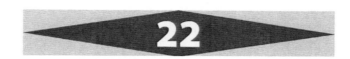

# An Overview of Sports Supplements

## Chris Lockwood

## OBJECTIVES

On the completion of this chapter you will be able to:

1. Understand the common reasons that individuals take different supplements.
2. Differentiate between various dietary supplements.
3. Determine the efficacy of using certain dietary supplements.
4. Understand the mechanisms of actions associated with common dietary supplements.
5. Appropriately determine supplementation protocols based on the scientific literature.
6. Know the various common names used to represent specific supplements.

## ABSTRACT

In this chapter, you will be provided an overview of some of the most frequently used sports nutrition and physique-augmenting dietary supplements. For quick reference, the supplements are presented in alphabetical order using their Common, or "street" Name. The information is further presented in a revised and abbreviated monograph format. Each monograph details the dietary supplement by, 1) **COMMON NAME**, 2) **OTHER NAMES** (including, if applicable, abbreviations, primary plant source, and commercially licensed trade name), 3) **COMMON USES** (as pertaining to sports nutrition and physique augmentation), 4) **REVIEW** (of the relevant clinical data), and 5) **DOSE** (as has either been recommended in the literature or could confidently be determined to be safe and elicit an efficacious response).

Note that because of inherent space limitations, supplements discussed in other chapters of this book, the scope of this chapter as it pertains to the context of the book's overall scope and purpose, as well as continuous advances in new products and clinical data, the list of supplements presented herein is in no way intended or implied to be an exhaustive list of all ingredients used by persons around the world for the purposes of athletic and/or physical improvement. Rather, the following is offered to provide a summation of only a select number of frequently used and readily available dietary supplements to date. It is also outside of the scope of this text to review, in detail, all contraindications, precautions, and possible adverse reactions of the ingredients listed. Therefore, only the most relevant substantiation data as they pertain to healthy, active populations and the subsequent use of each supplement have been included in this review. Lastly, please note that the section within each supplement monograph, entitled **COMMON USES**, refers *only* to the most generally

From: *Essentials of Sports Nutrition and Supplements*
Edited by J. Antonio, D. Kalman, J. R. Stout, M. Greenwood, D. S. Willoughby, and
G. G. Haff © Humana Press, a part of Springer Science+Business Media, Totowa, NJ

accepted uses of that supplement as is frequently propagated within the public; some uses, as you will soon find, are not substantiated by the available data nor are the common uses listed meant to serve as either a direct or implied recommendation for the use of a particular supplement.

*Key Words:* adaptogen, antioxidant, secretagogue, standardized, toxicity

**COMMON NAME:** **4-Hydroxyisoleucine**
**OTHER NAMES:** 4-OH-Ile; 4-Hydroxy; Fenugreek seed extract; *Trigonella foenum-graecum* extract; Promilin™
**COMMON USES:** Insulin Mimetic
Glucose Disposal
Glycogen Resynthesis
Glucose Loading
Improve Exercise Recovery
**REVIEW:** In vitro studies in isolated pancreatic β cells of rats and humans have shown that 4-OH-Ile increases insulin secretion in a glucose-dependent manner—the more glucose that is present, the more pronounced the insulinotropic effect of 4-OH-Ile.[1] Sauvaire et al. also noted that 4-OH-Ile was 25 and 15 times more effective than either leucine or isoleucine, respectively, at increasing the release of insulin. Similarly, in vivo coadministration of 4-OH-Ile and glucose, provided to normal and insulin-resistant rats and dogs, also resulted in improved glucose tolerance; again, an increased release of insulin was noted.[2] In a recent placebo-controlled, double-blind crossover trial, trained male cyclists consumed either 1.8 g/kg body weight (BW) glucose or 1.8 g/kgBW glucose + 5 mg/kgBW Promilin™ (a patent-pending Fenugreek seed extract consisting of 40% of the extract's total weight as 4-OH-Ile; or, approximately 2 mg/kgBW) immediately after the completion of a 90-minute, glycogen-depleting bike test. Muscle biopsies revealed that athletes consuming glucose + Promilin™ increased muscle glycogen resynthesis by a 63% greater rate than when consuming glucose alone.[3] It is plausible that 4-OH-Ile, provided immediately postworkout in the absence of exogenous glucose may also elicit an insulin mimetic response and, therefore, facilitate the transport of amino acids into muscle. For example, an acute infusion study involving rats revealed that 4-OH-Ile was capable of promoting an insulinotropic effect in the muscle and liver of healthy rats, as well as in the muscle of diabetic rats in the absence of supplemental glucose.[4] However, to date, no such human data exist to substantiate this frequently applied use of 4-OH-Ile within the bodybuilding community.
**DOSE:** *Glucose Disposal*: ≥2 mg/kgBW 4-OH-Ile (or as 5 mg/kgBW Promilin™); consume with each glucose-containing meal and/or with a preworkout glucose load
*Glycogen Resynthesis*: ≥2 mg/kgBW 4-OH-Ile (or as 5 mg/kgBW Promilin™); consume immediately postworkout with ≥1.8 g/kgBW glucose load

**COMMON NAME:** **5-Hydroxytryptophan**
**OTHER NAMES:** 5-HTP; L-5-HTP; L-5-hydroxytryptophan; Oxitriptan; L-2-amino-3-(5-hydroxy-l-*H*-indol-3-yl)propionic acid
**COMMON USES:** Increase Serotonin
Promote Restful Sleep
Improve Recovery

**REVIEW:**

Antistress/Anticatabolic

Appetite Control

5-HTP is an immediate precursor to the neurotransmitter, serotonin (5-HT), and is often found in dietary supplements in the form of *Griffonia simplicifolia* active extract. Although data are conflicting and more studies are needed, some evidence supports the use of 5-HTP to improve symptoms associated with fibromyalgia and mild insomnia. In addition, 5-HTP may function as a mild analgesic, antidepressant, and appetite suppressant.[5-7] Research has also shown that 5-HTP (200 mg) increases cortisol secretion in men, as well as luteinizing hormone (LH); the latter is believed to be the result of 5-HTP causing an increase in gonadotropin-releasing hormone (GnRH).[8,9] Although contradictory to current dogma surrounding cortisol, the ability of 5-HTP to support an increase in endogenous cortisol production may very well serve as its most anabolic function in athletes if validated—the greater the catabolic response generated during a heavy resistance training session, the greater the anabolic response to that training session. In other words, an increase in cortisol, above homeostatic levels, signals the body to release anabolic hormones, such as testosterone and insulin, in an effort to bring the body back into homeostasis. Thus, it could be surmised that consuming 5-HTP before heavy training may elicit a greater anabolic response as a result of a potentially increased catabolic state. Clearly, as a precursor to serotonin and likely to cause drowsiness, such use probably is not ideal. However, because cortisol presents its greatest steady-state diurnal rhythmic peak immediately upon awakening and is increased with bright, early morning sunlight, the consumption of 5-HTP before bedtime may be warranted to ensure proper hypothalamic-pituitary-adrenal axis function and avoid overtraining; "resetting" your body's natural anabolic alarm clock.

**DOSE:**

*Exercise Recovery and General Use*: 50–300 mg/d; consume approximately 30 minutes before bedtime, on an empty stomach

*Fibromyalgia*: 100 mg × 3/d; consume approximately 30 minutes before meals, on an empty stomach

*Appetite Control*: 8 mg/kg BW/d or 750 mg/d; consume approximately 30 minutes before meals on an empty stomach

*NOTE: May be most effective if consumed in the presence of a decarboxylase inhibitor and in the presence of low vitamin B6 levels.

**COMMON NAME:** **Adenosine Triphosphate**

**OTHER NAMES:** ATP; Adenosine 5′-triphosphate; Adenosine 5′-triphosphoric acid; Adenosine, 5′(tetrahydrogen triphosphate); Adenylpyrophosphoric acid; PEAK ATP™

**COMMON USES:** Increase Workout Volume

Increase Power Output

Increase Muscle Hypertrophy

Increase Muscle Strength

Increase Energy

Improve Recovery

Increase Mental Acuity

Promote Vasodilation

**REVIEW:** ATP is frequently referred to as the body's primary energy currency; without it (ATP), cellular energy within the human body and life itself would cease to exist. Inasmuch, its sports nutrition applications are vast and promising. In vivo studies in human neural stem cells, for example, have demonstrated that by introducing ATP into the extracellular medium, stem cell proliferation increases significantly; the action potential arising as a result of ATP directly stimulating the release of $Ca^{2+}$ from intracellular stores. Caffeine had no up-regulating or down-regulating effect on the action generated by ATP on neural cell.[10] This, however, is just one of several examples of in vitro data in support of the use of ATP, consistently revealing a direct and dose-dependent response between an increase in extracellular and intracellular ATP levels. Human use studies have been less optimistic, however. Jordan et al.[11] found no significant aerobic or anaerobic ergogenic effect in healthy men that received either 150 or 225 mg ATP, or placebo, for 14 days. The researchers did, however, note significant within-group differences in those consuming 225 mg ATP, per day. Specifically, 1 RM, number of repetitions to failure during the first set of exercise, and total lifting volume were all significantly improved in the 225-mg ATP group. It may simply be that the doses used have been too low to elicit an ergogenic response; however, more data are required before any recommendation can be made for the use of ATP as an efficacious sports supplement.

**DOSE:** Insufficient data

**COMMON NAME:** **Alanine**

**OTHER NAMES:** L-Alanine; Ala; 2-Aminopropionic acid; (S)-2-Aminopropanoic acid; alpha-Aminopropionic acid; L-alpha-Aminopropionic acid

**COMMON USES:** Increase Protein Synthesis
Anticatabolic
Glycogen Resynthesis
Glucose Sparing

**REVIEW:** Alanine is a nonessential amino acid produced from the transamination of pyruvate, and is the most important amino acid involved in carrying nitrogen from muscle to the liver where its carbon skeleton can be converted to glucose via gluconeogenesis and citrate synthesis. Thus, Alanine, similar to lactate and glycerol, acts as a glucose precursor during exercise or carbohydrate restriction, and is directly responsible for generating approximately 10% of the total energy requirements during exercise via its involvement in the tricarboxylic acid (TCA) cycle. In fact, Alanine release from muscle increases by approximately 2.5-fold during prolonged exercise.[12] Alanine is, therefore, critical in preserving muscle tissue and supporting healthy blood glucose levels, especially during prolonged periods of strenuous exercise or as part of a carbohydrate-restricted diet when glucose availability is compromised. Similarly, Alanine supplementation may be warranted for exercising persons possessing diabetic complications. Studies involving Alanine, at doses as high as 100 g consumed before, during, and/or after exercise, have, in fact, shown reduced ketosis and increased nitrogen uptake into muscle, postexercise, as well as revealing no gastrointestinal distress in healthy subjects.[13–17] For example, Korach-André et al.[17] found a significant increase in protein synthesis when they provided healthy subjects 1 g/kg Alanine, beginning 20 minutes before exercise and every 20 minutes thereafter for a total of 7 doses during a 180-minute, low-intensity cycling test. It seems, then, that the use of Alanine is warranted; however, with the necessity of such large doses to achieve an efficacious effect, its consistent use may simply be too impractical.

**DOSE:** *Glucose Sparing and Protein Synthesis*: Up to 1 g/kg BW/d; consume in divided doses, beginning 20 minutes preexercise and continue ingesting throughout the exercise event

**COMMON NAME:** **Alpha-Glyceryl Phosphoryl Choline**
**OTHER NAMES:** alpha-GPC; GPC; alpha-Glycerylphosphorylcholine; L-alpha-Glycerylphosphorylcholine; (R) 1,2-Glycero-3-Phosphatidylcholine; Choline Alfoscerate; Choline-glycerophosphate; Choline-hydroxide
**COMMON USES:** Growth Hormone Secretagogue
Increase Mental Acuity
Increase Energy
Cholinergic/Dopaminergic Agonist
**REVIEW:** Alpha-GPC, when hydrolyzed in the gut, produces, among other metabolites, the essential nutrient choline (discussed in more detail, later in this chapter). Choline is a water-soluble B vitamin that readily crosses the blood-brain barrier and is a precursor of the cholinergic (or dopaminergic) agonist, acetylcholine (ACh), as well as the membrane phospholipids, phosphatidylcholine and sphingomyelin. Increasing choline availability is likely the most important role attributed to alpha-GPC. Several Italian studies, involving healthy, aged, or diseased population groups have shown alpha-GPC to effectively increase human growth hormone (hGH), ACh, and improve cognitive function, memory and performance, as well as reaction time.[18-21]
**DOSE:** *Cognitive Function*: 400 mg × 3/d; consume between or with meals
*GH Secretagogue*: 1 g/d; consume approximately 20 minutes before exercise

**COMMON NAME:** **Alpha-Ketoglutarate**
**OTHER NAMES:** AKG; α-KG; 2-Oxoglutarate; 2-OG; Pentanedioic acid, 2-oxo-, ion(2-); 2-Oxopentanedioate; 2-Ketoglutarate; 2-Oxoglutaric acid; 2-Ketoglutaric acid; α-Ketoglutaric acid; 2-Oxopentanedioic acid
**COMMON USES:** Anticatabolic
Increase Glutamine Synthesis
**REVIEW:** AKG is both the carbon skeleton of glutamine catabolism and a precursor to its (glutamine) synthesis, and along with pyridoxal-5-phosphate (a B vitamin) is one of two critical cofactors used in the transamination of all amino acids. AKG's most recognized function, when administered orally, is to spare endogenous glutamine pools—increasing glutamine synthesis and availability. In patients having undergone total hip replacement surgery, 0.28 g/kgBW AKG + 2 g/kgBW glucose was equally as effective as 0.28 g/kgBW glutamine + 2 g/kgBW glucose at preventing protein catabolism and sparing muscle free glutamine concentrations in the 24 hours postsurgery.[22] In trained, but noncompetitive male subjects, 13.905 mg/kgBW AKG, in combination with

16.095 mg/kgBW pyridoxine, but neither ingredient separately, increased maximal oxygen uptake (VO₂ max) by 6% and significantly decreased peak blood lactate after supramaximal running workloads lasting less than 140 seconds.[23] A more effective and recent trend in delivering AKG, however, has been to form peptide bonds in attempt to address a rate-limiting step in amino acid transamination, attaching AKG to one or more amino acids, such as arginine, ornithine or glycine, just to name a few. A few of these AKG formulations will be briefly addressed later in this chapter.

**DOSE**: *Anticatabolic*: 0.28 g/kgBW/d; consume with glucose, immediately postexercise or in divided doses on non-training days

*General Ergogenic Aid*: 13.905 mg/kgBW; consume with a slightly greater dose of vitamin B6, at least 20 minutes before exercise

**COMMON NAME**: **Alpha-Ketoisocaproate**

**OTHER NAMES**: KIC; Ketoisocaproic acid; Ketoleucine; 2-Oxoisocaproic acid; 2-Ketoisocaproate; α-Ketoisocaproic acid; 4-methyl-2-Oxovaleric acid; 4-methyl-2-Oxopentanoic acid; 4-methyl-2-Oxopentanoate; 4-methyl-2-Oxovalerate

**COMMON USES**: Increase Protein Synthesis
Anticatabolic
Improve Recovery
Insulin Mimetic

**REVIEW**: KIC is referred to as a branched-chain keto acid (BCKA), which is essentially a branched-chain amino acid (BCAA) containing a "keto" group as opposed to an "amino." As such, BCKAs perform many of the same functions as BCAAs and are used both in the synthesis of BCAAs as well as are synthesized from the transamination of BCAAs. Specifically, KIC is the keto acid of the BCAA, leucine, and when ingested, about 50% of the consumed dose of KIC is converted into leucine. In fact, arterial KIC levels are often used to assess protein synthesis because it (arterial KIC) directly correlates to basal hepatic and intramuscular leucine concentrations.[24] KIC also acts as a direct precursor to the production of beta-hydroxy-beta-methylbutyrate (HMB) and has been shown to possess both anabolic and anticatabolic properties; believed to be independent and synergistic to its conversion to leucine.[25,26] Also, similar to glucose, KIC is capable of promoting a sustained release of insulin from pancreatic β cells. This is likely the result of KIC being exclusively transaminated within the mitochondria with glutamine or glutamate, and then being converted into both AKG and leucine.[27,28] Human ingestion studies, however, currently do not support the use of KIC as a dietary supplement for sports and/or physique augmentation when consumed isonitrogenously, primarily because such studies simply do not exist. It is interesting to note some recent comparative studies that found dipeptide forms of KIC more effective than other frequently used dipeptides. Specifically, in traumatized, starve-fed rat models, AKIC (Arginine-alpha-Ketoisocaproate) was more effective than both arginine and AAKG (Arginine-alpha-Ketoglutarate) at increasing nitrogen retention and weight gain; AKIC was also found to be more effective than OKIC (Ornithine-alpha-Ketoisocaproate) at increasing net protein synthesis.[29,30]

**DOSE:** *Exercise Recovery*: >0.10g/kgBW/d; consume immediately postworkout and/or in divided doses with meals

**COMMON NAME:** **Alpha-Lipoic Acid**

**OTHER NAMES:** ALA; Lipoic acid; LA; Thioctic acid; Lipoate; Alpha-lipoate; 5-(1,2-dithiolan-3-yl)pentanoic acid; 1,2-dithiolane-3-pentanoic acid; 1,2-ditholane-3-valeric acid; 6,8-thiotic acid; 5-[3-C1,2-dithiolanyl)]-pentanoic acid; delta-[3-(1,2-dithiacyclopentyl)] pentanoic acid; Acetate Replacing Factor; Pyruvate Oxidation Factor

**COMMON USES:** Insulin Mimetic
Glucose Disposal
Glycogen Resynthesis
Antioxidant

**REVIEW:** ALA is found in abundance in red meat and is in the *thiol* class of organic sulfur derivatives—an endogenously produced, nonessential nutrient in healthy humans with a wide array of biologic functions. As it relates to sports performance, ALA's primary functions are as an intra- and extracellular redox agent (e.g., antioxidant), cofactor in energy-producing reactions within cell mitochondria—principally, the oxidation of pyruvate, AKG, and of the BCAAs—and as an insulin mimetic. As an antioxidant, 600 mg/d × 8 weeks, in healthy adults, was shown to significantly inhibit low density lipoprotein (LDL) cholesterol oxidation, and was found superior to vitamin E in reducing plasma protein carbonyls.[31] In fact, ALA is often referred to as a "metabolic antioxidant" because of its unique ability to be accepted as a preferential reducing substrate, or cofactor, within cell mitochondria. As such, ALA can use a cell's metabolic energy to continuously recycle itself into its active form and, therefore, be readily available as a reducing cofactor again and again within the cell. Thus, the dose required to effectively enhance tissue glutathione (GSH) availability is relatively small. By sparing GSH, it is possible that ALA may delay fatigue and elicit an ergogenic effect during vigorous, long-duration aerobic exercise.[32] ALA is most frequently used by athletes, though, to promote an insulin mimetic effect, either in the absence of glucose or to increase the postexercise insulin response when ALA is coingested with glucose. A recent, randomized, controlled trial in healthy, nonexercising men support such an insulinotropic use: Subjects consuming 1g ALA, combined with 20g creatine monohydrate and 100g sucrose, per day for 5 days, revealed significantly greater increases in muscle phosphocreatine (PCr) and total creatine compared with subjects consuming creatine + sucrose, or creatine alone.[33] Bioavailability of ALA seems to be improved if delivered in its reduced, or R(+)-enantiomer, as opposed to its S(–)-enantiomer form.[34,35] It should also be noted that, as is common in reduction reactions, the availability of nicotinamide adenine dinucleotide and nicotinamide adenine dinucleotide phosphate (NADPH) are required for ALA to be reduced and may, therefore, be useful micronutrients to be coingested with ALA, especially if ALA is delivered in its nonreduced form.

**DOSE:** *Antioxidant*: 300–600 mg/d, as *R*-ALA; consume on an empty stomach in divided doses, or as a single bolus immediately postexercise
*Insulin Mimetic*: 1 g/d, as *R*-ALA; consumed with glucose immediately postexercise

**COMMON NAME:** **Androst-4-ene-3,6,17-trione**
**OTHER NAMES:** 3,6,17-androstenetrione; 6-keto-androstenedione; 4beta,5beta-epoxyandrosta-3,6,17,19-tetraone (6); 4beta,5beta-epoxy-19-oxo metabolite; 6-OXO™
**COMMON USES:** Aromatase Inhibitor
Increase Testosterone/Estrogen Ratio
**REVIEW:** Numazawa et al.[36] demonstrated, in vitro, that Androst-4-ene-3,6,17-trione irreversibly binds to the aromatase enzyme, inhibiting its action in a competitive and active site-directed manner—a biochemical reaction, sometimes referred to as "suicide inhibiting." No peer-reviewed, human use data have, however, been published to either confirm and/or refute the safety and current use of this supplement among bodybuilders as a "pro-testosterone" or "anti-estrogen."
**DOSE:** Insufficient data

**COMMON NAME:** **Arginine**
**OTHER NAMES:** L-Arginine; Arg; 2-Amino-5-guanidinopentanoic acid; (S)-2-amino-5-[(aminoiminomethyl)amino] pentaenoic acid; 1-Amino-4-guanidovaleric acid; L-alpha-Amino-delta-guanidinovaleric acid
**COMMON USES:** Increase Nitric Oxide
Increase Vasodilation
Growth Hormone Secretagogue
Increase Protein Synthesis
Anticatabolic
Increase Immune Function
Treat Erectile Dysfunction
**REVIEW:** Arginine is a conditionally essential amino acid, synthesized from ornithine and citrulline, and is used as a precursor to creatine phosphate, polyamines, and nitric oxide (NO), just to list a few. Via its NO-promoting action, Arginine is believed to derive much, although not all of its benefits. NO, considered an endogenous messenger molecule, performs a wide array of critical functions within the cardiovascular, immune and nervous systems, and is produced by all tissues in the body. For example, in iNOS knockout and injured mice, ornithine but not Arginine improved wound healing. Thus, whereas ornithine is capable of working through non-NO-specific mechanisms to support recovery, Arginine is largely NO dependent.[37] In supraphysiologic doses (200–500 mg/kgBW/d) and in otherwise healthy subjects, however, Arginine does seem to speed recovery from traumatic injury by increasing collagen synthesis, stimulating cell proliferation, increasing T cell response, and inhibiting platelet aggregation, as well as increasing growth hormone and insulin-like growth factor (IGF)-1 release.[38,39] Any GH-stimulating effect in healthy adults is unlikely, albeit may arise when doses of 250 mg/kgBW/d are used. For example, 5 g Arginine, consumed 30 minutes before exercise had no effect on GH, and may have actually compromised the GH response via the NO-GHRH feedback loop with somatotroph cells.[40,41] A large mass of clinical data does, however, support the ergogenic-enhancing actions of both short-term and chronic use of Arginine when provided in high doses (>6 g/d) to persons with mild-to-moderate heart disease.[42,42] This may simply be the result of Arginine promoting NO-mediated endothelial cell vasodilation, and thus decreasing blood pressure, although the improvement in exercise capacity and function may also be linked to Arginine's stimulatory actions

on the adrenal and pituitary glands. Aside from those mentioned previously, Arginine is also a major component involved in the synthesis of the antidiuretic hormone, vasopressin. Although very few data substantiate any performance-enhancing effect(s) in healthy populations, it should equally be noted that the data in this area are scarce and need more emphasis. From the information currently available, it seems likely that Arginine, when provided preexercise, is best utilized for aiding endurance and long-duration glycolytic exercise—otherwise, ingested postexercise to increase intracellular uptake of other key macro- and micronutrients to aid recovery. Additionally, the process by which Arginine is transported across cells seems to be ACh-dependent, and may warrant the coadministration of ACh agonists to improve Arginine's function(s).[44]

**DOSE:** *Exercise Recovery*: ~8 g/d; consume postexercise
*Endurance Performance*: 8–21 g/d; consume preexercise
*Erectile Dysfunction*: >5 g/d; consume approximately 30 minutes before "event," on an empty stomach
*GH Secretagogue*: >250 mg/kg BW/d; consume 30 minutes before bedtime and/or exercise

**COMMON NAME:** **Asparagine**
**OTHER NAMES:** L-Asparagine; Asn; 2-Amino-3-carbamoylpropanoic acid; (S)-2,4-Diamino-4-oxobutanoic acid; Aspartamic acid; Aspartic acid beta-amide; alpha-Aminosuccinamic acid
**COMMON USES:** Increase Protein Synthesis
Anticatabolic
**REVIEW:** Asparagine is a nonessential amino acid, chemically related to and synthesized from aspartate or the aspartate metabolite, oxaloacetate (a Krebs, or Citric Acid, or TCA cycle intermediate/cofactor). Asparagine assists in protein synthesis and contributes to a wide array of brain and nervous system functions; however, Asparagine is believed to hold no major physiologic function when available in its free amino acid state. A recent exercise study in rats, whereby the rodents were forced to swim to exhaustion on two occasions—first, without supplementation, and a second time after having received a combination of Asparagine (400 mM) and aspartate (350 mM) for 7 days—found that the Asparagine + aspartate bolus significantly reduced glycogen depletion in exercised muscle and liver, and increased exercising time to exhaustion. The researchers concluded that a shift to oxidative metabolism may have been what contributed to the improved exercise performance.[45] Considering the TCA cycle role of aspartate, it is questionable if Asparagine added any benefit to the aforementioned study outcome or if the same results would have been found simply using aspartate only. Collectively, the available data do not warrant the supplemental use of isocalorically provided Asparagine except in conditions of clinically low magnesium levels.

**DOSE:** Insufficient data

**NAME:** **Aspartic Acid**
**OTHER NAMES:** L-Aspartic acid; Asp; Aspartate; L-Aspartate; 2-Aminobutanedioic acid; L-Amino succinate
**COMMON USES:** Delay Muscle Fatigue
Increase Protein Synthesis
Anticatabolic
Glucose Sparing

**REVIEW:** Aspartate is a nonessential, dicarboxylic amino acid and is vital to the metabolism of amino acids and the production of cellular energy. Aspartate is a direct precursor to the TCA cycle intermediate/cofactor, oxaloacetate, and is responsible for the removal of ammonia created from transamination within the urea cycle. Inasmuch, Aspartate contributes heavily to protein synthesis and many brain and nervous system functions, as well as to the production of ATP, DNA, and RNA.[46] Despite such promise, early data (from the 1950s) that had shown Aspartate to delay muscle fatigue in humans have not been validated in subsequent and more recent studies. One reviewer theorized that the use of the D- or DL-Aspartic acid form may be required to elicit an ergogenic effect, as opposed to the use its L- isomer.[47] To date, this theory has not been tested. Similarly, other reviewers have discussed the increased need for oxaloacetate precursors to prevent muscle wasting, and to improve fat and glucose oxidation and utilization during periods of increased energy needs or protein catabolism.[48,49] Although, here again, no data in healthy adults support the use of additional Aspartate above that which may be obtained from increasing total protein intake to accommodate for any increase in caloric expenditure. Glycogen sparing in muscle and liver, and improved exercise time to exhaustion was, however, found to occur when rats were administered Aspartate.[32] Aspartate has also been shown to increase neurostimulatory amino acids in the brain of rats when coadministered with arginine.[50] It should also be noted that Aspartate is frequently used as a metal chelator to improve active mineral transport to subcellular sites; this use, too, is often debated, however, further research is warranted.

**DOSE:** Insufficient data

**COMMON NAME:** *Avena sativa*

**OTHER NAMES:** *Avena sativa* L.; Oat Straw; *Avena fatua*; Avenae stramentum; Oats; Green Oats; Green Tops; Oat herb; Wild Oat herb; Avenae herba; *Haferkraut*; Common Oat

**COMMON USES:**
Increase Testosterone
Increase Energy
Increase Muscle Strength
Increase Muscle Hypertrophy
Treat Erectile Dysfunction

**REVIEW:** *Avena sativa* is the Latin, or herbal name for the common oat; similar to store-bought rolled oats used in breakfast preparations albeit not stripped of its outer shell. Instead, traditional preparations use the whole plant; when washed in an alcohol solution and its actives extracted, the herb is said to act as a stimulant, antispasmodic, antifungal, antioxidant, aphrodisiac, and antiinflammatory (when applied externally to the skin), just to list a few of its reported uses. The only German Commission E approved use, however, is as an externally applied antiinflammatory (e.g., Aveeno® brand skincare products). Claims that *Avena sativa* increases LH are currently based solely on secondary findings from a study published in 1976, involving rats.[51] Although it is true that *Avena sativa* contains active steroid saponins, sterols, flavonoids, amino acids, silicic acid, and soluble oligo- and polysaccharides, unfortunately no substantiating data have since been presented to confirm or refute any LH-increasing action from *Avena sativa* supplementation. More importantly, even if *Avena sativa* elicits an increase in LH, is there a corresponding and significant increase in free testosterone? It does, however, look promising that *Avena sativa* may possess powerful antioxidant and possibly antifungal benefits, and if correct could be applied for use in sports performance.[52-55] Standardization is currently not established for this product, so any use of this herb as well as any claims made to substantiate the use of *Avena sativa* are speculative at best.

**DOSE:** Insufficient data

**COMMON NAME:** **Banaba**

**OTHER NAMES:** Banaba leaf; *Lagerstroemia speciosa* L.; Queen's flower; Pride of India; Queen's crape myrtle; Pyinma; *Lagerstroemia flos-reginae*; *Munchausia speciosa*; Glucosol™

**COMMON USES:** Insulin Mimetic
Increase Glycogen Resynthesis
Improve Exercise Recovery

**REVIEW:** Banaba is a tropical plant, grown primarily in the Philippines, and used traditionally as an antidiabetic. Although research on this plant is in its infancy and no established standardization has been approved, enough compelling evidence does exist to be fairly confident that the primary actives responsible for increasing glucose disposal are corosolic acid and/or lagerstroemin.[56,57] For example, Liu et al.[58] found that Banaba extract increased glucose uptake in adipocytes, in vitro, in a dose-dependent and selective response similar to that of insulin albeit to a lesser extent. In the presence of insulin, however, there was a decrease in glucose uptake, which points toward an antagonizing and/or competing response at the point of cellular uptake when Banaba is provided in concert with increased insulin levels. It was similarly noted that Banaba extract affected GLUT4 translocation and therefore possesses a direct or indirect action on PPARγ2 expression (a protein responsible for glucose uptake in to adipocytes). Interestingly, both the hot water and alcohol extracted forms of Banaba were equally effective, whereas Banaba extract from distilled water wash was ineffective at increasing glucose disposal. Thus, it was concluded that the active responsible for the insulin mimetic response was most likely not a protein.[58] In a recent, randomized, controlled study involving adult Type II diabetic humans provided 32 or 48 mg/d, for 2 weeks, of either a dry power capsule or soft gel form of the 1% corosolic acid-containing Banaba extract, Glucosol™, it was found that glucose disposal was dose-dependent and provided a reduction in blood glucose by 30% and 20% in those taking the gel caps versus regular dry powder encapsulation, respectively.[59] More recently, an acute oral dose of corosolic acid (10 mg/kg BW) was provided to Type II diabetic mice, and shown to significantly reduce blood glucose, without effecting insulin, and caused a significant translocation of the glucose transporter isoform, GLUT4, from micro- to plasma membrane locations. Thus, it was concluded that the hypoglycemic effect of corosolic acid is largely the result of an increased uptake of glucose into muscle.[60] Hattori et al.,[61] however, noted that the active ellagaitannin polyphenol, lagerstroemin, provides a wider insulin mimetic response than simply effecting glucose transport systems—lagerstroemin was shown to directly increase tyrosine phosphorylation of the insulin receptors, themselves. Although this study was performed in vitro, it does support the argument for a need to standardize Banaba leaf extract to more than just the presence of corosolic acid (corosolic acid is prevalent in many species of plants, whereas lagerstroemin is more specific to the Banaba plant). Another active Banaba leaf extract, valoneic acid, for example, was shown to be more potent than the xanthine oxidase-inhibiting drug, allopurinol, in vitro, and has also been shown to be a potent alpha-amylase inhibitor.[62,63] However, until more conclusive data are found to support the standardization of Banaba to several of its key actives, the use of a 1% corosolic acid-containing extract for glucose disposal seems warranted if consumed in the absence of glucose or other insulin-promoting compounds (e.g., BCAAs, KIC, or Leucine).

**DOSE:** *Insulin Mimetic:* >16 mg/dose corosolic acid (from Banaba leaf extract, standardized to contain not less than 1% corosolic acid); consume on an empty stomach, before meals and immediately postexercise, before consuming carbohydrates, protein, or other insulinotropic actives

**COMMON NAME:** **Bee Pollen**
**OTHER NAMES:** Pollen
**COMMON USES:** Increase Energy
Improve Endurance Performance
Promote Weight Gain
Improve Immune Function

**REVIEW:** Bee Pollen is derived from the male germ seeds of plants and is collected from honeybees as they enter their hive. Bee Pollen is considered high in B vitamins as well as a source of antioxidants, including the natural plant antioxidant, phytic acid.[64] Human performance studies of both aerobic and anaerobic type clearly dismiss any efficacious use of Bee Pollen as an ergogenic aid, and even those studies conducted in animals and in vitro are not compelling enough to support its use as an effective ergogenic aid. For example, Bee Pollen was only about 50% as effective as propolis at inhibiting fungal growth, in vitro.[65] One of the few substantiating trials involved pregnant rats that were provided either 10 or 20 g/kgBW/d Bee Pollen. The researchers found a dose-dependent increase in fetal birth weight and reduced death rates in newborns; the mother's body weight, hemoglobin, total protein, and serum iron and albumin also increased.[66] In light of the sport-specific, human studies to the contrary, Bee Pollen use in sports is not recommended.

**DOSE:** Insufficient data

**COMMON NAME:** **Beta-Alanine**
**OTHER NAMES:** βAlanine; beta-Ala; beta-aminopropionic acid; 3-aminopropionic acid; 3-aminopropanoic acid
**COMMON USES:** Increase Muscle Hypertrophy
Increase Muscle Strength
Increase Muscle Power Output
Proton Buffering
Anticatabolic

**REVIEW:**

Beta-Alanine is a naturally occurring beta-amino acid and is the rate-limiting pre-cursor of the histidine containing imidazole dipeptide, carnosine, as well as is a component of the B vitamin, pantothenic acid (B3). Supplementation in humans has largely been positive regarding the use of Beta-Alanine as an ergogenic aid in exercise of short-to-moderate duration and of high power output. For example, Stout et al[66a] reported that 34 g dextrose + 1.6 g Beta-Alanine × 4/d × 6 d and then 1.6 g × 2/d × 22 d was significantly more effective than 34 g dextrose + placebo at delaying neuromuscular fatigue in previously untrained men, as assessed by physical working capacity at neuromuscular fatigue threshold (PWC$_{FT}$) cycle ergometry. Stout et al also reported no significant difference between Beta-Alanine or Creatine groups (creatine groups received 34 g dextrose + 5.25 g Cr × 4/d × 6 d, then 5.25 g × 2 d × 22 d), and no additive effect when Beta-Alanine and Creatine were combined. The latter, confirming previously unpublished data by Hill et al[66b] that found no significant difference between 28 days of Beta-Alanine, Creatine, Beta-Alanine + Creatine, or Placebo supplementation in cycling times to exhaustion, working at 110% of estimated maximal power output. The latter, being an interesting point, in light of recent work by Derave et al.[66c] that reported a significant increase in isokinetic knee extension torque during the last two 30-rep sets (i.e. sets 4 and 5, of a 5-set bout) of maximal voluntary contractions (MVC) in 400-m sprint-trained competitive athletes, following four weeks of 4.8 g/d Beta-Alanine or placebo. Though 400-m race time and an endurance test of isokentic knee torque conducted at 45% MVC revealed no significant difference between Beta-Alanine or placebo groups, of interest is the finding that Beta-Alanine significantly increased muscle carnosine content in competitive sprinters by 47% and 37% in the soleus and gastrocnemius, respectively. One, confirming previous findings by Hill et al.[66d] that found significantly increased muscle carnosine levels in previously untrained subjects, in response to four weeks of 6.4 g/d Beta-Alanine, and two, suggestive that, unlike creatine that has been reported as having a "ceiling effect" with regards to intramuscular concentrations peaking after one week of loading, data has yet to find a similar such ceiling effect in response to Beta-Alanine supplementation and their respective effects on muscle carnosine concentrations in both previously untrained and highly trained subjects. Harris et al. has concluded that Beta-Alanine, because of its conversion to carnosine, likely improves power output by buffering accumulated hydrogen ions.[67] It should be noted, however, that Harris et al has similarly shown that whereas ingested Beta-Alanine results in a dose-dependent increase in plasma Beta-Alanine and muscle carnosine content, carnosine supplementation alone has been shown to provide no added benefit to that achieved by Beta-Alanine.[68] It should also be noted that Beta-Alanine and the beta-amino acid, Taurine, directly compete for transport, for example at glycine receptors located within the brain hippocampus region; that, in animal models, a disproportional increase in Beta-Alanine availability has been shown to reduce taurine uptake into the brain, myocardium and skeletal muscle tissue.[70,71] Harris et al.[68]

similarly showed that in humans, plasma taurine increased significantly in response to Beta-Alanine supplementation, however, they reported no significant loss of taurine via urine analysis. Although inconclusive, it is therefore warranted to recommend that taurine also be supplemented into the diet whenever Beta-Alanine is also being used. Lastly, because Beta-Alanine requires the release of histidine to be converted into the subsequent dipeptides, there exists the potential for Beta-Alanine supplementation to result in an allergic-type ("flushing") response because of the increase in histamine residues generated. A maximal threshold of 10 mg/kg/d BW of Beta-Alanine has been suggested as the uppermost amount not likely to elicit such an effect.

**DOSE:** *Proton Buffering*: 3.2–6.4 g/d; consume approximately 60 minutes before exercise, on an empty stomach

**COMMON NAME:** **Betaine**

**OTHER NAMES:** Trimethylglycine; TMG; *N*-trimethylglycine; Glycine betaine; Glycocoll betaine; Oxyneurine; Lycine; 1-carboxy-*N,N,N*-trimethylmethanaminium inner salt; Betaine HCL; Betaine Hydrochloride; Pluchine; 1-carboxy-*N,N,N*-trimethylmethanaminium chloride

**COMMON USES:** Increase Protein Utilization
Methyl Donor

**REVIEW:** A metabolite of choline, and the trimethylated form of glycine (hence the name, TMG), Betaine is present in large concentrations in wheat germ and bran, as well as in shrimp, spinach, beet juice, and other wheat products.[72] Betaine's two main functions in the body are as a methyl donor and osmolyte: As an osmolyte, Betaine protects proteins, cells, and enzymes from heat, dehydration, and other environmental and physiologic stresses, and as a methyl donor, Betaine is used to convert homocysteine to L-methionine and is, therefore, also a precursor to *S*-adenosylmethionine (SAMe) and creatine. Betaine availability has a key role in hepatic fat metabolism, and in its hydrochloride (HCL) form, Betaine HCL, is often used as a digestive aid for protein digestion.[73] In a thorough review by Craig,[74] it was concluded that Betaine "is an important nutrient for the prevention of chronic disease." Likely, the result of Betaine's role in "neutralizing" homocysteine levels from reaching cytotoxic levels on and within the tissues most affected by high homocysteine (e.g., liver cirrhosis and Alzheimer's disease have both been attributed to high levels of homocysteine). In healthy adults, 6 weeks of Betaine supplementation of 1.5, 3, and 6 g/d was shown to decrease homocysteine levels in a dose-dependent manner.[75] In a double-blind, placebo-controlled, randomized, parallel study, 6 g/d Betaine, for 12 weeks, provided to 42 obese men and women, also showed a significant reduction in homocysteine levels. However, Betaine supplementation resulted in no changes in body composition, body weight, or resting energy expenditure.[76] Data to substantiate an ergogenic effect are also limited, albeit two recent studies, currently only available in abstract form, provide evidence showing that when Betaine was coingested with a carbohydrate and electrolyte beverage, during and after exercise in hot climates, sprint time to exhaustion, as well as anaerobic and aerobic metabolism improved.[77,78]

**DOSE:**

Until these studies become available in their entirety and have been peer-reviewed, the methodology and conclusions remain suspect.

*Protein Utilization and General Use*: 600 mg/dose-6 g/d; consume with meals and/or immediately postexercise with protein

**COMMON NAME:** **Beta-Hydroxy-Beta-Methylbutyrate**

**OTHER NAMES:** HMB; Hydroxymethylbutyrate; Beta-Hydroxyisovalerate; 3-Hydroxyisovalerate; beta-Hydroxyisovaleric acid; 3-Hydroxy-3-methylbutyric acid; Beta Hydroxy-Methyl-Butyrate

**COMMON USES:** Anticatabolic
Increase Muscle Hypertrophy
Improve Exercise Recovery
Increase Muscle Strength
Increase Protein Synthesis

**REVIEW:** HMB is a natural metabolite of the essential and BCAA, L-leucine, and is formed directly from alpha-ketoisocaproate (KIC) transamination. One outcome of HMB metabolism is its conversion to beta-hydroxy-beta-methylglutaryl-CoA (HMG-CoA) within cell mitochondria where it (HMG-CoA) can be further broken down to acetyl-CoA and acetoacetate to support cholesterol synthesis, improve cell wall integrity, and perform a host of other metabolic functions. A recent meta-analysis involving several common sports supplements substantiates the proposed use of HMB as an effective sports supplement; collectively, detailing HMB as having been shown to improve strength and lean mass gains during anaerobic and aerobic training, and to work as an anticatabolic to spare muscle protein and speed recovery.[79] Additionally, when HMB is combined with creatine, the ergogenic benefits, as compared with what could otherwise be achieved by either compound independently, are significantly increased.[80] Evidence in the elderly, those with metabolic wasting disease, as well as in vitro data also lends support to the many anticatabolic and other metabolic effects of HMB.[81] For example, 3 g/d × 8 weeks of HMB was shown to be extremely safe, and significantly decrease LDL cholesterol and systolic blood pressure in older men and women.[82] Unfortunately, however, HMB has yet to show a clear benefit in previously trained, or competitive athletes—HMB has primarily been shown to provide an ergogenic and anticatabolic effect only in previously untrained subjects.[83,84] Kreider et al.,[85] for example, provided experienced weightlifters 3 or 6 g/d HMB × 28 d, in a double-blind, randomized, controlled trial and found no improvements in net protein synthesis, 1 RM strength, body composition, or other measures of anticatabolic or anabolic action. Although it is plausible that the doses used are simply too low for trained individuals or that as a result of HMB increasing ketone production, it may be most effective when consumed during carbohydrate- and/or calorie-restricted phases of dieting, the evidence thus far only supports the use of HMB in previously untrained or elderly populations.

**DOSE:** *Anticatabolic and Increased Muscle Strength*\*: 3–6 g/d; consume immediately postworkout or in two divided doses—one serving pre- and the second immediately postworkout

*Efficacious dose specific only to previously untrained and elderly persons engaged in physical fitness.

| | |
|---|---|
| **COMMON NAME**: | **Branched-Chain Amino Acids** |
| **OTHER NAMES**: | BCAAs; ʟ-Leucine, ʟ-Isoleucine, ʟ-Valine; Large Neutral Amino Acids; LNAAs |
| **COMMON USES**: | Improve Exercise Recovery |
| | Increase Protein Synthesis |
| | Anticatabolic |
| | Increase Muscle Hypertrophy |
| | Increase Muscular Endurance |
| | Insulin Mimetic/Glucose Disposal |
| | Increase Gluconeogenesis |
| | Increase Energy |
| **REVIEW**: | The essential amino acids Leucine, Isoleucine, and Valine, collectively form what is referred to as the BCAAs, comprising approximately 30% of the total muscle protein pool and acting as the primary nitrogen source for glutamine and alanine synthesis in muscle. BCAAs are found in high concentrations in dairy protein—whey protein isolate is approximately 26% BCAAs, and milk protein about 21%—and BCAAs, unlike most free-form amino acids, are not degraded in the liver (i.e., dietary intake of BCAAs directly increases plasma and tissue BCAA concentrations). BCAAs are, however, the primary amino acids oxidized in muscle during exercise and catabolic stress, and, therefore, have received much attention by athletes for the purpose of increasing muscle mass and/or performance. The sheer volume of studies on BCAA use is too expansive for discussion here; in addition, BCAAs have been discussed in detail in Chapter 12 of this text. However, in summary, BCAAs, whether consumed pre-, during, or postexercise, support muscle protein synthesis and decrease protein catabolism, and are vitally important to endogenous glucose production via the glucose-alanine cycle; by some accounts, contributing to greater than 40% of glucose production during sustained endurance exercise, as well as increasing insulin sensitivity.[86-90] Although BCAAs clearly support recovery from exercise, and therefore could be argued as indirectly ergogenic-enhancing, thus far there are no conclusive human findings that BCAAs have a direct performance-enhancing effect *during* exercise. The BCAA, Leucine, is amassing convincing evidence that it may be the most essential of the essential BCAAs, and will be discussed in greater length later in this chapter. Lastly, it is worth noting the importance of increased vitamin B6 (pyridoxine) availability when using a BCAA-containing supplement; B6 derives the essential cofactor, pyridoxal-5-phosphate, used to facilitate BCAA transamination reactions.[91] |
| **DOSE**: | *Anabolic, Anticatabolic, Glycogen Resynthesis, and Insulin Mimetic*: 6–20 g/d; consume pre-, during, and/or immediately postworkout, and/or in divided doses throughout the day |

*NOTE: There exists a wide variance of BCAA formula compositions within the available literature; however, a ratio of Leucine/Isoleucine/Valine of approximately 45%:25%:30% has been shown effective in multiple trials, and is recommended here.

| COMMON NAME: | **Carnosine** |
|---|---|
| OTHER NAMES: | L-Carnosine; Beta-Alanylhistidine; Beta-Alanyl-L-Histidine |
| COMMON USES: | Proton/Hydrogen Ion Buffering |
| | Increase Work Output/Volume |
| | Increase Power Output |
| | Increase Muscle Strength |
| | Increase Muscle Hypertrophy |
| | Improve Exercise Recovery |
| | Antioxidant |

REVIEW:    Carnosine is a naturally occurring histidine dipeptide, present primarily in type II (anaerobic/glycolytic) as opposed to type I (aerobic/oxidative) fibers. Skeletal muscle Carnosine concentrations are greatest in large-breed animals, such as cows, pigs, thoroughbred horses, and whales, as opposed to what is observed in human type II muscle fibers. Though in vitro data has identified a possible increased skeletal muscle sensitivy to $Ca^{2+}$ as a possible response to Carnosine, the more commonly addressed and researched area of focus is that increasing histidine dipeptide availability during exercise may increase intramyocellular pH buffering capabilities. The nitrogen containing imidazole ring of histidine dipeptides can be used to neutralize the unbound, highly charged hydrogen ions ($H^+$) generated during the splitting of ATP. If more histidine dipeptides are available to neutralize accumulating levels of intramuscular $H^+$, then high-intensity muscular contractions can be sustained for longer periods of time.[92] For example, Suzuki et al.,[93] in a recent muscle biopsy study, presented data showing that high levels of muscle Carnosine in the human vastus lateralis (a predominantly type II muscle) correlated strongly with maximal exercise performance in the latter stages of a 30-second all-out ergometer sprint test. Unfortunately, any ergogenic benefit of increasing exogenous Carnosine has thus far only been reported when its precursor, beta-alanine, is ingested (refer to Beta-Alanine). For example, as was reported earlier in the Beta-Alanine section, Derave et al has in fact shown that increasing skeletal muscle Carnosine concentrations, via 28 days of beta-alanine supplementation, increased dynamic knee extension torque in the final two sets of MVC, in competitive sprinters. Lastly, there is substantial in vitro evidence showing that Carnosine, as well as the other histidine dipeptide anserine, may function as site-specific, naturally occurring antioxidants within muscle, as well as act as potent heavy-metal chelating agents and free-radical scavengers.[94–96] Despite availability of in vivo data being limited to non-sports-specific use, there does exist a high level of safety of ingested Carnosine.[97]

DOSE:    *Proton Buffering*: 20–40 mg/kg BW/d; consume 30–90 minutes preexercise, on an empty stomach
*Antioxidant and General Use*: 1–3 g/d; consume on an empty stomach

| COMMON NAME: | **Choline** |
|---|---|
| OTHER NAMES: | 2-Hydroxy-*N,N,N*-trimethylethanaminum; (beta-hydroxyethyl) trimethylammonium; Bilineurine |
| COMMON USES: | Increase Mental Acuity |
| | Increase Energy |
| | Increase Endurance Performance |
| | Improve Exercise Recovery |

REVIEW:     Choline was recently categorized as an essential nutrient, and therefore is only now being fully recognized
publicly for its many vital functions in human development and health. Specifically, Choline is directly
required for the synthesis of cell membrane phospholipids [phosphatidylcholine (PC), phosphatidylserine (PS),
and PE], the methyl donor, betaine, and the cholinergic
neurotransmitter, ACh. Inasmuch, Choline has a key
role in cholinergic neurologic functions and transmem-
brane signaling, as well as in cell-structure integrity and
fat metabolism; particularly important in its lipid transport function, is its lipotropic activity in the liver.
Although Choline can be found in high concentrations
in a variety of foods (eggs and soy lecithin are the
two most common), it is most often present in its
phospholipid form as PC.[98,99] Despite its many essential
functions, as well as repeatedly validated findings
that Choline levels decrease significantly as a result of
strenuous exercise, and that supplementation with
Choline, PC, or lecithin can significantly increase
Choline availability, the available data studying Choline's effects on endurance performance have shown no
ergogenic benefit.[100-103] One glaring similarity in each
endurance-specific trial is that Choline was provided to
competitive athletes either immediately before an endurance event or no greater than 1 day before competition.
Thus, to conclude that Choline supplementation is
ineffective as an ergogenic aid would be premature and
dismissive of the direct correlation between reduced
exercise and/or mental performance and reduced choline
availability.

DOSE:       *General Use*: 300 mg/d–1.2 g/d as Choline bitartrate or
Choline citrate (or 3–9 g/d as PC): consume in divided
doses, with meals, and/or preexercise

COMMON NAME:     **Chondroitin Sulfate**
OTHER NAMES:     CS; Chondroitin; Chondroitin Sulfate A; Chondroitin
4-Sulfate;    Chondroitin    Sulfate    C;    Chondroitin
6-Sulfate; Chondroitin Sulfate B; Dermatan Sulfate;
Shark Cartilage
COMMON USES:     Reduce Inflammation
Alleviate Joint Pain
Inhibit Joint Degradation
Maintain Cartilage and Connective Tissue Elasticity
REVIEW:          Chondroitin sulfate functions as a glycosaminoglycan
(GAG) to form what are called proteoglycans; proteoglycans and collagen comprise the two most important components of connective tissue. In fact, proteoglycans form
the structural framework of collagen, not to mention
promote water retention within the joint structure, and
increase joint flexibility and resistance to compression
forces. It should further be noted that in similarly related
studies, long-term compressive loading and unloading,
as what frequently takes place at higher intensities in
most forms of exercise and weight training, reproduces
responses in articular cartilage similar to that seen in
degenerative joint diseases such as osteoarthritis (OA).[104]
Although long-term preventative use studies involving
Chondroitin supplementation in otherwise healthy and/
or younger athletes is currently not available, its high
level of safety and vital function to potentially mitigate
such joint degeneration seems prudent. There is, however,

a plethora of data to support the use of Chondroitin across a wide range of older and/or arthritic subjects, and dosing protocols. For example, a recent, double-blind, placebo-controlled, randomized, multicenter study involving 110 patients with knee OA confirmed that as little as 800 mg/d Chondroitin Sulfate, consumed orally, significantly decreased knee joint degeneration and improved measures of pain and joint function.[105] It has been speculated that the sulfur, and not Chondroitin itself, may be providing the analgesic and joint-protecting functions, and also that Chondroitin inhibits the enzymes that break down cartilage as opposed to Chondroitin directly rebuilding connective tissue.[106] Although frequently coadministered with glucosamine, there exist almost no data to substantiate that the combination of the two compounds is significantly more effective than either active delivered independent of the other. Preliminary data in animals support an improved effect of coadministration of Chondroitin Sulfate, glucosamine HCL and manganese ascorbate, as opposed to either ingredient delivered separately; the combination was shown to more significantly blunt the progression of cartilage degeneration.[107] This study was later reproduced in humans, however failed to compare the effects of the ingredients when delivered separately.[108]

**DOSE:** *Joint Health and Analgesic:* 800 mg/d–1.5 g/d as Chondroitin Sulfate; consume with food in one or divided doses

*NOTE: Chondroitin Sulfate may require chronic use for as long as 3 months before significant improvements in joint function can be measured and/or recognized.

**COMMON NAME:** **Chrysin**
**OTHER NAMES:** 5,7-Dihydroxy-2-phenyl-4*H*-1-benzopyran-4-one; 5,7-Dihydroxyflavone; Galangin flavanone; *Passiflora caerulea* L. extract; Blue Passionflower extract; Bluecrown Passionflower extract
**COMMON USES:** Anti-Estrogen/Anti-Aromatase
Increase Testosterone
**REVIEW:** Chrysin is a glucosidal plant flavone, commercially extracted most notably from the herb *Passiflora caerulea*; a member of the passion flower family. Chrysin is also common in most fruits and vegetables, as are most bioflavonoids, and is present in pine trees, honey, and propolis. In vitro tests have demonstrated that Chrysin, at concentrations of 50 nM and 1.1 μg/mL of solution does, indeed, possess a strong affinity to estrogen and inhibits aromatase activity. Also, the ability of Chrysin to either stimulate or suppress estrogen appears dose-dependent.[109,110] Human and animal data, however, reveal poor systemic absorption of Chrysin when consumed orally as either a single, active extract or from whole source material (e.g., honey and propolis), and thus far has been shown to possess no ability to increase testosterone or suppress endogenous estrogen conversion when provided in doses of 400 mg/d or 50 mg/kg/d.[111,112] Although 1%–7% of an oral dose has been shown to be metabolized systemically, as much as 98% of ingested Chrysin is excreted unmetabolized in feces, even when delivered as encapsulated within a phospholipid gel. Although standardization and dosing cannot totally be ruled out, there simply is not enough positive data to

support the recommended use of Chrysin as an anti-aromatase, at this time.

**DOSE:** Insufficient data

**COMMON NAME:** **Citrulline**

**OTHER NAMES:** L-Citrulline; Cit; L-Ornithine, $N^5$-(aminocarbonyl); $N^5$-(Aminocarbonyl)ornithine; $N$(delta)-Carbamylornithine; $N^5$-Carbamoyl-L-ornithine; Sitrulline; alpha-Amino-delta-ureidovaleric acid; delta-Ureidonorvaline; Stimol

**COMMON USES:**
Increase ATP Synthesis
Increase Aerobic Energy
Increase NO
Increase Protein Synthesis
Increase Power Output

**REVIEW:** Citrulline is a nonessential amino acid derived from arginine during NO synthase, but can itself be used to form arginine through a process called the Citrulline–NO cycle. As an NO and arginine precursor, there exists a multitude of potential uses of Citrulline (refer to the Arginine monograph presented earlier in this chapter), although most recently its actions within the TCA cycle have been more rigorously investigated because there exists, during exercise, an inverse relationship between intramuscular Citrulline and lactate—as exercise intensity increases, intramuscular Citrulline decreases whereas lactate increases. If free intramuscular lactate is not reabsorbed and reassimilated into the TCA cycle for ATP resynthesis, or released from the cell (a process requiring co-transport with a proton, or $H^+$) to be made available for use as fuel by other tissues, intracellular proton concentration [H+] will rise in a linear fashion. Briand et al.[113] demonstrated, in vitro, that Citrulline increased lactate reabsorption and an increase in ATP resynthesis. Similarly, Callis et al.[114] found that Citrulline preferentially increased bicarbonate reabsorption in renal tissue when provided to healthy men in a double-blind, placebocontrolled, randomized, crossover study that was specific to the metabolic effects of the compound within hepatic and renal tissue. In both studies, as well as is present in the majority of the literature, Citrulline was provided in the form of Citrulline Malate (L-Citrulline-DL-Malate). In fact, Briand et al. noted that the combination of Citrulline Malate was significantly more effective at increasing ATP resynthesis than either compound delivered independent of the other. In a more recent "exercise"-specific (finger flexion) study of the effects of 6g/d × 15 days, orally consumed Citrulline Malate, provided to 18 men, ATP production during exercise increased 34% and PCr resynthesis after exercise improved by 20%.[115] Similar improvements in measures of autonomic function have been found in men and women with arterial hypotension and receiving 6g/d Citrulline Malate.[116] It has been proposed that whereas Citrulline preferentially increases lactate reabsorption, DL-Malate facilitates ATP resynthesis via its role as a TCA cycle intermediate.

**DOSE:** *Delay Muscle Fatigue/Increase ATP Resynthesis*: 6g/d as Citrulline Malate (53.9% L-Citrulline; 46.1% DL-Malate)

**COMMON NAME:** **Coenzyme Q10**

**OTHER NAMES:** CoQ10; Coenzyme Q(50); CoQ(50); Ubiquinone 50; Ubidecarenone; 2,3-dimethyoxy-5-methyl-6-decaprenyll,4-benzoquinone; Ubiquinol-10; Tobacco leaf extract; Fermented Sugar Cane extract; Fermented Beet extract

**COMMON USES:** Increase Energy
Increase Endurance Performance
Antioxidant
Improve Exercise Recovery
Support Heart Health

**REVIEW:** CoQ10 is a fat-soluble ubiquinone—an essential cofactor involved in electron transport and energy production within cell mitochondria. As such, CoQ10 is involved in all oxygen-dependent (aerobic) metabolic functions and is, therefore, vital to all tissues within the human body. In a recent meta-analysis of the literature involving CoQ10 supplementation and exercise performance, six studies supported its ability to increase exercise capacity whereas an almost equal number (five) of studies found no improvement from CoQ10 supplementation. The same study did, however, confirm, via meta-analysis, the safe and effective use of CoQ10 in significantly lowering blood pressure in persons with hypertension.[117] In fact, the cardioprotective and antioxidant actions of CoQ10 are widely reported and accepted, and believed to be, at least in part, attributable to the ability of CoQ10 to prevent LDL cholesterol oxidation.[118] Inasmuch, the inconclusive findings in exercise-specific studies may simply be the result of a large majority of ingested CoQ10 being preferentially utilized in antioxidative functions. Of major interest, though, are the results of a recent, double-blind, placebo-controlled, randomized study whereby muscle biopsies of the vastus lateralis were collected from aged adults before their receiving 300 mg/d CoQ10 or placebo, for 4 weeks, before hip replacement surgery. When muscle biopsies were again analyzed after supplementation, it was reported that CoQ10 functioned as a second messenger that significantly increased gene expression and cellular metabolism. In fact, it was discovered that those taking CoQ10 had a significant shift from slow-twitch to fast-twitch muscle fibers, resulting in an increase in type IIb muscle tissue.[119]

**DOSE:** *Cardioprotective and General Use*: 50–300 mg/d; consume with fat-containing food or as a phospholipid encapsulated gel cap

**COMMON NAME:** **Conjugated Linoleic Acid**
**OTHER NAMES:** CLA; Octadecadienoic acid; 9,11 (or 10,12)-Octadecadienoic acid; 9,11 (or 10,12)-Linoleic acid; Ricineic acid; Ricinenic acid; Tonalin™
**COMMON USES:** Increase Muscle Hypertrophy
Decrease Body Fat
Improve Immune Function
Antioxidant

**REVIEW:** CLA occurs naturally—most prevalent in ruminant meats and dairy—as a group of isomers of the omega-6 fatty acid, linoleic acid. *Cis*-9, *trans*-11 and *trans*-10, *cis*-12 are the two most frequently used and studied isomers of CLA; *trans*-10, *cis*-12 is most often noted for its reported effects on lipid metabolism and body composition, whereas *cis*-9, *trans*-11 is frequently used as an anticarcinogenic and to increase body mass.[120,121] However, in humans, the effects of CLA supplementation on body composition or exercise performance have been highly inconclusive, especially when provided to otherwise healthy populations in eucaloric states. Thus, it could be surmised that CLA supplementation is most effective in calorie- and fat-restricted states; however, no meta-analysis exists to date to either confirm or refute such claims. It should also be noted that much of the available research from which to draw conclusions have been conducted in animal models, and that some studies have raised concerns regarding the potential negative effects on insulin sensitivity and blood lipids (CLA has been shown to reduce high density lipoprotein in some studies), whereas previous work on CLA showed promise in these areas.[122–126]

**DOSE:** Insufficient data

**COMMON NAME:** **Cordyceps**

**OTHER NAMES:** *Cordyceps sinesis*; Dong Chong Xia Cao; Chinese Caterpillar Fungus; Chinese Mushroom; *Cordyceps militaris*; *Cordyceps kyushuensis*; CordyMax Cs-4®

**COMMON USES:** Increase Oxygen Uptake
Increase Energy
Improve Endurance Performance
Increase Testosterone
Improve Immune Function

**REVIEW:** Cordyceps is a fungal parasite, or mushroom, used as an adaptogen to increase energy, lung and immune function, inhibit tumor growth, reduce blood pressure, improve liver metabolism and function, increase blood flow and sex drive, improve kidney function and glucose metabolism, and to increase Leydig cell steroidogenesis (apparently via PKA pathways), just to name a few of the many reported uses.[127–132] Its primary active components are cordycepin, adenosine, adenosine monophosphate (AMP), inosine, and its saccharides; principally glucose, mannose, and galactose.[133–137] Synthetic Cordyceps (those grown in vitro) seem to be as effective as natural forms, albeit the level of active extracts do vary considerably among species. A major limitation to substantiating the many reported uses of Cordyceps is that most of the research has been conducted on rodents or in vitro. A limited number of well-controlled human trials have studied the effects of Cordyceps supplementation on exercise performance. Those that do exist have used the commercially available Cordyceps product, CordyMax CS-4® (Pharmanex®), which uses *Cordyceps sinesis* standardized to 0.14% adenosine and <6% mannitol. Recently, CordyMax CS-4 was shown to provide no benefit on endurance performance or aerobic capacity in trained, male cyclists who consumed 3 g/d × 5 weeks.[138] Previous studies, however, have shown improvements in both trained athletes and sedentary populations. VO$_2$ max and anaerobic threshold were increased in elderly adults who consumed 3 g/d, for 4–12 weeks, and work output, VO$_2$ peak, and time to VO$_2$ peak increased, whereas respiratory exchange ratio was shown to decrease (indicative of a greater percentage of fuel coming from aerobic as opposed to anaerobic metabolism) when 110 sedentary adults consumed CordyMax CS-4 for 12 weeks.[139,140] When 4.5 g/d CordyMax CS-4 was provided to competitive athletes for 6 weeks, oxygen pulse increased during a submaximal running test, and respiratory exchange ratio and blood lactate decreased.[141] Although arguably inconclusive, the available data are compelling enough to warrant the use of Cordyceps as an adaptogenic with potential ergogenic properties.

**DOSE:**      *Adaptogen/General Use*: 4.5 g/d *Cordyceps sinesis* (standardized to no less than 0.14% adenosine); consume on an empty stomach, in divided doses
*Endurance Performance*: 4.5 g/d *Cordyceps sinesis* (standardized to no less than 0.14% adenosine); consume on an empty stomach, approximately 30 minutes before exercise

**COMMON NAME:**   **Cysteine**
**OTHER NAMES:**   Cys; L-Cysteine; L-2-amino-3-mercaptopropanoic acid; 2-amino-3-mercaptopropanoic acid; beta-mercaptoalanine; 2-amino-3-mercaptopropionic acid; alpha-amino-beta-thiolpropionic acid; Thioserine
**COMMON USES:**   Increase Protein Synthesis
Increase Muscle Strength and Power Output
Improve Exercise Recovery
Anticatabolic
Improve Immune Function
Antiinflammatory
**REVIEW:**    Cysteine, also often referred to by its oxidized and more stable, doubled-bonded form, Cystine, comprises a majority of the sulfur in food, and is especially prevalent in eggs and legumes. Cysteine is a conditionally essential amino acid that serves as a precursor to protein synthesis, as well as to the synthesis of taurine, coenzyme A, inorganic sulfate, and to the body's most powerful antioxidant, GSH. In fact, up to half of the body's total flux of Cysteine may be used to form GSH.[142] Exercise increases Cysteine release from muscle and decreases GSH in a linear manner; however, supplementation with free-form L-Cysteine is rapidly oxidized when consumed orally and is, therefore, not regarded as being capable of effectively increasing GSH. Instead, *N*-acetylcysteine (NAC) is most often used for this purpose and will be discussed at length, later in this chapter.
**DOSE:**      Insufficient data

**COMMON NAME:**   **Digestive Enzymes**
**OTHER NAMES:**   Enzymes; Alpha-Galactosidase; *Aspergillus niger* extract; Amylase; Alpha-amylase; *Aspergillus oryzae* extract; Amylolytic Enzymes; Bromelain; Proteolytic Enzymes; *Ananas sativus* extract; Cellulase; Chymotrypsin; Lipase; Lipolytic Enzymes; Lactase; Beta-Galactosidase; Pancreatin; Pancreatic Enzymes; Pancrelipase; Papain; *Carica papaya* extract; Pepsin; Trypsin
**COMMON USES:**   Improve Digestive Function
Improve Nutrient Absorption/Efficiency
Antiinflammatory
Pain Management
Improve Exercise Recovery
Increase Metabolism
**REVIEW:**    Digestive Enzymes are secreted primarily by the pancreas, small intestine, and, to a lesser extent, salivary glands and the stomach, and act as the catalysts responsible for efficiently converting ingested nutrients into their more useful form(s). Proteolytic Enzymes, such as Bromelain, Chymotrypsin, Papain, Pepsin, and Trypsin,

are necessary to break down proteins into amino acids and small (di- and tri-) peptide fragments; Amylolytic Enzymes, such as Alpha-Galactosidase, Amylase, Alpha-Amylase, Cellulase, Lactase, and Beta-Galactosidase are used to digest carbohydrates into monosaccharides; and, Lipolytic Enzymes, such as Lipase are used in the conversion of fats into free fatty acids and monoglycerides. Pancreatin, however, is a "complete" Enzyme and contains the three pancreatic Enzymes, Trypsin (for protein), Amylase (for carbohydrates), and Lipase (for fat). Athletes frequently consume Digestive Enzymes in an attempt to maximize protein uptake and efficiency, as well as increase metabolism when consuming excess calories and/or protein for weight gain, or when consuming a disproportionate amount of protein relative to total calories for the purpose of promoting fat loss. Food-restricted animal studies do, in part, support the aforementioned: Food-deprived animals supplemented with Digestive Enzymes have been shown to have significantly higher body weight increases than animals not provided Digestive Enzymes while calorie-restricted.[143] Cancer patients provided an enteric-coated Pancreatin Enzyme were shown to increase body weight by 1.2% whereas patients not receiving the supplement lost 3.7% bodyweight.[144] Another area of importance to athletes is the antiinflammatory and improved wound-healing results found in humans supplemented with Digestive Enzymes.[145] Orally ingested Digestive Enzymes, for example, were equally as effective as the nonsteroidal antiinflammatory drug (NSAID), Diclofenac, in alleviating pain in persons with OA of the knee.[146] The German Commission E Monographs do, in fact, approve the use of the Proteolytic Enzyme, Bromelain, for "acute post-operative and post-traumatic conditions of swelling."[147] It is also worth noting that plant tannins (a polyphenolic) have been shown to inhibit Digestive Enzymes, which may, in part, explain why diets high in plant tannins are often associated with reduced weight gain.[148,149]

**DOSE:**  *Nutrient Utilization and General Use*: Consume Digestive Enzymes approximately 30 minutes before meals

*Pancreatin*: 500 mg/dose (containing 25,000 USP of Trypsin; 20,000 USP of Amylase; and 4500 USP of Lipase)

*Alpha-Galactosidase*: 150 GalU/dose (GalU refers to galactose units)

*Bromelain*: 250–500 mg/dose

*Lactase*: 4500 ALU/dose (ALU refers to acid lactase units)

*NOTE: Evidence suggests that enteric-coated Digestive Enzymes may provide improved efficacy.

**COMMON NAME:**  **Dimethylaminoethanol**

**OTHER NAMES:**  DMAE; Deanol; 2-Dimethylaminoethanol; 2-(Dimethyl-amino)-1-ethanol; beta-Hydroxyethyldimethylamine; *N,N*-Dimethyl-2-aminoethanol; Dimethylmonoethanol-amine; Dimethyl(2-hydroxyethyl)amine; Bimanol

**COMMON USES:**  Increase Mental Acuity

Increase Energy

Decrease Symptoms of Attention Deficit Disorder (ADD/ADHD)

**REVIEW:** DMAE was first marketed in the 1960s under the drug name, Deaner (as, deanol acetamidobenzoate), and was later removed as a drug when additional clinical efficacy studies were not provided to the Food and Drug Administration. The claims are that DMAE acts as a cholinergic precursor that increases ACh synthesis in the brain, and could therefore affect brain and neurotransmitter function, as well as energy levels. It seems that extremely high doses of DMAE are required to promote an excitatory response, whereas low-dose DMAE use may have a reverse effect. For example, patients with tardive dyskinesia, a tremor-like disorder, showed no improvement with 1 g/d DMAE, but showed significant improvement in some measures when provided 2 g/d DMAE.[150] Inhalation studies also support the contention that DMAE must be delivered in high oral doses to promote a positive response.[151] Otherwise, DMAE has been shown to actually inhibit choline uptake into the brain and inhibits the production of betaine.[152,153] An area of promise, albeit also supporting the need for high doses of DMAE to effectively increase levels within the bloodstream, is that when DMAE was directly applied to serum-deprived fibroblasts, DNA synthesis increased dramatically as well as did the mitogenic action of insulin.[154]

**DOSE:** Insufficient data

**COMMON NAME:** D-**Pinitol**

**OTHER NAMES:** D-(+)-Pinitol; Pinit; Sennit; Sennitol; D-chiro-Inositol, 3-O-methyl- (9CI); Inositol, 3-O-methyl-, D-chiro- (8CI); Inzitol™

**COMMON USES:** Insulin Mimetic
Increase Glycogen Resynthesis
Improve Exercise Recovery

**REVIEW:** D-Pinitol is chemically similar to the sugar-like compound, inositol, and is found in high concentrations in various legumes, fruits, plants, and pine tree components, and seems to stimulate glucose uptake by directly acting upon the phosphatidylinositol 3-kinase (PI3K) enzyme. D-Pinitol is most effective at reducing blood glucose when consumed either in the absence of glucose or rather before a glucose-containing load, and has generally been found to have no direct effect on insulin or insulin sensitivity.[155–157] For this reason, D-Pinitol has become popular with bodybuilders and fitness athletes attempting to promote muscle cell loading and recovery (e.g., when provided in combination with creatine), especially when adhering to a carbohydrate-restricted diet. When 600 mg/d D-Pinitol, for 6–8 weeks, was provided to lean women with polycystic ovary syndrome, D-Pinitol supplementation did, in fact, result in a significant reduction in circulating insulin and plasma androgens, and improved metabolic functions frequently associated with syndrome X.[158] Evidence also points toward the potential use of D-Pinitol in the treatment of depression disorders.[159] Although quite expensive and its sports use still inconclusive, the available data involving D-Pinitol supplementation and its insulin mimetic effects in the absence of glucose do present a host of sports-specific applications if validated.

**DOSE:** *Glucose Disposal:* 200 mg/dose; consume approximately 30 minutes before meals

*Glycogen Resynthesis*: 600 mg/dose; consume immediately postexercise, before glucose

| | |
|---|---|
| **COMMON NAME:** | **Ecdysterone** |
| **OTHER NAMES:** | Beta-Ecdysterone; 20-hydroxyecdysone; 2-beta,3-beta, 14,20,22,25-Hexahydroxy-5-beta-cholet-7-en-6-one; Isoinokosterone; Viticosterone; Polypodine A; *Rhaponticum carthamoides* extract; *Leuzea carthamoides* extract; Leuzea extract; *Cyanotis vaga* extract; *Serratula coronata* extract; *Serratula strangulate* extract; Ecdisten; Ecdysten |
| **COMMON USES:** | Increase Protein Synthesis<br>Increase Muscle Hypertrophy<br>Increase Muscle Strength<br>Improve Exercise Recovery<br>Antioxidant |
| **REVIEW:** | Ecdysterone is an insect hormone, or ecdysteroid, that is active during the molting stage of development (e.g., maggot stage of a fly's life cycle), and is also present as a phytoecdysteroid in most plant species. For example, Adler and Grebenok[160] noted that of all of the phytoecdysteroids present in more than 100 species of plants, including a thorough review pertaining to spinach, 20-hydroxyecdysone ("Ecdysterone") was the most prevalent. Harmatha and Dinan[161] found that the synthetic form of Ecdysterone derived from insect metabolites, although clearly available as a natural phytoecdysteroid extract from plants or natural mycoecdysteroid from fungi, was most effective at increasing ligand binding in vitro. Most of the human and animal studies, however, have used the plant-derived Ecdysterone form. For example, in 1976, Russian researchers reported that Ecdysterone derived from *Rhaponticum carthamoides* significantly increased body weight and protein content in muscle and other organs in rats that had received 0.5 mg/100 g BW, per day for 7 days. The effect was most prevalent in younger, growing rats, and it was noted that the increased protein synthesis was not via an androgenic-anabolic pathway.[162] Significant, as well as dose-dependent, increases in growth were also noted in quails when provided Ecdysterone derived from *Leuzea carthamoides*. Interestingly, it was also noted that a greater anabolic response was achieved when quails were provided a pure Ecdysterone dose as opposed to that which was achieved with a comparable dose of Ecdysterone provided in the form of an active ingredient within whole Leuzea seeds.[163] Natural ecdysteroids derived from fly larvae was shown, in vitro, to be only about 12% as effective as epidermal growth factors at increasing human fibroblast growth. However, when pure Ecdysterone was added to the maggot ecdysteroid extract and epidermal growth factor-stimulated fibroblasts, a significant increase in growth rate was achieved.[164] Thus, this somewhat validated both that pure Ecdysterone is required to achieve an anabolic response, as well as that for a significant growth response to take place, a previous growth-enhancing environment must first be achieved. In other words, Ecdysterone may be best used in younger athletes or in combination with other anabolic agents. Several Eastern |

European studies exist that do, in fact, support such a theory. For example, when Ecdysterone was provided in combination with pure protein to aerobically and anaerobically trained subjects, for 3 weeks, muscle mass and total work increased, and body fat decreased; however, most of these studies are in Russian and available in translated form only as abstracts.[165] Similarly, increased erythropoietin (EPO) and improved sexual function, sleep, memory and learning, as well as antioxidant, antifungal, and immune-supporting effects have all been attributed to Ecdysterone.[166–171] Despite limitations in translation, pure Ecdysterone does seem to have enough supporting data to warrant its use in sports.

**DOSE:** *Protein Synthesis and General Use*: 0.5–10 mg/kg BW/d Ecdysterone (as, 20-hydroxyecdysone); consume in divided doses, with protein, and/or immediately post-workout with protein

**COMMON NAME:** **Epimedium**

**OTHER NAMES:** Horny Goat Weed; Herba Epimediia; Yin Yang Huo; *Epimedium brevicornum*; *Epimedium koreanum*; *Epimedium pubescens*; *Epimedium sagittatum*; *Epimedium wushanense*; *Epimedium acuminatum*; *Epimedium grandiflorum*; *Epimedium hunanense*; *Epimedium leptorrhizum*

**COMMON USES:** Anticatabolic
Increase Sex Hormone Release
Increase Energy
Treat Erectile Function
Improve Immune Support
Antioxidant

**REVIEW:** Epimedium is often categorized as an adaptogenic herb because of its broad range of uses, albeit sometimes conflicting biologic outcomes that arise from its use from one study to the next. Although quite possibly an adaptogen, another plausible explanation for the inconsistent findings is that Epimedium is a genus of more than 16 plant species, collectively containing more than 130 active compounds—the glycoside, icariin, seems to be the most important of the Epimedium active extracts. As such, effectiveness varies from one species to the next depending on the level of this active. Icariin has been shown to increase cAMP (adenosine cyclic monophosphate), decrease cGMP (cyclic guanosine monophosphate), inhibit cholinesterase enzyme,[172–174] restore endothelial nitric oxide synthase function, increase intracavernous pressure and erectile function,[175,176] improve immune function, decrease corticosterone (CORT) and adrenocorticotropic hormone (ACTH), as well as act as a powerful antioxidant.[177–180] Other Epimedium studies, whereby no standardization was noted, have revealed somewhat contradictory results—increased CORT, decreased T3 (triiodothyronine),[181] and increased estrogenic function, just to name a few. For example, the Epimedium compounds icaritin and desmethylicaritin were found to be dose-dependent and similarly as effective as estradiol at stimulating estrogen receptors, whereas icariin was found to have no effect.[182] Icariin, too, seems to work dose-dependently, and there is evidence that its racemic (reduced), or higher hydrogen-containing metabolites are more powerful than icariin, itself.[125,183] To find a high-icariin-containing, high-quality Epimedium, a Chinese study denotes *Epimedium koreanum*, grown in Northeast China, as possessing "the best quality," followed by *E. brevicornu* and *E. sagittatum*, respectively.[184] Also, the rhizome and roots of Epimedium contain higher quantities of the icariin active extract than are found in the plant's leaves and stem.[185]

**DOSE:** *Ergogenic Aid and General Use*: 5–10 mg/kg BW/d icariin active (from *Epimedium koreanum* rhizome and/or root extract); consume on an empty stomach, in divided doses, and/or pre- and/or postexercise

**COMMON NAME:** **Essential Amino Acids**

**OTHER NAMES:** EAA; EAAs; L-Isoleucine, L-Leucine, L-Lysine, L-Methionine, L-Phenylalanine, L-Threonine, L-Tryptophan, L-Valine

**COMMON USES:** Increase Protein Synthesis
Increase Muscle Hypertrophy
Increase Muscle Strength
Anticatabolic
Improve Exercise Recovery
Increase Energy/Delay Muscle Fatigue
Insulin Mimetic
Increase Immune Support

**REVIEW:** EAAs are alpha amino acids that the body cannot manufacture and, therefore, must be consumed within the diet. There are eight EAAs: Isoleucine, Leucine, Lysine, Methionine, Phenylalanine, Threonine, Tryptophan, and Valine. Two additional amino acids—Histidine and Arginine—are also often included. Inasmuch, EAA formulations vary; the results of clinical research should be interpreted with this discrepancy in mind. In general, however, the data involving EAAs suggest that EAAs dose-dependently contribute to protein synthesis, that EAA availability is more important for recovery from intense exercise than is the availability of total energy (calories), and that EAAs increase protein synthesis directly as opposed to reducing muscle breakdown. The mechanism by which EAAs stimulate protein synthesis is dependent on the availability and concentration(s) of extracellular EAAs; however, whether there is a need for all of the EAAs or just specific EAAs is not currently known.[186] Tipton et al.[187] showed that consuming 15 g of an EAA beverage immediately before, and another 15 g of EAAs 1 hour after a resistance training (30 g EAA, in total), provided a significant additive effect on net muscle protein balance (NB) over a 24-hour period when compared with NB at rest. This confirms that NB can be increased, and therefore readjusted, by exercise and EAA availability. Many of the same researchers collaborated on other EAA works. The outcomes of this, and other studies, show that: NEAAs (nonessential) are not required for protein synthesis; consuming EAAs preexercise may be more important than when consumed postexercise; EAA + carbohydrate (CHO) preexercise has a greater protein synthesis response than when consumed postexercise; the addition of CHO to EAAs, postexercise, has only a modest improvement in protein synthesis; and there may be a threshold of EAA intake and its protein synthesis response (i.e., more may not be better).[188–193] In light of all studies—specifically, those confirming that

EAA concentrations directly stimulate protein synthesis—there warrants support for the common practice of multiple daily dosing of EAAs (often derived from whey protein supplements) as a method of constantly readjusting concentration levels to promote increased protein synthesis. It is worth noting, however, that many of the EAA studies noted here used an EAA solution including the amino acid, Histidine, but was void of the amino acids Tryptophan and Arginine.

**DOSE:** *Protein Synthesis and Exercise Recovery*: 3–40 g/d; consume isocalorically and/or in combination with CHO acutely and/or in divided doses, as well as immediately preexercise and within 3 hours postexercise.

**COMMON NAME:** **Eurycoma**
**OTHER NAMES:** *Eurycoma longifolia* Jack; *Eurycoma longifolia*; Tongkat Ali; Malaysian ginseng; Longjack; TJ 100™
**COMMON USES:** Increase Testosterone
Increase Muscle Hypertrophy
Increase Muscle Strength
Treat Erectile Dysfunction
**REVIEW:** Eurycoma is indigenous to Southeast Asia, with a long history of use of its roots as an aphrodisiac, antimalarial, and infection-fighting medicine. Recently, a possible role in glucose disposal was discovered: 150 mg/kg BW of two different aqueous extracts of *Eurycoma longifolia* modestly reduced glucose levels in hyperglycemic-induced rats.[194] Although much work has been done on rodents, both normal and castrated, to support the use of Eurycoma for dose-dependently improving measures of sexual activity and vigor—most notably effective when provided in doses above 400 mg/kg BW/d of a 100:1 water-extracted solution[195–198]—there stands no peer-reviewed or published data that Eurycoma increases testosterone or has any ergogenic benefit when used in humans. A commercially available form of Eurycoma raw material, LJ100™, uses as its substantiation for use in bodybuilding and in promoting testosterone, two non-reviewed works involving doses of just 100 mg/d: one, an abstract that was presented in 2003 that involved 14 young, healthy men, engaged in a bodybuilding-type resistance training program for 8 weeks; the second, an independent study of five men, and their saliva-tested DHEA and SHBG (sex hormone binding globulin) response to 3 weeks of supplementation. Collectively, the data were modestly positive—increased lean body mass and arm circumference, and increased DHEA and reduced SHBG. However, these data should be viewed with extreme skepticism, in part because of the huge discrepancy in the dose used as compared with efficacious doses as detailed in other studies. Also, until peer reviewed, and the study designs fully disclosed, it would be prudent not to accept the manufacturer's claims.
**DOSE:** *General Use*: >150 mg/kg BW/d *Eurycoma longifolia* root (standardized to contain a 100:1 water extracted active extract); consume on an empty stomach, before meals, and/or immediately postexercise

**COMMON NAME:** **Flaxseed**
**OTHER NAMES:** Flax; Common Flax; Flax Oil; Flaxseed Oil; Linseed; Linseed Oil; *Linum usitatissimum*; Winterlien; Lint Bells

COMMON USES:    Increase Metabolism (during calorie-restricted dieting)
                Antiinflammatory
                Pain Relief
                Decrease Cholesterol

REVIEW:         Flaxseed is one of the oldest cultivated plants in history, and is one of the richest natural sources of the omega-3 fatty acid, alpha-linolenic acid; the fatty oils from Flaxseed contain 52%–76% linolenic acid esters. Flaxseed is also high in omega-6, or linoleic acid, and the lignan, secoisolariciresinol glycoside (SDG). Flaxseed contains 75–800 times as much SDG than was found present in 68 other common foods.[199] Flaxseed has been shown to reduce proinflammatory cytokines, tumore necrosis factor (TNF)-alpha and IL-1-beta, by up to 30% in healthy adults; however, fish oils were found to be more than 2.5 times as effective.[200] Flaxseed is, however, highly regarded for its anticarcinogenic and lipid-lowering abilities, but a word of caution to men: SDG is a phytoestrogen and there is supporting evidence that men on a low-fat diet, supplementing with 30 g of Flaxseed per day, may realize decreases in total testosterone by up to 15% within 30 days.[201] A follow-up study showed that total testosterone decreased over 6 months, but the decrease was not significant.[202,203] Thus, Flaxseed as a source of omega-3 and omega-6 fatty acids may be best realized in female athletes. The phytoestrogenic properties further support postmenopausal, physically active women.

DOSE:           *General Use*: 30–50 g/d Flaxseed as bruised or whole seed (or 3–5 tbsp./d as Flaxseed oil); consume in divided doses, with meals and/or protein supplements; do not exceed 50 g (or 5 tbsp.), per day

*NOTE: Overweight persons should consume Flaxseed as whole seed, and not as oil, to avoid potential overconsumption of fat calories.

COMMON NAME:    **Gamma-Aminobutyric Acid**
OTHER NAMES:    GABA; Butanoic acid; 4-Aminobutanoic acid; 4-Aminobutyric acid; Piperidic acid; Piperidinic acid; gamma-Amino-*n*-butyric acid; gamma-Amino-*N*-butyric acid; γ-Aminobutyric acid

COMMON USES:    Improve Exercise Recovery
                Increase Growth Hormone
                Promote Restful Sleep
                Antianxiety

REVIEW:         GABA is an amino acid, formed from glutamate (the salt form of glutamic acid) and present in high concentrations throughout the central nervous system (CNS), acting as an excitatory neurotransmitter antagonist. GABA became popular among bodybuilders when a study revealed acute supplementation resulted in an increase in GH within 3 hours after consuming a 5-g oral dose.[204] Two follow-up studies confirmed the efficacy of a 5-g oral dose in healthy adults, as well as revealing a dose-dependent increase when 10 g of GABA was ingested.[205,206] One of the studies did, however, reveal a curvilinear response—18 g of GABA, for 4 days, resulted in a blunted GH response. A more recent study in sheep, involving intravenous (i.v.) and intracerebroventricular (i.c.v.) injections of 10 and 100 mg of GABA, showed both the GH-increasing as well as the curvilinear dose dependency—i.v. doses significantly and rapidly increased GH, whereas the 10 mg i.c.v.

dose increased, but the 100 mg i.c.v. dose decreased plasma GH. [Note: i.c.v. injections are delivered directly into the cerebroventricular brain tissue and, therefore, do no undergo systemic metabolism across cell membranes.][207] Although supraphysiologic doses of GABA could be consumed to yield desired outcomes and overcome well-documented limitations of GABA crossing the blood-brain barrier, a potentially more efficient approach may be in the coadministration of GABA with PS; PC and phosphatidylinositol, however, have been shown ineffective as transport aides.[208] Benassi et al.,[209] for example, showed that when 740 mg/kg BW GABA and 740 mg/kg BW PS were intraperitoneally coinjected, there was a significantly increased passage across, and into, the blood and brain nerve endings. This result was significantly more pronounced than when the same doses were injected separately, although delivered separately did show significant results whereas GABA and PS injected without the other present was ineffective at entering nerve endings. Interestingly, despite the intimate role GABA has in sleep, there are currently no direct studies involving GABA supplementation and sleep promotion. Data in mildly hypertensive humans and rodents do, however, confirm both the acute and chronic use of GABA to reduce systolic blood pressure.[210–213] Although limited, these data do point toward a potential use of GABA as an antianxiety aide, and thus indirectly promote improved sleep.

**DOSE:** *GH Secretagogue*: 5–10 g/d; consume on an empty stomach, approximately 1 hour before bedtime
*Blood Pressure Reduction (possible antianxiety)*: ≥1.2 mg/kg BW/d for at least 2 weeks; consume on an empty stomach

*Note: GABA, as provided in a PS encapsulated gel cap, may offer improved absorption and efficacy.

| | |
|---|---|
| **COMMON NAME:** | **Ginger** |
| **OTHER NAMES:** | *Zingiber officinale*; Ginger root; *Zingiberis rhizome*; Canton ginger; *Amomum zingiber*; *Amomum angustifolium*; Garden Ginger |
| **COMMON USES:** | Improve Digestion |
| | Antiinflammatory |
| | Increase Blood Flow |
| | Improve Exercise Recovery |
| | Antioxidant |

**REVIEW:** Ginger is most frequently used to reduce symptoms associated with motion sickness and nausea; however, it has recently become a popular ingredient in many diet and energy products, and is found in many endurance and pain management formulations. Use within diet products is primarily attributable to claims that Ginger decreases transit time and speeds digestion. A German study, for example, found that 200 mg of Ginger rhizome extract increased digestive motility both when consumed on an empty stomach as well as when consumed after a meal.[214] A study in guinea pigs also showed an accelerated transit time; however, this study was specific only to the Ginger extract, 6-shogaol.[215] A more recent human study evaluated the use of Ginger in the presence of acute hyperglycemia—a common stimulus of stomach discomfort and delayed gastric emptying in healthy adults. One gram of Ginger root, consumed 30 minutes before receiving dextrose infusion, significantly reduced hyperglycemia-induced gastric disruption and significantly blunted prostaglandin production.[216] The latter effect may, in part, explain a potential role in the ability of Ginger to mitigate pain. For example, several Ginger extracts were found, in vitro, to significantly inhibit cyclooxygenase (COX)-1, and several of the extracts produced a more potent antiplatelet effect than aspirin. The most powerful of the Ginger constituents was shown to be 8-paradol.[217] In a similar in vitro study, 17 Ginger extracts were tested for their effect on COX-2 inhibition; 8-paradol and 8-shogaol were found to be the most effective actives.[218] Using the Bitter Ginger (*Zingiber zerumbet*) rhizome sesquiterpene extract, zerumbone, COX-2, prostaglandin E2 and TNF-alpha were all suppressed, whereas no change was seen in COX-1 in yet another in vitro study.[219] More research in humans will need to be conducted to determine if these laboratory results are duplicated in vivo.

**DOSE:** *Digestive Aide, Analgesic, and General Use*: 200–600 mg/dose, or up to 4 g/d as *Zingiber officinale* dried rhizome [standardized to contain not less than 1.5% (mL/g) volatile oil]; consume 30 minutes before, or immediately after meals

**COMMON NAME:** **Ginseng**

**OTHER NAMES:** *Panax ginseng*; Ginseng root; Ginseng radix; Asian ginseng; Oriental ginseng; *Panax schinseng*; Chinese ginseng; Korean ginseng; True ginseng; G115®; Ginsana®; *Panax notoginseng*; Noto-G™; Notoginseng; *Panax pseudoginseng*; Japanese ginseng; Bamboo ginseng; san-qi ginseng; Tienchi ginseng; *Panax japonicus*; *Panax quinquefolius*; American ginseng; *Eleutherococcus senticosus*; Eleuthero; Eleuthero root; *Acanthopanax senticosus*; Eleutherococci radix; Eleutherococcus; Siberian ginseng; Ussurian thorny pepperbush; Taiga root; *Panax sessiliflorus*; *Eleutherococcus sessiliflorus*; *Acanthopanax sessiliflorus*; Stalkless-flower eleuthero; Pseudostellaria; *Pseudostellaria heterophylla*; Lesser ginseng; Prince ginseng

**COMMON USES:** Increase Energy
Increase Endurance Performance/Delay Muscle Fatigue
Increase Sexual Performance and Fertility
Increase Testosterone
Improve Immune Function
Insulin Mimetic
Stimulant
Increase Mental Acuity/Mental Focus
Increase Vasodilation

**REVIEW:** There are many species of Ginseng; each is similar in its botany and most species function as an adaptogen. However, as with most herbs, there is considerable variation in chemical makeup between and even within Ginseng species, as was quantitatively presented in a recent literature review. Ginsenosides vary between species by 26%–103%, and the type of ginsenoside present within each species varies by 36%–112%.[220] *Panax ginseng* (or Asian Ginseng) and American Ginseng (or *Panax quinquefolius*) are the most common forms of Ginseng, and are believed to be effective because of their biologically active ginsenosides—Asian Ginseng, for its high concentration of the CNS-stimulating Rg1, and American Ginseng, which contains a higher concentration of the CNS-suppressing Rb1 ginsenoside. Siberian Ginseng (or Eleuthero), although debatable as to whether it belongs within the "true" Ginseng family, is often used in sports supplements, and contains active eleutherosides—B, B1, and E are believed to be the most important. With such diversity among species, one should not expect all forms of Ginseng to elicit similar performance or physiologic benefits. Bucci et al.,[221] in a comprehensive review of the clinical data relevant to Ginseng as an ergogenic aid, concluded that Asian Ginseng extracts, standardized to not less than 4% total ginsenosides, produced some ergogenic effect in 74% of the studies that were designed with high statistical power (adequate number of subjects) and of sufficient duration (4 weeks or more). Bucci et al. also concluded that Asian Ginseng was ineffective if used for fewer than 4 weeks, and that the data on American Ginseng and Eleuthero currently does not warrant their use as performance-enhancing supplements.[221] Respectfully, that may not be entirely true: Whereas Asian Ginseng, when consumed before exercise, can improve performance and act as a stimulant, American Ginseng has strong evidence to suggest its use in glucose disposal and recovery. For example, Vuksan et al.[223] provided healthy adults 1, 2, or 3 g of American Ginseng, standardized to 3.21% total ginsenosides and 1.53% Rb1, at 40, 20, 10, or 0 minutes before receiving a 25-g oral glucose load. All three doses were equally effective at reducing blood glucose levels, but only when consumed 40 minutes before receiving the glucose.[222] This confirmed a previous study, by the same researchers, that also showed a hypoglycemic response to American Ginseng when consumed 40 minutes before a glucose load. In a double-blind, randomized, multiple-crossover design study, eight different species of Ginseng were tested separately; healthy adults consumed 3 g of Ginseng, 40 minutes before receiving a 75-g oral glucose load. American and Vietnamese Ginseng lowered plasma glucose, whereas Asian, American-wild, and Siberian Ginsengs increased plasma glucose. The researchers concluded that the ratio of protopanaxadiol/protopanaxatriol ginsenosides (Rb1/Rg1) was strongly correlated to glycemic effect, albeit they could not entirely rule out other plant constituents as potentially contributing to a synergistic effect.[224] The claims that Ginseng increases testosterone are nonconclusive, and if such exists are likely to be an adaptogenic response to low levels of endogenous testosterone.

**DOSE:**  *Energy, Performance Enhancing, Adaptogen, and General Use*: 200 mg/d as *Panax ginseng* root (standardized to not less than 4% total ginsenosides, and containing not less than 1.5% total ginsenosides as ginsenoside Rg1); consumed in divided doses, once in the morning and again approximately 30–60 minutes before exercise

*Glucose Disposal, Adaptogen, and General Use*: 1–3 g/d as *Panax quinquefolius* root (standardized to not less than 3.21% total ginsenosides, and containing not less than 1.5% total ginsenosides as ginsenoside Rb1); consume in divided doses, 40 minutes before meals and/or glucose loads

COMMON NAME:     **Glucosamine**
OTHER NAMES:     2-Amino-2-deoxyglucose;     2-Amino-2-deoxy-D-glucose;
                 2-Amino-2-deoxy-beta-D-glucopyranose;     Chitosamine;
                 D-Glucosamine
COMMON USES:     Reduce Inflammation
                 Alleviate Joint Pain
                 Inhibit Joint Degradation
                 Maintain Cartilage and Connective Tissue Elasticity
REVIEW:          Glucosamine is an amino sugar, formed in the body as glucosamine 6-phosphate from the combination of glutamine to modified glucose. Glucosamine is found in the greatest concentrations within articular cartilage and is essential to forming GAGs and proteoglycans: proteoglycans form collagen and help to retain water within the joint to support flexibility and resistance to compressive forces; GAGs bind to water to form proteoglycans and, therefore, form the cartilage matrix itself. As such, the incredible popularity of Glucosamine as a preventative against overuse and degenerative joint diseases, such as OA, is largely associated with its ability to increase the synthesis of new proteoglycans and inhibit proteoglycan degradation.[225] To test this theory, Christgau et al.[226] conducted a 3-year double-blind, placebo-controlled trial in 212 subjects with knee OA. Daily use of Glucosamine (as Glucosamine Sulfate) reduced collagen type II degradation by 15.5% within 12 months in those with advanced OA. In a separate 3-year randomized, placebo-controlled study involving 202 patients with mild to moderate OA, 1500 mg/d Glucosamine Sulfate significantly improved symptoms by as much as 25%; severe joint space narrowing, a condition associated with the loss of cartilage, occurred in 14% of those taking the placebo but in only 5% of those consuming Glucosamine Sulfate.[227] An independent meta-analysis of the randomized, placebo-controlled clinical trials published between 1980–March 2002 concluded that Glucosamine "demonstrated a highly significant efficacy" against all structural and symptomatic (such as pain) measures, including evidence to support the use of Glucosamine to reduce joint space narrowing.[228] Glucosamine Sulfate (1500 mg/d) has also been determined to relieve joint pain associated with OA as effectively as 1200 mg/d ibuprofen.[229] This, as well as the overall effectiveness of Glucosamine Sulfate, has been proposed as being a synergistic effect between Glucosamine and sulfate, or simply having more to do with the role sulfur has in the body as opposed to the positive effects being solely attributable to Glucosamine. Sulfur is also essential to the synthesis of GAGs, and unlike Glucosamine supplementation, orally consumed sulfur directly affects its presence in serum whereas Glucosamine is almost entirely modified or degraded in the liver. NSAIDs, such as ibuprofen and acetaminophen, require sulfation in their metabolism and have, in fact, been shown to compromise GAG synthesis.[230] Hoffer et al.[231] tested this theory, in part, and found that 1 g of Glucosamine Sulfate increased serum and synovial fluid sulfate by 13% in healthy adults, but sodium sulfate was ineffective; coadministration with 1 g of acetaminophen reduced sulfate levels by approximately 11%. Recently, however, Glucosamine HCL is being used more often in commercially available formulations, although there are

far fewer data to substantiate the effects of its use being better than, or even comparable to that of Glucosamine Sulfate. Lastly, a thorough review of available clinical trials (3063 human subjects, in total) confirmed the wide range of safety (no adverse effects reported up to 2700 mg/ d × 12 months) and dispelled concerns that Glucosamine supplementation adversely affects glucose metabolism in humans. Slight, nonsignificant reductions in fasting plasma glucose have been shown to occur after 66 weeks of Glucosamine supplementation.[232]

**DOSE:**

*Joint Health and Analgesic*: 1500–2000 mg/d as Glucosamine Sulfate; consume as one dose or in divided doses for a minimum of 6 weeks

**COMMON NAME:** **Glutamic Acid/Glutamate**

**OTHER NAMES:** L-Glutamic acid; L-Glutamate; L-Glutamic acid, (ion)1-; 1-Aminopropane-1,3-dicarboxylic acid; 2-Aminopentane-dioic acid; Glusate; Glutacid; L-2-Aminoglutaric acid; L-Glutaminic acid; Pentanedioic acid, 2-amino-, (S)-; alpha-Aminoglutaric acid; Glutaton; Glutaminol

**COMMON USES:** Increase Protein Synthesis
Delay Onset of Muscle Fatigue
Increase Work Output
Improve Gut Integrity
Increase Insulin

**REVIEW:** Glutamic acid is one of nature's most abundant amino acids: animal protein contains 11%–22% Glutamate, and some plants contain as much as 40% Glutamate. In humans, Glutamate is one of the most abundant amino acids in the free amino acid pool in muscle, and is found in high concentration in the liver, kidney, and brain. The average daily turnover in sedentary humans is about 48 g/d, but despite such a high turnover, the average human only holds a mere 20 mg or so of Glutamate in the plasma. Such overwhelming disparity between intra- as opposed to extracellular concentrations is evidence of the many important functions Glutamate has within tissues. Specifically, Glutamate is the primary amino acid taken up into muscle, during rest and exercise. Glutamate is essential to the transamination of the BCAAs to AKG and the deamination of most amino acids during the synthesis of urea. Glutamate directly contributes to the synthesis of ammonia, aspartate, alanine, and glutamine, as well as GSH, and is generally regarded as the primary excitatory neurotransmitter within the central and peripheral nervous systems. Glutamate was shown to be active in signaling approximately one third of all CNS synapses.[233–236] These major roles in all brain and muscle (and liver and kidney) functions help explain why Glutamic acid is one of the three most prevalent free amino acids in human breast milk. Glutamic acid and taurine are the highest in colostrum; taurine then remains stable, whereas Glutamic acid increases 2.5× and glutamine increases 20×. In fact, Glutamic acid and glutamine collectively comprise greater than 50% of the total free amino acids in breast milk at 3-months lactation.[237] Yet, despite all of its functionality and specificity to supporting the TCA cycle, Glutamic acid remains a nonessential amino acid and has limited data of its use as a supplement during exercise. In a double-blind, cross-over study, Mourtzakis and Graham[236] provided active, healthy adult subjects 150 mg/kg BW Glutamate (as monosodium glutamate, or MSG), 40 minutes before exercising at 85% $VO_2$ max for 15 minutes on a cycle ergometer. Blood and $VO_2$ were measured before, during and after exercise. Glutamate significantly increased $VO_2$ during exercise (5.3%), but there was no shift in fuel utilization; REE (respiratory exchange) did not differ between groups. Plasma ammonia, which increases during exercise as amino acids within muscle are broken down, was almost 25% less during exercise in those taking Glutamate as compared with placebo. This was accompanied by a dramatic increase in plasma Glutamate ($>18\times$), aspartate, alanine, and taurine, with steady but only modest increases in plasma glutamine. It is also worth noting that this study supported previous work that demonstrated an immediate and dramatic increase in insulin upon ingestion of Glutamate. Graham et al. found that 150 mg/kg BW Glutamate (as MSG) tripled insulin, and that this increase in insulin occurred before any measurable increase in plasma Glutamate, thus providing evidence that hepatic Glutamate metabolism may directly stimulate insulin release. Animal data also provide evidence of an anabolic, anticatabolic, and potentially ergogenic benefit of orally consumed glutamate. However, more safety and human use studies are needed.[238-240]

**DOSE:**               Insufficient data

**COMMON NAME:**   **Glutamine**

**OTHER NAMES:**   L-Glutamine; Levoglutamide; L-2-Aminoglutaramidic acid; (S)-2,5-Diamino-5-oxopentanoic acid; 2-Aminoglutaramic acid, L-; Cebrogen; Glavamin; Glutamic acid 5-amide; L-Glutamic acid gamma-amide; L-Glutamide; Stimulina; Pentanoic acid, 2,5-diamino-5-oxo-, (S)-

**COMMON USES:**   Anticatabolic
Increase Muscle Hypertrophy
Increase Cell Volumization
Improve Immune Function
Improve Gut Integrity
Increase Glycogen Resynthesis
Improve Exercise Recovery

**REVIEW:**            Glutamine is the most prevalent free amino acid in plasma and one of the most prevalent in muscle. However, supplementation with this conditionally essential amino acid has, to date, yielded no improvement in body composition or sports performance when provided to otherwise healthy subjects. For example, Candow et al.[241] conducted a double-blind, placebo-controlled, randomized study in which 31 young, active adults consumed either 0.9 g/kg lean tissue mass/d Glutamine or a maltodextrin placebo for 6 weeks, while engaged in a controlled strength-training program. One repetition maximum squat and bench press strength, peak knee extension torque, lean tissue mass (as measured by dual-energy X-ray absorptiometry) and protein degradation were equally improved in both the Glutamine and placebo groups. Antonio et al.[242] also found no improvement in weightlifting performance in a double-blind, placebo-controlled, crossover study in resistance-trained men receiving an acute dose of 0.3 g/kg BW, 60 minutes before exercise. Haub et al.[243] also found no ergogenic effect of Glutamine supplementation when provided as an acute dose (0.03 g/kg body mass), 90 minutes before five, 60-second cycle ergometer tests at 100% $VO_2$ peak, separated by 60-second rest periods. Forming the conclusion that the dose in the Haub et al. study was too small to reveal a positive acute response to the TCA cycle-mediated exercise test does not seem warranted.[244] Bruce et al.[245] found a 31% greater increase in TCA intermediates (citrate, malate, fumarate, and succinate) within the vastus lateralis of well-trained cyclists after subjects had exercised for 10 minutes, cycling at 70% $VO_2$ max, 60 minutes after consuming 0.125 mg/kgBW Glutamine as opposed to placebo. However, no differences were observed between groups on measures of blood glucose, lactate, heart rate, REE, or expired ventilation. There is, however, supporting evidence that Glutamine increases glycogen resynthesis after exhaustive exercise and, therefore, may be useful for periods of dietary restriction of carbohydrates. Eight grams of Glutamine was equally as effective at increasing muscle glycogen resynthesis as was consuming a glucose polymer-containing beverage immediately postexercise. It was also noted that Glutamine + glucose polymer beverage provided no additional effect on muscle glycogen than Glutamine alone, but did increase whole-body glycogen resynthesis, presumably increasing hepatic glycogen levels. Moreover, Glutamine alone did not increase insulin, whereas insulin increased significantly in the other two glucose polymer–containing trials.[246] It should be stressed that the claims that Glutamine reduces protein breakdown and supports immune function are somewhat misleading. Several independent reviews of the literature have come to much of the same conclusion—Glutamine supplementation is required in very high (at least 20 g/d), sustained doses (consumed immediately upon injury, as well as fed continuously/chronically thereafter) to be effective in influencing net protein balance and physiologically measured immune function. Additionally, it is glutamate (or glutamic acid), and not glutamine, that preferentially improves gut mucosa.[247–250]

**DOSE:** *Glycogen Resynthesis*: 8 g/dose; consume immediately postexercise

*Anticatabolic and General Use*: ≥20 g/d; consume immediately postexercise or in divided doses

**COMMON NAME:** **Glycerol**

**OTHER NAMES:** Glycerine; Glycerin; 1,2,3-Propanetriol; 1,2,3-Trihydroxypropane; Glyceritol; Glycyl alcohol; Ophthalgan; Osmoglyn; Propanetriol; Trihydroxypropane; Vitrosupos

**COMMON USES:** Promote Hyperhydration
Increase Blood Volume
Improve Endurance Performance
Rehydration
Diuretic

**REVIEW:** Glycerol is one of the most prevalent alcohols in the body, produced during the breakdown of triglycerides, glucose, proteins, pyruvate, and other sugar alcohols, and is used as the backbone of triacylglycerols (triglycerides, or fat) and phospholipids. Most notorious for its use within high-protein or low-carbohydrate nutrition bars, Glycerol is marketed as a sugar alcohol that does not affect blood sugar or increase insulin. That is and is not entirely true. Trimmer et al.[251] concluded that when

Glycerol was coadministered with glucose at rest and then continuously infused during a 90-minute cycle ergometer test of light and moderate intensities, as much as 75%–100% of the rate of removal of Glycerol from serum could be accounted for by its conversion to glucose. However, Glycerol did not increase hepatic glucose production during exercise, nor did Glycerol have a glucose-sparing or glucose-altering effect either during rest or exercise. In other words, Glycerol did not affect insulin, but did convert into glucose, presumably via pyruvate. Burelle et al.[252] performed a similar test, but instead of constant infusion, Glycerol and glucose were provided as a single oral bolus immediately before 120 minutes of moderate-intensity exercise. Similarly, Glycerol did not disrupt glucose absorption or oxidation, but did convert to glucose and therefore decreased endogenous glucose oxidation. No muscle glycogen-sparing or ergogenic effects were found, however. A review, published in 2000, concluded as much: Glycerol supplementation seems "to have no meaningful advantage." The researchers' assessment was based on available controlled studies whereby hyperhydration with Glycerol (Glycerol has been shown to increase total body water by up to 700 mL) was unable to lower core or skin temperatures, improve sweating efficiency, or reduce heart rate while exercising in hot temperatures.[253] Two, more recent, randomized, controlled, double-blind studies, do however reveal that 1 or 1.2 g/kg BW Glycerol added to 20 or 25 mL/kg BW of a 6% CHO-containing beverage (Gatorade®), respectively, consumed 1–2 hours preexercise, has significant and notable results on endurance-trained and competitive Olympic distance triathletes while exercising in hot climates. Specifically, hyperhydration or water retention was improved, plasma volume increased, exercising heart rate was reduced, performance times improved, and rectal temperature decreased.[254,255]

**DOSE:** *Endurance Performance, Hydration, and Heat Tolerance*: 1 g : 20 mL–1.2 g : 25 mL, per kg BW, of a Glycerol : 6% carbohydrate-containing fluid; consume slowly, beginning 2 hours before endurance event

*Note: 20–25 mL/kg BW of a 6% CHO-containing beverage is approximately equivalent to 0.75 g/kg BW CHO to be contained per milliliter of fluid to be consumed.

**COMMON NAME:** **Ipriflavone**

**OTHER NAMES:** 7-Isopropoxyisoflavone; 7-(1-Methylethoxy)-3-phenyl-4*H*-1-benzopyran-4-one; 4*H*-1-Benzopyran-4-one, 7-(1-methylethoxy)-3-phenyl-; 7-isopropoxy-3-phenylchromone; Osten; Yambolap; Ostivone™

**COMMON USES:** Improve Bone Health
Antiinflammatory
Support Healthy Sex Hormone Levels (Pro-Estrogen and Anti-Estrogen)
Increase Protein Synthesis

**REVIEW:** Ipriflavone, a plant isoflavone derivative that was once believed to bind directly to estrogen receptor cells has since been shown to possess no discernable affinity for binding to estrogen receptors and therefore has no direct estrogenic or antiestrogenic effect.[256,257] Instead, Ipriflavone seems to selectively modulate the effects of estrogen as opposed to increasing or blocking estrogen output.[258–260]

As noted in a 1999 review by Messina,[261] "The prevailing hypothesis has been that isoflavones exert antiestrogenic effects when placed in a high-estrogen environment... and estrogenic effects when in a low-estrogen environment." In other words, Ipriflavone can improve the beneficial effects of estrogen when estrogen levels are low (Ipriflavone has clearly been shown to improve bone density and reduce fracture risks in postmenopausal women) or can reduce deleterious effects of abnormally high estrogen levels, as has been confirmed in postmenopausal women undergoing estrogen replacement therapy.[262–264] In fact, supplementation with Ipriflavone reduces the estrogen dose required in women receiving estrogen replacement therapy.[265,266] Any claims of an androgenic effect in men are, at best, misleading. Another isoflavone, genistein, was shown in vitro to inhibit 5-α-reductase, the enzyme that converts testosterone to dihydrotestosterone.[267] Isoflavones from red clover were also found to inhibit dihydrotestosterone production and reduce prostate growth in mice.[268] Ipriflavone may elicit the same response if consumed; however, even so it is unlikely to have any notable benefit outside of reducing the chances of prostate growth and/or cancer. Isoflavones deposit in far greater concentration in prostatic fluid than in plasma.[269] Likewise, Ipriflavone showed no androgenic or androgenic-augmenting effects in castrated rats. It was only when Ipriflavone was combined with androgen therapy that improvements were seen in bone mineral content.[270] The very reason Ipriflavone is currently being used in older adults, may also be its most beneficial use in the remainder of the active population—building stronger, denser bones. Ipriflavone seems to increase the beneficial effects that both calcium and vitamin K have on bone, and Ipriflavone has also been shown to be more effective than calcium at preserving bone density; 600 mg/d Ipriflavone, for 12 months, was more effective than 500 mg/d of calcium at decreasing bone loss in postmenopausal women.[271–273] Another area of interest is a reported ability of Ipriflavone to work as both a COX-2 inhibitor and to promote COX-1 cytoprotective effects, thus working as both an antiinflammatory and analgesic. A recent in vitro study reported that Ipriflavone was one of several potential supplements to possess such actions on COX-2 and COX-1, but Kuzuna et al. previously showed that an acute dose of 50–300 mg/kg BW Ipriflavone offered no analgesic effect in male and female mice. A pain-inhibiting effect was, however, found in estrogen-deficient and arthritic female mice after 3 weeks of chronic ingestion of 100 mg/kg BW Ipriflavone.[274,275] Further research in this area is needed to determine if an oral dose may have similar analgesic and/or antiinflammatory effects when provided to active, healthy adults.

**DOSE:** *Bone Support*: 600 mg/d; consume with food or in the form of a lipid-suspended gel cap

**COMMON NAME:** **Leucine**
**OTHER NAMES:** L-Leucine; Leu; 2-Amino-4-methylpentanoic acid (L); 2-Amino-4-methylvaleric acid (L); L-Norvaline, 4-methyl-; L-alpha-Aminoisocaproic acid; Pentanoic acid, 2-amino-4-methyl-, (S)-; Valeric acid, 2-amino-4-methyl-, (S)-
**COMMON USES:** Increase Protein Synthesis
Insulin Mimetic/Glucose Disposal

Increase Muscle Hypertrophy
Anticatabolic
Improve Exercise Recovery
Increase Endurance Performance

**REVIEW:** The essential and BCAA, Leucine, is amassing evidence that it may very well be the most anabolic and essential of all the amino acids. Infusion studies were among the first to identify Leucine's potentially superior ability to increase protein synthesis and inhibit muscle catabolism in humans. For example, Nair et al.[276] infused 154 mmol/kgBW of either L-Leucine or saline into healthy males for a period of 1 hour. Plasma Leucine and KIC increased by almost 3.3- and 1.5-fold, respectively, with no changes in circulating insulin. Significant shifts in improving net protein balance and reduced protein degradation did occur, however. Orally ingested Leucine has since been shown to promote similar results as would be expected because Leucine, as with the other two BCAAs, is not oxidized in the liver. Ingestion of Leucine directly affects plasma and tissue concentrations of the amino acid.[277] To determine the lowest dose of Leucine capable of stimulating muscle protein synthesis in food-deprived rats, 0.068–1.35 g/kgBW of L-Leucine was administered in an oral bolus 30 minutes before a battery of tests. The results were dose-dependent, with 0.135 g/kgBW proving to be the lowest possible dose of Leucine capable of eliciting a significant increase in muscle protein synthesis.[278] Koopman et al.[279] recently demonstrated, in humans, that coingesting carbohydrates + protein + L-Leucine (CHO + PRO + Leu) stimulates protein synthesis and improves whole-body protein balance more than CHO alone or CHO + PRO when ingested immediately after 45 minutes of resistance exercise. Plasma insulin response from the CHO + PRO + Leu was also shown to be 240% and 77% greater than for CHO and CHO + PRO, respectively. In fact, the synergistic action and signaling between Leucine and insulin is at the forefront of explaining Leucine's powerful anabolic and metabolic roles in the human body. Escobar et al.[280] described the anabolic response from Leucine as being "insulin-independent, substrate-dependent, and tissue-specific." As is evident from the studies of Escobar et al., Koopman et al., and others, Leucine is capable of amplifying an insulin response, enhancing the anabolic effects of insulin, signaling the release of insulin, or simply mimicking its (insulin) actions altogether.[281–284] In what was, at the time, one of the most thorough investigations of Leucine's metabolic effects, Xu et al.[285] more precisely identified the insulin-independent and rapamycin-sensitive signaling pathway by which Leucine availability stimulates phosphorylation of the mRNA binding translational regulator, p70[s6k], and therefore effects protein synthesis and proliferation, and enhances pancreatic β-cell function. The researchers concluded that the aforementioned anabolic and metabolic effects likely arise as a result of Leucine's involvement as a key substrate in oxidative decarboxylation and glutamate dehydrogenase activation within the mitochondria. In fact, Leucine, when combined with glutamine, was found to be equally as effective as a complete amino acid formula at increasing p70[s6k] phosphorylation; Leucine by itself was almost as effective. This intramitochondrial mechanism was further elucidated in vitro when it was shown that 1-week, but not acute Leucine availability up-regulated glucose-induced ATP synthase and increased ATP in rat pancreatic β cells, resulting in increased $Ca^{2+}$ and insulin release.[286] Collectively, this supports the purported use of Leucine to increase muscle protein content, improve insulin sensitivity and function, and support energy production and efficiency. However, to date, no *direct* performance-enhancing effects have been shown in studies involving supplementation with isocalorically supplemented Leucine. It is worth noting, however, that, 1) very few ergogenic-enhancing studies on Leucine exist, and 2) those that have been performed were acute dosing protocols only.[287,288]

**DOSE:** *Protein Synthesis/Anabolic, Insulin Mimetic, and General Use:* ≥0.05 g/kg BW/d; consume before, during, and/or immediately after exercise, and/or in divided doses throughout the day

**COMMON NAME:** *N*-Acetylcysteine

**OTHER NAMES:** NAC; *N*-Acetyl cysteine; *N*-Acetyl-L-cysteine; *N*-Acetyl-3-mercaptoalanine; Acetylcysteine; Acetadote; L-alpha-Acetamido-beta-mercaptopropionic acid; Mercapturic acid; Parvolex

**COMMON USES:** Antioxidant
Anticatabolic
Increase Endurance Performance/Delay Muscle Fatigue
Improve Exercise Recovery
Free Radical Scavenger
Improve Liver Function
Improve Lung Function
Increase Vasodilation

**REVIEW:** NAC, used extensively to treat acetaminophen-induced hepatotoxicity as well as a variety of respiratory illnesses, is categorized as a thiol compound and, similar to ALA, is a powerful redox agent capable of reducing oxidative stress and improving immune function, most likely resulting from an ability to significantly increase GSH availability.[289–291] NAC, however, promotes GSH in a more direct up-regulating, as opposed to ALA's apparent GSH-sparing mechanism. Specifically, orally consumed NAC absorbs rapidly and is then metabolized almost entirely during first-pass digestion across the small intestine and in the liver. In fact, despite that about 97% of an orally consumed dose of NAC is absorbed, less than 1% of that dose enters the bloodstream as intact NAC.[292–294] Instead, almost all of the NAC consumed goes toward building peptide bonds (e.g., insulin) and increasing tissue availability of NAC metabolites; the most important of the metabolites to arrive in the liver seems to be the amino acid, cysteine, as well as inorganic phosphate. A primary result of this process has proved to be the ability of NAC to significantly increase intracellular biosynthesis of GSH when oxidative stress exceeds immediate GSH availability. The acute effects of exercise is one such stress that results in both a dramatic decrease in intramuscular and hepatic GSH, as well as an inversely related increase in circulating GSH. If demand continuously exceeds supply, muscle catabolism and contraction-induced fatigue increase, and insulin sensitivity and fat burning decrease, to state just a few of the downstream biologic outcomes of a compromised GSH system.[295–297] The use of NAC to support GSH homeostasis, and therefore elicit an ergogenic benefit when administered preexercise, has been positive albeit variable-specific. Collectively, NAC dose-dependently increases intracellular cysteine, hepatic GSH, and whole-body free radical scavenging ability, but only condition-specifically increases intramuscular GSH and whole-body GSH.[298–300] Increased $VO_2$ peak is directly correlated with an improved NAC response, and it could therefore be surmised that the beneficial effects of NAC will increase as a person increases his or her aerobic fitness level.[301] Similarly, NAC supplementation preferentially and more significantly increases intramuscular GSH in slow-, as opposed to fast-twitch fibers. As a result, either acute or chronic ingestion of NAC is capable of delaying muscle fatigue during prolonged aerobic and moderately glycolytic exercise; however, no direct ergogenic benefit during short-duration (<3 minutes) or maximal anaerobic contractions in healthy or athletic populations has been demonstrated.[302–304] In older persons, however, NAC has been shown to increase contractile strength and resistance to fatigue during short-duration, moderate exercise.[305] Such effects in aerobically compromised subjects supports recent findings that NAC may signal up-regulation of EPO, as well as aid performance under hypoxic conditions (e.g., high altitude).[306] Likewise, the use of NAC supplementation is warranted in persons who smoke or are chronically subjected to secondhand smoke, have or are predisposed to cardiopulmonary disorders, are of older age, are chronically subjected to high levels of heavy metals [note: nonchelated minerals, such as boron and chromium, are also capable of becoming heavy metal contaminants in the body], chronically consume alcohol, and/or chronically consume NSAIDs such as acetaminophen.[307–312] Whether all of these beneficial functions of NAC are the direct result of increased GSH is not entirely clear. For example, there is good evidence that NAC may work by acting upon adrenergic pathways. NAC has been shown to stimulate NO and improve blood flow without competing with, or increasing beta-adrenergically induced vasodilation.[313,314] In rats that were subjected to traumatic skeletal muscle damage of the lower limb, 400 mg/kg BW provided immediately posttrauma dramatically improved erythrocyte flux into the damaged tissue, and significantly reduced creatine kinase and edema (swelling).[315] Whether the same can be said for postexercise use in anaerobic-specific exercise (e.g., weight training) or, more importantly, if such actions improve anthropometric and/or sport-specific outcomes requires further investigation.

**DOSE:**  *Endurance Performance and Delaying Muscle Fatigue*: 600–1500 mg/d; consume with food, approximately 60–120 minutes before aerobic exercise, with food
*Antioxidant, Vasodilation, and General Use*: 600 mg/d–4 g/d; consume in divided doses, with meals

**COMMON NAME:**  **Ornithine-alpha-Ketoglutarate**
**OTHER NAMES:**  OKG; Ornicetil; Di-L-ornithine-alpha-ketoglutarate; Ornithine 2-oxoglutarate; OGO; Ornithine oxoglutarate; L-Ornithine, mixt. with 2-oxopentanedioic acid

**COMMON USES**:

Anabolic
Anticatabolic
Increase Muscle Hypertrophy
Increase Muscle Strength
Increase Vasodilation
Improve Exercise Recovery
Increase Insulin
Increase Growth Hormone

**REVIEW**:

OKG—a combination of two molecules of the nonessential amino acid, ornithine, bound to the cofactor, alpha-ketoglutarate (αKG)—has been studied for the past 25 years, in France, to treat severely traumatized burn and other hypermetabolic patients. Collectively, and most compelling to our discussion, is that OKG has been shown to stimulate a dose-dependent increase in arginine, plasma glutamate, and intramuscular glutamine, as well as stimulate a dose-dependent increase in insulin secretion (whether in the presence or absence of glucose), NO synthesis, and decrease in plasma glucose, while also increasing plasma hGH, IGF-1, and glucagon.[316,317] One of the mechanisms by which OKG is believed to be able to promote an anabolic and anticatabolic response is attributed to ornithine and αKG sharing similar metabolic pathways. Therefore, when coingested as OKG, the two compounds saturate receptor sites, increasing the availability of its unbound metabolites. The dose-dependent increase in insulin secretion resulting from OKG seems to be via a direct, and nonglucose-mediated mechanism within the pancreas, likely resulting from the conversion of ornithine to arginine, and then subsequent release of NO.[318,319] The aforementioned, combined with a direct secretory effect on TNF-alpha cells may explain the anabolic/anticatabolic effects resulting from OKG administration in patients experiencing hypercatabolic states, however, so too and/or in combination with the increase in glutamine availability from OKG has been directly linked to improved nitrogen retention and recovery rates.[320–323] Cursory review of the results from Bruce et al.[324] would conflict with the conclusion that OKG stimulates glutamine availability. However, Bruce et al. found that glutamine significantly increased glutamine availability, whereas OKG was not significantly effective. It should be noted that this study involved male cyclists who ingested either 0.125 g/kgBW OKG or glutamine, 1 hour before a 10-minute cycle test; the subjects were also provided a preexercise meal consisting of approximately 1400 CALS (35% from CHO, and 11% as PRO). Although muscle glycogen and TCA cycle intermediates may have been compromised as a result of the protocol used, it is unlikely that glutamine availability was significantly depleted and could, therefore, explain the non-effect of OKG.[324,325] In fact, Vaubourdolle et al.[326] had previously shown in human fibroblasts that OKG was most anabolic when delivered in a glutamine-free environment. Both the effect on arginine and glutamine synthesis, as well as many of the resulting metabolic outcomes discussed previously are not as simple as assuming the consumption of ornithine and/or αKG may derive similar results.[327] Instead, OKG has been found significantly more effective than when either ornithine or αKG is consumed separately or coingested, but unbound as OKG. Although contradictory to the results of Bruce et al., OKG has also been shown to increase intramuscular glutamine more so than glutamine itself, when OKG is consumed in equimolar quantities as ingested glutamine.[328–331] Lastly, a randomized, controlled trial involving 54 critically ill burn patients, with burns covering 20%–50% surface area, provides additional dosing protocol discoveries. Patients were randomly assigned to receive either continuous infusions of multiple OKG doses, or assigned to receive a single daily bolus of an OKG dose for approximately 3 weeks, beginning on the second day after admission to the hospital. Doses were 10, 20, and/or 30 g/d, administered as either single boluses or in divided doses. An isonitrogenous amount and dosing protocol using soy protein isolate was provided as a control. It was concluded that 30 g/d OKG, provided as a single bolus as opposed to multiple, smaller doses, was the most effective protocol for improving wound healing.[332] These results confirm the previously discussed metabolic pathway saturation that OKG elicits, thereby enabling OKG to more directly effect hepatic conversion into OKG's more active metabolites.[333] Additional research involving healthy populations is warranted to determine if acute and/or chronic OKG use offers any direct or indirect ergogenic and/or anthropometric benefit. However, despite such limitations in available research, healthy adult metabolic response data warrant the use of high-dose OKG consumed immediately after high-intensity training as a potential anabolic/anticatabolic hormone-stimulating vehicle, consumed in the presence or absence of glucose.

**DOSE:** *Anabolic, Anticatabolic, and Insulin Secretagogue*: ≥20–30 g/d OKG (as 64% Ornithine and 36% αKG); consume as a single dose, immediately postexercise

**COMMON NAME:** **Phosphatidylserine**
**OTHER NAMES:** PS; 1,2-diacyl-*sn*-glycerol-(3)-L-phosphoserine
**COMMON USES:** Anticortisol (antistress)
Increase Mental Acuity
Increase Mental Energy
Improve Exercise Recovery
Improve Immune Function
Improve Cell Integrity
Promote Fat Loss

**REVIEW:** PS is a major phospholipid of all cell membranes. For example, PS is synthesized directly on the mitochondrial-associated membrane (an area just outside of the mitochondria) of a cell's endoplasmic reticulum. This newly formed PS may either enter the mitochondria or simply accumulate within and traverse the mitochondrial-associated membrane where it is largely believed to be involved in a variety of signal-transduction activities. In fact, PS may function more as a carrier into, or signaling mechanism of a cell than having any specific direct metabolite-derived effect on the cell itself. For example, PS has previously been shown to be an effective liposomal delivery medium for improving the absorption of GABA into the blood and synaptosomes (brain nerve endings), and improving the anticonvulsant effect of GABA in epileptic rodents. Even when injected separately, the bioavailability of GABA was improved.[334,335] More profoundly, the accumulation and exposure of PS on the outer surface of mitochondria-associated membranes functions as a trigger of cell apoptosis (death and removal), whereas ATP depletion is characterized by a reduced translocation of PS into the mitochondria.[336-338] Similarly, PS has been shown to improve glucose concentrations within the brain, as well as improve $Na^+$, $K^+$-adenosine triphosphatase activity and ACh release from brain synaptosomes in aged rats that were orally fed 60 mg/kgBW/d PS, for 60 days.[339,340] Such actions may explain why PS has shown promise in mitigating the deleterious effects of dementia, as well as improving cognitive function in elderly patients. Mitochondrial ATP capabilities are reduced with age and may likely be a major contributing factor to age-related neurodegenerative disorders.[341] Any nootropic effect of PS, however, may simply be the result of the aforementioned ability to act as a delivery vehicle for other, more active compounds that require transport across the blood-brain barrier. PS has, however, been shown to significantly blunt the exercise-induced increase in ACTH and cortisol in healthy adults.[342,343] Some caution, however, should be afforded the use of PS consumed preexercise—anabolic recovery is directly correlated to the catabolic environment created during an exercise bout; reducing the body's catabolic response to exercise may, in fact, reduce the anabolic cascade. Thus, consumption of an "anticatabolic," delivered preexercise, is not strongly advocated.

**DOSE:** *Anticatabolic*: 800 mg/d; consume postexercise

**COMMON NAME:** **Rhodiola**

**OTHER NAMES:** *Rhodiola rosea* L., Crassulaceae; Golden root; Roseroot; *R. rosea*; *rodia riza*; Artic root; *Sedum roseum*; *S. rhodiola*; *hong jing tian*; Artic rose; King's crown; Rosewort; Snowdown rose; SHR-5

**COMMON USES:** Increase Oxygen Uptake and Utilization
Increase Energy
Delay Muscle and Mental Fatigue
Increase Muscular Endurance
Increase Muscle Power
Improve Exercise Recovery
Improve Acclimatization
Stimulate Fat Loss
Antioxidant
Support General Health
Increase Fertility

**REVIEW:** *R. rosea* was one of five herbs, of 189 medicinal plants reviewed in 1968 by Soviet pharmacologists, identified as meeting all of the necessary criteria for classification as an adaptogen.[344] Indicative of its role as an adaptogenic herb, *R. rosea* has been shown to promote a wide variety of benefits and uses—neurostimulant, antidepressant, antifatigue, antihypoxic, antioxidant, immunostimulant, sex hormone stimulant, antistress, antiinflammatory, and anticancer, just to list a few.[345-352] For example, De Bock et al.[353] recently conducted a double-blind, placebo-controlled, randomized trial whereby 24 active, healthy men and women were tested against a series of performance measures to determine the effects of both an acute (1-hour preexercise test) and chronic (4 weeks) daily dose of 200 mg of *R. rosea* extract (standardized to contain 3% rosavin and 1% salidroside). Time to exhaustion during a 30-minute endurance test was found to increase significantly (~3%), as did VO$_2$ peak and expired VCO$_2$ peak (~5%) in those taking *R. rosea* during the acute phase of the test. No significant differences were noted, however, between groups in measures of muscle strength, reaction time, speed, or attention, nor did the 4-week phase elicit any significant differences between groups.[353] Although the exact mechanism(s) by which *R. rosea* produces its effects is still a matter of debate, its three cinnamyl-D-glycosides—rosavin, rosin, and rosarin (collectively referred to as "rosavins")—are almost certainly at the root of the herb's beneficial use.[354] It should also be noted that these three rosavins are unique only to the *R. rosea* species and are not present in other Rhodiola plants such as *R. crenulata*, *R. kirilowii*, *R. sacra*, or *R. sachalinensis*, just to name a few of the more than 50 species of Rhodiola plant that are known to exist.[355,356] As such, not all Rhodiola data can, or should be grouped collectively as indicative of a single species' value as a dietary supplement. For example, Abidov et al.[357] presented evidence that showed when rats were subjected to an exhaustive swimming test after receiving an oral dose of either 50 mg/kg BW *R. rosea* or *R. crenulata* extract, that those consuming *R. rosea* prolonged swimming time to exhaustion by 24.6% more than those taking *R. crenulata*, and that skeletal muscle mitochondrial ATP content was resynthesized faster after intense exercise in those receiving *R. rosea*. Researchers at the University of Utah (Salt Lake City, UT) presented data showing that the species *R. rosca* was ineffective at increasing blood oxygenation in healthy volunteers subjected to high altitude, hypoxic conditions, whereas a similar study was conducted 1 year prior that found *R. rosea* was, in fact, effective at increasing blood oxygen saturation in healthy males living at high altitude (5380 m).[358,359] Such discrepancies within the Rhodiola genus were made more evident by Ruan et al.,[360] who identified the wide range of differences among just six species of Rhodiola, all grown within the same region of China. Wide variances existed for nine of the major trace elements tested, and species contained between 8–18 amino acids and 3–7 indispensable amino acids. *R. rosea* was noted as containing the most complete profile of the plants assayed.

**DOSE:** *Adaptogen and General Use (chronic)*: 100–600 mg/d as *Rhodiola rosea* L. root extract (standardized to provide 3.6–21.6 mg/d rosavin); consume on an empty stomach

*Adaptogen and General Use (acute)*: 300–1800 mg as *Rhodiola rosea* L. root extract (standardized to provide 10.8–64.8 mg rosavin); consume on an empty stomach, approximately 30–60 minutes before exercise or competition

*NOTE: *Rhodiola rosea* L. is frequently standardized to yield an approximate 3:1 extract of rosavin/salidroside. However, the most widely studied *R. rosea* product, SHR-5, is standardized to 3.6% rosavin, 1.6% salidroside, and <0.1% *p*-tyrosol.

**COMMON NAME:** Ribose
**OTHER NAMES:** D-Ribose; alpha-D-ribofuranoside; alpha-D-ribofuranose; Pentose; D-ribo-Pentose; D-Rib; Ribo-2,3,4,5-tetrahydroxyvaleraldehyde, D-

**COMMON USES:**  Increase ATP Resynthesis
Increase Muscle Power
Increase Muscle Strength
Increase Muscle Hypertrophy
Improve Exercise Recovery
Increase Energy
Increase Muscular Endurance

**REVIEW:**  As the creatine kinase system can no longer maintain ATP requirements during high-intensity exercise, intramuscular adenosine diphosphate increases and is eventually reduced to both AMP and IMP (inosine 5'-monophosphate). IMP generally remains within the cell for eventual rephosphorylation to ATP once exercise ceases, but some of the reduced IMP—adenine and hypoxanthine—is released from the cell, decreasing the availability of intramuscular nucleotides required for ATP resynthesis. To replenish lost nucleotides, a slow process referred to as de novo nucleotide synthesis is required. The formation of phosphoribosyl pyrophosphate, which is derived from ribose 5-phosphate (i.e., ribose that has been phosphorylated), determines the rate at which de novo nucleotide synthesis occurs. The aforementioned process is at the core of the bioenergetic rationale for sports supplementation with Ribose—a naturally occurring 5-carbon monosaccharide. Although inconclusive, it does seem Ribose supplementation accelerates ATP resynthesis. For example, when 4.75 mM Ribose was perfused into rat calf muscles immediately after an ATP-depleting (average loss of 50%), high-intensity bout of exercise, nucleotide recovery rates were five- to sevenfold faster in Ribose-perfused than in non-Ribose controls when measured 60 minutes postexercise. A repeated exercise bout after 60 minutes rest showed that, despite improved ATP recovery, there was no positive effect on muscle force output in those receiving Ribose versus control.[361] Similarly, Hellsten et al.[362] showed that when eight healthy subjects orally consumed 600 mg/kg BW/d D-Ribose, muscle ATP recovery was significantly improved versus placebo. Mean and peak power output, and total work, however, were unaffected by supplementation with Ribose. A lack of consistent anaerobic ergogenic benefit was similarly shown in repeated cycle sprint tests by Berardi and Ziegenfuss[363] (subjects received 8 g oral D-Ribose every 8 hours, for 36 hours), repeated 30-second Wingate anaerobic sprint tests by Kreider et al.[364] (subjects received 10 g/d × 5 d oral D-Ribose), and tests for muscle power and force output by Op't Eijnde et al.[365] (subjects received 16 g/d × 5 d oral D-Ribose). Interestingly, Op't Eijnde et al. presented data that showed Ribose provided no ATP nucleotide recovery rate–improving effect; Hellsten et al. would later refute the accuracy of those findings. Additional long-term studies are required before a more conclusive assessment of the sport-specific application(s) of Ribose can be made, if, in fact, one does exist. Of note, there seems to be merit in both the acute and chronic use of Ribose for improving quantitative and qualitative performance and functional measures in patients experiencing episodes of myocardial ischemia, although the doses reported were substantial—up to 60 g/d.[366,367]

**DOSE:**  Insufficient data

**COMMON NAME:** Sodium Bicarbonate

**OTHER NAMES:** Sodium Bicarb; Baking soda; Bicarbonate of soda; Carbonic acid monosodium salt; Acidosan; Monosodium carbonate; Monosodium hydrogen carbonate; Sodium hydrogencarbonate; Soda Mint; Sodium acid carbonate

**COMMON USES:**
Delay Muscle Fatigue
Reduce Lactic Acid
Increase Endurance Performance
Increase Power Output
Increase Training Volume
Improve Bone Health

**REVIEW:** As ATP is reduced during muscular contractions, unbound, or positively charged protons (also referred to as hydrogen ions, or H+) are released into the cellular space. Assuming there is an adequate supply of PCr to bind with these highly charged H+, the muscle can continue contracting without interruption (e.g., aerobic exercise). However, during high-intensity, anaerobic contractions, PCr availability is dramatically reduced and H+ builds within the cell, decreasing the intracellular pH and therefore reducing a muscle's firing capacity. Similarly, acidosis increases the oxidation of BCAAs, and in severe metabolic acidosis is associated with reduced muscle mass.[368] Sodium Bicarb, however, is extremely alkaline (low acidity/high pH) and has generally been shown effective at increasing intra- and extracellular pH, delaying the onset of muscle fatigue, and improving recovery from events requiring high-intensity bursts of anaerobic contractions of large muscle groups.[369–374] For example, when equimolar doses of Sodium Bicarb, sodium citrate, sodium lactate, or placebo were orally and randomly provided to 15 competitive endurance runners 90 minutes before an exhaustive sprint test, Sodium Bicarb was found to be 1%, 2.2%, and 2.7% more effective at delaying fatigue than sodium lactate, sodium citrate, and placebo, respectively.[375] McNaughton and Thompson[376] also found an improved anaerobic response from a 500 mg/kg BW dose of Sodium Bicarb provided either acutely or daily, for 6 days before a 90-second max cycle ergometer test, and also noted a more significant improvement from chronic as opposed to acute supplementation. This confirms more direct trials that found improved recovery between bouts of high-intensity intermittent bouts of exercise, as well as the use of Sodium Bicarb to increase muscle force and power output.[377] There does not, however, seem to be an ergogenic benefit when Sodium Bicarb is consumed before endurance events.[378–382] Indirectly, however, endurance athletes may benefit from the use of Sodium Bicarb for its possible use in improving bone and connective tissue. In vitro and animal models have shown both an increased synthesis and accumulation of proteoglycans, and improved bone mineral content and density from the administration of Sodium Bicarb.[383,384] This is likely a result of the stimulating effect Sodium Bicarb has on the release of parathyroid hormone.[385] Lastly, the use of Potassium Bicarbonate may prove to offer advantages over Sodium Bicarb, but more data are required before a more accurate recommendation can be made.[386–388]

**DOSE**:

*Delay Anaerobic Muscle Fatigue*: 300 mg/kg BW/d as Sodium Bicarbonate diluted in 1 L of water; consume 1–2 hours before exercise or competition

**COMMON NAME**: **Taurine**

**OTHER NAMES**: L-Taurine; Tau; Aminoethanesulfonic acid; beta-Aminoethylsulfonic acid; 2-Sulfoethylamine; 2-Aminoethanesulfonic acid; 2-Aminoethylsulfonic acid; Ethanesulfonic acid, 2-amino-

**COMMON USES**: Increase Energy
Antifatigue
Insulin Mimetic
Increase Protein Synthesis

**REVIEW**: Taurine is a beta-amino acid containing a sulfonic acid group off of the bea-carbon, in place of the carboxylic acid group found in other amino acids. Thus, Taurine is not an amino acid in the classic definition, nor is it incorporated into other proteins (i.e., protein synthesis). Instead, Taurine is the most abundant free amino acid in excitable tissues, such as in the muscle, heart, and brain, and its synthesis in the liver, from cysteine and methionine, is dependent on the availability of pyridoxal-5'-phosphate (the active coenzyme form of vitamin B6).[389] Beta-agonists, exercise, oxidative stress, as well as low vitamin B6 have all been shown to reduce whole-body Taurine, whereas choline supplementation that acts as a methyl donor increases endogenous Taurine synthesis.[390–393] The exercise-induced increase in cortisol dramatically increases Taurine transport into muscle, whereas NO down-regulates its transport. Similarly, IGF-1 up-regulates the cortisol- and exercise-induced increase in Taurine transport, but IGF-1 alone is ineffective at increasing Taurine transport.[394–396] Although nonessential, Taurine is responsible for many vital functions within the body, notably its conjugation of bile acids, cell-volume regulation, detoxification of xenobiotics, modulation of neuronal excitability, cell membrane stabilization, and control of calcium flux into and from a cell.[397–405] Of particular concern to human development is that low-plasma Taurine in infants is directly related to reduced neurodevelopment and increased insulin-resistant disorders (Type II diabetes).[406–409] Interestingly, Taurine is still not found in all brands of infant formula. Taurine has also been shown to support cardiovascular function in persons with cardiovascular disease, prevent epileptic seizures, and protect against a wide range of oxidative damage, such as exercise, cigarette smoking, alcohol abuse, and chronic acetaminophen use.[410–418] The importance of Taurine in exercising muscle was clearly expressed in a recent study whereby Taurine transporter knockout mice (i.e., mice that were incapable of transporting Taurine across the cell membrane) were exercised on a treadmill to exhaustion; the exercise capacity was reduced by more than 80% in knockout mice compared with their age-matched wild-type controls. Unexpectedly, the researchers noted no significant deficit in $VO_2$ or $VCO_2$ (cardiac function). Instead, they found that in a Taurine-depleted state, the heart is capable of utilizing other organic solutes whereas muscle cannot.[419] Matsuzaki et al.[420] reported that intramuscular Taurine concentrations decrease as a result of exhaustive exercise lasting 30, 60, or 100 minutes, and the deficit is more specific to fast-twitch muscle fibers. A similar muscle fiber specificity was shown by Dawson et al. who supplemented rats with either Taurine or the Taurine transport inhibitor, beta-alanine, for 1 month, and then tested the rats against a 90-minute downhill treadmill test. Aside from noting that Taurine supplementation significantly increased plasma and intramuscular Taurine, except within the slow-twitch predominant soleus muscles, the researchers showed that beta-alanine decreased intramuscular Taurine by approximately 50% and also resulted in a significant loss in body weight. Furthermore, Taurine was shown to attenuate exercise-induced injury.[421] Likewise, when 500 mg/kg BW Taurine was fed to rats for 2 weeks, intramuscular Taurine and running time to exhaustion increased significantly.[422] In healthy, young adults supplemented with Taurine for 1 week before an exhaustive exercise bout, it was found that Taurine significantly improved exercise time to exhaustion, $VO_2$ max, and maximal workload, and Taurine supplementation significantly reduced exercise-induced white blood cell DNA damage (as measured 24 hours after exercise) and improved preexercise cellular protective properties (shown as a reduction in plasma thiobarbituric acid reactive substances).[423] Such cytoprotective actions are likely a combined result of Taurine's ability to control calcium flux and regulate cell volume, and its functioning as a hepatoprotective and GSH-sparing antioxidant. For example, Duchenne muscular dystrophy (MD) is characterized by an increase in intracellular calcium which leads to muscle degeneration and cell death. IGF-1 is a common drug used to treat MD; however, when either creatine or Taurine, in combination with exercise, was provided to MD mice, for up to 8 weeks, Taurine > creatine > IGF-1 counteracted exercise-induced muscle weakness and it was also shown that whereas IGF-1 restored muscle conductance across all muscles tested, Taurine's effects were muscle-specific.[424] Taurine has also been shown to be involved in the regulation of core body temperature, and its use may prevent heat stress and stroke.[425] The antioxidant and hepatic functions of Taurine have been widely studied, collectively showing that increased Taurine availability decreases oxidative stress, increases GSH availability, improves pancreatic beta-cell function, and increases glucose utilization.[426–434] These data confirm the often overlooked fact that the amino acid Taurine is one of the body's most abundant, tissue-specific, and naturally occurring antioxidants.

**DOSE:** *Antioxidant, Glucose Disposal, Ergogenic Aid, and General Use*: 100–500 mg/kg BW/d; consume before meals and/or glucose-containing solutions

**COMMON NAME:** **Tribulus**
**OTHER NAMES:** *Tribulus terrestris*; Gokshura; Ji li (fruit); Yingjili; Puncturevine caltrop; Small caltrops; Caltrop; Goathead; Land Caltrops; Trikanta; Al-Gutub; Devil's-weed; Devil's-thorn; Cat's-head; Tribestan®
**COMMON USES:** Increase Testosterone
Increase Strength
Increase Protein Synthesis
Treat Erectile Dysfunction
Increase Energy

**REVIEW**:    Tribulus is a native ground cover to many parts of the world and probably best recognized as an annoying nuisance to mountain bikers in the western United States for its ability to puncture tires as Tribulus' flowering fruits dry out, beginning in late Spring. Thus, it is deserving of its common name, puncturevine or Devil's thorn. Bodybuilders, however, have long used Tribulus to increase endogenous testosterone, strength, and muscularity, but thus far the clinical data in humans are conflicting. Much of the lay data in circulation have been provided by the manufacturer of a Bulgarian-derived, high protodioscin-containing Tribulus product, called Tribestan®. The manufacturer, Sopharma AD, references a wide array of published animal data, but only in-house beta-tests to support the use of Tribestan® in humans and therefore the data should be viewed as suspect until peer reviewed. Antonio et al.[435] randomly provided Tribulus or placebo to 15 resistance-trained males who consumed a daily dose equal to 3.21 mg/kgBW for 8 weeks. Tribulus was found to offer no performance-enhancing or physique-altering benefit compared with placebo. Whereas, more recently, Rogerson et al (J Strength Cond Res. 2007;21(2):348–53) reported that 450 mg/d, *T. terrestris* extract, for five weeks, had no significant effect on strength, lean muscle mass or testosterone/epitestosterone (T/E) urinary ratio, versus placebo, in preseason training rugby players. It cannot, however, be ruled out that the dose used in the aforementioned trials was too low to elicit an ergogenic response, and/or that the Tribulus material used was simply of poor quality. For example, Gauthaman et al.[436] showed a statistically significant and dose-specific response in rats receiving oral daily doses of 5 and 10 mg/kgBW/d, but not 2.5 mg/kgBW/d active protodioscin (from *Tribulus terrestris* extract) for 8 weeks. Body weight increased by 23%, 18%, and 9%, respectively. Deng et al.[437] discovered a similar dose-specific response to Tribulus, noting that higher doses promoted the proliferation of human melanocytes whereas a smaller dose inhibited the growth. Gauthaman et al. also reported that a 5 mg/kgBW/d oral daily dose of active protodioscin (from *Tribulus terrestris* extract) for 8 weeks significantly increased androgen receptor (AD) and NADPH-diaphorase (NADPH-d) immunoreactivity in mice by 58% and 67%, respectively. Both AD and NADPH-d are known to increase in response to androgens.[438–440] Further clarifying the dose-specific response, Gauthaman et al. noted that only the 5 and 10 mg/kgBW/d active protodioscin (from *Tribulus terrestris* extract) doses significantly increased intracavernous pressure (43% and 26%, respectively) and mounting frequency (27% and 24%), and only the 5 mg/kgBW/d dose significantly reduced the time between sexual events (20%) in rats receiving oral, daily doses of Tribulus. The 2.5 mg/kgBW/d was determined to be no more effective than the control. Thus, there seems to be both a minimally and maximally effective dose. Although Tribulus' mechanism of action is of debate—the Tribestan manufacturer claims that Tribulus increases LH in men and follicle-stimulating hormone (FSH) in women—the available, published data show that Tribulus possesses a hypoglycemic effect, possibly attributable to a direct insulin secretory effect on pancreatic beta cells or reduction in hepatic enzyme action. Tribulus has also been shown to increase smooth muscle contractions, possibly via COX-2 and/or angiotensin-converting enzyme inhibition.[441-449] Thus, Tribulus may support testosterone release via indirect actions arising from insulin-dependent pathways, or Tribulus may be of benefit as an anti-inflammatory if its COX-2–inhibiting functions are found to be accurate. Irrespective, quality assurance of the primary active, protodioscin, will likely affect a user's response to Tribulus. Ganzera et al.[450] found a significant variance in protodioscin content of Tribulus products purchased from retail shelves or otherwise obtained directly from Tribulus raw material suppliers. Protodioscin content varied by 0.024%–6.492% per 100 g of Tribulus, depending on the sample tested. Tribulus raw material derived from Bulgaria generally contained the highest concentration of active steroidal saponins, whereas materials from India and China the lowest (0.024% and 0.063%, respectively). Of the products purchased from store shelves, the Bulgarian-derived Tribulus was highest in protodioscin (6.492%) whereas the two other samples contained concentrations of only 0.176% and 0.847% active saponins. Although it could be argued that the steroidal saponin, protodioscin, is not the only active extract of *Tribulus terrestris*—harmane, norharmane, tribulosin, and D-pinitol have also been identified, just to name a few—such findings do provide further evidence of an industry-wide standardization problem whereby products are often being marketed using claims that are not compatible with the raw materials that are substantiated within the literature. It should also be noted that protodioscin is frequently found in several plant species, and that protodioscin alone has not been found to be as effective as equivalent doses consumed as naturally occurring *Tribulus terrestris*.

**DOSE:** *General Use*: 5–10 mg/kg BW/d active protodioscin (from *Tribulus terrestris* L above ground parts); consume in divided doses, with meals, or as a single dose immediately before exercise

**COMMON NAME:** **Tyrosine**

**OTHER NAMES:** L-Tyrosine; 4-Hydroxy-L-phenylalanine; L-2-Amino-3-*p*-hydroxyphenylpropanoic acid; (*S*)-alpha-Amino-4-hydroxybenzenepropanoic acid; lpha-Amino-beta-(4-hydroxyph-enyl)propionic acid; beta-(*p*-Hydroxyphenyl)alanine; (–)-alpha-Amino-*p*-hydroxyhydrocinnamic acid

**COMMON USES:** Increase Energy
Increase Mental Acuity
Increase Fat Burning
Decrease Fatigue
Increase Power Output
Increase Muscle Strength

**REVIEW:** Tyrosine is an aromatic, conditionally essential amino acid that is endogenously produced as a result of hydroxylation of the essential amino acid, phenylalanine. Tyrosine is a well-documented precursor to the thyroid hormone, thyroxine, as well as has a direct role in the production of melanin (responsible for skin pigmentation). Some studies have addressed a link between

Tyrosine and increased gonadotropin-releasing hormone (and therefore increased LH), but the data in this area are far from conclusive.[451,452] Tyrosine's primary role in the body is as the direct precursor to thyroxine and to the catecholaminergic neurotransmitters (or hormones), dopamine, epinephrine, and norepinephrine (NE), and thus it is plausible that Tyrosine supplementation may improve both endurance and anaerobic performance via metabolic and/or neurotransmitter (hormone) upregulation. Sutton et al.[453] recently conducted a double-blind, placebo-controlled crossover study whereby men received an acute dose of either 150 mg/kgBW Tyrosine or placebo, 30 minutes before a battery of tests to measure endurance, muscle strength, and anaerobic performance. Despite a significant increase in plasma Tyrosine, the researchers found no ergogenic benefit, nor did they report a significant increase in plasma NE. Troy et al.[454] found similar results in competitive cyclists consuming, as fluid, 25 mg/kgBW Tyrosine; 25 mg/kgBW Tyrosine +70 g/L dextrose; 70 g/L dextrose; or placebo beverage. Previous studies, however, have shown that supplemental Tyrosine not only increases plasma Tyrosine, but also catecholamines and measures of performance in both humans and animals.[455–459] In sleep-deprived subjects, 150 mg/kgBW Tyrosine improved memory, reasoning, mathematical processing, tracking, and visual vigilance when compared against D-amphetamine, phentermine, or high-dose caffeine (approximately 300 mg).[460] Researchers at the Naval Aerospace Medical Research Laboratory, in Pensacola, FL, also reported that a dose of 150 mg/kgBW Tyrosine, when provided to sleep-deprived subjects, ameliorated the typical psychomotor performance declines associated with mental fatigue.[461] A dose of 400 mg/kgBW, administered intraperitoneally 30 minutes before induced hypothermia completely abolished behavioral depression in humans, whereas an identical dose administered to mice before induced heat stress was found to sustain NE release and improve behavioral coping; the opposite occurred in the control groups.[462,463] Avraham et al.[464] administered 100 mg/kgBW Tyrosine or saline solution to rats, and subjected them to significant food restriction and increased exercise. Rats receiving saline lost 27% body weight and further decreased food consumption by 22%, whereas the Tyrosine-supplemented group lost no weight, and actually increased exercise activity by 22% and restored food consumption to baseline. In another diet-restricted study, Tyrosine supplementation was again shown to have a significant benefit. Tyrosine significantly increased choline uptake, cholinergic and beta-adrenergic receptor function, cognitive function, and decreased alpha-adrenergic function in mice that were fed just 40% of their daily requirements for calories as compared with mice fed 60% daily requirements, or control-fed mice.[465] Because food and sleep deprivation, as well as hypoxia (e.g., high-altitude training), are well-established stressors that result in an initial increase in endogenous catecholamines, it is plausible that Tyrosine is capable of offering an added catecholaminergic effect. It is well documented that Tyrosine prolongs and augments a previously, or separately stimulated increase, in catecholamines, but by itself is a weak stimulant in normative states.[466–471] The most likely explanation for the latter nonresponse in normative states is that, in rested conditions, Tyrosine availability exceeds the capacity of the rate-limiting enzyme, tyrosine hydroxylase (TH), required to convert Tyrosine to dopamine. As catecholamines are reduced, TH is upregulated and can accommodate more Tyrosine. A critical cofactor in TH function is tetrahydrobiopterin, and the same actions that up-regulate TH also up-regulate tetrahydrobiopterin—insulin-induced hypoglycemia and catecholamine depletion, to name a few.[472] Thus, reduced glucose availability and prior sympathetic nervous system stimulation are key to increasing Tyrosine's potential use in sports, as is avoiding the coingestion of Tyrosine with large amino acids, particularly the BCAAs and tryptophan, which compete with Tyrosine for uptake across the cellular wall.[473,474] Therefore, the use, by Sutton et al., of 70 g of glucose (in the form of apple sauce) as a carrier for Tyrosine, as well as Troy et al. providing subjects a pretest meal containing 1300–1330 kcal (73% of kcals as CHO) may very well have negated any potential benefit these researchers may otherwise have found from preexercise ingestion of Tyrosine.

**DOSE:** *Exercise Performance and Mental Acuity*: 50–150 mg/kg BW; consume on an empty stomach, approximately 60–90 minutes before exercise. Coingest with a faster-acting and more potent catecholaminergic agonist, such as caffeine, and do not consume with BCAAs or glucose

*Energy and General Use*: 50–150 mg/kg BW/d; consume on an empty stomach, in divided doses; consume at least one dose immediately upon waking in the morning. Coingest with a faster-acting and more potent catecholaminergic agonist, such as caffeine, and do not consume with BCAAs or glucose

**COMMON NAME:** **Vanadium**

**OTHER NAMES:** IV; Vanadate; V; Vanadyl Sulfate; VSO5; VO(SO4); Vanadic sulfate; Vanadium sulfate; Vanadium oxysulfate; Vanadium oxide sulphate; Peroxovanadium; Metavanadate; Panchromium; Vanadis

**COMMON USES:** Insulin Mimetic
Increase Muscle Hypertrophy
Increase Endurance Performance
Improve Exercise Recovery

**REVIEW:** In 1985, the trace element Vanadium (a trace element, because the total amount found in the human body is about 0.1–0.3 mg) was shown to possess both insulin-mimetic and antidiabetic actions when chronically administered to diabetic-induced mice, as 100 mg/kg BW/d Sodium Orthovanadate. More importantly, the results occurred without effecting endogenous production and/or release of insulin.[475] Since then, a large body of evidence has amassed to support the use of Vanadium in the form of either its organic salts (e.g., Vanadyl Sulfate) or other synthetic compounds [e.g., BMOV, or Bis(maltolato)oxovanadium(IV)], as potent actives to ameliorate and/or reverse the effects of insulin resistance and hyperglycemia in diabetics.[476–478] In fact, chronic administration of Vanadyl Sulfate to diabetic rats or humans has revealed that many of the positive effects can sustain long after dosing has ceased,[479,480] possibly because Vanadium has a direct and/or indirect protective function on pancreatic β cells. This may, in part, explain why Vanadium has been shown more effective at treating Type II diabetes than the Type I, insulin-dependent form of the disease. Nevertheless, aside from the occasional in vitro study, Vanadium complexes have shown no such insulin mimetic effect in healthy animals or subjects.[481–484] Jentjens and Jeukendrup, for example, demonstrated that an oral dose of 100 mg/d Vanadyl Sulfate offered no acute or chronic (6 days) benefit in healthy adults subjected to a glucose tolerance test administered the morning after supplementation.[485] Similarly, no improvements in body composition or weight training performance were found by Fawcett et al.[486,487] after an oral dose of 0.5 mg/kgBW/d × 12 weeks Vanadyl Sulfate was provided to 31 resistance-trained men, in a double-blind, placebo-controlled trial. The researchers also measured red and white blood cells for potential toxicity, as well as tested for blood viscosity and found no significant changes resulting from the Vanadyl Sulfate treatment. However, it should be noted that the dose used was quite small and only equivalent to about 40 mg/d for a person weighing 175 lbs. Although even at such a low dose, two subjects did, in fact, withdraw from the test because of side effects. Diarrhea, dehydration, and other such side effects are unfortunately extremely common with the use of Vanadyl Sulfate and Vanadium complexes, and could be argued as indicative of a compound with drug-like effects. It should also be noted that MAO inhibitors antagonize the effects of Vanadium, whereas Vanadium itself, whether in normal or hypertensive subjects, increases intracellular free magnesium.[488,489] Collectively, the use of Vanadium or its "less-toxic" synthesized complexes as a glucose disposal agent in otherwise healthy persons is not recommended, and instead is best used by active persons with diagnosed diabetic complications.[490–493]

**DOSE**: *Glucose Disposal (Diabetic Athletes only)*: 150–300 mg/d as enteric coated Vanadyl Sulfate[494,495]

---

## Sidebar 22.1. Adaptogen Classification

To be classified as an "adaptogen," herbs such as *Rhodiola rosea* and several species of *Panax ginseng* had to meet three defining criteria. An adaptogenic herb must:

1. Be innocuous and cause minimal disturbance in normal physiologic functions of an organism
2. Increase resistance to a wide range of harmful physical, chemical, and biologic assaults
3. Promote normalizing actions in body systems that are over- or underproducing in relation to steady-state function (e.g., if testosterone levels are low, an adaptogen has been shown to bring levels back to normal)

*Adaptogenic Irony: The Catch-22*

An adaptogenic herb will likely provide statistically significant acute and/or short-term benefits against physical and environmental stresses. However, because of its inherent "normalizing" properties, it will likely not elicit continued improvements, beyond those initially achieved, if chronically consumed. Therefore, it has been proposed that athletes may benefit most from the use of adaptogens if consumed in a periodized ("cycling") approach, although no specific data have yet been conducted to assess any such cycling between various adaptogenic herbs for short to moderate durations.

## Sidebar 22.2. Standardization and Quality Assurance of Herbs— At the Root of an Herb's Effect

To say that Ginseng and Ginger are as different from the other as Glutamine is to Glycine, would not surprise too many people. However, all too often, all species within a plant genus (Ginseng, for example) are not afforded the same species-specific judgment each individual plant deserves (e.g., American Ginseng versus Asian Ginseng versus Siberian Ginseng). It is the equivalent of assuming that an athlete consuming 1 g/d *Rhodiola crenulata*, before traveling to a high-altitude event, will derive the same oxygenation benefits as those that have been reported in the literature in support of *R. rosea*. Rarely is the same generalization made in other areas of sports science. Few strength coaches would agree that an athlete that performs isometric contractions will derive equal muscle hypertrophy as an athlete utilizing dynamic contractions. Essentially similar . . . but far from the same.

Despite the propensity to frequently refer to and judge the efficacy of all species sharing the same common genus name, one should instead always be reminded that no two species within the same genus share an identical fingerprint. Similarly, identical species harvested from different regions, even if from within the same general region, also do not share the same chemical make-up. The part, or parts, of the plant used in an herbal preparation is also of primary importance. To simplify and to say there is no difference between species is to assume all plants are grown within a vacuum. Instead, herbs depend on rain, soil, sunlight, and a host of other environmental factors to derive their specific chemical composition. Therefore, ingestion of a *Tribulus terrestris* tincture derived from puncturevine collected from a bike's tires after a mountain bike trip in Salt Lake City, UT, is not likely to provide a similar effect as a tincture comprised of *Tribulus terrestris*, harvested from its native, arid regions of Bulgaria.

Just as the specific species, location of harvest, and part(s) used are important in identifying the value of an herb, so too are the extraction methods used by the manufacturer. Most herbs are treated with an extracting solvent containing both ethanol and water. However, the exact method and/or percentages used are wholly based on the lipophilic and/or hydrophilic nature of the plant constituents. In other words, if a clinical study of an herb reports positive findings and, within the study methodology, the researchers note that the plant extract used was derived via an ethanol solution, then subsequent and conflicting data from studies using an aqueous extract should be suspect.

This, too, points to a larger discussion on standardization of materials. The American Botanical Council defines standardization: "A standardized extract is manufactured to contain a consistent level of one or more phytochemical constituents that are derived from the original starting material." The American Herbal Products Association provides an expanded definition, stating that: "Standardization refers to the body of information and controls necessary to produce material of reasonable consistency. This is achieved through minimizing the inherent variation of natural product composition through quality assurance practices applied to agricultural and manufacturing processes."

Although it is the "best practice" currently available, standardization has its own inherent flaws: 1. standardizing an herb to one active ingredient has led to "spiking" of lesser-quality bulk materials with the known, standardized active, 2. standardization is only as valid as the method used for detection of that active compound, and 3. standardizing an herb to one marker compound does not necessarily confirm its complete profile.[496] *R. rosea*, for example, was previously standardized to its salidroside content until it was later discovered that a wide array of other plants also contain high amounts of salidrosides. The active rosavins, however, seem to be unique only to *R. rosea*, and are now used in concert with salidroside content to more precisely identify the quality of the species used. The need for standardization to more than one active extract applies to almost all herbs. Only using the actives protodioscin and corosolic acid, for example, as standardization for *Tribulus terrestris* and Banaba leaf, respectively, ignores the fact that these active compounds are also very common in several other species of plants and can, therefore, be used as "spiking" ingredients in lesser-quality species of the intended herb. In other words, if, for example, a Rhodiola-containing product lists that it contains rosavins, but does not list *R. rosea* as its source plant, then it is very possible that the manufacturer is either intentionally misleading its customers and/or has "spiked" its lesser Rhodiola species with rosavins from *R. rosea*. However, the same cautionary measures are almost impossible to apply to an herb such as Tribulus that uses no unique active to more clearly identify the efficacious species.

Despite the inherent flaws in existing standardization methodologies, its use as a minimal marker of product quality and efficacy, when combined with the proper use of the specific herb as presented in the literature, is currently the best established guidelines available to practitioners to use when recommending herbs to their clients.

## PRACTICAL APPLICATIONS

Just as the supplements presented here represent only a small percentage of an otherwise vast pool of active compounds used in modern sports nutrition, so too should it be glaringly obvious that there is limited human use, sports-specific clinical data to fully substantiate the common uses of many of these substances. Despite such obvious limitations, however, one simply cannot and should not overlook the potential benefits, uses, and applications of a supplement based solely on the mere lack of directly applicable study designs. Doing so would be to assume 1) that all that can and needs to be learned of an ingredient has already been determined, and/or 2) that anything that has not been directly studied would be of no added value in expanding of our knowledge of a substance's effects within and on the human body. Nowhere in the field of science should such definitive and ignorant judgments be rendered; to do so is in direct defiance of the very principles and practices of research itself.

That is not to say that all dietary supplements are, in fact, effective and/or have safe and direct application for use in sports and body transformation. Androst-4-ene-3,6,17-trione, for example, is widely revered within the body-building community as an antiaromatase and is often consumed by men that have recently discontinued use of an anabolic steroid or similar androgen-enhanced drug cycle. Based on theory, chemistry, and in vitro data, it is easy to see how such a leap of applied faith could be made. However, with absolutely no peer-reviewed data in humans or animals to confirm efficacy, and more importantly safety, the use of this compound could not be recommended at this time. It is the hope of this reviewer that products such as this one, as well as all finished goods being sold by dietary supplement companies are not provided to the public based solely on a company's own presumption of the product's safety and efficacy, but are, instead, based on validated, well-controlled trials.

Vanadyl Sulfate, for example, has an overwhelming abundance of data specific to its use in humans. However, its questionable safety and potential toxicity, as has been clearly documented in the literature, raises serious doubts about the benefits/risk ratio of Vanadyl Sulfate use in otherwise healthy adults. In defense of Vanadyl Sulfate, one could argue that the widespread use and commercial availability, dating back to the early 1990s, shows a history of safe use and, therefore, Vanadyl Sulfate should not be so quickly overlooked. That argument, however, assumes there currently exists a thoroughly accurate and nearly 100% compliant adverse events reporting system within the dietary supplement industry and among its many thousands of companies that market such products, just within the United States alone. Unfortunately, no such level of compliance likely exists with the current adverse events reporting system. Therefore, when combined with the available data (although, arguably limited) that has shown Vanadyl Sulfate, even when provided in reasonably safe doses, ineffective as an insulin mimetic and ergogenic aid, it can logically be concluded that, given the availability of other supplements that have shown similarly desired effects with fewer side effects, there are clearly better, safer, more effective alternatives for deriving an insulin mimetic response than to simply use Vanadyl Sulfate.

Alpha-Lipoic Acid, Banaba leaf extract, D-Pinitol, American Ginseng, and Leucine, for example, have each been shown to be quite safe and efficacious as insulin mimetics, as well as it is likely that the Fenugreek seed-derived form of 4-Hydroxyleucine possesses similar, promising actions with regard to increasing the effects of insulin. Increasing insulin or deriving an insulin-like response serves many purposes, but is usually manipulated for the purpose of delivering other active compounds into muscle. Nowhere is this practice more obvious than during the postworkout "window." Of the many active compounds presented in this chapter that could significantly aid postworkout recovery, none seems more anabolic or more "essential" than the essential and BCAA, Leucine. Other strong candidates for supporting anabolic recovery from intense training are Arginine, BCAAs, EAAs, OKG, AKG, KIC, or high-dose Glutamine, just to list a few. Similarly, providing powerful antioxidants, postworkout, could promote an indirect anabolic and/or ergogenic response; one such antioxidant stack would be NAC, ALA, Taurine, and an adaptogenic herb such as American Ginseng. Carnosine, as well as the other histidine dipeptide, anserine (not currently available), may also provide added muscle-specific protection from exercise-induced damage.

Aside from the use of stimulants and glucose-loading, the pre- and during-workout window has largely and unfortunately been overlooked until recent years. Although NO-promoting products, such as AAKG, have become a class of bodybuilding supplements all their own, the clinical data in exercising adults clearly point toward a more substantiated use when NO-promoting compounds are consumed preendurance exercise. The use of such products in bodybuilding, however, is to attain transient hypertrophy, or "the pump;" a practice that has not been shown to promote increased ergogenic and/or physique-augmentation benefits, and instead is dependant upon a pathway that runs counter to promoting a training environment consistent with eliciting progressive overload. It is just the recommendation of this author, but the best application for NO-type products may be found to be within the immediate postworkout window to help increase insulin response and promote vasodilation for improved delivery of key nutrients into damaged tissue. In lieu of using NO-type products to simply achieve a transient "pump," it would be of greater sustained benefit to a weight-training individual if he or she supplemented with any one of the following, consumed pre-and/or during exercise: Leucine, Carnosine, Beta-Alanine, BCAAs, EAAs, Asian Ginseng, NAC, Tyrosine, Sodium Bicarbonate, *Rhodiola rosea*, Cordyceps, or Citrulline Malate, to name a few.

However, just knowing the right product to take is not enough: equally as important as the ingredient itself is the dose, timing, and coingestion requirements and/or contraindications, as well as the standardization, if applicable (Table 22.1). As is almost always the case, each supplement requires a precise environment to be optimally effective. For example, the beneficial effects of CoQ10 could very well be lost if not coingested with a modest amount of fat. For Tyrosine to sustain and/or increase the release of catecholamines, it appears necessary that it be consumed in a hypoglycemic state and requires that a catecholaminergic response first be stimulated by something other than Tyrosine itself. *R. rosea*, but none of the other Rhodiola species have been shown to reduce the hypoxic effects of high-altitude transition; however, the dose used requires that *R. rosea* be standardized to contain not less than 3.6 mg rosavins per 100 mg of total *R. rosea* root extract. Similarly, the same specificity of source materials, standardization, and proper use and conditions is applicable to virtually all dietary supplements and drugs, in order to render a positive product response.

Lastly, a reminder should be made that, as is almost always the case with therapeutic drugs, clinical trials to measure efficacy and safety are first presented in vitro and then eventually progress to studies measuring the effects of the active compound within various animal models. Once a clear measure of safety has been established, studies then advance to, and are conducted on human populations. It is this progression and compiling of analytical data that enables scientists to formulate a hypothesis of the proposed mechanisms, as well as expected outcomes likely to arise when an active ingredient is introduced into humans. In the case of dietary supplements, however, the aforementioned steps are not required and are often not performed at all. As such, it is not uncommon to find a wide range of supplements boasting an invertible cornucopia of structure/function claims with little more than data from cell culture tests and biophysiologic inferences as substantiation. Although such theoretical extrapolation functions as a good starting point for research and discovery, the field of sports nutrition will simply not advance unless more rigorous trials are conducted on both the finished products available today and the discovery of the products of tomorrow.

# SUMMARY

**TABLE 22.1. Summary of sports supplements.**

| Common name | Recommended use(s) | Recommended dose(s) | Pre-exercise | During exercise | Post-exercise | Other | Special notes |
|---|---|---|---|---|---|---|---|
| 4-Hydroxyisoleucine | Glucose disposal, Glycogen resynthesis | ≥2 mg/kg b.w. (or, as 5 mg/kg b.w. Promilin™) | √ | | √ | With meals | Consume with glucose |
| 5-Hydroxytryptophan | Exercise recovery, Fibromyalgia | 50–300 mg/d | | | | 30 min before meals and/or bedtime | Consume on an empty stomach |
| Adenosine Triphosphate | n/a | n/a | | | | | Insufficient data |
| Alanine | Glucose sparing, Protein synthesis | Up to 1 g/kg b.w./d | √ | √ | | | Consume in divided doses beginning 20 min preexercise and continue ingesting throughout exercise session |
| Alpha-glyceryl Phosphoryl Choline | Cognitive function, GH secretagogue | 1–1.2 g/d | √ | | | Between or with meals | Consume approximately 20 min preexercise |
| Alpha-Ketoglutarate | Anticatabolic, Ergogenic aid | 13.905 mg/kg b.w.–0.28 g/kg b.w./d | √ | | √ | With meals | Consume with glucose and vitamin B6 |
| Alpha-Ketoisocaproate | Exercise recovery | >0.10 g/kg b.w./d | | | √ | With meals | |
| Alpha-Lipoic Acid | Antioxidant, Insulin mimetic | 300 mg/d–1 g/d as R-ALA | | | √ | Between or with meals | Consume with or in the absence of glucose |
| Androst-4-ene-3,6,17-trione | n/a | n/a | | | | | Insufficient data |
| Arginine | Exercise recovery, Endurance performance, Erectile dysfunction, GH secretagogue | 5–21 g/d | √ | | √ | 30 min before bedtime or sexual "event" | |
| Asparagine | n/a | n/a | | | | | Insufficient data |
| Aspartic Acid | n/a | n/a | | | | | Insufficient data |
| Avena sativa | n/a | n/a | | | | | Insufficient data |
| Banaba | Insulin mimetic | >16 mg Corosolic acid (from Banaba leaf extract, standardized to ≥1% corosolic acid) | | | √ | Before meals | Consume on an empty stomach |
| Bee Pollen | n/a | n/a | | | | | Insufficient data |
| Beta-Alanine | Proton buffering | 3.2–6.4 g/d | √ | | | | Consume on an empty stomach |
| Betaine | Protein utilization, General use | 600 mg/serving–6 g/d | | | √ | With meals | Consume with meals and protein |
| Beta-Hydroxy-Beta-Methylbutyrate | Anticatabolic, Increased muscle strength | 3–6 g/d | √ | | √ | | Only applies to previously untrained and/or elderly athletes |

*(Continued)*

**TABLE 22.1.** *Continued*

| Common name | Recommended use(s) | Recommended dose(s) | Pre-exercise | During exercise | Post-exercise | Other | Special notes |
|---|---|---|---|---|---|---|---|
| Branched-Chain Amino Acids | Anabolic<br>Anticatabolic<br>Glycogen resynthesis<br>Insulin mimetic | 6–20 g/d | √ | √ | √ | With meals | Consume as 45% : 25% : 30% ratio of Leu/Iso/Val |
| Carnosine | Proton buffering<br>General use<br>Antioxidant | 20–40 mg/kg b.w./d | √ | | | Between meals | Consume on an empty stomach |
| Choline | General use | 300 mg/d–1.2 g/d as Choline Bitartrate or Choline Citrate | √ | | | With meals | May be substituted with 3–9 g/d Phosphotidylcholine |
| Chondroitin Sulfate | Joint health<br>Analgesic | 800 mg/d–1.5 g/d | | | | With meals | |
| Chrysin | n/a | n/a | | | | | Insufficient data |
| Citrulline | Delay muscle fatigue<br>Increase ATP resynthesis | 6 g/d as Citrulline Malate | √ | √ | | Between or with meals | Consume as 53.9% L-Citrulline and 46.1% DL-Malate |
| Coenzyme Q10 | Cardioprotective<br>General use | 50–300 mg/d | √ | | √ | With meals | Consume with fat or as phospholipid gel cap |
| Conjugated Linoleic Acid | n/a | n/a | | | | | Insufficient data |
| Cordyceps | Endurance performance<br>Adaptogen<br>General use | 4.5 g/d as *Cordyceps sinesis* (standardized to ≥0.14% adenosine) | √ | | | Between meals | Consume on an empty stomach |
| Cysteine | n/a | n/a | | | | | Insufficient data |
| Digestive Enzymes | Nutrient utilization<br>General use | Pancreatin: 500 mg/dose<br>Alpha-Galactosidase: 150 GalU/dose<br>Bromelain: 250–500 mg/dose<br>Lactase: 4500 ALU/dose | | | | With meals | Consume 30 min before meals |
| Dimethylaminoethanol | n/a | n/a | | | | | Insufficient data |
| D-Pinitol | Glucose disposal<br>Glycogen resynthesis | 200–600 mg/dose | √ | | √ | Before meals | |
| Ecdysterone | Protein synthesis<br>General use | 0.5–10 mg/kg b.w./d as 20-Hydroxyecdysone | | | √ | With meals | Consume with protein |
| Epimedium | Ergogenic aid<br>General use | 5–10 mg/kg b.w./d Icariin active (from *Epimedium koreanum* rhizome and/or root) | √ | | √ | Between or with meals | Consume on an empty stomach |

518

| Supplement | Uses | Dosage | | | Timing | Comments |
|---|---|---|---|---|---|---|
| Essential Amino Acids | Protein synthesis, Exercise recovery | 3–40 g/d | ✓ | ✓ | Between or with meals | Consume on an empty stomach or in combination with CHO |
| Eurycoma | General use | >150 mg/kg b.w./d as *Eurycoma longifolia* root (standardized to contain a 100:1 water/active extract) | ✓ | | Before meals | Consume on an empty stomach |
| Flaxseed | General use | 30–50 g/d as bruised or whole seed | | | With meals and/or protein 1h before bedtime | May be substituted with 3–5 tbsp./d Flaxseed oil |
| Gamma-Aminobutyric Acid | GH secretagogue, Blood pressure reduction, Possible antianxiety | 1.2 mg/kg b.w./d–10 g/d | | | | Consume on an empty stomach |
| Ginger | Digestive aid, Analgesic, General use | 200 mg/dose–4 g/d as *Zingiber officinale* dried rhizome [standardized to ≥1.5% (mL/g) volatile oil] | ✓ | ✓ | Before or after meals | |
| Ginseng | Performance enhancing, Energy, Glucose disposal, Adaptogen, General use | 200 mg/d as *Panax ginseng* root [standardized to ≥4% total ginsenosides, and ≥1.5% total ginsenosides as Rg1] 1–3g/d as *Panax quinquefolius* root (standardized to ≥3.21% total ginsenosides, and ≥1.5% total ginsenosides as Rb1) | ✓ | ✓ | Before meals and/or glucose | |
| Glucosamine | Joint health, Analgesic | 1500–2000 mg/d as Glucosamine Sulfate | | | With meals | |
| Glutamic Acid/Glutamate | n/a | n/a | | | | |
| Glutamine | Glycogen resynthesis, Anticatabolic, General use | 8g/dose–≥20g/d | ✓ | | Between meals | Insufficient data |

*(Continued)*

TABLE 22.1. *Continued*

| Common name | Recommended use(s) | Recommended dose(s) | Pre-exercise | During exercise | Post-exercise | Other | Special notes |
|---|---|---|---|---|---|---|---|
| Glycerol | Endurance performance<br>Hydration<br>Heat tolerance | 1 g:20 mL–1.2 g:25 mL, per kg b.w. (as Glycerol/6% CHO-containing fluid) | √ | √ | √ | | Consume slowly |
| Ipriflavone | Bone support | 600 mg/d | | | √ | With meals | Consume with food |
| Leucine | Protein synthesis/anabolic<br>Insulin mimetic<br>General use | ≥0.05 g/kg b.w./d | √ | √ | √ | Before or after meals | |
| N-Acetylcysteine | Endurance performance<br>Delay muscle fatigue<br>Vasodilation<br>Antioxidant<br>General use | 600 mg/d–4 g/d | √ | | √ | With meals | Consume with food |
| Ornithine-alpha-Ketoglutarate | Anabolic<br>Anticatabolic<br>Insulin secretagogue | ≥20–30 g/d | | | √ | | Consume in one dose, as 64% Orn/36% AKG |
| Phosphatidylserine | Anticatabolic | 800 mg/d | | | √ | | |
| Rhodiola | Adaptogen<br>General use (chronic)<br>General use (acute) | 100–1800 mg/d as *Rhodiola rosea* root (standardized to ≥3.6–64.8 mg/d rosavin, respectively) | √ | | | Between meals | Consume on an empty stomach |
| Ribose | n/a | n/a | | | | | Insufficient data |
| Sodium Bicarbonate | Delay anaerobic muscle fatigue | 300 mg/kg.b.w./d | √ | | | | Dilute in 1 L of water |
| Taurine | Glucose disposal<br>Antioxidant<br>Ergogenic aid<br>General use | 100–500 mg/kg.b.w./d | √ | | √ | Before meals and/or glucose | Consume on an empty stomach, before glucose |
| Tribulus | General use | 5–10 mg/kg.b.w./d<br>Protodioscin active (from *Tribulus terrestris* above ground parts) | √ | | | With meals | |
| Tyrosine | Exercise performance<br>Mental acuity<br>Energy<br>General use | 50–150 mg/kg.b.w./d | √ | | | Immediately upon waking in the morning | Consume on an empty stomach with more potent catecholaminergic agonist(s); do not consume with BCAAs or glucose |
| Vanadium | Glucose disposal | 150–300 mg/d as enteric coated Vanadyl Sulfate | | | √ | With meals | Diabetic athletes ONLY |

## QUESTIONS

1. Which of the following is NOT one of the three BCAAs?
   a. Valine
   b. Isoleucine
   c. Leucine
   d. Glycine

2. Which of the following is NOT recommended for use as an insulin mimetic in healthy adults?
   a. D-Pinitol
   b. Leucine
   c. Vanadium
   d. Alpha-Lipoic Acid

3. Which of the following has NOT been shown to directly promote protein synthesis in humans?
   a. Taurine
   b. HMB
   c. EAAs
   d. OKG

4. Which of the following is NOT an adaptogen?
   a. Asian Ginseng
   b. *Avena sativa*
   c. *Rhodiola rosea*
   d. *Cordyceps sinesis*

5. Which of the following should be consumed before or with Tyrosine?
   a. Glucose
   b. OKG
   c. Caffeine
   d. BCAAs

6. Which of the following has NOT been shown to function as a muscle-specific antioxidant?
   a. Taurine
   b. Carnosine
   c. Anserine
   d. Glutamine

7. 200 mg 5-HTP was shown to increase which two hormones in man?
   a. LH and CORT
   b. CORT and GH
   c. IGF-1 and CORT
   d. CORT and FSH

8. 20-Hydroxyecdysone will likely work best if consumed with:
   a. Glucose
   b. Glycerol
   c. Taurine
   d. Whey protein

9. HMB will likely work best if consumed by:
   a. Endurance athletes
   b. Competitive bodybuilders
   c. Previously untrained weightlifters
   d. Carbohydrate-depleted fitness competitors

10. Which of the following has NOT been shown to function as a GH secretagogue?
    a. alpha-GPC
    b. Arginine
    c. Epimedium
    d. GABA

11. AKG and KIC are members of what family of acids?
    a. BCKA
    b. BCAA
    c. NEAA
    d. DEA

12. *Avena sativa* is the Latin name for what common grocery item?
    a. Brown rice
    b. Couscous
    c. Rolled oats
    d. Wild yams

13. Banaba extract is not as likely to reduce blood glucose if the active extract has been:
    a. Distilled water-extracted
    b. Hot water-extracted
    c. Alcohol-extracted

14. Betaine functions as a ____ donor, used to convert homocysteine to methionine.
    a. Nitrogen
    b. Hydrogen
    c. Methyl
    d. Organ

15. HMB is formed from:
    a. Leucine and KIC
    b. Valine and Glycine
    c. Glutamine and AKG

16. Which of the following products has NOT been shown to support bone and/or joint health?
    a. Ipriflavone
    b. Sodium Bicarbonate
    c. Glycerol
    d. Glucosamine

17. Which of the following is MOST LIKELY to offer the greatest benefit when consumed pre- and/or during resistance training exercise?
    a. Phosphatidylserine (PS)
    b. 5-Hydroxytryptophan (5-HTP)
    c. Arginine alpha-Ketoglutarate (AAKG)
    d. Citrulline Malate

18. Which of the following is MOST LIKELY to offer the greatest benefit when consumed as a muscle tissue-specific anti-oxidant?
    a. Carnosine
    b. Tribulus terrestris
    c. Vanadyl Sulfate
    d. Androst-4-ene-3,6,17-trione

19. Which of the following is MOST LIKELY to offer the greatest benefit when consumed immediately post-workout?
    a. BCAAs
    b. OKG
    c. KIC
    d. All of the above

20. Which of the following is MOST LIKELY to provide an ergogenic effect?
    a. L-Leucine
    b. Beta-Alanine
    c. Citrulline Malate
    d. All of the above

## ACKNOWLEDGMENTS

This chapter is dedicated in loving memory to the best friend, companion, and teacher with whom I was ever so blessed to have been provided the opportunity to share 13-plus years. Max: your mother, brother, and I, love and miss you deeply. I also thank my wife, Beth, for her incredible display of both patience and support throughout this year-long exercise into insanity. Without her love and friendship, I would not have been able to accomplish such an undertaking. And to our newest addition—the greatest joy God has ever afforded me—Avery, I love you.

## REFERENCES

1. Sauvaire Y, et al. 4-Hydroxyisoleucine: a novel amino acid potentiator of insulin secretion. Diabetes 1998;47(2):206–210.
2. Broca C, et al. 4-Hydroxyisoleucine: experimental evidence of its insulinotropic and antidiabetic properties. Am J Physiol Endocrinol Metab 1999;277(40):E617–E623.
3. Ruby B, et al. The addition of fenugreek extract (Trigonella foenum-graecum) to glucose feeding increases muscle glycogen resynthesis after exercise. Amino Acids 2005;28(1):71–76.
4. Broca C, et al. Insulinotropic agent ID-1101 (4-hydroxyisoleucine) activates insulin signaling in rat. Am J Physiol Endocrinol Metab 2004;287(3):E463–E471.
5. Caruso I, et al. Double-blind study of 5-hydroxytryptophan versus placebo in the treatment of primary fibromyalgia syndrome. J Int Med Res 1990;18(3):201–209.
6. Birdsall TC. 5-Hydroxytryptophan: a clinically-effective serotonin precursor. Altern Med Rev 1998;3(4):271–280.
7. Cangiano C, et al. Effects of oral 5-hydroxy-tryptophan on energy intake and macronutrient selection in non-insulin dependent diabetic patients. Int J Obes Relat Metab Disord 1998;22(7):648–654.
8. Lee MA, et al. Inhibitory effect of ritanserin on the 5-hydroxytryptophan-mediated cortisol, ACTH and prolactin secretion in humans. Psychopharmacology (Berl) 1991;103(2):258–264.
9. Lado-Abeal J, et al. L-5-hydroxytryptophan does not stimulate LH secretion directly from the pituitary in patients with gonadotrophin releasing hormone deficiency. Clin Endocrinol (Oxf) 1998;49(2):203–207.
10. Ryu JK, et al. Adenosine triphosphate induces proliferation of human neural stem cells: role of calcium and p70 ribosomal protein S6 kinase. J Neurosci Res 2003;72(3):352–362.
11. Jordan AN, et al. Effects of oral ATP supplementation on anaerobic power and muscular strength. Med Sci Sports Exerc 2004;36(6):983–990.
12. Williams BD, et al. Alanine and glutamine kinetics at rest and during exercise in humans. Med Sci Sports Exerc 1998;30:1053–1058.
13. Carlin JI, et al. The effects of post-exercise glucose and alanine ingestion on plasma carnitine and ketosis in humans. J Physiol 1987;390:295–303.
14. Koeslag JH, et al. Postexercise ketosis in post-prandial exercise: effect of glucose and alanine ingestion in humans. J Physiol 1985;358:395–403.
15. Koeslag JH, et al. The effects of alanine, glucose and starch ingestion on the ketosis produced by exercise and by starvation. J Physiol 1982; 325:363–376.
16. Tipton KD, et al. Postexercise net protein synthesis in human muscle from orally administered amino acids. Am J Physiol Endocrinol Metab 1999;276:E628–E634.
17. Korach-André M, et al. Differential metabolic fate of the carbon skeleton and amino-N of 13C- and [15N]alanine ingested during prolonged exercise. J Appl Physiol 2002;93:499–504.
18. Ceda GP, et al. Alpha-glycerylphosphorylcholine administrations increases the GH responses to GHRH of young and elderly subjects. Horm Metab Res 1992;24(3):119–121.
19. Lopez CM, et al. Effect of a new cognition enhancer, alpha-glycerylphosphorylcholine, on scopolamine-induced amnesia and brain acetylcholine. Pharmacol Biochem Behav 1991;39:835–840.
20. Frattola L, et al. Multicenter clinical comparison of the effects of choline alfoscerate and cytidine diphosphocholine in the treatment of multi-infarct dementia. Curr Ther Res 1991;49(4):683–693.
21. Abbati C, et al. Nootropic therapy of cerebral aging. Adv Ther 1991;8(6):268–276.

22. Blomqvist BI, et al. Glutamine and alpha-ketoglutarate prevent the decrease in muscle free glutamine concentration and influence protein synthesis after total hip replacement. Metabolism 1995;44(9):1215–1222.

23. Marconi C, et al. The effect of an alpha-ketoglutarate-pyridoxine complex on human maximal aerobic and anaerobic performance. Eur J Appl Physiol Occup Physiol 1982;49(3):307–317.

24. Barazzoni R, et al. Arterial KIC as marker of liver and muscle intracellular leucine pools in healthy and type I diabetic humans. Am J Physiol Endocrinol Metab 1999;277(40):E238–E244.

25. Flakoll PJ, et al. Influence of α-ketoisocaproate on lamb growth, feed conversion, and carcass composition. J Anim Sci 1991;69:1461–1467.

26. Gao Z, et al. Distinguishing features of leucine and α-ketoisocaproate sensing in pancreatic β-cells. Endocrinology 2003;144:1949–1957.

27. Bränström R, et al. Direct inhibition of the pancreatic β-cell ATP-regulated potassium channel by α-ketoisocaproate. J Biol Chem 1998;273(23):14113–14118.

28. Lembert N, Idahl L. α-Ketoisocaproate is not a true substrate for ATP production by pancreatic β-cell mitochondria. Diabetes 1998;47:339–344.

29. Jeevanandam M, et al. Nutritional and metabolic effects and significance of mild orotic aciduria during dietary supplementation with arginine or its organic salts after trauma injury in rats. Metabolism 1997;46(7):785–792.

30. Jeevanandam M, et al. Relative nutritional efficacy of arginine and ornithine salts of alpha-ketoisocaproic acid in traumatized rats. Am J Clin Nutr 1993;57(6):889–896.

31. Marangon K, et al. Comparison of the effect of alpha-lipoic acid and alpha-tocopherol supplementation on measures of oxidative stress. Free Radic Biol Med 1999;27(9–10):1114–1121.

32. Sen CK, Packer L. Thiol homeostasis and supplements in physical exercise. Am J Clin Nutr 2000;72(Suppl):653S–669S.

33. Burke DG, et al. Effect of alpha-lipoic acid combined with creatine monohydrate on human skeletal muscle creatine and phosphagen concentration. Int J Sport Nutr Exerc Metab 2003;13(3):294–302.

34. Hermann R, et al. Enantioselective pharmacokinetics and bioavailability of different racemic alpha-lipoic acid formulations in healthy volunteers. Eur J Pharmaceut Sci 1996;4:167–174.

35. Hermann R, et al. Gastric emptying in patients with insulin dependent diabetes mellitus and bioavailability of thioctic acid-enantiomers. Eur J Pharmaceut Sci 1998;6:27–37.

36. Numazawa M, et al. Mechanism for aromatase inactivation by a suicide substrate, androst-4-ene-3,6,17-trione. The 4 beta, 5 beta-epoxy-19-oxo derivative as a reactive electrophile irreversibly binding to the active site. Biochem Pharmacol 1996;52(8):1253–1259.

37. Shi H, et al. Effect of supplemental ornithine on wound healing. J Surg Res 2002;106:299–302.

38. Appleton J. Arginine: clinical potential of a semi-essential amino acid. Altern Med Rev 2002;7(6):512–522.

39. Witte MB, Barbul A. Arginine physiology and its implication for wound healing. Wound Rep Reg 2003;11:419–423.

40. Besset A, et al. Increase in sleep related GH and Prl secretion after chronic arginine aspartate administration in men. Acta Endocrinol 1982;99:18–23.

41. Marcell TJ, et al. Oral arginine does not stimulate basal or augment exercise-induced GH secretion in either young or old adults. J Gerontol A Biol Sci Med Sci 1999;64:M395–M399.

42. Wu G, Meininger CJ. Arginine nutrition and cardiovascular function. J Nutr 2000;130:2626–2629.

43. Bronisław B, et al. L-Arginine supplementation prolongs duration of exercise in congestive heart failure. Kardiol Pol 2004;60(4):348–353.

44. Parnell MM, et al. In vivo and in vitro evidence for ACh-stimulated L-arginine uptake. Am J Physiol Heart Circ Physiol 2004;287:H395–H400.

45. Marquezi ML, et al. Effect of aspartate and asparagine supplementation on fatigue determinants in intense exercise. Int J Sport Nutr Exerc Metab 2003;13(1):65–75.

46. Stegink LD. Absorption, utilization, and safety of aspartic acid. J Toxicol Environ Health 1976;2(1):215–242.

47. Di Pasquale M. Amino Acids and Proteins for the Athlete: The Anabolic Edge. Boca Raton, FL: CRC Press; 1997.

48. Dioguardi FS. Wasting and the substrate-to-energy controlled pathway: a role for insulin resistance and amino acids. Am J Cardiol 2004;93(8A):6A–12A.

49. Gibala MJ. Regulation of skeletal muscle amino acid metabolism during exercise. Int J Sport Nutr Exer Metab 2001;11:87–108.

50. Campistron G, et al. Pharmacokinetics of arginine and aspartic acid administered simultaneously in the rat: II. Tissue distribution. Eur J Drug Metab Pharmacokinet 1982;7(4):315–322.
51. Fukushima M, et al. Extraction and purification of a substance with luteinizing hormone releasing activity from the leaves of Avena sativa. Tohoku J Exp Med 1976; 119(2):115–122.
52. Czerwinski J, et al. Oat (Avena sativa L.) and amaranth (Amaranthus hypochondriacus) meals positively affect plasma lipid profile in rats fed cholesterol-containing diets. J Nutr Biochem 2004;15(10):622–629.
53. Emmons CL, et al. Antioxidant capacity of oat (Avena sativa L.) extracts. 2. In vitro antioxidant activity and contents of phenolic and tocol antioxidants. J Agric Food Chem 1999;47(12):4894–4898.
54. Handelman GJ, et al. Antioxidant capacity of oat (Avena sativa L.) extracts. 1. Inhibition of low-density lipoprotein oxidation and oxygen radical absorbance capacity. J Agric Food Chem 1999;47(12):4888–4893.
55. Li SS, Claeson P. Cys/Gly-rich proteins with a putative single chitin-binding domain from oat (Avena sativa) seeds. Phytochemistry 2003;63(3):249–255.
56. Kakuda T, et al. Hypoglycemic effect of extracts from Lagerstroemia speciosa L. leaves in genetically diabetic KK-AY mice. Biosci Biotechnol Biochem 1996;60: 204–208.
57. Suzuki Y, et al. Antiobesity activity of extracts from Lagerstroemia speciosa L. leaves on female KK-AY mice. J Nutr Sci Vitaminol 1999;45:791–795.
58. Liu F, et al. An extract of Lagerstroemia speciosa L. has insulin-like glucose uptake-stimulatory and adipocyte differentiation-inhibitory activities in 3T3-L1 cells. J Nutr 2001;131:2242–2247.
59. Judy WV, et al. Antidiabetic activity of a standardized extract (Glucosol) from Lagerstroemia speciosa leaves in Type II diabetics. A dose-dependence study. J Ethnopharmacol 2003;87(1):115–117.
60. Miura T, et al. Corosolic acid induces GLUT4 translocation in genetically Type 2 diabetic mice. Biol Pharm Bull 2004;27(7):1103–1105.
61. Hattori K, et al. Activation of insulin receptors by lagerstroemin. J Pharmacol Sci 2003;93:69–73.
62. Unno T, et al. Xanthine oxidase inhibitors from the leaves of Lagerstroemia speciosa (L.) Pers. J Ethnopharmacol 2004;93(2–3):391–395.
63. Hosoyama H, et al. Isolation and quantitative analysis of the alpha-amylase inhibitor in Lagerstroemia speciosa (L.) Pers. (Banaba). Yakugaku Zasshi 2003;123(7): 599–605.
64. Campos MG, et al. Age-induced diminution of free radical scavenging capacity in bee pollens and the contribution of constituent flavonoids. J Agric Food Chem 2003; 51(3):742–745.
65. Ozcan M, et al. Inhibitory effect of pollen and propolis extracts. Nahrung 2004;48(3):188–194.
66. Xie Y, et al. Effect of bee pollen on maternal nutrition and fetal growth. Hua Xi Yi Ke Da Xue Xue Bao 1994;25(4):434–437.
66a. Stout JR, et al. Effects of twenty-eight days of beta-alanine and creatine monohydrate supplementation on the physical working capacity at neuromuscular fatigue threshold. J Strength Cond Res 2006;20(4):928–932.
66b. Hill et al. (Med Sci Sports Exerc. 2005;37(Suppl):S348.
66c. Derave W, et al. Beta-alanine supplementation augments muscle carnosine content and attenuates fatigue during repeated isokinetic contraction bouts in trained sprinters. J Appl Physiol 2007;103(5):1736–1743.
66d. Hill CA, et al. Influence of beta-alanine supplementation on skeletal muscle carnosine concentrations and high intensity cycling capacity. Amino Acids 2007;32(2): 225–233.
67. Harris RC, et al. Effect of combined beta-alanine and creatine monohydrate supplementation on exercise performance. Med. Sci. Sports Exerc. 2003;35(Suppl.): S218.
68. Harris RC, et al. The absorption of orally supplied beta-alanine and its effect on muscle carnosine synthesis in human vastus lateralis. Amino Acids. 2006;30(3): 279–289.
70. Mori M, et al. β-Alanine and taurine as endogenous agonists at glycine receptors in rat hippocampus in vitro. J Physiol 2002;539(1):191–200.
71. Abebe W, Mozaffari MS. Taurine depletion alters vascular reactivity in rats. Can J Physiol Pharmacol 2003;81(9):903–909.
72. Zeisel SH, et al. Concentrations of choline-containing compounds and betaine in common foods. J Nutr 2003;133:1302–1307.
73. Monograph: betaine. Altern Med Rev 2003;8(2):193–196.
74. Craig S. Betaine in human nutrition. Am J Clin Nutr 2004;80:539–549.

75. Olthof MR, et al. Low dose betaine supplementation leads to immediate and long term lowering of plasma homocysteine in healthy men and women. J Nutr 2003; 133(12):4135–4138.

76. Schwab U, et al. Betaine supplementation decreases plasma homocysteine concentrations but does not affect body weight, body composition, or resting energy expenditure in human subjects. Am J Clin Nutr 2002;76:961–967.

77. Roti MW, et al. Homocysteine, lipid and glucose responses to betaine supplementation during running in the heat [abstract]. Med Sci Sports Exerc 2003;35:S271.

78. Armstrong LE, et al. Rehydration with fluids containing betaine: running performance and metabolism in a 31 C environment [abstract]. Med Sci Sports Exerc 2003;35:S311.

79. Nissen SL, Sharp RL. Effect of dietary supplements on lean mass and strength gains with resistance exercise: a meta-analysis. J Appl Physiol 2003;94:651–659.

80. Jowko E, et al. Creatine and beta-hydroxy-beta-methylbutyrate (HMB) additively increase lean body mass and muscle strength during a weight-training program. Nutrition 2001;17(7–8):558–566.

81. Smith HJ, et al. Mechanism of the attenuation of proteolysis-inducing factor stimulated protein degradation in muscle by beta-hydroxy-beta-methylbutyrate. Cancer Res 2004;64(23):8731–8735.

82. Nissen S, et al. β-Hydroxy-β-methylbutyrate (HMB) supplementation in humans is safe and may decrease cardiovascular risk factors. J Nutr 2000;130:1937–1945.

83. Slater GJ, Jenkins D. Beta-hydroxy-beta-methylbutyrate (HMB) supplementation and the promotion of muscle growth and strength. Sports Med 2000;30(2):105–116.

84. Thomson JS. Beta-hydroxy-beta-methylbutyrate (HMB) supplementation of resistance trained men. Asia Pac J Clin Nutr 2004;13(Suppl):S59.

85. Kreider RB, et al. Effects of calcium beta-hydroxy-beta-methylbutyrate (HMB) supplementation during resistance-training on markers of catabolism, body composition and strength. Int J Sports Med 1999;20(8):503–509.

86. Shimomura Y, et al. Exercise promotes BCAA catabolism: effects of BCAA supplementation on skeletal muscle during exercise. J Nutr 2004;134(6 Suppl):1583S–1587S.

87. Karlsson HK, et al. Branched-chain amino acids increase p70S6k phosphorylation in human skeletal muscle after resistance exercise. Am J Physiol Endocrinol Metab 2004;287(1):E1–E7.

88. Blomstrand E, Bengt S. BCAA intake affects protein metabolism in muscle after but not during exercise in humans. Am J Physiol Endocrinol Metab 2001;281:E365–E374.

89. Fryburg DA, et al. Insulin and insulin-like growth factor-I enhance human skeletal muscle protein anabolism during hyperaminoacidemia by different mechanisms. J Clin Invest 1995;96(4):1722–1729.

90. Ahlborg G, et al. Substrate turnover during prolonged exercise in man. J Clin Invest 1974;53:1080–1090.

91. Eiduson S, et al. The effect of pyridoxine deficiency on L-aromatic amino acid decarboxylase and tyrosine aminotransferase in developing brain. Adv Biochem Psychopharmacol 1972;4:63–80.

92. Abe H. Role of histidine-related compounds as intracellular proton buffering constituents in vertebrate muscle. Biochemistry (Moscow) 2000;65(7):757–765.

93. Suzuki Y, et al. High level of skeletal muscle carnosine contributes to the latter half of exercise performance during 30-s maximal cycle ergometer sprinting. Jpn J Physiol 2002;52(2):199–205.

94. Quinn PJ, et al. Carnosine: its properties, functions and potential therapeutic applications. Molec Aspects Med 1992;13:379–444.

95. Wu H, et al. Antioxidant activities of carnosine, anserine, some free amino acids and their combination. J Food Drug Anal 2003;11(2):148–153.

96. Decker EA, et al. A re-evaluation of the antioxidant activity of purified carnosine. Biochemistry (Moscow) 2000;65(7):766–770.

97. Boldyrev AA, Severin SE. The histidine-containing dipeptides, carnosine and anserine: distribution, properties and biological significance. Adv Enzyme Regul (Moscow). 1990;30:175–194.

98. Zeisel SH. Choline: needed for normal development of memory. J Am Coll Nutr 2000;19(5):528S–531S.

99. Wurtman RJ, et al. Precursor control of neurotransmitter synthesis. Pharmacol Rev 1980;32(4):315–335.

100. Babb SM, et al. Oral choline increases choline metabolites in human brain. Psychiatry Res 2004;130(1):1–9.

101. Spector SA, et al. Effect of choline supplementation on fatigue in trained cyclists. Med Sci Sports Exerc 1995;27(5):668–673.

102. Buchman AL, et al. The effect of lecithin supplementation on plasma choline concentrations during a marathon. J Am Coll Nutr 2000;19(6):768–770.

103. Warber JP, et al. The effects of choline supplementation on physical performance. Int J Sport Nutr Exerc Metab 2000;10(2):170–181.

104. Sauerland K, et al. The sulfation pattern of chondroitin sulfate from articular cartilage explants in response to mechanical loading. Biochim Biophys Acta 2003; 1638(3):241–248.

105. Uebelhart D, et al. Intermittent treatment of knee osteoarthritis with oral chondroitin sulfate: a one-year, randomized, double-blind, multicenter study versus placebo. Osteoarthritis Cartilage 2004;12(4):269–276.

106. Parcell S. Sulfur in human nutrition and applications in medicine. Altern Med Rev 2002;7(1):22–44.

107. Lippiello L, et al. In vivo chondroprotection and metabolic synergy of glucosamine and chondroitin sulfate. Clin Orthop 2000;381:229–240.

108. Leffler CT, et al. Glucosamine, chondroitin, and manganese ascorbate for degenerative joint disease of the knee or low back: a randomized, double-blind, placebo-controlled pilot study. Mil Med 1999;164(2):85–91.

109. Han D, et al. Relationship between estrogen receptor-binding and estrogenic activities of environmental estrogens and suppression by flavonoids. Biosci Biotechnol Biochem 2002;66(7):1479–1487.

110. Jeong HJ, et al. Inhibition of aromatase activity by flavonoids. Arch Pharm Res 1999;22(3):309–312.

111. Gambelunghe C, et al. Effects of chrysin on urinary testosterone levels in human males. J Med Food 2003;6(4):387–390.

112. Saarinen N, et al. No evidence for the in vivo activity of aromatase-inhibiting flavonoids. J Steroid Biochem Mol Biol 2001;78(3):231–239.

113. Briand J, et al. Use of a microbial model for the determination of drug effects on cell metabolism and energetics: study of citrulline-malate. Biopharm Drug Dispos 1992;13(1):1–22.

114. Callis A, et al. Activity of citrulline malate on acid-base balance and blood ammonia and amino acid levels. Study in the animal and in man. Arzneimittelforschung 1991;41(6):660–663.

115. Bendahan D, et al. Citrulline/malate promotes aerobic energy production in human exercising muscle. Br J Sports Med 2002;36:282–289.

116. Oknin Vlu, et al. Use of citrulline malate (stimol) in patients with autonomic dystonia associated with arterial hypotension. Zh Nevrol Psikhiatr Im S S Korsakova 1999;99(1):30–33.

117. Rosenfeldt F, et al. Systematic review of effect of coenzyme Q10 in physical exercise, hypertension and heart failure. Biofactors 2003;18(1–4):91–100.

118. Monograph: Coenzyme Q10. Altern Med Rev 1998;3(1):58–61.

119. Linnane AW, et al. Cellular redox activity of coenzyme Q10: effect of CoQ10 supplementation on human skeletal muscle. Free Radic Res 2002;36(4):445–453.

120. Pariza MW. The biologically active isomers of conjugated linoleic acid. Prog Lipid Res 2001;40(4):283–298.

121. Kelly GS. Conjugated linoleic acid: a review. Altern Med Rev 2001;6(4):367–382.

122. Riserus U, et al. Treatment with dietary trans10cis12 conjugated linoleic acid causes isomer-specific insulin resistance in obese men with the metabolic syndrome. Diabetes Care 2000;25:1516–1521.

123. Terpstra AHM. Effect of conjugated linoleic acid on body composition and plasma lipids in humans: an overview of the literature. Am J Clin Nutr 2004;79:352–361.

124. Kelley DS, Erickson KL. Modulation of body composition and immune cell functions by conjugated linoleic acid in humans and animal models: benefits vs. risks. Lipids 2003;38(4):377–386.

125. Noone EJ, et al. The effect of dietary supplementation using isomeric blends of conjugated linoleic acid on lipid metabolism in healthy human subjects. Br J Nutr 2002;88(3):243–251.

126. Tricon S, et al. Opposing effects of cis-9,trans-11 and trans-10,cis-12 conjugated linoleic acid on blood lipids in healthy humans. Am J Clin Nutr 2004;80(3):614–620.

127. Hsu C, et al. Regulatory mechanism of Cordyceps sinensis mycelium on mouse Leydig cell steroidogenesis. FEBS Lett 2003;543:140–143.

128. Koh JH, et al. Antifatigue and antistress effect of the hot-water fraction from mycelia of Cordyceps sinensis. Biol Pharm Bull 2003;26(5):691–694.

129. Yoo HS, et al. Effects of Cordyceps militaris extract on angiogenesis and tumor growth. Acta Pharmacol Sin 2004;25(5):657–665.

130. Koh J, et al. Hypocholesterolemic effect of hot-water extract from mycelia of Cordyceps sinensis. Biol Pharm Bull 2003;26(1):84–87.

131. Manabe N, et al. Effects of the mycelial extract of cultured Cordyceps sinensis on in vivo hepatic energy metabolism and blood flow in dietary hypoferric anaemic mice. Br J Nutr 2000;83:197–204.

132. Shin KH, et al. Anti-tumour and immuno-stimulating activities of the fruiting bodies of Paecilomyces japonica, a new type of Cordyceps spp. Phytother Res 2003;17(7):830–833.

133. Ikumoto T, et al. Physiologically active compounds in the extracts from tochukaso and cultured mycelia of Cordyceps and Isaria. Yakugaku Zasshi 1991;111(9):504–509.

134. Kuo YC, et al. Growth inhibitors against tumor cells in Cordyceps sinensis other than cordycepin and polysaccharides. Cancer Invest 1994;12(6):611–615.

135. Yu KW, et al. Pharmacological activities of stromata of Cordyceps scarabaecola. Phytother Res 2003;17(3):244–249.

136. Sun YJ, et al. Nucleoside from Cordyceps kyushuensis and the distribution of two active components in its different parts. Yao Xue Xue Bao 2003;38(9):690–694.

137. Gong YX, et al. Simultaneous determination of six main nucleosides and bases in natural and cultured Cordyceps by capillary electrophoresis. J Chromatogr A 2004;1055(1–2):215–221.

138. Parcell AC, et al. Cordyceps sinensis (CordyMax Cs-4) supplementation does not improve endurance exercise performance. Int J Sport Nutr Exerc Metab 2004; 14(2):236–242.

139. Xio Y, et al. Increased aerobic capacity in healthy elderly humans given a fermentation product of Cordyceps Cs-4. Med Sci Sports Exerc 1999;31:S174.

140. Talbott SM, et al. CordyMax Cs-4 enhances endurance in sedentary individuals. Am J Clin Nutr 2002;75:401S.

141. Nicodemus KJ, et al. Supplementation with Cordyceps Cs-4 fermentation product promotes fat metabolism during prolonged exercise. Med Sci Sports Exerc 2001;33: S164.

142. Fukagawa NK, et al. Plasma methionine and cysteine kinetics in response to an intravenous glutathione infusion in adult humans. Am J Physiol 1996;270(2 Pt 1): E209–E214.

143. Pinheiro DF, et al. Effect of early feed restriction and enzyme supplementation on digestive enzyme activities in broilers. Poult Sci 2004;83(9):1544–1550.

144. Bruno MJ, et al. Placebo controlled trial of enteric coated pancreatin microsphere treatment in patients with unresectable cancer of the pancreatic head region. Gut 1998;42:92–96.

145. Walker AF, et al. Bromelain reduces mild acute knee pain and improves well-being in a dose-dependent fashion in an open study of otherwise healthy adults. Phytomedicine 2002;9(8):681–686.

146. Klein G, Kullich W. Reducing pain by oral enzyme therapy in rheumatic diseases. Wien Med Wochenschr 1999;149(21–22):577–580.

147. Blumenthal M, et al. The Complete German Commission E Monographs: Therapeutic Guide to Herbal Medicines. Austin, TX: American Botanical Council. 1998:94–95.

148. Griffiths DW. The inhibition of digestive enzymes by polyphenolic compounds. Adv Exp Med Biol 1986;199:509–516.

149. Kandra L, et al. Inhibitory effects of tannin on human salivary alpha-amylase. Biochem Biophys Res Commun 2004;319(4):1265–1271.

150. George J, et al. Double blind controlled trial of deanol in tardive dyskinesia. Aust N Z J Psychiatry 1981;15(1):68–71.

151. Lukoshko SO, et al. The effect of dimethylethanolamine on the summation capacity of the central nervous system and on the work capacity of animals in a chronic experiment. Fiziol Zh 1997;43(1–2):19–22.

152. Fisher MC, et al. Inhibitors of choline uptake and metabolism cause developmental abnormalities in neurulating mouse embryos. Teratology 2001;64(2):114–122.

153. Lohr J, Acara M. Effect of dimethylaminoethanol, an inhibitor of betaine production, on the disposition of choline in the rat kidney. J Pharmacol Exp Ther 1990; 252(1):154–158.

154. Kiss Z, Crilly KS. Ethanolamine analogues stimulate DNA synthesis by a mechanism not involving phosphatidylethanolamine synthesis. FEBS Lett 1996; 381(1–2):67–70.

155. Fonteles MC, et al. Antihyperglycemic effects of 3-O-methyl-D-chiro-inositol and D-chiro-inositol associated with manganese in streptozotocin diabetic rats. Horm Metab Res 2000;32(4):129–132.

156. Bates SH, et al. Insulin-like effect of pinitol. Br J Pharmacol 2000;130(8):1944–1948.

157. Davis A, et al. Effect of pinitol treatment on insulin action in subjects with insulin resistance. Diabetes Care 2000;23:1000–1005.

158. Iuorno MJ, et al. Effects of d-chiro-inositol in lean women with the polycystic ovary syndrome. Endocr Pract 2002;8(6):417–423.

159. Taylor MJ, et al. Inositol for depressive disorders. Cochrane Database Syst Rev 2004;(2):CD004049.

160. Adler JH, Grebenok RJ. Biosynthesis and distribution of insect-molting hormones in plants: a review. Lipids 1995;30(3):257–262.

161. Harmatha J, Dinan L. Biological activity of natural and synthetic ecdysteroids in the BII bioassay. Arch Insect Biochem Physiol 1997;35(1–2):219–225.

162. Syrov VN, Kurmukov AG. Anabolic activity of phytoecdysone-ecdysterone isolated from Rhaponticum carthamoides (Willd.) Iljin Farmakol Toksikol 1976;39(6):690–693.

163. Slama K, et al. Insect hormones in vertebrates: anabolic effects of 20-hydroxyecdysone in Japanese quail. Experientia 1996;52(7):702–706.

164. Prete PE. Growth effects of Phaenicia sericata larval extracts on fibroblasts: mechanism for wound healing by maggot therapy. Life Sci 1997;60(8):505–510.

165. Gadzhieva RM, et al. A comparative study of the anabolic action of ecdysten, leveton and Prime Plus, preparations of plant origin. Eksp Klin Farmakol 1995;58(5):46–48.

166. Syrov VN, et al. The results of experimental study of phytoecdysteroids as erythropoiesis stimulators in laboratory animals. Eksp Klin Farmakol 1997;60(3):41–44.

167. Mirzaev IuR, et al. Effect of ecdysterone on parameters of the sexual function under experimental and clinical conditions. Eksp Klin Farmakol 2000;63(4):35–37.

168. Mosharrof AH. Effects of extract from Rhaponticum carthamoides (Willd) Iljin (Leuzea) on learning and memory in rats. Acta Physiol Pharmacol Bulg 1987;13(3):37–42.

169. Trenin DS, Volodin VV. 20-Hydroxyecdysone as a human lymphocyte and neutrophil modulator: in vitro evaluation. Arch Insect Biochem Physiol 1999;41(3):156–161.

170. Cai YJ, et al. Antioxidative and free radical scavenging effects of ecdysteroids from Serratula strangulata. Can J Physiol Pharmacol 2002;80(12):1187–1194.

171. Kokoska L, et al. Screening of some Siberian medicinal plants for antimicrobial activity. J Ethnopharmacol 2002;82(1):51–53.

172. Zhao Y, et al. Effects of icariin on the differentiation of HL-60 cells. Zhonghua Zhong Liu Za Zhi 1997;19(1):53–55.

173. Xin ZC, et al. Effects of icariin on cGMP-specific PDE5 and cAMP-specific PDE4 activities. Asian J Androl 2003;(5):15–18.

174. Oh MH, et al. Screening of Korean herbal medicines used to improve cognitive function for anti-cholinesterase activity. Phytomedicine 2004;11(6):544–548.

175. Tian L, et al. Effects of icariin on the erectile function and expression of nitrogen oxide synthase isoforms in corpus cavernosum of arteriogenic erectile dysfunction rat model. Zhonghua Yi Xue Za Zhi 2004;84(11):954–957.

176. Tian L, et al. Effects of icariin on intracavernosal pressure and systematic arterial blood pressure of rat. Zhonghua Yi Xue Za Zhi 2004;84(2):142–145.

177. Mao H, et al. Experimental studies of icariin on anticancer mechanism. Zhong Yao Cai 2000:23(9):554–556.

178. Iinuma M, et al. Phagocytic activity of leaves of Epimedium species on mouse reticuloendothelial system. Yakugaku Zasshi 1990;110(3):179–185.

179. Cai D, et al. Clinical and experimental research of Epimedium brevicornum in relieving neuroendocrino-immunological effect inhibited by exogenous glucocorticoid. Zhongguo Zhong Xi Yi Jie He Za Zhi 1998;18(1):4–7.

180. Liu ZQ, et al. The antioxidative effect of icariin in human erythrocytes against free-radical-induced haemolysis. J Pharm Pharmacol 2004;56(12):1557–1562.

181. Kuang AK, et al. Effects of yang-restoring herb medicines on the levels of plasma corticosterone, testosterone and triiodothyronine. Zhong Xi Yi Jie He Za Zhi 1989;9(12):737–738, 710.

182. Wang ZQ, Lou YJ. Proliferation-stimulating effects of icaritin and desmethylicaritin in MCF-7 cells. Eur J Pharmacol 2004;504(3):147–153.

183. Chiba K, et al. Neuritogenesis of herbal (+)- and (−)-syringaresinols separated by chiral HPLC in PC12h and Neuro2a Cells. Biol Pharm Bull 2002;25(6):791–793.

184. Guo BL, Xiao PG. Comment on main species of herba epimedii. Zhongguo Zhong Yao Za Zhi 2003;28(4):303–307.

185. Guo B, Xiao P. Determination of flavonoids in different parts of five epimedium plants. Zhongguo Zhong Yao Za Zhi 1996;21(9):523–525, 574.

186. Wolfe RR. Effects of amino acid intake on anabolic processes. Can J Appl Physiol 2001;26(Suppl):S220–S227.

187. Tipton KD, et al. Acute response of net muscle protein balance reflects 24-h balance after exercise and amino acid ingestion. Am J Physiol Endocrinol Metab 2002;284:E76–E89.

188. Borsheim E, et al. Essential amino acids and muscle protein recovery from resistance exercise. Am J Physiol Endrocrinol Metab 2002;283:E648–E657.

189. Levenhagen DK, et al. Postexercise nutrient intake timing in humans is critical to recovery of leg glucose and protein homeostasis. Am J Physiol Endocrinol Metab 2001;280:E982–E993.

190. Miller SL, et al. Independent and combined effects of amino acids and glucose ingestion on muscle protein metabolism following resistance exercise. Med Sci Sports Exerc 2003;35(3):449–455.

191. Rasmussen BB, et al. An oral essential amino acid-carbohydrate supplement enhances muscle protein anabolism after resistance exercise. J Appl Physiol 2000;88:386–392.

192. Tipton KD, et al. Postexercise net protein synthesis in human muscle from orally administered amino acids. Am J Physiol Endocrinol Metab 1999;276:E628–E634.

193. Tipton KD, et al. Timing of amino acid-carbohydrate ingestion alters anabolic response of muscle to resistance exercise. Am J Physiol Endocrinol Metab 2001;281:E197–E206.

194. Husen R, et al. Screening for antihyperglycaemic activity in several local herbs of Malaysia. J Ethnopharmacol 2004;95(2–3):205–208.

195. Ang HH, et al. Effects of Eurycoma longifolia Jack (Tongkat Ali) on the initiation of sexual performance of inexperienced castrated male rats. Exp Anim 2000;49(1):35–38.

196. Ang HH, et al. Eurycoma longifolia Jack enhances sexual motivation in middle-aged male mice. J Basic Clin Physiol Pharmacol 2003;14(3):301–308.

197. Ang HH, Sim MK. Eurycoma longifolia JACK and orientation activities in sexually experienced male rats. Biol Pharm Bull 1998;21(2):153–155.

198. Bedir E, et al. Eurycomaoside: a new quassinoid-type glycoside from the roots of Eurycoma longifolia. Chem Pharm Bull 2003;51(11):1301–1303.

199. Haggerty W. Flax: ancient herb and modern medicine. HerbalGram 1999;45:51–56.

200. Caughey GE, et al. The effect on human tumor necrosis factor and interleukin-1: production of diets enriched in n-3 fatty acids from vegetable oil and fish oil. Am J Clin Nutr 1996;63(1):116–122.

201. Demark-Wahnefried W, et al. Pilot study of dietary fat restriction and flaxseed supplementation in men with prostate cancer before surgery: exploring the effects on hormonal levels, prostate-specific antigen, and histopathologic features. Urology 2001;58:47–52.

202. Demark-Wahnefried W, et al. Pilot study to explore effects of low-fat, flaxseed-supplemented diet on proliferation of benign prostatic epithelium and prostate-specific antigen. Urology 2004;63(5):900–904.

203. Ipatova OM, et al. Biological activity of linseed oil as the source of omega-3 alpha-linolenic acid. Biomed Khim 2004;50(1):25–43.

204. Cavagnini F, et al. Effect of acute and repeated administration of gamma aminobutyric acid (GABA) on growth hormone and prolactin secretion in man. Acta Endocrinol (Copenh) 1980;93(2):149–154.

205. Cavagnini F, et al. Effect of gamma-aminobutyric acid on growth hormone and prolactin secretion in man: influence of pimozide and domperidone. J Clin Endocrinol Metab 1980;51(4):789–792.

206. Cavagnini F, et al. Effects of gamma aminobutyric acid (GABA) and muscimol on endocrine pancreatic function in man. Metabolism 1982;31(1):73–77.

207. Spencer GS, et al. Neuroendocrine regulation of growth hormone secretion in sheep. VII. Effects of GABA. Regul Pept 1994;52(3):181–186.

208. Toffano G, et al. Synergistic effect of phosphatidylserine with gamma-aminobutyric acid in antagonizing the isoniazid-induced convulsions in mice. Neurochem Res 1984;9(8):1065–1073.

209. Benassi E, et al. Evaluation of the mechanisms by which gamma-amino-butyric acid in association with phosphatidylserine exerts an antiepileptic effect in the rat. Neurochem Res 1992;17(12):1229–1233.

210. Inoue K, et al. Blood-pressure-lowering effect of a novel fermented milk containing gamma-aminobutyric acid (GABA) in mild hypertensives. Eur J Clin Nutr 2003;57(3):490–495.

211. Hayakawa K, et al. Mechanism underlying gamma-aminobutyric acid-induced antihypertensive effect in spontaneously hypertensive rats. Eur J Pharmacol 2002;438(1–2):107–113.

212. Hayakawa K, et al. Effect of a gamma-aminobutyric acid-enriched dairy product on the blood pressure of spontaneously hypertensive and normotensive Wistar-Kyoto rats. Br J Nutr 2004;92(3):411–417.

213. Aoki H, et al. Effect of γ-aminobutyric acid-enriched tempeh-like fermented soybean (GABA-Tempeh) on the blood pressure of spontaneously hypertensive rats. Biosci Biotechnol Biochem 2003;67(8):1806–1808.

214. Micklefield GH, et al. Effects of ginger on gastroduodenal motility. Int J Clin Pharmacol Ther 1999;37(7):341–346.

215. Hashimoto K, et al. Component of Zingiber officinale that improves the enhancement of small intestinal transport. Planta Med 2002;68(10):936–939.

216. Gonlachanvit S, et al. Ginger reduces hyperglycemia-evoked gastric dysrhythmias in healthy humans: possible role of endogenous prostaglandins. J Pharmacol Exp Ther 2003;307(3):1098–1103.

217. Nurtjahja-Tjendraputra E, et al. Effective anti-platelet and COX-1 enzyme inhibitors from pungent constituents of ginger. Thromb Res 2003;111(4–5):259–265.

218. Tjendraputra E, et al. Effect of ginger constituents and synthetic analogues on cyclo-oxygenase-2 enzyme in intact cells. Bioorg Chem 2001;29(3):156–163.

219. Murakami A, et al. Zerumbone, a Southeast Asian ginger sesquiterpene, markedly suppresses free radical generation, proinflammatory protein production, and cancer cell proliferation accompanied by apoptosis: the alpha,beta-unsaturated carbonyl group is a prerequisite. Carcinogenesis 2002;23(5):795–802.

220. Sievenpiper JL, et al. A systematic quantitative analysis of the literature of the high variability in ginseng (Panax spp.): should ginseng be trusted in diabetes? Diabetes Care 2004;27(3):839–840.

221. Bucci LR, et al. Nutritional Ergogenic Aids. Boca Raton, FL: CRC Press; 2004: 379–410.

222. Vuksan V, et al. American ginseng (Panax quinquefolius L.) attenuates postprandial glycemia in a time-dependent but not dose-dependent manner in healthy individuals. Am J Clin Nutr 2001;73:753–758.

223. Vuksan V, et al. American ginseng reduces postprandial glycemia in nondiabetic and diabetic individuals. Arch Intern Med 2000;160:1009–1013.

224. Sievenpiper JL, et al. Decreasing, null and increasing effects of eight popular types of ginseng on acute postprandial glycemic indices in healthy humans: the role of ginsenosides. J Am Coll Nutr 2004;23(3):248–258.

225. Kelly GS. The role of glucosamine sulfate and chondroitin sulfates in the treatment of degenerative joint disease. Altern Med Rev 1998;3(1):27–39.

226. Christgau S, et al. Osteoarthritic patients with high cartilage turnover show increased responsiveness to the cartilage protecting effects of glucosamine sulphate. Clin Exp Rheumatol 2004;22(1):36–42.

227. Pavelka K, et al. Glucosamine sulfate use and delay of progression of knee osteoarthritis: a 3-year, randomized, placebo-controlled, double-blind study. Arch Intern Med 2002;162(18):2113–2123.

228. Richy F, et al. Structural and symptomatic efficacy of glucosamine and chondroitin in knee osteoarthritis: a comprehensive meta-analysis. Arch Intern Med 2003; 163(13):1514–1522.

229. Ruane R, Griffiths P. Glucosamine therapy compared to ibuprofen for joint pain. Br J Community Nurs 2002;7(3):148–152.

230. Parcell S. Sulfur in human nutrition and applications in medicine. Altern Med Rev 2002;7(1):22–44.

231. Hoffer LJ, et al. Sulfate could mediate the therapeutic effect of glucosamine sulfate. Metabolism 2001;50(7):767–770.

232. Anderson JW, et al. Glucosamine effects in humans: a review of effects on glucose metabolism, side effects, safety considerations and efficacy. Food Chem Toxicol 2005;43(2):187–201.

233. Garattini S. Glutamic acid, twenty years later. J Nutr 2000;130:901S–909S.

234. Brosnan JT. Glutamate, at the interface between amino acid and carbohydrate metabolism. J Nutr 2000;130:988S–990S.

235. Graham TE, et al. Glutamate ingestion: the plasma and muscle free amino acid pools of resting humans. Am J Physiol Enodcrinol Metab 2000;278:E83–E89.

236. Mourtzakis M, Graham TE. Glutamate ingestion and its effects at rest and during exercise in humans. J Appl Physiol 2002;93:1251–1259.

237. Agostoni C, et al. Free glutamine and glutamic acid increase in human milk through a three-month lactation period. J Pediatr Gastroenterol Nutr 2000;31(5):508–512.

238. Kumar D, et al. Improved high altitude hypoxic tolerance and amelioration of anorexia and hypophagia in rats on oral glutamate supplementation. Aviat Space Environ Med 1999;70(5):475–479.

239. Hasebe M, et al. Glutamate in enteral nutrition: can glutamate replace glutamine in supplementation to enteral nutrition in burned rats? J Parenter Enteral Nutr 1999;23(5 Suppl):S78–S82.

240. de Souza CT, et al. Insulin secretion in monosodium glutamate (MSG) obese rats submitted to aerobic exercise training. Physiol Chem Phys Med NMR 2003; 35(1):43–53.

241. Candow DG, et al. Effect of glutamine supplementation combined with resistance training in young adults. Eur J Appl Physiol 2001;86(2):142–149.

242. Antonio J, et al. The effects of high-dose glutamine ingestion on weightlifting performance. J Strength Cond Res 2002;16(1):157–160.

243. Haub MD, et al. Acute l-glutamine ingestion does not improve maximal effort exercise. J Sports Med Phys Fitness 1998;38(3):240–244.

244. Rennie MJ, et al. Interaction between glutamine availability and metabolism of glycogen, tricarboxylic acid cycle intermediates and glutathione. J Nutr 2001; 131:2488S–2490S.

245. Bruce M, et al. Glutamine supplementation promotes anaplerosis but not oxidative energy delivery in human skeletal muscle. Am J Physiol Endocrinol Metab 2001;280: E669–E675.

246. Bowtell JL, et al. Effect of oral glutamine on whole body carbohydrate storage during recovery from exhaustive exercise. J Appl Physiol 1999;86:1770–1777.

247. Buchman AL. Glutamine: commercially essential or conditionally essential? A critical appraisal of the human data. Am J Clin Nutr 2001;74:25–32.

248. Novak F, et al. Glutamine supplementation in serious illness: a systematic review of the evidence. Crit Care Med 2002;30(9):2022–2029.

249. Garcia-de-Lorenzo A, et al. Critical evidence for enteral nutritional support with glutamine: a systematic review. Nutrition 2003;19(9):805–811.

250. Castell L, et al. Glutamine supplementation in vitro and in vivo, in exercise and in immunodepression. Sports Med 2003;33(5):323–345.

251. Trimmer JK, et al. Autoregulation of glucose production in men with a glycerol load during rest and exercise. Am J Physiol Endocrinol Metab 2001;280:E657–E668.

252. Burelle Y, et al. Oxidation of [C]glycerol ingested along with glucose during prolonged exercise. J Appl Physiol 2001;90:1685–1690.

253. Latzka WA, Sawka MN. Hyperhydration and glycerol: thermoregulatory effects during exercise in hot climates. Can J Appl Physiol 2000;25(6):536–545.

254. Anderson MJ, et al. Effect of glycerol-induced hyperhydration on thermoregulation and metabolism during exercise in heat. Int J Sport Nutr Exerc Metab 2001;11(3): 315–333.

255. Coutts A, et al. The effect of glycerol hyperhydration on Olympic distance triathlon performance in high ambient temperatures. Int J Sport Nutr Exerc Metab 2002; 12(1):105–119.

256. Petilli M, et al. Interactions between ipriflavone and the estrogen receptor. Calcif Tissue Int 1995;56:160–165.

257. Miyauchi A, et al. Novel ipriflavone receptors coupled to calcium influx regulate osteoclast differentiation and function. Endocrinology 1996;137:3544–3550.

258. Melis GB, et al. Lack of any estrogenic effect of ipriflavone in postmenopausal women. J Endocrin Invest 1992;15:755–761.

259. Yamazaki I, Kinoshita M. Calcitonin secreting property of ipriflavone in the presence of estrogen. Life Sci 1986;38:1535–1541.

260. Yamazaki I. Effect of ipriflavone on the response of uterus and thyroid to estrogen. Life Sci 1986;38:757–764.

261. Messina MJ. Legumes and soybeans: overview of their nutritional profiles and health effects. Am J Clin Nutr 1999;70(Suppl):439S–450S.

262. Agnusdei D, Bufalino L. Efficacy of ipriflavone in established osteoporosis and long-term safety. Calcif Tissue Int 1997;61(Suppl):S23–S27.

263. Reginster JY. Ipriflavone: pharmacological properties and usefulness in postmenopausal osteoporosis. Bone Miner 1993;23(3):223–232.

264. Somekawa Y, et al. Efficacy of ipriflavone in preventing adverse effects of leuprolide. J Clin Endocrinol Metab 2001;86(7):3202–3206.

265. Agnusdei D, et al. Prevention of early postmenopausal bone loss using low doses of conjugated estrogens and the non-hormonal, bone-active drug ipriflavone. Osteoporos Int 1995;5:462–466.

266. Melis GB, et al. Ipriflavone and low doses of estrogen in the prevention of bone mineral loss in climacterium. Bone Miner 1992;19:S49–S56.

267. Evans BA, et al. Inhibition of 5 alpha-reductase in genital skin fibroblasts and prostate tissue by dietary lignans and isoflavonoids. J Endocrinol 1995;147(2): 295–302.

268. Jarred RA, et al. Anti-androgenic action by red clover-derived dietary isoflavones reduces non-malignant prostate enlargement in aromatase knockout (ArKo) mice. Prostate 2003;56(1):54–64.

269. Morton MS, et al. Measurement and metabolism of isoflavonoids and lignans in human male. Cancer Lett 1997;114:145–151.

270. Yamazaki I. Effect of ipriflavone on accessory sexual organs and bone metabolism in male rats. Bone Miner 1987;2(4):271–280.

271. Head KA. Ipriflavone: an important bone-building isoflavone. Altern Med Rev 1999;4(1):10–22.

272. Notoya K, et al. Similarities and differences between the effects of ipriflavone and vitamin K on bone resorption and formation in vitro. Bone 1995;16:S349–S353.

273. Gambacciani M, et al. Effects of ipriflavone administration on bone mass and metabolism in ovariectomized women. J Endocrinol Invest 1993;16(5):333–337.

274. Seaver B, Smith JR. Inhibition of COX isoforms by nutraceuticals. J Herb Pharmacother 2004;4(2):11–18.

275. Kuzuna S, et al. Effects of ipriflavone (TC-80, an anti-osteoporotic drug) on acute and chronic pain. Nippon Yakurigaku Zasshi 1986;88(1):9–17.

276. Nair KS, et al. Leucine as a regulator of whole body and skeletal muscle protein metabolism in humans. Am J Physiol 1992;263(5 Pt 1):E928–E934.

277. Mero A, et al. Leucine supplementation and serum amino acids, testosterone, cortisol and growth hormone in male power athletes during training. J Sports Med Phys Fitness 1997;37(2):137–145.

278. Crozier SJ, et al. Oral leucine administration stimulates protein synthesis in rat skeletal muscle. J Nutr 2005;135(3):376–382.

279. Koopman R, et al. Combined ingestion of protein and free leucine with carbohydrate increases postexercise muscle protein synthesis in vivo in male subjects. Am J Physiol Endocrinol Metab 2005;288(4):E645–E653.

280. Escobar J, et al. A physiological rise in plasma leucine stimulates muscle protein synthesis in neonatal pigs by enhancing translation initiation factor activation. Am J Physiol Endocrinol Metab 2005;288(5):E914–E921.

281. Layman DK. Role of leucine in protein metabolism during exercise and recovery. Can J Appl Physiol 2002;27(6):646–663.

282. Layman DK. The role of leucine in weight loss diets and glucose homeostasis. J Nutr 2003;133:261S–267S.

283. Hinault C, et al. Amino acids and leucine allow insulin activation of the PKB/mTOR pathway in normal adipocytes treated with wortmannin and in adipocytes from db/db mice. FASEB J 2004;18(15):1894–1896.

284. Anthony JC, et al. Signaling pathways involved in translational control of protein synthesis in skeletal muscle by leucine. J Nutr 2001;131:856S–860S.

285. Xu G, et al. Metabolic regulation by leucine of translation initiation through the mTOR-signaling pathway by pancreatic β-cells. Diabetes 2001;50:353–360.

286. Yang J, et al. Leucine culture reveals that ATP synthase functions as a fuel sensor in pancreatic β-cells. J Biol Chem 2004;279(52):53915–53923.

287. Mero A, et al. Leucine supplementation and intensive training. Sports Med 1999;27(6):347–358.

288. Pitkanen HT, et al. Leucine supplementation does not enhance acute strength or running performance but affects serum amino acid concentrations. Amino Acids 2003;25(1):85–94.

289. Kelly GS. Clinical applications of N-acetylcysteine. Alt Med Rev 1998;3(2):114–127.

290. Patrick L. Nutrients and HIV. Part 3. n-Acetylcysteine, alpha-lipoic acid, l-glutamine, and l-carnitine. Altern Med Rev 2000;5(4):290–305.

291. Sen CK, Packer L. Thiol homeostasis and supplements in physical exercise. Am J Clin Nutr 2000;72(Suppl):653S–669S.

292. De Caro L, et al. Pharmacokinetics and bioavailability of oral acetylcysteine in healthy volunteers. Arzneim Forsch 1989;39:382–385.

293. Borgstrom L, et al. Pharmacokinetics of N-acetylcysteine in man. Eur J Clin Pharmacol 1986;31:217–222.

294. Holdiness MR. Clinical pharmacokinetics of N-acetylcysteine. Clin Pharmacokinet 1991;20(2):123–134.

295. Kinscherf R, et al. Low plasma glutamine in combination with high glutamate levels indicate risk of loss of body cell mass in healthy individuals: the effect of N-acetylcysteine. J Mol Med 1996;74(7):393–400.

296. Quadrilatero J, Hoffman-Goetz L. N-acetyl-L-cysteine prevents exercise-induced intestinal lymphocyte apoptosis by maintaining intracellular glutathione levels and reducing mitochondrial membrane depolarization. Biochem Biophys Res Commun 2004;319(3):894–901.

297. Quadrilatero J, Hoffman-Goetz L. N-acetyl-L-cysteine inhibits exercise-induced lymphocyte apoptotic protein alterations. Med Sci Sports Exerc 2005;37(1):53–56.

298. Sen CK, et al. Oxidative stress after human exercise: effect of N-acetylcysteine supplementation. J Appl Physiol 1994;76(6):2570–2577.

299. Mariotti F, et al. Acute ingestion of dietary proteins improves post-exercise liver glutathione in rats in a dose-dependent relationship with their cysteine content. J Nutr 2004;134(1):128–131.

300. Wessner B, et al. Effect of single and combined supply of glutamine, glycine, N-acetylcysteine, and R,S-alpha-lipoic acid on glutathione content of myelomonocytic cells. Clin Nutr 2003;22(6):515–522.

301. Medved I, et al. Effects of intravenous N-acetylcysteine infusion on time to fatigue and potassium regulation during prolonged cycling exercise. J Appl Physiol 2004; 96:211–217.

302. Medved I, et al. N-acetylcysteine enhances muscle cysteine and glutathione availability and attenuates fatigue during prolonged exercise in endurance-trained individuals. J Appl Physiol 2004;97(4):1477–1485.

303. Medved I, et al. N-acetylcysteine infusion alters blood redox status but not time to fatigue during intense exercise in humans. J Appl Physiol 2003;94:1572–1582.

304. Reid MB. N-acetylcysteine inhibits muscle fatigue in humans. J Clin Invest 1994; 94:2468–2474.

305. Hauer K, et al. Improvement in muscular performance and decrease in tumor necrosis factor level in old age after antioxidant treatment. J Mol Med 2003;81(2): 118–125.

306. Hildebrandt W, et al. Effect of N-acetyl-cysteine on the hypoxic ventilatory response and erythropoietin production: linkage between plasma thiol redox state and $O_2$ chemosensitivity. Blood 2002;99(5):1552–1555.

307. De Flora S, et al. Mechanisms of N-acetylcysteine in the prevention of DNA damage and cancer, with special reference to smoking-related end-points. Carcinogenesis 2001;22(7):999–1013.

308. Alhamdan AA. The effects of dietary supplementation of N-acetyl-L-cysteine on glutathione concentration and lipid peroxidation in cigarette smoke-exposed rats fed a low-protein diet. Saudi Med J 2005;26(2):208–214.

309. MacNee W, et al. The effects of N-acetylcysteine and glutathione on smoke-induced changes in lung phagocytes and epithelial cells. Am J Med 1991;91(3C):60S–66S.

310. De Benedetto F, et al. Long-term oral n-acetylcysteine reduces exhaled hydrogen peroxide in stable COPD. Pulm Pharmacol Ther 2005;18(1):41–47.

311. Grattagliano I, et al. Effect of dietary restriction and N-acetylcysteine supplementation on intestinal mucosa and liver mitochondrial redox status and function in aged rats. Exp Gerontol 2004;39(9):1323–1332.

312. Duong MH, et al. N-acetylcysteine prophylaxis significantly reduces the risk of radiocontrast-induced nephropathy: comprehensive meta-analysis. Catheter Cardiovasc Interv 2005;64(4):471–479.

313. Girouard H, et al. N-acetylcysteine improves nitric oxide and alpha-adrenergic pathways in mesenteric beds of spontaneously hypertensive rats. Am J Hypertens 2003;16(7):577–584.

314. Song D, et al. Chronic N-acetylcysteine prevents fructose-induced insulin resistance and hypertension in rats. Eur J Pharmacol 2005;508(1–3):205–210.

315. Schaser KD, et al. Acute effects of N-acetylcysteine on skeletal muscle microcirculation following closed soft tissue trauma in rats. J Orthop Res 2005;23(1):231–241.

316. Cynober L, et al. Kinetics and metabolic effects of orally administered ornithine alpha-ketoglutarate in healthy subjects fed with a standardized regimen. Am J Clin Nutr 1984;39(4):514–519.

317. Jeevanandam M, Petersen SR. Substrate fuel kinetics in enterally fed trauma patients supplemented with ornithine alpha ketoglutarate. Clin Nutr 1999;18(4):209–217.

318. Cynober L. Ornithine alpha-ketoglutarate as a potent precursor of arginine and nitric oxide: a new job for an old friend. J Nutr 2004;134(10 Suppl):2858S–2862S.

319. Schneid C, et al. Effects of ornithine alpha-ketoglutarate on insulin secretion in rat pancreatic islets: implication of nitric oxide synthase and glutamine synthetase pathways. Br J Nutr 2003;89(2):249–257.

320. Moinard C, et al. Involvement of glutamine, arginine, and polyamines in the action of ornithine alpha-ketoglutarate on macrophage functions in stressed rats. J Leukoc Biol 2000;67(6):834–840.

321. Coudray-Lucas C, et al. Ornithine alpha-ketoglutarate improves wound healing in severe burn patients: a prospective randomized double-blind trial versus isonitrogenous controls. Crit Care Med 2000;28(6):1772–1776.

322. Schneid C, et al. In vivo induction of insulin secretion by ornithine alpha-ketoglutarate: involvement of nitric oxide and glutamine. Metabolism 2003;52(3): 344–350.

323. Pernet P, et al. Dose dependency of the effect of ornithine alpha-ketoglutarate on tissue glutamine concentrations and hypercatabolic response in endotoxaemic rats. Br J Nutr 2004;92(4):627–634.

324. Bruce M, et al. Glutamine supplementation promotes anaplerosis but not oxidative energy delivery in human skeletal muscle. Am J Physiol Endocrinol Metab 2001;280: E669–E675.

325. Bowtell JL, Bruce M. Glutamine: an anaplerotic precursor. Nutrition 2002;18(3): 222–224.

326. Vaubourdolle M, et al. Action of ornithine alpha ketoglutarate on DNA synthesis by human fibroblasts. In Vitro Cell Dev Biol 1990;26(2):187–192.

327. Vaubourdolle M, et al. Fate of enterally administered ornithine in healthy animals: interactions with alpha-ketoglutarate. Nutrition 1989;5(3):183–187.

328. De Bandt JP, et al. Metabolism of ornithine, alpha-ketoglutarate and arginine in isolated perfused rat liver. Br J Nutr 1995;73(2):227–239.

329. Cynober L, et al. Action of ornithine alpha-ketoglutarate, ornithine hydrochloride, and calcium alpha-ketoglutarate on plasma amino acid and hormonal patterns in healthy subjects. J Am Coll Nutr 1990;9(1):2–12.

330. Jeevanandam M, et al. Ornithine-alpha-ketoglutarate (OKG) supplementation is more effective than its component salts in traumatized rats. J Nutr 1996;126(9): 2141–2150.

331. Le Boucher J, et al. Enteral administration of ornithine alpha-ketoglutarate or arginine alpha-ketoglutarate: a comparative study of their effects on glutamine pools in burn-injured rats. Crit Care Med 1997;25(2):293–298.

332. De Bandt JP, et al. A randomized controlled trial of the influence of the mode of enteral ornithine α-ketoglutarate administration in burn patients. J Nutr 1998; 128:563–569.

333. Cynober LA. The use of alpha-ketoglutarate salts in clinical nutrition and metabolic care. Curr Opin Clin Nutr Metab Care 1999;2(1):33–37.

334. Toffano G, et al. Synergistic effect of phosphatidylserine with gamma-aminobutyric acid in antagonizing the isoniazid-induced convulsions in mice. Neurochem Res 1984;9(8):1065–1073.

335. Benassi E, et al. Evaluation of the mechanisms by which gamma-amino-butyric acid in association with phosphatidylserine exerts an antiepileptic effect in the rat. Neurochem Res 1992;17(12):1229–1233.

336. Kuypers FA, de Jong K. The role of phosphatidylserine in recognition and removal of erythrocytes. Cell Mol Biol (Noisy-le-grand) 2004;50(2):147–158.

337. Vance JE, Shiao YJ. Intracellular trafficking of phospholipids: import of phosphatidylserine into mitochondria. Anticancer Res 1996;16(3B):1333–1339.

338. Vance JE. Molecular and cell biology of phosphatidylserine and phosphatidylethanolamine metabolism. Prog Nucleic Acid Res Mol Biol 2003;75:69–111.

339. Bruni A, et al. Pharmacological effects of phosphatidylserine liposomes. Nature 1976;260(5549):331–333.

340. Suzuki S, et al. Oral administration of soybean lecithin transphosphatidylated phosphatidylserine improves memory impairment in aged rats. J Nutr 2001;131: 2951–2956.

341. Cenacchi T, et al. Cognitive decline in the elderly: a double-blind, placebo-controlled multicenter study on efficacy of phosphatidylserine administration. Aging Clin Exp Res 1993;5:123–133.

342. Monteleone P, et al. Effects of phosphatidylserine on the neuroendocrine response to physical stress in humans. Neuroendocrinology 1990;52(3):243–248.

343. Monteleone P, et al. Blunting by chronic phosphatidylserine administration of the stress-induced activation of the hypothalamo-pituitary-adrenal axis in healthy men. Eur J Clin Pharmacol 1992;42(4):385–388.

344. Brekhman II, Dardymov IV. New substances of plant origin which increase nonspecific resistance. Ann Rev Pharmacol 1968;(9):419–430.

345. Brown RP, et al. Rhodiola rosea: a phytomedicinal overview. HerbalGram 2002; 56:40–52.

346. Kelly GS. Rhodiola rosea: a possible plant adaptogen. Altern Med Rev 2001; 6(3):293–302.

347. Monograph: Rhodiola rosea. Altern Med Rev 2002;7(5):421–423.

348. Shevtsov VA, et al. A randomized trial of the two different doses of a SHR-5 Rhodiola rosea extract versus placebo and control of capacity for mental work. Phytomedicine 2003;10(2–3):95–105.

349. Maslova LV, et al. The cardioprotective and antiadrenergic activity of an extract of Rhodiola rosea in stress. Exsp Klin Farmakol 1994;57(6):61–63.

350. Abidov M, et al. Extract of Rhodiola rosea radix reduces the level of C-reactive protein and creatinine kinase in the blood. Bull Exp Biol Med 2004;138(1):63–64.

351. Pogorelyi VE, Makarova LM. Rhodiola rosea extract for prophylaxis of ischemic cerebral circulation disorder. Eksp Klin Farmakol 2002;65(4):19–22.

352. De Sanctis R, et al. In vitro protective effect of Rhodiola rosea extract against hypochlorous acid-induced oxidative damage in human erythrocytes. Biofactors 2004;20(3):147–159.

353. De Bock K, et al. Acute Rhodiola rosea intake can improve endurance exercise performance. Int J Sport Nutr Exerc Metab 2004;14(3):298–307.

354. Furmanowa M, et al. Phytochemical and pharmacological properties of Rhodiola rosea L. Herba Polonica. 1999;95(2):108–113.

355. Tolonen A, et al. Phenylpropanoid glycosides from Rhodiola rosea. Chem Pharm Bull 2003;51(4):467–470.

356. Ganzera M, et al. Analysis of the marker compounds of Rhodiola rosea L. (Golden Root) by reversed phase high performance liquid chromatography. Chem Pharm Bull 2001;49(4):465–467.

357. Abidov M, et al. Effect of extracts from Rhodiola rosea and Rhodiola crenulata (Crassulaceae) roots on ATP content in mitochondria of skeletal muscles. Bull Exp Biol Med 2003;136(6):585–587.

358. Wing SL, et al. Lack of effect of Rhodiola or oxygenated water supplementation on hypoxemia and oxidative stress. Wilderness Environ Med 2003;14(1):9–16.

359. Ha Z, et al. The effect of rhodiola and acetazolamide on the sleep architecture and blood oxygen saturation in men living at high altitude. Zhonghua Jie He He Hu Xi Za Zhi 2002;25(9):527–530.

360. Ruan X, et al. Analysis on the trace elements and amino acid content in xinjiang 6 series Rhodiola L. plant. Guang Pu Xue Yu Guang Pu Fen Xi 2001;21(4):542–544.

361. Zarzeczny R, et al. Influence of ribose on adenine salvage after intense muscle contractions. J Appl Physiol 2001;91:1775–1781.

362. Hellsten L, et al. Effect of ribose supplementation on resynthesis of adenine nucleotides after intense intermittent training in humans. Am J Physiol Regul Integr Comp Physiol 2004;286:R182–R188.

363. Berardi JM, Ziegenfuss TN. Effects of ribose supplementation on repeated sprint performance in men. J Strength Cond Res 2003;17(1):47–52.

364. Kreider RB, et al. Effects of oral D-ribose supplementation on anaerobic capacity and selected metabolic markers in healthy males. Int J Sport Nutr Exerc Metab 2003;13(1):76–86.

365. Op't Eijnde B, et al. No effects of oral ribose supplementation on repeated maximal exercise and de novo ATP resynthesis. J Appl Physiol 2001;91:2275–2281.

366. Pliml W, et al. Effects of ribose on exercise-induced ischaemia in stable coronary artery disease. Lancet 1992;340(8818):507–510.

367. Omran H, et al. D-Ribose improves diastolic function and quality of life in congestive heart failure patients: a prospective feasibility study. Eur J Heart Fail 2003; 5(5):615–619.

368. Kooman JP, et al. The influence of bicarbonate supplementation on plasma levels of branched-chain amino acids in haemodialysis patients with metabolic acidosis. Nephrol Dial Transplant 1997;12:2397–2401.

369. Matson LG, Tran ZV. Effects of sodium bicarbonate ingestion on anaerobic performance: a meta-analytic review. Int J Sport Nutr 1993;3(1):2–28.

370. Requena B, et al. Sodium bicarbonate and sodium citrate: ergogenic aids? J Strength Cond Res 2005;19(1):213–224.

371. Tiryaki GR, Atterbom HA. The effects of sodium bicarbonate and sodium citrate on 600 m running time of trained females. J Sports Med Phys Fitness 1995;35(3): 194–198.

372. Bird SR, et al. The effect of sodium bicarbonate ingestion on 1500-m racing time. J Sports Sci 1995;13(5):399–403.

373. Price M, et al. Effects of sodium bicarbonate ingestion on prolonged intermittent exercise. Med Sci Sports Exerc 2003;35(8):1303–1308.

374. Kolkhorst FW, et al. Effects of sodium bicarbonate on VO2 kinetics during heavy exercise. Med Sci Sports Exerc 2004;36(11):1895–1899.

375. Van Montfoort MC, et al. Effects of ingestion of bicarbonate, citrate, lactate, and chloride on sprint running. Med Sci Sports Exerc 2004;36(7):1239–1243.

376. McNaughton L, Thompson D. Acute versus chronic sodium bicarbonate ingestion and anaerobic work and power output. J Sports Med Phys Fitness 2001;41(4): 456–462.

377. Verbitsky O, et al. Effect of ingested sodium bicarbonate on muscle force, fatigue, and recovery. J Appl Physiol 1997;83(2):333–337.

378. Kozak-Collins K, et al. Sodium bicarbonate ingestion does not improve performance in women cyclists. Med Sci Sports Exerc 1994;26(12):1510–1515.

379. Heck KL, et al. Sodium bicarbonate ingestion does not attenuate the VO2 slow component during constant-load exercise. Int J Sports Nutr 1998;8(1):60–69.

380. McNaughton L, et al. Sodium bicarbonate can be used as an ergogenic aid in high-intensity, competitive cycle ergometry of 1 h duration. Eur J Appl Physiol Occup Physiol 1999;80(1):64–69.

381. Stephens TJ, et al. Effect of sodium bicarbonate on muscle metabolism during intense endurance cycling. Med Sci Sports Exerc 2002;34(4):614–621.

382. Santalla A, et al. Sodium bicarbonate ingestion does not alter the slow component of oxygen uptake kinetics in professional cyclists. J Sports Sci 2003;21(1):39–47.

383. Waldman SD, et al. Effect of sodium bicarbonate on extracellular pH, matrix accumulation, and morphology of cultured articular chondrocytes. Tissue Eng 2004; 10(11–12):1633–1640.

384. Rico H, et al. Effects of sodium bicarbonate supplementation on axial and peripheral bone mass in rats on strenuous treadmill training exercise. J Bone Miner Metab 2001;19(2):97–101.

385. Iwasaki Y, et al. Sodium bicarbonate infusion test: a new method for evaluating parathyroid function. Endocr J 2003;50(5):545–551.

386. Lemann J, et al. Potassium bicarbonate, but not sodium bicarbonate, reduces urinary calcium excretion and improves calcium balance in healthy men. Kidney Int 1989;35(2):688–695.

387. Gougeon-Reyburn R, et al. Effects of bicarbonate supplementation on urinary mineral excretion during very low energy diets. Am J Med Sci 1991;302(2):67–74.

388. Lindinger MI, et al. NaHCO3 and KHCO3 ingestion rapidly increases renal electrolyte excretion in humans. J Appl Physiol 2000;88:540–550.

389. Stipanuk MH. Role of the liver in regulation of body cysteine and taurine levels: a brief review. Neurochem Res 2004;29(1):105–110.

390. Shin HK, Linkswiler HM. Tryptophan and methionine metabolism of adult females as affected by vitamin B6 deficiency. J Nutr 1974;104:1348–1355.

391. Waterfield CJ, et al. Effect of treatment with beta-agonists on tissue and urinary taurine levels in rats. Mechanism and implications for protection. Adv Exp Med Biol 1996;403:233–245.

392. Inoue M, Arias IM. Taurine transport across hepatocyte plasma membranes: analysis in isolated rat liver sinusoidal plasma membrane vesicles. J Biochem (Tokyo) 1988;104(1):155–158.

393. Boelens PG, et al. Plasma taurine concentrations increase after enteral glutamine supplementation in trauma patients and stressed rats. Am J Clin Nutr 2003;77:250–256.

394. Park SH, et al. Cortisol and IGF-1 synergistically up-regulate taurine transport by the rat skeletal muscle cell line, L6. Biofactors 2004;21(1–4):403–406.

395. Roos S, et al. Human placental taurine transporter in uncomplicated and IUGR pregnancies: cellular localization, protein expression, and regulation. Am J Physiol Regul Integr Comp Physiol 2004;287(4):R886–R893.

396. Oja SS, Saransaari P. Modulation of taurine release by glutamate receptors and nitric oxide. Prog Neurobiol 2000;62(4):407–425.

397. Birdsall TC. Therapeutic applications of taurine. Alt Med Rev 1998;3(2):128–136.

398. Huxtable RJ. Physiological actions of taurine. Physiol Rev 1992;72:101–163.

399. Monograph: Taurine. Altern Med Rev 2001;6(1):78–82.

400. Petrosian AM, Haroutounian JE. Taurine as a universal carrier of lipid soluble vitamins: a hypothesis. Amino Acids 2000;19(2):409–421.

401. Messina SA, Dawson R Jr. Attenuation of oxidative damage to DNA by taurine and taurine analogs. Adv Exp Med Biol 2000;483:355–367.

402. Schaffer S, et al. Role of osmoregulation in the actions of taurine. Amino Acids 2000;19(3–4):527–546.

403. El Idrissi A, Trenkner E. Taurine as a modulator of excitatory and inhibitory neurotransmission. Neuorchem Res 2004;29(1):189–197.

404. Conte Camerino D, et al. Taurine and skeletal muscle disorders. Neurochem Res 2004;29(1):135–142.

405. El Idrissi A, Trenkner E. Taurine regulates mitochondrial calcium homeostasis. Adv Exp Med Biol 2003;526:527–536.

406. Aerts L, Van Assche FA. Taurine and taurine-deficiency in the perinatal period. J Perinat Med 2002;30(4):281–286.

407. Wharton BA, et al. Low plasma taurine and later neurodevelopment. Arch Dis Child Fetal Neonatal Ed 2004;89:F497–F498.

408. Arany E, et al. Taurine supplement in early life altered islet morphology, decreased insulitis and delayed the onset of diabetes in non-obese diabetic mice. Diabetologia 2004;47(10):1831–1837.

409. Franconi F, et al. Is taurine beneficial in reducing risk factors for diabetes mellitus? Neurochem Res 2004;29(1):143–150.

410. Zhang M, et al. Beneficial effects of taurine on serum lipids in overweight or obese non-diabetic subjects. Amino Acids 2004;26(3):267–271.

411. Schaffer SW, et al. Interaction between the actions of taurine and angiotensin II. Amino Acids 2000;18(4):305–318.

412. Militante JD, Lombardini JB. Treatment of hypertension with oral taurine: experimental and clinical studies. Amino Acids 2002;23(4):381–393.

413. Kingston R, et al. The therapeutic role of taurine in ischaemia-reperfusion injury. Curr Pharm Des 2004;10(19):2401–2410.

414. Yamori Y, et al. Fish and lifestyle-related disease prevention: experimental and epidemiological evidence for anti-atherogenic potential of taurine. Clin Exp Pharmacol Physiol 2004;31(Suppl 2):S20–S23.

415. El Idrissi A, et al. Prevention of epileptic seizures by taurine. Adv Exp Med Biol 2003;526:515–525.

416. Sener G, et al. Taurine treatment protects against chronic nicotine-induced oxidative changes. Fundam Clin Pharmacol 2005;19(2):155–164.

417. Olive MF. Interactions between taurine and ethanol in the central nervous system. Amino Acids 2002;23(4):345–357.

418. Lee JY, et al. Effect of taurine on biliary excretion and metabolism of acetaminophen in male hamsters. Biol Pharm Bull 2004;27(11):1792–1796.

419. Warskulat U, et al. Taurine transporter knockout depletes muscle taurine levels and results in severe skeletal muscle impairment but leaves cardiac function uncompromised. FASEB J 2004;18(3):577–579.

420. Matsuzaki Y, et al. Decreased taurine concentration in skeletal muscles after exercise for various durations. Med Sci Sports Exerc 2002;34(5):793–797.

421. Dawson R Jr, et al. The cytoprotective role of taurine in exercise-induced muscle injury. Amino Acids 2002;22(4):309–324.

422. Yatabe Y, et al. Effects of taurine administration in rat skeletal muscles on exercise. J Orthop Sci 2003;8(3):415–419.

423. Zhang M, et al. Role of taurine supplementation to prevent exercise-induced oxidative stress in healthy young men. Amino Acids 2004;26(2):203–207.

424. De Luca A, et al. Enhanced dystrophic progression in mdx mice by exercise and beneficial effects of taurine and insulin-like growth factor-1. J Pharmacol Exp Ther 2003;304(1):453–463.

425. Bouchama A, et al. Alteration of taurine homeostasis in acute heatstroke. Crit Care Med 1993;21(4):551–554.

426. Miyazaki T, et al. Optimal and effective oral dose of taurine to prolong exercise performance in rat. Amino Acids 2004;27(3–4):291–298.

427. Kaplan B, et al. Effects of taurine in glucose and taurine administration. Amino Acids 2004;27(3–4):327–333.

428. Nandhini ATA, et al. Effect of taurine on biomarkers of oxidative stress in tissues of fructose-fed insulin-resistant rats. Singapore Med J 2005;46(2):82–87.

429. Manabe S, et al. Decreased blood levels of lactic acid and urinary excretion of 3-methylhistidine after exercise by chronic taurine treatment in rats. J Nutr Sci Vitaminol (Tokyo) 2003;49(6):375–380.

430. Harada N, et al. Taurine alters respiratory gas exchange and nutrient metabolism in type 2 diabetic rats. Obes Res 2004;12(7):1077–1084.

431. Han J, et al. Taurine increases glucose sensitivity of UCP2-overexpressing beta-cells by ameliorating mitochondrial metabolism. Am J Physiol Endocrinol Metab 2004;287(5):E1008–E1018.

432. Sang-Hoon L, et al. Enhancing effect of taurine on glucose response in UCP2-overexpressing beta-cells. Diabetes Res Clin Pract 2004;66(Suppl 1):S69–S74.

433. Brons C, et al. Effect of taurine treatment on insulin secretion and action, and on serum lipid levels in overweight men with a genetic predisposition for type II diabetes mellitus. Eur J Clin Nutr 2004;58(9):1239–1247.

434. Boujendar S, et al. Taurine supplementation of a low protein diet fed to rat dams normalizes the vascularization of the fetal endocrine pancreas. J Nutr 2003;133:2820–2825.

435. Antonio J, et al. The effects of Tribulus terrestris on body composition and exercise performance in resistance-trained males. Int J Sport Nutr Exerc Metab 2000;10(2):208–215.

436. Gauthaman K, et al. Sexual effects of puncturevine (Tribulus terrestris) extract (Protodioscin): an evaluation using a rat model. J Altern Complement Med 2003;9(2):257–265.

437. Deng Y, et al. Effect of Tribulus terrestris L decoction of different concentrations on tyrosinase activity and the proliferation of melanocytes. Di Yi Jun Yi Da Xue Xue Bao 2002;22(11):1017–1019.

438. Cauthaman K, Adaikan PG. Effect of Tribulus terrestris on nicotinamide adenine dinucleotide phosphate-diaphorase activity and androgen receptors in rat brain. J Ethnopharmacol 2005;96(1–2):127–132.

439. Gauthaman K, et al. Aphrodisiac properties of Tribulus terrestris extract (Protodioscin) in normal and castrated rats. Life Sci 2002;71(12):1385–1396.

440. Adaikan PG, et al. Proerectile pharmacological effects of Tribulus terrestris extract on the rabbit corpus cavernosum. Ann Acad Med Singapore 2000;29(1):22–26.

441. Li M, et al. Hypoglycemic effect of saponin from Tribulus terrestris. Zhong Yao Cai 2002;25(6):420–422.

442. Chu S, et al. Effect of saponin from Tribulus terrestris on hyperlipidemia. Zhong Yao Cai 2003;26(5):341–344.

443. Squires PE, et al. The putative imidazoline receptor agonist, harmane, promotes intracellular calcium mobilization in pancreatic beta-cells. Eur J Pharmacol 2004;501(1–3):31–39.

444. Sangeeta D, et al. Effect of Tribulus terrestris on oxalate metabolism in rats. J Ethnopharmacol 1994;44(2):61–66.

445. Wang B, et al. 406 cases of angina pectoris in coronary heart disease treated with saponin of Tribulus terrestris. Zhong Xi Yi Jie He Za Zhi 1990;10(2):85–87, 68.

446. Arcasoy HB, et al. Effect of Tribulus terrestris L. saponin mixture on some smooth muscle preparations: a preliminary study. Boll Chim Farm 1998;137(11):473–475.

447. Al-Ali M, et al. Tribulus terrestris: preliminary study of its diuretic and contractile effects and comparison with Zea mays. J Ethnopharmacol 2003;85(2–3):257–260.

448. Hong CH, et al. Evaluation of natural products on inhibition of inducible cyclooxygenase (COX-2) and nitric oxide synthase (iNOS) in cultured mouse macrophage cells. J Ethnopharmacol 2002;83(1–2):153–159.

449. Sharifi AM, et al. Study of antihypertensive mechanism of Tribulus terrestris in 2K1C hypertensive rats: role of tissue ACE activity. Life Sci 2003;73(23):2963–2971.

450. Ganzera M, et al. Determination of steroidal sapoinins in Tribulus terrestris by reversed-phase high-performance liquid chromatography and evaporative light scattering detection. J Pharm Sci 2001;90:1752–1758.

451. Stevenson JS, et al. Luteinizing hormone release and reproductive traits in anestrous, estrus-cycling, and ovariectomized cattle after tyrosine supplementation. J Anim Sci 1997;75:2754–2761.

452. Zurek E, et al. Metabolic status and interval to first ovulation in postpartum dairy cows. J Dairy Sci 1995;78:1909–1920.

453. Sutton EE, et al. Ingestion of tyrosine: effects on endurance, muscle strength, and anaerobic performance. Int J Sport Nutr Exerc Metab 2005;15:173–185.

454. Troy D, et al. Effects of L-tyrosine and carbohydrate ingestion on endurance exercise performance. J Appl Physiol 2002;93:1590–1597.

455. Benedict CR, et al. The influence of oral tyrosine and tryptophan feeding on plasma catecholamines in man. Am J Clin Nutr 1983;38(3):429–435.

456. Alonso R, et al. Elevation of urinary catecholamines and their metabolites following tyrosine administration in humans. Biol Psychiatry 1982;17(7):781–790.

457. Agharanya JC, et al. Changes in catecholamine excretion after short-term tyrosine ingestion in normally fed human subjects. Am J Clin Nutr 1981;34(1):82–87.

458. Gibson CJ. Increase in norepinephrine turnover after tyrosine or DL-threo-3,4-dihydroxyphenylserine (DL-threo-DOPS). Life Sci 1988;42(1):95–102.

459. Acworth IN, et al. Tyrosine: effects on catecholamine release. Brain Res Bull 1988;21(3):473–477.

460. Magill RA, et al. Effects of tyrosine, phentermine, caffeine D-amphetamine, and placebo on cognitive and motor performance deficits during sleep deprivation. Nutr Neurosci 2003;6(4):237–246.

461. Neri DF, et al. The effects of tyrosine on cognitive performance during extended wakefulness. Aviat Space Environ Med 1995;66(4):313–319.

462. Rauch TM, Lieberman HR. Tyrosine pretreatment reverses hypothermia-induced behavioral depression. Brain Res Bull 1990;24(1):147–150.

463. Lieberman HR, et al. Tyrosine prevents effects of hyperthermia on behavior and increases norepinephrine. Physiol Behav 2005;84(1):33–38.

464. Avraham Y, et al. Tyrosine improves appetite, cognition, and exercise tolerance in activity anorexia. Med Sci Sports Exerc 2001;33(12):2104–2110.

465. Avraham Y, et al. Diet restriction in mice causes a decrease in hippocampal choline uptake and muscarinic receptors that is restored by administration of tyrosine: interaction between cholinergic and adrenergic receptors influencing cognitive function. Nutr Neurosci 2001;4(2):153–167.

466. Hayashi Y, et al. Enhancement of in vivo tyrosine hydroxylation in the rat adrenal gland under hypoxic conditions. J Neurochem 1990;54(4):1115–2111.

467. Melamed E, et al. Tyrosine administration increases striatal dopamine release in rats with partial nigrostriatal lesions. Proc Natl Acad Sci USA 1980;77(7):4305–4309.

468. Asbach S, et al. Effects of corticotrophin-releasing hormone on locus coeruleus neurons in vivo: a microdialysis study using a novel bilateral approach. Eur J Endocrinol 2001;145:359–363.

469. Agharanya JC, Wurtman RJ. Studies on the mechanism by which tyrosine raises urinary catecholamines. Biochem Pharmacol 1982;31(22):3577–3580.

470. Jaskiw GE, et al. Tyrosine augments clozapine-induced dopamine release in the medial prefrontal cortex of the rat in vivo: effects of access to food. Neurosci Lett 2004;357(1):5–8.

471. Jaskiw GE, et al. Tyrosine augments acute clozapine- but not haloperidol-induced dopamine release in the medial prefrontal cortex of the rat: an in vivo microdialysis study. Neuropsychopharmacology 2001;25(1):149–156.

472. Martha M, et al. Tetrahydrobiopterin increases in adrenal medulla and cortex: a factor in the regulation of tyrosine hydroxylase. Proc Natl Acad Sci USA 1981; 78(5):2703–2706.

473. Fernstrom MH, et al. In vivo inhibition of tyrosine uptake into rat retina by large neutral but not acidic amino acids. Am J Physiol 1986;251(4 Pt 1):E393–E399.

474. Oishi T, Szabo S. Effect of tyrosine administration on duodenal ulcer induced by cysteamine in the rat. J Pharmacol Exp Ther 1987;240(3):879–882.

475. Heyliger CE, et al. Effect of vanadate on elevated blood glucose and depressed cardiac performance of diabetic rats. Science 1985;227:1474–1477.

476. Verma S, et al. Nutritional factors that can favorably influence the glucose/insulin system: vanadium. J Am Coll Nutr 1998;17(1):11–18.

477. Poucheret P, et al. Vanadium and diabetes. Mol Cell Biochem 1998;188(1–2):73–80.

478. Srivastava AK, Mehdi MZ. Insulino-mimetic and anti-diabetic effects of vanadium compounds. Diabet Med 2005;22(1):2–13.

479. Cam MC, et al. Concentration-dependent glucose lowering effects of vanadyl are maintained following treatment withdrawal in streptozotocin diabetic rats. Metabolism 1995;44:332–339.

480. Cohen N, et al. Oral vanadyl sulfate improves hepatic and peripheral insulin sensitivity in patients with non-insulin dependent diabetes mellitus. J Clin Invest 1995;95:2501–2509.

481. Marzban L, et al. Mechanisms by which bis(maltolato)oxovanadium(IV) normalizes phosphoenolpyruvate carboxykinase and glucose-6-phosphatase expression in streptozotocin-diabetic rats in vivo. Endocrinology 2002;143(12):4636–4645.

482. Xie M, et al. A new orally active antidiabetic vanadyl complex—bis(alpha-furancar boxylato)oxovanadium(IV). J Inorg Biochem 2005;99(2):546–551.

483. Brownsey RW, Dong GW. Evidence for selective effects of vanadium on adipose cell metabolism involving actions on cAMP-dependent protein kinase. Mol Cell Biochem 1995;153(1–2):131–137.

484. Rehder D, et al. In vitro study of the insulin-mimetic behavior of vanadium(IV, V) coordination compounds. J Biol Inorg Chem 2002;7(4–5):384–396.

485. Jentjens RL, Jeukendrup AE. Effect of acute and short-term administration of vanadyl sulphate on insulin sensitivity in healthy active humans. Int J Sport Nutr Exerc Metab 2002;12(4):470–479.

486. Fawcett JP, et al. The effect of oral vanadyl sulfate on body composition and performance in weight-training athletes. Int J Sport Nutr 1996;6(4):382–390.

487. Fawcett JP, et al. Oral vanadyl sulphate does not affect blood cells, viscosity or biochemistry in humans. Pharmacol Toxicol 1997;80(4):202–206.

488. Marti L, et al. Tyramine and vanadate synergistically stimulate glucose transport in rat adipocytes by amine oxidase-dependent generation of hydrogen peroxide. J Pharmacol Exp Ther 1998;285(1):342–349.

489. Barbagallo M, et al. Insulin-mimetic action of vanadate: role of intracellular magnesium. Hypertension 2001;38(2):701–704.

490. McNeill JH, et al. Increased potency of vanadium using organic ligands. Mol Cell Biochem 1995;153(1–2):175–180.

491. Reul BA, et al. Effects of vanadium complexes with organic ligands on glucose metabolism: a comparison study in diabetic rats. Br J Pharmacol 1999;126:467–477.

492. Conconi MT, et al. Effects of some vanadyl coordinating compounds on the in vitro insulin release from rat pancreatic islets. Horm Metab Res 2003;35(7):402–406.

493. Elberg G, et al. Vanadium activates or inhibits receptor and non-receptor protein tyrosine kinases in cell-free experiments, depending on its oxidation state. J Biol Chem 1994;269(13):9521–9527.

494. Goldfine AB, et al. Metabolic effects of vanadyl sulfate in humans with non-insulin-dependent diabetes mellitus: in vivo and in vitro studies. Metabolism 2000; 49(3):400–410.

495. Fugono J, et al. Enteric-coating capsulation of insulinomimetic vanadyl sulfate enhances bioavailability of vanadyl species in rats. J Pharm Pharmacol 2002; 54(5):611–615.

496. Bone K. Standardized extracts: neither poison nor panacea. HerbalGram 2001; 53:50–55.

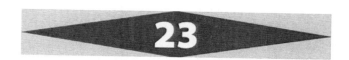

# Hormonal Supplements
## Legal and Illegal

### Jamie Landis and Tim N. Ziegenfuss

## OBJECTIVES

On the completion of this chapter you will be able to:

1. Understand the basic types of endogenous hormones and how they are synthesized.
2. Discuss why anabolic-androgenic steroids may be used by athletes.
3. Explain how anabolic-androgenic steroids work.
4. Understand the ramifications of using anabolic androgenic steroids.
5. Differentiate between anabolic-androgenic steroids and prohormones.
6. Discuss the two major prohormones and their effects.
7. Explain the role of the thyroid hormones and why they might be used by athletes.
8. Understand the physiologic effects of using growth hormone.
9. Discuss the physiologic effects of insulin.
10. Explain the clinical uses of a variety of drugs that have been abused by athletes.
11. Understand the ergogenic effects of erythropoietin and discuss the potential contraindications to using this drug.
12. Explain the potential benefits and ramifications of using corticosteroids.
13. Discuss the potential future abuse of gene technologies.

## ABSTRACT

Numerous hormones and hormone supplements are used by athletes in the hope of improving performance. Often, the marketing claims and gym lore regarding the utility of a given supplement do not agree with empirically obtained evidence. It is incumbent upon those who work with athletes to maintain a solid knowledge base regarding the science of hormone supplementation, as well as cultivate a process of critically appraising the current literature regarding hormone supplements. Indeed, it is likely that the science of hormonal manipulation will continue to evolve, and the rules and records will change to reflect modern athletes and their drive to succeed.

Key Words: anabolic androgenic, prohormones, corticosteroids, IGF-1, steroids

Most athletes are familiar with the training adage, "Bigger, faster, stronger," however, less widely acknowledged is the inclusion (for some) of "doper" in that phrase. The root of the word doping is believed to have come from the Dutch word, "dop," which was an alcoholic drink consumed by Zulu warriors before battle.[1] Indeed, the phenomenon of seeking physical and performance enhancement through the use chemical and biologic substances is clearly not

From: *Essentials of Sports Nutrition and Supplements*
Edited by J. Antonio, D. Kalman, J. R. Stout, M. Greenwood, D. S. Willoughby, and G. G. Haff © Humana Press, a part of Springer Science+Business Media, Totowa, NJ

an invention of modern society. The roots of such supplementation may be traced across time and geography to include examples from many aboriginal cultures in which the organs, particularly the hearts, of revered competitors were consumed in order to gain their strength. The athletes of today have thankfully refined this approach, and instead of relying on spiritual notions, they have taken inspiration from the biologic sciences.

As the following sections illustrate, physiologic and chemical knowledge of human hormones and exercise response has helped define the rationale for hormonal manipulation in athletic performance enhancement. It is a field of interest that continues to expand, both on the level of scientific investigation and the use among athletes. However, even as the body of scientific knowledge increases, many athletes may not be taking advantage of a fully informed decision-making process. Any consideration by an athlete regarding the use of hormone supplements must include the caveats of side effect and contraindication, as well as the legal aspects of usage. As it is with people in general, an educated athlete is a more complete athlete, and more likely to make responsible decisions. The end result, one hopes, is that those in pursuit of "Bigger, faster, stronger," continually train "smarter."

## WHAT IS A HORMONE?

Classically, hormones have been defined as chemicals produced in the endocrine tissues of the body that will exert an effect on a target tissue via an interaction with a cellular receptor [2] (Table 23.1). Many of the endocrine tissues of the body, and the hormones they produce, are influenced by an axis of control that involves the hypothalamus and pituitary (Figure 23.1).

Growth and development are chief among the essential functions influenced by hormones. The method of influence varies with both the type of hormone, and the mechanisms of receptor action (Figure 23.2). For example, protein hormones generally bind with cell surface receptors. The interaction with these cell surface receptors results in a cascade of post receptor chemical reactions that ultimately create an interaction within the target cell. Alternatively, the steroid hormones are fat-soluble and thus easily diffuse through cell membranes to bind with receptors inside of cells. Once bound, these hormone–receptor complexes then interact with the genetic machinery of the cell to stimulate a response. These general interactions are complicated to some extent by the evidence of coactivator and repressor molecules, and the apparent interaction of different molecules at the same genetic regions.

TABLE 23.1. Endogenously produced hormones used as supplements by athletes.

| Hormone name | Hormone type | Main tissue of origin |
|---|---|---|
| Adrenocorticotropic hormone | Peptide | Corticotrophic cells of anterior pituitary |
| Androstenedione | Steroid | Zona fasciculata and zona reticularis of adrenal cortex |
| Cortisol | Steroid | Zona Fasiculata of adrenal cortex |
| Dehydroepiandrosterone | Steroid | Zona fasciculata and zona reticularis of adrenal cortex |
| Erythropoietin | Peptide | Peritubular cells of renal cortex |
| Growth hormone | Peptide | Somatotrophic cells of anterior pituitary |
| Human chorionic gonadotropin | Peptide | Trophoblastic cells of placenta |
| Insulin | Peptide | Beta cells of pancreatic islets |
| Insulin-like growth factor | Peptide | Liver |
| Testosterone | Steroid | Leydig cells of testicle |
| Thyroxine and triiodothyronine | Amine (dipeptide) | Follicular cells of thyroid gland |

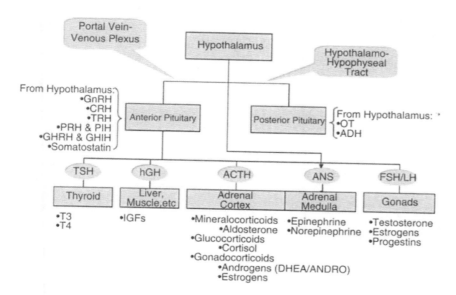

**FIGURE 23.1.** Hormonal control vectoring on the hypothalamic-pituitary axis. The release of many hormones of the body are regulated by central control from the hypothalamus of the brain.

## HORMONES AND SPORT

In relation to athletic performance, certain hormones garner far more attention than others. In general, hormones that exhibit either a positive (anabolic), or negative (catabolic), influence are the most widely sought and utilized. There are obvious reasons for this, and although the utility of each hormone may not be well established in the world of sport, these types of hormones may have the potential to promote recovery from vigorous exercise, enhance the development of lean muscle mass, and alter the ratio of macronutrient fuel.

Athletes have utilized several methods of hormonal manipulation, including the stimulation or suppression of hormone release, as well as the concomitant attempts to mask their use and avoid detection. However, the most direct tactic involves hormone supplementation to supraphysiologic levels through either the consumption or injection of manufactured hormones or hormone analogs.

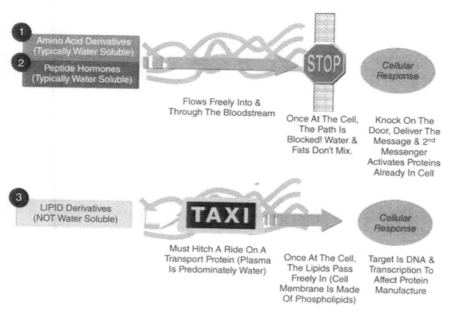

**FIGURE 23.2.** Hormone transport and cellular response. The chemical nature of hormones affects their transport in blood and interaction with target tissues.

## HORMONES AND HORMONE SUPPLEMENTS

The following section represents an overview of the notable hormones and hormone supplements used by athletes to putatively improve performance. The information presented reflects the current body of peer-reviewed empiric literature. Students are encouraged to explore this body of literature, as well as participate in and attend International Society of Sports Nutrition meetings and proceedings, in order to maintain an up-to-date perspective of the subject matter.

## ANABOLIC-ANDROGENIC STEROIDS

### Overview of Use

Anabolic-androgenic steroids (AASs) can be administered via injection, oral ingestion, or as skin patches and gel preparations for transdermal absorption.[3] They have been used medically in the treatment of several conditions including certain forms of anemia, breast cancer, endometriosis, constitutional delay in puberty, hypogonadism, and a number of wasting syndromes such as those caused by major burns and infectious diseases (AIDS). Recently, studies have demonstrated a positive influence of AASs in the healing from muscle contusion injury, and a reduction in immobilization-induced muscular atrophy. AASs have also been noted to improve muscle mass and bone mineral density, as well as functional ability in elderly women recovering from hip fracture. AAS use by athletes has traditionally been motivated by a desire to improve lean muscular mass, power, and strength.

## Sidebar 23.1. The Use of Banned Substances

*Christopher McKinley Heben*
*United States Navy SEAL, PA-C*

The desire to enhance human performance through the use of foreign or forbidden substances has been undertaken since the earliest recordings of man. For illustration, one needs to look no further than the biblical account of Adam and Eve eating from the "forbidden fruit" in the Garden of Eden. Since that time, however, a cat and mouse game has unfolded within the ranks of organized athletics to rival that of the actual sporting events themselves.

To be certain, analytical chemists have much on their plates. The International Olympic Committee (IOC) has placed more than 150 substances on the illegal list—150 molecular milieus that chemists must try to extract and identify from blood and urine. In the future, hair may be added to this. Public enemy number one are AASs that increase muscle and strength. Next are the peptide hormones, to include erythropoietin (EPO). EPO increases the production of oxygen-carrying red blood cells. Additionally, the IOC also bans stimulants, pain killers, and urine-altering agents used to hide the presence of these illegal substances. Because concentrations of certain compounds on this list do exist naturally in the urine and blood of most athletes, laboratory technicians are forced to invent clever methods of discerning the true source (endogenous versus exogenous) of the performance-enhancing agent(s) in question.

Initially, when athletes were exposed to drug testing, they were caught off guard. The subjects of Organic and

Analytical chemistry were not the types of curriculum that athletes generally specialized in. Both coaches and athletes soon realized, after speaking with more qualified personnel, that simply going off of AASs and other agents, in a timely manner, would result in a negative drug test. However, a systematic approach needed to be followed. This was done by simply submitting urine samples to a laboratory outfitted with the proper analytical equipment. The results of the previous day's submission of urine would be revealed to the coach and athlete. At some point all parties would know exactly how many "clean" days it would take to pass a drug test. Consequently, going into a meet, the athlete would feel confident that he/she would be submitting a negative sample. This worked well until the advent of slightly more sophisticated methods for detection of AASs and other blood-doping agents.

The uncertainty of not knowing the exact type of equipment to be used or the precise methods that would be followed, served to create a demand by athletes for alternative methods of avoiding detection. Diuretic use was one such strategy. Diuretics have been predominantly used in sports having weight classes and are used to shed pounds quickly via massive dehydration. After a successful weigh-in, an athlete would receive equally aggressive intravenous fluid replacement. Diuretics were also used to increase urine dilution, thus making small quantities of banned substances more difficult to detect. Although drug testing by the IOC was started in 1967, it was not until 1988 that testing for diuretics began. Accordingly, with diuretics on the banned list, other alternatives had to be found. Namely, physical methods such as transfusions, catheterization, and urine substitution began to be utilized.

Beyond diuretics, renal blocking agents were used. The premise is a simple one: If one cannot eliminate the metabolites of anabolics/androgens out of one's system, then a person cannot get caught. Probenecid was the most common offender of the blocking agents. Medically, Probenecid is used in the prevention of gout and in the reduction of high uric acid levels, as well as an adjunct to antibiotic therapy by blocking renal excretion and thereby allowing for increased serum levels. This latter role is responsible for it being on the list of banned substances by the IOC, for if it retards the excretion of antibiotics, it follows that AASs and other doping agents would be blocked as well. Athletes taking Probenecid could, conceivably, continue using doping agents closer to competition and still deliver a clean test. Further success was achieved through the combination of multiple techniques: The Bulgarian weightlifting team would routinely fast about 2–3 days before a competition. Fasting lowers the amplitude and pulsatility of leuteinizing hormone (LH). Accordingly, endogenous production of testosterone (T) from the Leydig cells of the testes would also be lowered. Additionally, fasting also causes an increase in the excretion of steroids. In summation, the athlete's urine samples would exhibit lower levels of T and other aids because by the time they were sampled, they had eliminated most of the illegal substance(s) away. Add Probenecid to this technique, and a further benefit is achieved. When it became known that athletes were using Probenecid and other blocking agents, these drugs were promptly added to the banned list.

Relative to T, differentiating between endogenous and exogenous or pharmaceutical T is another problem. Although the IOC instituted a test for the 1984 Olympic Games, athletes have always found ways to counter this procedure. The test involves measuring the ratio of T metabolites found in urine to a second naturally occurring androgen: epitestosterone (E). To circumvent this, athletes inject with E—attainable via a Food and Drug Administration (FDA)-authorized prescription—in addition to T, thereby leaving this acceptable ratio unchanged. Naturally, the IOC placed E on the banned list.

In an effort to thwart this, technicians at the University of Iowa proposed measuring the ratio of T to that of LH. LH also controls the natural release of T; however, unlike E, it is currently unavailable in any FDA-approved formulation. In one study, the scientists showed that in measuring the concentration of LH in serum (blood) by immunoassay, and combining the value with gas chromatography and mass spectrometry levels of T in urine, a greater sensitivity for detecting T abuse was achieved when compared with the standard measure of T to E. Alternatively, athletes self-administer human chorionic gonadotropin (hCG) which stimulates the body to manufacture both T and E in the proper ratio.

Researchers at UCLA's Olympic Analytical Laboratory offered another weapon for detecting illicit T doping. In one study, scientists relied on subtle differences in ratios of carbon isotopes $^{12}C$ and $^{13}C$ to distinguish between endogenous T and exogenous T. Exogenously administered T, which is normally synthesized from plant sources, differs in the carbon isotope ratios from endogenous T. Athletes, with help from those in the know, stayed ahead of the game through the use of equine, bovine, and porcine extrapolations of T which contain isotopes with very similar ratios to endogenous human T.

The recent identification of tetrahydrogestrinone (THG), the first known "designer androgen," as a sports doping agent reflects both a sophisticated illicit manufacturing facility and an underground network of androgen abusers in elite sports. Never marketed, THG was apparently developed by BALCO (Bay Area Laboratory Cooperative) as a potent androgen that was undetectable by conventional IOC–mandated urinary sports doping tests. This was achieved by the built-in degradation quality of its chemical "signature" or structure when subjected to blood or urine sample analysis. Not entirely without benefit, this, and other "designer" AASs also offer the possibility of tissue-specific effects enhancing the beneficial medical effects of androgens while mitigating the undesirable ones.

In brief summation, it is evident that much research has been done and continues to be done on a variety of fronts to prohibit and terminate the use of banned substances. Yet, not surprisingly, even before said tests become used, the athletes are aware of the means to circumvent them. With this in mind, a proposition has arisen that the gathering of a longitudinal hormonal database profile of the athlete (a "Hematologic Passport") be attained in order to be used as a template for testing purposes. Although the idea seems far fetched, consider the concept of stem cells only a few short years ago.

## Chemistry/Physiology

The steroid T was first isolated from a bull in the 1930s, and the chemically modified analogs of T, the AASs, were synthesized shortly after.[4] T is the primary androgen secreted by the Leydig cells of the testes in males, and is secreted in small amounts by the theca cells of the ovaries, the adrenal cortex, and placenta. Pharmacologic development of AASs has focused on maximizing anabolic effects while minimizing androgenic effects (Table 23.2). An additional effect of these modifications to the T molecule has also resulted in a slower metabolic clearance of the hormone, and thus a prolonged time of action.

Physiologically, AASs are suspected to act in much the same way as endogenous T. The effects of T in humans (both males and females have androgen

**TABLE 23.2. Frequently used anabolic-androgenic steroids.**

| Name | Dosage form | Anabolic/androgenic activity |
|---|---|---|
| Dromostanolone | Injectable | 3:1 to 6:1 |
| Fluoxymesterone | Oral | 1:1 to 2:1 |
| Methyltestosterone | Oral | 1:1 |
| Nandrolone esters (decanoate, phenpropionate) | Injectable | 2.5:1 to 4:1 |
| Oxymetholone | Oral | 2.5:1 to 6:1 |
| Stanozolol | Oral | 3:1 to 6:1 |
| Testosterone esters (cypionate, enanthate, propionate) | Injectable | 1:1 |

receptors) generally occur through two main mechanisms[5]: first, by activation of the androgen receptor (either directly or as dihydrotestosterone [DHT]); second, the effects may be mediated by the conversion of T to estradiol (aromatization) and the subsequent activation of certain estrogen receptors. In the body, free and albumin-bound T traverses the plasma membrane of target tissue cells, where it may bind to an androgen receptor, or be reduced to 5α-DHT by a 5α-reductase enzyme. DHT may bind to the androgen receptor in a way which creates a potency of about 2.5 times that of T. The bound androgen-receptor complex undergoes a structural change that allows it to move into the nucleus and bind directly to specific nucleotide sequences of the chromosomal DNA. The areas of binding are called hormone response elements, and influence transcriptional activity of certain genes, producing androgenic effects including the promotion of protein synthesis, growth of muscle mass and strength, increased bone density and maturation, and numerous virilizing effects such as growth of the penis (enlargement of the clitoris in females), formation of the scrotum, and deepening of the voice, as well as beard and torso hair (the secondary male sexual characteristics).

As previously mentioned, T may also convert into estradiol via an enzymatic process known as aromatization. This conversion is essential during different periods of development, and estradiol has been demonstrated as a necessary stimulus for both bone maturation and brain development.[6] The latter effect is intriguing on several levels, because it represents a prenatal masculinization, with estradiol organizing the sexually dimorphic areas of the brain that will later account for male sexual behavior.

Finally, it has also been suggested that T and AASs may exert anabolic effects through a competition for receptor binding with the major catabolic steroid of the body (cortisol). In this latter role, androgens would be considered "anticatabolic" agents.[7]

## Effects on Performance

Because a fair amount of early published data on AASs relied on case reports and athletes who self-administered therapeutic doses of AASs, the validity of these studies is questionable. Certainly, it is well known that athletes often use more than one AAS concurrently (a practice known as "stacking," or more properly, polypharmacy) at dose levels and dose patterns vastly different from those studied by researchers. Also, AASs tend to have easily recognized side effects (thus making blinded placebo controls very difficult). Collectively, this makes the interpretation of scientific studies on AASs difficult to evaluate. That said, a meta-analysis published in 1999[8] considered 48 different studies, aggregating them into seven different outcomes. The authors concluded from their analysis that the majority of studies did not use sufficient numbers of participants to assess the effects they were hoping to measure. In short, most studies did not account for the influence of weight training alone, suggesting that any true phenomenon of AASs has yet to be accurately detected statistically. However, a number of studies have attempted to address these issues of study design, and have simultaneously demonstrated beneficial changes in body composition, and increases in strength concurrent with supraphysiologic (i.e., >300 mg/week of injectable T ester) doses of AASs.[9,10] Bhasin and colleagues have produced a number of published reports detailing the effects of T administration in humans.[11] Indeed, this research has been seminal in demonstrating T-associated increases in lean body mass and decreases in fat mass in both young and aged men.[12] Interestingly, the muscles of older men are as responsive to the anabolic effects of T as are the muscles of young men. Additionally, their work has also helped explain the observed androgen-induced changes in lean mass by substantiating the hypothesis that androgens promote the change of pluripotent mesenchymal cells into myogenic cells (muscle precursors),[13] and increase the number of resident muscle satellite cells which in turn leads to larger myofibers.[14]

## Side Effects/Contraindications

Assessing the side effects of AAS use by athletes has proven similarly difficult to the study of primary effects. However, numerous anecdotal reports exist. Indeed, any passing of a strength athlete seems to be received by some with a raised eyebrow. Several studies have actually attempted to estimate mortality rates and causes among both known and suspected users of AASs.[15,16] Mortality rates for AAS users have been estimated to be fourfold higher than age-matched controls, with causes of death varied but notable for the presence of violence. Both suicide and homicide are often implicated in the deaths of AAS users. Because other studies have documented an increased exhibition of aggressive and impulsive personality traits in AAS users, the suggestion has been made that the increased risk of violent death in AAS users is related to the propensity for impulsive, aggressive, or depressive behavior. These assertions, however, remain unproven empirically.

In addition to psychologic disturbances, numerous studies have shown AAS use as a correlate of virilization of females, liver damage, testicular atrophy, increased blood pressure, atherogenic blood lipid profiles, and cardiovascular disease. However, a 3-month post-AAS use follow-up study revealed a return to normal-range liver enzyme levels, lipid profiles, and blood pressure.[17] These results suggest that some of the AAS-associated effects may be reversible with discontinuation. Indeed, recent reviews[18,19] as well have concluded that the side effects from AASs have been historically overstated.

One clearly irreversible consequence of AAS usage reflects the poor hygiene sometimes associated with parenteral drug use.[20] Sadly, both hepatitis and human immunodeficiency viruses have been noted in needle-sharing AAS users.

Finally, increased levels of AASs or T in children have been associated with precocious puberty and premature epiphyseal closure, leading to a diminished potential adult height.[21]

## Banned

Although there are medical indications for the use of AASs, they are currently banned by the World Anti-Doping Agency (WADA), the IOC, the National Collegiate Athletic Association (NCAA), and all major North American professional sports leagues—the National Football League, Major League Baseball, the National Hockey League, the National Basketball Association, and Major League Soccer (MLS). Banning regulations and testing procedures have been recently complicated by the ongoing development of newer, "designer" steroids. These compounds do not always fall within the language of the regulations, nor do they necessarily result in a positive drug test.

## Legality

AASs are legally available with a physician's prescription when used for treatment of an approved indication.

## Sidebar 23.2. The Rule of Law—A Brief History of the Legalities of Anabolic Steroids and Their Precursors

### Richard D. Collins

The legislative history of anabolic steroids and their metabolic precursors demonstrates the complexities of classifying ergogenic substances and distinguishing drugs from dietary supplements.

In the 1980s, anabolic steroids were regulated by the FDA as prescription drugs. Although the IOC had banned anabolic steroids since 1975, Canadian sprinter Ben Johnson's highly publicized 1988 doping violation suggested that sports bodies needed help in ensuring a level playing field. Congress held hearings as to whether steroids should be scheduled as controlled substances such as cocaine, heroin, and LSD. Most of the witnesses who testified, including representatives of the American Medical Association, FDA, Drug Enforcement Administration (DEA), and National Institute on Drug Abuse, recommended against scheduling, maintaining that steroid abuse does not lead to the physical or psychologic dependence required under the Controlled Substances Act.

Congress voted nevertheless to schedule anabolic steroids, placing them under DEA authority. The Anabolic Steroids Control Act of 1990 (ASCA) inserted 27 steroids, along with their muscle-building salts, esters, and isomers, in the same legal class—Schedule III—as barbiturates, LSD precursors, ketamine, and narcotic painkillers such as Vicodin. Simple possession of any Schedule III substance is a federal offense punishable by up to 1 year in prison and/or a minimum fine of $1000 for a first offense. Distributing steroids, or possessing them with intent to distribute, is a federal felony punishable by up to 5 years in prison (10 years for a prior drug offender) and/or a $250,000 fine.

The ASCA diverted anabolic steroids almost exclusively to the burgeoning black market, increasing demand for legally available muscle-building alternatives. Dietary supplements containing androstenedione (andro) were introduced in the mid-1990s and were promoted as a natural way to help increase strength and muscle mass. Andro opened the door for many other "prohormone" and "prosteroid" products to be developed that were not listed, and could not be barred, under the ASCA. They were instead marketed as dietary supplements under the Dietary Supplement Health and Education Act of 1994 (DSHEA), even though not all of the products seemed to be in compliance.

As these products proliferated, sometimes hawked with outlandish claims, critics suggested that some were actually anabolic steroids masquerading as supplements, citing loopholes in both DSHEA and the ASCA. Sports bodies and legislators began decrying the availability of these products, particularly to young athletes.

Although DSHEA provides the FDA ample enforcement authority to protect the public health and remove noncompliant supplements, legislative solutions were explored in an effort to redefine "anabolic steroids" to encompass these products. Congress passed a bill in October 2004 that will expand the list of anabolic steroids to include many of the precursor products currently marketed. Once in effect, the law will subject possessors and distributors of these products to the same penalties as possessors and distributors of traditional anabolic steroids.

Editors' note: The Anabolic Steroid Control Act of 2004 made practically all precursors ("prohormones"), excluding DHEA, illegal.

Rick Collins is a practicing lawyer (www.cmgesq.com), and serves as counsel to organizations including the International Society of Sports Nutrition and the United Supplement Freedom Association.

## STEROID PROHORMONES

### Overview of Use

The steroid prohormones exist as a class of compounds that have been putatively marketed as precursors of either T or one of the AASs. Some of the compounds are modified in such a way that metabolic conversion in the liver should theoretically yield an anabolic product. The list of available compounds increased yearly throughout the 1990s; however, the most frequently studied compounds have been andro and dehydroepiandrosterone (DHEA). Andro has been modified and marketed in a number of differing molecular configurations, but none has gained particular notoriety for an accepted medical or ergogenic use.[22,23] Only DHEA has found some acceptance among the medical community as a replacement for T decreases in aged men, and the suggestion from in vitro research that it may convey some degree of immune system enhancement.[24,25] However, physician reports of clinical observations regarding DHEA are varied and do not suggest a pattern of efficacy. The extent of the use of prohormones by athletes is unknown; however, the use of these preparations seems to be based on the intuitive notion that AAS-like improvements in strength and lean body mass will be consequent.

## Chemistry/Physiology

Although not true of all prohormone compounds, both andro and DHEA are endogenous weakly androgenic steroid products of the adrenal cortex. As previously mentioned, the marketing claim is based on the potential to bio-convert prohormones into either T or an AAS, thus allowing them to have similar physiologic effects to the former compounds. Several studies have attempted to examine this assertion by examining the effects of andro supplementation. Only a few investigators have demonstrated modest increases in T in males,[23,26] although it is well established that T levels may significantly increase in females.[27] The ironic finding in many studies with andro is that whereas T levels may remain statistically unchanged in males, the level of serum estrogens is significantly increased. For a more detailed review of prohormones, see Ziegenfuss et al.[28]

## Effects on Performance

Because the majority of studies have used andro as the prototypical prohormone, no generalized conclusions can be made regarding performance effects for all prohormone preparations. However, the authors are unaware of any published studies that have demonstrated a significant improvement in muscle mass, strength, or other markers of performance enhancement from andro supplementation.

Several researchers have demonstrated positive effects of DHEA in rats.[29–31] An important issue overlooked in some promotional marketing is that rats do not normally have appreciable concentrations of DHEA, and thus their biologic responses may be different than those in humans. Furthermore, the initially promising in vitro effects of DHEA on immune function do not seem to be manifest in vivo. In younger, physically active men and women, no study has demonstrated a DHEA-associated increase in serum T concentration, reduction in body fat, or performance enhancement.

## Side Effects/Contraindications

Because prohormones share metabolites with T and many of the AASs, the side effect profiles and contraindications are reasoned to be similar. Indeed, decreased high density lipoprotein levels and gonadal axis disruption have been demonstrated with the use of some prohormones.[22] It is recommended that women in particular avoid using prohormones because of the androgen-induced increase in virilization. Furthermore, as previously noted, sustained elevated androgen levels in children have been associated with precocious puberty and premature epiphyseal closure.

## Banned

Andro and DHEA are banned by the same sport governing bodies as AASs. Because the many chemical analogs of andro share metabolites with certain AASs (such as nandrolone decanoate), most sport governing bodies consider them to be AASs.

## Legality

Except for DHEA, prohormones are illegal to possess.

## THYROID HORMONES

### Overview of Use

The thyroid hormones are dipeptide molecules that have attached either 3 (triiodothyronine or T3) or 4 (tetraiodothyronine, thyroxine, or T4) iodines.[2] The general metabolic stimulant activity of the thyroid hormones has been known, and used therapeutically, since the 1800s in the form of desiccated animal thyroid gland. Current medical uses are principally directed at using synthetic forms of thyroid hormone to treat an underactive thyroid gland (hypothyroidism). The use of thyroid hormones among athletes seems to be predicated upon their effects as metabolic stimulants, and therefore are taken to enhance weight loss.

### Chemistry/Physiology

The physiology of the thyroid is interdependent with the functioning of both the hypothalamus and pituitary. The hypothalamus is responsible for synthesizing thyrotropin-releasing hormone (TRH), which passes through the hypophyseal portal venous system to reach the anterior pituitary. At the anterior pituitary, thyroid-stimulating hormone (TSH) production and release is provoked by TRH. TSH, once released into the general circulation, will reach the thyroid gland and cause both an increase in production and release of the thyroid hormones (T3 and T4). The control loop is regulated by negative feedback of the thyroid hormones on the pituitary.

The thyroid hormones originate in the follicular cells of the thyroid gland as thyroid colloid, which is a glycoprotein comprised largely of thyroglobulin.[2] Thyroglobulin is mainly composed of iodinated tyrosine residues, which are the direct precursors of the thyroid hormone. Proteolysis of thyroglobulin creates the active hormones T3 and T4, which are then secreted into the blood. Whereas T3 is the more metabolically potent hormone (3–5×), approximately 90% of the released thyroid hormone is in the form of T4. However, T3 still has an important role because the majority of biologically active T3 (80%–90%) is produced by the peripheral conversion of T4 via a 5'-deiodinase enzyme.

The mechanism of action of T3 is somewhat unusual considering that the hormone is peptide based.[32] It acts at the level of the DNA, much like that of the steroid hormones. Interaction of T3 inside cells produces increases in basal metabolic consumption of oxygen, increased metabolism of macronutrients, modulation of other hormone effects, and it seems to have an essential role in growth and maturation of the central nervous system.

### Effects on Performance

Although supplementation with thyroid hormones has not been exclusively studied in athletes, and no evidence supporting their use as performance enhancers currently exists, there are a number of documented effects that may have substantiated their use by sport competitors. Indeed, T3 has demonstrated an important thermogenic function, and has been used as a therapeutic intervention with selected obese individuals.[33] Furthermore, the thyroid hormones have been shown to up-regulate more than 380 genes critical for skeletal muscle function.[34] Among the affected genes are those concerned with a wide range of cellular functions including transcriptional control, mRNA maturation, protein turnover, signal transduction, cellular trafficking, and energy metabolism. Finally, thyroid hormone levels have previously been shown to directly regulate the sarcoplasmic reticulum protein levels.[35] Research in this area has led to the speculation that thyroid hormones may alter calcium concentration, and thus influence the process of excitation-contraction coupling in skeletal muscles.

## Side Effects/Contraindications

In general, unwanted side effects of thyroid hormone usage appear in the same constellation of symptoms as hyperthyroidism (overactive thyroid gland).[36] Typical among those are complaint of headache, irritability, nervousness, sweating, cardiac arrhythmia (especially tachycardia), increased body temperature, increased bowel motility, and menstrual irregularities. If symptoms such as cardiac arrhythmia and increased body temperature become fulminant, a life-threatening condition known as thyroid storm may develop. Thyroid hormones are also well known for their potential to alter or accelerate the metabolism of numerous pharmacologic compounds. Anyone supplementing with thyroid hormones and taking other medications should seek consultation with a knowledgeable physician or other qualified healthcare provider.

## Banned

The thyroid hormones are not currently banned by any sporting organization.

## Legality

The thyroid hormones are legally available via a physician's prescription for treatment of an approved indication.

# GROWTH HORMONE

## Overview of Use

Human growth hormone (hGH), a 191 amino acid protein secreted by the anterior pituitary (adenohypophysis), is sometimes also referred to as somatotropin. It was identified in the 1920s as a growth-promoting factor, and for many years pharmacologic hGH consisted of a purified derivative of cadaverous pituitary glands. Since the 1980s, hGH produced in bacteria using recombinant DNA technology has been available for use, eliminating concerns about potential contamination with prions or viruses. Available only by physician prescription, therapeutic uses of growth hormone include children and adults with short stature or growth hormone deficiency, and individuals afflicted with diseases characterized by muscle wasting and weakness (such as AIDS). Because of the association between hGH treatment and syndromes of short stature or muscle wasting, athletes have attempted to use hGH to stimulate growth and enhance performance.

## Chemistry/Physiology

hGH is secreted into the blood from the somatotrope cells of the adenohypophysis.[2] Control of hGH release resides largely in several hypothalamic nuclei which release factors into the venous portal system which drains down through the pituitary. Growth hormone–releasing hormone from the arcuate nucleus, and the gut hormone ghrelin promote hGH secretion, and somatostatin (or growth hormone release inhibiting hormone) from the periventricular nucleus suppresses hGH release. The balance of the releasing and inhibiting hormones is in turn affected by many physiologic or constitutional factors. hGH release may be positively influenced by sleep, heavy weightlifting exercise, states of hypoglycemia, and dietary protein/amino acid supplementation. Inhibition of hGH secretion may be influenced by high dietary carbohydrate and increased serum glucocorticoids (both endogenous and exogenous).

hGH secretion tends to occur in several pulses of pituitary release every day.[37] Pulses generally last between 10–30 minutes. However, the largest pulses usually occur shortly after (1–4 hours) the onset of sleep. The amount and pattern of GH secretion change throughout life, with the greatest basal levels during childhood, the highest pulses during adolescence, and a gradual decline throughout adulthood.

As its name implies, growth and anabolism are the effects generally ascribed to hGH.[38] These effects seem to be stimulated via two main mechanisms. First, hGH can directly stimulate epiphyseal chondrocytes to divide and multiply, thus laying the groundwork for growth of the long bones. Second, hGH will also stimulate the production of insulinlike growth factor 1 (IGF-1, also known as somatomedin C) in the liver. hGH in synergy with IGF-1 has growth-stimulating effects on a wide variety of tissues (see IGF-1 section).

Overall, hGH stimulates a host of body processes, including increases in calcium retention, the mineralization of bone, and increases in muscle mass.[39] It favors protein synthesis and as a result, helps create a positive nitrogen balance (or more accurately, nitrogen "status") within the body. These latter muscle-building effects make it an attractive "partitioning agent" when used in the cattle industry to produce leaner beef. However, where human athletes are concerned, the potentially positive effects of hGH on muscle hypertrophy are not matched by increases in strength. Indeed, individuals with acromegaly (oversecretion of hGH in the adult) may actually have a myopathy in which there are larger but functionally weaker muscles.[40] hGH also decreases the liver uptake of glucose, and promotes lipolysis, functions that make it something of an antagonist to the hormone insulin. However, it has previously been demonstrated that for the normal physiologic actions of hGH, insulin must also be present.

## Effects on Performance

There is a paucity of research concerning the effects of hGH in athletes. Most research regarding the effects of hGH supplementation has been accomplished with elderly men. Presently, supplementation in the hGH-deficient elderly has not demonstrated any effect on muscular strength. Other investigators have noted modest improvements in nitrogen balance, but this effect seems to be transient, lasting only a few weeks into hGH therapy. Supplementation with hGH has demonstrated increases in lean body mass, but these changes occurred in nonmuscular tissues. Furthermore, in a study involving weightlifters, no increases in amino acid incorporation into skeletal muscle were noted. Currently, there is no published evidence to support an hGH-associated improvement in athletic performance. That said, some athletes have suggested that the benefits of hGH are only manifested when it is combined with AASs. This is yet another untested assertion.

## Side Effects/Contraindications

As previously noted, hGH administration can lead to a myopathy characterized by functionally weaker muscles. Additionally, chronic use of hGH may lead to insulin resistance, effectively producing a diabetes-like state. Additional documented side effects include abnormal growth of bones (acromegaly) and internal organs such as the heart, kidneys, and liver, accelerated atherosclerosis (hardening of the arteries), and hypertension (high blood pressure). Less frequently, repeated use of hGH has resulted in nerve entrapments such as carpal tunnel syndrome (median neuropathy at the wrist).

## Banned

hGH is banned by all the major North American sport governing bodies.

## Legality

hGH is legally available via a physician's prescription for treatment of an approved indication.

# INSULIN

## Overview of Use

First isolated in the 1920s, insulin is a 51 amino acid peptide hormone that is released from the beta cells of the pancreatic islets in response to hyperglycemia (high blood glucose). It has been used extensively as an injectable replacement hormone in the treatment of diabetes mellitus. Previously, the most often used insulin preparation was from bovine and porcine sources. However, modern preparations are actually human insulin cultivated from bacteria engineered with recombinant DNA technology. Insulin is administered via an intramuscular or intravenous delivery, usually more than once per day, in response to monitored blood glucose levels. Use of insulin by athletes has emerged because of the role it has in facilitating the uptake of glucose and amino acids by numerous body tissues.

## Chemistry/Physiology

Insulin is a small protein hormone that exists as two peptide chains held together by disulfide bonds. Its structure is highly conserved across vertebrate species, thus allowing for the use of bovine and porcine insulin in humans. Insulin is synthesized and secreted from the beta cells of the pancreatic islets. Originally synthesized as a single polypeptide chain, it undergoes posttranslational processing to achieve the final disulfide linked form.

The secretion of insulin is primarily in response to elevated blood concentrations of glucose.[41] However, increased blood concentrations of other macronutrient molecules, including certain amino acids and fatty acids, may also promote insulin secretion.

In nearly all body tissues except brain and liver, insulin binds to a surface receptor that activates cytoplasmic glucose transporters to fuse with the cell membrane and allow for an increase in glucose uptake by the cell, thus lowering the blood glucose level.[42] Although insulin is not necessary for glucose uptake by the liver, it is stimulatory of a number of other functions including glucose storage in the form of glycogen, and increased fatty acid synthesis. Furthermore, because insulin drives most cells to preferentially use carbohydrates, it has an overall fat-sparing effect on the body. Insulin will also stimulate the uptake of amino acids, a role that complements its overall anabolic effect. A final, although sometimes clinically important, role of insulin is the positive effect it has on the sodium-potassium ATPase (pump), causing a cellular influx of potassium.

## Effects on Performance

Although it has been known for some time that insulin-treated diabetics have an increase in lean body mass as compared with matched controls, insulin supplementation has not been studied in the context of sport.[43] However, a number of case reports do exist documenting its use among nondiabetic athletes.[44,45] These case studies suggest that insulin is being used in conjunction with AASs, to create a potential synergy between steroid-influenced muscle building and insulin-facilitated muscle uptake of glucose and amino acids. This presumption is grounded in a reported phenomenon, known as the hyperinsulinemic clamp, in which hyperinsulinemia (high insulin level in the blood) can stimulate bulk glycogen and protein synthesis in the presence of hyperglycemia (high level of glucose in the blood) and hyperaminoacidemia (high amino acid level in the blood), however this has not yet been empirically demonstrated in athletes.

## Side Effects/Contraindications

Although insulin may interact with a number of other pharmacologic preparations, the cautionary side effect of note is a potentially lethal hypoglycemic reaction.[46] Indeed, this is one of the most frequent adverse effects experienced by diabetic users of insulin. It is generally a consequence of either taking too much insulin, eating too little, presence of an infection, or engaging in additional exercise near the regular time of dosing. Symptoms of hypoglycemia may occur suddenly, and can include sweating, dizziness, palpitation, anxiety, blurred vision, slurred speech, unsteady movement, headache, personality changes, disorientation, seizures, and unconsciousness. If such a condition is rapidly assessed, it can be helped by administering fruit juice, or other carbohydrate-containing drink.

### Banned

Insulin supplementation is currently banned by the IOC and WADA.

### Legality

Insulin is legally available over the counter in many states, and via a physician's prescription, for treatment of an approved indication.

## INSULINLIKE GROWTH FACTOR 1

### Overview of Use

IGF-1 (or somatomedin C) is a single-chain polypeptide of 70 amino acids that is secreted mainly by the liver in response to stimulation by hGH.[2] It seems to work in conjunction with hGH as a trophic factor; however, its present clinical use is as a marker in the diagnosis of human growth disorders. It has gained interest among athletes because of its putative anabolic and lipolytic activities.

### Chemistry/Physiology

Although the main source of production of IGF-1 is the liver, many other tissues are capable of synthesizing it.[47] It is thought that IGF-1 exerts anabolic effects through induction of amino acid transporters in the cell membrane. However, more scrutiny has been focused on the apparent influence IGF-1 has on neuronal structure and function. For example, IGF-1 has demonstrated an ability to preserve nerve cell function and promote nerve growth in experimental studies. As a result of this research, recombinant human IGF-1 is in clinical trials for the treatment of the neurodegenerative disease, amyotrophic lateral sclerosis. Alternatively, its mitogenic activity has created interest in a possible role for IGF-1 in cancer growth, particularly prostate cancer.

### Effects on Performance

There is a paucity of research concerning both the physiologic effects of IGF-1, and the claims made in the marketing of supplemental IGF-1. Indeed, no substantive research exists for most of the putative benefits of IGF-1 supplementation. Among the claims are anti-aging effects, enhancement of lean muscle mass, improved athletic and sexual performance, protection of joints, immune system enhancement, and neuroprotection. Recent research in the rat model has demonstrated that treatment with direct injection of IGF-1 significantly decreased the time until functional recovery and diminished the maximal functional deficit incurred after transection of the Achilles tendon.[48] Rodents have also demonstrated improvements in muscle mass.[49] However, regarding the use of supplemental IGF-1 for improvement of lean muscle mass in humans, research involving high-dose administration failed to produce more than very modest anabolic effects in AIDS patients.[50] Furthermore, orally administered supplemental IGF-1 has very poor bioavailability. As yet, there is no credible evidence that IGF-1 is absorbed from the oral mucosa, and the amounts that are ingested are probably digested like any other protein would be in the gut. As research continues, it is possible that some clinical indications for the use of IGF-1 will emerge. However, whatever therapeutic promise IGF-1 ultimately shows, its utility will depend on the validity of its association with an elevated risk of several cancers, most notably cancer of the prostate.[51]

## Side Effects/Contraindications

There are no documented acute adverse reactions or interactions for IGF-1 supplementation. However, given its functional similarities to hGH, it is possible that any side effect profile that might emerge would be similar to that of hGH. Additionally, given the mitogenic potential of IGF-1, its use is not recommended for those with any evidence of active malignancy.

## Banned

IGF-1 is banned by the IOC and WADA.

## Legality

Recombinant human IGF-1 is currently undergoing clinical trials, and is not available to the general public. Naturally sourced (often extracted from deer antler velvet) IGF-1 is available and marketed as a dietary supplement, usually in the form of an oral spray.

# HUMAN CHORIONIC GONADOTROPHIN

## Overview of Use

hCG is a glycoprotein composed of an alpha subunit and a beta subunit, and is secreted by the trophoblast (layer of cells which gives rise to the placenta). Structurally similar to the gonadotropins, LH, and follicle-stimulating hormone (FSH), hCG acts in much the same way. With females it has been used clinically in both urinary-derived and recombinant human forms to enhance assisted reproductive technologies such as oocyte harvesting which precedes in vitro fertilization. hCG has been used in hypogonadic males to stimulate T production. Similarly, male athletes have also used hCG as a potentiator of endogenous T production, often after down-regulating their own testicular T production with the prolonged use of AASs.

## Chemistry/Physiology

In pregnant females, the trophoblastic cells (chorionic villi) surrounding the implanted ovum secrete hCG, which serves to prolong the existence of the corpus luteum.[2] This results in the continued production of estrogen and progesterone, and therefore the continued maintenance of the endometrium. During early pregnancy, hCG appears in maternal blood and is excreted in the urine, allowing for the rapid diagnosis of pregnancy by testing for hCG, in particular its unique beta subunit. The alpha subunit of hCG shares significant homology with the alpha subunits of LH, FSH, and TSH.

## Effects on Performance

Although no direct assessment of specific performance markers in participants taking only hCG has been attempted, a number of other investigations concerning hCG effects have been undertaken. A study involving both trained and untrained males demonstrated a significant increase in the basal plasma T levels in response to repeated hCG stimulation of the trained participants.[52] Furthermore, in an additional study, androgen response was analyzed before and after a single dose of hCG in six power athletes, who had used high doses of AASs for 3 months.[53] Although the hCG was administered 3 weeks after the cessation of AAS use, the study subjects were still characterized by hypogonadism. After hCG injection, serum T and DHT concentrations increased significantly. These results demonstrate that during transient hypogonadism in adult men, there is testicular responsiveness to a single injection of hCG.

Anecdotal evidence suggests that many users of AASs will also supplement concurrently with hCG in the hope that the latter will maintain gonadal function. A study examining the effects of combined AASs/hCG was accomplished using a cohort of such male users.[54] The study revealed that the concomitant abuse of hCG and supraphysiologic AAS dosages may cause transient impairment on semen quality in males, while maintaining spermatogenesis.

## Side Effects/Contraindications

At clinically used doses, other than possible interference with pregnancy testing, no major side effects or contraindications have been reported. However, given that hCG may be used to enhance endogenous T production, it is possible that a side-effect profile similar to AAS use may emerge, particularly gynecomastia.

## Banned

hCG is banned by the IOC, WADA, and the NCAA.

## Legality

hCG is legally available with a physician's prescription when used for treatment of an approved indication.

# ERYTHROPOIETIN

## Overview of Use

EPO is a protein hormone made primarily in the cortex of the kidneys that can stimulate the production of erythrocytes (red blood cells).[55] Although not isolated until the 1950s, the existence of EPO had been postulated for some 50 years prior when it was noted that injection of plasma from a previously bled animal into a normal recipient caused reticulocytosis (increase in immature erythrocytes in circulation). Pharmacologic human EPO is manufactured using recombinant DNA technology. It has been used clinically to treat individuals with failing kidneys, who lose their ability to produce EPO and ultimately become anemic. EPO has also been used to treat the anemia that is often consequent to certain drug therapies (i.e., chemotherapy of cancer, AIDS). EPO may also be used to improve circulatory function after blood loss for individuals whose religion forbids the use of blood transfusion (Jehovah's Witnesses). Because of EPO's effect on red cell indices, it has also been used by endurance athletes to improve their oxygen delivery and ultimately enhance their performance.

## Chemistry/Physiology

EPO is a glycoprotein produced by peritubular cells in the kidneys of the adult, and in liver cells (hepatocytes) in the fetus. Small amounts of extrarenal EPO are produced by the liver and brain of adults.

The primary action of EPO seems to be the rescue of erythroid cells from apoptosis (programmed cell death), thus increasing their survival time in circulation.[55] EPO also acts in synergy with a number of cytokine growth factors to promote maturation and proliferation of erythroid progenitor cells, thus creating more erythrocytes. Regulation of EPO production is thought to be oxygen-dependent, with relative and absolute hypoxia acting as stimulants.

## Effects on Performance

Use of EPO can be traced to a practice known as "blood doping," which has been in use by endurance athletes since the 1960s.[56] Blood doping involved the intravascular infusion of either donated, or the athlete's own, packed red blood cells. This immediate increase in hematocrit was shown to increase both the oxygen-carrying capacity and the time until exhaustion. EPO works in much the same way, but without the necessity of transfusion and storing of blood products.

The few studies that have examined the ergogenic potential of EPO have demonstrated improvements in performance similar to those noted for blood doping.[57,58] Indeed, a quick PubMed search will reveal numerous studies illustrating the positive effects of EPO on hematocrit, maximal oxygen uptake, and aerobic performance.

## Side Effects/Contraindications

Because EPO increases the erythrocyte concentration (hematocrit) beyond physiologically normal levels, this leads to an increase in blood viscosity. The increase in viscosity creates additional risk for both cardiac failure and intravascular clotting (thrombosis), which in turn increases the possibility of stroke or tissue infarction. Indeed, since 1987, the year pharmacologic EPO was initially released to the European market, a number of long-distance cyclists have died from thrombotic/embolic causes, such as stroke, myocardial infarction, and pulmonary embolism.[59]

## Banned

EPO is banned by the IOC, WADA, NCAA, MLS, and the International Cycling Union.

## Legality

EPO is legally available with a physician's prescription when used for treatment of an approved indication.

# ADRENOCORTICOTROPIC HORMONE AND CORTISOL

## Overview of Use

Adrenocorticotropic hormone (ACTH) and cortisol are products of the anterior pituitary-adrenal cortex axis, with ACTH acting as the stimulus for cortisol release.[60] Several manufactured derivatives of cortisol exist (e.g., prednisone, hydrocortisone, dexamethasone), and are used to provide relief of injury or illness-induced inflammation and allergic/hypersensitivity reactions. They are also used as part of the chemotherapy of cancer, asthma, certain forms of arthritis, and autoimmune diseases. The administration of ACTH is largely limited to its use as a testing agent for adrenal sensitivity and response. Endurance athletes have attempted to use both ACTH and corticosteroids to increase maximal performance by increasing the availability of glucose to exercising muscles, and through a psychologic component described as a "feeling of well-being" or euphoria.

## Chemistry/Physiology

The physiologic corticosteroid of greatest importance in human beings is cortisol.[61] It is mainly produced in the middle zone of the adrenal cortex, the zona fasciculata, in response to ACTH released from the anterior pituitary. The secretion of ACTH is stimulated by the release of corticotropin-releasing factor from the hypothalamus, which in turn is influenced by a number of physiologic or psychologic stressors (fear, pain, exhaustion, low blood sugar, strenuous exercise, infections). Both ACTH and cortisol levels rise and fall in a circadian cycle, with cortisol levels generally highest in the waking hours of the morning (post-fasting).

Cortisol serves many functions, including participation in the regulation of the body's use of proteins, carbohydrates, and fats.[61] Indeed, cortisol may stimulate the breakdown of muscle protein, leading to a use of the released amino acids in the synthesis of new glucose in the liver (i.e., gluconeogenesis). This "new glucose" is subsequently released into the circulation for distribution to the tissues of the body. Cortisol may also prompt the release of fatty acids into the circulation. Both processes help ensure that circulating levels of macronutrients will be maintained, thus assuring the availability of energy during times of stress.

## Effects on Performance

Although the claims that ACTH and corticosteroids will enhance maximal performance have apparently been accepted by many athletes, they have never been empirically established. Indeed, very little research exists on the topic of corticosteroid effects on performance. However, at least one study has attempted to distinguish between physiologic and psychologic aspects of performance enhancement.[62] In one study, 1 mg of either ACTH or placebo was injected into 16 professional cyclists. After cycling, no increase of maximal performance was observed with ACTH, on either the day of administration, or on the subsequent day. Subjective complaint of fatigue was diminished only during submaximal exercise (during the ACTH trial).

## Side Effects/Contraindications

Corticosteroids are well known, and widely utilized, for their immunosuppressive effects. However, although this attribute may be effective in the treatment of certain immunopathies, it will often lead to a decreased resistance to disease and infection. Because of the corticosteroid effects on elevating circulating glucose levels, it is effectively an antagonist to insulin. The release of insulin will increase to compete with the corticosteroids, in an effort to maintain homeostatic levels of blood glucose. Abruptly discontinuing the use of corticosteroids will result in an "over-secretion" of insulin, and subsequent hypoglycemia. This phenomenon, along with disruption of the adrenal axis, accounts for the reason corticosteroids are often prescribed in a descending dose pattern. Obviously, the use of corticosteroids in hypoglycemic or hyperglycemic (diabetic) individuals requires careful monitoring. Prolonged use of corticosteroids may lead to an "insulin insensitivity" or even "beta cell burnout," in which the ability to produce insulin is exhausted (effectively creating a new diabetic patient).

Corticosteroids have also been known to cause fluid and electrolyte disturbances, muscle weakness and loss of muscle mass, ulcerative esophagitis and peptic ulcer, impaired wound healing, and suppression of growth in children.[61]

Chronic use of ACTH may lead to anterior pituitary atrophy (because it replaces the normal pituitary output), which may lead to an "empty sella syndrome" and subsequent decreases in output of all the anterior pituitary hormones.[63]

## Banned

Corticosteroids are banned by the IOC, WADA, and the NCAA. Topical application, inhalation, and intraarticular or local injection are permitted by IOC/WADA, although reporting is mandatory.

## Legality

Corticosteroids are legally available over the counter in many topical lotion preparations, and via a physician's prescription, for treatment of an approved indication. ACTH is available only via a physician's prescription.

## Sidebar 23.3. The Brave New World—Gene Doping

*Rita Mengerink*

According to WADA, gene or cell doping is defined as "the non-therapeutic use of cells, genes, genetic elements, or the modulation of gene expression, having the capacity to enhance athletic performance."[64] Originally developed for therapeutic uses in conditions such as anemia and muscular dystrophy, gene doping is now referenced in the list of banned substances and methods in sports by the IOC, in collaboration with WADA.[64] Gene-transfer technology presents a new threat to the integrity of fair sports competition, because detection of its use requires methods exceedingly more complex than those of current pharmacologic means.

Discovery of genetic mutations that enhance physical parameters have been demonstrated in both human and animal populations. The phenomena of hyperplasia, increased muscular hypertrophy, and decreased body fat have been documented in cattle, particularly with the higher frequencies seen in the Belgian Blue and Piedmontese breeds.[65–68] These traits make a significant impact on meat yield and quality, both important economic aspects to beef production.[65] Recent studies have discovered that a defective myostatin (or growth/differentiation factor 8 [GDF-8]) gene is at least partly responsible for such findings in cattle,[66] and that purposeful disruption of the gene in mice produces similar phenotypes.[67] Myostatin controls muscle cell number and size by inhibiting myoblast proliferation. Therefore, if this gene is disrupted, muscle cell hyperplasia and hypertrophy can continue unchecked. Previously undocumented in humans, a myostatin mutation was recently revealed in a child developing extreme muscularity.[68]

While scientists are closely following the changes in "Baby Superman" as he matures, pharmaceutical companies have already designed a protein (MYO-029) putatively capable of disrupting myostatin (currently in clinical trials).[69] The confirmation of myostatin's role as a negative regulator of muscle growth in humans sparks interest for its potential in treating muscular dystrophy, yet also opens the door for myostatin-blocked athletes with strength and power capabilities far beyond those seen today.

Illicit use of exogenous EPO has been possible since 1989, when it was made available commercially for treatment of anemia. The 1998 Tour de France brought attention to its use in elite cyclists, as a team masseur was caught with EPO among other illegal performance-enhancing substances. Gene-doping technology might be able to turn the ordinary distance runner into another Eero Mäntyranta, the Finnish cross-country skier who won two gold metals at the 1964 Winter Olympics. Mäntyranta and his family had a genetic mutation that caused a defect in the EPO receptor, preventing the inhibitory feedback needed to turn off RBC production. Consequently the oxygen-carrying capacity of his blood was significantly higher (25%–50%) than that of his peers, giving him a distinct advantage in the endurance-oriented sport.[70]

IGF-1 might also be an appealing target for gene doping, because its actions might delay the effects of aging on elite athletes. Mechano Growth Factor (MGF-1), an isoform of IGF-1, might also be in athletes' crosshairs, because it is activated by the intense physical activity common to all athletes' training programs.[71] Research has demonstrated the ability of IGF-1 in increasing muscle mass and strength in young mice, as well as increasing strength in older muscles.[72] A proposed theory of age-related skeletal muscle loss is that the ability to repair damage caused by muscular activity decreases over time. By stimulating satellite cells to build new muscle tissue, gene therapy with IGF-1 and/or MGF-1 could be beneficial to patients with accelerated muscle loss, but might also lead to abuse in the athletic arena.

The well-publicized Human Genome Project remains at the forefront in solving many mysteries of human disease, yet it undoubtedly holds the key to enhanced athletic performance through manipulation of the same principles. Anti-doping technology will likely struggle to keep pace with an emerging technology that promises to change the very essence of the athlete: the DNA.

## SUMMARY

Numerous hormones and hormone supplements are used by athletes in the hope of improving performance (Table 23.3). Often, the marketing claims and gym lore regarding the utility of a given supplement do not agree with empirically obtained evidence. It is incumbent upon those who work with athletes to maintain a solid knowledge base regarding the science of hormone supplementation, as well as cultivate a process of critically appraising the current literature regarding hormone supplements. Indeed, it is likely that the science of hormonal manipulation will continue to evolve (literally, see Sidebar 23.3), and the rules and records will change to reflect modern athletes and their drive to succeed.

TABLE 23.3. Hormone supplements: putative effects, documented effects, and associated sports.

| Hormone supplement | Putative effects in athletes | Documented effects | Athlete/sport association |
|---|---|---|---|
| Adrenocorticotropic hormone and cortisol | Improve endurance performance and psychologic sense of well-being | No improvements in performance, but did decrease complaint of fatigue during submaximal exercise | Endurance athletes: distance runners and cyclists |
| Androstenedione and dehydroepiandrosterone | Increases muscle mass and strength, reduction in body fat | No significant improvement in muscle mass or strength or reduction in body fat | Power athletes; weightlifters, sprinters, throwers, football and hockey players, and wrestlers |
| Erythropoietin | Increase in endurance performance | Improves both oxygen-carrying capacity of the blood and time until exhaustion | Endurance athletes; distance runners and cyclists |
| Growth hormone | Increases muscle mass and strength, reduction in body fat | Increases in nonmuscular lean body mass, but no improvements in performance | Power athletes; weightlifters, sprinters, throwers, football and hockey players, and wrestlers |
| Human chorionic gonadotropin | Increases muscle mass and strength via increasing testosterone production, maintain testicular function while using anabolic-androgenic steroids | Increases testosterone levels, maintains spermatogenesis, but previous anabolic-androgenic steroid users still qualify as hypogonadal even with human chorionic gonadotropin use | Power athletes; weightlifters, sprinters, throwers, football and hockey players, and wrestlers |
| Insulin | Increases muscle mass | No empiric demonstration of effects as yet in athletes | Power athletes; weightlifters, sprinters, throwers, football and hockey players, and wrestlers |
| Insulin-like growth factor | Increases muscle mass and strength, reduction in body fat | Improves muscle mass and recovery from injury in rodents | Power athletes; weightlifters, sprinters, throwers, football and hockey players, and wrestlers |
| Testosterone and anabolic-androgenic steroids | Increases muscle mass and strength | Improves lean body mass and strength | Power athletes; weightlifters, sprinters, throwers, football and hockey players, and wrestlers |
| Thyroxine and triiodothyronine | Increase overall rate of metabolism, reduction in body fat | Improved weight loss in certain obese individuals, but no known effects on athletic performance | Power athletes; weightlifters, sprinters, throwers, football and hockey players, and wrestlers |

# QUESTIONS

1. All of the following are considered anabolic hormones, EXCEPT:
   a. Testosterone
   b. Growth hormone
   c. Cortisol
   d. Insulin

2. Which of the following is used by athletes to increase the oxygen-carrying capacity of their blood?
   a. Growth hormone
   b. Erythropoietin
   c. Cortisol
   d. Thyroxine

3. Which of the following hormone supplements is conditionally banned by the International Olympic Committee/World Anti-Doping Agency?
   a. Testosterone
   b. Growth Hormone
   c. Insulinlike growth factor 1
   d. Corticosteroids

4. Which of the following hormones may have the effect of muscle wasting?
   a. Insulinlike growth factor 1
   b. Anabolic-androgenic steroids
   c. Cortisol
   d. Erythropoietin

5. Which of the following hormones may produce the effect of pituitary wasting (empty sella syndrome)?
   a. Adrenocorticotropic hormone
   b. Insulinlike growth factor 1
   c. Erythropoietin
   d. Androstenedione

6. Which athlete may be most likely to be interested in taking supplemental erythropoietin?
   a. Weightlifter
   b. Cyclist
   c. Sprinter
   d. Football player

7. Thus far, insulinlike growth factor 1 has proven to decrease recovery time after injury in:
   a. Sedentary humans
   b. Rodents
   c. Human athletes
   d. No species as yet

8. Anabolic-androgenic steroids have demonstrated an effect of improving muscle mass and strength.
   a. T
   b. F

9. Insulin is legally available as an over-the-counter drug.
   a. T
   b. F

10. Erythropoietin is made in the adrenal gland.
    a. T
    b. F

11. Some prohormones may ultimately be converted to estrogen.
    a. T
    b. F

12. Some prohormones may ultimately be converted to dihydrotestosterone.
    a. T
    b. F

13. An approved use for corticosteroids is treatment of asthma.
    a. T
    b. F

14. An approved use for erythropoietin is in the treatment of certain forms of anemia.
    a. T
    b. F

15. An approved use of testosterone is in the treatment of certain forms of anemia.
    a. T
    b. F

# REFERENCES

1. World Anti-Doping Agency. A Brief History of Anti-Doping. Montreal: WADA. Available at: www.wada-ama.org/en/dynamic.ch2?pageCategory_id=20. Accessed June 30, 2005.
2. Greenspan FS, Gardner DG. Basic & Clinical Endocrinology. 7th ed. New York: McGraw-Hill Medical; 2003.
3. Thiblin I, Petersson A. Pharmacoepidemiology of anabolic androgenic steroids: a review. Fundam Clin Pharmacol 2005;19(1):27–44.
4. Gooren LJ, Bunck MC. Androgen replacement therapy: present and future. Drugs 2004;64(17):1861–1891.

5. Black BE, Paschal BM. Intranuclear organization and function of the androgen receptor. Trends Endocrinol Metab 2004;15(9):411–417.

6. Giammanco M, Tabacchi G, Giammanco S, Di Majo D, La Guardia M. Testosterone and aggressiveness. Med Sci Monit 2005;11(4):RA136–145.

7. Danhaive PA, Rousseau GG. Binding of glucocorticoid antagonists to androgen and glucocorticoid hormone receptors in rat skeletal muscle. J Steroid Biochem 1986; 24(2):481–487.

8. Spence J. Effects of anabolic-androgenic steroids on muscular strength: a meta-analysis. Med Sci Sport Exerc 1999;31(5):Suppl abstract 2071.

9. Bhasin S, Storer TW, Berman N, et al. The effects of supraphysiologic doses of testosterone on muscle size and strength in normal men. N Engl J Med 1996;335(1): 1–7.

10. Giorgi A, Weatherby RP, Murphy PW. Muscular strength, body composition, and health responses to the use of testosterone enanthate: a double blind study. J Sci Med Sport 1999;2:341–355.

11. Herbst KL, Bhasin S. Testosterone action on skeletal muscle. Curr Opin Clin Nutr Metab Care 2004;7(3):271–277.

12. Bhasin S, Woodhouse L, Casaburi R, et al. Older men are as responsive as young men to the anabolic effects of graded doses of testosterone on the skeletal muscle. J Clin Endocrinol Metab 2005;90(2):678–688.

13. Bhasin S, Taylor WE, Singh R, et al. The mechanisms of androgen effects on body composition: mesenchymal pluripotent cell as the target of androgen action. J Gerontol A Biol Sci Med Sci 2003;58(12):M1103–1110.

14. Sinha-Hikim I, Taylor WE, Gonzalez-Cadavid NF, Zheng W, Bhasin S. Androgen receptor in human skeletal muscle and cultured muscle satellite cells: up-regulation by androgen treatment. J Clin Endocrinol Metab 2004;89(10):5245–5255.

15. Parssinen M, Kujala U, Vartiainen E, Sarna S, Seppala T. Increased premature mortality of competitive powerlifters suspected to have used anabolic agents. Int J Sports Med 2000;21(3):225–227.

16. Thiblin I, Lindquist O, Rajs J. Cause and manner of death among users of anabolic androgenic steroids. J Forensic Sci 2000;45:16–23.

17. Hartgens F, Rietjens G, Keizer HA, Kuipers H, Wolffenbuttel BH. Effects of androgenic-anabolic steroids on apolipoproteins and lipoprotein (a). Br J Sports Med 2004;38(3):253–259.

18. Evans NA. Current concepts in anabolic-androgenic steroids. Am J Sports Med 2004;32(2):534–542.

19. Hartgens F, Kuipers H. Effects of androgenic-anabolic steroids in athletes. Sports Med 2004;34(8):513–554.

20. Rich JD, Foisie CK, Towe CW, Dickinson BP, McKenzie M, Salas CM. Needle exchange program participation by anabolic steroid injectors, United States 1998. Drug Alcohol Depend 1999;56(2):157–160.

21. Abu EO, Horner A, Kusec V, Triffitt JT, Compston JE. The localization of androgen receptors in human bone. J Clin Endocrinol Metab 1997;82(10):3493–3497.

22. Broeder CE, Quindry J, Brittingham K, et al. The Andro Project: physiological and hormonal influences of androstenedione supplementation in men 35 to 65 years old participating in a high-intensity resistance training program. Arch Intern Med 2000;160(20):3093–3104.

23. Brown GA, Martini ER, Roberts BS, Vukovich MD, King DS. Acute hormonal response to sublingual androstenediol intake in young men. J Appl Physiol 2002; 92:142–146.

24. Brown GA, Vukovich MD, Sharp RL, Reifenrath TA, Parsons KA, King DS. Effect of oral DHEA on serum testosterone and adaptations to resistance training in young men. J Appl Physiol 1999;87:2274–2283.

25. Khorram O, Vu L, Yen SS. Activation of immune function by dehydroepiandrosterone (DHEA) in age-advanced men 2. J Gerontol A Biol Sci Med Sci 1997;52: M1–M7.

26. Leder BZ, Longcope C, Catlin DH, Ahrens B, Schoenfeld DA, Finkelstein JS. Oral androstenedione administration and serum testosterone concentrations in young men. JAMA 2000;283(6):779–782.

27. Kicman AT, Bassindale T, Cowan DA, Dale S, Hutt AJ, Leeds AR. Effect of androstenedione ingestion on plasma testosterone in young women: a dietary supplement with potential health risks. Clin Chem 2003;49(1):167–169.

28. Ziegenfuss TN, Berardi JM, Lowery LM. Effects of prohormone supplementation in humans: a review. Can J Appl Physiol 2002;27(6):628–646.

29. Kurata K, Takebayashi M, Morinobu S, Yamawaki S. beta-Estradiol, dehydroepiandrosterone, and dehydroepiandrosterone sulfate protect against N-methyl-D-aspartate-induced neurotoxicity in rat hippocampal neurons by different mechanisms. J Pharmacol Exp Ther 2004;311(1):237–245.

30. MacLusky NJ, Hajszan T, Leranth C. Effects of dehydroepiandrosterone and fluta-mide on hippocampal CA1 spine synapse density in male and female rats: implications for the role of androgens in maintenance of hippocampal structure. Endocrinology 2004;145(9):4154–4161.

31. Celebi F, Yilmaz I, Aksoy H, Gumus M, Taysi S, Oren D. Dehydroepiandrosterone prevents oxidative injury in obstructive jaundice in rats. J Int Med Res 2004; 32(4):400–405.

32. Bassett JH, Harvey CB, Williams GR. Mechanisms of thyroid hormone receptor-specific nuclear and extra nuclear actions. Mol Cell Endocrinol 2003;213(1): 1–11.

33. Krotkiewski M. Thyroid hormones in the pathogenesis and treatment of obesity. Eur J Pharmacol 2002;440(2–3):85–98.

34. Clement K, Viguerie N, Diehn M, et al. In vivo regulation of human skeletal muscle gene expression by thyroid hormone. Genome Res 2002;12(2):281–291.

35. Hudecova S, Vadaszova A, Soukup T, Krizanova O. Effect of thyroid hormones on the gene expression of calcium transport systems in rat muscles. Life Sci 2004; 75(8):923–931.

36. Ralph CT. Finding and treating the cause of hyperthyroidism. JAAPA 2004;17(2):20, 23–26, 29, 30.

37. Rogol AD. Gender and hormonal regulation of growth. J Pediatr Endocrinol Metab 2004;17(Suppl 4):1259–1265.

38. Rosenfeld RG. The IGF system: new developments relevant to pediatric practice. Endocr Dev 2005;9:1–10.

39. Svensson J, Johannson G. Long-term efficacy and safety of somatropin for adult growth hormone deficiency. Treat Endocrinol 2003;2(2):109–120.

40. Arosio M, Ronchi CL, Epaminonda P, di Lembo S, Adda G. New therapeutic options for acromegaly. Minerva Endocrinol 2004;29(4):225–239.

41. Gagliardino JJ. Physiological endocrine control of energy homeostasis and post-prandial blood glucose levels. Eur Rev Med Pharmacol Sci 2005;9(2):75–92.

42. Plum L, Schubert M, Bruning JC. The role of insulin receptor signaling in the brain. Trends Endocrinol Metab 2005;16(2):59–65.

43. Santeusanio F, Di Loreto C, Lucidi P, et al. Diabetes and exercise. J Endocrinol Invest 2003;26(9):937–940.

44. Evans PJ, Lynch RM. Insulin as a drug of abuse in body building. Br J Sports Med 2003;37:356–357.

45. Rich JD, Dickinson BP, Merriman NA, Thule PM. Insulin use by bodybuilders. JAMA 1998;279(20):1613.

46. Bates N. Overdose of insulin and other diabetic medication. Emerg Nurse 2002; 10(7):22.

47. Carro E, Nuñez A, Busiguina S, Torres-Aleman I. Circulating insulin-like growth factor 1 mediates effects of exercise on the brain. J Neurosci 2000;20:2926–2933.

48. Kurtz CA, Loebig TG, Anderson DD, DeMeo PJ, Campbell PG. Insulin-like growth factor I accelerates functional recovery from Achilles tendon injury in a rat model. Am J Sports Med 1999;27(3):363–369.

49. Song YH, Godard M, Li Y, Richmond SR, Rosenthal N, Delafontaine P. Insulin-like growth factor I-mediated skeletal muscle hypertrophy is characterized by increased mTOR-p70S6K signaling without increased Akt phosphorylation. J Investig Med 2005;53(3):135–142.

50. Waters D, Danska J, Hardy K, et al. Recombinant human growth hormone, insulin-like growth factor 1, and combination therapy in AIDS-associated wasting. A randomized, double-blind, placebo-controlled trial. Ann Intern Med 1996;125(11): 865–872.

51. Platz EA, Pollak MN, Leitzmann MF, Stampfer MJ, Willett WC, Giovannucci E. Plasma insulin-like growth factor-1 and binding protein-3 and subsequent risk of prostate cancer in the PSA era. Cancer Causes Control 2005;16(3):255–262.

52. Jezova D, Komadel L, Mikulaj L. Plasma testosterone response to repeated human chorionic gonadotropin administration is increased in trained athletes. Endocrinol Exp 1987;21(2):143–147.

53. Martikainen H, Alen M, Rahkila P, Vihko R. Testicular responsiveness to human chorionic gonadotrophin during transient hypogonadotrophic hypogonadism induced by androgenic/anabolic steroids in power athletes. J Steroid Biochem 1986;25(1): 109–112.

54. Karila T, Hovatta O, Seppala T. Concomitant abuse of anabolic androgenic steroids and human chorionic gonadotrophin impairs spermatogenesis in power athletes. Int J Sports Med 2004;25(4):257–263.

55. Fisher JW. Erythropoietin: physiology and pharmacology update. Exp Biol Med (Maywood) 2003;228(1):1–14.

56. Scott J, Phillips GC. Erythropoietin in sports: a new look at an old problem. Curr Sports Med Rep 2005;4(4):224–226.

57. Birkeland KI, Stray-Gundersen J, Hemmersbach P, Hallen J, Haug E, Bahr R. Effect of rhEPO administration on serum levels of sTfR and cycling performance. Med Sci Sports Exerc 2000;32(7):1238–1243.

58. Ekblom B, Berglund B. Effect of erythropoietin administration on maximal aerobic power. Scand J Med Sci Sports 1991;1:88–93.

59. Sawka MN, Joyner MJ, Miles DS, Robertson RJ, Spriet LL, Young AJ. American College of Sports Medicine position stand. The use of blood doping as an ergogenic aid. Med Sci Sports Exerc 1996;28(6):i–viii.

60. Jacobson L. Hypothalamic-pituitary-adrenocortical axis regulation. Endocrinol Metab Clin North Am 2005;34(2):271–292, vii.

61. Arlt W, Stewart PM. Adrenal corticosteroid biosynthesis, metabolism, and action. Endocrinol Metab Clin North Am 2005;34(2):293–313, viii.

62. Soetens E, De Meirleir K, Hueting JE. No influence of ACTH on maximal performance. Psychopharmacology 1995;118(3):260–266.

63. Hanberg A. Common disorders of the pituitary gland: hyposecretion versus hypersecretion. J Infus Nurs 2005;28(1):36–44.

64. World Anti-Doping Agency. The World Anti-Doping Code. The 2005 Prohibited List: International Standard. Available at: http://www.wada-ama.org. Accessed November 4, 2004.

65. Pringle TD, West RL, Williams SE, Johnson DD. The Role of the Calpain/Calpastatin System in Muscle Hypertrophy Associated with Double-Muscling in Beef. UGA Animal & Dairy Science Annual Report. Gainesville: The University of Florida; 1995:61–65. Available at: http://www.ads.uga.edu/annrpt/1995/95_061.htm. Accessed November 4, 2004.

66. Grobet L, Martin LJ, Poncelet D, et al. A deletion in the bovine myostatin gene causes the double-muscled phenotype in cattle. Nat Genet 1997;17:71–74.

67. McPherron AC, Lee SJ. Double muscling in cattle due to mutations in the myostatin gene. Proc Natl Acad Sci USA 1997;94:12457–12461.

68. Schuelke M, Wagner KR, Stolz LE, et al. Myostatin mutation associated with gross muscle hypertrophy in a child. N Engl J Med 2004;350(26):2682–2688.

69. The Seattle Times. Muscular 4-year-old may power medical advances. The Associated Press and Baltimore Sun. Available at: http://seattletimes.nwsource.com/text/2001963965_muscleboy24.html. Accessed November 5, 2004.

70. Aschwanden C. Gene cheats. New Scientist 15 January 2000:24–29.

71. Goldspink G. Changes in muscle mass and phenotype and the expression of autocrine and systemic growth factors by muscle in response to stretch and overload. J Anat 1999;194(3):323–324.

72. Barton-Davis ER, Shoturma DI, Musaro A, et al. Viral mediated expression of insulin-like growth factor I blocks the aging-related loss of skeletal muscle function. Proc Natl Acad Sci USA 1998;95(26):15603–15607.

# PART V

# Special Topics

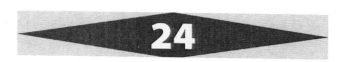

# Special Legal Review

## The Androstenedione Ban and the Criminalization of Steroid Precursors—Implications for the Sports Nutritional Supplement Market

### Richard D. Collins and Alan H. Feldstein

## OBJECTIVES

On the completion of this chapter you will be able to:

1. List the major laws and acts that affect the supplement industry.
2. Discuss in detail the ramifications and guidelines presented in the laws and acts that affect the supplement industry.
3. Understand the changes made in 2004 to the 1990 Anabolic Steroid Control Act.
4. Discuss the legal ramifications of possession or distribution of anabolic-androgenic steroids.
5. Explain the levels of oversight for the supplement industry.

## ABSTRACT

The Food and Drug Administration's action on androstenedione suggested a new interest in utilizing the authority provided by the Dietary Supplement Health and Education Act, and a heightened enforcement policy against what the agency deems to be adulterated new dietary ingredients. This pronouncement on androstenedione is illustrative of the lack of cooperation and communication that exists between the Food and Drug Administration and the sports nutrition industry. The industry must conduct and publish safety studies and police itself against unscrupulous marketers who make false or unsubstantiated claims. At the same time, representatives and government officials must take a close look at the inherent and institutionalized bias that exists against dietary supplements within our government and begin to find ways to undo the existing bias by promoting productive and meaningful dialogue between respective groups. The purpose of this chapter is to discuss various sensationalized media reports and anti-supplement positions by some members of Congress while illustrating the general institutionalized bias against

From: *Essentials of Sports Nutrition and Supplements*
Edited by J. Antonio, D. Kalman, J. R. Stout, M. Greenwood, D. S. Willoughby, and G. G. Haff © Humana Press, a part of Springer Science+Business Media, Totowa, NJ

alternative health approaches that creates an environment for less than honorable marketers and at the same time compromises the freedoms of Americans to make their own health choices under the Dietary Supplement Health and Education Act.

*Key Words:* **noncompliant, legislative, enforcement, structure and function claims, FDA, DSHEA**

On March 11, 2004, the Food and Drug Administration (FDA) pronounced that dietary supplement products containing androstenedione ("andro") were adulterated new dietary ingredients under the Dietary Supplement Health and Education Act of 1994 (DSHEA). Despite the lack of evidence of an imminent health hazard and instead of the formal administrative procedure of issuing a proposed rule and inviting public comment, FDA took unilateral action, issued a press release, held a news conference, and sent warning letters to 23 companies that had manufactured, marketed, or distributed the products containing androstenedione. In its warning letters, FDA threatened possible enforcement actions for noncompliance. The effect was to cause retailers, manufacturers, and distributors alike to cease selling products containing androstenedione without FDA having had meaningful dialogue with the industry before taking action.

FDA's pronouncement helped pave the way for more expansive Congressional action. On October 22, 2004, a bill criminalizing a long list of steroid precursors was passed. Many of these precursors, including androstenedione, had been sold in the United States as ingredients in sports nutrition products. Efficacy aside, androstenedione was a popular product consumed by many and did not have a single adverse event report filed with FDA that would have raised safety concerns. The new law, which took effect on January 20, 2005, was an effort to demonstrate strong Congressional disapproval of the notion of drugs being sold as supplements, and went far beyond a ban on sales, making not only distribution but mere possession of the substances a federal drug offense.

The FDA pronouncement on androstenedione is illustrative of the lack of cooperation and communication that exists between FDA and the sports nutrition industry. The sports nutrition industry, in failing to take an aggressive role in conducting research and publishing studies, has contributed to the situation. FDA's antagonistic attitude toward dietary supplements in general and the sports and fitness category in particular could result in an increasing encroachment upon DSHEA. This attitude, combined with sensationalized media reports, anti-supplement leanings by some members of Congress, the sensationalism of the steroids in sports issue, and a general institutionalized bias against alternative health approaches, has created an environment that compromises the freedoms of Americans to make their own health choices under DSHEA.

## PUBLIC HEALTH PROTECTIONS ON DIETARY SUPPLEMENTS PROVIDED UNDER THE DIETARY SUPPLEMENT HEALTH AND EDUCATION ACT

In 1994, DSHEA[1] was passed with the unanimous consent of Congress. As discussed in a 2002 law review article, FDA's anti-supplement tactics provoked a groundswell of legislative criticism ultimately leading to DSHEA[2]:

> DSHEA was enacted because FDA was viewed as distorting the law that existed before DSHEA to try improperly to deprive the public of safe and popular dietary supplement products. . . . In its official report about the need for DSHEA to curtail excessive regulation of dietary supplements by FDA, the Senate Committee on Labor and Human Resources . . . stated explicitly "in fact, FDA has been distorting the law in its actions to try to prevent the marketing of safe dietary supplement substances."[3] The Senate Committee also concluded, "FDA has attempted to twist the statute [i.e., the provisions of the FDCA, as it then existed] in what the Committee sees as a result-oriented effort to impede the manufacture and sale of dietary supplements."[4]

DSHEA represented a sharp rebuke to FDA's unreasonable regulatory tactics. It was FDA's own actions that brought about the need for DSHEA. However, DSHEA did not leave FDA paralyzed. Despite media statements to the contrary, the industry is not an unregulated industry. In fact, DSHEA ensured FDA's authority to provide legitimate protections for the public health. The Food, Drug, and Cosmetic Act (FDCA)[5] prohibits introducing adulterated products into interstate commerce.[6] The penalties for a first conviction can include a fine of up to $1000, imprisonment for up to 1 year, or both.[7] Subsequent convictions, or convictions for offenses committed with the intent to defraud or mislead, can include fines of up to $10,000, imprisonment of up to 3 years, or both.[8]

Several grounds exist by which unsafe dietary supplements can be deemed "adulterated."[9] Whereas the Secretary of Health and Human Services has the power to declare a dangerous supplement to be an "imminent hazard" to public health or safety and suspend sales of the product,[10] FDA also has the authority to protect consumers from dietary supplements that do not present an imminent hazard to the public but do present certain risks of illness or injury to consumers. Two provisions are relevant.

The first provision, which applies to all dietary supplements, states that a supplement shall be deemed adulterated if it presents "a significant or unreasonable risk of illness or injury under . . . conditions of use recommended or suggested in labeling, or . . . if no conditions of use are suggested or recommended in the labeling, under ordinary conditions of use."[11] The standard does not require proof that consumers have actually been harmed, or even that a product will harm anyone. It was under this provision that FDA, after 7 years, numerous criticisms including a negative report from the General Accountability Office,[12] and a storm of public debate, concluded that dietary supplements containing ephedra presented an unreasonable risk. However, the conclusion FDA drew and its reasoning to declare products containing ephedra adulterated utilized a new and novel approach that distorts the definition of significant or unreasonable risk. In the case of ephedra, FDA did an analysis of whether the product's known or reasonably likely risks outweigh its known or reasonably likely benefits. Thus, this is no longer a straight safety analysis, but is now a risk/benefit analysis, which is not what is called for in the statute. Even though ephedra had been shown beneficial for short-term weight loss, FDA used this standard to conclude that these benefits did not outweigh the risks that FDA believed ephedra products posed.[13] Litigation was instituted challenging FDA's actions. After a reversal in the lower court, FDA's position was upheld in the appellate courts and is now valid precedent for FDA to unilaterally change a statute without the need for a legislative amendment. There is now a danger that many popular and less-controversial supplements will also be at risk of being removed from the market.

# DIETARY SUPPLEMENT HEALTH AND EDUCATION ACT PROTECTIONS AGAINST ADULTERATED "NEW DIETARY INGREDIENTS"

The second provision addresses only dietary supplements containing new dietary ingredients, for which FDA believes there may be inadequate information to provide a reasonable assurance that the ingredient does not present a significant risk of illness or injury. Recognizing that new and untested dietary supplement products may pose unknown health issues, DSHEA distinguishes between products containing dietary ingredients that were already on the market and products containing new dietary ingredients that were not marketed before the enactment of the law.[15] A "new dietary ingredient" or "NDI" is defined as a dietary ingredient that was not marketed in the United States before October 15, 1994.[16]

DSHEA grants FDA greater control over supplements containing new dietary ingredients. A new dietary ingredient is deemed adulterated and subject to FDA enforcement sanctions unless it meets one of two exemption criteria: either 1) the supplement in question contains "only dietary ingredients which have been present in the food supply as an article used for food in a form in which the food has not been chemically altered"; or 2) there is a "history of use or other evidence of safety" provided by the manufacturer or distributor to FDA at least 75 days before introducing the product into interstate commerce.[17] The first criterion is silent as to how and by whom presence in the food supply as food articles without chemical alteration is to be established. The second criterion—applicable only to new dietary ingredients that have not been present in the food supply—requires manufacturers and distributors of the product to take certain actions. Those actions include submitting, at least 75 days before the product is introduced into interstate commerce, information that is the basis on which a product containing the new dietary ingredient will "reasonably be expected to be safe."[18] That information would include: a) the name of the new dietary ingredient and, if it is an herb or botanical, the Latin binomial name; b) a description of the dietary supplement that contains the new dietary ingredient, including the i) level of the new dietary ingredient in the product; ii) conditions of use of the product stated in the labeling, or if no conditions of use are stated, the ordinary conditions of use; and iii) history of use or other evidence of safety establishing that the dietary ingredient, when used under the conditions recommended or suggested in the labeling of the dietary supplement, will be reasonably expected to be safe.

There is no guidance as to what evidence is required to establish a reasonable expectation of safety.[19] In fact, although FDA has recently requested comments on its NDI process,[20] FDA specifically states that the person submitting the application is responsible for determining what information provides the basis for the conclusion that the product will be reasonably expected to be safe. By not providing guidance one could argue that FDA is giving itself a wide berth to arbitrarily decide what ingredients to approve or disapprove. The only hint given is that FDA expects the applicant to "consider the evidence of safety found in the scientific literature, including an examination of adverse effects associated with the use of the substance."[19] Thus, it seems that the question should be one of safety alone as opposed to a safety and efficacy analysis, which in turn naturally progresses to a risk/benefit analysis. This is a much different and more difficult, if not impossible, standard for a NDI to meet.

## FOOD AND DRUG ADMINISTRATION'S ACTION AGAINST ANDROSTENEDIONE

Supplements containing androstenedione were introduced in the mid-1990s and were promoted as a natural way to help increase strength and muscle mass and to combat the effects of the aging process in older men, much of which is attributed to declining testosterone levels. Androstenedione is a naturally derived precursor to testosterone, which converts directly to testosterone in the metabolic pathway. The fact that it is naturally derived and, as described below, present in the food supply, is important in relation to the action taken by FDA.

In its press release[21] and warning letters,[22] FDA declared androstenedione to be an adulterated new dietary ingredient based on its position that no evidence demonstrates "that androstenedione was lawfully marketed as a dietary ingredient in the United States before October 15, 1994."[22] It would seem to be correct that androstenedione was not marketed before 1994, given that the first commercial marketing of products containing androstenedione seems to have been in 1996. Furthermore, a review of FDA's electronic database indicates no submission of an application for a new dietary ingredient involving androstenedione.[23] Interestingly, however, FDA goes beyond the words of the statute and uses the term "lawfully marketed" in their letters instead of simply "marketed." The implication is that to receive "grandfathered" status into DSHEA as a pre-1994 supplement ingredient, the product must not only have been marketed but must have met the additional requirement of having been *lawfully* marketed. At least one commentator has interpreted this language to impose a burden on the industry to prove the product was generally regarded as safe pre-1994—an impossible standard for any product that was not explicitly affirmed as such by FDA before the enactment of DSHEA.[24]

Assuming that androstenedione is indeed a new dietary ingredient, FDA could determine that products containing androstenedione are adulterated under DSHEA unless they meet either of the two exemption criteria stated above. Accordingly, it seems that the question of exemption turns on a) whether or not androstenedione is present in the food supply as an article used for food without chemical alteration, and b) if not, could the product satisfy the requirement of reasonable expectation of safety.

With respect to the first exemption, according to scientific journals, androstenedione is indeed present in the food supply without chemical alteration.[25-27] Had there been open communication between FDA and the sports nutrition industry, the scientific evidence that androstenedione is present in the foods we eat could have been presented and discussed with FDA. Moreover, until 1998, which is the date for the most recent information, there were no reports of adverse events reported on FDA's database.[28] Adverse events are one of the few specific pieces of information that FDA sets forth in their "information" about what safety data they require.[19]

FDA's policy creates a nearly impossible procedure to demonstrate safety. FDA's requirements to show safety have never been articulated. On FDA's Web site, the following statement appears:

> You are not limited in what evidence you may rely on in determining whether the use of a new dietary ingredient will reasonably be expected to be safe. (See section 413(a)(2) of the act (21 U.S.C. 350b(a)(2)). You must provide a history of use or other evidence of safety establishing that the dietary ingredient, when used under the conditions recommended or suggested in the labeling of the dietary supplement, will reasonably be expected to be safe. *To date, we have not published guidance defining the specific information that the submission must contain. Thus, you are responsible for determining what information provides the basis for your conclusion.* Nonetheless, we expect that—in making a determination that a new dietary ingredient is reasonably expected to be safe,—you will consider the evidence of safety found in the scientific literature, including an examination of adverse effects associated with the use of the substance.[19] [emphasis added]

First, no mention is made of efficacy, the necessary component for a risk/benefit analysis. Second, a lack of guidance by FDA has created a circular process whereby at any time the agency can declare that the product does not satisfy its unspoken standards and deem the product adulterated.

Both FDA and the industry must take responsibility for this acrimonious and hostile environment. FDA must rid itself of its institutionalized bias against supplements and have meaningful and cooperative discussions with the industry. The industry must take it upon itself to conduct further safety research of its products and police itself with respect to unscrupulous marketers who make false or unsubstantiated claims. If this had been done, the fate of androstenedione might have been decidedly different. It is too late to have fruitful cooperation between the agency and the industry once there are press conferences, press releases, warning letters, and products pulled from store shelves.

How would FDA have responded if the sports nutrition industry had submitted the scientific literature on androstenedione to FDA? What FDA would have done is implied in its warning letters. After citing androstenedione as an adulterated new dietary ingredient, FDA directly addresses the safety issue:

> Even if the required notification had been submitted, based on what we know now, we know of no evidence that would establish that your product is not adulterated. In the absence of a history of use or other evidence of safety establishing that androstenedione, when used under the conditions recommended or suggested in the labeling of your product, will reasonably be expected to be safe, a product containing andro is adulterated under 21 U.S.C. 342(f)(1)(B) and 350b(a) as a dietary supplement that contains a new dietary ingredient for which there is inadequate information to provide reasonable assurance that such ingredient does not present a significant or unreasonable risk of illness or injury.[22]

Thus, FDA suggests that even if the industry had provided proper notification pursuant to statute, its position is that there exists inadequate information from which to conclude that androstenedione could be reasonably expected to be safe as a dietary ingredient. In fact, FDA believes to the contrary according to its androstenedione "Questions and Answers" Web page:

> Based on a limited number of studies of androstenedione's actions in humans and existing knowledge about steroid hormone metabolism and action in the body, FDA believes that the use of dietary supplements containing androstenedione may increase the risk of serious health problems because of their conversion in the body to active hormones with androgenic and estrogenic properties.[29]

A review of the "limited number" of androstenedione studies and a scientific analysis of their meaning is beyond the scope of this article.[30] However, if the sports nutrition industry desires to continue to develop and market innovative new dietary products, it is going to have to adopt a more aggressive role in conducting research and publishing studies. It is going to have to forge stronger and more extensive relationships with the scientific community to analyze its products and their effects, and must ensure that those studies are brought to the attention of FDA and others.

## THE NEW ANABOLIC STEROID CONTROL ACT

In the 1980s, anabolic steroids were regulated by FDA as prescription drugs. Although the International Olympic Committee had banned anabolic steroids since 1975, Canadian sprinter Ben Johnson's highly publicized 1988 doping violation suggested that sports bodies needed help in ensuring a level playing field. Congress held hearings as to whether steroids should be scheduled as controlled substances. Most of the witnesses who testified, including representatives of the American Medical Association, FDA, the Drug Enforcement Administration (DEA), and the National Institute on Drug Abuse, recommended against scheduling, maintaining that steroid abuse does not lead to the physical or psychologic dependence required under the Controlled Substances Act.[31]

Congress voted nevertheless to schedule anabolic steroids, placing them under DEA authority. The Anabolic Steroid Control Act (ASCA)[32] of 1990 inserted 27 steroids, along with their muscle-building salts, esters, and isomers, in the same legal class—Schedule III—as barbiturates, LSD precursors, ketamine, and narcotic painkillers such as Vicodin. Simple possession of anabolic steroids is a federal crime punishable by up to 1 year in prison and/or a minimum fine of $1000 for a first offense.[33] Distributing steroids, or possessing them with intent to distribute, is a federal felony punishable by up to 5 years in prison (10 years for a prior drug offender) and/or a $250,000 fine.[34]

The restraints imposed by the ASCA increased the demand for legally available alternatives for building size and strength and improving athletic performance. It was onto this landscape that androstenedione was introduced. Androstenedione was followed by other naturally occurring steroid precursor or "prohormone" products. Later, edgier precursor products were brought to market, including some for which there was no evidence of existence within the human food supply and some which were clearly chemically altered.

As these products proliferated, critics claimed that loopholes in DSHEA and the ASCA were allowing anabolic steroids to masquerade as supplements. Sports bodies and legislators began decrying the availability of these products, particularly to young athletes. Various federal bills were introduced to expand the definition of an anabolic steroid to include precursor products. FDA's position that androstenedione might increase the risk of serious health problems helped spur the bills. On October 22, 2004, new legislation was passed.

The ASCA of 2004[35] took effect on January 20, 2005, revising and expanding the ASCA that had been passed in 1990. The new law provides $15 million for educational programs for children about the dangers of anabolic steroids, and directs the U.S. Sentencing Commission to consider revising federal guidelines to increase the penalties for steroid and steroid precursor possession and distribution. The law adds 26 new steroid compounds, including many steroid precursors, to the previous list of substances that are legally defined as "anabolic steroids." [The new compounds are androstanediol; androstanedione; androstenediol; androstenedione; bolasterone; calusterone; λ-dihydrotestosterone (a.k.a. "1-testosterone"); furazabol; 13β-ethyl-17α-hydroxygon-4-en-3-one; 4-hydroxytestosterone; 4-hydroxy-19-nortestosterone; mestanolone; 17α-methyl-3β,17β-dihydroxy-5α-androstane; 17α-methyl-3α,17β-dihydroxy-5α-androstane; 17α-methyl-3β,17β-dihydroxyandrost-4-ene; 17α-methyl-4-hydroxynandrolone; methyldienolone; methyltrienolone; 17α-methyl-λ-dihydrotestosterone (a.k.a. "17-α-methyl-1-testosterone"); norandrostenediol; norandrostenedione; norbolethone; norclostebol; normethandrolone; stenbolone; and tetrahydrogestrinone.] Some of these new substances have been widely marketed as dietary supplements, such as androstenedione, norandrostenedione, norandrostenediol, 1-testosterone, and 4-hydroxytestosterone. Others, such as bolasterone, calusterone, furazabol, and stenbolone, are actually very old pharmaceutical steroids that were missed in the original federal law (note, however, that some states, among them California, did include some of these compounds in their own steroid laws). These compounds were likely included after the highly publicized reemergence of norbolethone (also added to the list) in an Olympic urine sample. Also listed is tetrahydrogestrinone (THG), the alleged "designer steroid" involved in the BALCO scandal. However, after a protracted battle on the issue among members of Congress, the law permits the continued sale of dehydroepiandrosterone (DHEA) as a dietary supplement by adding it to the list of other excluded hormonal substances (estrogens, progestins, and corticosteroids).

The law also changes the general requisite elements of an anabolic steroid. The "promotes muscle growth" language that preceded the list of compounds in the 1990 steroid act is now removed from the statute. Ironically, an anabolic steroid, under the new law, need *not* be *anabolic*. It simply needs to be chemically and pharmacologically related to testosterone, and either on the new list of substances, or any salt, ester, or ether of a substance on the list.

The new law is far more than a ban on precursor supplement sales. An extensive list of new steroids and steroid precursors are now classified as *controlled substances*. This categorization lacks a basis in fact, given that there is no scientific evidence that these prohormone products meet the test of a controlled substance. Controlled substances are drugs—such as cocaine, heroin, and LSD—or other substances with addictive qualities that may lead to physical or psychologic dependence.[36] There is not a scintilla of evidence that these products have been exerting addictive effects or leading to dependency issues. Nevertheless, the newly listed prohormones are now Schedule III drugs, and persons who possess them face arrest and prosecution, with the same penalties as those applied to pharmaceutical anabolic steroids. As is the case with steroids, some new prohormone drug crimes could trigger forfeiture laws permitting the government to seize assets. And a drug conviction—even for mere possession—can be a bar to certain licenses and—significantly to students—even a bar to federal school financial aid. It should be noted that although the law may be helpful in remedying some of the headaches for drug-testing authorities, criminalizing the products through a "drug war" approach also affects fitness-minded, otherwise law-abiding consumers who do not compete in any sports at all.

## RAMIFICATIONS FOR THE SPORTS NUTRITION INDUSTRY

The next question that must be asked is what does this mean for other dietary supplements? The loss of ephedra and androstenedione are strong signals of FDA's intent to reach as far as possible in their attempt to regulate supplements. Anyone attuned to what is transpiring in this industry is aware that there is a movement to undo most of the framework of DSHEA. The fallout may have ramifications far beyond the sports and fitness nutrition community, impacting the mainstream vitamin industry and traditional herbalists.

Senator Richard Durbin of Illinois, a long-time critic and opponent of the dietary supplement industry, recently addressed Congress in promoting a bill he is sponsoring that would put safety burdens on the supplement market and criminalize certain supplements:

> People unsuspectingly go into these health food stores, vitamin stores, and see the dietary supplements with all sorts of claims on them; they buy them, they use them, and the consumers of America become the guinea pigs. . . .
>
> [I]f they are dangerous, if they hurt someone, clearly then the Government will take them off the shelf, right? No, I am sorry, that is not right because understand that the law we passed at the request of the industry does not require dietary supplement manufacturers to report to the Government when people are literally dying from the products they sell. . . .
>
> I am happy to see the Institute of Medicine creating momentum for Congress to finally make a decision. I am happy to see the administration, after more than a year of urging, finally banning ephedra, but more has to be done. Today as we speak, innocent children and consumers across America are buying products which they presume to be safe and they are not.[37]

The Senator's statement about the Institute of Medicine of the National Academies refers to a recent publication suggesting a new framework for evaluating the safety of dietary supplement ingredients,[38] using a "spectrum of concern" model more appropriate to the review of prescription drugs. Although the effort is a noble one, the sports nutrition industry should be careful that such an approach is not the first step backward toward a pre-DSHEA environment and a movement to define many dietary supplement ingredients as drugs.

No one can or should object that manufacturers and distributors of products should be able to substantiate the claims they make about their products. No one can argue that safety research on products should be conducted. Any company that manufactures or distributes dietary supplements should have a comprehensive policy for handling reports of serious adverse health events. Finally, any manufacturer or distributor should have proper labels on their products with appropriate cautions and warnings.

There also needs to be more rational reporting within the media. An extreme example of the media bias against sports supplements involved the reported story of a 22-year-old "would-be bodybuilder" who claimed that his use of creatine monohydrate at recommended doses for three and a half months caused liver and kidney failure and the loss of the full use of his legs.[39] The story begins by describing the "deep blue and red scar [that] carves the skin on the outside of both of [his] legs, from his hips to his ankles. Orthopedic surgeons' scalpels have sliced them open again and again over the past five months to save his life and legs." It continues with: "'After the fourth day they wanted to amputate both legs at the hip,' he said. 'They were afraid the decay would spread to my lower intestines.'" Finally, the story proceeds to: "What caused all the problems? 'The doctors . . . told me it was the creatine,' he said. 'My body wouldn't process it.' It ended up poisoning him." The story was tossed to the public without any comments from nutrition experts or even the doctors who supposedly attributed the horrific symptoms to creatine. This disconnect between the fitness community's experience with these products and the questionable scare stories reported by the media does nothing but perpetuate an atmosphere of confusion and mistrust.

More importantly, FDA must also assume some responsibility for this state of affairs. If the nutritional supplement market is going to be compelled to institute policies and procedures, then there must also be changes within FDA. This means a change in attitude toward supplements, hiring people within the FDA Center for Food Safety and Applied Nutrition (CFSAN) responsible for supplements whom understand and support the use of supplements, and the appointment of an ombudsman within CFSAN as there are in other centers within FDA.

This lack of guidance and communication with FDA makes it very difficult for anyone to know whether or not they could even comply with FDA's requirements. As was evidenced by the process in ephedra, FDA did not, in any meaningful way, communicate with the supplement industry to learn about the industry's experiences. Even after the industry compiled a marketing study,[40] FDA did not communicate with industry representatives about the findings.* The lack of communication between FDA and the nutritional supplement industry fosters an atmosphere of frustration and suspicion that benefits neither FDA nor the industry, and most importantly is a detriment to the American public. Until there are better cooperation and communication between FDA and the sports nutrition industry and until there are people within FDA who support the use of dietary supplements, this will continue to be a problem.

It is hoped that before FDA takes any other actions or makes any other pronouncements about dietary supplement ingredients, a mutually cooperative dialogue can take place. Even if that were to occur, however, there is another issue to consider. Although FDA enforcement against other dietary supplement ingredients is possible, future action may be legislative rather than regulatory.

## CONCLUSION

FDA's action on androstenedione suggests a new interest in utilizing the authority provided by DSHEA, and a heightened enforcement policy against what the agency deems to be adulterated new dietary ingredients. Products brought to market that do not meet either of the two exemption criteria of 21USC 350(b) may not be overlooked in the future. If a new dietary ingredient is exempted from adulterated status because it is present in the food supply as an article used for food in a form in which the food has not been chemically altered, it is prudent to document that information before marketing the product or even to communicate that information to FDA. If a new dietary ingredient is not exempted from adulterated status based on the food supply exemption, then premarket notification of history of use or other evidence of safety establishing that the dietary ingredient, when used under the conditions recommended or suggested in the labeling of the dietary supplement, will be reasonably expected to be safe must be provided to FDA at least 75 days before the product is introduced into interstate commerce.

The sports nutrition industry as regulated by DSHEA is still a relatively new industry. Like any new industry, it is going through growing pains. The marketing of pro-steroid products that were noncompliant with DSHEA caused further damage to a tenuous relationship between FDA and the industry. For this industry to survive, it must earnestly resolve to comply with the evolving requirements of DSHEA, and begin to attempt to establish communication with legislative representatives and administrative agencies such as FDA. It must begin an era of cooperation among its members, no matter how competitive they may be in business, to establish procedures and to develop and publish science. Failure to do so will result in constantly being buffeted by the winds of public opinion and sensationalistic journalism. At the same time, our representatives and government officials must take a close look at the inherent and institutionalized bias that exists against dietary supplements within government and begin to find ways to undo that bias so that productive and meaningful dialogue can take place. Until that happens, the American public will be disadvantaged.

---

*One of the authors, Alan Feldstein, was head of the Ephedra Committee of the American Herbal Products Association which was responsible for arranging for the Arthur Anderson Survey. The Committee was never contacted after the survey was released and submitted to FDA.

## QUESTIONS

1. The Dietary Supplement Health and Education Act (DSHEA) of 1994 was enacted in order to:
   a. Restrict sales of androstenedione and steroid precursors
   b. Curtail FDA's excessive regulation of supplements
   c. Educate the public on the dangers of anabolic steroids
   d. Regulate supplements in the same way as prescription drugs

2. A dietary supplement that presents a significant or unreasonable risk of illness or injury under recommended or ordinary conditions of use is deemed to be:
   a. Adulterated
   b. Safe
   c. Deadly
   d. A new dietary ingredient

3. A new dietary ingredient is defined as one that:
   a. Presents an imminent hazard to public safety
   b. Is exempt from regulation under DSHEA
   c. Was not marketed before the enactment of DSHEA
   d. Contains androstenedione and hormone precursors

4. One goal of DSHEA was to:
   a. Preempt FDA's authority over imminent safety hazards
   b. Render the supplement industry totally unregulated
   c. "Grandfather" adulterated supplements
   d. Ensure FDA's authority to provide legitimate protections for the public health

5. A new dietary ingredient is deemed adulterated unless:
   a. The supplement contains only dietary ingredients found in the food supply as an article used for food without chemical alteration
   b. There is a "history of use or other evidence of safety" provided to FDA at least 75 days before introducing the product into interstate commerce
   c. Both a and b
   d. Either a or b

6. Androstenedione is:
   a. A synthetic anabolic steroid
   b. A naturally derived precursor to testosterone
   c. An imminent hazard to public health under DSHEA
   d. A prescription drug

7. The relationship between FDA and the nutritional supplement industry has been:
   a. Open and trusting
   b. Fruitful
   c. Hostile and acrimonious
   d. Mutually cooperative

8. FDA removed androstenedione from the market because:
   a. Androstenedione was deemed to be an adulterated new dietary ingredient
   b. There had been no information as to "history of use or other evidence of safety" provided to FDA at least 75 days before introducing the product into interstate commerce
   c. FDA believed that androstenedione might increase the risk of serious health problems because of its conversion in the body to active hormones with androgenic and estrogenic properties
   d. All of the above

9. Before the enactment of the Anabolic Steroid Control Act (ASCA) of 1990, anabolic steroids were:
    a. Prescription drugs
    b. Controlled substances
    c. Dietary supplements
    d. Deemed to be adulterated

10. Simple unlawful possession of anabolic steroids is:
    a. A violation of DSHEA
    b. A federal crime punishable by up to 1 year in prison
    c. A federal felony punishable by up to 5 years in prison
    d. Lawful for mature adults

11. The ASCA of 2004:
    a. Reduced the list of anabolic steroids
    b. Expanded the list of anabolic steroids
    c. Provided no funds for educational programs
    d. Directed consideration of an decrease in federal steroid punishments

12. The ASCA explicitly excludes certain hormonal substances, including:
    a. Corticosteroids
    b. Estrogens
    c. Dehydroepiandrosterone (DHEA)
    d. All of the above

13. Norandrostenediol, once an ingredient in popular prohormone supplements, is now:
    a. A Schedule III controlled substance under federal law
    b. Available as a prescription drug in U.S. pharmacies
    c. Sold only in expensive American supplement products
    d. None of the above

14. The Institute of Medicine of the National Academies suggested a new framework for evaluating the safety of dietary supplement ingredients, using a "spectrum of concern" model which would:
    a. Prevent FDA from targeting dangerous products
    b. Classify all supplements as controlled substances
    c. Treat supplements more like prescription drugs
    d. All of the above

15. To ensure a successful future for the sports nutritional supplement community:
    a. FDA must change its attitudes about dietary supplements
    b. The industry must resolve to comply with the evolving requirements of DSHEA
    c. Government officials must examine the institutionalized bias against dietary supplements within government
    d. All of the above

## ACKNOWLEDGMENTS

Mr. Collins practices in the firm of Collins, McDonald & Gann, P.C., primarily in the areas of nutritional supplement law, performance drugs, and criminal defense. A former certified personal trainer, he is the author of the popular book *Legal Muscle*, a monthly columnist for *Muscular Development* magazine, and the legal advisor to the International Federation of BodyBuilders. Mr. Feldstein is of counsel to Collins, McDonald & Gann. He concentrates in the area of nutritional supplement law, having served as general counsel for a dietary supplement company for seven years. In the 1990s, he was the catalyst for assembling several industry associations in the effort to educate the public, legislators, and administration officials on the facts and science regarding dietary supplements containing ephedra.

# REFERENCES

1. Pub L No. 103-417, 108 Stat 4325 (1994) (codified at 21USC 301 et seq.) (signed by the President October 25, 1994).

2. McNamara S, Siegner W. FDA Has Substantial and Sufficient Authority to Regulate Dietary Supplements. 57 Food & Drug L.J. 15, 2002; referencing 140 Congressional Record-House of Representatives 11173-11179 (Oct. 6, 1994); 140 Congressional Record-Senate 14798-14800 (Oct. 7, 1994).

3. Ibid, citing Senate Report No. 103-410, 103d Congress, 2nd Sess, Committee on Labor and Human Resources (Oct. 8, 1994), at page 16.

4. Ibid, citing Senate Report No. 103-410, at page 22.

5. Pub L No. 75-717, 52 Stat 1040 (1938) (1994) (codified as amended 21USC 301 et seq.).

6. 21USC §331(a) and (v).

7. 21USC §333(a)(1).

8. 21USC §333(a)(2).

9. 21USC §342(f)(1) and 350b(a).

10. Provided that the Secretary then initiates on-the-record rulemaking to affirm or withdraw the declaration. See, 21USC §342(f)(1).

11. 21USC §342(f)(1)(A).

12. GAO Report. Dietary Supplements: Uncertainties in Analyses Underlying FDA's Proposed Rule on Ephedrine Alkaloids. June 25, 1999. Available at: www.gao.gov/archive/1999/h299090.pdf.

13. See, Final Rule Declaring Dietary Supplements Containing Ephedrine Alkaloids Adulterated Because They Present an Unreasonable Risk. 69 Federal Register 6788 (Feb. 11, 2004). Available at: http://www.cfsan.fda.gov/~lrd/fr040211.html.

14. See, NVE, Inc. v. Dept. of Health and Human Services, et al., No. 2:04-cv-00999-JAP-MCA, D. N.J. (2004).

15. A "dietary ingredient" may be a vitamin, a mineral, an herb or other botanical, an amino acid, a dietary substance for use by man to supplement the diet by increasing the total dietary intake, or a concentrate, metabolite, constituent, extract, or combination of any of these. See, 21USC 321(ff)(1).

16. 21USC §350b(c).

17. 21USC §350b(a).

18. See, FDA, Center for Food Safety & Applied Nutrition (CFSAN). New Dietary Ingredients in Dietary Supplements. Available at: http://www.cfsan.fda.gov/~dms/ds-ingrd.html#whatis. See also, 21CFR §190.6.

19. "To date, we have not published guidance defining the specific information that the submission must contain. Thus, you are responsible for determining what information provides the basis for your conclusion." FDA, CFSAN. Available at: http://www.cfsan.fda.gov/~dms/ds-ingrd.html.

20. See, FDA, CFSAN. Notice of Dietary Supplement Public Meeting Pre-Market Notification Program for New Dietary Ingredients. Available at: http://www.cfsan.fda.gov/~dms/ds-ndi.html. In response, the authors co-authored "Comments on FDA's Pre-Market Notification for New Dietary Ingredients," presented to the Food and Drug Administration in Washington, DC, on Nov. 15, 2004.

21. FDA, CFSAN. Androstenedione Press Release. Available at: http://www.fda.gov/bbs/topics/news/2004/hhs_031104.html.

22. FDA, CFSAN. Androstenedione Warning Letters. Available at: http://www.cfsan.fda.gov/~dms/andrlist.html#letter.

23. FDA, CFSAN. Update to FDA's Table of New Dietary Ingredient Notifications. Sept. 10, 2001. Available at: http://www.cfsan.fda.gov/~dms/dsingrd.html#whatis.

24. Siegner W. FDA's Actions on Ephedra and Androstenedione: Understanding How They Erode the Protections of DSHEA. Paper for FDLI's 47th Annual Conference. Apr. 16, 2004.

25. Johnson SK, Lewis PE, Inskeep EK. Steroids and CAMP in follicles of postpartum beef cows treated with norgestomet. J Anim Sci 1991;69(9):3747–3753.

26. Braden TD, King ME, Odde KG, Niswender GD. Development of preovulatory follicles expected to form short-lived corpora lutea in beef cows. J Reprod Fertil 1989;85(1):97–104.

27. Wise TH, Caton D, Thatcher WW, Lehrer AR, Fields MJ. Androstenedione, dehydroepiandrosterone and testosterone in ovarian vein plasma and androstenedione in peripheral arterial plasma during the bovine oestrous cycle. J Reprod Fertil 1982; 66(2):513–518.

28. Margolis M. Dietary Supplements: Caveat Athlete. Available at: http://www.law.uh.edu/healthlawperspectives/Food/980910Dietary.html. Also, the authors have filed a FOIA request to FDA to determine the number, if any, of adverse event reports associated with androstenedione which have been reported to FDA.

29. FDA, CFSAN. Questions and Answers: Androstenedione. Available at: http://www. cfsan.fda.gov/~dms/androqa.html.

30. For a primer with extensive references, see Antonio J, Chromiak J, Street J. Androgens and GH releasers. In: Antonio, J, Stout JR, eds. Sports Supplements. Baltimore: Lippincott Williams & Wilkins; 2001:160–178.

31. 21USC §812(b).

32. Pub L No. 101-647, 04 Stat. 4851 (1990), amending 21USC §812(c) (1981) to include anabolic steroids.

33. 21USC §844(a).

34. 21USC §841(b)(1)(D).

35. Pub L No. 108-358, 118 Stat. 1661 (2004), amending 21USC §802 to clarify the definition of anabolic steroids and to provide for research and education activities relating to steroids and steroid precursors.

36. See, 21USC §812(b)(3); 21USC § 811(c).

37. Comments of Senator Richard Durbin. Congressional Record (Senate). Apr. 1, 2004; S3545-48. Available at: http://thomas.loc.gov/cgi-bin/query/R?r108:FLD001: S53548.

38. Institute of Medicine (IOM) report. Dietary Supplements: A Framework for Evaluating Safety. Available at: http://www.iom.edu/report.asp?id=19578.

39. Archbold M. Bigger, stronger . . . but at a terrible cost: bodybuilder undergoes battery of surgeries to save life, legs. The King County Journal, Apr. 2, 2004. Available at: http://www.kingcountyjournal.com/sited/story/html/160240.

40. Ephedra Survey Results: 1995–1999. Food & Drug Administration Docket 1995-N-0304.

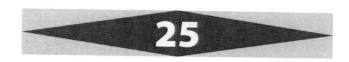

# Very-Low-Carbohydrate Diets

Jeff S. Volek and Cassandra Forsythe

## OBJECTIVES

On the completion of this chapter you will be able to:

1. Explain the basic metabolism of ketone bodies.
2. Describe the different ketone bodies and how they are synthesized.
3. Relate ketone body production to very-low-carbohydrate "ketogenic" diets (VLCKDs).
4. Understand the mechanisms used to regulate ketone body synthesis and utilization.
5. Explain the different metabolic adaptations that occur in response to VLCKDs.
6. Compare and contrast weight loss and body-composition changes in VLCKDs with low-fat diets.
7. Describe why many individuals believe VLCKDs increase cardiovascular disease risk and refute these claims.
8. Understand the effects of VLCKDs on total cholesterol, high-density lipoprotein cholesterol, low-density lipoprotein cholesterol, and triacylglycerols.
9. Describe the effects of VLCKDs on markers of inflammation.
10. Relate VLCKDs to exercise performance and weight loss.

## ABSTRACT

Recently, much interest has surfaced on the value of very low daily carbohydrate diets. Therefore, the primary purpose of this chapter is to provide an overview of this topic while examining relevant scientific research concerning the metabolic responses to very-low-carbohydrate "ketogenic" diets (VLCKDs). Our focus is on studies that have limited carbohydrate ingestion to <50g of carbohydrates per day. From a clinical point of view, a discussion of the effects of VLCKDs on body-weight regulation, lipoprotein metabolism, and cardiovascular disease risk factors is presented. The issue of participating in physical activity and exercise performance while on a VLCKD is also discussed. Additional studies are warranted to further validate the physiologic effects of VLCKDs over longer periods of time including studies that look at modifying the quality of macronutrients and the interaction with other interventions such as exercise, dietary supplements, and drugs.

*Key words:* Low carbohydrate, ketogenic, performance, metabolic syndrome

From: *Essentials of Sports Nutrition and Supplements*
Edited by J. Antonio, D. Kalman, J. R. Stout, M. Greenwood, D. S. Willoughby, and
G. G. Haff © Humana Press, a part of Springer Science+Business Media, Totowa, NJ

The popularity of diets that limit intake of carbohydrate has increased dramatically in recent years. Extreme dietary restriction of carbohydrate (i.e., <40–50 g per day) results in a metabolic state of ketosis, and these diets are frequently referred to as "ketogenic" diets. These diets are gaining acceptance because of an increasing number of scientific studies supporting their health-promoting effects on fat loss and a myriad of clinical risk factors for cardiovascular disease and diabetes. Because there are many misconceptions regarding the metabolic state of ketosis, particularly when induced by carbohydrate restriction in healthy individuals, this chapter overviews ketone metabolism and discusses the factors regulating ketone production and disposal. Much "recent" research has been generated in the last 5 years, so a primary purpose is to provide an overview of scientific studies that have examined the metabolic responses to very-low-carbohydrate "ketogenic" diets (VLCKDs). A focus is on studies that have limited carbohydrate to <50 g per day. From a clinical point of view, a discussion of the effects of VLCKDs on body-weight regulation, lipoprotein metabolism, and cardiovascular disease risk factors is provided. We also discuss the issue of performing physical activity and exercise performance while on a VLCKD.

## REVIEW OF THE LITERATURE

### Overview of Ketone Body Metabolism

Several scientific reviews discussing ketone body metabolism in health and disease have been published over the last two decades.[1–6] The presence of ketones has generally been viewed as negative, perhaps a result of the association with diabetic hyperketoacidosis, which is a serious condition for persons with uncontrolled diabetes. The presence of low levels of ketones, such as during fasting or carbohydrate restriction, is quite different. In fact, there is ongoing research into the therapeutic potential of ketones in a variety of clinical states including: 1) diseases of substrate insufficiency or insulin resistance, 2) diseases resulting from free radical damage, and 3) diseases resulting from hypoxia.[7,8] In fact, ketones have been referred to as "super fuels" because they are about 25% more efficient at producing adenosine triphosphate (ATP) than glucose or fatty acid.[9]

During prolonged fasting or dietary carbohydrate restriction, whole-body metabolism gradually shifts toward oxidizing a greater percentage of energy from lipid sources. High rates of triacylglycerol (TAG) lipolysis and increased delivery of fatty acids to the liver subsequently lead to the accumulation of substantial amounts of acetyl-coenzyme A (CoA) and formation of ketone bodies (acetoacetate and β-hydroxybutyrate) in the mitochondrial matrix of the liver. The carbons used in ketone body production are preferentially obtained from acetyl-CoA derived from fatty acid oxidation rather than glucose, the latter being directed toward metabolism in the citric acid cycle. Biosynthesis of ketones in the liver is shown in Figure 25.1. The only known reaction involving β-hydroxybutyrate is interconversion with acetoacetate. Very small quantities of acetone are also formed by decarboxylation of acetoacetate and volatilized in the lungs. Clinically, ketone body production indicates that lipolysis has been accelerated and that all the enzymes involved in metabolic pathways of lipid metabolism (e.g., lipolysis, fatty acid transport, β-oxidation, and ketogenesis) are operational.

On a VLCKD, adipocyte lipolysis is enhanced, free fatty acid concentrations in the blood increase, and ketone body production in the liver increases. Ketone bodies produced in the liver are soluble in the blood and travel to extrahepatic tissues where they are used as fuel substrates after conversion back to acetyl-CoA. Unique to ketone bodies is the wide range of blood concentrations that span more than four orders of magnitude ($10^{-2}$ to $10^{-5}$ mol/L).[10] This range is in contrast to the tightly regulated and narrow limits imposed on other energy-providing substrates such as glucose, lactate, fatty acids, alanine, and glycerol. The concentration of blood ketones (β-hydroxybutyrate plus acetoacetate) in healthy individuals in the fed state is about 0.1 mmol/L and increases to about 0.3 mmol/L after an overnight fast.[10] Prolonged fasting up to 20 days can increase

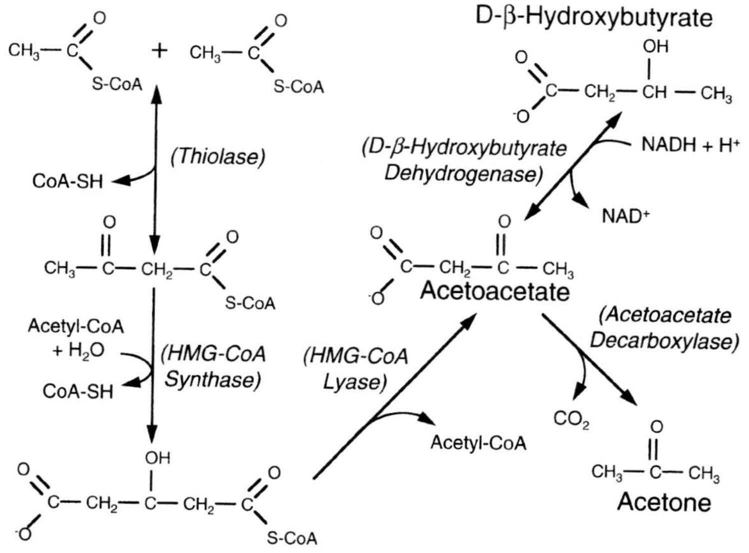

**FIGURE 25.1.** Biosynthesis of ketone bodies (acetoacetate, β-hydroxybutyrate, and acetone) from acetyl-coenzyme A (CoA) in the mitochondrial matrix of the liver. Thiolase catalyzes the condensation of two acetyl-CoA molecules to acetoacetyl-CoA. Mitochondrial 3-hydroxy-3-methyglutaryl (HMG)-CoA synthase catalyzes the condensation of acetoacetyl-CoA with another acetyl-CoA forming HMG-CoA. Acetoacetate is formed by cleavage of acetyl-CoA by mitochondrial HMG-CoA lyase. β-Hydroxybutyrate is formed from acetoacetate via reduction of acetoacetate by β-hydroxybutyrate dehydrogenase. Acetone is also formed in small amounts by spontaneous loss of a carboxyl group or by the action of acetoacetate decarboxylase.

ketone bodies to >10 mmol/L. In healthy men, an isocaloric VLCKD (<20 g carbohydrate/day) resulted in β-hydroxybutyrate >2 mmol/L after 2 weeks and 3 mmol/L by 4 weeks.[11] The extent of ketosis achievable with dietary carbohydrate restriction is well below the levels that occur in uncontrolled diabetes, which often exceed 20 mmol/L. Thus, the level of ketosis on a VLCKD is a "physiologic" ketosis and not comparable to that associated with diabetic hyperketoacidosis.

## Regulation of Ketone Production

Regulation of ketogenesis is controlled at three levels, the first being extrahepatic and the remaining two occurring in the liver: 1) the extent of TAG hydrolysis in adipocytes, 2) the extent of free fatty acid transport across the inner mitochondrial membrane, and 3) partitioning of acetyl-CoA between the ketogenic pathway and oxidation via the citric acid cycle inside the mitochondrial matrix (Figure 25.2). The enzymes hormone-sensitive lipase (HSL), carnitine palmitoyl transferase-I (CPT-I), and mitochondrial 3-hydroxy-3-methyglutaryl (HMG)-CoA synthase regulate these three levels of regulation, respectively.

The extent of hepatic ketogenesis is dependent on the amount of fatty acids passing through the liver. In turn, fatty acid delivery to the liver is largely a reflection of the rate of lipolysis in adipocytes. Many hormones influence adipose tissue metabolism, the most notable of which is insulin during resting

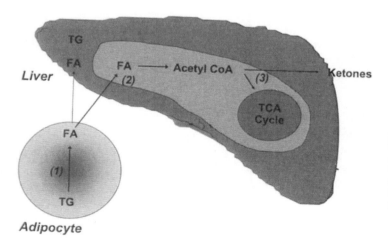

**FIGURE 25.2.** Regulation of ketone production occurs at three levels: 1) triacylglycerol (TG) hydrolysis in adipocytes leads to increased levels of fatty acids (FA). This step is primarily regulated by the activity of hormone-sensitive lipase. 2) Fatty acids passing through the liver will be either taken up into the mitochondria or esterified into TG. Entry into the mitochondria is regulated by the enzyme carnitine palmitoyl transferase I. 3) Fatty acids in the mitochondria are oxidized to acetyl-coenzyme A (CoA) via β-oxidation. Partitioning of acetyl-CoA between the citric acid cycle (oxidation) and production of ketones is regulated by the enzyme 3-hydroxy-3-methyglutaryl CoA synthase.

conditions. At rest, the rate of lipolysis is exquisitely sensitive to physiologic levels of insulin.[12] Insulin reduces cyclic AMP levels in the cell and inactivates the primary hormone involved in TAG hydrolysis, HSL. Insulin also promotes glucose uptake into adipocytes and activates several lipogenic enzymes (e.g., fatty acid synthase), thus further reducing the release of fatty acids from adipose tissue.

In the liver, fatty acids may be either esterified into TAG in the cytosol or transported into the mitochondria. Once inside the mitochondrial matrix, the fatty acyls are committed to oxidation and subsequent formation of acetyl-CoA. Thus, the rate of fatty acid entry into the mitochondria also determines the extent of ketogenesis. Long-chain fatty acids in the cytosol are activated by the enzyme acyl-CoA synthetase on the outer mitochondria membrane in the presence of CoA and ATP. However, the inner mitochondrial membrane is impermeable to these activated fatty acids. Transport across the inner mitochondrial is achieved via a carnitine-dependent process that involves formation of acylcarnitine from free carnitine and acyl-CoA. The reaction is catalyzed by the enzyme CPT-I, located on the outer mitochondrial membrane.[13] Acylcarnitine is transported through the carnitine-acyl/carnitine transporter into the mitochondrial matrix. Within the mitochondria matrix, acylcarnitine is reconverted to the respective acyl-CoA by another enzyme, CPT-II, located on the inner leaflet of the inner mitochondrial membrane. Once inside the matrix, acyl-CoAs are committed to $\beta$-oxidation. CPT-I is inhibited by malonyl-CoA, the first intermediate in the biosynthesis of long-chain fatty acids. Thus, biosynthesis and oxidation of long-chain fatty acids are regulated by the concentration of malonyl-CoA. Malonyl-CoA is up-regulated by insulin. Thus, when insulin levels are increased, as in the fed condition or when carbohydrates are in abundance, malonyl-CoA is activated leading to a decrease in the transport of long-chain fatty acids into the mitochondrial matrix and subsequent inhibition of fatty acid oxidation. Conversely, when insulin levels are low, as during starvation or carbohydrate restriction, malonyl-CoA levels increase and activate CPT-I. Thus, transport of long-chain fatty acids into the mitochondria is increased, leading to higher rates of fatty acid oxidation. Additionally, low insulin concentrations release the normal inhibition of TAG hydrolysis in adipocytes, thus enhancing delivery of fatty acids to the liver.

The last regulatory step for ketogenesis is the partitioning of acetyl-CoA between the ketogenic pathway and oxidation to $CO_2$ via the citric acid cycle. Proportionally more acetyl-CoA enters the ketogenic pathway (diverted away from citrate synthase and entry into the citric acid cycle) as the level of serum fatty acids increases, thus allowing the liver to oxidize greater quantities of fatty acids. A reduction in the concentration of oxaloacetate in the mitochondria has been hypothesized to impair the citric acid cycle metabolism of acetyl-CoA leading to greater production of ketones. The importance of mitochondrial HMG-CoA synthase, which catalyzes the condensation of acetoacetyl-CoA with another molecule of acetyl-CoA to form HMG-CoA, as a regulatory element in the ketogenic pathway has been emphasized.[14] Both short-term regulation of HMG-CoA synthase by succinylation-desuccinylation and long-term regulation via changes in mRNA levels have been reported.[15] HMG-CoA synthase mRNA and protein levels were increased in rats under ketogenic conditions of starvation, diabetes, fat feeding, and injection of cyclic AMP whereas it was decreased by insulin and refeeding.[14] The same effectors that increase HMG-CoA synthase mRNA levels also desuccinylate and activate the enzyme.

## Utilization of Ketones

Comprehensive reviews describing various physiologic roles of ketone bodies have been written.[1,5] During starvation or periods of a VLCKD, ketone bodies serve as an alternative oxidative fuel for peripheral tissues to spare carbohydrate. Oxidation of ketone bodies occurs in many extrahepatic tissues. Skeletal muscle contributes a large portion to total ketone body consumption because of its large mass and capacity to increase blood flow, especially during exercise. Extrahepatic tissues generally oxidize ketones in proportion to their concentration in the blood. However, tissues become saturated as the concentration increases.[4] There are three enzymes involved in ketone oxidation: β-hydroxybutyrate dehydrogenase which forms acetoacetate from β-hydroxybutyrate; succinyl CoA-oxoacid transferase (SCOT) which catalyzes the formation of acetoacetyl-CoA from acetoacetate; and methylacetoacetyl-CoA thiolase (MAT) which catalyzes the formation of two acetyl-CoAs from acetoacetyl-CoA. As ketone body production increases, urinary excretion will be increased in direct proportion to the plasma concentration[4,16] and may represent 10%–20% of ketone body production.[17] Thus, increased circulating ketones is primarily a reflection of increased ketone body production that is complemented by a progressive decrease in the ability of tissues to remove ketones from plasma as the concentration increases.[16]

## Metabolic Adaptations

An increase in the capacity to oxidize lipid substrates is an important adaptation when carbohydrate intake and availability are low. Hormonal and metabolic adaptations to a VLCKD mirror many of the responses usually seen with fasting.[18,19] Although the exact stimuli for such adaptations have not been elucidated, an increase in sympathoadrenal activity and subsequent metabolic alterations favoring oxidation of fat and ketone bodies are frequently observed.

VLCKDs influence the storage and utilization of energy substrates. Many of the studies examining the effects of VLCKDs on metabolism have used exercise as a model. Physical activity requires accelerated rates of ATP hydrolysis, thus placing an enhanced demand on metabolic pathways to supply the required energy. When muscle and liver glycogen are depleted or reduced, cells (in particular skeletal muscle fibers) must adapt to using circulating fatty acids, ketones, and TAG in very low-density lipoproteins (VLDLs) and/or use muscle TAG stores as alternative fuels. Because the ultimate oxidation of fat in skeletal muscle is subject to complex regulation at multiple levels, to optimally switch over from carbohydrate to lipid requires a complex set of metabolic adaptations that originate at the level of gene expression.[20]

Many animal and human studies have consistently demonstrated that high-fat/low-carbohydrate diets consumed for >7 days decrease muscle glycogen content and carbohydrate oxidation, which is compensated for by markedly increased rates of fat oxidation,[21–26] even in well-trained endurance athletes who already demonstrate increased fat oxidation.[23] The source of enhanced fat oxidation seems to be circulating fatty acids, ketones, and TAG-derived VLDLs,[22,25,27] the latter probably resulting from enhanced skeletal muscle lipoprotein lipase (LPL) activity.[28] The enhanced capacity for fat oxidation and muscle glycogen sparing after a high-fat diet persist even when carbohydrate is provided before exercise (e.g., one study carbohydrate loaded for 7 days) or when glucose is ingested during exercise.[29] Compared with a conventional diet, this so-called carbohydrate loading after adaptation to a high-fat diet has been shown to enhance performance during ultraendurance exercise challenges,[24,30] but others studies have failed to show a clear benefit despite increased fat oxidation.[29,31,32]

The increase in fat oxidation and decrease in carbohydrate oxidation on a high-fat diet are associated with robust metabolic and enzymatic adaptations (see Table 25.1). These adaptations are to some extent fiber-type specific and depend on the increase in dietary fat. The time course of metabolic adaptations remains unclear. Some lipolytic adaptations occur within a week (e.g., gene expression of FAT/CD36 and β-HAD) whereas others take longer (e.g., FABP and CPT-I). Thus, at least several weeks are necessary for complete switch over to optimal fat utilization.

## Weight Loss

Obesity is a fast-growing epidemic that is primarily the result of environmental influences. Nutrition and exercise represent modifiable factors with a major impact on energy balance. The basic principle on which weight-loss diets are

**TABLE 25.1. Metabolic and enzymatic adaptations to low-carbohydrate/high-fat diets.**

Fat metabolism:
↑ fat oxidation
↑ muscle TAG storage
↑ muscle TAG utilization during exercise
↑ VLDL catabolism during exercise
↑ fatty acid bind protein and fatty acid translocase (FAT/CD36)
↑ ketone body production and utilization
↑ muscle lipoprotein lipase
↑ β-hydroxyacyl-CoA dehydrogenase
↑ carnitine acyltransferase I
↑ 3-oxoacid CoA thiolase

Carbohydrate metabolism:
↓ carbohydrate oxidation
↓ muscle glycogen storage
↓ muscle glycogen rate of utilization during exercise
↑ gluconeogenesis
↑ phosphoenolpyruvate carboxykinase
↓ hexokinase
↓ pyruvate dehydrogenase

TAG = triacylglycerol, VLDL = very low-density lipoprotein, CoA = coenzyme A.

based is to reduce dietary energy intake below energy expenditure. Whether the relative composition of macronutrients can influence the magnitude or composition of weight loss achieved on an energy-restricted diet has been a point of contention. Despite considerable research, there remains continued debate regarding the macronutrient distribution of effective weight-loss diets. Low-fat (LF) diets have been and continue to be advised by the standard medical and nutrition establishment to reduce obesity. However, their effectiveness has recently been challenged because the prevalence of obesity continues to increase despite reductions in fat intake.[33] Research strongly supports the notion that VLCKDs may have advantages over conventional LF diets.

There was much interest in studying VLCKDs in the 1960s and 1970s. In lieu of favorable studies published during this time,[34,35] there was a virtual absence of studies for the next two decades. A resurgence in this area of research is evident by the publication of several studies that compared weight loss between VLCKDs and LF diets in the last few years.[36–42] Each of these studies showed a greater weight loss with a free-living VLCKD than a LF diet after 3–6 months. In fact, weight loss was about twofold greater in each of these studies (Figure 25.3). Although in two studies weight loss was not statistically different between a VLCKD and a LF diet after 1 year,[37,40] numerically the VLCKD still resulted in twofold greater weight loss over the LF diet and improved surrogate markers of cardiovascular disease.

**FIGURE 25.3.** Weight loss in studies comparing very-low-carbohydrate "ketogenic" diets (VLCKDs) and low-fat diets in overweight/obese individuals. All studies were 6 months in duration with the exception of Sondike et al.,[39] which was 3 months.

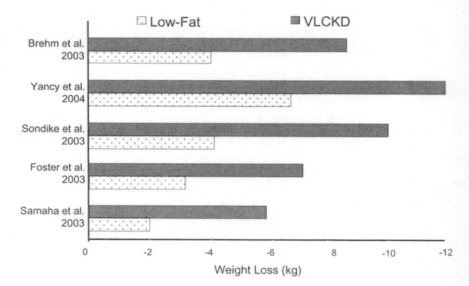

What is the reason for the greater weight loss with VLCKDs? There are many possibilities. One argument is that the greater weight loss on an ad libitum VLCKD is primarily a result of subjects spontaneously reducing their energy intake,[43] and this has been reported previously.[44] A reduction in energy intake on a VLCKD has a logical physiologic basis and could account for a portion of the greater weight loss observed in studies that involved free-living ab libitum VLCKD. Ketone levels increase several-fold on a VLCKD, and β-hydroxybutyrate has been shown to directly inhibit appetite.[45] Also, the low glycemic nature of a VLCKD may prevent transient dips in blood glucose, which can occur with higher-carbohydrate diets. Thus, avoidance of hypoglycemic episodes may reduce appetite.[46] Because food was not provided in these studies, it is possible less dietary energy was consumed during the VLCKD. However, dietary analysis of self-recorded food records indicated that energy intake was similar between VLCKDs and LF diets, or higher during the VLCKD and there is no reason to believe subjects systematically over-reported during the VLCKD or under-reported during the LF diet. Furthermore, other studies that compared formula-based isocaloric VLCKDs and LF diets still showed greater weight loss on a VLCKD.[35,47] Thus, other mechanisms are likely operating to explain the greater weight loss seen with VLCKDs.

Differential weight loss with isocaloric diets differing in macronutrient distribution is the underlying basis of metabolic advantage. Nutritionists have long held that "a calorie is a calorie" and that weight loss on hypocaloric diets is independent of the macronutrient distribution, invoking the first law of thermodynamics to defend this principle.[43] The first law is a conservation law stating that the form of energy may change, but the total is always the same. The second law is important in this respect too, and states that in any irreversible process, the entropy (i.e., disorder or high probability) must increase. In other words, balance is not expected. Feinman and Fine[48] have argued and clearly defended their stance, that acceptance of "a calorie is a calorie" is actually a violation of this second law of energy. Given such evidence, it is difficult to understand the alternate position claiming a calorie must be a calorie in order to satisfy the first law of thermodynamics.[49] There is widespread misunderstanding of the laws of thermodynamics among many nutrition researchers and dietitians. Indeed, many studies have been published to establish the existence of metabolic advantage and eloquent reviews have clearly explained that there are no theoretical violations of laws of thermodynamics.[48,50] Furthermore, there are many theoretical mechanisms to explain the phenomenon. Diets very low in carbohydrate use different chemical pathways that vary in efficiency. Thermogenesis also differs between the macronutrients with protein exhibiting a several-fold-higher energy cost than carbohydrate and fat.[51] This difference alone could explain the greater weight loss on VLCKDs and support metabolic advantage. A metabolic advantage on a VLCKD may also be driven by increased protein turnover to fuel gluconeogenesis.[52] Not all studies have shown greater weight loss with a VLCKD diet[53] and the specific conditions that are required to elicit a metabolic advantage remain unknown.

## Body Composition

Although several studies have shown that VLCKDs result in greater reductions in body mass, how these diets affect the composition/distribution of weight loss continues to be debated. A common criticism of VLCKDs is that the weight loss is mainly water and lean body mass, not fat mass. However, the evidence clearly indicates this is not true. In fact, the opposite may occur. That is, VLCKDs may enhance fat loss and spare losses in lean body mass. Some loss in lean body mass is expected with weight loss. In a meta-analysis, Garrow and Summerbell[54] predict from regression analysis that for a weight loss of 10 kg by dieting alone the expected loss of fat mass is about 71%. Studies that have measured body composition on VLCKDs are shown in Table 25.2 and expressed as the amount of fat lost relative to total weight lost. Although variable, these studies do not provide any evidence of a preferential loss of lean tissue. In fact, several studies are indicative of a preservation of lean tissue.

TABLE 25.2. Very-low-carbohydrate ketogenic diet studies that assessed weight loss and fat loss.

| Reference | Weight loss (kg) | Fat loss (kg) | Fat loss/weight loss (%) | Duration | Method |
|---|---|---|---|---|---|
| Benoit et al.[55] | −6.6 | −6.4 | 97 | 10 d | UWW |
| Young et al.[56] | −15.6 | −14.9 | 96 | 9 wk | K40 |
| Phinney et al.[57] | −10.6 | −7.1 | 67 | 6 wk | UWW |
| Willi et al.[58] | −15.4 | −16.6 | 109 | 8 wk | DEXA |
| Volek et al.[59] | −2.2 | −3.3 | 150 | 6 wk | DEXA |
| Meckling et al.[60] | −5.0 | −4.0 | 80 | 8 wk | BIA |
| Meckling et al.[53] | −6.0 | −4.2 | 68 | 10 wk | BIA |
| Brehem et al.[36] | −6.8 | −4.8 | 71 | 6 mo | BIA |
| Yancy et al.[38] | −12.0 | −9.9 | 83 | 24 wk | BIA |
| Volek et al.[42] | −6.0 | −4.3 | 73 | 6 wk | DEXA |
| Volek et al. (unpublished) | −7.2 | −5.8 | 80 | 12 wk | DEXA |

UWW = underwater weighing, K40 = potassium 40 counting, DEXA = dual-energy X-ray absorptiometry, BIA = bioelectrical impedance analysis.

We recently reported that a free-living 6-week VLCKD prescribed to be isocaloric resulted in significant decreases in fat mass and increases in lean body mass in normal-weight men.[59] In a follow-up study, we showed that a VLCKD resulted in twofold greater whole-body fat loss and threefold greater fat loss in the trunk region compared with a LF diet.[42] This study was a crossover design (subjects were randomized to both a VLCKD and a LF diet). Fat loss in the trunk region was greater during the VLCKD in 12 of 15 men and 12 of 13 women. This could be of important clinical significance because accumulation of fat in the abdominal area is associated with insulin resistance, diabetes, dyslipidemias, and atherosclerosis.[61]

Although the mechanisms by which VLCKDs increase fat loss have not been elucidated, a reduction in insulin is probably important in explaining a portion of the greater fat loss. Inhibition of lipolysis occurs at relatively low concentrations of insulin with a half-maximal effect occurring at a concentration of 12 pmol/L and a maximal effect at a concentration of about 200–300 pmol/L.[12] Thus, even small reductions in insulin may be permissive to mobilization of body fat on a VLCKD.

## Cardiovascular Disease Risk

Atherosclerotic disease and its major complications are still a major health problem in the Western world. Atherosclerosis (hardening of the arteries) has long been considered a disease characterized merely by accumulation of cholesterol in the arterial wall. This has led to a focus on measuring cholesterol levels to assess the efficacy of drug and lifestyle interventions such as diet. There is also substantial evidence revealing the important role of inflammation at all stages of atherosclerosis,[62,63] and this has led to a number of additional markers shown to predict future cardiovascular events (e.g., C-reactive protein).[62]

Because VLCKDs are inherently high in total fat, saturated fat, and cholesterol, there has been concern that cholesterol levels and other standard markers of cardiovascular disease may be adversely affected. There has been a rather large number of studies that have examined the effects of VLCKDs on lipids. Although these studies differ somewhat in respect to a number of design aspects (e.g., total energy intake, macronutrient distribution, weight loss, type of fat, subject characteristics, length of dietary intervention), they share the common element that all involved prescription of a very-low-carbohydrate intake.

## Metabolic Syndrome

The metabolic syndrome is a highly prevalent, multifaceted clustering of cardiovascular disease risk factors with key features of central obesity, insulin resistance, dyslipidemia, and hypertension, as well as chronic inflammation, procoagulation, and impaired fibrinolysis.[64,65] Although the precise definition varies, it is estimated that almost one quarter of adults >20 years and 40% of adults >40 years have metabolic syndrome in the United States.[66] Therefore, metabolic syndrome has been described as a health care crisis of epidemic proportions.[67] The basis of therapies at this time is interventions promoting weight loss and physical activity,[68] but diet represents another behavioral aspect that could have an important impact on the risk factors associated with metabolic syndrome. The lipid disorders of metabolic syndrome classically include increased fasting TAG (>150 mg/dL) and low high-density lipoprotein cholesterol (HDL-C) (<40 or 50 mg/dL for men and women, respectively), but also is characterized by enhanced postprandial lipemia (i.e., an exaggerated and prolonged increase in TAG after a meal) and a predominance of small low-density lipoprotein (LDL) particles. Other characteristics include increased fasting glucose (>120 mg/dL), waist circumference (>102 or 88 cm for men and women, respectively), and increased systolic blood pressure (>130 mm Hg). As described next, VLCKDs seem to favorably affect these metabolic abnormalities.

## Total Cholesterol

There is a strong association between plasma concentrations of total cholesterol (TC) and LDL-C with the severity of coronary atherosclerosis and rates of coronary artery disease (CAD).[69] Consequently, dietary strategies aimed at improving blood lipid profiles and the risk of CAD have focused on reducing TC and LDL-C as main targets for therapy.

The majority of VLCKD studies conducted have been in subjects who lost weight. The general response in these studies is a moderate reduction (>5%) in TC,[11,34,57,58,60,70–74] which is probably driven primarily by the beneficial effect of weight loss on lipoproteins.[75] However, some studies have reported no change or small increases in TC even with weight loss.[37,41,74,76,77] The reduction in TC on a VLCKD is usually not as great in magnitude compared with a LF diet.[34,39,74,77] In subjects receiving isocaloric VLCKDs that result in minimal changes in body weight, TC generally increases.[78,79] The type of fat has an important impact on TC in standard mixed diets, but few studies have addressed this issue on a VLCKD. There is some evidence that an isocaloric VLCKD low in saturated fat and rich in either polyunsaturated[80] or monounsaturated[81] fat attenuates the increase in TC, indicating that the type of fat in a VLCKD may also have a small role in determining cholesterol responses.

The increases in TC on a VLCKD in the absence of weight loss may be transient with concentrations peaking after 2–4 weeks and gradually returning toward baseline levels after 6–8 weeks.[78,81] It should also be noted that much intersubject variability in TC responses exists. Figure 25.4 shows the variability in TC responses in 90 subjects we have studied in our laboratory. Approximately half the subjects show a decrease and half an increase in TC in response to a VLCKD. Future research should be directed at understanding what biologic and genetic factors contribute to this variability. This variability is partially (about 27%) explained by the change in body weight, indicating that other factors also contribute to the diverse TC responses.

## Low- and High-Density Lipoprotein Cholesterol

TC is composed of both LDL-C and HDL-C. There is strong evidence implicating increased LDL-C in the causation of CAD.[69] In contrast, a low HDL-C level is strongly and inversely associated with risk for CAD and a high level of HDL-C is associated with reduced risk.[82] A high HDL-C value ≥60 mg/dL is considered a negative risk factor, and its presence evokes removal of one risk factor from the total count used for setting treatment goals for LDL-C.[68]

Although TC responses to a VLCKD are sometimes increased, nearly all studies indicate that this is a result of increases in both LDL-C and HDL-C. In fact, most studies report that the increase in HDL-C is proportionally greater than the increase in LDL-C such that the TC/HDL-C ratio actually decreases.[36,37,39,60,70–72,74,78,79,81] The response is particularly evident in studies that

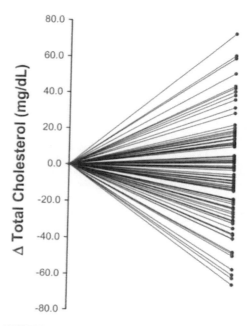

**FIGURE 25.4.** Individual total cholesterol responses to a very-low-carbohydrate ketogenic diet. Subjects are from studies conducted in our laboratory and include overweight men,[74] overweight women,[77] normal-weight men,[78,81] and normal-weight women.[79]

reported minimal weight loss. This is probably because active weight loss is associated with significant reductions in HDL-C,[75] at least if induced by a LF diet, whereas VLCKD tends to prevent this decrease. Although women have higher HDL-C compared with men, their response to a VLCKD is similar, or in some cases higher in magnitude, than men.[78,79] One study showed an increase in the mean size of HDL particles after a 6-week VLCKD in patients with atherosclerotic cardiovascular disease.[73] Larger particles correspond to the $HDL_2$ subfraction, which is believed to be the specific subclass responsible for the cardioprotective effects of HDL-C.[83]

## Fasting Triacylglycerols

A recent meta-analysis of prospective studies indicated that an increase in fasting TAGs is associated with a significant increase in the incidence of cardiovascular disease in men and women, and the effect is independent of HDL-C concentrations.[84] The most consistent response to a VLCKD is a moderate to large reduction in TAGs,[11,34,36,37,39,41,57,60,70-74,76,77,85] which is independent of weight loss.[78,79] The largest reductions in TAGs (–55%) were reported in healthy men who consumed a VLCKD supplemented with fish oils,[81] indicating supplementation may work in concert with carbohydrate restriction to maximize TAG-lowering. Although nearly all subjects experience a reduction in TAGs, those with higher levels seem to experience the greatest reductions. In fact, 72% of the variability in TAG responses to a VLCKD in our studies is explained by baseline (starting) values (Figure 25.5). This finding is of particular relevance for people with the highly prevalent metabolic syndrome.

## Postprandial Lipemia

The atherogenicity of TAG-rich lipoproteins in the postprandial state, either directly or indirectly, may have a greater role than fasting values in CAD risk and has been the topic of several studies and review articles.[86,87] Patsch et al.[88] demonstrated a greater lipemia after a fat load test in patients with severe CAD compared with control subjects without CAD. Fasting TAG failed to be an independent risk factor using multivariate logistic-regression analysis whereas postprandial TAG was the most accurate variable among several other accepted risk factors for predicting the presence or absence of CAD.[88]

Our laboratory group has demonstrated that a VLCKD decreases postprandial lipemia on the order of one third to half in normal-weight men,[78,81] normal-weight women,[79] overweight men,[74] and overweight women.[77] Individuals that exhibit an exaggerated postprandial TAG response (i.e., peak postmeal values >400 mg/dL) demonstrate the largest improvements after a VLCKD. The sig-

**FIGURE 25.5.** Association between individual triacylglycerol (TAG) responses to a very-low-carbohydrate ketogenic diet (VLCKD) and baseline TAG values. Subjects are from studies conducted in our laboratory and include overweight men,[74] overweight women,[77] normal-weight men[78,81] and normal-weight women.[79]

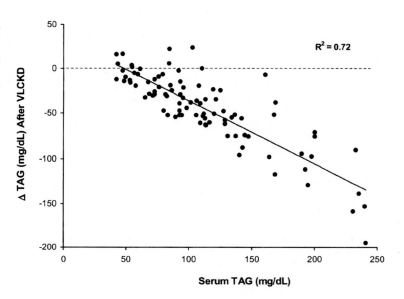

nificant reductions in both fasting and postprandial TAGs could be attributable to a combination of a reduced hepatic VLDL-TAG production rate, which has been shown to increase on a high-carbohydrate diet[89] and/or an increase in TAG removal because low-carbohydrate/high-fat diets (46%–65% of total energy) significantly increase post-heparin plasma LPL activity and skeletal muscle LPL activity in humans.[90,91]

## Low-Density Lipoprotein Subclass Distribution

Although the significant reductions in fasting and postprandial TAG and the increases in HDL-C in response to VLCKDs are favorable in terms of CAD risk, the moderate increases in LDL-C in some people could be interpreted as unfavorable. However, there seems to be changes in the size and composition of LDL-C that may counteract any adverse effect on CAD. The existence of different subclasses of LDL-C has been known for many years. Distinct LDL subclasses can be separated out based on their diameter, which range in size from approximately 21.8 nm for the small, dense LDL particles to 27.8 nm for the larger, more buoyant LDL particles.[92] Individuals with a predominance of large, buoyant LDL-C have been classified as "pattern A" whereas those with a predominance of small, dense LDL particles are termed "pattern B," the latter being associated with a greater than threefold risk of CAD.[93]

Switching from a high-fat (46% of energy) to a LF (26% of energy) diet resulted in an increase in small, dense LDL particles in a subset of men (33%) with large, buoyant LDLs.[94] In a follow-up study, a further reduction in fat to 10% of energy increased small, dense LDLs in men with increased TAGs,[95] suggesting that individuals with increased TAGs are more prone to alterations in LDL subclass toward small, dense particles in response to reductions in dietary fat. Reducing dietary carbohydrate, however, decreases fasting and postprandial TAGs and thereby increases HDL-C and formation of larger, less-atherogenic LDL particles.[93,96] We have shown that a VLCKD results in increased peak LDL size and shifts in particle distribution from pattern B to pattern A in normal-weight[78] and overweight[74] men. We did not report the same effect in women,[77] but this was likely because of the larger starting particle sizes in the women. In these studies, there was an inverse correlation between baseline peak LDL size and the change in LDL size to the VLCKD, indicating that both men and women who have smaller, more atherogenic LDL particles increase LDL size in response to a VLCKD. One other study has also shown that a VLCKD results in significantly increased mean LDL size in patients with cardiovascular disease and a high prevalence of metabolic syndrome.[73] Collectively, these studies indicate that when carbohydrate is increased and fat is decreased the distribution of LDL moves toward a smaller, more dense particle and when dietary carbohydrate is reduced, the distribution of LDL moves toward larger, less-atherogenic particles.

## Inflammatory Markers

It is now known that inflammatory processes have a pivotal role in the pathogenesis of atherosclerosis and mediate many of the stages of atheroma development from initial leukocyte recruitment to eventual rupture of the unstable atherosclerotic plaque.[62] The primary proinflammatory cytokines and oxidatively modified LDL (oxLDL) both activate the endothelium and increase the expression of adhesion molecules that are crucial to the recruitment of inflammatory cells from the blood stream and can serve as markers of vascular inflammation.[97,98] Increased plasma levels in humans of these inflammatory biomarkers can provide information about the inflammatory status in individuals at high risk for cardiovascular disease. Currently, very limited data exist on the effects of VLCKDs on markers of inflammation such as proinflammatory cytokines and cellular adhesion molecules (CAMs).

Our laboratory has examined the effects of VLCKDs on inflammatory biomarkers in various populations. In one study looking at the effects of an isoenergetic VLCKD in normal-weight, normolipidemic women for 4 weeks,[79] we found no significant effects on high sensitivity C-reactive protein (hs-CRP), interleukin (IL)-6, or tumor necrosis factor (TNF)-α. In a recent study examining a hypoenergetic 6-week VLCKD in overweight men, we observed significant reductions in hs-CRP (–48%), TNF-α (–42%), IL-6 (–46%), and soluble intercellular cell-adhesion molecule-1 (–20%).[99] These decreases were similar to that achieved by our control who consumed a LF weight-loss diet and are consistent with several other studies showing favorable effects of weight loss on inflammatory markers.[100,101] We have observed similar beneficial effects in women too. Thus, there does not seem to be any support for VLCKDs being proinflammatory.

## PRACTICAL APPLICATION

### Exercise

For more than 30 years, dietary recommendations for active individuals have emphasized high-carbohydrate levels and discouraged VLCKDs.[102] The origin of this position is unclear, but clearly the work after the advent of the percutaneous needle biopsy in the 1960s that allowed measurement of glycogen and other intramuscular fuel sources during exercise was important. These studies of short-term diet manipulation led to the paradigm that still pervades sports nutritionists today: that high-carbohydrate diets are necessary to maintain adequate muscle glycogen during exercise, and the popular carbohydrate loading approach to optimize performance.[103] Given the potential widespread benefits of VLCKDs on weight/fat loss and clinical risk factors for heart disease, it is worth investigating the strength of evidence for high-carbohydrate diets, and perhaps more importantly, answering the question of whether VLCKDs are detrimental to performance.

In an excellent review, Phinney[104] eloquently overviewed the topic of ketogenic diets and exercise performance including a discussion of some of the oversights made in studies that concluded VLCKDs are detrimental to exercise capacity. Historically, entire physically demanding, hunting-based populations lived and thrived on diets virtually devoid of carbohydrate (e.g., Inuit people of the Canadian and Alaskan Arctic regions). There are also descriptive accounts of explorers surviving on VLCKDs and scientific studies replicating these experiences in the literature (overviewed in Phinney[104]). A major limitation in the studies linking reduced carbohydrate intake with impaired performance was that inadequate time was allowed for complete adaptation to the diet. Most studies usually investigate the effects of dietary manipulations on exercise performance for a few days or <1 week. At least several weeks are necessary for complete metabolic adaptation to occur on a VLCKD. When adequate time is allowed for these metabolic adaptations, performance does not seem to be impaired.[21,25,57]

Only a few longitudinal studies have researched VLCKDs (that actually induced ketosis) and the effects on exercise capacity. More than 20 years ago, Phinney et al.[11,25,57] conducted a series of experiments in obese individuals and athletes to examine the effects of VLCKDs on biochemical adaptations and exercise performance. In the first study, six moderately obese, untrained subjects (five female and one male) were adapted to a hypocaloric (500–750 kcal/day), ketogenic diet. For 6 weeks, the subjects consumed a diet that consisted of lean meat, fish, or fowl which provided 1.2 g protein/kg/day ideal body weight and <10 g carbohydrate/day.[57] The diets were also supplemented with sodium and potassium. At the end of weeks 1 and 6, the subjects ran on a treadmill until exhaustion at 70% of maximal oxygen consumption. Subjects performed the postdiet tests with a backpack equal in weight to the amount of weight loss. Compared with endurance time at baseline (168 minutes), there was a significant decrease after 1 week (130 minutes) followed by a significant increase after 6 weeks (249 minutes). Peak aerobic power was not affected. In a follow-up study, Phinney et al.[25] studied five elite cyclists who performed an exhaustive submaximal endurance test (60%–65% of maximal oxygen consumption) on a cycle ergometer after 1 week of a normal, balanced diet and after 4 weeks of an isocaloric VLCKD. There was no change in aerobic performance after 4 weeks. Metabolic measures in both of these studies indicated that the majority of energy was derived from fat oxidation with a subsequent marked reduction in carbohydrate oxidation. These studies confirm that VLCKDs can adversely affect performance for the first week but longer adaptation to the diet does not significantly impair physical performance. These studies[25,57] have not been refuted since their publication more than 2 decades ago.

Our laboratory group investigated the effects of a 6-week VLCKD on several measures of exercise capacity (peak oxygen consumption, endurance capacity, and anaerobic capacity) in normal-weight, relatively untrained but recreationally active men. The VLCKD resulted in moderate ketosis and there was a small, but significant amount of weight loss (−2.2 kg). Peak oxygen consumption was reduced (absolute L/min) but was unchanged when expressed relative to body mass (mL/kg/min). There were small reductions in peak and mean power output during 30-second all-out cycling bouts, as well as work performed during a 45-minute timed cycling ride. We think the small deleterious effects on anaerobic performance in particular may be accounted for in part by a reduction in body mass and/or increased perceived exertion. Nevertheless, the subjects were able to reproduce their efforts very close to the prediet performance, indicating that VLCKDs are compatible with a physically active lifestyle. Subsequent anecdotal claims from younger and older subjects in recent VLCKD studies in our laboratory reveal that subjects do feel some impairment in exercise capacity during the initial week of the diet but have no problems performing physical labor, recreational activities, or structured exercise programs including both endurance training and weight training after this initial period.

In summary, adaptation to a VLCKD does not seem to inhibit submaximal endurance capacity even in highly trained athletes, but may not be optimal for higher-intensity exercise. The use of VLCKDs is proving to be most beneficial for individuals who present characteristics indicative of metabolic syndrome and risk for diabetes and cardiovascular disease. These individuals are not those likely to participate in high-intensity exercise, but are those who more often engage in moderate-intensity physical activity. Physical activity recommendations for prevention of CAD are to participate in 30–60 minutes of moderate-intensity exercise on most days of the week.[105] With this knowledge, sports nutritionists should have no inhibitions recommending a VLCKD to these individuals because of fear that it will harm physical ability, especially because the combination of proper diet prescription and exercise acts synergistically to prevent CAD, diabetes, and combat obesity. In the realm of athletics, certain athletes may benefit from VLCKDs to maximize fat loss without compromising lean tissue mass and strength. The aesthetic potential of VLCKDs was shown during a 6-week VLCKD intervention in young men who actually increased lean body mass while decreasing fat mass.[59] Thus, in certain sports in which the emphasis is on body composition, VLCKDs may have advantages over other diets.

## SUMMARY

In recent years, restriction of carbohydrate intake has become widespread and has led to a revolution in the food industry to meet the demand of consumers trying to restrict carbohydrate (Table 25.3). It is critical that researchers, clinicians, and perhaps most important, dietitians and sports nutritionists on the grass root level, understand the metabolic adaptations and the potential impact of VLCKDs on clinical end points. The dramatic change in macronutrient distribution associated with restriction of carbohydrate results in robust and powerful metabolic adaptation that improves a person's ability to mobilize and utilize noncarbohydrate energy sources. The metabolic adaptations to VLCKDs are comparable to those seen during fasting with the major exception that the body is not operating under a major energy deficit. This could have theoretical advantages for mobilizing and utilizing TAGs stored in adipocytes and thus weight loss and weight control. A major adaptation is the production of ketones, which serve as an alternative fuel for nonhepatic cells and thus reduce the

**TABLE 25.3. Comparison of a very-low-carbohydrate ketogenic diet (VLCKD) versus a traditional high-carbohydrate diet (sample 1-day menu).**

**One-day low-fat meal plan:**
**Breakfast**
1 cup Bran Flakes cereal
1 cup skim milk
6 ounces fat-free yogurt

**Snack**
1 apple

**Lunch**
Tuna salad sandwich with light mayonnaise on whole wheat bread
15 baby carrots
1/2 cup strawberries
1 cup skim milk

**Snack**
8 low-fat whole-wheat crackers
1 fat-free cheese slice

**Dinner**
4 ounces baked cod with lemon
1/2 cup steamed brown rice with low-sodium soy sauce
3/4 cup frozen mixed vegetables
1 small whole-wheat dinner roll with 1 tsp. nonhydrogenated margarine
1 cup apple juice

**Snack**
1/2 cup fat-free chocolate pudding
OR
2 cups low-fat popcorn

**One-day VLCKD meal plan:**
**Breakfast**
1 slice Canadian bacon
2 scrambled eggs
1 ounce cheddar cheese
2 Tbsp. salsa
1 cup low-carbohydrate milk

**Snack**
6 ounces low-carbohydrate yogurt

**Lunch**
Green salad with low-carbohydrate dressing
3/4 can pink salmon
1.5 ounces almonds
1 cup hot tea with 1 package Splenda

**Snack**
1/2 cup zucchini sticks
1 ounce mozzarella cheese

**Dinner**
4 ounces grilled pork chop
1 cup steamed asparagus with garlic powder
1/2 cup low-carbohydrate coleslaw
1 cup sugar-free lemonade

**Snack**
1/2 cup sugar-free chocolate mousse
OR
1/2 cup broccoli florets with sour cream dip

demand for glucose that must be met primarily through gluconeogenesis. This "physiologic" ketosis is not dangerous. In most studies, weight loss is greater on a VLCKD than an LF diet. The effects of VLCKDs on circulating lipoproteins have been assessed in a number of studies in different populations. The most consistent effect is an improvement in fasting and postprandial TAGs, HDL-C, and the distribution of LDL-C subclasses. These are the lipid abnormalities of the metabolic syndrome and thus carbohydrate restriction seems to be quite suited for this highly prevalent condition. Additional studies are needed to further validate the physiologic effects of VLCKDs over longer periods of time including studies that look at modifying the quality of macronutrients (i.e., the type of fat and protein) and the interaction with other interventions (e.g., exercise, dietary supplements, drugs). In conclusion, studies support the notion that short-term VLCKDs are safe and effective in terms of promoting weight/fat loss, improving metabolic and cardiovascular risk factors, and are compatible with a physically active lifestyle. No one diet is ideal or even preferred by everyone. There is sufficient scientific research to safely prescribe a VLCKD as an option to those people who prefer this approach or for those who have not responded to other diets. In this respect, VLCKDs should be considered another option and need not be avoided because of unsubstantiated concerns regarding their safety in healthy individuals.

## Sidebar 25.1. Implication of Postprandial Lipemia in Coronary Artery Disease

The postprandial state refers to the period after food ingestion during which metabolic changes occur in the body that last 4–6 hours (or longer in some cases) and include shifts in blood flow, insulin secretion, dietary-induced thermogenesis, and changes in respiratory exchange ratio. Underlying processes include lymph production, nutrient oxidation and/or storage, synthesis of both chylomicrons and VLDL TAGs, their release into the circulation, and their clearance. During this time, the metabolic priority of the body is "storage" rather than "production," and both hormonal and cardiovascular responses to the digestion and absorption of food dictate differences within each individual. Most humans spend the majority of their day in the postprandial period because of the ingestion of regularly consumed meals.

After consuming a meal that includes fat, there is a dramatic increase in the amount of TAGs in the blood carried by chylomicrons and chylomicron remnants; this metabolic state is known as postprandial lipemia. VLDL production also increases, in response to dietary lipid reaching the liver via the portal vein or from chylomicron delivery. In healthy, normolipidemic individuals, plasma TAG levels do not increase to the same extent as individuals with certain dyslipidemic conditions, and their TAG levels normalize within 4–6 hours.[106] A prolonged postprandial lipemia in dyslipidemic individuals is the subject of many investigations, and is suggested to promote increased risk of atherosclerosis.

Prolonged postprandial lipemia is associated with a constellation of potentially atherogenic lipoprotein changes, including: a) an increase in the plasma concentration of intestinally derived chylomicrons and their remnants, b) an increase in the level of hepatic VLDLs and their remnants, c) a decrease in HDL-C because of increase in cholesteryl ester transfer from HDL to postprandial chylomicrons by cholesteryl ester transfer protein (CETP), and d) a decrease in LDL size associated with increased susceptibility of LDLs to oxidation.[107]

Chylomicron remnants are considered to be atherogenic because they can penetrate arterial tissue and become trapped within the subendothelial space. Furthermore, chylomicron remnants can induce substantial lipid uptake by macrophages, a hallmark feature of atherogenesis.[108] Schaefer[109] noted that after a high-fat meal, the influx of TAGs carried by chylomicrons competed with VLDL TAGs for breakdown by lipoprotein lipase (in adipose and muscle), and in turn, increased availability of TAGs and free fatty acids to promote an increase in hepatic synthesis of VLDLs. Thus, plasma VLDL TAG concentration increased and its residency was prolonged by decreased clearance and increased production in the postprandial state. These extended periods of increase in TAGs could facilitate the formation of intermediate density particles and the higher-density, small LDL.

Although it is generally unclear to what extent VLDL TAGs and their remnants contribute to the formation of atherosclerotic lesions, evidence from several sources have shown that these lipoproteins are potentially atherogenic and thrombogenic.[107] VLDLs and their remnants have been found in human atherosclerotic plaques and their uptake by macrophages in culture has been shown to result in the formation of lipid-loaded cells resembling the foam cells of atherosclerotic lesions.[107]

The relationship between chylomicrons and HDLs is best reflected by the inverse relationship between the magnitude of postprandial lipemia and the plasma concentration of fasting HDL-C. Individuals who have an increased plasma TAG response to a fat meal tend to have a reduced level of HDL-C in the fasting state. When TAG catabolism is inhibited, TAG concentration increases and HDL-C levels decrease.[107] Two mechanisms have been proposed to explain this effect of TAG metabolism on plasma HDL levels: 1) defective clearance of postprandial chylomicrons and VLDLs could result in diminished generation of surface components (free cholesterol, phospholipid, and C-apolipoproteins) that would reduce the rate of formation of HDL particles, and 2) alternatively, increased formation and transfer of cholesteryl esters from HDLs to chylomicrons and VLDLs—mediated by CETP—could result in a reduced amount of plasma HDL.[107]

In conclusion, through the consumption of regular meals, most people are in a postprandial state throughout the majority of a day. Atherosclerosis and CAD must therefore be viewed as processes that occur when plasma lipoproteins are derived from, or under the influence of, lipids from a recently consumed meal. Investigations of dietary manipulations on CAD risk should focus on metabolic events that occur during the postprandial period and recognize that improvements in postprandial lipemia have significant therapeutic implications.

## Sidebar 25.2. Case Study

S.B. was a male subject in a recent study investigating physiologic responses to a VLCKD in our laboratory. He was 57 years of age and weighed 179.5 lbs. and 24.2% body fat assessed using dual-energy X-ray absorptiometry (DEXA). He switched from his habitual diet, which was very low in fat and high in carbohydrate to a VLCKD consisting of <10% carbohydrate. The VLCKD was followed for a period of 12 weeks. S.B. was very active, routinely training for marathons and triathlons. He maintained this high level of activity (>2 hours/day) throughout the VLCKD. S.B. was very meticulous in following the diet as shown by his high level of ketones recorded during the study on a daily basis. He lost a total of 17.6 lbs. after 12 weeks, which was about average for the group. His change in body composition was most remarkable. S.B. went from 24.2% to 12.7% body fat. He lost almost 23 lbs. of fat mass while gaining just over 6 lbs. of lean body mass. These measures were assessed using DEXA, the most accurate method for determining body composition. He also experienced significant improvements in his plasma lipids and was able to set personal records in his training.

## ACKNOWLEDGMENTS

Dr. Volek has received research support from the Dr. Robert C. Atkins Foundation.

## QUESTIONS

1. In the absence of significant dietary carbohydrate, which fuel does the body primarily use for energy?
   a. Blood glucose
   b. Adipocyte triacylglycerol
   c. Skeletal amino acids
   d. Liver glycogen

2. How does insulin decrease the rate of hepatic ketogenesis?
   a. It decreases the rate of adipocyte lipolysis
   b. It up-regulates malonyl-CoA
   c. It increases the rate of adipocyte lipogenesis
   d. All of the above

3. What is the common millimole concentration of ketones found in the blood during a VLCKD?
   a. >20 mmol/L
   b. <0.1 mmol/L
   c. 10–15 mmol/L
   d. 1–3 mmol/L

4. Which enzyme facilitates fatty acid transport across the inner mitochondrial membrane?
   a. Hormone-sensitive lipase
   b. Carnitine palmitoyl transferase-II
   c. Carnitine palmitoyl transferase-I
   d. Lipoprotein lipase

5. How may a VLCKD favorably affect body composition?
   a. It does not affect body composition
   b. It can decrease fat mass
   c. It can decrease bone mineral density
   d. It can decrease lean muscle mass

6. Ketolysis means:
   a. Fatty acid oxidation
   b. Ketone oxidation

c. Triacylglycerol breakdown

d. Glycogen breakdown

7. When muscle glycogen is reduced from low-carbohydrate intake, the activity of which enzyme is decreased?
   a. 3 Oxoacid CoA thiolase
   b. β-Hydroxyacyl-CoA dehydrogenase
   c. Lipoprotein lipase
   d. Hexokinase

8. Which dietary approach has been shown to benefit ultraendurance performance?
   a. A high-fat diet followed by carbohydrate loading
   b. A high-protein diet followed by fat loading
   c. A high-carbohydrate diet followed by protein loading
   d. None of the above

9. Protein is a thermogenic macronutrient because:
   a. It is inefficient; it takes more energy to metabolize it than other macronutrients
   b. It is efficient; it takes less energy to metabolize it than other macronutrients
   c. It is converted easily to glucose via gluconeogenesis
   d. It increases lean muscle mass

10. A "calorie is not a calorie" because:
    a. Most isocaloric diets of different macronutrient composition do not result in equal amounts of weight loss
    b. More calories are lost as heat as carbohydrate intake decreases
    c. Protein, carbohydrate, and fat all have different effects on the hormone profile and enzyme activity in the body
    d. All of the above

11. In which area of the body is fat accumulation most likely to increase the risk of chronic disease?
    a. The abdominal region
    b. The thigh region
    c. The triceps region
    d. The subscapularous region

12. This condition refers to hardening of the arteries and can increase the risk for heart attack and/or stroke:
    a. Diabetes
    b. Cancer
    c. Hypercholesterolemia
    d. Atherosclerosis

13. Characteristics of the metabolic syndrome are:
    a. High fasting plasma HDL cholesterol levels
    b. Hypotension
    c. Insulin sensitivity
    d. High fasting plasma triacylglycerol levels

14. Individuals characterized with "pattern B" LDL cholesterol have:
    a. Large, buoyant LDL cholesterol particles
    b. Large HDL cholesterol particles
    c. Small, dense LDL cholesterol particles
    d. Prolonged postprandial lipemia

15. This proinflammatory cytokine is a powerful inducer of local inflammation in blood vessels:
    a. Interleukin-6
    b. Oxidized LDL cholesterol
    c. Insulin
    d. Acetoacetate

16. This measure of exercise performance has not shown to be significantly impaired by VLCKD:
   a. Peak oxygen consumption
   b. Peak aerobic power
   c. Time to exhaustion
   d. All of the above

17. VLCKDs may be very beneficial for certain athletes because:
   a. They reduce fat mass while preserving lean muscle mass
   b. They do not decrease muscular strength
   c. They reduce risk factors for cardiovascular disease
   d. All of the above

18. Physiologic levels of ketones in the blood are harmful.
   a. True
   b. False

19. Dietary protein is less thermogenic than carbohydrate.
   a. True
   b. False

20. During VLCKDs, most of the weight loss is attributable to water losses.
   a. True
   b. False

21. Atherosclerosis results partly from increased inflammation.
   a. True
   b. False

22. Individuals with metabolic syndrome are characterized by low fasting HDL cholesterol levels.
   a. True
   b. False

23. Dietary polyunsaturated fat can prevent increases in total cholesterol when dietary saturated fat intake is high.
   a. True
   b. False

24. VLCKDs may prevent cardiovascular disease because they result in reduced triacylglycerol concentrations.
   a. True
   b. False

25. VLCKDs are always detrimental to exercise performance.
   a. True
   b. False

26. All athletes need to eat a high-carbohydrate diet.
   a. True
   b. False

27. After adaptation to VLCKD, physical activity is not hindered.
   a. True
   b. False

## REFERENCES

1. Robinson AM, Williamson DH. Physiological roles of ketone bodies as substrates and signals in mammalian tissues. Physiol Rev 1980;60:143–187.
2. McGarry JD, Foster DW. Regulation of hepatic fatty acid oxidation and ketone body production. Annu Rev Biochem 1980;49:395–420.
3. McGarry JD, Woeltje KF, Kuwajima M, Foster DW. Regulation of ketogenesis and the renaissance of carnitine palmitoyltransferase. Diabetes Metab Rev 1989;5:271–284.
4. Balasse EO, Fery F. Ketone body production and disposal: effects of fasting, diabetes, and exercise. Diabetes Metab Rev 1989;5:247–270.

5. Mitchell GA, Kassovska-Bratinova S, Boukaftane Y, et al. Medical aspects of ketone body metabolism. Clin Invest Med 1995;18:193–216.

6. Nosadini R, Avogaro A, Doria A, Fioretto P, Trevisan R, Morocutti A. Ketone body metabolism: a physiological and clinical overview. Diabetes Metab Rev 1989;5:299–319.

7. Veech RL. The therapeutic implications of ketone bodies: the effects of ketone bodies in pathological conditions—ketosis, ketogenic diet, redox states, insulin resistance, and mitochondrial metabolism. Prostaglandins Leukot Essent Fatty Acids 2004;70:309–319.

8. Veech RL, Chance B, Kashiwaya Y, Lardy HA, Cahill GF Jr. Ketone bodies, potential therapeutic uses. IUBMB Life 2001;51:241–247.

9. Cahill GF Jr, Veech RL. Ketoacids? Good medicine? Trans Am Clin Climatol Assoc 2003;114:149–161; discussion 162–163.

10. Rich AJ. Ketone bodies as substrates. Proc Nutr Soc 1990;49:361–373.

11. Phinney SD, Bistrian BR, Wolfe RR, Blackburn GL. The human metabolic response to chronic ketosis without caloric restriction: physical and biochemical adaptation. Metabolism 1983;32:757–768.

12. Jensen MD, Caruso M, Heiling V, Miles JM. Insulin regulation of lipolysis in non-diabetic and IDDM subjects. Diabetes 1989;38:1595–1601.

13. Kerner J, Hoppel C. Fatty acid import into mitochondria. Biochim Biophys Acta 2000;1486:1–17.

14. Serra D, Casals N, Asins G, Royo T, Ciudad CJ, Hegardt FG. Regulation of mitochondrial 3-hydroxy-3-methylglutaryl-coenzyme A synthase protein by starvation, fat feeding, and diabetes. Arch Biochem Biophys 1993;307:40–45.

15. Thumelin S, Forestier M, Girard J, Pegorier JP. Developmental changes in mitochondrial 3-hydroxy-3-methylglutaryl-CoA synthase gene expression in rat liver, intestine and kidney. Biochem J 1993;292(Pt 2):493–496.

16. Fery F, Balasse EO. Ketone body production and disposal in diabetic ketosis. A comparison with fasting ketosis. Diabetes 1985;34:326–332.

17. Garber AJ, Menzel PH, Boden G, Owen OE. Hepatic ketogenesis and gluconeogenesis in humans. J Clin Invest 1974;54:981–989.

18. Galbo H, Christensen NJ, Mikines KJ, et al. The effect of fasting on the hormonal response to graded exercise. J Clin Endocrinol Metab 1981;52:1106–1112.

19. Pequignot JM, Peyrin L, Peres G. Catecholamine-fuel interrelationships during exercise in fasting men. J Appl Physiol 1980;48:109–113.

20. Cameron-Smith D, Burke LM, Angus DJ, et al. A short-term, high-fat diet up-regulates lipid metabolism and gene expression in human skeletal muscle. Am J Clin Nutr 2003;77:313–318.

21. Fleming J, Sharman MJ, Avery NG, et al. Endurance capacity and high-intensity exercise performance responses to a high fat diet. Int J Sport Nutr Exerc Metab 2003;13:466–478.

22. Helge JW, Watt PW, Richter EA, Rennie MJ, Kiens B. Fat utilization during exercise: adaptation to a fat-rich diet increases utilization of plasma fatty acids and very low density lipoprotein-triacylglycerol in humans. J Physiol 2001;537:1009–1020.

23. Goedecke JH, Christie C, Wilson G, et al. Metabolic adaptations to a high-fat diet in endurance cyclists. Metabolism 1999;48:1509–1517.

24. Rowlands DS, Hopkins WG. Effects of high-fat and high-carbohydrate diets on metabolism and performance in cycling. Metabolism 2002;51:678–690.

25. Phinney SD, Bistrian BR, Evans WJ, Gervino E, Blackburn GL. The human metabolic response to chronic ketosis without caloric restriction: preservation of submaximal exercise capability with reduced carbohydrate oxidation. Metabolism 1983;32:769–776.

26. Lambert EV, Speechly DP, Dennis SC, Noakes TD. Enhanced endurance in trained cyclists during moderate intensity exercise following 2 weeks adaptation to a high fat diet. Eur J Appl Physiol Occup Physiol 1994;69:287–293.

27. Schrauwen P, Wagenmakers AJ, van Marken Lichtenbelt WD, Saris WH, Westerterp KR. Increase in fat oxidation on a high-fat diet is accompanied by an increase in triglyceride-derived fatty acid oxidation. Diabetes 2000;49:640–646.

28. Kiens B, Essen-Gustavsson B, Gad P, Lithell H. Lipoprotein lipase activity and intramuscular triglyceride stores after long-term high-fat and high-carbohydrate diets in physically trained men. Clin Physiol 1987;7:1–9.

29. Burke LM, Hawley JA, Angus DJ, et al. Adaptations to short-term high-fat diet persist during exercise despite high carbohydrate availability. Med Sci Sports Exerc 2002;34:83–91.

30. Lambert EV, Goedecke JH, Zyle C, et al. High-fat diet versus habitual diet prior to carbohydrate loading: effects of exercise metabolism and cycling performance. Int J Sport Nutr Exerc Metab 2001;11:209–225.

31. Burke LM, Angus DJ, Cox GR, et al. Effect of fat adaptation and carbohydrate restoration on metabolism and performance during prolonged cycling. J Appl Physiol 2000;89:2413–2421.

32. Carey AL, Staudacher HM, Cummings NK, et al. Effects of fat adaptation and carbohydrate restoration on prolonged endurance exercise. J Appl Physiol 2001;91: 115–122.

33. Kuczmarski RJ, Flegal KM, Campbell SM, Johnson CL. Increasing prevalence of overweight among US adults. The National Health and Nutrition Examination Surveys, 1960 to 1991. JAMA 1994;272:205–211.

34. Rabast U, Kasper H, Schonborn J. Comparative studies in obese subjects fed carbohydrate-restricted and high carbohydrate 1,000-calorie formula diets. Nutr Metab 1978;22:269–277.

35. Rabast U, Schonborn J, Kasper H. Dietetic treatment of obesity with low and high-carbohydrate diets: comparative studies and clinical results. Int J Obes 1979;3: 201–211.

36. Brehm BJ, Seeley RJ, Daniels SR, D'Alessio DA. A randomized trial comparing a very low carbohydrate diet and a calorie-restricted low fat diet on body weight and cardiovascular risk factors in healthy women. J Clin Endocrinol Metab 2003;88: 1617–1623.

37. Foster GD, Wyatt HR, Hill JO, et al. A randomized trial of a low-carbohydrate diet for obesity. N Engl J Med 2003;348:2082–2090.

38. Yancy WS Jr, Olsen MK, Guyton JR, Bakst RP, Westman EC. A low-carbohydrate, ketogenic diet versus a low-fat diet to treat obesity and hyperlipidemia: a randomized, controlled trial. Ann Intern Med 2004;140:769–777.

39. Sondike SB, Copperman N, Jacobson MS. Effects of a low-carbohydrate diet on weight loss and cardiovascular risk factor in overweight adolescents. J Pediatr 2003;142:253–258.

40. Stern L, Iqbal N, Seshadri P, et al. The effects of low-carbohydrate versus conventional weight loss diets in severely obese adults: one-year follow-up of a randomized trial. Ann Intern Med 2004;140:778–785.

41. Samaha FF, Iqbal N, Seshadri P, et al. A low-carbohydrate as compared with a low-fat diet in severe obesity. N Engl J Med 2003;348:2074–2081.

42. Volek JS, Sharman MJ, Gomez AL, et al. Comparison of energy-restricted very low-carbohydrate and low-fat diets on weight loss and body composition in overweight men and women. Nutr Metab (Lond) 2004;1:13.

43. Bray GA. Low-carbohydrate diets and realities of weight loss. JAMA 2003;289: 1853–1855.

44. Yudkin J, Carey M. The treatment of obesity by the "high-fat" diet: the inevitability of calories. Lancet 1960:939–941.

45. Arase K, Fisler JS, Shargill NS, York DA, Bray GA. Intracerebroventricular infusions of 3-OHB and insulin in a rat model of dietary obesity. Am J Physiol 1988;255: R974–981.

46. Melanson KJ, Westerterp-Plantenga MS, Saris WH, Smith FJ, Campfield LA. Blood glucose patterns and appetite in time-blinded humans: carbohydrate versus fat. Am J Physiol 1999;277:R337–345.

47. Volek JS, Westman EC. Very-low-carbohydrate weight-loss diets revisited. Cleve Clin J Med 2002;69:849, 853, 856–858 passim.

48. Feinman RD, Fine EJ. "A calorie is a calorie" violates the second law of thermodynamics. Nutr J 2004;3:9.

49. Buchholz AC, Schoeller DA. Is a calorie a calorie? Am J Clin Nutr 2004;79: 899S–906S.

50. Feinman RD, Fine EJ. Thermodynamics and metabolic advantage of reducing diets. Metab Syndr Rel Disord 2003;1:209–219.

51. Jequier E. Pathways to obesity. Int J Obes Relat Metab Disord 2002;26(Suppl 2): S12–17.

52. Bisschop PH, Pereira Arias AM, Ackermans MT, et al. The effects of carbohydrate variation in isocaloric diets on glycogenolysis and gluconeogenesis in healthy men. J Clin Endocrinol Metab 2000;85:1963–1967.

53. Meckling KA, O'Sullivan C, Saari D. Comparison of a low-fat diet to a low-carbohydrate diet on weight loss, body composition, and risk factors for diabetes and cardiovascular disease in free-living, overweight men and women. J Clin Endocrinol Metab 2004;89:2717–2723.

54. Garrow JS, Summerbell CD. Meta-analysis: effect of exercise, with or without dieting, on the body composition of overweight subjects. Eur J Clin Nutr 1995;49: 1–10.

55. Benoit FL, Martin RL, Watten RH. Changes in body composition during weight reduction in obesity. Balance studies comparing effects of fasting and a ketogenic diet. Ann Intern Med 1965;63:604–612.

56. Young CM, Scanlan SS, Im HS, Lutwak L. Effect of body composition and other parameters in obese young men of carbohydrate level of reduction diet. Am J Clin Nutr 1971;24:290–296.

57. Phinney SD, Horton ES, Sims EA, Hanson JS, Danforth E Jr, LaGrange BM. Capacity for moderate exercise in obese subjects after adaptation to a hypocaloric, ketogenic diet. J Clin Invest 1980;66:1152–1161.

58. Willi SM, Oexmann MJ, Wright NM, Collop NA, Key LL Jr. The effects of a high-protein, low-fat, ketogenic diet on adolescents with morbid obesity: body composition, blood chemistries, and sleep abnormalities. Pediatrics 1998;101:61–67.

59. Volek JS, Sharman MJ, Love DM, et al. Body composition and hormonal responses to a carbohydrate-restricted diet. Metabolism 2002;51:864–870.

60. Meckling KA, Gauthier M, Grubb R, Sanford J. Effects of a hypocaloric, low-carbohydrate diet on weight loss, blood lipids, blood pressure, glucose tolerance, and body composition in free-living overweight women. Can J Physiol Pharmacol 2002;80:1095–1105.

61. Gasteyger C, Tremblay A. Metabolic impact of body fat distribution. J Endocrinol Invest 2002;25:876–883.

62. Blake GJ, Ridker PM. Novel clinical markers of vascular wall inflammation. Circ Res 2001;89:763–771.

63. Ross R. Atherosclerosis is an inflammatory disease. Am Heart J 1999;138:S419–420.

64. Haffner S, Taegtmeyer H. Epidemic obesity and the metabolic syndrome. Circulation 2003;108:1541–1545.

65. Sakkinen PA, Wahl P, Cushman M, Lewis MR, Tracy RP. Clustering of procoagulation, inflammation, and fibrinolysis variables with metabolic factors in insulin resistance syndrome. Am J Epidemiol 2000;152:897–907.

66. Ford ES, Giles WH, Dietz WH. Prevalence of the metabolic syndrome among US adults: findings from the third National Health and Nutrition Examination Survey. JAMA 2002;287:356–359.

67. Kereiakes DJ, Willerson JT. Metabolic syndrome epidemic. Circulation 2003;108:1552–1553.

68. National Cholesterol Education Program Expert Panel on Detection, Evaluation, and Treatment of High Blood Cholesterol in Adults (Adult Treatment Panel III). Bethesda, MD: National Heart, Lung and Blood Institute and National Institutes of Health; 2001.

69. Gordon T, Kannel WB, Castelli WP, Dawber TR. Lipoproteins, cardiovascular disease, and death. The Framingham study. Arch Intern Med 1981;141:1128–1131.

70. Newbold HL. Reducing the serum cholesterol level with a diet high in animal fat. South Med J 1988;81:61–63.

71. Westman EC, Yancy WS, Edman JS, Tomlin KF, Perkins CE. Effect of 6-month adherence to a very low carbohydrate diet program. Am J Med 2002;113:30–36.

72. Dashti HM, Bo-Abbas YY, Asfar SK, et al. Ketogenic diet modifies the risk factors of heart disease in obese patients. Nutrition 2003;19:901–902.

73. Hays JH, DiSabatino A, Gorman RT, Vincent S, Stillabower ME. Effect of a high saturated fat and no-starch diet on serum lipid subfractions in patients with documented atherosclerotic cardiovascular disease. Mayo Clin Proc 2003;78:1331–1336.

74. Sharman MJ, Gomez AL, Kraemer WJ, Volek JS. Very low-carbohydrate and low-fat diets affect fasting lipids and postprandial lipemia differently in overweight men. J Nutr 2004;134:880–885.

75. Dattilo AM, Kris-Etherton PM. Effects of weight reduction on blood lipids and lipoproteins: a meta-analysis. Am J Clin Nutr 1992;56:320–328.

76. Larosa JC, Fry AG, Muesing R, Rosing DR. Effects of high-protein, low-carbohydrate dieting on plasma lipoproteins and body weight. J Am Diet Assoc 1980;77:264–270.

77. Volek JS, Sharman MJ, Gomez AL, et al. Comparison of a very low-carbohydrate and low-fat diet on fasting lipids, LDL subclasses, insulin resistance, and postprandial lipemic responses in overweight women. J Am Coll Nutr 2004;23:177–184.

78. Sharman MJ, Kraemer WJ, Love DM, et al. A ketogenic diet favorably affects serum biomarkers for cardiovascular disease in normal-weight men. J Nutr 2002;132:1879–1885.

79. Volek JS, Sharman MJ, Gomez AL, Scheett TP, Kraemer WJ. An isoenergetic very low carbohydrate diet improves serum HDL cholesterol and triacylglycerol concentrations, the total cholesterol to HDL cholesterol ratio and postprandial pipemic responses compared with a low fat diet in normal weight, normolipidemic women. J Nutr 2003;133:2756–2761.

80. Fuehrlein BS, Rutenberg MS, Silver JN, et al. Differential metabolic effects of saturated versus polyunsaturated fats in ketogenic diets. J Clin Endocrinol Metab 2004;89:1641–1645.

81. Volek JS, Gomez AL, Kraemer WJ. Fasting lipoprotein and postprandial triacylglycerol responses to a low-carbohydrate diet supplemented with n-3 fatty acids. J Am Coll Nutr 2000;19:383–391.

82. Wilson PW, Garrison RJ, Castelli WP, Feinleib M, McNamara PM, Kannel WB. Prevalence of coronary heart disease in the Framingham Offspring Study: role of lipoprotein cholesterols. Am J Cardiol 1980;46:649–654.

83. Katzel LI, Busby-Whitehead MJ, Rogus EM, Krauss RM, Goldberg AP. Reduced adipose tissue lipoprotein lipase responses, postprandial lipemia, and low high-density lipoprotein-2 subspecies levels in older athletes with silent myocardial ischemia. Metabolism 1994;43:190–198.

84. Austin MA, Hokanson JE, Edwards KL. Hypertriglyceridemia as a cardiovascular risk factor. Am J Cardiol 1998;81:7B–12B.

85. Rickman F, Mitchell N, Dingman J, Dalen JE. Changes in serum cholesterol during the Stillman diet. JAMA 1974;228:54–58.

86. Karpe F, Steiner G, Uffelman K, Olivecrona T, Hamsten A. Postprandial lipoproteins and progression of coronary atherosclerosis. Atherosclerosis 1994;106:83–97.

87. Krauss RM. Atherogenicity of triglyceride-rich lipoproteins. Am J Cardiol 1998;81:13B–17B.

88. Patsch JR, Miesenbock G, Hopferwieser T, et al. Relation of triglyceride metabolism and coronary artery disease. Studies in the postprandial state. Arterioscler Thromb 1992;12:1336–1345.

89. Chen YD, Coulston AM, Zhou MY, Hollenbeck CB, Reaven GM. Why do low-fat high-carbohydrate diets accentuate postprandial lipemia in patients with NIDDM? Diabetes Care 1995;18:10–16.

90. Jackson RL, Yates MT, McNerney CA, Kashyap ML. Relationship between post-heparin plasma lipases, triglycerides and high density lipoproteins in normal subjects. Horm Metab Res 1990;22:289–294.

91. Campos H, Dreon DM, Krauss RM. Associations of hepatic and lipoprotein lipase activities with changes in dietary composition and low density lipoprotein subclasses. J Lipid Res 1995;36:462–472.

92. Krauss RM, Burke DJ. Identification of multiple subclasses of plasma low density lipoproteins in normal humans. J Lipid Res 1982;23:97–104.

93. Austin MA, King MC, Vranizan KM, Krauss RM. Atherogenic lipoprotein phenotype. A proposed genetic marker for coronary heart disease risk. Circulation 1990;82:495–506.

94. Dreon DM, Fernstrom HA, Miller B, Krauss RM. Low-density lipoprotein subclass patterns and lipoprotein response to a reduced-fat diet in men. FASEB J 1994;8:121–126.

95. Dreon DM, Fernstrom HA, Williams PT, Krauss RM. A very low-fat diet is not associated with improved lipoprotein profiles in men with a predominance of large, low-density lipoproteins. Am J Clin Nutr 1999;69:411–418.

96. Griffin BA, Freeman DJ, Tait GW, et al. Role of plasma triglyceride in the regulation of plasma low density lipoprotein (LDL) subfractions: relative contribution of small, dense LDL to coronary heart disease risk. Atherosclerosis 1994;106:241–253.

97. Libby P, Ridker PM. Novel inflammatory markers of coronary risk: theory versus practice. Circulation 1999;100:1148–1150.

98. Hwang SJ, Ballantyne CM, Sharrett AR, et al. Circulating adhesion molecules VCAM-1, ICAM-1, and E-selectin in carotid atherosclerosis and incident coronary heart disease cases: the Atherosclerosis Risk In Communities (ARIC) study. Circulation 1997;96:4219–4225.

99. Sharman MJ, Volek JS. Weight loss leads to reductions in inflammatory biomarkers after a very-low-carbohydrate diet and a low-fat diet in overweight men. Clin Sci (Lond) 2004;107:365–369.

100. Ziccardi P, Nappo F, Giugliano G, et al. Reduction of inflammatory cytokine concentrations and improvement of endothelial functions in obese women after weight loss over one year. Circulation 2002;105:804–809.

101. Heilbronn LK, Noakes M, Clifton PM. Energy restriction and weight loss on very-low-fat diets reduce C-reactive protein concentrations in obese, healthy women. Arterioscler Thromb Vasc Biol 2001;21:968–970.

102. Position of Dietitians of Canada, the American Dietetic Association, and the American College of Sports Medicine: Nutrition and Athletic Performance. Can J Diet Pract Res 2000;61:176–192.

103. Bergstrom J, Hermansen L, Hultman E, Saltin B. Diet, muscle glycogen and physical performance. Acta Physiol Scand 1967;71:140–150.

104. Phinney SD. Ketogenic diets and physical performance. Nutr Metab (Lond) 2004;
     1:2.
105. Haennel RG, Lemire F. Physical activity to prevent cardiovascular disease. How
     much is enough? Can Fam Physician 2002;48:65–71.
106. Yu KC, Cooper AD. Postprandial lipoproteins and atherosclerosis. Front Biosci
     2001;6:D332–354.
107. Cohn JS. Postprandial lipemia: emerging evidence for atherogenicity of remnant
     lipoproteins. Can J Cardiol 1998;14(Suppl B):18B–27B.
108. Smith D, Watts GF, Dane-Stewart C, Mamo JC. Post-prandial chylomicron response
     may be predicted by a single measurement of plasma apolipoprotein B48 in the
     fasting state. Eur J Clin Invest 1999;29:204–209.
109. Schaefer EJ. Lipoproteins, nutrition, and heart disease. Am J Clin Nutr 2002;75:
     191–212.

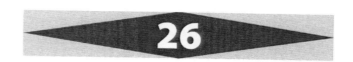

# Eating to Improve Body Composition

Jose Antonio and Anssi H. Manninen

## OBJECTIVES

On the completion of this chapter you will be able to:

1. Understand the scientific literature about the effectiveness of various dietary strategies that have been used for weight loss.
2. Explain specific details about various studies that have investigated specific dietary practices.
3. Discuss the concept of metabolic advantage and how it relates to different dietary practices.
4. Understand the concept of metabolic advantage and the components that contribute to it.
5. Explain the effects of nutrient-timing practices and how they relate to training adaptations and or physiologic changes.
6. Discuss the concept of meal frequency and how this may impact weight loss or gain.
7. Understand the effects of coupling protein supplements with resistance training on physiologic adaptations.
8. Differentiate the physiologic adaptations associated with soy, casein, and whey protein supplements.

## ABSTRACT

For optimal health and athletic performance, gaining lean skeletal muscle mass and losing body fat mass is one ideal outcome of a nutritional/exercise intervention desired by athletes and fitness competitors alike. While achieving a lean muscular physique based on proper diet and intense training may be a goal of bodybuilding and fitness populations, it may not be the primary goal of competitive athletes. Athletes training and competing for specific events are often judged on sport-specific performance affected by a number of interactive variables including but not limited to excellent body composition (i.e. high degree of muscularity and low body fat levels). With these elements in mind, this chapter focuses on various clinical trials that have examined body composition changes through various diet and/or exercise interventions. Issues surrounding the mechanisms governing why substituting carbohydrate for protein and/or fat can enhance body composition are also discussed.

*Key Words:* **Mediterranean, ketogenic, satiety, calorie, thermodynamics**

For optimal health and athletic performance, gaining lean body mass (i.e., primarily skeletal muscle mass) and losing fat mass is the ideal outcome of a

From: *Essentials of Sports Nutrition and Supplements*
Edited by J. Antonio, D. Kalman, J. R. Stout, M. Greenwood, D. S. Willoughby, and G. G. Haff © Humana Press, a part of Springer Science+Business Media, Totowa, NJ

nutritional/exercise intervention. There may be few exceptions to this such as sumo wrestling[1,2] in which very high body mass is a premium (even if a large percentage of the sumo's body weight is fat) and long-distance, open-water swimming in which carrying substantive subcutaneous fat may indeed help swimming performance, particularly in cold environments, because of the insulation provided by subcutaneous fat.[3]

Nonetheless, achieving a lean physique is often the outcome of proper diet and exercise although it may not be the primary goal of competitive athletes. Bodybuilders and fitness competitors are perhaps the only "athletes" who are judged solely on looks (i.e., muscle hypertrophy, definition, symmetry, etc). However, athletes in track and field, football, baseball, and other sports would perform optimally if they achieved low levels of body fat and a significant degree of muscularity. Certainly, it would challenge common sense that carrying body fat somehow conferred a performance advantage. This chapter focuses on the clinical trials that have examined body composition changes vis a vis diet and/or exercise interventions.

It should be noted that there are no studies utilizing elite athletes as subjects. For the science purist, one might conclude that none of the following studies (many of them done on overweight or unhealthy subjects) are pertinent to the athletic population. We disagree inasmuch as, from a practical standpoint, elite athletes (at the national or international level) would likely never participate in a study knowing a priori that perhaps one of the interventions may be less effective. Thus, we as sports nutritionists are left to glean whatever useful information we can from the various clinical trials and in essence experiment with these interventions in real life.

Physique athletes such as bodybuilders and fitness/figure competitors already know what science is now showing. Replacing carbohydrate (especially processed carbohydrate) with protein and unsaturated fat is an effective way in promoting significant losses of fat mass while sparing lean body mass.

## REVIEW OF LITERATURE

In 1965, Benoit et al.[4] published the first systematic study of the effect of a very-low-carbohydrate (ketogenic) diet on composition of weight loss. They observed that when a 1000-kcal ketogenic diet (10 g of carbohydrates/day) was fed for 10 days, their seven male subjects lost an average of 600 g/day, of which 97% was fat. However, the energy value of the tissue loss reported by Benoit et al. is about 7000 kcal/day, a highly improbable level of energy expenditure for subjects confined to a metabolic chamber. Young et al.[5] compared three isoenergetic (1800 kcal/day) and isoprotein (115 g/day) diets differing in carbohydrate content (30, 60, and 104 g/day). After 9 weeks on the 30-, 60-, and 104-g carbohydrate diets, weight loss was 16.2, 12.8, and 11.9 kg and fat accounted for 95%, 84%, and 75% of the weight loss, respectively.

Investigators evaluated a moderate-fat diet (i.e., Mediterranean diet) versus an isoenergetic standard low-fat diet. In a randomized, prospective, 18-month trial in a free-living population, 101 overweight men and women [body mass index (BMI) range of 26.5–46] consumed either a moderate-fat diet (35% of energy) or a low-fat diet (20% of energy). In the moderate-fat group, there were mean decreases in body weight of 4.1 kg, BMI of 1.6 kg/m², and waist circumference of 6.9 cm, compared with increases in the low-fat group of 2.9 kg, 1.4 kg/m², and 2.6 cm, respectively; $p \leq 0.001$ between the groups (Figure 26.1). According to the authors, "A moderate-fat, Mediterranean-style diet, controlled in energy, offers an alternative to a low-fat diet with superior long-term participation and adherence, with consequent improvements in weight loss."[6]

Consuming protein at the expense of carbohydrates (at least in the short term) is associated with increased satiety, increased thermogenesis, sparing of muscle protein loss, and enhanced glycemic control. This could be attributable to a lower postprandial increase in blood glucose and lower insulin response, and higher protein providing increased branched-chain amino acid leucine levels and gluconeogenic substrates.[7] Another unique feature of these diets seems to be the higher intake of branched-chain amino acid leucine with unique regulatory actions on muscle protein synthesis, modulation of the

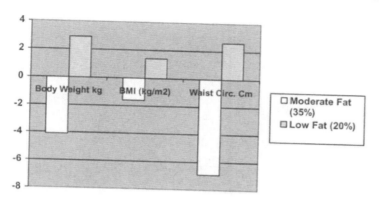

**Figure 26.1.** McManus et al.[6] showed that an isocaloric diet higher in fat content is superior to a low-fat diet with respect to body weight, body mass index (BMI), and waist circumference.

insulin signal, and sparing of glucose use by stimulation of the glucose-alanine cycle.[7]

Layman et al.[8] examined the efficacy of two weight-loss diets with modified carbohydrate (CHO)/protein ratios on body composition and blood lipids in adult women. Women (n = 24; 45–56 years old) with body mass indices >26 kg/m² were assigned to either a CHO group consuming a diet with a CHO/protein ratio of 3.5 (68 g protein/day) or a protein group with a ratio of 1.4 (125 g protein/day). Diets were isoenergetic, providing 7100 kJ/day, and similar amounts of fat (~50 g/day). After consuming the diets for 10 weeks, the CHO group lost 6.96 ± 1.36 kg body weight and the protein group lost 7.53 ± 1.44 kg. The protein group lost more fat and less lean body mass (fat/lean ratio: 6.3 ± 1.2 g/g) compared with the CHO group (3.8 ± 0.9). Both groups had significant reductions in serum cholesterol (approximately 10%), whereas the protein group also had significant reductions in triacylglycerols (21%) and the ratio of triacylglycerols/high density lipoprotein cholesterol (23%) (Figure 26.2). Thus, increasing the proportion of protein to carbohydrate in the diet of adult women has positive effects on body composition, blood lipids, glucose homeostasis, and satiety during weight loss.

Another investigation compared the effects of a low-carbohydrate, ketogenic diet program with those of a low-fat, low-cholesterol, and reduced-calorie diet. There were 120 overweight, hyperlipidemic volunteers from the community. The diet interventions were: 1) low-carbohydrate diet (initially, <20 g of carbohydrate daily) plus nutritional supplementation, exercise recommendation, and group meetings; and 2) low-fat diet (<30% energy from fat, <300 mg of cholesterol daily, and deficit of 500–1000 kcal/day) plus exercise recommendation and group meetings. They found that a greater proportion of the low-carbohydrate diet group than the low-fat diet group completed the study (76% versus 57%; p = 0.02). At 24 weeks, weight loss was greater in the low-carbohydrate diet group than in the low-fat diet group (mean change, −12.9% versus −6.7%; p < 0.001). Patients in both groups lost substantially more fat mass (change, −9.4 kg with the low-carbohydrate diet versus −4.8 kg with the low-fat diet) than fat-free mass (FFM) (change, −3.3 kg versus −2.4 kg, respectively) (Figure 26.3). According to the investigators, "compared with a low-fat

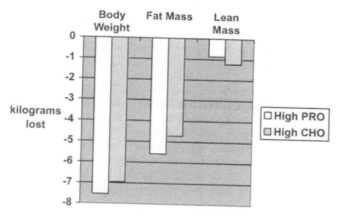

**FIGURE 26.2.** Layman et al.[8] showed that a high-protein (PRO) diet is superior to a low-carbohydrate (CHO) diet with respect to overall body composition.

**FIGURE 26.3.** Yancy et al.[9] showed improvement in body composition using a lower carbohydrate (CHO) approach.

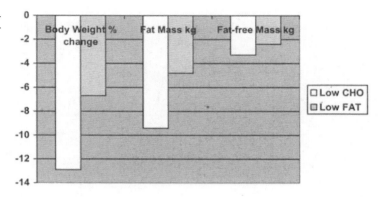

diet, a low-carbohydrate diet program had better participant retention and greater weight loss. During active weight loss, serum triglyceride (TG) levels decreased more and high-density lipoprotein cholesterol level increased more with the low-carbohydrate diet than with the low-fat diet."[9]

Samaha et al.[10] randomly assigned 132 severely obese subjects to a low-carbohydrate or calorie- and fat-restricted (low-fat) diet. Seventy-nine subjects completed this 6-month study. It should be noted that the difference in consumption of energy from carbohydrate was quite narrow: 51% in the low-fat group and 37% in the low-carbohydrate group. Total energy intake at the 6-month mark was 1567 kcal/day in the low-fat group and 1630 kcal/day in the low-carbohydrate group. Thus, the low-carbohydrate group consumed 54 extra kcal/day. Nevertheless, the low-carbohydrate group lost 5.8 kg (and was still losing weight at 6 months) versus 1.9 kg (leveled off) in the low-fat group.[11]

Brehm et al.[12] designed a randomized, controlled trial to determine the effects of a very-low-carbohydrate diet on body composition and cardiovascular risk factors. Subjects were randomized to 6 months of either an ad libitum very-low-carbohydrate diet or a calorie-restricted diet with 30% of the calories as fat. Fifty-three healthy, obese female volunteers were randomized; 42 completed the trial. Both groups were free-living and had reduced energy intake by similar amounts at 3 and 6 months, but the low-carbohydrate group lost more weight (8.5 versus 3.9 kg) and more body fat (4.8 versus 2.0 kg). According to authors, "It is difficult to explain the differences in weight loss between the two groups primarily as a function of differing caloric intake."

In a randomized, controlled, 12-week trial, Sondike et al.[13] compared the effects of a low-carbohydrate diet with those of a low-fat diet on weight loss and serum lipids in overweight adolescents. The low-carbohydrate group (n = 16) was instructed to consume <20 g of carbohydrate per day for 2 weeks, then <40 g/day for 10 weeks, and to eat low-carbohydrate foods according to hunger. The low-fat group (n = 14) was instructed to consume <30% of energy from fat. The results indicated that the low-carbohydrate group lost 9.9 kg versus 4.1 kg for the low-fat group, despite both lower initial weight of the low-carbohydrate group (92.1 versus 99.5 kg) and disparity in calories in favor of the high-carbohydrate group.

Greene et al.[14] found that people eating an extra 300 kcal a day on a very-low-carbohydrate diet lost a similar amount of weight during a 12-week study as those on a low-fat diet. Over the course of the study, subjects consumed an extra 25,000 kcal that should have added up to about a 7-pound weight gain; it did not. The study was unique because all the food was prepared at an upscale Italian restaurant, so the researchers knew exactly what they ate, and one could not argue that diets were not palatable.

A recent randomized, balanced, two-diet study compared effects of isocaloric, energy-restricted ketogenic and low-fat diets on weight loss and body composition in overweight/obese men (n = 15) and women (n = 13).[15] Despite significantly greater calorie intake (1855 versus 1562 kcal/day), both between and within group comparison revealed a distinct advantage of a ketogenic diet over a low-fat diet for weight loss/fat loss for men. In fact, five men showed more than 10 pounds difference in weight loss. The majority of women also

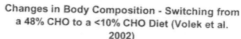

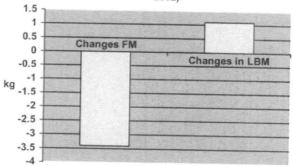

**FIGURE 26.4.** Volek et al.[16] showed that switching from a higher-carbohydrate diet (48%) to a very-low-carbohydrate diet (<10%) improves body composition. FM = fat mass, LBM = lean body mass.

responded more favorably to the ketogenic diet, especially in terms of trunk fat loss. Furthermore, the individual responses revealed that three men and four women who did the ketogenic diet first, regained body mass and fat mass after the switch to the low-fat, whereas no subjects regained weight or fat mass after switching to the ketogenic diet.

Volek et al.[16] examined the effects of 6-week very-low-carbohydrate diet on total and regional body composition. Interestingly, their results indicated that fat mass was significantly decreased (–3.4 kg) and lean body mass significantly increased (+1.1 kg) at week 6 (Figure 26.4).

A recent paper intended as a systematic review concluded, "Weight loss while using low-carbohydrate diets was principally associated with decreased caloric intake and increased diet duration, not with reduced carbohydrate content."[17] As pointed out by Kauffman,[18] however, in the true low-carbohydrate group in the study, the mean weight loss in trials was 17 kg, whereas in the higher-carbohydrate group it was only 2 kg. Oddly enough, the authors did not consider this significant. As Kauffman pointed out, "The conclusions should have been that low-carbohydrate diets are both safe and effective." Only by intermingling trials of low to medium and high-carbohydrate diets could the authors reach the misleading conclusion quoted above. Nonetheless, it is evident that with a growing number of published clinical trials, the provision of protein and/or fat in place of carbohydrate (isoenergetically) produces more favorable changes in body composition.

Foster et al.[19] conducted a 1-year, multicenter, controlled trial involving 63 obese men and women who were randomly assigned to either a low-carbohydrate, high-protein, high-fat diet or a low-calorie, high-carbohydrate, low-fat diet. The results indicated that the low-carbohydrate diet produced a greater weight loss than did the conventional diet for the first 6 months, but the differences were not significant at 1 year. As pointed out by Kauffman, however, "the absolute weight loss difference was actually 3% between groups, favouring the low-carbohydrate group, at 12 months, among those actually completing the study."

## POSSIBLE MECHANISMS BEHIND THE METABOLIC ADVANTAGE

According to Feinman and Fine,[20] the principle of "a calorie is a calorie," violates the second Law of Thermodynamics. The *metabolic advantage* in low-carbohydrate diets (i.e., greater weight loss compared with isocaloric diets of different composition) can be explained in large part by the enhanced thermogenesis (seen with low-carbohydrate diets) as sufficient to predict metabolic advantage. The hormonal changes associated with a low-carbohydrate diet include a reduction in the circulating levels of insulin along with increased levels of glucagons, leading to activation of phosphoenolpyruvate carboxykinase, fructose 1,6-biphosphatase, and glucose 6-phosphatase and inhibition of pyruvate kinase, 6-phosphofructo-1-kinase, and hexokinase, favoring gluconeogenesis over glycolysis. Gluconeogenesis is an energy-consuming process because 6 mol of adenosine triphosphate (ATP) are consumed for the synthesis of 1 mol of glucose from pyruvate or lactate. The transformation of gluconeogenic amino acids into glucose requires even more energy because ATP is needed to dispose of the nitrogen as urea.[21]

In addition, a low-carbohydrate diet increases turnover of body proteins; and the energy-dependent processes of maintaining the turnover of proteins including synthesis, folding, targeting, regulatory processes, and protein breakdown have an overall cost to body energy homeostasis that is significantly higher than previously appreciated. Also, a low-carbohydrate diet is often high in protein and a recent study demonstrated that postprandial thermogenesis was increased 100% on a high-protein/low-fat diet versus a high-carbohydrate/low-fat diet in healthy subjects.[22]

Furthermore, the ketogenic diets are characterized by elevations of free fatty acids, leading to the increased transcription of mitochondrial uncoupling proteins (UCPs) and of peroxisomal β-oxidation. UCPs allow the proton gradient generated by the respiratory chain to reenter the mitochondria by pathways, which bypass the F1 adenosine triphosphatase generating heat rather than ATP. Also, fatty acids undergoing β-oxidation with peroxisomes have no mechanism for energy conservation and result solely in heat production.[23] The important bottom line is that this leads to metabolic inefficiency.

Finally, there is evidence that hyperinsulinemia increases fat mass without a concomitant increase in energy intake. For example, Carlson and Campbell[24] studied six adult patients with diabetes on conventional insulin therapy and after 2 months of intensive insulin therapy while maintaining constant caloric intake and were compared with a group of six matched nondiabetic volunteers. Not surprisingly, the results indicated that 2 months of intensive insulin therapy improved glycemic control dramatically. However, this improvement was achieved at a cost of a weight gain of about 2.6 kg over the 2-month treatment as the result of an increase in fat mass and not lean body tissue.

Of the weight gain, 70% could be accounted for by elimination of glycosuria and 30% by reduction in daily energy expenditure. Although elimination of glycosuria is not relevant to healthy, nondiabetic individuals, daily energy expenditure decreased 5% (approximately 120 kcal/day). The authors concluded that the reduction in the energy expenditure was the result of the decrease in TG/free fatty acid cycling and nonoxidative glucose and protein metabolism. The TG/free fatty acid cycling represents those free fatty acids that are hydrolyzed from TG stores and are subsequently re-esterified back to TG rather than being oxidized. Nonoxidative glucose metabolism refers to glycogen synthesis, Cori cycling, and urinary glucose loss. Nonoxidative protein metabolism represents protein synthesis and the amino acid contribution to gluconeogenesis.

## ROLE OF NUTRIENT TIMING IN BODY-COMPOSITION ALTERATIONS

There is a growing body of evidence that shows the importance of consuming a combination of protein and carbohydrate immediately pre- or postexercise vis a vis skeletal muscle protein synthesis and glycogen restoration (for a more thorough review of the literature, we suggest you read the chapters written by John Ivy, PhD and Chris Rasmussen, MS in this text).[25–55]

For instance, scientists investigated the importance of immediate (P0) or delayed (P2) intake of an oral protein supplement upon muscle hypertrophy and strength over a period of resistance training in elderly males. Thirteen men [age, $74 \pm 1$ years; BMI, $25 \pm 1 \, kg \, m^{-2}$ (means ± SEM)] completed a 12-week resistance-training program (3 times per week) receiving oral protein in liquid form (10 g protein, 7 g carbohydrate, 3 g fat) immediately after (P0) or 2 hours after (P2) each training session. In response to training, the cross-sectional area of quadriceps femoris muscle (54.6 to 58.3 cm$^2$) and mean fiber area (4047–5019 μm$^2$) increased in the P0 group, whereas no significant increase was observed in P2. For P0, both dynamic and isokinetic strength increased, by 46% and 15%, respectively ($p < 0.05$), whereas P2 only improved in dynamic strength, by 36% ($p < 0.05$). No differences in glucose or insulin response were observed between protein intake at 0 and 2 hours postexercise. The authors concluded that consuming an oral protein supplement after resistance training produced muscle hypertrophy in this group of elderly men.[45]

Chromiak et al.[56] investigated whether postexercise consumption of a supplement containing whey protein, amino acids, creatine, and carbohydrate combined with a strength-training program promoted greater gains in FFM, muscle strength and endurance, and anaerobic performance compared with an isocaloric, carbohydrate-only control drink combined with strength training. Forty-one males (n = 20 in control group, n = 21 in the supplement group; mean age, 22.2 years) participated in a 4 days/week, 10-week periodized strength-training program. They found that across groups, FFM increased during 10 weeks of strength training. FFM increased in the supplement group by 3.4 kg compared with a 1.5-kg increase in the control group ($p = 0.077$). According to this investigation, the supplemented grouped trended toward a greater increase in FFM, although one might argue that it was not statistically significant (i.e., $p > 0.05$); future work should perhaps look at longer treatment durations.[56]

## MEAL FREQUENCY

Although anecdotal reports show that many bodybuilders and physique athletes eat frequent meals (e.g., ≥6 meals per day) with the goal of improving body composition, the data are sparse in this regard. According to one study, there tends to be an inverse relationship between people's habitual frequency of eating and body weight (i.e., greater meal frequency is associated with lower body weight). Thus, the notion that "grazing" is a better way to eat than "gorging" has been suggested as a way to regulate body weight.[57] Data on feeding patterns (i.e., grazing versus gorging) show that the thermic effect of feeding is higher when an isoenergetic test load is divided into multiple small meals; however, other studies show no effect. It has been suggested that the effect of feeding frequency on body-weight regulation is probably mediated through effects on the food intake side of the energy-balance equation.[57] For instance, healthy young men with a high habitual meal frequency showed lower 24-hour energy intake compared with those with a low habitual meal frequency.[58]

The role of meal frequency in regulating plasma hormone levels might have a role in regulating body composition. In a randomized, crossover trial with two phases of 14 days each, subjects consumed their normal diet on either 6 occasions per day (regular) or by following a variable meal frequency (3–9 meals/day, irregular). In phase 2, subjects followed the alternative meal pattern to that followed in phase 1, after a 2-week (washout) period. The data revealed that fasting glucose and insulin values were not affected by meal frequency, but peak insulin and AUC of insulin responses to the test meal were higher after the irregular compared with the regular eating patterns. The irregular meal frequency was also associated with higher fasting total and low density lipoprotein cholesterol. Thus, it seems plausible that by habitually consuming frequent meals (i.e., 6 meals per day), one can better regulate plasma insulin concentrations. In fact, one might posit that irregular meal frequency seems to decrease insulin sensitivity.[59] This same group investigated the impact of irregular meal frequency on body weight, energy intake, appetite, and resting energy expenditure in healthy, lean women (18–42 years) using a randomized, crossover design consisting of 3 phases over a total of 43 days. Subjects attended the laboratory at the start and end of phases 1 and 3. In phase 1 (14 days), subjects were asked to consume similar things as normal, but either on 6 occasions per day (regular meal pattern) or follow a variable predetermined meal frequency (between 3 and 9 meals/day) with the same total number of meals over the week. During phase 2 (14 days), subjects continued their normal diet as a washout period. In phase 3 (14 days), subjects followed the alternative meal pattern to that followed in phase 1. They found no significant differences in body weight and 3-day mean energy intake between the regular and irregular meal pattern. Interestingly, during the irregular period, the mean energy intake on the day when 9 meals were consumed was significantly greater than when 6 or 3 meals were consumed. There was no significant difference between the 3 days of the regular meal pattern. Subjective appetite measurement showed no significant differences before and after the test meal in all visits. Fasting resting metabolic state showed no significant differences over the experiment. However, the overall thermic effect of food (TEF) over the 3 hours after the test meal (milkshake: 50% CHO, 15% protein, and 35% fat of energy content) was significantly lower after the irregular meal pattern. What does this mean? Certainly, having variable eating patterns may have a negative effect on thermogenesis. According to the authors, "The reduced TEF with the irregular meal frequency may lead to weight gain in the long term."[60]

Another report examined the effects of meal frequency on changes in body composition in trained individuals. Twelve boxers were divided between a two-meals day (2M) and a six-meals day (6M). Both groups ingested 5.02 MJ (1200 kcal) daily for 2 weeks. Although there was no difference in change of body weight by food restriction between the two groups, the decrease in lean body mass was significantly greater in the 2M group than in the 6M group. The decrease in urinary 3-methylhistidine/creatinine was significantly greater in the 6M group than in the 2M group. Thus, at least in boxers who are calorically restricted, spreading meals over six feeding periods (even when isoenergetic) has a protein-sparing or anticatabolic effect.[61]

## PROTEIN SUPPLEMENTATION PLUS EXERCISE

The use of protein supplements as a means of augmenting the hypertrophic response to exercise is common. One investigation compared the effects of a 12-week moderate hypocaloric, high-protein diet and resistance training, using two different protein supplements, versus hypocaloric diet alone on body compositional changes in overweight police officers. The groups were divided as follows: one group (n = 10) was placed on a nonlipogenic, hypocaloric diet alone (80% of predicted needs). A second group (n = 14) was placed on the hypocaloric diet plus resistance exercise plus a high-protein intake (1.5 g/kg/day) using a casein protein hydrolysate. In the third group (n = 14), treatment was identical to the second, except for the use of a whey protein hydrolysate.

Investigators found that weight loss was approximately 2.5 kg in all three groups. Mean percent body fat with diet alone decreased from a baseline of 27% ± 1.8% to 25% ± 1.3% at 12 weeks. With diet, exercise, and casein the decrease was from 26% ± 1.7% to 18% ± 1.1% and with diet, exercise, and whey protein the decrease was from 27% ± 1.6% to 23% ± 1.3%. Lean mass gains in the three groups did not change for diet alone, versus gains of 4 ± 1.4 and 2 ± 0.7 kg in the casein and whey groups, respectively. Mean increase in strength for chest, shoulder, and legs was 59% ± 9% for casein and 29% ± 9% for whey, a significant group difference. Thus, at least with this investigation, differing protein sources have different anabolic effects (casein > whey) and that protein supplementation in conjunction with resistance training can improve body composition.[62]

Another study examined the effect of protein bar supplementation on body composition alterations in young males from a university weight-training class. All subjects were considered experienced weightlifters with at least 1 year or more experience. They were given daily servings of micronutrient-fortified protein bars containing soy or whey protein (33 g protein/day, 9 weeks, n = 9 for each protein treatment group). Subjects were randomly assigned in a double-blind manner to a soy, whey, or control group. The controls did the exercise program but did not consume a protein product (n = 9/each group). Each subject was instructed to consume three bars per day for the 9-week training period. Their daily diet was otherwise not altered. The strength-training protocol was 3 sets of 4–6 repetitions for 14 exercises that targeted major muscle groups: 1) chest press; 2) chest fly; 3) incline press; 4) lat pull-down; 5) seated row;

6) military press; 7) lateral raise for the deltoids; 8) preacher curls; 9) bicep curl; 10) supine triceps extension; 11) seated triceps extension; 12) leg press; 13) calf raise; and 14) abdominal crunches. Both the soy and whey treatment groups showed a gain in lean body mass, but the training-only group did not. According to the authors, "soy and whey protein bar products both promoted exercise training-induced lean body mass gain."[63] A 6-month clinical trial on overweight individuals found that a high soy protein and low-fat diet can induce significant fat loss in overweight and obese people while preserving muscle mass.[64] Soy protein has been shown in well-controlled animal studies to prevent exercise-induced protein degradation in skeletal muscle via the inhibition of calpain-mediated proteolysis.[65] Furthermore, there are data that whey protein supplementation (20 g/day for 3 months) in humans can increase peak power and 30-second work capacity and augment antioxidant defenses.[66]

It should be mentioned that many clinicians claim that "high protein" intakes may have deleterious effects; unfortunately, this has no basis in fact. Protein intakes up to 2.8 g daily per kilogram body weight does not impair renal function in well-trained athletes.[67] Also, increasing protein intake from 0.78 to 1.55 g of protein daily per kilogram of body weight with meat supplements in combination with reducing carbohydrate intake does not alter urine calcium excretion and may have a favorable impact on the skeleton in healthy older men and women[68] (Figure 26.5).

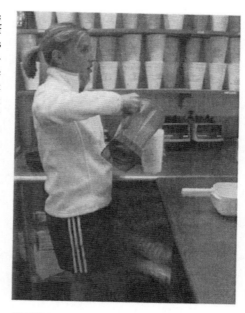

**FIGURE 26.5.** Athletes often use meal replacement powders or protein powders to get additional calories and/or protein for the express purpose of augmenting muscle hypertrophy. (Photograph courtesy of Athletes' Performance, Tempe, AZ.)

## SUMMARY

It is increasingly clear that the notion of "a calorie is a calorie" is a very simplistic (and incorrect) approach to body composition alterations vis a vis caloric restriction and macronutrient manipulation. The preponderance of evidence strongly suggests that the substitution of carbohydrate for protein or fat will lead to more favorable changes in body composition. The mechanisms governing why substituting carbohydrate for protein and/or fat can enhance body composition include: increased satiety, stabilization of plasma insulin, as well as the thermic effect of feeding (i.e., protein's high thermic effect).

Certainly, it is the opinion of the authors of this chapter that for optimal improvement in body composition, it would be wise for most individuals to not follow the guidelines of the American Heart Association.[69] The AHA recommends consuming approximately 50%–60% of one's total calories as carbohydrate. It should be evident that for most individuals, it is not necessary nor is it an effective strategy to consume such a high percentage of one's calories as carbohydrates.

Recently, Feinman and Fine[20] have concluded that the "metabolic advantage with low-carbohydrate diets is well established in the literature. . . . Attacking the obesity epidemic will involve giving up many old ideas that have not been productive. 'A calorie is a calorie' might be a good place to start." However, there will be metabolic accommodations and one cannot assume that the metabolic advantage (i.e., greater weight loss compared with isocaloric high-carbohydrate diet) will stay the same over a long term.

Furthermore, it is evident that consuming the proper macronutrients pre- and postexercise can profoundly affect skeletal muscle protein synthesis and body composition. This applies only for exercising individuals. However, it would behoove any individual seeking to positively alter his/her body composition to not only utilize the proper dietary strategy, but an exercise strategy as well.

Meal frequency also may have an important role in body composition regulation. It is likely a better strategy to eat frequent meals habitually (e.g., six meals or more per day) because of the beneficial effects on plasma insulin as well the enhanced thermic effect (or at worst, a neutral effect on thermogenesis). One also cannot discount the effect of high meal frequencies in regulating appetite, particularly on the intake side of the energy balance equation.

The ideal weight-loss diet, if it exists, remains to be determined; however, a high-carbohydrate/low-protein diet may be unsatisfactory for individuals who seek to improve body composition in the most effective manner.

## PRACTICAL APPLICATION

For sports nutritionists, one should be cognizant of the fact that the preponderance of scientific and anecdotal data strongly suggest that replacing carbohydrate with an isoenergetic amount of protein and/or fat is a effective approach to improving body composition.

However, one cannot assume that just because a strategy works in the short term, that it will have the same effect in the long term. One could speculate that there will be metabolic accommodations and perhaps the metabolic advantage (i.e., greater weight loss compared with isocaloric high-carbohydrate diet) may not apply in the long term. Many athletes now undertake a periodized approach to nutrition (i.e., akin to periodized exercise training) in which athletes, with the help of their sports nutritionist, alter their nutrition program depending on the type of training they are doing at the time.

It would be wise to experiment with several approaches to see which approach works best for the *individual* athlete. It is likely that there are a minority of individuals who respond best to a higher carbohydrate intake. However, we would suggest that a general approach that may be efficacious for most individuals is to restrict or substitute the intake of carbohydrate (especially processed carbohydrate) and replace it with lean protein foods and unsaturated fat.

## QUESTIONS

1. A ketogenic diet can be described best as:
   a. High fat, high carbohydrate
   b. High fat, low carbohydrate
   c. High protein
   d. High protein, high carbohydrate

2. The Mediterranean diet is best described as:
   a. Low fat
   b. Moderate fat
   c. High protein

3. Consuming protein at the expense of carbohydrates (at least in the short term) is associated with:
   a. Increased satiety
   b. Increased thermogenesis
   c. Sparing of muscle protein loss
   d. Enhanced glycemic control
   e. All of the above

4. Increasing the proportion of protein to carbohydrate in the diet of adult women generally has ____ effects on body composition, blood lipids, glucose homeostasis, and satiety during weight loss.
   a. Beneficial
   b. Detrimental

5. Low-carbohydrate diets (≤40% carbohydrate) tend to produce a ____ in serum triglycerides in comparison to high-carbohydrate diets.
   a. Increase
   b. Decrease
   c. Neither a or b

6. Switching from a higher-carbohydrate to a very-low-carbohydrate diet (isoenergetic diets) tends to promote ____ in lean body mass.
   a. Gains
   b. Decreases
   c. No effect

7. The notion of "a calorie is just a calorie" means that:
   a. Regardless of the food source, your body will treat dietary energy identically

    b. The thermic effect of different foods in reality does not exist

    c. Neither a nor b

8. The hormonal changes associated with a low-carbohydrate diet include:

    a. Reduction in the circulating levels of insulin

    b. Increased levels of glucagons

    c. Increased level of testosterone

    d. Two of the above are correct

9. Which of the following produces the greatest thermic effect when consumed?

    a. Carbohydrate

    b. Protein

    c. Fat

10. The ketogenic diets are further characterized by:

    a. Elevations of free fatty acids

    b. Increased transcription of mitochondrial uncoupling proteins (UCPs)

    c. Increased oxidation of free fatty acids

    d. All of the above

11. There is evidence that hyperinsulinemia increases ____ without a concomitant increase in ____ intake.

    a. Fat mass, energy

    b. Muscle mass, fat

    c. Fat mass, protein

    d. Energy, fat

12. In older men who consumed an oral protein supplement (10g protein, 7g carbohydrate, and 3g fat) in conjunction with heavy resistance training, investigators found that consuming the supplement ____ was effective in promoting gains in lean body mass.

    a. Immediately postexercise

    b. Two hours postexercise

    c. Four hours postexercise

13. Data on feeding patterns (i.e., grazing versus gorging) show that the thermic effect of feeding is ____ when an isoenergetic test load is divided into multiple small meals or that there is no difference.

    a. Higher

    b. Lower

14. An irregular meal frequency is associated with ____ fasting total and low density lipoprotein cholesterol.

    a. Higher

    b. Lower

    c. No change

15. In a study in boxers, spreading meals over six feeding periods compared with an isoenergetic three feeding periods has a ____ effect.

    a. Protein-sparing

    b. Catabolic

    c. Proteolytic

16. Another unique feature of these restricted carbohydrate diets seems to be the higher intake of branched-chain amino acid ____ with unique regulatory actions on muscle protein synthesis, modulation of the insulin signal, and sparing of glucose use by stimulation of the glucose-alanine cycle.

    a. Leucine

    b. Valine

    c. Glutamine

17. According to Feinman and Fine, the principle of "a calorie is a calorie," violates the:

    a. Second Law of Thermodynamics

    b. Law of Gravity

    c. Murphy's Law

18. The *metabolic advantage* in low-carbohydrate diets refers to:
   a. The greater weight loss compared with isocaloric diets of different composition
   b. How great you feel when you are in ketosis
   c. Is a term coined by a "diet guru" selling nutrition books

19. A low-carbohydrate diet ____ turnover of body proteins.
   a. Increases
   b. Decreases

20. Postprandial thermogenesis was ____ 100% on a high-protein/low-fat diet versus a high-carbohydrate/low-fat diet in healthy subjects according to a study by Johnston et al.
   a. Increased
   b. Decreased

21. Mediterranean-style diet, controlled in energy, offers an alternative to a low-fat diet with superior long-term participation and adherence, with consequent improvements in weight loss.
   a. True
   b. False

22. The use of protein supplements as a means of augmenting the hypertrophic response to exercise is common.
   a. True
   b. False

23. A study by Demling and Desanti found that differing protein sources have different anabolic effects (casein>whey) and that protein supplementation in conjunction with resistance training can improve body composition.
   a. True
   b. False

24. According to one study, there tends to be an inverse relationship between people's habitual frequency of eating and body weight (i.e., greater meal frequency is associated with lower body weight).
   a. True
   b. False

25. It has been suggested that the effect of feeding frequency on body weight regulation is probably mediated through effects on the food intake side of the energy balance equation.
   a. True
   b. False

26. There is a reduced thermic effect of feeding with the irregular meal frequency.
   a. True
   b. False

27. There are published data that show that soy and whey protein bar supplementation may promote exercise training–induced lean body mass gain.
   a. True
   b. False

28. Soy protein has been shown in well-controlled animal studies to prevent exercise-induced protein degradation in skeletal muscle via the inhibition of calpain-mediated proteolysis.
   a. True
   b. False

29. There are data that whey protein supplementation (20 g/day for 3 months) in humans can increase peak power and 30-second work capacity and augment antioxidant defenses.
   a. True
   b. False

30. Protein intakes of up to 2.8 g daily per kilogram body weight do not impair renal function in well-trained athletes.
    a. True
    b. False

## REFERENCES

1. Kanehisa H, Kondo M, Ikegawa S, Fukunaga T. Characteristics of body composition and muscle strength in college Sumo wrestlers. Int J Sports Med 1997;18(7):510–515.
2. Kanehisa H, Kondo M, Ikegawa S, Fukunaga T. Body composition and isokinetic strength of professional Sumo wrestlers. Eur J Appl Physiol Occup Physiol 1998;77(4):352–359.
3. Frisch RE, Hall GM, Aoki TT, et al. Metabolic, endocrine, and reproductive changes of a woman channel swimmer. Metabolism 1984;33(12):1106–1111.
4. Benoit FL, Martin RL, Watten RH. Changes in body composition during weight reduction in obesity. Balance studies comparing effects of fasting and a ketogenic diet. Ann Intern Med 1965;63(4):604–612.
5. Young CM, Scanlan SS, Im HS, Lutwak L. Effect of body composition and other parameters in obese young men of carbohydrate level of reduction diet. Am J Clin Nutr 1971;24(3):290–296.
6. McManus K, Antinoro L, Sacks F. A randomized controlled trial of a moderate-fat, low-energy diet compared with a low-fat, low-energy diet for weight loss in overweight adults. Int J Obes Relat Metab Disord 2001;25(10):1503–1511.
7. Layman DK, Baum JI. Dietary protein impact on glycemic control during weight loss. J Nutr 2004;134(4):968S–973S.
8. Layman DK, Boileau RA, Erickson DJ, et al. A reduced ratio of dietary carbohydrate to protein improves body composition and blood lipid profiles during weight loss in adult women. J Nutr 2003;133(2):411–417.
9. Yancy WS Jr, Olsen MK, Guyton JR, Bakst RP, Westman EC. A low-carbohydrate, ketogenic diet versus a low-fat diet to treat obesity and hyperlipidemia: a randomized, controlled trial. Ann Intern Med 2004;140(10):769–777.
10. Samaha FF, Iqbal N, Seshadri P, et al. A low-carbohydrate as compared with a low-fat diet in severe obesity. N Engl J Med 22 2003;348(21):2074–2081.
11. Kauffman JM. Low-carbohydrate diets. J Sci Exploration 2004;18:83–134.
12. Brehm BJ, Seeley RJ, Daniels SR, D'Alessio DA. A randomized trial comparing a very low carbohydrate diet and a calorie-restricted low fat diet on body weight and cardiovascular risk factors in healthy women. J Clin Endocrinol Metab 2003;88(4):1617–1623.
13. Sondike SB, Copperman N, Jacobson MS. Effects of a low-carbohydrate diet on weight loss and cardiovascular risk factor in overweight adolescents. J Pediatr 2003;142(3):253–258.
14. Greene P, Willett W, Devecis, J, et al. Pilot 12-week feeding weight loss comparison: low-fat vs. low-carbohydrate (ketogenic) diets [abstract]. Obes Res 2003;11:A23.
15. Volek JS, Sharman MJ, Gomez AL, et al. Comparison of energy-restricted very low-carbohydrate and low-fat diets on weight loss and body composition in overweight men and women. Nutr Metab (Lond) 2004;1(1):13.
16. Volek JS, Sharman MJ, Love DM, et al. Body composition and hormonal responses to a carbohydrate-restricted diet. Metabolism 2002;51(7):864–870.
17. Bravata DM, Sanders L, Huang J, Krumholz HM, Olkin I, Gardner CD. Efficacy and safety of low-carbohydrate diets: a systematic review. JAMA 2003;289(14):1837–1850.
18. Kauffman JM. Bias in recent papers on diet and drugs in peer-reviewed medical journals. J Am Phys Surg 2004;9:11–14.
19. Foster GD, Wyatt HR, Hill JO, et al. A randomized trial of a low-carbohydrate diet for obesity. N Engl J Med 2003;348(21):2082–2090.
20. Feinman RD, Fine EJ. "A calorie is a calorie" violates the second law of thermodynamics. Nutr J 2004;3(1):9.
21. Hue L. Regulation of gluconeogenesis in liver. In: Handbook of Physiology—Section 7: The Endocrine System—Volume II: The Endocrine Pancreas and Regulation of Metabolism. L. S. Jefferson and A. Cherrington(eds). Oxford: Oxford University Press; 2001:649–657.
22. Johnston CS, Day CS, Swan PD. Postprandial thermogenesis is increased 100% on a high-protein, low-fat diet versus a high-carbohydrate, low-fat diet in healthy, young women. J Am Coll Nutr 2002;21(1):55–61.

23. Veech RL. The therapeutic implications of ketone bodies: the effects of ketone bodies in pathological conditions: ketosis, ketogenic diet, redox states, insulin resistance, and mitochondrial metabolism. Prostaglandins Leukot Essent Fatty Acids 2004;70(3):309–319.

24. Carlson MG, Campbell PJ. Intensive insulin therapy and weight gain in IDDM. Diabetes 1993;42(12):1700–1707.

25. Biolo G, Tipton KD, Klein S, Wolfe RR. An abundant supply of amino acids enhances the metabolic effect of exercise on muscle protein. Am J Physiol 1997;273(1 Pt 1): E122–129.

26. Flakoll PJ, Judy T, Flinn K, Carr C, Flinn S. Postexercise protein supplementation improves health and muscle soreness during basic military training in marine recruits. J Appl Physiol 2004;96(3):951–956.

27. Burke LM, Kiens B, Ivy JL. Carbohydrates and fat for training and recovery. J Sports Sci 2004;22(1):15–30.

28. Borsheim E, Aarsland A, Wolfe RR. Effect of an amino acid, protein, and carbohydrate mixture on net muscle protein balance after resistance exercise. Int J Sport Nutr Exerc Metab 2004;14(3):255–271.

29. Borsheim E, Cree MG, Tipton KD, Elliott TA, Aarsland A, Wolfe RR. Effect of carbohydrate intake on net muscle protein synthesis during recovery from resistance exercise. J Appl Physiol 2004;96(2):674–678.

30. Williams MB, Raven PB, Fogt DL, Ivy JL. Effects of recovery beverages on glycogen restoration and endurance exercise performance. J Strength Cond Res 2003;17(1): 12–19.

31. Tipton KD, Borsheim E, Wolf SE, Sanford AP, Wolfe RR. Acute response of net muscle protein balance reflects 24-h balance after exercise and amino acid ingestion. Am J Physiol Endocrinol Metab 2003;284(1):E76–89.

32. Miller SL, Tipton KD, Chinkes DL, Wolf SE, Wolfe RR. Independent and combined effects of amino acids and glucose after resistance exercise. Med Sci Sports Exerc 2003;35(3):449–455.

33. Ivy JL, Res PT, Sprague RC, Widzer MO. Effect of a carbohydrate-protein supplement on endurance performance during exercise of varying intensity. Int J Sport Nutr Exerc Metab 2003;13(3):382–395.

34. Roy BD, Luttmer K, Bosman MJ, Tarnopolsky MA. The influence of post-exercise macronutrient intake on energy balance and protein metabolism in active females participating in endurance training. Int J Sport Nutr Exerc Metab 2002;12(2): 172–188.

35. Phillips SM, Parise G, Roy BD, Tipton KD, Wolfe RR, Tamopolsky MA. Resistance-training-induced adaptations in skeletal muscle protein turnover in the fed state. Can J Physiol Pharmacol 2002;80(11):1045–1053.

36. Levenhagen DK, Carr C, Carlson MG, Maron DJ, Borel MJ, Flakoll PJ. Postexercise protein intake enhances whole-body and leg protein accretion in humans. Med Sci Sports Exerc 2002;34(5):828–837.

37. Ivy JL, Goforth HW Jr, Damon BM, McCauley TR, Parsons EC, Price TB. Early postexercise muscle glycogen recovery is enhanced with a carbohydrate-protein supplement. J Appl Physiol 2002;93(4):1337–1344.

38. Borsheim E, Tipton KD, Wolf SE, Wolfe RR. Essential amino acids and muscle protein recovery from resistance exercise. Am J Physiol Endocrinol Metab 2002; 283(4):E648–657.

39. Tipton KD, Wolfe RR. Exercise, protein metabolism, and muscle growth. Int J Sport Nutr Exerc Metab 2001;11(1):109–132.

40. Tipton KD, Rasmussen BB, Miller SL, et al. Timing of amino acid-carbohydrate ingestion alters anabolic response of muscle to resistance exercise. Am J Physiol Endocrinol Metab 2001;281(2):E197–206.

41. Tipton KD. Gender differences in protein metabolism. Curr Opin Clin Nutr Metab Care 2001;4(6):493–498.

42. Tipton KD. Muscle protein metabolism in the elderly: influence of exercise and nutrition. Can J Appl Physiol 2001;26(6):588–606.

43. Levenhagen DK, Gresham JD, Carlson MG, Maron DJ, Borel MJ, Flakoll PJ. Postexercise nutrient intake timing in humans is critical to recovery of leg glucose and protein homeostasis. Am J Physiol Endocrinol Metab 2001;280(6):E982–993.

44. Jentjens RL, van Loon LJ, Mann CH, Wagenmakers AJ, Jeukendrup AE. Addition of protein and amino acids to carbohydrates does not enhance postexercise muscle glycogen synthesis. J Appl Physiol 2001;91(2):839–846.

45. Esmarck B, Andersen JL, Olsen S, Richter EA, Mizuno M, Kjaer M. Timing of postexercise protein intake is important for muscle hypertrophy with resistance training in elderly humans. J Physiol 2001;535(Pt 1):301–311.

46. Doi T, Matsuo T, Sugawara M, et al. New approach for weight reduction by a combination of diet, light resistance exercise and the timing of ingesting a protein supplement. Asia Pac J Clin Nutr 2001;10(3):226–232.

47. van Loon LJ, Kruijshoop M, Verhagen H, Saris WH, Wagenmakers AJ. Ingestion of protein hydrolysate and amino acid-carbohydrate mixtures increases postexercise plasma insulin responses in men. J Nutr 2000;130(10):2508–2513.

48. van Loon LJ, Saris WH, Kruijshoop M, Wagenmakers AJ. Maximizing postexercise muscle glycogen synthesis: carbohydrate supplementation and the application of amino acid or protein hydrolysate mixtures. Am J Clin Nutr 2000;72(1):106–111.

49. Rennie MJ, Tipton KD. Protein and amino acid metabolism during and after exercise and the effects of nutrition. Annu Rev Nutr 2000;20:457–483.

50. Rasmussen BB, Tipton KD, Miller SL, Wolf SE, Wolfe RR. An oral essential amino acid-carbohydrate supplement enhances muscle protein anabolism after resistance exercise. J Appl Physiol 2000;88(2):386–392.

51. Tipton KD, Ferrando AA, Phillips SM, Doyle D Jr, Wolfe RR. Postexercise net protein synthesis in human muscle from orally administered amino acids. Am J Physiol 1999;276(4 Pt 1):E628–634.

52. Phillips SM, Tipton KD, Ferrando AA, Wolfe RR. Resistance training reduces the acute exercise-induced increase in muscle protein turnover. Am J Physiol 1999;276(1 Pt 1):E118–124.

53. Tipton KD, Wolfe RR. Exercise-induced changes in protein metabolism. Acta Physiol Scand 1998;162(3):377–387.

54. Phillips SM, Tipton KD, Aarsland A, Wolf SE, Wolfe RR. Mixed muscle protein synthesis and breakdown after resistance exercise in humans. Am J Physiol 1997;273(1 Pt 1):E99–107.

55. Ferrando AA, Tipton KD, Bamman MM, Wolfe RR. Resistance exercise maintains skeletal muscle protein synthesis during bed rest. J Appl Physiol 1997;82(3):807–810.

56. Chromiak JA, Smedley B, Carpenter W, et al. Effect of a 10-week strength training program and recovery drink on body composition, muscular strength and endurance, and anaerobic power and capacity. Nutrition 2004;20(5):420–427.

57. Bellisle F, McDevitt R, Prentice AM. Meal frequency and energy balance. Br J Nutr 1997;77(Suppl 1):S57–70.

58. Westerterp-Plantenga MS, Kovacs EM, Melanson KJ. Habitual meal frequency and energy intake regulation in partially temporally isolated men. Int J Obes Relat Metab Disord 2002;26(1):102–110.

59. Farshchi HR, Taylor MA, Macdonald IA. Regular meal frequency creates more appropriate insulin sensitivity and lipid profiles compared with irregular meal frequency in healthy lean women. Eur J Clin Nutr 2004;58(7):1071–1077.

60. Farshchi HR, Taylor MA, Macdonald IA. Decreased thermic effect of food after an irregular compared with a regular meal pattern in healthy lean women. Int J Obes Relat Metab Disord 2004;28(5):653–660.

61. Iwao S, Mori K, Sato Y. Effects of meal frequency on body composition during weight control in boxers. Scand J Med Sci Sports 1996;6(5):265–272.

62. Demling RH, DeSanti L. Effect of a hypocaloric diet, increased protein intake and resistance training on lean mass gains and fat mass loss in overweight police officers. Ann Nutr Metab 2000;44(1):21–29.

63. Brown EC, Disilvestro RA, Babaknia A, Devor ST. Soy versus whey protein bars: effects on exercise training impact on lean body mass and antioxidant status. Nutr J 2004;3(1):22.

64. Deibert P, Konig D, Schmidt-Trucksaess A, et al. Weight loss without losing muscle mass in pre-obese and obese subjects induced by a high-soy-protein diet. Int J Obes Relat Metab Disord 2004;28(10):1349–1352.

65. Nikawa T, Ikemoto M, Sakai T, et al. Effects of a soy protein diet on exercise-induced muscle protein catabolism in rats. Nutrition 2002;18(6):490–495.

66. Lands LC, Grey VL, Smountas AA. Effect of supplementation with a cysteine donor on muscular performance. J Appl Physiol 1999;87(4):1381–1385.

67. Poortmans JR, Dellalieux O. Do regular high protein diets have potential health risks on kidney function in athletes? Int J Sport Nutr Exerc Metab 2000;10(1):28–38.

68. Dawson-Hughes B, Harris SS, Rasmussen H, Song L, Dallal GE. Effect of dietary protein supplements on calcium excretion in healthy older men and women. J Clin Endocrinol Metab 2004;89(3):1169–1173.

69. American Heart Association. Step I, Step II and TLC Diets (January 2006) http://www.americanheart.org/presenter.jhtml?identifier=4764.

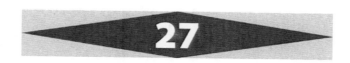

# Nutrition Before, During, and After Exercise for the Endurance Athlete

## John L. Ivy

## OBJECTIVES

On the completion of this chapter you will be able to:

1. Understand the consequences of dehydration.
2. Discuss the mechanisms by which the body regulates body temperature and how this affects dehydration.
3. Explain the role of carbohydrate stores in the body and how they affect exercise performance.
4. Understand the relationship between muscle glycogen and exercise performance.
5. Discuss the effects of endurance exercise on muscle damage, soreness, and immune responses.
6. Define the effects of hyperhydration on performance.
7. Talk about the process of glycogen loading and the effects of this practice on performance.
8. Clarify the role of pre-event carbohydrate feedings and outline the basic guidelines for endurance athletes.
9. Discuss the role of fluid, electrolyte, and carbohydrate supplementation during an endurance bout of exercise.
10. Talk about the relationships among cortisol, carbohydrates, and immunosuppression.
11. Appreciate the value of a postexercise fluid and carbohydrate replacement regime.

## ABSTRACT

Although it is understood that nutritional supplementation improves performance and enhances training adaptations, it is also vital to grasp how inadequate nutritional practices limit endurance performance. Therefore, in the first section of this chapter, major physiologic factors that result in fatigue during prolonged aerobic exercise are discussed. Adverse consequences of strenuous exercise over time such as muscle damage and immune system suppression are also discussed in this section. In section two, nutritional recommendations in preparation for exercise are presented, whereas nutritional supplementation during exercise is provided in section three. Nutritional strategies for rapid recovery and enhancement of training adaptation are subsequently discussed, whereas the summary section of the chapter consists of practical applications in which nutritional supplementation guidelines are provided to promote endurance performance.

***Key Words:*** **aerobic, dehydration, recovery, glycogen, hyperhydration, protein synthesis, nutrient timing**

From: *Essentials of Sports Nutrition and Supplements*
Edited by J. Antonio, D. Kalman, J. R. Stout, M. Greenwood, D. S. Willoughby, and G. G. Haff © Humana Press, a part of Springer Science+Business Media, Totowa, NJ

The endurance athlete is generally a very dedicated and compulsive individual willing to train for many hours each day. Although a well-balanced, healthy diet is essential for optimum performance and quality-training sessions day after day, it is also true that endurance athletes have very special nutritional needs that go beyond a well-balanced diet. Numerous studies have documented that endurance athletes can improve their exercise performance during competition and enhance their training sessions with nutritional supplements.

Nutritional supplementation can prevent or slow dehydration, provide additional fuel to drive muscle contraction, reduce muscle damage and inflammation, and speed recovery. However, supplementation is only as effective as the appropriateness of the nutrients provided, as well as the timing of their ingestion. Supplementing with the appropriate nutrients at the appropriate time can have a significant impact on exercise performance and training adaptation.

To understand how nutritional supplementation can improve performance and enhance training adaptation, it is first necessary to understand what limits endurance performance. Therefore, the first section of this review discusses the major physiologic factors that result in fatigue during prolonged, aerobic exercise. Strenuous exercise also can result in physiologic changes that do not initially limit performance, but can have adverse consequences over time. These changes include muscle damage and immune system suppression, and they are discussed in the first section as well. In section two, nutritional recommendations in preparation for exercise are discussed. This is followed in section three with a discussion of nutritional supplementation during exercise. In section four, nutrition for rapid recovery and enhancement of training adaptation is discussed. Section five is the chapter summary, and the last section consists of practical applications in which nutritional supplementation guidelines are provided.

## CAUSES OF FATIGUE DURING AEROBIC EXERCISE

The causes of fatigue during prolonged, aerobic exercise will vary according to the type of exercise and the environmental conditions in which the exercise is performed. However, fatigue will typically result from either thermal stress caused by dehydration, muscle glycogen depletion, or limited blood glucose availability caused by a decline in liver glucose output.

### Dehydration

The most critical physiologic change that occurs during prolonged exercise is fluid loss. For optimal exercise performance, body temperature must be tightly controlled. There are several mechanisms that the body can use to maintain a stable temperature. For example, during running or cycling, excess body heat can be dissipated by convection, which occurs when cool air moves over the surface of the body. During swimming, excess body heat can be dissipated by the transfer of heat to the water by conduction. However, direct transfer to the environment is generally not an efficient means of dissipating heat, particularly when environmental conditions are hot and humid. During exercise, the primary means of heat dissipation is by sweat evaporation. Evaporation accounts for about 80% of the total heat loss during physical activity. For each liter of water that evaporates, 580 kcal of heat are dissipated from the body and transferred to the environment.

During exercise, heat is generated in relation to exercise intensity. To rapidly dissipate this heat, it is transferred to the blood vessels surrounding the muscles and carried by the blood to vessels just below the surface of the skin. Sweat glands are activated resulting in perspiration, which then evaporates, cooling both the skin and the blood just below the skin. The cooled blood can then be returned to the muscles to help dissipate additional heat. The need to move blood from the muscles to the skin to dissipate heat, however, can put a strain on the heart and cardiovascular system because of the requirement to pump blood to the skin as well as the working muscles. The warmer and more

**TABLE 27.1. Normal concentrations (mmol·L$^{-1}$) of the major electrolytes in sweat and plasma.**

| Electrolytes | Sweat | Plasma |
|---|---|---|
| Sodium | 20.0–80.0 | 130.0–155.0 |
| Potassium | 4.0–8.0 | 3.2–5.5 |
| Calcium | 0.0–1.0 | 2.1–3.0 |
| Magnesium | 0.1–0.2 | 0.7–1.5 |
| Chloride | 20.0–60.0 | 96.0–110.0 |

humid the environment, the greater the sweat rate and skin blood flow required to dissipate the heat generated by the muscles.

As body water is lost, blood volume declines, which limits the capacity of the circulatory system to carry oxygen and nutrients to and remove metabolic byproducts such as lactic acid as well as heat from the exercising muscles. A loss of body fluid equal to as little as 1% body weight (approximately 1.5 lbs. for a 150-lb. athlete) can significantly reduce blood volume, putting stress on the cardiovascular system and limiting physical performance.[1–3] As dehydration increases, performance will continue to decrease. Reduction in performance can occur in the form of reduced strength, endurance, fine motor skills such as eye–hand coordination, and mental alertness. When dehydration approaches 4%, athletes can experience heat cramps and heat exhaustion.[4–6] When dehydration approaches 6%, there may be cessation of sweating, a rapid increase in body temperature followed by heat stoke.[7] Heat stroke is life-threatening and requires immediate medical attention.

A second consequence of dehydration can be the loss or imbalance in electrolytes. Electrolytes are charged minerals that are necessary for many metabolic functions such as muscle contraction, nerve transmission, and hormonal secretion. Significant losses of electrolytes can occur when large volumes of sweat are produced. The electrolyte composition of sweat is variable, but the major electrolytes in sweat are sodium and chloride. Typically, the plasma sodium and chloride concentrations will range between 130 and 155 mmol·L$^{-1}$ and 96 to 110 mmol·L$^{-1}$, respectively. It is important that the sodium and chloride concentrations in the plasma be maintained within these ranges to keep the tissues and organs of the body functioning properly. During exercise, sodium losses can range from 20 to 80 mmol·L$^{-1}$ of sweat and chloride losses can range between 20 to 60 mmol·L$^{-1}$ of sweat.[6] Other electrolytes such as potassium and magnesium are also lost, but in much smaller amounts (Table 27.1).

## Depletion of Carbohydrate Stores

Depletion of carbohydrate is now considered one of the primary causes of fatigue during exercise that is sustained for long periods of time. Relative to the amount of fat and protein, your body has a limited supply of carbohydrate. About 300–500 g of glycogen is stored in the muscles and another 75–100 g is stored in the liver.[8] This is enough carbohydrate to run at a moderate intensity for about 20 miles. However, the utilization of carbohydrate by the muscle can be greatly altered by exercise intensity. With an increase in exercise intensity, the rate of carbohydrate utilization is exponentially increased with the major contribution coming from muscle glycogen.[9]

During low-intensity aerobic exercise [40%–50% maximal oxygen uptake (VO$_2$ max)], such as brisk walking, the major fuel for muscle contraction is fat. Carbohydrate use is low and primarily comes from blood glucose.[10] Exercise can be performed for many hours at this low intensity because the liver can continually supply glucose to maintain the blood glucose concentration. When the aerobic exercise intensity is moderate (60%–75% VO$_2$ max), 40% of the energy requirements of exercise must come from carbohydrate.[10] If carbohydrate availability is compromised such that it cannot contribute 40% of the energy requirement, fatigue will occur.[11–13] As exercise intensity increases, the percentage of carbohydrate necessary to sustain muscle contraction also increases.

Reduction in either muscle glycogen or blood glucose can limit carbohydrate availability. At moderate exercise intensities (60%–75% VO$_2$ max) the carbohydrate needs of the muscle can come from blood glucose and muscle glycogen. At the start of exercise, muscle glycogen is preferentially used, but as muscle glycogen declines and its rate of utilization decreases, there is an increased reliance on blood glucose by the exercising muscles.[8,14] At moderate exercise intensities, glucose uptake can support the carbohydrate needs of the muscle in the event of muscle glycogen depletion as long as the blood glucose concentration is maintained within a normal range. However, when blood glucose decreases below 3.5 mM, fatigue will soon occur.[11–13]

## Depletion of Muscle Glycogen

At high aerobic exercise intensities (75%–85% VO$_2$ max), the contribution of carbohydrate to total energy expenditure is in excess of 70%, with muscle glycogen contributing approximately 85% of the carbohydrate requirements.[9,10] At these exercise intensities, fatigue is directly related to muscle glycogen depletion because muscle glucose uptake is too slow to support the carbohydrate needs of the exercising muscles even when blood glucose levels are normal.[15,16] At exercise intensities of more than 85% VO$_2$ max, fatigue is generally associated with an accumulation of lactic acid caused by the rapid hydrolysis of muscle glycogen, or reduction in the high-energy phosphates. There is also evidence of central nervous system limitations at high intensities.[17]

Although depletion of muscle glycogen is normally associated with fatigue during continuous aerobic exercises such as marathon running, it is important to recognize its impact for team and skill sports that require bursts of speed or powerful movements. Without adequate muscle glycogen it becomes impossible for the basketball player to continually sprint up and down the court or the tennis player to move quickly to the net. Adequate muscle glycogen stores are critical for top athletic performance.

## Other Consequences of Endurance Exercise

### MUSCLE DAMAGE AND SORENESS

Muscle damage can be an unfortunate consequence of exercise. This generally occurs when training intensity is increased or during competition when maximal effort is given. During training, some of the muscle damage may be beneficial because mild muscle damage stimulates the rebuilding process resulting in new and stronger muscle proteins. However, more severe damage can result in muscle stiffness and soreness, limited recovery, and reduced performance. This type of damage is attributable to disruption of the muscle membrane and contractile proteins and inflammation.

Three primary causes of muscle damage are contractile stress, hormonal shifts, and free radical reactions. It is important to understand how each of these contributes to muscle damage because it is now known that nutritional intervention, when performed properly, can greatly limit muscle damage, enhancing muscle training adaptations and limiting recovery time between intense training sessions.

Initial damage occurs as a result of the physical forces acting on the muscles. Muscle contraction, particularly the eccentric phase, places great stress on the muscles, which can lead to small tearing of the muscle fiber membranes and contractile proteins.[18,19] Muscle injury triggers an acute inflammatory response and within hours specific cells migrate to the site of the damage and begin removing tissue debris. This process causes swelling, which can further damage muscle cell membranes. The acute inflammatory response does not peak for up to 24 hours, which is one reason why muscle soreness is often not felt until well after the exercise is completed.[20]

The second cause of muscle soreness is hormonal related. This is attributable to the release of the catabolic hormone cortisol.[20] Cortisol is released from the adrenal glands when blood glucose is low or during high-intensity exercise. The primary function of cortisol during exercise is to generate fuel for working muscles by activating gluconeogenesis, lipolysis, and proteolysis. The activation of proteolysis, however, can result in muscle damage.

The third cause of muscle damage is the formation of excess free radicals.[21,22] Free radicals are highly reactive molecules that can damage muscle protein and membranes and may even inactivate enzymes associated with the proper functioning of the immune system. During aerobic metabolism, free radicals are generated and must be neutralized by antioxidants such as vitamins C and E.

### IMMUNE SYSTEM SUPPRESSION

Athletes when training intensely or competing are often more susceptible to colds and infections than the general population. For example, Nieman et al.[23] reported a much higher incidence of self-reported symptoms of upper respiratory tract infections in runners who completed long-distance races compared with runners who did not compete in the events. The frequency of infections is increased with added stress such as a demanding travel schedule, frequent competition, or personal problems. The result is that in the latter stages of a season, athletes are far more prone to infection and chronic fatigue. Normally, moderate-intensity exercise stimulates the immune system. Strenuous exercise and mental stress, however, can actually suppress immune function thereby increasing susceptibility to infection and disease.

There are several reasons for the immunosuppressive effects of strenuous exercise. These include an increase in blood cortisol and other stress hormones, and a decrease in blood glutamine and glucose. Research has shown that most of the immunosuppressive responses of exercise are caused by an increase in blood cortisol.[24,25] Cortisol lowers the concentration and activities of many of the important immune cells that fight infection. As discussed previously, blood cortisol levels increase during strenuous exercise or when blood glucose decreases. Cortisol also increases during periods of mental stress, thus provoking an even greater immunosuppressive response during strenuous exercise when also confronted with unpleasant or critical life situations. Immune system suppression can last up to 72 hours after exercise and significantly increase susceptibility to infection.[26]

## PREPARING THE BODY FOR EXERCISE AND COMPETITION

There are several considerations when preparing for prolonged, intense training or competition. Athletes should first try to be fully hydrated. Second, they should try to have adequate muscle and liver glycogen stores.

### Hyperhydration

Because of the need to minimize the impact of sweat loss on exercise performance, it is important to ensure that athletes are fully hydrated before exercise. In addition, some studies have suggested that increasing total body water above normal or hyperhydrating may increase sweat rate and improve thermoregulation during exercise in the heat.[27,28] The benefits of hyperhydration are somewhat controversial, however.[29,30] The controversy may have arisen because of differences in experimental designs and not hyperhydration per se. Studies that reported no benefit of hyperhydration replaced fluid lost during exercise, whereas studies that found a benefit did not maintain hydration status during exercise. These results suggest that hyperhydrating before exercise may be of benefit when fluid consumption during exercise is limited, but may not be essential when sufficient fluid can be ingested. Most athletes, however, do not consume sufficient fluid during competition even when available. Therefore, hyperhydration would seem to be a good strategy when exercise is anticipated to occur during environmental conditions that present a substantial thermal load on the body.

Attempts to hyperhydrate before exercise are usually thwarted by the prompt diuretic response that ensues when the body water content is increased. This is primarily attributable to the dilution of the blood sodium concentration and plasma osmolality. To overcome this effect, it is recommended that fluids containing sodium concentrations of 100 mmol·L⁻¹ or more be consumed.[31] When preparing for competition, hyperhydration should start several days before competition and be sufficient to result in light-colored urine. Consuming approximately 500 mL of fluid 2 hours before and again 15 minutes before exercise is also recommended.

## Glycogen Loading

The importance of muscle glycogen as a fuel source for muscle contraction has been known for more than a century. Over the years, research has shown that with increasing intensity of exercise there is an increased reliance on muscle glycogen and that the increasing perception of fatigue during prolonged, strenuous exercise parallels the decrease in muscle glycogen concentration.[15,16,32] It has also been noted that the rate of muscle glycogen utilization is directly related to the initial muscle glycogen stores.[33,34] However, despite a greater reliance on muscle glycogen when preexercise levels are elevated, increasing the muscle glycogen stores before competition has generally been found to improve performance when competition lasts in excess of 90 minutes.[15,16,35] Muscle glycogen stores normally range between 90 to 100 μmol·g⁻¹ wet muscle wt. Endurance training can increase the average muscle glycogen concentration to 120–130 μmol·g⁻¹ wet muscle wt, and consuming a high-carbohydrate diet can elevate the glycogen stores to 140–150 μmol·g⁻¹ wet muscle wt during training. However, because of the importance of muscle glycogen as a fuel source, means of maximizing the glycogen stores or "glycogen loading" before competition have been investigated for many years.

Bergström and colleagues[15] were the first to investigate muscle glycogen loading and its effect on endurance performance. These investigators found that the most effective means of increasing the muscle glycogen stores was first to deplete these stores by exercise; second, to maintain a low glycogen concentration by consuming a carbohydrate-free, high-protein and high-fat diet for 3 days; and third, to follow with a second glycogen-depleting exercise bout and a 3-day, high-carbohydrate diet. This procedure was found to increase the muscle glycogen stores twofold above normal levels. However, this is a very stressful and difficult process because of the two glycogen-depletion exercises, and many athletes found that it frequently resulted in chronic fatigue, muscle soreness, and injury.

Sherman et al.,[33] however, found that a less-extreme diet–exercise regimen could be equally as effective in elevating the preexercise muscle glycogen stores as the traditional protocol of Bergström et al.[15] The protocol of Sherman et al.[33] made the loading procedure more compatible with the normal training routine used by endurance athletes before competition (Figure 27.1). The protocol starts with a hard training session to lower the muscle glycogen stores. During the subsequent 3 days, a mixed diet composed of 45%–50% carbohydrate is consumed, and a natural training taper is started. On days 4–6, the training taper is continued, but the dietary carbohydrate concentration is increased to approximately 70%. This protocol was found to increase muscle glycogen to levels in excess of 200 μmol·g⁻¹ wet muscle wt, which is similar to that demonstrated by Bergström et al.[15]

More recently, Fairchild et al.[36] reported that trained athletes could substantially increase their muscle glycogen stores in less than 24 hours by performing only 3 minutes of supramaximal exercise followed by a high-carbohydrate diet. In addition, Bussau et al.[37] reported that trained athletes could increase their muscle glycogen to 180 μmol·g⁻¹ wet muscle wt in 24 hours after glycogen-depleting exercise if they remained inactive during recovery and ingested 10 g of carbohydrate·kg⁻¹ of body wt.

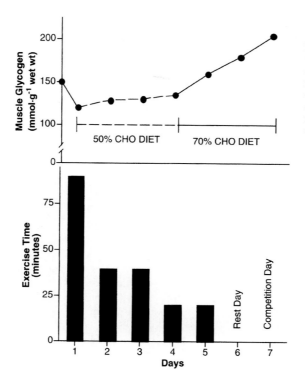

**FIGURE 27.1.** An illustration of the glycogen loading protocol as designed by Sherman et al.[33] During the loading process, an exercise training taper follows an initial hard exercise bout. The exercise intensity is maintained at approximately 75% VO$_2$ max. During the first 3 days of the taper, a mixed diet consisting of 50% carbohydrate (CHO) is consumed. During the final days of the taper and before competition, a high-carbohydrate diet is consumed.

## Preexercise Carbohydrate Feedings

### FOUR TO SIX HOURS BEFORE EXERCISE

The ingestion of 200–300 g of carbohydrate 4–6 hours before exercise has been found to increase the muscle glycogen levels of fasted subjects, increase carbohydrate oxidation, and blunt free fatty acid mobilization and fat oxidation.[38] These metabolic changes can persist for up to 6 hours, but do not seem to be detrimental to exercise performance. On the contrary, despite a greater reliance on carbohydrate as a fuel source after its ingestion, exercise performance is normally improved.[39,40] In fact, it has been suggested that a high-carbohydrate meal 3–4 hours before exercise may be as beneficial as supplementing with carbohydrate during exercise.[39] The enhanced performance observed is likely related to small increases in both muscle and liver glycogen stores. Furthermore, it has been reported that supplementing before and during exercise can have an additive effect on performance.[41] From a practical perspective, a light meal consisting of 150–200 g of carbohydrate 4–5 hours before training or competition may be a good strategy to ensure adequate carbohydrate available during competition if carbohydrate availability is limited or not available.

### ONE HOUR BEFORE EXERCISE

The ingestion of carbohydrate in the hour immediately before competition or exercise has been controversial. Carbohydrates ingested 30–60 minutes before exercise increases the level of plasma insulin, which has a strong effect on metabolism. The increase in plasma insulin reduces liver glucose output by inhibiting liver glycogenolysis and gluconeogenesis and stimulates muscle glucose uptake.[42] As a consequence, blood glucose rapidly declines during exercise as muscle contraction and insulin function additively increase muscle glucose uptake while liver glucose output is restricted. Fat oxidation is also reduced because of insulin inhibition of lipolysis in adipocytes and muscle.[42,43] In addition, some studies have reported an increased reliance on muscle glycogen as a fuel source because of a reduced availability of blood-borne fuels.[43,44]

Foster et al.[45] reported that a carbohydrate supplement consumed 30 minutes before exercise at 80% VO$_2$ max caused a significant reduction in blood glucose levels within 15 minutes after the start of exercise. The reliance on carbohydrate as a fuel source was increased, and a 19% reduction in time to fatigue occurred. Most studies, however, have failed to demonstrate a reduction in exercise performance after a preexercise carbohydrate meal or supplement,[46] and several studies actually found that performance was improved although carbohydrate oxidation was increased.[47]

Research studies by Hargreaves et al.[46] and Goodpaster et al.[47] are examples of studies that have found that preexercise carbohydrate feedings have no effect or a positive effect on performance, respectively. Hargreaves et al.[46] investigated the effects of 75 g glucose and fructose supplements on cycling time to exhaustion. The exercise intensity was 75% $VO_2$ max and the carbohydrate supplements, taken 75 minutes before exercise, were compared with a placebo. No differences were found between treatments in time to exhaustion or muscle glycogen use despite blood glucose levels being significantly lower during the glucose treatment compared with the placebo and fructose treatments. Goodpaster et al.[47] compared preexercise supplements composed of different forms of carbohydrate and an artificially sweetened placebo. Carbohydrate ($1\,g\cdot kg^{-1}$ body wt) was ingested 30 minutes before exercise and consisted of waxy starch, resistant starch, or glucose. Compared with placebo, performance was improved when glucose or waxy starch was ingested. Performance also tended to be improved when the resistance starch was ingested, although statistical significance was not reached ($p < 0.09$).

In summary, carbohydrate supplementation in the hours before exercise will result in a reduced rate of lipolysis and fatty acid oxidation and increased reliance of blood glucose and possibly muscle glycogen at the onset of exercise. Despite these metabolic alterations, endurance performance does not seem to be diminished. On the contrary, if a sufficient amount of carbohydrate is consumed, it may actually improve performance. However, individual responses to preexercise carbohydrate supplementation are quite variable and therefore supplementation practices should be based on individual experiences.

## SUPPLEMENTATION DURING EXERCISE

Supplementation during exercise can have a profound effect on endurance performance. Many types of supplements have been tested, but the ones that have been found to be safe and most effective and even necessary under some environmental conditions are fluid replacement with electrolytes and carbohydrate supplementation.

### Fluid and Electrolyte Supplementation

During exercise, one should try to fully replace fluid losses that occur. The amount of fluid lost during exercise by sweating is going to depend on a number of factors, but the most important are exercise intensity, ambient temperature, and individual sweat characteristics. Therefore, it is important to determine one's sweat rate for different ambient temperatures. Furthermore, sweat rate during exercise can reach $3.0\,L\cdot h^{-1}$[6] and far exceed the maximum rate of gastric emptying. Gastric emptying is the rate at which fluid enters the intestines from the stomach. Maximal rates of gastric emptying during exercise range from 1.0 to $1.2\,L\cdot h^{-1}$.[48] As a general rule, when sweat rates are high, one should try to consume as much fluid as can be tolerated during workouts and competition. This should be done with small volumes of fluid consumed frequently rather than a few large volumes of fluid occasionally. For example, a general strategy is to consume 150–200 mL every 15 minutes of exercise. Thirst is not a good indicator of fluid requirements or the degree of dehydration. It has been observed that athletes left to voluntarily drink during exercise will replace only 30%–50% of the fluid lost. Therefore, it is essential that a plan of fluid replacement be established and maintained throughout exercise (Table 27.2).

Sodium chloride is the major salt lost in sweat, and sodium is the most important electrolyte to replace. Although the sodium concentration of sweat is hypotonic to plasma, it is beneficial to replace some of this electrolyte when

**TABLE 27.2.** Average sweat rates per hour at moderate exercise intensity for different ambient temperatures.

| Temperature | Light sweaters | | Moderate sweaters | | Heavy sweaters | |
|---|---|---|---|---|---|---|
| 40°F (4.4°C) | 12 oz. | 355 mL | 17 oz. | 503 mL | 31 oz. | 917 mL |
| 55°F (12.8°C) | 15 oz. | 444 mL | 22 oz. | 650 mL | 35 oz. | 1035 mL |
| 70°F (21.1°C) | 22 oz. | 650 mL | 27 oz. | 798 mL | 47 oz. | 1390 mL |
| 90°F (32.2°C) | 31 oz. | 917 mL | 37 oz. | 1095 mL | 75 oz. | 2218 mL |

hydrating during exercise. First, it helps to maintain body fluid balance and the drive to drink.[49] Drinking only water can quickly quench thirst but limit fluid consumption. Second, absorption of fluid that enters the intestines is more rapid when sodium is present, and it also can hasten intestinal glucose absorption. Third, sodium replacement prevents developing hyponatremia.[50] Hyponatremia is characterized by a plasma sodium concentration of $125 \, mmol \cdot L^{-1}$ or lower. It occurs when plasma volume increases faster than the electrolyte concentration, usually because of excess water consumption. This is not typically seen during exercise, but can occur when water consumption is substantial during prolonged exercise in the heat. Symptoms include bloating, headaches, nausea, vomiting, muscle weakness, cramping, and seizures. Acute hyponatremia has a mortality rate of about 50% and must be taken seriously.

Other electrolytes found in significant amounts in the sweat include potassium and magnesium. These electrolytes can generally be replaced adequately after exercise with well-balanced meals. However, most sports drinks are formulated to provide the proper ratio of electrolytes lost in sweat. The sodium concentration of sports drinks is usually between $15-30 \, mmol \cdot L^{-1}$ and the potassium concentration between $3-6 \, mmol \cdot L^{-1}$.

## Carbohydrate Supplementation

One of the first studies to address the effects of carbohydrate supplementation during exercise was conducted by Dill et al.[51] They found that feeding a dog 20 g of carbohydrate every hour during exercise prevented a decline in blood glucose and enabled the dog to run at an intense pace for 13 hours without fatiguing. When only water was provided, the dog was unable to run for more than 6 hours continuously. Since this early study, many researchers have confirmed the benefits of carbohydrate supplementation on endurance capacity and performance. Beneficial effects of carbohydrate supplementation have been demonstrated during prolonged, continuous exercise of constant or similar intensity[11-13]; continuous exercise of varying intensities[52]; prolonged, intermittent exercise[53]; and even intense exercise lasting only 45–60 minutes.[54] In fact, carbohydrate supplementation has been found to improve the performance of participates in team sports, particularly late in the event.[55] The mechanism by which carbohydrate supplementation improves performance is not always obvious and seems to depend on the type and intensity of exercise.

The ingestion of carbohydrate during prolonged, moderate-intensity exercise helps prevent the decline in blood glucose and carbohydrate oxidation. Liver glucose output is reduced with possible liver glycogen sparing, and muscle glucose uptake is increased. Carbohydrate supplementation does not seem to improve performance by sparing muscle glycogen, at least not during steady-state cycling.[11] Instead, supplementation improves performance by preventing a decline in blood glucose thereby ensuring an adequate carbohydrate oxidation rate even under conditions of muscle glycogen depletion. However, during intermittent or variable-intensity cycling, decreases in muscle glycogen utilization have been observed when supplementation occurs and this seems to contribute to an improvement in endurance performance.[52] Likewise, recent research indicates that carbohydrate supplementation during running spares muscle glycogen and improves endurance capacity.[56]

## AMOUNT OF CARBOHYDRATE

The main objective of supplementing with carbohydrate during prolonged, strenuous exercise is to maintain normal blood glucose concentration or euglycemia. When muscle glycogen stores are low and euglycemic conditions prevail, the maximal rate of blood glucose oxidation has been estimated to be 1.0 and 1.2 g·min[-1].[12] The maximal oxidation rate, however, has recently been found to depend on the carbohydrate composition of the supplement. For example, exogenous carbohydrate oxidation rates in excess of 1.2 g·min[-1] late in exercise have been observed after the ingestion of a mixture of glucose and fructose or glucose and sucrose.[57] Whether increasing the exogenous carbohydrate oxidation rate beyond 1.2 g·min[-1] will improve endurance performance has not been determined. Regardless, the amount of exogenous carbohydrate required for best results still seems to be between 30–60 g·h[-1].[12,53]

The average rate of gastric emptying of a glucose solution is approximately 0.5–1.0 g·min[-1].[58] This, however, is dependent on the concentration of the glucose supplement and the volume of fluid ingested. Costill[48] reported that when 120 mL of a glucose solution was provided every 15 minutes during exercise, the amount of glucose emptied from the stomach increased proportionately as the glucose concentration of the solution increased from 2% to 10%. The volume of fluid emptied remained constant at approximately 11 mL·min[-1]. When the glucose concentration exceeded 10%, the amount of glucose emptied from the stomach plateaued at approximately 1.0 g·min[-1], whereas the volume of fluid emptied started to decrease as the glucose concentration increased. This suggests that glucose solutions up to 10% can be used without substantially impeding fluid replacement. Glucose concentrations in excess of 10%, however, seem to delay gastric emptying and compromise fluid replacement (Figure 27.2).

The appropriate percent glucose solution to use will depend on the imposing thermal stress of the activity and the type of exercise. When thermal stress is high, sweat rate can exceed 1200 mL·h[-1], and fluid replacement becomes important to prevent dehydration and hyperthermia. Cyclists can empty from the stomach up to 1000 mL of fluid per hour, and therefore 40–60 g of carbohydrate can be easily ingested while consuming a large volume of fluid.[2] Runners, however, generally consume less than 500 mL of fluid per hour.[59] This is because of the difficulty of drinking on the run and the discomfort of running with a large gastric volume. Therefore, runners must use more concentrated solutions than do cyclists if they are to consume the recommended amount of carbohydrate. For cyclists, a carbohydrate solution of 4%–6% is generally sufficient when fluid replacement is important. For runners, this concentration may have to be 8%–10% to provide the appropriate amount of carbohydrate.

**FIGURE 27.2.** The effect of carbohydrate (CHO) concentration on the rate of gastric emptying of fluids and carbohydrate from the stomach during exercise. Carbohydrate concentrations of between 8%–10% maximize carbohydrate gastric emptying without substantially reducing fluid delivery. (Adapted from Costill.[48])

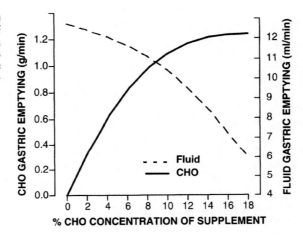

### Timing of Carbohydrate Ingestion

Researchers have found that fatigue can be delayed and performance improved when carbohydrate supplements are provided periodically throughout exercise or when they are ingested 30–40 minutes before the onset of fatigue.[12,13] Therefore, the supplement schedule can vary greatly and still enhance performance. The important consideration is whether the ingested carbohydrate is capable of supplementing the blood glucose stores at a rate of more than $1.0\,g\cdot min^{-1}$ by the time liver and muscle glycogen stores are severely depleted. Under normal conditions, muscle and liver glycogen stores are sufficient for a minimum of 1 hour of moderate-intensity exercise. Therefore, supplements do not necessarily have to be administered immediately upon the start of exercise. If fluid replacement is of concern, however, it may be necessary to start the supplement as soon as possible and consume a diluted carbohydrate supplement periodically throughout the course of the exercise. For example, during hot and humid conditions, consuming 250 mL of a 5% carbohydrate solution every 15 minutes would provide 50 g of carbohydrate and 1000 mL of fluid per hour. Starting supplementation early and continuing throughout exercise is also advisable when the exercise intensity is anticipated to vary considerably or be interrupted by periodic rest periods. Supplementing during this type of exercise has been found to increase the blood glucose and insulin levels and increase muscle glucose uptake, thereby sparing muscle glycogen during the periods of low exercise intensity or increasing its rate of synthesis when muscle fibers are inactive.

### Types of Carbohydrates

Many different types of carbohydrates have been evaluated against glucose for their ergogenic effects. Maltose, sucrose, and maltodextrins are metabolized at rates comparable to glucose. The oxidation rates of starches depend on their composition. Starches consisting of high concentrations of amylopectin are oxidized rapidly, whereas those with high amylose content are oxidized slowly.[47] Fructose and galactose are oxidized much slower than glucose because they must first be converted into glucose by the liver before the skeletal muscle can effectively metabolize them.[60] In addition, fructose is absorbed slowly from the intestines into the blood and when consumed alone in high concentration can cause gastrointestinal discomfort and diarrhea. As discussed previously, however, if a combination of glucose and fructose is ingested, carbohydrate is absorbed into the blood faster and exogenous carbohydrate oxidation rates can exceed $1.2\,g\cdot min^{-1}$.[57] Interestingly, when high amounts of fructose are combined with glucose, gastrointestinal problems are limited.

### Addition of Protein to a Carbohydrate Supplement

Recent research has suggested that adding small amounts of protein to a carbohydrate supplement can increase the effectiveness of the supplement.[61,62] For example, in one study, trained cyclists exercised on three separate occasions at intensities that varied between 45% and 75% $VO_2$ max for 3 hours and then at 85% $VO_2$ max until fatigued. Supplements (200 mL) were provided every 20 minutes and consisted of placebo, a 7.75% carbohydrate solution, and a 7.75% carbohydrate/1.94% protein solution (Figure 27.3). Carbohydrate supplementation significantly increased time to exhaustion, whereas the addition of protein enhanced the effect of the carbohydrate supplement by approximately 35%.[61] The addition of protein to a carbohydrate supplement was also found to enhance aerobic endurance by 30% when trained cyclists rode to exhaustion at 75% $VO_2$ max.[62]

## Supplementation in Support of the Immune System

After intense exercise, the immune system is generally suppressed and its effectiveness to combat pathogens is reduced for up to 72 hours postexercise. This is attributed in part to elevations in plasma cortisol and other stress hormones that suppress immune function. The stress hormones can be modulated

**FIGURE 27.3.** The effect of carbohydrate (CHO) and carbohydrate/protein supplementation during exercise on endurance performance at 85% VO₂ max. The subjects cycled at intensities that alternated between 45%–75% VO₂ max for 180 minutes and then at 85% VO₂ max to fatigue. Liquid supplements (200 mL) were provided every 20 minutes and consisted of placebo, 7.75% carbohydrate, or 7.75% carbohydrate/1.94% protein solution. (Adapted from Ivy et al.[61])

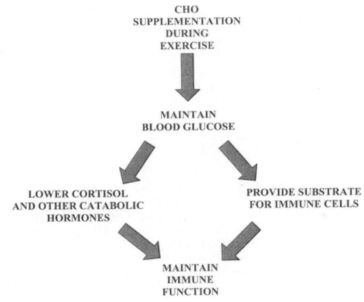

during exercise by controlling glucose availability. Bishop et al.[63] demonstrated that providing a 6% carbohydrate solution during exercise lowered plasma cortisol levels by 80% (Figure 27.4). Nieman et al.[23] has also found that carbohydrate supplementation will lower the cortisol response to exercise and limit immune system suppression. Nieman[64] reported that, aside from a reduced cortisol response, there was less of a reduction in T cells and natural killer cells after carbohydrate supplementation. Furthermore, cytokine response such as interleukin (IL)-6 and IL-1β were lowered with carbohydrate supplementation. Thus, carbohydrate supplementation during exercise has a protective effect on the immune system postexercise, while also maintaining an adequate supply of energy substrate for the immune system during exercise.

Although blood glucose is the primary substrate of the immune cells, providing protein during exercise may also benefit the immune system.[65] Inadequate intake of protein impairs the immune system with particular detrimental effects on the T lymphocytes. Supplementing with antioxidant vitamins, glutamine, zinc, and probiotics, however, have not proven to be immunoprotective.

**FIGURE 27.4.** The effect of carbohydrate (CHO) supplementation on cortisol and the immune system. PRO = protein.

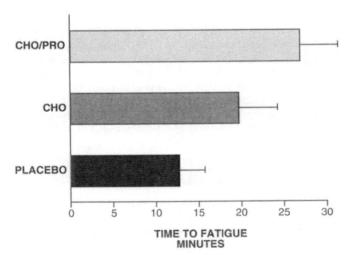

## Sidebar 27.1. Is Caffeine an Effective Ergogenic Aid?

Caffeine has been used by athletes for decades as an ergogenic aid, but its popularity escalated dramatically about 25 years ago when Costill and colleagues reported that caffeine ingestion before exercise could enhance endurance performance. The improvement was thought to be attributable to caffeine's ability to increase fat oxidation and spare the use of muscle glycogen, although it was also noted that caffeine altered perception of effort. In this regard, it is of interest to note that caffeine has been found to increase the concentration of hormone-like substances in the brain called β-endorphins during exercise. The endorphins affect mood, reduce perception of pain, and create a sense of well-being. Caffeine has also been reported to delay fatigue during exercise by blocking adenosine receptors in the brain. Adenosine is produced during exercise and inhibits the release of the brain neurotransmitter dopamine. Decreases in dopamine, along with increases in serotonin, another brain neurotrans-

mitter, have been linked to central nervous system fatigue during exercise. A decrease in the dopamine–serotonin ratio has been shown to reduce arousal, induce sleep, and suppress spontaneous activity of animals.

The concentrations of caffeine found to enhance endurance performance have ranged between 3–13 mg·kg$^{-1}$ body wt. The effect of caffeine on endurance performance does not seem to be compromised by carbohydrate supplementation. Research has shown that caffeine-induced increases in performance are not limited by carbohydrate supplementation before or during exercise, but that they are additive. There is a wide range of individual responses to caffeine, however, with some athletes being very sensitive to the metabolic actions of caffeine and others being insensitive. Moreover, regular users of caffeine often develop a tolerance over time that will minimize any potential impact on performance it might otherwise provide.

## NUTRITION FOR RAPID EXERCISE RECOVERY

### Rehydration

Beginning exercise in a hypohydrated state will significantly limit endurance performance. Efforts should therefore be made to completely rehydrate before the next training session or competition. The opportunities for replacement may be limited, as when several rounds of competition are scheduled on the same day. The ingestion of water after exercise-induced dehydration causes a large decrease in serum osmolality and sodium concentration with a subsequent diuresis. However, if an electrolyte-containing solution is ingested, plasma osmolality is better maintained, diuresis is reduced, and fluid retention increased. As mentioned previously, the decrease in serum osmolality and sodium concentration will also reduce the drive to drink. Therefore, fluid-replacement drinks should contain sodium and possibly other electrolytes lost during exercise. The amount of sodium should be similar to that lost in the sweat. This is between 20–80 mmol·L$^{-1}$. The higher the sodium content, the greater the fluid retention. However, there is little need to consume sodium in excess of 65 mmol·L$^{-1}$ unless trying to hyperhydrate. Potassium should also be considered and its concentration in a fluid-replacement solution should be between 2–6 mmol·L$^{-1}$.

The amount of fluid to consume needs to also be considered. Shirreffs et al.[66] found that after exercise-induced dehydration to about 2% body weight, the amount of diuresis during a 6-hour recovery period was directly related to the volume of fluid consumed. It was also found that whether solutions of low (23 mmol·L$^{-1}$) or high (61 mmol·L$^{-1}$) sodium concentration were used, simply replacing the volume of water loss was not sufficient to restore hydration. Ingesting fluid volumes equal to 150% and 200% of sweat loss of the low-sodium solution was also not quite sufficient for complete rehydration. However, when the 150% and 200% of the high-sodium solution was ingested, enough fluid was retained to result in euhydration after recovery.

### Muscle Glycogen Repletion

The amount of carbohydrate consumed has a significant effect on the rate of glycogen storage after exercise. Unless sufficient carbohydrate is ingested, muscle glycogen will not be normalized on a day-to-day basis if training intensely.[67] In general, with an increase in carbohydrate ingestion, there is an increase in muscle glycogen storage. Costill et al.[68] reported that consuming 150–650 g of carbohydrate per day resulted in a proportionately greater muscle glycogen synthesis during the initial 24 hours after exercise, which amounted to 7–10 g of carbohydrate per kilogram of body weight. Consumption of more than 650 g of carbohydrate per day was of no additional benefit. However, these findings are derived from studies when glycogen storage occurred during passive recovery. Daily carbohydrate requirements therefore may be higher for athletes who train more frequently than once per day, or may be less if their daily training program does not substantially deplete their muscle glycogen stores. Burke et al.[69] recommend consuming 5–7 g carbohydrate·kg$^{-1}$ body wt per day if training duration is moderate and intensity is low, 7–12 g carbohydrate·kg$^{-1}$ body wt per day if training duration is moderate and intensity is high, and 10–12 g carbohydrate·kg$^{-1}$ body wt per day if exercise training is extreme.

Because of the ever-increasing level of competition, many athletes feel the necessity to train more intensely and frequently to remain competitive. Moreover, many athletes may be required to compete in several different contests over subsequent days or even on the same day. Recent research has suggested that for these situations, athletes benefit from the rapid resynthesis of their muscle glycogen stores even when incomplete restoration occurs. Many factors will affect the rate of muscle glycogen storage after exercise. These include the timing of carbohydrate consumption, the amount and frequency of carbohydrate consumption, and the addition of protein to a carbohydrate supplement.

### TIMING OF SUPPLEMENTATION

It has been found that muscle glycogen synthesis is more rapid if carbohydrate is consumed immediately after exercise as opposed to waiting several hours.[70] When carbohydrate is consumed immediately after exercise, the rate of glycogen synthesis averages between 6–8 mmol·kg$^{-1}$ wet wt·h$^{-1}$;[70,71] whereas, if the supplement is delayed several hours, the rate of synthesis is reduced 50%.[70] The increased synthesis immediately postexercise is attributed in part to a faster rate of muscle glucose uptake as a result of an increase in muscle insulin sensitivity.[72,73] With time, however, the increase in insulin sensitivity declines resulting in a slower rate of muscle glucose uptake and glycogen storage.

It should also be pointed out that after exercise that depletes the body's carbohydrate stores, there is little if any increase in muscle glycogen storage until adequate carbohydrate is made available.[70,74,75] Therefore, early intake of carbohydrate after strenuous exercise is essential because it provides an immediate source of substrate to the muscle, while also taking advantage of the increased muscle insulin sensitivity. Furthermore, supplementing immediately after exercise seems to delay the decrease in insulin sensitivity, and with frequent supplementation, a relatively rapid rate of glycogen storage can be maintained for up to 8 hours postexercise.[71,74]

### AMOUNT AND FREQUENCY OF CARBOHYDRATE SUPPLEMENTATION

When provided immediately postexercise, the rate of glycogen storage will decline as glucose availability decreases.[70] However, Blom et al.[71] demonstrated that this decline could be attenuated for up to 8 hours if supplements were continually provided at 2-hour intervals. They also found that supplementing with 0.7 g glucose·kg$^{-1}$ body wt seemed to maximize muscle glycogen storage, as there was no difference found between supplements containing 0.7 and 1.4 g glucose·kg$^{-1}$ body wt. However, subsequent research suggested that when providing carbohydrate supplementation at 2-hour intervals, 1.2–1.4 g of glucose·kg$^{-1}$ body wt (0.6–0.7 g carbohydrate·kg$^{-1}$ body wt·h$^{-1}$) is required to maximize muscle glycogen storage.[70,74]

The rate of glycogen synthesis that is maintained by supplementing at 2-hour intervals, approximately 7 mmol·kg$^{-1}$ wet wt·h$^{-1}$, does not seem to be the highest rate of muscle glycogen synthesis possible. Some studies have found that supplementing at increased frequency can positively influence the rate of synthesis.[76,77]

When carbohydrate supplementation occurs at frequent intervals such as every 15–30 minutes and in high amounts, the rate of muscle glycogen storage has been found to be approximately 30% higher than when supplementing every 2 hours.[76,77] For example, Doyle et al.[76] reported glycogen storage rates of $10\,mmol \cdot kg^{-1}$ wet wt·h$^{-1}$ during the first 4 hours of recovery from exercise when subjects received $1.2\,g \cdot kg^{-1}$ body wt·h$^{-1}$ every 15 minutes. Thus, supplementing at 15- to 30-minute intervals with carbohydrate ($1.2$–$1.6\,g \cdot kg^{-1}$ body wt·h$^{-1}$) may be preferable to supplementing every 2 hours for the rapid restoration of the muscle glycogen stores postexercise.

### ADDITION OF PROTEIN TO A CARBOHYDRATE SUPPLEMENT

Several studies have also documented that the addition of protein to a carbohydrate supplement will enhance the rate of muscle glycogen synthesis.[75,78,79] Zawadzki et al.[75] found that providing a 3:1 carbohydrate/protein supplement at 2-hour intervals increased the rate of glycogen storage by 38%. Controversy arose, however, because the carbohydrate and carbohydrate/protein supplements used were not isocaloric, and subsequent research by others failed to confirm these findings.[80,81] The conflicting results, however, can probably be attributed to differences in experimental design such as the frequency of supplementation and the amount and types of carbohydrate and protein provided. Support for this supposition comes from a recent study comparing carbohydrate supplements of equal carbohydrate content or caloric equivalency when supplementing immediately and 2 hours postexercise.[79] After several hours of intense cycling to deplete the muscle glycogen stores, subjects received a carbohydrate protein (80 g carbohydrate, 28 g protein, 6 g fat), iso-carbohydrate (80 g carbohydrate, 6 g fat), or isocaloric carbohydrate (108 g carbohydrate, 6 g fat) supplement. After 4 hours of recovery, muscle glycogen was 54% and 40% greater for the carbohydrate/protein treatment when compared with the iso-carbohydrate and isocaloric treatments, respectively. Glycogen storage did not differ significantly between the iso-carbohydrate and isocaloric treatments. Of interest was the very large difference in glycogen storage between treatments during the first 40 minutes of recovery. Glycogen storage was twice as fast after the carbohydrate/protein treatment than after the isocaloric treatments, and four times faster than after the iso-carbohydrate treatment. This trend was also noted after the second feeding 2 hours into recovery.

These studies suggest that maximum rates of glycogen storage can be achieved by consuming $1.0$–$1.2\,g$ carbohydrate·h$^{-1}$ at frequent intervals. However, the coingestion of protein with carbohydrate greatly increases the efficiency of muscle glycogen storage when supplementing at intervals greater than 1 hour apart, or when the amount of carbohydrate ingested is below the threshold for maximal glycogen synthesis. These results have important implications for athletes who wish to limit their carbohydrate intake in an effort to control body weight and for those athletes who participate in sports that have very short recovery periods during competition such as basketball, ice hockey, and soccer. The ingestion of protein with carbohydrate also has the added benefit of stimulating muscle protein synthesis and tissue repair.

## Initiating Muscle Protein Synthesis and Limiting Muscle Tissue Damage

During prolonged strenuous exercise there is generally damage to the active muscles and this damage can continue long after exercise because of an acceleration in protein degradation. For complete recovery, it is important to initiate protein synthesis and limit protein degradation as quickly as possible. Similar to glycogen storage, muscle protein synthesis and degradation are affected by the type, amount, and timing of nutrient supplementation. Appropriate supplementation postexercise has been found to limit muscle damage, increase protein synthesis, and increase training adaptation.

### TYPES OF SUPPLEMENTATION AFFECTING PROTEIN SYNTHESIS AND DEGRADATION

Although the muscle can have residual catabolic activity after exercise, it is primed to shift into an anabolic state in the presence of the right nutrients.

This is attributed, in part, to an increase in muscle insulin sensitivity. Insulin increases muscle amino acid uptake and protein synthesis and reduces protein degradation. After exercise, increasing the plasma insulin level is key to limiting muscle damage and stimulating protein accretion.

Roy et al.[82] investigated the effect of carbohydrate supplementation on the fractional rate of protein synthesis after resistance exercise using one leg, with the opposite leg serving as a control. The subjects received 1 g of carbohydrate·kg$^{-1}$ body wt or a placebo immediately after and 1 hour after exercise. Exercise alone did not result in a significant increase in protein synthesis. Carbohydrate supplementation, however, significantly increased the plasma insulin level and increased protein synthesis by 36% in the exercised leg as compared with the nonexercised leg. Furthermore, urinary nitrogen and 3-methlyhistidine were significantly reduced after carbohydrate supplementation, suggesting a reduction in muscle tissue damage and protein degradation.

Supplementation of a mixture of essential amino acids or protein will also increase protein synthesis.[83,84] Increasing the plasma amino acid levels postexercise by infusion or oral supplementation has been reported to transition the muscle from a negative protein balance to a positive protein balance by stimulating protein synthesis.[85] When blood amino acid levels are reduced below normal, amino acids are released from the muscle and protein synthesis declines. Increasing the essential amino acid levels above normal, however, increases muscle amino acid uptake and muscle protein synthesis.[86]

Whereas supplementing with either carbohydrate or protein postexercise may limit muscle damage and stimulate protein synthesis, there is increasing evidence that the combination can have an additive effect.[87–89] For example, Miller et al.[88] found that both the plasma insulin response and protein synthesis rate were highest in response to a carbohydrate/amino acid supplement compared with providing carbohydrate or amino acid supplements separately. The effect of the carbohydrate/amino acid supplement on net muscle protein synthesis was approximately equivalent to the sum of the independent effects of either the carbohydrate or amino acid supplement alone.

The type of protein to consume might also be considered. Boirie et al.[90] found that protein synthesis increased 68% with whey supplementation and 32% with a casein supplement. The anabolic response, however, was longer lasting with casein. Because whey is fast-acting and casein's response more sustained, it might be most beneficial to consume a combination of whey and casein when supplementing postexercise.

## NUTRIENT TIMING ON PROTEIN SYNTHESIS AND DEGRADATION

There are a limited number of studies that have investigated the timing of supplementation on postexercise protein synthesis.[91,92] Levenhagen et al.[92] studied the effects of a carbohydrate/protein supplement on protein synthesis and degradation after a 60-minute moderate-intensity exercise bout of cycling. Subjects were given the supplement immediately or 3 hours after exercise. Protein degradation was unaffected by supplement timing, but leg protein synthesis was increased approximately threefold above basal when supplementation occurred immediately postexercise. No increase in protein synthesis occurred when the supplement was delayed 3 hours, and only when the supplement was immediately provided after exercise was there a positive protein balance (the rate of protein synthesis exceeded the rate of protein degradation). It was also of interest to note that when supplementation occurred immediately compared with 3 hours after exercise, there was a greater muscle glucose uptake and fat oxidation. Levenhagen et al.[92] concluded that ingesting a carbohydrate/protein supplement early after exercise increases protein accretion as well as muscle glycogen storage. Evidence of reduced muscle damage was provided in a recent report by Saunders et al.[62] These investigators found that 15 hours postexercise muscle damage, as determined by blood creatine phosphokinase levels, was significantly attenuated after carbohydrate/protein supplementation compared with carbohydrate supplementation.

## Sidebar 27.2.  Whole Foods or Liquid Supplements—Which Is Better for Exercise Recovery?

There is no debating that a well-balanced diet should be developed around complete, unprocessed whole foods. However, for exercise recovery nutrition, liquid supplements are more practical and often superior nutritionally to whole floods. Nutrient timing is critical for a rapid and complete recovery. In the first 30–45 minutes after exercise there is a metabolic window of opportunity (Figure 27.5). Although the muscle has residual catabolic activity after exercise, it will rapidly shift from a catabolic state to an anabolic state if the right nutrients are ingested soon after exercise. If the appropriate nutrients are not provided, muscle cells will remain in a catabolic state for hours. Once the metabolic window of opportunity has closed, nutrient supplementation will not be nearly as effective in shifting the muscles into an anabolic state resulting in a slow recovery and limited training adaptation. At no other time during the course of the day can nutrition make such a major difference in the overall training program.

Immediately after intense exercise, most individuals find it difficult to eat whole foods. Liquid supplements are palatable, easy to consume, and rapidly digested. They are formulated to provide the nutrients essential for a rapid postexercise recovery, and because liquid supplements are readily digested, they can provide the muscles with these nutrients at the most critical period of recovery. It may take several hours, however, for whole foods to be digested and provide sufficient nutrients that will impact muscle recovery.

Liquid supplements are specifically formulated to provide the appropriate types and amounts of nutrients for a complete recovery. Preparation is minimal and the volume of liquid supplement required for adequate recovery nutrition is far less than if trying to support one's nutritional needs with whole foods.

Nutrients that are essential for a rapid and complete recovery are fast-digesting proteins such as whey, certain amino acids, electrolytes, and high-glycemic carbohydrates in the appropriate ratio. The only way to ensure that these nutrients are present in the right amounts is to formulate a specific liquid blend or buy a commercially available one. Whole foods may miss the mark, providing too much or not enough of a given nutrient.

In addition, consuming a liquid supplement as the postexercise recovery nutrition helps to start the rehydration process. This can be a critical issue if recovery time is limited. Consuming whole foods as the recovery meal will slow gastric emptying and severely delay rehydration.

## Carbohydrate/Protein Supplementation and Immune Response

Recent research suggests that the ingestion of a carbohydrate/protein supplement postexercise can reduce muscle inflammation and positively impact the immune system. Flakoll et al.[93] provided a placebo, carbohydrate, or carbohydrate/protein supplement to U.S. Marine recruits immediately postexercise during 54 days of basic training. Compared with the placebo and carbohydrate groups, the carbohydrate/protein group had 33% fewer total medical visits, 28% fewer visits for bacterial/viral infections, 37% fewer visits for muscle and

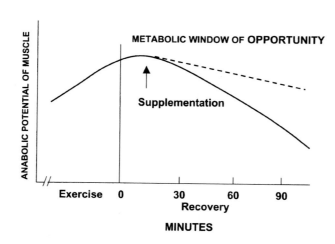

**FIGURE 27.5.** The metabolic window of opportunity is the time after exercise in which the muscle is highly capable of responding to the anabolic effects of insulin if sufficient substrate is made available. Without nutrient intervention, the metabolic window begins to close within 45 minutes after exercise.

joint problems, and 83% for heat exhaustion. Muscle soreness was reduced immediately postexercise by carbohydrate/protein supplementation. The researchers suggested that postexercise supplementation might not only enhance muscle protein accretion, but also have a significant impact on the immune system, muscle and joint soreness, and tissue hydration.

## SUMMARY

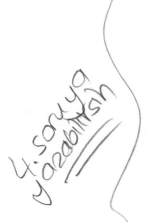

Fatigue during prolonged, endurance exercise is generally a result of hyperthermia caused by dehydration, a low blood glucose concentration, or muscle glycogen depletion. Other factors that may limit performance are muscle soreness and damage, and illness caused by exercise-induced suppression of the immune system. Proper nutrition and nutrient supplementation at the appropriate time can significantly delay the onset of fatigue, improve quality of training and response to training, and limit muscle tissue damage and other physiologic conditions that limit physical performance.

Preparation for competition should start several days before with glycogen loading. If the competition is going to present a thermal stress, it is also recommended that measures be taken to hyperhydrate. In the hours before exercise or competition, nutritional measures should also be taken to assure adequate hydration and muscle glycogen status. These should include consuming an adequate amount of fluid with appropriate electrolytes in the hours before exercise, and consuming several hundred grams of carbohydrate as part of a rehydration drink or a light meal consisting of easily digested carbohydrates. These measures become very important if supplementation is limited or not possible during exercise.

During exercise or competition, fluid replacement should ideally keep pace with fluid loss caused by sweating. Sweat rate can exceed the rate of gastric emptying. Therefore, when exercising in a hot and humid environment, it is important to start drinking as soon as possible. It is also advisable to consume a fluid-replacement drink that contains sodium to protect against hyponatremia. Furthermore, carbohydrate supplementation during exercise has been found to significantly improve endurance performance. The addition of small amounts of protein to a carbohydrate supplement might also be considered because this has recently been found to increase the effectiveness of the supplement and extend time to fatigue during prolonged, endurance exercise.

Nutrition during the immediate hours postexercise is also of importance. Recovery from exercise is a complex process requiring rehydration, replenishment of muscle glycogen stores, the repair of damaged muscle tissue, and the initiation of training adaptations. To initiate these processes effectively requires that the proper nutrients be consumed, and that they be consumed at the appropriate time. Nutrients essential for complete recovery include water, electrolytes, carbohydrate, and protein. In general, the sooner these nutrients can be ingested after exercise, the more effective they will be in promoting a rapid and full recovery.

## PRACTICAL APPLICATIONS

- In preparation for competition, athletes should strive to fully hydrate. Full hydration requires that fluids containing moderate concentrations of sodium be ingested regularly starting several days before competition.
- Athletes should also try and maximize their muscle glycogen stores. This can be accomplished during the training taper by consuming 7–10 g carbohydrates·kg$^{-1}$ body wt daily.
- In the immediate hours before competition, it is recommended that 500–1000 mL of fluid be ingested. It may also be beneficial to consume 200–300 g of carbohydrate if supplementation during exercise is limited or not possible.
- During exercise, athletes should try to fully replace fluid losses that occur, although during hot and humid conditions this may not be possible.

- It is best to consume small volumes of fluid frequently (150–250 mL every 15 minutes) rather than consuming high volumes of fluid occasionally (400 mL every 30 minutes).
- Electrolyte replacement should also be considered. Most sports drinks are formulated to adequately replace electrolyte losses caused by sweating.
- To maximize endurance performance, 45–60 g·h$^{-1}$ of carbohydrate should be ingested during exercise. Carbohydrate solutions should not exceed 10% if maintaining hydration is of consequence.
- Carbohydrate supplementation can be delayed until about 30–40 minutes before the onset of fatigue and still be effective. However, if fluid replacement is of concern, it is recommended that supplementation with a dilute carbohydrate solution start as soon as possible and continue periodically throughout exercise.
- The addition of small amounts of protein to a carbohydrate supplement may also increase the effectiveness of the supplement.
- For rapid rehydration after exercise, it is important to start fluid consumption early and replace at least 150% of the fluid lost during exercise with a dilute sodium solution.
- Requirements for the daily recovery of muscle glycogen will depend on the exercise intensity and duration. If the training duration is moderate and the intensity low, 5–7 g of carbohydrate·kg$^{-1}$ body wt per day should be consumed. If the training duration is moderate and the intensity is high, 7–12 g carbohydrate·kg$^{-1}$ body wt per day should be consumed, and if the training is extreme (4–6 hours per day) 10–12 g carbohydrate·kg$^{-1}$ body wt per day should be consumed.
- If there is only limited time to replenish the muscle glycogen stores, 1.0–1.2 g carbohydrate·kg$^{-1}$ body wt·h$^{-1}$ should be consumed at frequent intervals starting within the first 30 minutes postexercise.
- The addition of protein to the carbohydrate supplement will promote additional glycogen storage when carbohydrate intake is suboptimal or when frequent supplementation is not possible.
- Postexercise supplements composed of carbohydrate and protein have the added benefit of limiting muscle tissue damage, stimulating protein accretion, and protecting the immune system from exercise-induced immune suppression.

## QUESTIONS

1. Which of the following solutions has been shown to restore complete hydration after an exercise-induced dehydration of 2% body weight?
   a. A 23 mmol·L$^{-1}$ low-sodium fluid that replaces the volume of water loss
   b. A 61 mmol·L$^{-1}$ high-sodium fluid that replaces the volume of water loss
   c. A 23 mmol·L$^{-1}$ low-sodium fluid that replaces a volume equal to 150%–200% of sweat loss
   d. A 61 mmol·L$^{-1}$ high-sodium fluid that replaces a volume equal to 150%–200% of sweat loss

2. What is the daily carbohydrate requirement for an elite athlete who trains multiple times per day at an extreme intensity?
   a. 5–7 g carbohydrate·kg$^{-1}$ body wt
   b. 7–12 g carbohydrate·kg$^{-1}$ body wt
   c. 10–12 g carbohydrate·kg$^{-1}$ body wt
   d. Just a normal mixed diet will suffice

3. An increased glycogen synthesis rate immediately postexercise is attributable to:
   a. Increased muscle insulin sensitivity
   b. Low blood glucagon levels
   c. Increased glucose availability
   d. Both a and c

4. What is the main benefit of adding protein to a postexercise carbohydrate supplement?
   a. Increases blood glucose
   b. Decreases insulin sensitivity
   c. Increases glycogen synthesis
   d. Adds more calories to the supplement

5. Studies have shown that carbohydrate supplementation improves performance during prolonged continuous exercise. The latest a supplement can be taken to enhance performance is:
   a. At the onset of exercise
   b. During the first 30 minutes of exercise
   c. 30 minutes before the onset of fatigue
   d. At the start of fatigue

6. The maximum rate of gastric emptying is approximately:
   a. $500\,mL\cdot h^{-1}$
   b. $1200\,mL\cdot h^{-1}$
   c. $2400\,mL\cdot h^{-1}$
   d. $3000\,mL\cdot h^{-1}$

7. Which factor will influence the rate of gastric emptying of a solution?
   a. Concentration of carbohydrate
   b. Sweat rate
   c. Flavor of solution
   d. Taste

8. All are characteristics of fructose except:
   a. Fructose must be converted into glucose by the liver
   b. High amounts of fructose can cause gastrointestinal discomfort and diarrhea
   c. Compared with glucose, fructose is absorbed slowly from the intestines into the blood
   d. All of the above

9. An athlete weighs 150 lbs. before exercise. After exercise, he weighs 144 lbs. How much body fluid did he lose and what are the possible consequences of this loss?
   a. 4% of body fluid, stress only on cardiovascular system, limiting performance
   b. 6% of body fluid, rapid increase in body temperature followed by heat stroke
   c. 4% of body fluid, stress on cardiovascular system and possibly heat cramps and heat exhaustion
   d. 2% of body fluid, stress on cardiovascular system, limiting performance

10. An athlete running at 80% of $VO_2$ max for 2 hours expends 1600 kcal. Carbohydrates contribute ____ kcal of the energy expended, with muscle glycogen contributing approximately ____% of the carbohydrate requirements.
    a. 800, 85
    b. 1120, 50
    c. 1360, 70
    d. 1120, 85

11. Muscle damage as a result of exercise:
    a. May be beneficial because mild muscle damage stimulates the rebuilding process
    b. Can occur as a result of the physical forces acting on the muscle
    c. Results in stiffness and soreness, reducing performance
    d. All of the above

12. Cortisol during high-intensity exercise is released from the adrenal glands resulting in:
    a. Activation of many of the important immune cells that fight infection
    b. Generation of fuel for working muscle by activating gluconeogenesis, lipolysis, and proteolysis

    c. Results in muscle damage
    d. a and b
    e. b and c

13. Normal plasma sodium concentrations will range between:
    a. 130 and 155 mmol·L$^{-1}$
    b. 20 and 80 mmol·L$^{-1}$
    d. 96 and 110 mmol·L$^{-1}$
    e. 20 and 60 mmol·L$^{-1}$

14. Addition of which of the following to fluid ingested during prolonged endurance exercise in severe climatic conditions is most important for preventing the adverse effects of dehydration?
    a. Sodium
    b. Magnesium
    c. Calcium
    d. Vitamin C

15. An endurance athlete attempting to prevent dehydration during exercise would be advised to ingest fluid at what rate?
    a. 1 mL·min$^{-1}$
    b. 10 mL·min$^{-1}$
    c. 1000 mL·h$^{-1}$
    d. 2 L·h$^{-1}$

16. An individual's rate of fluid loss during aerobic exercise is most influenced by:
    a. Gender, climate, and age
    b. Exercise intensity and climate
    c. Climate and gender
    d. Age and weight

17. Which of the following combinations of exercise and supplementation is most likely to result in a temporary suppression of immune system function?
    a. 30-minute walk without carbohydrate supplementation
    b. 30-minute walk with carbohydrate supplementation
    c. Marathon with carbohydrate supplementation
    d. Marathon without carbohydrate supplementation

18. A carbohydrate/protein supplement provided immediately after a 60-minute, moderate-intensity exercise bout leads to:
    a. Increase in protein degradation with no change in protein synthesis
    b. Decrease in protein degradation with no change in protein synthesis
    c. No change in protein degradation and an increase in protein synthesis
    d. No change in protein degradation or in protein synthesis

19. Supplementation with a mixture of essential amino acids or protein post-exercise will result in:
    a. Release of amino acids from the muscle
    b. Increase in muscle protein synthesis
    c. Decrease in muscle glucose uptake
    d. No change in muscle protein synthesis

20. Which fluid supplement would be the best to consume during a prolonged run in hot and humid conditions?
    a. 250 mL of a 5% carbohydrate solution consumed every 15 minutes
    b. 150 mL of a 10% carbohydrate solution consumed every 15 minutes
    c. 1000 mL of a 5% solution consumed after the first hour of the run
    d. All the supplements will be equally as effective

21. For each liter of water that evaporates on the skin, how many kilocalories of heat are dissipated from the body?
    a. 320 kcal
    b. 580 kcal
    c. 1000 kcal
    d. 2000 kcal

22. The ergogenic effect of carbohydrate supplementation during exercise is in part attributable to the maintenance of carbohydrate availability for muscle energy substrate.
   a. True
   b. False

23. Drinking water after exercise-induced dehydration is associated with a decrease in serum osmolality and subsequent loss of thirst.
   a. True
   b. False

24. Ingesting carbohydrates every 15–30 minutes after exercise may be better for promoting muscle glycogen resynthesis than every 2 hours.
   a. True
   b. False

25. Muscle contraction, particularly the eccentric phase, places great stress on the muscles which can result in muscle damage.
   a. True
   b. False

26. About 100 g of glycogen is normally stored in the muscles.
   a. True
   b. False

27. Sensations of thirst do not provide an endurance athlete with an effective means of monitoring hydration status during prolonged exercise.
   a. True
   b. False

28. The functioning of the immune system is often enhanced temporarily after a bout of intense exercise.
   a. True
   b. False

29. Carbohydrate supplementation during prolonged endurance exercise will increase plasma cortisol and suppress immune function temporarily.
   a. True
   b. False

30. Muscle catabolic activity can be limited after exercise by increasing plasma insulin levels.
   a. True
   b. False

31. To promote muscle protein synthesis, provision of a carbohydrate/protein supplement 3 hours after a prolonged exercise is as effective as supplementing within the first 15 minutes postexercise.
   a. True
   b. False

32. Hyperhydration is an effective strategy for thermal regulation during exercise even when euhydration can be maintained.
   a. True
   b. False

33. Sports drinks that have a high sodium content will quench thirst faster than water.
   a. True
   b. False

## ACKNOWLEDGMENTS

John L. Ivy is Chair and Margie Gurley Seay Centennial Professor in the Department of Kinesiology and Health Education at the University of Texas at Austin. He is also a member of the Scientific Advisory Board for Experimental and Applied Sciences, Inc. and a consultant for Pacific Health Laboratories, Inc.

# REFERENCES

1. Coyle EF, Montain SJ. Benefits of fluid replacement with carbohydrate during exercise. Med Sci Sports Exerc 1992;24:S324–330.
2. Coyle EF, Montain SJ. Carbohydrate and fluid ingestion during exercise: are there trade-offs? Med Sci Sports Exerc 1992;24:671–678.
3. Gonzalez-Alonso J, Teller C, Andersen SL, Jensen FB, Hyldig T, Nielse B. Influence of body temperature on the development of fatigue during prolonged exercise in the heat. J Appl Physiol 1999;86:1032–1039.
4. Armstrong LE, Costill DL, Fink WJ. Influence of diuretic-induced dehydration on competitive running performance. Med Sci Sports Exerc 1985;17:456–461.
5. Craig EN, Cummings EG. Dehydration and muscular work. J Appl Physiol 1966; 21:670–674.
6. Maughan RJ. Fluid and electrolyte loss and replacement in exercise. J Sports Sci 1991;9:117–147.
7. Sutton JR, Bar-Or O. Thermal illness in fun running. Am Heart J 1980;100: 778–781.
8. Björkman O, Wahren J. Glucose homeostasis during and after exercise. In: Horton ES, Terjung RL, eds. Exercise, Nutrition, and Energy Metabolism. New York: Macmillan; 1988:80–89.
9. Saltin B, Karlsson J. Muscle glycogen utilization during work of different intensities. In: Pernow P, Saltin B, eds. Muscle Metabolism During Exercise. New York: Plenum Press; 1971:289–297.
10. Romijin JA, Colye EF, Sidossis LS, et al. Regulation of endogenous fat and carbohydrate metabolism in relation to exercise intensity and duration. Am J Physiol 1993;265:E380–E391.
11. Coyle EF, Coggan AR, Hemmert MK, Ivy JL. Muscle glycogen utilization during prolonged strenuous exercise when fed carbohydrate. J Appl Physiol 1986;61: 165–172.
12. Coggan AR, Coyle EF. Reversal of fatigue during prolonged exercise by carbohydrate ingestion late in exercise. J Appl Physiol 1987;63:2388–2395.
13. Coggan AR, Coyle EF. Metabolism and performance following carbohydrate ingestion late in exercise. Med Sci Sports Exerc 1989;21:59–65.
14. Saltin B, Gollnick PD. Fuel for muscular exercise: role of carbohydrate. In: Horton ES, Terjung RL, eds. Exercise, Nutrition, and Energy Metabolism. New York: Macmillan; 1988:45–53.
15. Bergström J, Hermansen L, Hultman E, Saltin B. Diet, muscle glycogen and physical performance. Acta Physiol Scand 1967;71:140–150.
16. Hermansen L, Hultman E, Saltin B. Muscle glycogen during prolonged severe exercise. Acta Physiol Scand 1967;71:129–139.
17. Carter JM, Jeukendrup AE, Jones DA. The effect of carbohydrate mouth rinse on 1-h cycle time trial performance. Med Sci Sports Exerc 2004;36:2107–2111.
18. Clarkson PM, Hubal MJ. Exercise-induced muscle damage in humans. Am J Phys Med Rehabil 2002;81(Suppl 11):S52–69.
19. Evans WJ. Effects of exercise on senescent muscle. Clin Orthop 2002;403(Suppl): S211–220.
20. Pedersen BK, Bruunsgaard H, Kolkker M, et al. Exercise-induced immunomodulation: possible roles of neuroendocrine and metabolic factors. Int J Sports Med 1997;18(Suppl 1):S2–7.
21. Tidball JG. Inflammatory processes in muscle injury and repair. Am J Physiol 2005;288:R345–353.
22. Peake J, Suzuki K. Neutrophil activation, antioxidant supplements and exercise-induced oxidative stress. Exerc Immunol Rev 2004;10:129–141.
23. Nieman DC, Johanssen LM, Lee JW, Arabatzis K. Infectious episodes in runners before and after the Los Angeles Marathon. J Sports Med Phys Fitness 1990;30: 316–328.
24. Shinkai S, Watanabe S, Asai H, Shek PN. Cortisol response to exercise and post-exercise suppression of blood lymphocyte subset counts. Int J Sports Med 1996; 17:597–603.
25. Berk LS, Nieman DC, Youngberg WS, et al. The effect of long endurance running on natural killer cells in marathoners. Med Sci Sports Exerc 1990;22:207–212.
26. Lakier Smith L. Overtraining, excessive exercise, and altered immunity: is this a T helper-1 versus T helper-2 lymphocyte response? Sports Med 2003;33:347–364.
27. Moroff SV, Bass DE. Effects of overhydration on man's physiological responses to work in the heat. J Appl Physiol 1965;20:267–270.
28. Neilsen B. Effects of changes in plasma volume and osmolarity on thermoregulation during exercise. Act Physiol Scand 1974;90:725–730.

29. Greenleaf JE, Castle BL. Exercise temperature regulation in man during hypohydration and hyperhydration. J Appl Physiol 1971;30:847–853.

30. Nadel ER, Fortney SM, Wenger CB. Effect of hydration state on circulatory and thermal regulations. J Appl Physiol 1980;49:715–721.

31. Fortney SM, Wenger CB, Bove JR, Nadel ER. Effect of hyperosmolality on control of blood flow and sweating. J Appl Physiol 1984;29:1688–1695.

32. Ahlborg B, Bergström J, Ekelund LG, Hultman E. Muscle glycogen and muscle electrolytes during prolonged physical exercise. Acta Physiol Scand 1967;70:129–142.

33. Sherman WM, Costill DL, Fink WJ, Miller JM. Effect of exercise-diet manipulation on muscle glycogen and its subsequent utilization during performance. Int J Sports Med 1981;2:114–118.

34. Hargreaves M, McConell GM, Proietto J. Influence of muscle glycogen on glycogenolysis and glucose uptake during exercise. J Appl Physiol 1995;78:288–292.

35. Walker JL, Heigenhauser GJ, Hultman E, Spriet LL. Dietary carbohydrate, muscle glycogen content, and endurance performance in well-trained women. J Appl Physiol 2000;88:2151–2158.

36. Fairchild TJ, Flectcher S, Steele P, Goodman C, Dawson B, Fournier PA. Rapid carbohydrate loading after a short bout of near maximal-intensity exercise. Med Sci Sports Exerc 2002;34:980–986.

37. Bussau VA, Fairchild TJ, Rao A, Steele P, Fournier PA. Carbohydrate loading in human muscle: an improved 1 day protocol. Eur J Appl Physiol 2002;87:290–295.

38. Coyle EF, Coggan AR, Hemmert MK, Lowe RC, Walters TJ. Substrate usage during prolonged exercise following a preexercise meal. J Appl Physiol 1985;59:429–433.

39. Chryssanthopoulos C, Williams C, Wilson W, Asher L, Hearne L. Comparison between carbohydrate feedings before and during exercise on running performance during a 30-km treadmill time trial. Int J Sport Nutr 1994;4:374–386.

40. Casey A, Mann R, Banister K, Fox J, Morris PG, MacDonald IA, Greenhaff PL. Effect of carbohydrate ingestion on glycogen resynthesis in human liver and skeletal muscle, measured by 13C MRS. Am J Physiol 2000;278:E65–75.

41. Chryssanthopoulos C, Williams C. Pre-exercise carbohydrate meal and endurance capacity when carbohydrates are ingested during exercise. Int J Sports Med 1997;18:543–548.

42. Marmy-Conus N, Fabris S, Proietto J, Hargreaves M. Preexercise glucose ingestion and glucose kinetics during exercise. J Appl Physiol 1996;81:853–857.

43. Costill DL, Coyle E, Dalsky G, Evans W, Fink W, Hoopes D. Effects of elevated plasma FFA and insulin on muscle glycogen usage during exercise. J Appl Physiol 1977;43:695–699.

44. Hargreaves M, Costill DL, Katz A, Fink WJ. Effect of fructose ingestion on muscle glycogen usage during exercise. Med Sci Sports Exerc 1985;17:360–363.

45. Foster C, Costill DL, Fink WJ. Effects of pre-exercise feedings on endurance performance. Med Sci Sports 1979;11:1–5.

46. Hargreaves M, Costill DL, Fink WJ, King DS, Fielding RA. Effect of pre-exercise carbohydrate feedings on endurance cycling performance. Med Sci Sports Exerc 1987;19:33–36.

47. Goodpaster BH, Costill DL, Fink WJ, et al. The effects of pre-exercise starch ingestion on endurance performance. Int J Sport Med 1996;17:366–372.

48. Costill DL. Gastric emptying of fluids during exercise. In: Gisolfi CV, Lamb DR, eds. Fluid Homeostasis During Exercise (Perspectives in Exercise Science and Sports Medicine). Vol 3. Indianapolis: Benchmark Press; 1990:97–121.

49. Wilk B, Bar-Or O. Effect of drink flavor and NaCl on voluntary drinking and hydration in boys exercising in the heat. J Appl Physiol 1996;80:1112–1117.

50. Coyle EF. Fluid and fuel intake during exercise. J Sport Sci 2004;22:39–55.

51. Dill DB, Edwards HT, Talbott JH. Studies in muscular activity. VII. Factors limiting the capacity to work. J Physiol (Lond) 1932;77:49–55.

52. Yaspelkis BB, Patterson JG, Anderla PA, Ding Z, Ivy JL. Carbohydrate supplementation spares muscle glycogen during variable-intensity exercise. J Appl Physiol 1993;75:1477–1485.

53. Hargreaves M, Costill DL, Coggan AR, Fink WJ, Nishibata I. Effect of carbohydrate feedings on muscle glycogen utilization and exercise performance. Med Sci Sports Exerc 1984;16:219–222.

54. Below P, Mora-Rodriguez R, Gonzalez-Alonso J, Coyle EF. Fluid and carbohydrate ingestion independently improve performance during 1 h of intense exercise. Med Sci Sports Exerc 1995;27:200–210.

55. Leatt PB, Jacobs I. Effect of glucose polymer ingestion on glycogen depletion during a soccer match. Can J Sports Sci 1989;14:112–116.

56. Tsintzas OK, Williams C, Boobis L, Greenhaff P. Carbohydrate ingestion and glycogen utilization in different muscle fibre types in man. J Physiol 1995;489:243–250.

57. Jeukendrup AE. Carbohydrate intake during exercise and performance. Nutrition 2004;20:669–677.

58. Hunt JN, Smith JL, Jiang CL. Effect of meal volume and energy density on the gastric emptying of carbohydrate. Gastroenterology 1985;89:1326–1330.

59. Noakes TD, Myburgh KH, Du Plessia J, et al. Metabolic rate, not percent dehydration, predicts rectal temperature in marathon runners. Med Sci Sports Exerc 1991;23:443–449.

60. Cori CF. The fate of sugar in the animal body. III. The rate of glycogen formation in the liver of normal and insulinized rats during the absorption of glucose, fructose, and galactose. J Biol Chem 1926;70:577–584.

61. Ivy JL, Res PT, Sprague RC, Widzer MO. Effect of a carbohydrate-protein supplement on endurance performance during exercise of varying intensity. Int J Sport Nutr Exerc Metab 2003;13:382–395.

62. Saunders MJ, Kane MD, Todd MK. Effects of a carbohydrate-protein beverage on cycling endurance and muscle damage. Med Sci Sports Exerc 2004;36:1233–1238.

63. Bishop NC, Blannin AK, Rand L, Johnson R, Gleeson M. Effects of carbohydrate and fluid intake on the blood leukocyte responses to prolonged exercise. J Sports Sci 1999;17:26–27.

64. Nieman DC. Nutrition, exercise, and immune system function. In: Wheeler KB, Lombardo JA, eds. Clinics in Sports Medicine: Nutritional Aspects of Exercise. Vol 18. Philadelphia: WB Saunders; 1999:537–538.

65. Bassit RA, Sawada LA, Bacurau RFP, et al. Branched-chain amino acid supplementation and immune response of long-distance athletes. Nutrition 2002;18:376–379.

66. Shirreffs SM, Taylor AJ, Leiper JB, Maughan RJ. Post-exercise rehydration in man: effects of volume consumed and drink sodium content. Med Sci Sports Exerc 1996;28:1260–1271.

67. Costill DL, Bowers R, Branam G, Sparks K. Muscle glycogen utilization during prolonged exercise on successive days. J Appl Physiol 1971;31:834–838.

68. Costill DL, Sherman WM, Fink WJ, Maresh C, Witten M, Miller J. The role of dietary carbohydrate in muscle glycogen resynthesis after strenuous running. Am J Clin Nutr 1981;34:1831–1836.

69. Burke LM, Kiens B, Ivy JL. Carbohydrate and fat for training and recovery. J Sport Sci 2004;22:15–30.

70. Ivy JL, Katz AL, Cutler CL, Sherman WM, Coyle EF. Muscle glycogen synthesis after exercise: effect of time of carbohydrate ingestion. J Appl Physiol 1988;64:1480–1485.

71. Blom PCS, Høstmark AT, Vaage O, Kardel KR, Mæhlum, S. Effect of different post-exercise sugar diets on the rate of muscle glycogen synthesis. Med Sci Sports Exerc 1987;19:491–496.

72. Garetto LP, Richter EA, Goodman MN, Ruderman NB. Enhanced muscle glucose metabolism after exercise in the rat: the two phases. Am J Physiol 1984;246:E471–475.

73. Richter EA, Garetto LP, Goodman MN, Ruderman NB. Enhanced muscle glucose metabolism after exercise: modulation by local factors. Am J Physiol 1984;246:E476–482.

74. Ivy JL, Lee MC, Brozinick JT, Reed MJ. Muscle glycogen storage after different amounts of carbohydrate ingestion. J Appl Physiol 1988;65:2018–2023.

75. Zawadzki KM, Yaspelkis BB III, Ivy JL. Carbohydrate-protein complex increases the rate of muscle glycogen storage after exercise. J Appl Physiol 1992;72:1854–1859.

76. Doyle JA, Sherman WM, Strauss RL. Effects of eccentric and concentric exercise on muscle glycogen replenishment. J Appl Physiol 1993;74:1848–1855.

77. van Hall G, Shirreffs SM, Calbet JAL. Muscle glycogen resynthesis during recovery from cycle exercise: no effect of additional protein ingestion. J Appl Physiol 2000;88:1631–1636.

78. van Loon LJ, Saris WH, Kruijshoop M, Wagenmakers AJ. Maximizing postexercise muscle glycogen synthesis: carbohydrate supplementation and the application of amino acid or protein hydrolysate mixtures. Am J Clin Nutr 2000;72:106–111.

79. Ivy JL, Goforth HW, Damon BD, McCauley TR, Parsons EC, Price TB. Early postexercise muscle glycogen recovery is enhanced with a carbohydrate-protein supplement. J Appl Physiol 2002;93:1337–1344.

80. Carrithers JA, Williamson DL, Gallagher PM, Godard MP, Schulze KE, Trappe SW. Effects of postexercise carbohydrate-protein feedings on muscle glycogen restoration. J Appl Physiol 2000;88:1976–1982.

81. Jentjents RLPG, van Loon LJC, Mann CH, Wagenmakers AJM, Jeukendrup AE. Addition of protein and amino acids to carbohydrates does not enhance postexercise muscle glycogen synthesis. J Appl Physiol 2001;91:839–846.

82. Roy BD, Tarnopolsky MA, MacDougall JD, Fowles J, Yarasheski KE. Effect of glucose supplement timing on protein metabolism after resistance training. J Appl Physiol 1997;82:1882–1888.

83. Biolo G, Tipton KD, Klein S, Wolfe RR. An abundant supply of amino acids enhances the metabolic effect of exercise on muscle protein. Am J Physiol 1997;273:E122–129.

84. Tipton KD, Ferrando AA, Phillips SM, Doyle D Jr, Wolfe RR. Postexercise net protein synthesis in human muscle from orally administered amino acids. Am J Physiol 1999;276:E628–634.

85. Rasmussen BB, Tipton KD, Miller SL, Wolf SE, Wolfe RR. An oral essential amino acid-carbohydrate supplement enhances muscle protein anabolism after resistance exercise. J Appl Physiol 2000;88:386–393.

86. Wolfe RR. Effects of amino acid intake on anabolic processes. Can J Appl Physiol 2001;26(Suppl):S220–227.

87. Suzuki M, Doi T, Lee SJ, et al. Effect of meal timing after resistance exercise on hind limb muscle mass and fat accumulation in trained rats. J Nutr Sci Vitaminol 1999;45:401–409.

88. Miller SL, Tipton KD, Chinkes DL, Wolf SE, Wolfe RR. Independent and combined effects of amino acids and glucose after resistance exercise. Med Sci Sports Exerc 2003;35:449–455.

89. Levenhagen DK, Carr C, Carlson MG, Maron DJ, Borel MJ, Flakoll PJ. Postexercise protein intake enhances whole-body and leg protein accretion in humans. Med Sci Sports Exerc 2002;34: 828–837.

90. Boirie Y, Dangin M, Gachon P, Vasson MP, Maubois JL, Beaufrere B. Slow and fast dietary proteins differently modulate postprandial protein accretion. Proc Natl Acad Sci USA 1997;94:14930–14935.

91. Okamura K, Doi T, Hamada K, et al. Effect of amino acid and glucose administration during postexercise recovery on protein kinetics in dogs. Am J Physiol 1997;272: E1023–1030.

92. Levenhagen DK, Gresham JD, Carlson MG, Maron DL, Borel MJ, Flakoll PJ. Postexercise nutrient intake timing in humans is critical to recovery of leg glucose and protein homeostasis. Am J Physiol 2001;280:E982–E993.

93. Flakoll PJ, Judy T, Flinn K, Carr C, Flinn S. Postexercise protein supplementation improves health and muscle soreness during basic military training in Marine recruits. J Appl Physiol 2004;96:951–956.

# Nutrition Before, During, and After Exercise for the Strength/Power Athlete

## Christopher J. Rasmussen

## OBJECTIVES

On the completion of this chapter you will be able to:

1. Understand the physiologic effects of strength/power training and how they relate to nutritional interventions.
2. Discuss the importance of preexercise nutrition.
3. Outline a preexercise nutrition intervention that targets the specific needs of the strength/power athlete.
4. Provide a rationale for a nutrition intervention strategy that is used during a bout of strength/power training.
5. Recommend a nutrition intervention that can be used during training by strength/power athletes.
6. Appreciate the importance of postexercise nutrition.
7. Formulate a postexercise intervention that targets the specific needs of a strength/power athlete.

## ABSTRACT

Proper training, maintaining a positive energy balance, adhering to proper nutrient timing, and obtaining adequate rest and recovery form the foundation for optimal performance. Therefore, this chapter begins with a description of factors associated with optimal performance of the strength/power athlete. Section two focuses on preexercise nutrition and how it can prepare the athlete for action and enhance the training response whereas section three addresses the nutritional importance in delaying fatigue. The next section addresses the importance of postexercise nutrition and how it can aid in recovery and prepare the athlete for subsequent exercise sessions, and the final section provides training and nutritional recommendations that serve as the foundation for a successful strength/power athlete.

*Key Words:* **glycemic index, amino acids, protein, carbohydrate, soy, casein, whey, anabolic, catabolic**

The strength/power athlete has special nutritional needs that go above and beyond those of the normal sedentary individual. To optimize performance, the strength/power athlete needs a solid foundation that includes proper training and nutrition. Proper training should be based on the principles of training and largely depends on the goals of the individual athlete and the point in time within the training cycle (preseason, in-season, postseason). Proper nutrition should focus on a variety of whole foods that adequately meet the demands of

From: *Essentials of Sports Nutrition and Supplements*
Edited by J. Antonio, D. Kalman, J. R. Stout, M. Greenwood, D. S. Willoughby, and G. G. Haff © Humana Press, a part of Springer Science+Business Media, Totowa, NJ

the athlete. In addition, supplementing the diet with additional nutrients is becoming increasingly important for those engaged in heavy training because oftentimes it is difficult to obtain the proper amount of macronutrients through whole foods alone. This chapter largely addresses the specific nutritional needs of the strength/power athlete before, during, and after exercise. Several studies have documented that strength/power athletes can improve their training sessions and performance with a combination of both proper everyday nutrition and supplementation.[1-3]

Proper nutrition can prepare the athlete for intense exercise, provide the energy for muscular contractions, help reduce postexercise muscle damage, and enhance recovery in anticipation of the next workout. The effectiveness of these processes is largely based on the types of macronutrients selected and the timing of their ingestion. It has been well established that there are preferred types of macronutrients that aid this process based on their quality and speed of digestion. Ingesting the proper nutrients can make a distinct difference on performance and training sessions.

To gain a better understanding of how proper nutrition can improve performance for the strength/power athlete, it is important to realize what drives their performance. This chapter thus begins with a description of the factors associated with optimal performance of the strength/power athlete. The second section focuses on preexercise nutrition and how it can prepare the athlete for action and enhance the training response. The third section discusses nutrition during exercise and its importance in delaying fatigue. The fourth section dives into postexercise nutrition and how it can aid in recovery and prepare the athlete for subsequent exercise sessions. Finally, a brief summary reviews the most important points and brings the chapter to a close.

## FACTORS ASSOCIATED WITH OPTIMAL PERFORMANCE OF THE STRENGTH/POWER ATHLETE

The mode of exercise most often utilized by the strength/power athlete to improve strength, power, and thus overall performance is resistance training. Varieties of resistance training such as power lifting, Olympic lifting, and traditional bodybuilding are utilized depending on the goals of the individual athlete. Manipulating the principles of training depending on objectives while coinciding with the respective training season will help optimize training and subsequent performance. Actin and myosin are the two major types of muscle protein and during contraction these two proteins slide back and forth over each other. Building muscle is a result of increasing the amount of actin and myosin in the muscles. Muscle fibers thus increase in diameter, get stronger and more powerful. Adenosine triphosphate (ATP) molecules provide the needed energy for these muscle fibers during a resistance-training workout. The breakdown of ATP into adenosine diphosphate drives muscle contraction. However, there is only enough ATP stored in the muscle for a few seconds of intense effort. ATP thus has to be rapidly and continuously replenished in order to continue with subsequent muscle contractions.

Creatine phosphate (CP) and muscle glycogen are the primary sources used for rapid repletion of ATP during an intense resistance-training workout. CP levels within the muscle are also limited and can be depleted after 10–15 seconds of maximal intensity effort. The rapid restoration of ATP and CP involves the anaerobic breakdown of muscle glycogen known as glycolysis. Most strength/power athletes do not realize how much muscle glycogen is used during a typical training session. One set of 10 biceps curls can result in a 12% loss of muscle glycogen, 3 sets can result in 35% depletion, and 6 sets can result in 40% depletion.[4] The benefits of habitual resistance training are endless and include enhanced glucose control, increased metabolic rate, decreased body fat percentage, increased strength, and increased bone mineral density.

Resistance training is not without its damaging effects. Intense resistance training, especially the eccentric phase, essentially causes microscopic tears in muscle fibers leading to muscle damage.[5,6] Delayed onset muscle soreness can set in at least 24 hours after a workout because of the subsequent inflammatory response to the intense training bout.[7] The body responds to the training by making bigger and stronger muscle fibers in order to sustain future demands. In addition to the microscopic tears, the catabolic hormone cortisol is released from the adrenal cortex during high-intensity exercise such as resistance training. Cortisol is the most potent glucocorticoid produced by the adrenal cortex and is a major stress hormone that acts to supply the exercising muscles with fuel through gluconeogenesis, lipolysis, and even proteolysis. The breakdown of body protein can also contribute to muscle damage and eventual muscle soreness.[7]

To combat the damaging and depleting effects of intense resistance training and further help the body respond to training, a well-planned diet that meets energy-intake needs and incorporates proper timing of essential nutrients is vital. Athletes that do not consume enough calories and/or do not consume enough of the right type of macronutrients may hinder training adaptations and subsequent performance. However, athletes who consume a well-planned diet during training can help the body adapt to training and will likely notice improved performance. Furthermore, maintaining a diet that is deficient of the essential macronutrients over time may lead to a loss of body mass, muscle mass, an increased susceptibility to illness, and an increase in the symptoms associated with overtraining. Practicing good dietary habits day after day is essential to help optimize training adaptations and subsequent performance. The following sections discuss nutritional strategies before, during, and after exercise for the strength/power athlete.

## Sidebar 28.1. What Do Sleep and Stress Have to Do with Training and Nutrition?

A combination of training and nutrition is essential for those athletes striving for optimal performance. Although nutrition is the primary focus of this review, the principles of training (i.e., overload, progression, specificity, rest/recovery, etc.) should not be forgotten. The principle of rest/recovery is one that is often overlooked by the strength/power athlete. This principle often goes hand in hand with the amount of sleep the athlete gets. To make the most of the nutrients ingested, proper rest/recovery must be recognized or a decrease in performance is likely to follow. A lack of sleep can impair energy levels and thus adversely affect training. Sleep deprivation can even affect the body's ability to metabolize glucose and has been shown to negatively affect leptin and grehlin levels leading to weight gain.

The persistent drive to get ahead in today's society in combination with the classic type A personality is largely to blame for the lack of sleep. Nearly a quarter of the adult population is sleep deprived getting an average of only 6 hours of sleep per night (8–9 hours is recommended). Tips to enhance sleep and thus the rest/recovery process include maintaining a regular exercise program; limiting alcohol, nicotine, and caffeine before bed; maintaining a regular sleep/wake schedule; and avoiding emotional stress.

Although the human stress response was designed as a survival mechanism to combat physical stressors, we rarely use it in that context in today's society. The cascade of catabolic hormones, specifically cortisol, that follow a stress response are more often left to wreak havoc on our physiologic systems and thus impair possible gains in training. This is especially true if the stressor is of the psychointrapersonal type and lingers for prolonged periods. It is for this reason that different types of relaxation and sleep therapy are now entering the realm of common stress-management programs hoping to decrease the negative effects these catabolic hormones can have on the body, including those in training.

## PREEXERCISE NUTRITION FOR THE STRENGTH/POWER ATHLETE

Preexercise nutrition should consist largely of moderate to low glycemic index (GI) foods/supplements that provide a slow, sustained release of carbohydrates and protein necessary to fuel a workout. It generally takes about 4 hours for dietary carbohydrate to be digested and begin to be stored as muscle and liver glycogen. Thus, preexercise meals should be consumed about 4–6 hours before exercise.[8] Putting this into an average everyday scenario means that if an athlete trains in the afternoon, breakfast is the most important meal to top off muscle and liver glycogen levels. If the athlete trains first thing in the morning, the meal the evening before is vital. The choice of foods/supplements selected is largely up to the individual athlete and their personal preferences. It is recommended that the strength/power athlete consume something familiar on the day of competition as opposed to experimenting with a new food/supplement.

## Sidebar 28.2. What Is the Glycemic Index?

The GI is a ranking of foods based on their actual postprandial blood glucose response compared with a reference food, either glucose or white bread. The GI concept was first developed in 1981 to help determine which foods were best for people with diabetes. The GI of a food is based on several factors including the physical form of the food, the amylose-to-amylopectin ratio (two different types of starch), sugar content, fiber content, fat content, and the acidity of a food. The index consists of a scale from 0 to 100 with 0 (water) representing the lowest ranking and 100 (pure glucose) the highest ranking. The GI is obtained through the use of an oral glucose tolerance test using 50 g of carbohydrate from the test food. Subsequent blood draws are taken periodically throughout a 2-hour time period, glucose levels are measured, and the area under the curve is calculated.

The GI of a carbohydrate has a profound effect on subsequent glucose and insulin responses. The high GI carbohydrates, i.e., dextrose and maltose, produce large increases in glucose and insulin levels. The moderate GI carbohydrates, i.e., sucrose and lactose, traditionally produce only modest increases in glucose and insulin. And finally, the low GI carbohydrates, i.e., fructose and maltodextrin (depending on the individual length of the glucose chain) have very little if any effect on glucose and insulin responses. It has been suggested that manipulating the GI of a sports supplement may optimize carbohydrate availability for exercise, particularly prolonged, intense exercise.

Caution should be used when applying the GI to whole foods that contain several ingredients. The GI is more accurate for individually packed foods/supplements because of the fewer number of ingredients and the standardization that exists with the processing of these snacks/supplements. The GI is not as applicable to whole foods/meals and has not been established for many of these whole foods/meals (Table 28.1).

Recent research has indicated that ingesting a light carbohydrate and protein snack 30–60 minutes before exercise (e.g., 50 g of carbohydrate and 5–10 g of protein) serves to further increase carbohydrate availability toward the end of an intense exercise bout because of the slight increase in glucose and insulin levels.[9,10] This can serve to increase the availability of amino acids and decrease exercise-induced protein catabolism.[9-11] Insulin inhibits protein degradation and apparently offsets the catabolic effects of other hormones, namely cortisol.[12] Anabolic actions of insulin seem to be related to its nitrogen-sparing effects and promotion of nitrogen retention.[12] In addition, resistance training in combination with immediate amino acid administration has been shown to augment protein synthesis acutely.[13,14] One would thus expect more pronounced muscle hypertrophy over a prolonged period.

A limited number of investigators have administered a carbohydrate–protein supplement before a strength/power workout. Tipton et al.,[15] put six subjects through two random trials to determine whether an oral essential amino acid–carbohydrate (EAC) supplement would be a more effective stimulator of muscle protein anabolism if given immediately before or immediately after an ~45-minute lower-body resistance-exercise bout. Ingestion of EAC changed net muscle protein balance from negative values, i.e., net release, to positive net uptake, in both trials. However, the total response to the consumption of EAC immediately before exercise was greater than the response when EAC was consumed immediately after exercise. Total net phenylalanine uptake, an indicator of muscle protein synthesis, across the leg over 3 hours was greater when the supplement was administered before as opposed to when the supplement was administered after exercise. Furthermore, the authors concluded that the change from a catabolic state in the muscle to an anabolic state seemed to be primarily attributable to an increase in muscle protein synthesis. This was likely the result of an elevated blood flow during exercise which maximizes delivery to the muscle. This study demonstrated that the acute effects of protein supplementation on muscle anabolism are even greater if protein is ingested before the training bout.

**TABLE 28.1. Partial list of the glycemic index (GI) of foods using glucose as the standard.**

| Low GI | | Moderate GI | | High GI | |
|---|---|---|---|---|---|
| Food | GI | Food | GI | Food | GI |
| Chana dal | 8 | Apple juice | 40 | Life Savers™ | 70 |
| Peanuts | 14 | Snickers™ | 41 | White bread | 70 |
| Plain yogurt | 14 | Peach | 42 | Bagel | 72 |
| Soy beans | 18 | Pudding | 43 | Watermelon | 72 |
| Rice bran | 19 | Pinto beans | 45 | Graham crackers | 74 |
| Peas | 22 | Orange juice | 46 | French fries | 75 |
| Cherries | 22 | Baked beans | 48 | Total™ | 76 |
| Barley | 25 | Strawberry jam | 51 | Vanilla wafers | 77 |
| Grapefruit | 25 | Sweat potato | 54 | Gatorade™ | 78 |
| Kidney beans | 27 | Pound cake | 54 | Fava beans | 79 |
| Link sausages | 28 | Popcorn | 55 | Jelly beans | 80 |
| Black beans | 30 | Brown rice | 55 | Tapioca pudding | 81 |
| Lentils | 30 | Fruit cocktail | 55 | Rice cakes | 82 |
| Butter beans | 31 | Pita bread | 57 | Team Flakes™ | 82 |
| Soy milk | 31 | PowerBar™ | 58 | Pretzels | 83 |
| Lima beans | 32 | Honey | 58 | Corn Chex™ | 83 |
| Skim milk | 32 | Blueberry muffin | 59 | Corn flakes™ | 84 |
| Split peas | 32 | Shredded wheat | 62 | Baked white potato | 85 |
| Fettucini | 32 | Black bean soup | 64 | Mashed potatoes | 86 |
| Chickpeas | 33 | Macaroni & cheese | 64 | Dark rye | 86 |
| Peanut M&Ms™ | 33 | Raisins | 64 | Instant rice | 87 |
| Chocolate milk | 34 | Cantaloupe | 65 | Crispix™ | 87 |
| Vermicelli | 35 | Mars Bar™ | 65 | Boiled Sebago | 87 |
| Whole wheat spaghetti | 37 | Rye bread | 65 | Rice Chex™ | 89 |
| Apple | 38 | Pineapple | 66 | Gluten-free bread | 90 |
| Pear | 38 | Grapenuts™ | 67 | Baked red potato | 93 |
| Tomato soup | 38 | Angel food cake | 67 | French baguette | 95 |
| Ravioli | 39 | Stoned wheat thins | 67 | Peeled Desiree | 101 |
| Pinto beans | 39 | Taco shells | 68 | Dates | 103 |
| Plums | 39 | Whole wheat bread | 69 | Tofu frozen dessert | 115 |

In another study, Andersen et al.[16] studied 22 males throughout a 14-week lower-body weight-training regime combined with timed ingestion of isoenergetic protein versus carbohydrate supplementation on muscle fiber hypertrophy and mechanical muscle performance. Supplementation was administered before and immediately after each training bout and, in addition, in the morning on nontraining days. Muscle biopsy specimens were obtained from the vastus lateralis muscle pre/post and analyzed for muscle fiber cross-sectional area (fCSA). After 14 weeks of resistance training, the protein group showed hypertrophy of type I and type II muscle fibers, whereas no change above baseline occurred in the carbohydrate group (Figure 28.1). Squat jump height increased

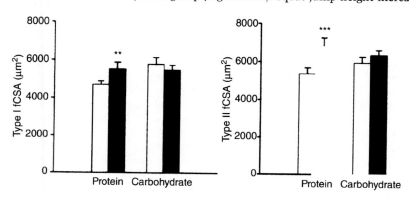

**FIGURE 28.1.** Fiber cross-sectional area (fCSA) of type I (left) and type II (right) muscle fibers at pretraining (open bars) and posttraining (filled bars). Only the protein group increased muscle fCSA in response to resistance training. Asterisks indicate significant difference from pretraining values: **$p < 0.01$; ***$p < 0.001$.

only in the protein group, whereas countermovement jump height and peak torque during slow isokinetic muscle contraction increased similarly in both groups. Thus, resistance training combined with protein supplementation resulted in 18% and 26% increased type I and type II muscle fCSA, respectively, over a prolonged training period. The authors concluded that the underlying metabolic explanation for muscle fiber hypertrophy is that protein synthesis is stimulated to a rate that exceeds muscle protein breakdown.

These two studies demonstrate both the acute and long-term benefits of carbohydrate/protein administration before exercise. Theoretically, a combination of amino acids, to increase amino acid availability, and carbohydrates, to stimulate insulin release, should prove to be a potent stimulator of net muscle protein synthesis.[17] Moreover, an acute strength/power exercise session increases muscle protein synthesis more than breakdown, so that net muscle protein balance (synthesis minus breakdown) is increased.[18-20] Combining all of these factors should thus lead to an optimal environment in which to train and foster increases in performance.

## NUTRITION DURING EXERCISE FOR THE STRENGTH/POWER ATHLETE

Nutrition during an intense resistance-training session can aid in the quality of the workout, especially if the workout exceeds 60–90 minutes. Nutrition during exercise for the strength/power athlete usually centers on supplementation more so that pre- and postexercise nutrition if for no other reason than the convenience supplements provide. Convenience supplements include meal replacement powders, ready to drink supplements, energy bars, energy gels, and fitness waters. They are typically fortified with differing amounts of vitamins and minerals and differ on the amount of carbohydrate, protein, and fat they contain. The beneficial effects of solid and liquid carbohydrate/protein supplements are similar when thermal stress is not a factor. Liquid supplements do provide the added benefits of aiding rehydration and tend to digest easier for most athletes while exercising. Rapid nutrient availability is especially important during a workout in order to maintain energy levels and training intensity. Thus, high GI sources should make up the majority of supplements ingested during a strength/power workout. The athlete should experiment with different formulations to find the one that works best for them before competition.

The three macronutrients all have the potential to provide calories to drive muscular contraction. However, the body prefers to burn carbohydrate during exercise and depending on the exercise intensity and duration will burn carbohydrate at a very quick rate during a strength/power exercise session. At low exercise intensities, the energy needed is provided mostly by the oxidation of plasma fatty acids.[21] As exercise intensity increases, plasma fatty acid turnover does not increase and the additional energy is obtained by the utilization of muscle glycogen, blood glucose, and intramuscular triglyceride. Further increases in exercise intensity are fueled mostly by increases in muscle glycogen utilization with some additional increase in blood glucose oxidation.[21] Recently, glycogenolysis has been demonstrated to be an important energy supplier during high-intensity, intermittent exercises, such as resistance training.[22] Resistance training that centers on higher repetition schemes (8–12 repetitions) and moderate loads may have an even greater effect on muscle glycogen concentration than those of lower repetition schemes.[22]

Fluids and electrolytes can be lost especially in hot and humid conditions. When a resistance-training session lasts more than 1 hour, the strength/power athlete should ingest a glucose/electrolyte solution in order to maintain blood glucose levels, spare muscle glycogen, help prevent dehydration, and reduce the immunosuppressive effects of intense exercise.[8,23-28] Many athletes do not replenish fluids and carbohydrates at a fast enough rate during exercise for a couple of reasons. A lack of accessibility, a personal preference, and the gastrointestinal discomfort that nutrient ingestion can cause during exercise can discourage supplementation while exercising. In addition, intense training often suppresses appetite and/or alters hunger patterns so that many athletes do not feel like eating.[29] However, supplementation during a strength/power exercise session can have a profound effect on performance, especially if the workout is longer than 60 minutes. Sucrose, starches, and maltodextrins, when taken separately or in combination, seem to have similar effects on performance and exhibit similar metabolic effects to glucose.[30–32] It is recommended that fructose be avoided. Fructose is absorbed from the intestines half as fast as glucose and fructose produces a lower blood glucose and insulin response than glucose.[33,34] When large concentrations of fructose are consumed during exercise, this can result in gastrointestinal discomfort, diarrhea, and an inadequate rate of glucose availability.

It is now well established that with prolonged continuous exercise, time to fatigue at moderate, submaximal exercise intensities is related to preexercise muscle glycogen concentrations, thus the importance of everyday nutrition along with preexercise nutrition.[35] In addition, a glucose/electrolyte solution has been the recommended supplement of choice for decades during exercise in order to preserve muscle glycogen and maintain blood glucose levels. With short-term, high-intensity exercise, the relation between the availability of muscle glycogen and performance is less clear. One study that utilized 15 high-intensity, 6-second bouts on a cycle ergometer concluded that a higher-carbohydrate regimen over 48 hours helped subjects maintain a higher power output compared with the exercise and dietary regimen that included the low-carbohydrate content.[36] This study demonstrated the importance of a high-carbohydrate diet in relation to short-term, high-intensity exercise.

However, Haub et al.[37] found that carbohydrate ingestion after maximal exercise does not seem to influence subsequent short-duration, maximal-effort exercise in competitive cyclists. Significant changes between treatments for plasma glucose did exist as the levels significantly decreased during a 60-minute recovery for the placebo group. The lack of performance difference supports the rationale that results gained from the investigations using moderately trained subjects[38] and non–sport-specific protocols[39] cannot be generalized to competitive athletes. The authors concluded that trained cyclists are likely to rely on factors other than the bioavailability of circulating fuels to influence subsequent short-duration, high-intensity exercise, such as changes in the central nervous system.[40]

Although the mode of exercise most frequently studied in relation to carbohydrate supplementation is aerobic in nature, Haff et al.[41] examined the effects of carbohydrate supplementation on muscle glycogen and resistance exercise using eight resistance-trained males. The exercise bout consisted of an initial isokinetic leg exercise before and after a lower-body, isotonic-resistance exercise session lasting ~39 minutes. Subjects consumed a carbohydrate (CHO) or placebo (PLC) treatment before and every 10 minutes during the isotonic resistance (IRT) exercise session. Muscle tissue was obtained from the vastus lateralis after a supine rest immediately after the initial isokinetic test (post-ISO) and immediately after the IRT (post-IRT). The CHO treatment elicited significantly less muscle glycogen degradation from the post-ISO to post-IRT compared with PLC (Figure 28.2). Although the results indicated no enhancement in the performance of the isokinetic leg exercise, the consumption of a CHO beverage did attenuate the decrease in muscle glycogen associated with isotonic resistance exercise. Furthermore, the authors concluded that because typical resistance exercise is intermittent in nature, the consumption of a carbohydrate beverage may inhibit muscle glycogenolysis and or result in some glycogen synthesis occurring during the rest intervals. This inhibition of glycogenolysis probably results from the elevation of insulin that occurs in response to the increased availability of glucose as a substrate when there is an exogenous consumption of a carbohydrate beverage. In addition, the lack of performance enhancement could be attributed to the performance test selected. It is also possible that attenuation of muscle glycogen may result in an enhanced performance of resistance exercise even when no performance gains are noted with an isokinetic test.[41]

Recent research has also shown that the addition of protein can have added benefits to a supplement ingested during exercise by reducing muscle protein degradation and speeding postexercise recovery. Carbohydrate and protein intake significantly alters circulating metabolites and the hormonal milieu (i.e., insulin, testosterone, growth hormone, and cortisol), as well as the response

**FIGURE 28.2.** Muscle glycogen response to carbohydrate and placebo treatments (mean + SEM). Open bars = carbohydrate (CHO); filled bars = placebo (PLC). *Significant difference between resting and post-isokinetic test (ISO) (p < 0.01). #Significant difference between post-ISO and post-isotonic resistance (IRT) (p < 0.01). +Significant difference between CHO and PLC (p < 0.01).

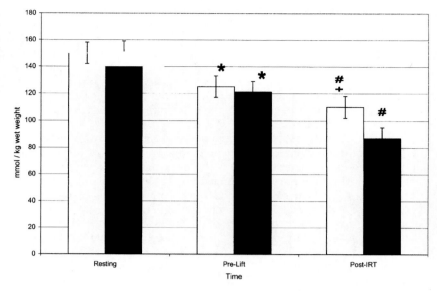

of muscle protein and glycogen balance.[42] Furthermore, the addition of protein to a carbohydrate supplement will enhance the insulin response of a carbohydrate supplement compared with a placebo[43] which can ultimately lead to performance gains.[44]

Saunders et al.[45] examined the effects of a carbohydrate–protein beverage on cycling endurance and muscle damage. Fifteen male cyclists were randomly administered either a carbohydrate or carbohydrate–protein beverage (4 : 1 ratio) every 15 minutes during exercise and immediately upon completion of a ride to volitional exhaustion. The carbohydrate–protein beverage produced significant improvements in time to fatigue and reductions in muscle damage in the selected endurance athletes. The authors concluded that the benefits observed were either the result of a higher total caloric content of the carbohydrate–protein beverage or of specific protein-mediated mechanisms. Controversy exists with numerous studies examining the addition of protein because the addition of protein increases the total caloric content of the supplement. Anytime a greater amount of calories is consumed, the athlete is likely to perform and recover quicker. Thus, careful consideration should be followed when examining studies that are not isocaloric.

Whey is the preferred protein to ingest during exercise because of its rapid absorption rates and the fact that it contains all of the essential amino acids as well as a high percentage of leucine and glutamine, which are two amino acids that the body uses during sustained exercise.[46] High GI carbohydrates (glucose, sucrose, and maltodextrin) should be combined with the protein in a 4 : 1 ratio to provide optimal benefits. Table 28.2 gives an example of the ideal nutrient composition for a sports drink during exercise.[47] A sports drink such as that shown in Table 28.2 should be ingested every 20 minutes during a strength/power training session to help improve performance and reduce muscle protein breakdown.

**TABLE 28.2. Ideal nutrient composition for a sports drink during exercise.**

| Nutrient objectives | Ideal composition (per 12 oz. water) |
| --- | --- |
| • Replace fluids and electrolytes<br>• Preserve muscle glycogen<br>• Maintain blood glucose levels<br>• Minimize cortisol increases<br>• Set the stage for a faster recovery | • High-glycemic carbohydrates, such as glucose, sucrose, and maltodextrin: 20–26 g<br>• Whey protein: 5–6 g<br>• Vitamin C: 30–120 g<br>• Vitamin E: 20–60 IU<br>• Sodium: 100–250 mg<br>• Potassium: 60–120 mg<br>• Magnesium: 60–120 mg |

# Sidebar 28.3. Which "Whey" to Go?

Protein is an essential macronutrient for the strength/power athlete before, during, and after exercise. It is easy to get confused amid the constant waves of information available today on the different types of proteins, especially whey, casein, and soy. There are two main components of milk protein: 1) whey and 2) casein protein. Whey is a byproduct of hard cheese manufacture and has greater similarities with human milk than either soy or casein. Casein protein is the predominant protein found in cow's milk making up approximately 80% of the protein whereas the remaining 20% is whey protein. Whey and casein are the two most popular types of protein found in supplements today.

When protein is removed from defatted soy flakes from the soybean the result is soy protein isolates, the most highly refined soy protein. Soy protein can be incorporated into foods although it has been reported to impart a bean-like flavor, and can give a gritty texture to drinks and a powdery texture to foods. In contrast, casein and whey have comparatively bland tastes and can easily be incorporated into foods. When used in nutrition bars, casein typically provides a softer texture than whey. However, whey's greater solubility makes it ideal for instant mixing drinks.

Whey protein's versatility is driving its use in a wide spectrum of foods and beverages, from nutrition bars, snacks, and sauces to frozen novelties and beverages. In addition to being highly versatile, whey protein is a nutritionally dense ingredient that may deliver significant health and nutritional benefits. The functional characteristics of whey protein also make it an ideal ingredient for postworkout nutritional supplements. Its faster digestion relative to casein and soy results in faster rates of protein synthesis for the first 3–4 hours after ingestion (Table 28.3). The high concentration of branched-chain amino acids may be of even greater importance during exercise. Whey protein has even been shown to produce greater satiety than the slower-digesting casein. The duration of the satiety response ultimately determines how long after eating the athlete desires the next snack or meal. This could have weight-control applications for those wishing to lose weight.

## POSTEXERCISE NUTRITION FOR THE STRENGTH/POWER ATHLETE

Postexercise nutrition for the strength/power athlete is vital to restore muscle glycogen stores, enhance skeletal muscle fiber repair and growth, and maintain overall health and wellness. This is especially important for those athletes engaging in prolonged training or competition sessions on the same or

**TABLE 28.3. Typical amino acid composition of whey, casein, and soy isolates.**

| Amino acid | Whey | Casein | Soy |
|---|---|---|---|
| Alanine | 4.6 | 2.7 | 3.8 |
| Arginine | 2.3 | 3.7 | 6.7 |
| Aspartic acid | 9.6 | 6.4 | 10.2 |
| Cysteine/cystine | 2.8 | 0.3 | 1.1 |
| Glutamic acid | 15.0 | 20.2 | 16.8 |
| Glycine | 1.5 | 2.4 | 3.7 |
| Histidine* | 1.6 | 2.8 | 2.3 |
| Isoleucine*† | 4.5 | 5.5 | 4.3 |
| Leucine*† | 11.6 | 8.3 | 7.2 |
| Lysine* | 9.1 | 7.4 | 5.5 |
| Methionine* | 2.2 | 2.5 | 1.1 |
| Phenylalanine* | 3.1 | 4.5 | 4.6 |
| Proline | 4.4 | 10.2 | 4.5 |
| Serine | 3.3 | 5.7 | 4.6 |
| Threonine* | 4.3 | 4.4 | 3.3 |
| Tryptophan* | 2.3 | 1.1 | 1.1 |
| Tyrosine | 3.3 | 5.7 | 3.3 |
| Valine*† | 4.5 | 6.5 | 4.5 |

*Note:* Values are expressed per 100 g of product.

*Essential amino acid.

†Branched-chain amino acid.

successive days. Multiple training sessions on the same day have now become the norm more than the exception for the elite strength/power athlete because of the ever-increasing level of competition and pressure to perform at optimal levels. An example could be a bodybuilder working one muscle group in the morning and an opposing muscle group that evening. In addition, athletes involved with team sports (e.g., football, basketball, and soccer) that hold multiple practices throughout the day and week are especially susceptible to nutrient deficiencies and performance decrements if proper postexercise nutrition is not followed. Although it is unlikely that muscle glycogen stores can be completely resynthesized within a few hours by nutritional supplementation alone, it would behoove all athletes to maximize the rate of muscle glycogen storage postexercise. This will ultimately result in faster recovery from training, thus possibly allowing for a greater training volume.[22]

After an intense exercise bout, the body is in a catabolic state and thus key muscle nutrients are being broken down. However, the opportunity exists to alter the catabolic state into a more anabolic hormonal profile in which the athlete actually begins to rebuild muscle and thus initiate a much faster recovery. Exercise that results in glycogen depletion will activate glycogen synthase, the enzyme responsible for controlling the transfer of glucose from UDP-glucose to an amylase chain.[48,49] This also happens to be the rate-limiting step of glycogen formation. The degree of glycogen synthase activation is influenced by the extent of glycogen depletion.[48] The complete resynthesis of muscle glycogen, however, is ultimately dependent on adequate carbohydrate intake.

Carbohydrates composed of glucose or glucose polymers are the most effective for replenishment of muscle glycogen, whereas fructose is most beneficial for the replenishment of liver glycogen.[50,51] Glucose and fructose are metabolized differently. They have different gastric emptying rates and are absorbed into the blood at different rates.[49,52] Furthermore, the insulin response to a glucose supplement is generally much greater than that of a fructose supplement.[53] The fact that approximately 79% and 14% of total carbohydrate is stored in skeletal muscle and the liver, respectively, is further indication of the importance of consuming glucose or glucose polymers postexercise.[8]

Blom et al.[54] found that ingestion of glucose and sucrose was twice as effective as fructose for restoration of muscle glycogen. The maximal stimulatory effect of oral glucose intake on postexercise muscle glycogen synthesis was reached at a dose of 0.70 g/kg taken every second hour after exercise in which the muscle glycogen concentration was reduced by an average of 80%. In addition, the rate of postexercise muscle glycogen synthesis increases with increasing oral glucose intake, up to a maximum rate of approximately 6 mmol/kg/hour. They indicated that the differences between glucose and fructose supplementation were the result of the way the body metabolized these sugars. Fructose metabolism takes place predominantly in the liver whereas the majority of glucose seems to bypass the liver and be stored or oxidized by the muscle.[51]

Subsequent research by Burke and associates[55] found that the intake of high GI carbohydrate foods after prolonged exercise produces significantly greater glycogen storage than consumption of low GI carbohydrate foods 24 hours postexercise. Although the meal immediately after exercise elicited exaggerated blood glucose and plasma insulin responses that were similar for the low GI and high GI meals, for the remainder of the 24 hours, the low GI meals elicited lower glucose and insulin responses than the high GI meals.[55]

Costill et al.[56] reported that a diet of simple carbohydrates (glucose/fructose/sucrose) was as effective in restoring muscle glycogen levels 24 hours after exercise depletion as a diet based on "starch" or complex carbohydrate foods. However, after 48 hours, the complex carbohydrate diet resulted in greater muscle glycogen gains than the simple carbohydrate diet. It can be theorized that simple carbohydrate foods (high GI) are absorbed quickly and may be useful as an immediate substrate in the early stages of glycogen restoration.[55–57] They tend to be less useful in the later stages when they may be stored as fat rather than glycogen. Complex carbohydrate foods (low GI) are absorbed slower and thus are more valuable during the latter stages of glycogen storage.[55–57] The underlying theme is that one should not wait to take full advantage of the postexercise window of opportunity. Figure 28.3 clearly shows this to be

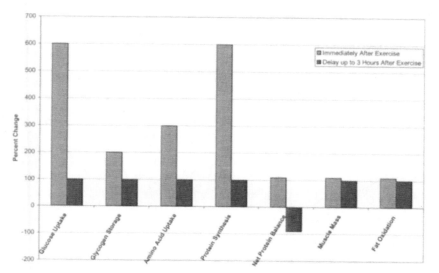

**FIGURE 28.3.** An illustration of the effect of nutrient delay on muscle anabolic processes. A delay in nutrient supplementation of up to 3 hours can dramatically decrease important anabolic activities including glycogen storage and protein balance. (Adapted from Chandler et al.[1])

the case. This chart summarizes the effects of delayed nutrient supplementation on muscle anabolic activities. As is clearly shown, nearly every important anabolic process is reduced after 3 hours.

Although several studies have focused on carbohydrate administration after exercise, less is known concerning the timing of postexercise nutrient supplementation and protein homeostasis. Levenhagen et al.[58] decided to examine how the timing of postexercise nutrient ingestion affects whole-body and leg protein dynamics in healthy adults. They studied 10 subjects twice with the same oral supplement (10 g protein, 8 g carbohydrate, 3 g fat) being administered either immediately (early) or 3 hours after (late) 60 minutes of moderate-intensity exercise. Whether taken immediately or 3 hours after exercise, consumption of this supplement resulted in similar plasma glucose and insulin concentrations in the plasma for the 3 hours after ingestion. Although the substrate and hormonal milieu were similar whether the supplement was given immediately or 3 hours after exercise, the leg uptake of glucose and amino acids was greater when the supplement was given immediately after exercise. More substrate and energy were thus available within the leg for protein synthesis. Even though leg proteolysis was not significantly different between the two treatments, leg protein synthesis was increased more than threefold for early versus late. In other words, there was a net accretion of leg protein when nutrients were ingested early in contrast to the net loss of leg protein when nutrients were given late.

The addition of protein to the postexercise supplement or snack has been shown to have additive effects to that of carbohydrate alone in regard to muscle glycogen resynthesis. The addition of protein to a carbohydrate supplement increases insulin levels greater than that produced by carbohydrate or protein alone.[59] Tarnopolsky et al.[60] showed that postexercise carbohydrate and carbohydrate-protein-fat nutritional supplements can increase glycogen resynthesis in the first 4 hours after exercise to a greater extent than placebo for both men and women. The supplements administered were both isoenergetic and isonitrogenous. Insulin has been demonstrated to have profound anabolic effects on skeletal muscle. In the resting state, insulin has been demonstrated to decrease the rate of muscle protein degradation.[61]

To further test the anabolic effects of a postexercise supplement, Borsheim et al.[62] studied the effects of a protein, amino acid (AA) and carbohydrate (CHO) (PAAC) mixture compared with an isoenergetic CHO placebo (CON) on net muscle protein synthesis after resistance exercise. In addition, the authors wanted to see if the stimulatory effect of the PAAC would last beyond the first hour after intake. Eight subjects participated in two trials in which they ingested the PAAC or CON 1 hour after a resistance exercise bout. The net protein balance response to the PAAC consisted of two components, one rapid, immediate response, and a smaller, delayed response about 90 minutes after the drink. In contrast, the CON only elicited a small, delayed response. After resistance exercise, the PAAC stimulated muscle protein synthesis to a greater extent than isoenergetic CON alone. The addition of protein to an AA + CHO mixture seemed to extend the anabolic effect.

Additional support of the anabolic properties of adding protein to a postexercise supplement was demonstrated again by Levenhagen et al.,[63] who studied five men and five women throughout a 30-minute basal, a 60-minute exercise (bicycle at 60% maximal oxygen uptake), and a 180-minute recovery period. An oral supplement was administered immediately after exercise in random order: NO = 0, 0, 0; SUPP = 0, 8, 3; or SUPP + PRO = 10, 8, 3 g of protein, carbohydrate, and lipid, respectively. SUPP + PRO increased plasma essential amino acids 33%, leg fractional extraction of phenylalanine fourfold, leg uptake of glucose 3.5-fold, and leg and whole-body protein synthesis sixfold and 15%, respectively. The authors concluded that although these data support the hypothesis that postexercise leg muscle protein synthesis is limited by the availability of amino acids, they do not support the hypothesis that energy availability per se controls postexercise muscle protein synthesis. Therefore, amino acid availability seems to be more limiting than energy for muscle protein synthesis after exercise.

A strength/power exercise session can have a profound effect on muscle growth only if muscle protein synthesis exceeds muscle protein breakdown. The exercise can improve muscle protein balance but in the absence of food intake, the balance remains negative inducing a catabolic state.[17] The response of muscle protein metabolism to a strength/power exercise session lasts for 24–48 hours. Amino acid availability is an important regulator of muscle protein metabolism. The interaction of postexercise metabolic processes and increased amino acid availability maximize the stimulation of muscle protein synthesis and results in even greater muscle anabolism than when dietary amino acids are not present.[17,64] Thus, athletes should consume carbohydrate and protein foods/supplements (e.g., 1 g/kg of carbohydrate and 0.5 g/kg of protein) within 30 minutes after exercise as well as consume a high-carbohydrate meal within 2 hours after exercise.[11,65,66]

To summarize, in addition to the macronutrients selected, the timing of nutrient ingestion can impact recovery. Research has clearly shown that muscle glycogen resynthesis occurs more quickly if carbohydrate is consumed immediately after exercise as opposed to waiting for several hours.[67] Whereas the majority of the everyday diet for the strength/power athlete should be a low to moderate GI diet, the postexercise diet should be centered on moderate to high GI sources. This nutritional approach has been found to accelerate glycogen resynthesis as well as promote a more anabolic hormonal state that may speed recovery.[60,68,69] The increased protein and glycogen synthesis is believed to be the result of insulin secretion from the pancreas combined with an increase in muscle insulin sensitivity.[70,71] This was shown in a study (Figure 28.4) showing

**FIGURE 28.4.** The effect of protein and carbohydrate alone and in combination on protein synthesis after exercise. (Adapted from Tarnopolsky et al.[60])

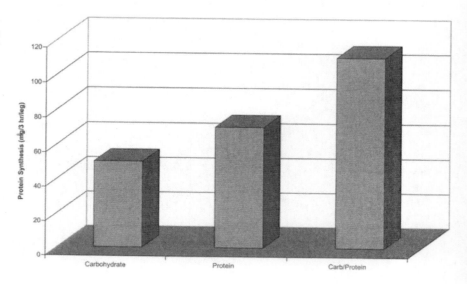

a carbohydrate/protein combination was 38% more effective in stimulating protein synthesis than a protein supplement and more than twice as effective as a carbohydrate supplement.[72] Insulin seems to stimulate biosynthetic pathways that lead to increased glucose utilization, increased carbohydrate and fat storage, and increased protein synthesis. This metabolic pattern is characteristic of the absorptive state. The increase in insulin secretion during this state is responsible for shifting metabolic pathways to net anabolism.[8] In contrast, when insulin secretion is low, the opposite effect occurs. The rate of glucose entry into the cells is reduced and net catabolism rather than net synthesis of glycogen, triglycerides, and protein occurs. This pattern is reminiscent of the postabsorptive state.[73]

Finally, Flakoll et al.[74] provided a placebo, carbohydrate, or carbohydrate/protein supplement to U.S. Marine recruits immediately postexercise during 54 days of basic training to test the long-term impact of postexercise carbohydrate/protein supplementation on variables such as health, muscle soreness, and function. Compared with the placebo and carbohydrate groups, the combined carbohydrate/protein group had 33% fewer total medical visits, 28% fewer visits as a result of bacterial/viral infections, 37% fewer visits because of muscle and joint problems, and 83% because of heat exhaustion. Muscle soreness was also reduced immediately postexercise by the carbohydrate/protein supplement. The authors further postulated that postexercise carbohydrate/protein supplementation may not only enhance muscle protein deposition but also has significant potential to positively impact health, muscle soreness, and tissue hydration during prolonged, intense exercise training, suggesting a potential therapeutic approach for the prevention of health problems in severely stressed exercising populations.

## SUMMARY

Proper training, maintaining a positive energy balance, adhering to proper nutrient timing, and obtaining adequate rest and recovery form the foundation for optimal performance. Training for the strength/power athlete should be based on the proper utilization of the principles of training depending on individual goals and the training season (preseason, in-season, postseason). The nutritional base should focus on an everyday diet that emphasizes whole foods. The types of macronutrients selected are of the utmost importance for developing a well-refined everyday diet. The use of nutritional supplements that research has shown can help improve energy availability (e.g., sports drinks, carbohydrate) and/or promote recovery (carbohydrate, protein) can provide additional benefits in certain situations. The strength/power athlete should habitually follow a low to moderate GI diet to optimize training, maintain weight, and promote good health. Preexercise nutrition should be composed of primarily low GI sources. The preexercise meal should be consumed 4–6 hours before exercise with an additional snack recommended 30–60 minutes before exercise. Moderate to high GI foods/supplements containing both carbohydrate and protein should be ingested every 20 minutes during exercise to maintain energy levels and reduce muscle protein breakdown. Moderate to high GI foods/supplements containing both carbohydrate and protein are also the foods of choice after exercise. These foods/supplements should be consumed within 30 minutes after the completion of a workout to take full advantage of the anabolic hormonal profile that exists postexercise. Finally, to allow training and nutrition to exert their effects, adequate rest and recovery must be allowed. Following these training and nutritional recommendations can serve as the foundation for a successful strength/power athlete.

## QUESTIONS

1. After intense exercise, athletes should consume:
   a. A combination of carbohydrate and protein 2 hours after exercise
   b. A combination of carbohydrate and fat immediately after exercise

    c. A combination of carbohydrate and protein immediately after exercise

    d. Water

2. How many hours does it generally take for dietary carbohydrates to be digested and begin to be stored as muscle and liver glycogen?

    a. 2

    b. 6

    c. 4

    d. 8

3. How many hours of sleep per night are recommended for the average adult?

    a. 10–11

    b. 6–7

    c. 5–6

    d. 8–9

4. Amino acids plus carbohydrates stimulate net protein synthesis:

    a. By increasing amino acid availability and glycogen release, respectively

    b. By decreasing glycogen breakdown and protein breakdown, respectively

    c. By increasing amino acid availability and insulin release, respectively

    d. By decreasing muscle protein breakdown and increasing glycogen breakdown, respectively

5. When was the glycemic index first developed?

    a. 1971

    b. 1986

    c. 1981

    d. 1991

6. Which protein is the predominant protein found in cow's milk?

    a. Colostrum

    b. Casein

    c. Whey

    d. Soy

7. Which principle of training allows for the replacement and growth of body tissue, yet is often overlooked?

    a. Rest/recovery

    b. Overload

    c. Progression

    d. Specificity

8. One way the addition of protein augments performance and recovery is:

    a. By accelerating muscle protein breakdown

    b. By decreasing the glycemic index of the supplement

    c. Through enhanced release of cortisol

    d. Through added calories

9. What helps accelerate muscle glycogen resynthesis postexercise?

    a. Refraining from nutrient intake until at least 2 hours postexercise

    b. A predominately low glycemic index food/supplement

    c. An increased muscle insulin sensitivity

    d. Maintaining blood glucose levels

10. The consumption of carbohydrate and protein immediately postexercise:

    a. Augments muscle protein synthesis, repair, and growth

    b. Decreases muscle protein synthesis

    c. Enhances cardiac output

    d. Decreases muscle glycogen resynthesis

11. Where is the majority of total carbohydrate stored in the body?

    a. Kidney

    b. Blood

    c. Liver

    d. Skeletal muscle

12. The nutritional needs of the strength/power athlete:
    a. Are the same as the traditional weekend warrior
    b. Go above and beyond those of the normal sedentary individual
    c. Fall well below those of the normal sedentary individual
    d. Coincide with those of the normal sedentary individual

13. Total net phenylalanine uptake is a good indicator of:
    a. Muscle protein synthesis
    b. Glycogenolysis
    c. Muscle protein proteolysis
    d. Lipid breakdown

14. Which of the following is likely to have the lowest glycemic index?
    a. Kidney beans
    b. Sweet potato
    c. Pretzels
    d. Brown rice

15. Which of the following combinations maximizes protein synthesis postexercise?
    a. Carbohydrate/fat
    b. Protein/fat
    c. Carbohydrate/protein
    d. Vitamin/protein

16. All of the following serve as nutrient objectives for a postexercise nutritional supplement except:
    a. Replenishing muscle glycogen stores
    b. Promoting a catabolic hormonal profile
    c. Reducing muscle damage and supporting the immune system
    d. Initiating tissue repair and setting the stage for muscle growth

17. Which type of protein is recommended during and after exercise because of its faster rate of digestion?
    a. Casein
    b. Soy
    c. Colostrum
    d. Whey

18. What type of foods/supplements should be consumed immediately postexercise?
    a. High-glycemic carbohydrate
    b. Fast-absorbing protein such as whey
    c. Liquid form of supplement
    d. All of the above

19. Which monosaccharide should be avoided during exercise because of the possibility of gastrointestinal discomfort, diarrhea, and inadequate energy availability?
    a. Glucose
    b. Fructose
    c. Sucrose
    d. Galactose

20. Which of the following provides the needed energy to directly drive muscular contractions?
    a. Adenosine triphosphate (ATP)
    b. Creatine phosphate
    c. Protein
    d. Muscle glycogen

21. In general what is the glycemic index of pure glucose?
    a. 91
    b. 100
    c. 0
    d. 50

22. Glycogen synthase is the enzyme responsible for transferring:
    a. Lipid to glucose
    b. Glycogen to glucose
    c. Glucose to protein
    d. Glucose to glycogen

23. How many hours after a strength/power workout does it usually take for delayed onset muscle soreness to set in?
    a. 12
    b. 24
    c. 6
    d. 18

24. Which two amino acids does the body frequently use during sustained exercise?
    a. Leucine and glutamine
    b. Alanine and tryptophan
    c. Proline and serine
    d. Methionine and phenylalanine

25. At low exercise intensities, the energy needed to fuel muscular contractions is mostly provided by which of the following substrates?
    a. Muscle proteins
    b. Blood glucose
    c. Plasma fatty acids
    d. Muscle glycogen

26. Which type of carbohydrates consumed after exercise produce significantly greater glycogen storage up to 24 hours postexercise?
    a. No glycemic index carbohydrates
    b. Low glycemic index carbohydrates
    c. Moderate glycemic index carbohydrates
    d. High glycemic index carbohydrates

27. What type of carbohydrate should be consumed during exercise?
    a. High glycemic index
    b. Moderate glycemic index
    c. Moderate to low glycemic index
    d. Low glycemic index

28. In their study, Andersen et al. compared the consumption of 25 g of protein (pre- and postexercise) versus an isocaloric carbohydrate supplement (in conjunction with resistance training over 14 weeks). The protein group experienced:
    a. A greater increase in slow-twitch muscle fiber size
    b. A greater increase in type II muscle fiber size
    c. A greater improvement in squat jump height
    d. All of the above

29. The catabolic hormone cortisol is released from which of the following glands?
    a. Adrenal medulla
    b. Pituitary
    c. Adrenal cortex
    d. Thymus

30. Which type of muscle contraction is to blame for the majority of the microscopic tears and subsequent muscle soreness experienced after weight training?
    a. Eccentric
    b. Concentric
    c. Isometric
    d. Isokinetic

# REFERENCES

1. Chandler RM, Byrne HK, Patterson JG, Ivy JL. Dietary supplements affect the anabolic hormones after weight-training exercise. J Appl Physiol 1994;76:839–845.

2. Kreider RB, Klesges RC, Harmon K, et al. Effects of ingesting supplements designed to promote lean tissue accretion on body composition during resistance training. Int J Sport Nutr 1996;6:234–246.

3. Kreider RB, Klesges RC, Lotz D, et al. Effects of nutritional supplementations during off-season college football training on body composition and strength. J Exerc Physiol online 1999;2.

4. Ivy J, Portman R. Nutrient Timing. North Bergen, NJ: Basic Health Publications; 2004:34, 61.

5. Clarkson PM, Hubal MJ. Exercise-induced muscle damage in humans. Am J Phys Med Rehabil 2002;81(Suppl 11):S52–69.

6. Evans WJ. Effects of exercise on senescent muscle. Clin Orthop 2002;403(Suppl): S211–220.

7. Pedersen BK, Bruunsgaard H, Kolkker M, et al. Exercise-induced immunomodulation: possible roles of neuroendocrine and metabolic factors. Int J Sports Med 1997;18(Suppl 1):S2–7.

8. Sherman WM, Jacobs KA, Leenders N. Carbohydrate metabolism during endurance exercise. In: Kreider R, Fry AC, O'Toole ML, eds. Overtraining in Sport. Champaign, IL: Human Kinetics Publishers; 1998:289–308.

9. Carli G, Bonifazi M, Lodi L, Lupo C, Martelli G, Viti A. Changes in the exercise-induced hormone response to branched chain amino acid administration. Eur J Appl Physiol Occup Physiol 1992;64(3)272–277.

10. Cade JR, Reese RH, Privette RM, Hommen NM, Rogers JL, Fregly MJ. Dietary intervention and training in swimmers. Eur J Appl Physiol Occup Physiol 1991; 63(3–4):210–215.

11. Kreider RB. Dietary supplements and the promotion of muscle growth with resistance exercise. Sports Med 1999;27(2):97–110.

12. Kraemer WJ. Hormonal mechanisms related to the expression of muscular strength and power. In: Komi PV, ed. Strength and Power in Sport. Cambridge, MA: Blackwell Scientific; 1992, 64–76.

13. Biolo G, Tipton KD, Klein S, et al. An abundant supply of amino acids enhances the metabolic effect of exercise on muscle protein. Am J Physiol 1997;273: E122–E129.

14. Rasmussen BB, Tipton KD, Miller SL, et al. An oral essential amino acid-carbohydrate supplement enhances muscle protein anabolism after resistance exercise. J Appl Physiol 2000;88:386–392.

15. Tipton KD, Rasmussen BB, Miller SL, et al. Timing of amino acid-carbohydrate ingestion alters anabolic response of muscle to resistance exercise. Am J Physiol Endocrinol Metab 2001;281:E197–E206.

16. Andersen LL, Tufekovic G, Zebis MK, et al. The effect of resistance training combined with timed ingestion of protein on muscle fiber size and muscle strength. Metabolism 2005;54(2):151–156.

17. Tipton KD, Wolfe RR. Exercise, protein metabolism, and muscle growth. Int J Sports Med 2110;11:109–132.

18. Biolo G, Maggi SP, Williams BD, Tipton KD, Wolfe RR. Increased rates of muscle protein turnover and amino acid transport after resistance exercise in humans. Am J Physiol Endocrinol Metab 1995;268:E514–520.

19. Phillips SM, Tipton KD, Aarsland A, Wolf SE, Wolfe RR. Mixed muscle protein synthesis and breakdown after resistance exercise in humans. Am J Physiol Endocrinol Metab 1997;273:E99–107.

20. Phillips SM, Tipton KD, Ferrando AA, Wolfe RR. Resistance training reduces the acute exercise-induced increase in muscle protein turnover. Am J Physiol Endocrinol Metab 1999;276:E118–124.

21. Coyle E. Substrate utilization during exercise in active people. Am J Clin Nutr 1995;61(Suppl):968S–979S.

22. Haff GG, Lehmkuhl MJ, McCoy LB, Stone MH. Carbohydrate supplementation and resistance training. J Strength Cond Res 2003;7(1):187–196.

23. Nieman DC, Fagoaga OR, Butterworth DE, et al. Carbohydrate supplementation affects blood granulocyte and monocyte trafficking but not function after 2.5h of running. Am J Clin Nutr 1997;66(1):153–159.

24. Nieman DC. Influence of carbohydrate on the immune response to intensive, prolonged exercise. Exerc Immunol Rev 1998;4:64–76.

25. Nieman DC, Pedersen BK. Exercise and immune function. Recent developments. Sports Med 1999;27(2):73–80.

26. Burke LM. Nutritional needs for exercise in the heat. Comp Biochem Physiol A Mol Integr Physiol 2001;128(4):735–748.

27. Burke LM. Nutrition for post-exercise recovery. Aust J Sci Med Sport 1997;29(1): 3–10.

28. Maughan RJ, Noakes TD. Fluid replacement and exercise stress. A brief review of studies on fluid replacement and some guidelines for the athlete. Sports Med 1991;12(1):16–31.

29. Berning JR. Energy intake, diet and muscle wasting. In: Kreider R, Fry AC, O'Toole ML, eds. Overtraining in Sport. Champaign, IL: Human Kinetics Publishers; 1998: 275–288.

30. Coggan AR, Coyle EF. Reversal of fatigue during prolonged exercise by carbohydrate infusion or ingestion. J Appl Physiol 1987;63:2388.

31. Coyle EF, Coogan AR, Hemmert MK, et al. Muscle glycogen utilization during prolonged strenuous exercise when fed carbohydrate. J Appl Physiol 1986;61:165.

32. Goodpaster BH, Costill DL, Fink WJ, et al. The effects of pre-exercise starch ingestion on endurance performance. Int J Sports Med 1996;17:366.

33. Cori CF. The fate of sugar in the animal body III. The rate of glycogen formation in the liver of normal and insulinized rats during the absorption of glucose, fructose, and galactose. J Biol Chem 1926;70:577.

34. Levine C, Evans WJ, Cadarett BS, et al. Fructose and glucose ingestion and muscle glycogen use during submaximal exercise. J Appl Physiol 1983;55:1761.

35. Bergstrom J, Hermansen L, Hultman E, Saltin B. Diet, muscle glycogen and physical performance. Acta Physiol Scand 1967;71:140–150.

36. Balsom PD, Gaitanos GC, Soderlund K, Ekblom B. High-intensity exercise and muscle glycogen availability in humans. Acta Physiol Scand 1999;165:337–345.

37. Haub MD, Haff GG, Potteiger JA. The effect of liquid carbohydrate ingestion on repeated maximal effort exercise in competitive cyclists. J Strength Cond Res 2003;17(1):20–25.

38. Haub MD, Potteiger JA, Jacobsen DJ, Nau KL, Magee LA, Comeau MJ. Glycogen replenishment and repeated maximal effort exercise: effect of liquid carbohydrate. Int J Sport Nutr 1999;9:406–415.

39. Bangsbo J, Graham TE, Kiens B, Saltin B. Elevated muscle glycogen and anaerobic energy production during exhaustive exercise in man. J Physiol 1992;451:205–227.

40. McConell G, Kloot K, Hargreaves M. Effect of timing of carbohydrate ingestion on endurance exercise performance. Med Sci Sports Exerc 1996;28:1300–1304.

41. Haff GG, Koch AJ, Potteiger JA, et al. Carbohydrate supplementation attenuates muscle glycogen loss during acute bouts of resistance exercise. Int J Sports Nutr Exerc Metab 2000;10:326–339.

42. Volek JS. Influence of nutrition on responses to resistance training. Med Sci Sports Exerc 2004;36(4):689–696.

43. Ivy JL, Res PT, Sprague RC, Widzer MO. Effect of a carbohydrate-protein supplement on endurance performance during exercise of varying intensity. Int J Sports Nutr Exerc Metab 2003;13:382–395.

44. Andersen LL, Tufekovic G, Zebis MK, et al. The effect of resistance training combined with timed ingestion of protein on muscle fiber size and muscle strength. Metabolism 2005;54(2):151–156.

45. Saunders MJ, Kane MD, Todd MK. Effects of a carbohydrate-protein beverage on cycling endurance and muscle damage. Med Sci Sports Exerc 2004;36(7): 1233–1238.

46. Dangin M, Boirie Y, Garcia-Rodenas C, et al. The digestion rate of protein is an independent regulating factor of postprandial protein retention. Am J Physiol Endocrinol Metab 2001;280:E340–348.

47. Ivy J, Portman R. The Performance Zone. North Bergen, NJ: Basic Health Publications; 2004:35, 54.

48. Costill D, Hargreaves M. Carbohydrate nutrition and fatigue. Sports Med 1992;13: 86–92.

49. Ivy J. Muscle glycogen synthesis before and after exercise. Sports Med 1991;11: 6–11.

50. Houston M. Biochemistry Primer for Exercise Science. Champaign, IL: Human Kinetics Publishers; 1995:52–53.

51. Ivy J. Glycogen resynthesis after exercise: effect of carbohydrate intake. Int J Sports Med 1998;19:S142–145.

52. Haymond M. Hypoglycemia in infants and children. Endocrinol Metab Clin North Am 1989;18:211–252.

53. Gastelu D, Hatfield F. Dynamic Nutrition for Maximum Performance. Garden City Park, NY: Avery Publishing Group; 1997:45–46.

54. Blom P, Hostmark A, Vaage O, Kardel K, Maehlum S. Effects of different post-exercise sugar diets on the rate of muscle glycogen synthesis. Med Sci Sports Exerc 1987;19:491–496.

55. Burke L, Collier G, Hargreaves M. Muscle glycogen storage after prolonged exercise: effect of the glycemic index of carbohydrate feedings. J Appl Physiol 1993;75:1019–1023.

56. Costill D, Sherman W, Fink W, Maresh C, Witten M, Jiller J. The role of dietary carbohydrates in muscle glycogen synthesis after strenuous running. Am J Clin Nutr 1981;34:1821–1836.

57. Burke L, Collier G, Hargreaves M. Glycemic index: a new tool in sport nutrition. Int J Sport Nutr 1998;8:401–415.

58. Levenhagen DK, Gresham JD, Carlson MG, Maron DJ, Borel MJ, Flakoll PJ. Postexercise nutrient intake timing in humans is critical to recovery of leg glucose and protein homeostasis. Am J Physiol Endocrinol Metab 2001;280:E982–993.

59. Jentjens RLPG, van Loon LJC, Mann CH, Wagenmakers AJM, Jeukendrup AE. Addition of protein and amino acids to carbohydrates does not enhance post-exercise muscle glycogen synthesis. J Appl Physiol 2001;91:839–846.

60. Tarnopolsky MA, Bosman M, Macdonald JR, Vandeputte D, Martin J, Roy BD. Postexercise protein-carbohydrate and carbohydrate supplements increase muscle glycogen in men and women. J Appl Physiol 1997;83:1877–1883.

61. Evans WJ. Protein nutrition and resistance exercise. Can J Appl Physiol 2001;26(Suppl): S141–152.

62. Borsheim E, Aarsland A, Wolfe RR. Effect of an amino acid, protein, and carbohydrate mixture on net muscle protein balance after resistance exercise. Int J Sports Nutr Exerc Metab 2004;14:255–271.

63. Levenhagen DK, Carr C, Carlson MG, Maron DJ, Borel MJ, Flakoll PJ. Postexercise protein intake enhances whole-body and leg protein accretion in humans. Med Sci Sports Exerc 2002;34(5):828–837.

64. Rasmussen BB, Tipton KD, Miller SL, Wolf SE, Wolfe RR. An oral essential amino acid-carbohydrate supplement enhances muscle protein anabolism after resistance exercise. J Appl Physiol 2000;88:386–392.

65. Leutholtz B, Kreider R. Exercise and sport nutrition. In: Wilson T, Temple N, eds. Nutritional Health. Totowa, NJ: Humana Press; 2001:207–239.

66. Kreider RB. Nutritional considerations of overtraining. In: Stout JR, Antonio J, eds. Sports Supplements: A Complete Guide to Physique and Athletic Enhancement. Baltimore: Lippincott, Williams & Wilkins; 2001:199–208.

67. Ivy JL, Katz AL, Cutler CL, Sherman WM, Coyle EF. Muscle glycogen synthesis after exercise: effect of time of carbohydrate ingestion. J Appl Physiol 1988;64: 1480–1485.

68. Zawakzki KM, Yaspelkis BB, Ivy JL. Carbohydrate-protein complex increases the rate of muscle glycogen storage after exercise. J Appl Physiol 1992;72(5):1854–1859.

69. Kraemer WJ, Volek JS, Bush JA, Putukian M, Sebastianelli WJ. Hormonal responses to consecutive days of heavy-resistance exercise with or without nutritional supplementation. J Appl Physiol 1998;85(4):1544–1555.

70. Garetto OP, Richter EA, Goodman MN, Ruderman NB. Enhanced muscle glucose metabolism after exercise in the rat: the two phases. Am J Physiol 1984;246: E471–475.

71. Richter EA, Garetto LP, Goodman MN, Ruderman NB. Enhanced muscle glucose metabolism after exercise: modulation by local factors. Am J Physiol 1984;246: E476–482.

72. Miller SL, Tipton KD, Chinkes DL, et al. Independent and combined effects of amino acids and glucose after resistance exercise. Med Sci Sports Exerc 2003;35:449–455.

73. Sherwood L. Human Physiology: From Cells to Systems. St. Paul, MN: West Publishing; 1993:667–679.

74. Flakoll PJ, Judy T, Flinn K, Carr C, Flinn S. Postexercise protein supplementation improves health and muscle soreness during basic military training in marine recruits. J Appl Physiol 2001;96:951–956.

# Answer Key

**CHAPTER 1**

**Thermodynamics**

1. b
2. a, b
3. c
4. a
5. d
6. a
7. c
8. a
9. a
10. b

**Biochemistry**

1. b
2. d
3. a
4. c
5. a, d
6. d
7. c
8. a
9. b
10. b

**Energy Expenditure**

1. a
2. a
3. c
4. d
5. d
6. a

7. d
8. a
9. b
10. a

**CHAPTER 2**

1. a
2. c
3. d
4. b
5. b
6. c
7. b
8. b
9. c
10. c
11. e
12. c
13. a
14. c
15. a
16. a
17. a
18. a
19. d
20. b
21. a
22. b
23. d
24. a
25. c

26. d

27. c

28. b

29. d

30. a

## CHAPTER 3

1. a

2. d

3. c

4. e

5. a

6. d

7. a

8. e

9. e

10. b

11. b

12. b

13. e

14. e

15. a

16. a

17. a

18. c

19. c

20. e

21. a

22. a

23. b

24. b

25. a

26. a

27. b

28. b

29. b

30. a

## CHAPTER 4

1. a

2. a

3. e

4. b

5. c

6. b

7. a

8. c

9. b

10. e,

11. d

12. d

13. d

14. a

15. c

16. d

17. b

18. b

19. b

20. a

21. e

22. e

23. c

24. c

25. c

26. b

27. b

28. c

29. e

30. e

## CHAPTER 5

1. d

2. c

3. a

4. c

5. a

6. b

7. b

8. c

9. c

10. c

11. c

12. a

13. c
14. d
15. d
16. c
17. b
18. a
19. c
20. b
21. a
22. d
23. b
24. b
25. d
26. b
27. d
28. a
29. b
30. a

## CHAPTER 6

1. c
2. d
3. a
4. d
5. d
6. d
7. a
8. b
9. c
10. d
11. b
12. a
13. a
14. d
15. d
16. d
17. d
18. c
19. a
20. c
21. a

22. b
23. a
24. a
25. b
26. a
27. a
28. a
29. b
30. a

## CHAPTER 7

1. d
2. b
3. c
4. c
5. b
6. a
7. d
8. d
9. d
10. b
11. c
12. b
13. c
14. b
15. d
16. a
17. b
18. c
19. a
20. d
21. a
22. b
23. b
24. a
25. b
26. b
27. a
28. b
29. a
30. b

## CHAPTER 8

1. d
2. c
3. e
4. d
5. a
6. e
7. d
8. a
9. c
10. d
11. b
12. e
13. a
14. c
15. b
16. c
17. b
18. c
19. b
20. d

## CHAPTER 9

1. b
2. c
3. a
4. c
5. d
6. b
7. a
8. c
9. d
10. d
11. c
12. d
13. a
14. c
15. c
16. c
17. b
18. b

19. c
20. b
21. b
22. b
23. a
24. a
25. b
26. b
27. a
28. b
29. b
30. b
31. a

## CHAPTER 10

1. d
2. b
3. c
4. a
5. b
6. d
7. c
8. c
9. a
10. b
11. a
12. d
13. b
14. b
15. a
16. c
17. b
18. d
19. c
20. a
21. b
22. a
23. b
24. b
25. a
26. b

27. a

28. b

29. a

30. b

## CHAPTER 11

1. d

2. d

3. b

4. a

5. c

6. d

7. b

8. a

9. d

10. c

11. c

12. d

13. c

14. d

15. c

16. b

17. c

18. d

19. b

20. b

21. a

22. b

23. a

24. b

25. a

26. b

27. b

28. a

29. a

30. a

## CHAPTER 12

1. c

2. b

3. c

4. a

5. b

6. b

7. d

8. b

9. d

10. d

11. b

12. d

13. c

14. a

15. c

16. c

17. c

18. c

19. c

20. c

21. a

22. a

23. a

24. b

25. a

26. a

27. a

28. a

29. b

30. a

## CHAPTER 13

1. b

2. b

3. d

4. d

5. a

6. c

7. b

8. a

9. a

10. b

11. c

12. d

13. a

14. a

15. b

16. b

17. d

18. d

19. a

20. c

21. b

22. b

23. b

24. b

25. a

26. b

27. a

28. b

29. b

30. a

## CHAPTER 14

1. c

2. c

3. c

4. b

5. b

6. d

7. b

8. d

9. b

10. d

11. c

12. a

13. c

14. a

15. b

16. b

17. c

18. b

19. d

20. a

21. a

22. b

23. a

24. b

25. a

26. c

27. b

28. a

29. a

30. a

31. b

32. b

33. a

34. b

35. a

36. b

37. b

38. a

39. a

40. b

41. a

42. b

43. a

44. a

45. b

46. a

47. a

48. a

49. a

50. b

## CHAPTER 15

1. c

2. d

3. c

4. b

5. b

6. b

7. b

8. d

9. a

10. d

11. b

12. c

13. c
14. a
15. a
16. b
17. a
18. a
19. b
20. d
21. a
22. a
23. b
24. a
25. b
26. a
27. b
28. b
29. a
30. a

## CHAPTER 16

1. d
2. a
3. d
4. d
5. b
6. d
7. a
8. b
9. d
10. b
11. b
12. b
13. c
14. d
15. b
16. c
17. d
18. c
19. a
20. c
21. b

22. b
23. a
24. a
25. a
26. b
27. b
28. b
29. a
30. b

## CHAPTER 17

1. c
2. b
3. d
4. d
5. d
6. b
7. a
8. d
9. b
10. b
11. c
12. d
13. e
14. b
15. c
16. b
17. a
18. d
19. c
20. b
21. a
22. a
23. a
24. a
25. b
26. b
27. b
28. a
29. a
30. a

## CHAPTER 18

1. c
2. d
3. c
4. b
5. a
6. b
7. c
8. c
9. d
10. d
11. b
12. d
13. a
14. a
15. b
16. b
17. c
18. b
19. a
20. d
21. b
22. b
23. a
24. a
25. b
26. a
27. a
28. b
29. b
30. b
31. b
32. a
33. b
34. b
35. a

## CHAPTER 19

1. e
2. a
3. d
4. d
5. d
6. b
7. e
8. d
9. e
10. c
11. a
12. b
13. a
14. a
15. a
16. d
17. c
18. d
19. d
20. a
21. b
22. a
23. b
24. b
25. b
26. a
27. a
28. a
29. b
30. a

## CHAPTER 20

1. a
2. d
3. b
4. b
5. d
6. c
7. a
8. b
9. d
10. c
11. e
12. a

13. b

14. c

15. d

16. b

17. c

18. c

19. d

20. e

21. b

22. a

23. a

24. a

25. b

26. b

27. b

28. a

29. a

30. b

## CHAPTER 21

1. c

2. c

3. d

4. c

5. a

6. a

7. b

8. d

9. a

10. d

11. d

12. f

13. b

14. a

15. e

16. c

17. e

18. e

19. d

20. d

21. b

22. b

23. b

24. a

25. a

26. b

27. b

28. b

29. a

30. b

## CHAPTER 22

1. d

2. c

3. a

4. b

5. c

6. d

7. a

8. d

9. c

10. c

11. a

12. c

13. a

14. c

15. a

16. c

17. d

18. a

19. d

20. d

## CHAPTER 23

1. c

2. b

3. c

4. c

5. a

6. b

7. b

8. a

9. a
10. b
11. a
12. a
13. a
14. a
15. a

## CHAPTER 24

1. b
2. a
3. c
4. d
5. d
6. b
7. c
8. d
9. a
10. b
11. b
12. d
13. a
14. c
15. d

## CHAPTER 25

1. b
2. d
3. d
4. b
5. a
6. b
7. d
8. a
9. a
10. d
11. a
12. d
13. d
14. c

15. a
16. d
17. d
18. b
19. b
20. b
21. a
22. a
23. a
24. a
25. b
26. b
27. a

## CHAPTER 26

1. b
2. b
3. e
4. a
5. b
6. a
7. a
8. d
9. b
10. d
11. a
12. a
13. a
14. a
15. a
16. a
17. a
18. a
19. a
20. a
21. a
22. a
23. a
24. a
25. a
26. a

27. a
28. a
29. a
30. a

31. b
32. b
33. b

## CHAPTER 27

1. d
2. c
3. d
4. c
5. c
6. b
7. a
8. d
9. c
10. d
11. d
12. e
13. a
14. a
15. c
16. b
17. d
18. c
19. b
20. a
21. b
22. a
23. a
24. a
25. a
26. b
27. a
28. b
29. b
30. a

## CHAPTER 28

1. c
2. c
3. d
4. c
5. c
6. b
7. a
8. d
9. c
10. a
11. d
12. b
13. a
14. a
15. c
16. b
17. d
18. d
19. b
20. a
21. b
22. d
23. b
24. a
25. c
26. d
27. a
28. d
29. c
30. a

# Index

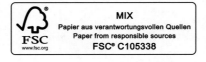

Printed by Books on Demand, Germany